Surgery of the
GALLBLADDER and BILE DUCTS

Lawrence W. Way, M.D.

Professor of Surgery
University of California School of Medicine
San Francisco
Chief, Surgical Service
V.A. Medical Center
San Francisco, California

Carlos A. Pellegrini, M.D.

Associate Professor of Surgery
University of California School of Medicine
San Francisco
Chief of Surgical Clinics
V.A. Medical Center
San Francisco, California

1987
W. B. SAUNDERS COMPANY
Philadelphia • London • Toronto • Mexico City
Rio de Janeiro • Sydney • Tokyo • Hong Kong

W. B. Saunders Company: West Washington Square
Philadelphia, PA 19105

Library of Congress Cataloging-in-Publication Data

Main entry under title:

Surgery of the gallbladder and bile ducts.

1. Gall-bladder—Surgery. 2. Bile-ducts—Surgery.
I. Way, Lawrence W. II. Pellegrini, Carlos A.
[DNLM: 1. Gallbladder—surgery. 2. Bile Ducts—surgery.
WI 750 S9613]

RD546.S947 1987 617′.556 85–2028

ISBN 0–7216–9139–0

Editor: Dean Manke
Designer: Terri Siegel
Production Manager: Bob Butler
Manuscript Editor: Constance Burton
Illustration Coordinator: Walt Verbitski
Indexer: Barbara Farabaugh

Surgery of the Gallbladder and Bile Ducts ISBN 0–7216–9139–0

Last digit is the print number: 9 8 7 6 5 4 3 2 1

CONTRIBUTORS

JOHN ALEXANDER-WILLIAMS, M.D., F.A.C.S.

Chief of Surgery and Consultant Surgeon, The General Hospital, University of Birmingham, Birmingham, England.

Bacteriology of Biliary Disease

S. AUSTIN JONES, M.D.*

Professor of Surgery, Emeritus, University of California, School of Medicine, Irvine, California.

The Use of Transduodenal Sphincteroplasty in Biliary Tract Disease

ROBERT N. BERK, M.D.

Professor and Chairman, Department of Radiology, University of California, San Diego, School of Medicine; Chief, Department of Radiology, University of California, San Diego, Medical Center, San Diego, California.

Oral Cholecystography, IV Cholangiography

L. H. BLUMGART, M.D., F.R.C.S.

Professor of Surgery, Royal Postgraduate Medical School; Director of Surgery, Hammersmith Hospital, London, England.

Postcholecystectomy Syndrome

PETER W. CALLEN, M.D.

Associate Professor of Radiology and of Obstetrics, Gynecology, and Reproductive Sciences, University of California, San Francisco, School of Medicine, San Francisco, Calfornia.

Ultrasonography of the Gallbladder and Bile Ducts

*Deceased

JOHN L. CAMERON, M.D.

Professor of Surgery, Johns Hopkins University School of Medicine; Chairman, Department of Surgery, Johns Hopkins Hospital, Baltimore, Maryland.

Acute Cholangitis

PETER B. COTTON, M.D., F.R.C.P.

Director, Department of Gastroenterology, The Middlesex Hospital and Medical School, London, England.

Transendoscopic Therapeutic Techniques

ALFRED A. DE LORIMIER, M.D.

Professor of Surgery, University of California, San Francisco, School of Medicine; Attending Surgeon, University of California Hospital, Mount Zion Hospital, Children's Hospital, Kaiser Permenente Hospital, San Francisco, California.

Congenital Biliary Atresia

LAWRENCE DENBESTEN, M.D.

Professor of Surgery, University of California, Los Angeles, School of Medicine, Los Angeles, California.

Choledocholithiasis

ROY A. FILLY, M.D.

Professor of Radiology and of Obstetrics, Gynecology, and Reproductive Sciences; Chief, Section of Diagnostic Ultrasonography; Vice Chairman, Diagnostic Radiology, University of California, San Francisco, School of Medicine, San Francisco, California.

Ultrasonography of the Gallbladder and Bile Ducts

ERIC W. FONKALSRUD, M.D.

Professor and Chief of Pediatric Surgery; Vice-Chairman, Department of Surgery, University of California, Los Angeles, School of Medicine, Los Angeles, California.

Biliary Cystic Disease in Children and Adults

JAMES H. FOSTER, M.D.

Professor of Surgery, University of Connecticut School of Medicine; Chief of Surgery, John Dempsey Hospital, University of Connecticut Health Center, Farmington, Connecticut.

Carcinoma of the Gallbladder

HENRY I. GOLDBERG, M.D.

Professor of Radiology, University of California, San Francisco, School of Medicine, San Francisco, California.

Computed Tomography and Magnetic Resonance Imaging of the Gallbladder and Bile Ducts

MICHAEL R. HARRISON, M.D.

Associate Professor of Surgery, University of California, San Francisco, School of Medicine; Attending Surgeon, University of California Hospital, Mount Zion Hospital, Children's Hospital, Kaiser Permenente Hospital, San Francisco, California.

Congenital Biliary Atresia

ROBERT E. HERMANN, M.D.

Chairman, Department of General Surgery, Cleveland Clinic; Clinical Professor of Surgery, Case Western Reserve University, Cleveland, Ohio.

Choledochoduodenostomy

STANLEY O. HOERR, M.D.

Emeritus Staff, Cleveland Clinic Foundation, Cleveland, Ohio.

Choledochoduodenostomy

PAUL B. HOFFER, M.D.

Professor of Diagnostic Radiology, Yale University School of Medicine; Director, Section of Nuclear Medicine, Yale–New Haven Hospital, New Haven, Connecticut.

Radioisotopic Evaluation of Biliary Function

ROBERT K. KERLAN, Jr., M.D.

Assistant Professor of Radiology, University of California, San Francisco, School of Medicine; Staff, Moffitt-Long Hospital, San Francisco, California.

Percutaneous Transhepatic Cholangiography and Interventional Radiology of the Gallbladder and Bile Ducts

HAROLD H. LINDNER, M.D., F.A.C.S.

Clinical Professor of Surgery and Topographic Anatomy, University of California, San Francisco, School of Medicine; Attending Staff, University of California, San Francisco Affiliated Hospitals, San Francisco, California.

Embryology and Anatomy of the Biliary Tree

SIR JOHN LOEWENTHAL, C.M.G., E.D., M.B., F.R.C.S.*

Formerly, Professor and Chairman, Department of Surgery, The University of Sydney, Sydney, Australia.

Echinococcosis

JAN H. LOUW, M.D., Ch.M., F.R.C.S., F.A.C.S.(Hon.)

Emeritus Professor of Surgery, University of Cape Town; Senior Surgeon, Red Cross War Memorial Children's Hospital; Honorary Consultant Surgeon, Groote Schuur Hospital, Cape Town, Republic of South Africa.

Ascariasis

CHARLES E. LUCAS, M.D.

Professor of Surgery, Wayne State University; Senior Attending Surgeon, Detroit Receiving Hospital, Harper Hospital, Hutzel Hospital, Detroit, Michigan.

Trauma to the Biliary Tract

R. F. McCLOY, B.Sc., M.D., F.R.C.S.

Senior Lecturer and Consultant Surgeon, Manchester Royal Infirmary, Manchester, England.

Postcholecystectomy Syndrome

CHARLES K. McSHERRY, M.D.

Professor of Surgery, Mount Sinai School of Medicine; Director of Surgery, Beth Israel Medical Center, New York, New York.

Cholecystostomy and Cholecystectomy

MAURICE P. MERCADIER, M.D.

Professor and Chairman, Department of Surgery, Pitié-Salpétrière Hospital; Chief-Surgeon, American Hospital of Paris, Paris, France.

Intrahepatic Strictures and Malformations of the Bile Ducts in the Adult; Carcinoma of the Bile Duct: Surgical Therapy

LEON MORGENSTERN, M.D.

Clinical Professor of Surgery, University of California, Los Angeles, School of Medicine; Direc-

*Deceased

tor of Surgery, Cedars-Sinai Medical Center, Los Angeles, California.

Exploration of the Common Bile Duct for Stones

DAVID L. NAHRWOLD, M.D.

Loyal and Edith Davis Professor of Surgery and Chairman, Department of Surgery, Northwestern University Medical School; Surgeon-in-Chief, Northwestern Memorial Hospital, Chicago, Illinois.

Benign Tumors and Pseudotumors of the Biliary Tract

G. B. ONG, D.Sc.

Professor of Surgery and Head, University of Hong Kong, Queen Mary Hospital, Hong Kong.

Recurrent Pyogenic Cholangitis

MARCO G. PATTI, M.D.

Research Fellow, Gastrointestinal Surgery, University of California, San Francisco, School of Medicine, San Francisco, California.

Motility of the Gallbladder and Bile Ducts and the Kinetics of Bile Flow

CARLOS A. PELLEGRINI, M.D.

Associate Professor, University of California, San Francisco, School of Medicine; Attending Surgeon, University of California, San Francisco Medical Center; Staff Surgeon and Chief, Outpatient Clinics, VA Medical Center, San Francisco, California.

Motility of the Gallbladder and Bile Ducts and the Kinetics of Bile Flow; Pathophysiology of Biliary Obstruction; Acute Cholecystitis; Biliary Pancreatitis

GERALD PESKIN, M.D.

Clinical Professor of Surgery, Yale University School of Medicine; Chairman, Department of Surgery, Hospital of St. Raphael, New Haven, Connecticut.

Biliary Fistula

HENRY A. PITT, M.D.

Associate Professor of Surgery, Johns Hopkins University School of Medicine; Vice Chairman, Department of Surgery, Johns Hopkins Hospital, Baltimore, Maryland.

Acute Cholangitis

JOHN H. C. RANSON, B.M., B.Ch., F.A.C.S.

Professor of Surgery, New York University School of Medicine; Attending Surgeon, New York University Hospital, Bellevue Hospital, New York, New York.

Perforation of the Gallbladder

ERNEST J. RING, M.D.

Professor, Department of Radiology; Chief, Interventional Radiology; Adjunct Professor, Department of Surgery, University of California, San Francisco, School of Medicine; Staff, Moffitt-Long Hospital, San Francisco, California.

Percutaneous Transhepatic Cholangiography and Interventional Radiology of the Gallbladder and Bile Ducts

HEINZ RODE, M.Med.(Chir.), F.C.S.(S.A.), F.R.C.S. (Edinburgh)

Senior Lecturer, Department of Paediatric Surgery, University of Cape Town; Senior Paediatric Surgeon, Red Cross War Memorial Children's Hospital, Cape Town, Republic of South Africa.

Ascariasis

PHILIP SANDBLOM, M.D., Ph.D., F.R.C.S., F.R.C.J., F.R.C.S.J., F.A.C.J.(Hon.)

Professor Emeritus of Surgery and Past President, University of Lund, Sweden; Guest Professor Emeritus of Surgery, University of Lausanne, Switzerland.

Hemobilia

BRUCE F. SCHARSCHMIDT, M.D.

Associate Professor of Medicine, University of California, San Francisco, School of Medicine; Attending Physician, University of California, San Francisco Affiliated Hospitals, San Francisco, California.

Bile Secretion, Intestinal Lipid Absorption, and the Enterohepatic Circulation of Bile Salts; The Jaundiced Patient: Differential Diagnosis and Clinical Approach

RUDI SCHMID, M.D., Ph.D.

Professor of Medicine and Dean, University of California, San Francisco, School of Medicine; Attending Physician, University of California, San Francisco Affiliated Hospitals, San Francisco, California.

Bile Secretion, Intestinal Lipid Absorption, and the Enterohepatic Circulation of Bile Salts

SEYMOUR I. SCHWARTZ, M.D.

Professor of Surgery, University of Rochester School of Medicine; Senior Surgeon, Strong Memorial Hospital, Rochester, New York.

Sclerosing Cholangitis

HOWARD SHAPIRO, M.D.

Clinical Professor of Medicine, University of California, San Francisco, School of Medicine, San Francisco, California.

Endoscopic Retrograde Cholangiography

SIR RODNEY SMITH, K.B.E., Hon. D.Sc., M.S., F.R.C.S., Hon. F.R.A.C.S., Hon. F.R.C.S. (Edinburgh), Hon. F.A.C.S., Hon. F.R.C.S. (Canada), Hon. F.R.C.S. (I), Hon. F.D.S.

The Rodney Smith Method of Biliary Stricture Repair

ROBERT C. STADALNIK, M.D.

Professor of Radiology; Chief, Division of Nuclear Medicine, University of California, Davis, School of Medicine, Sacramento, California.

Radioisotopic Evaluation of Biliary Function

J. TERBLANCHE, Ch.M., F.R.C.S.(Eng.), F.C.S.(S.A.), F.R.C.P.S.(Glasgow).

Professor and Head, Department of Surgery, University of Cape Town; Co-Director, Medical Research Council, Liver Research Group; Surgeon in Chief, Groote Schuur Hospital, Cape Town, Republic of South Africa; Visiting Professor and Hon. Consultant Surgeon, Royal Free Hospital, London, England.

Tumors of the Hepatic Duct Bifurcation: Stent Therapy

MARTIN TINDEL, M.D.

Instructor of Surgery, State University of New York (Stony Brook); Staff Surgeon (Voluntary Status), Long Island Jewish Medical Center, New Hyde Park, New York.

Carcinoma of the Ampulla of Vater

JAMES TOOULI, Ph.D., M.B., F.R.A.C.S.

Senior Lecturer, School of Medicine, Flinders University of South Australia; Visiting Specialist, Repatriation General Hospital, Daw Park; Senior Staff Specialist, Flinders Medical Centre, Adelaide, South Australia.

The Formation and Dissolution of Gallstones

ANDREW L. WARSHAW, M.D.

Associate Professor of Surgery, Harvard Medical School; Visiting Surgeon, Massachusetts General Hospital, Boston, Massachusetts.

Miscellaneous Causes of Bile Duct Obstruction

JAMES McK. WATTS, M.B., B.S., F.R.A.C.S.

Formerly, Foundation Professor of Surgery, School of Medicine, Flinders University of South Australia; Visiting Specialist, Repatriation General Hospital, Daw Park; Senior Visiting Specialist, Flinders Medical Centre, Adelaide, South Australia.

The Formation and Dissolution of Gallstones

LAWRENCE W. WAY, M.D.

Professor of Surgery, University of California, San Francisco, School of Medicine; Chief, Surgical Service, VA Medical Center, San Francisco, California.

The Jaundiced Patient: Differential Diagnosis and Clinical Approach; Cholelithiasis and Chronic Cholecystitis; Acute Cholecystitis; Gallstone Ileus; Biliary Stricture; Echinococcosis

MALCOLM J. WHITING, Ph.D.

Lecturer and Principal Hospital Scientist, School of Medicine, Flinders Medical Centre, Adelaide, South Australia.

The Formation and Dissolution of Gallstones

LESLIE WISE, M.D.

Professor of Surgery, The State University of New York (Stony Brook); Chairman, Department of Surgery, Long Island Jewish Medical Center, New Hyde Park, New York.

Carcinoma of the Ampulla of Vater

PREFACE

Diseases of the biliary tree have always occupied a central role in general surgery, and they continue to do so today. In the average surgical practice one can expect to encounter biliary diseases resulting from metabolic disorders (gallstones), infections, neoplasms, parasites, congenital anomalies, autoimmune conditions, and so forth.

In the last two decades progress in the understanding of biliary disease and biliary surgery has been remarkable. For example, owing to advances of just the past 15 years, the origin, epidemiology, natural history, and treatment of gallstone disease have had to be thoroughly rewritten. The advent of so many new diagnostic tests for lesions of the bile ducts has created the need to define the strategy of testing for different syndromes to avoid the risk of expensive overtesting.

Although biliary disease was once almost the exclusive province of surgeons, it now has attracted gastroenterologists, radiologists, oncologists, specialists in nuclear medicine, and others. The growing involvement of these other specialists has been a boon to the surgeon. Their techniques provide previously unavailable information about the patient's condition and additional modes of treatment, which often are useful in patients for whom surgery is risky or of limited value. Consequently, a team approach involving surgeons, gastroenterologists, and interventional radiologists, in particular, is often the most effective way to manage patients with complex biliary problems.

In some instances, however, new nonsurgical approaches have threatened to supplant established surgical methods of proven efficacy and safety. The debates generated by these conflicts inevitably have produced additional insights into disease mechanisms, challenged accepted theories, and stimulated clinical trials, which in turn have produced more information to be sifted and then put into practice.

This book is meant to serve as an authoritative reference work that covers in detail biliary tract disease and these recent dynamic changes. It should prove to be useful to anyone, regardless of specialty, who is responsible for treating patients with disease of the gallbladder or bile ducts. The chapter authors are well known for their important contributions to knowledge about this subject. They include nonsurgeons as well as surgeons, and have been selected from throughout the world. The text is thoroughly referenced so that readers can trace arguments back to the original data.

In a multiauthored book such as this there will inevitably be differences of opinion and overlap of coverage. The former reflects a lack of consensus on specific issues and is considered by the editors to be important to reflect the state of affairs. On the other hand, overlap has been retained only when its deletion would disrupt the context of the discussion.

We wish to acknowledge our debt to the late Dr. J. Englebert Dunphy, our wise and much beloved teacher, who participated in the inception of this project. We also give thanks to Mr. Dean Manke and others at the W.B. Saunders Company who have provided excellent support at every step.

LAWRENCE W. WAY
CARLOS A. PELLEGRINI
San Francisco

CONTENTS

SECTION II

SECTION III

SECTION I

ANATOMY—PHYSIOLOGY—PATHOPHYSIOLOGY

HAROLD H. LINDNER, M.D.

1

Embryology and Anatomy of the Biliary Tree

The extrahepatic biliary tree probably has more anomalous structures and relationships than any other area of the anatomy. This plethora of unusual findings and relationships is also found in the vascular structures supplying the liver and the biliary tree. The young or inexperienced surgeon may be confused by these aberrant structures and their anomalous relationships, and even the seasoned surgeon must be constantly on the lookout for them. This review of the embryologic development and anatomy of the biliary tree should assist the operating surgeon in understanding and recognizing the anomalies that may be encountered.

EMBRYOLOGY OF THE BILIARY TREE[10]

At about the 3 mm stage (fifth week of intrauterine life) the embryo shows the beginning of an outpouching from the ventral surface of the primitive gastrointestinal tract just distal to the junction of the foregut and midgut. The outpouching penetrates the primitive ventral mesogastrium and ultimately results in the formation of the two lobes of the liver, the intra- and extrahepatic biliary tree, the gallbladder and cystic duct, and the dorsal posterior half of the head of the pancreas and the uncinate process (Fig. 1–1). Also at this time a dorsal sacculation leaves the primitive bowel tube at a slightly more superior level to become the anlage of the remainder of the pancreatic head as well as the neck, the body, and the tail of the pancreas.[1]

As the ventral sacculation pushes its way ventrally and superiorly between the two leaves of the ventral mesogastrium, its distal or advancing tip divides into a superior and an inferior bud. Growing from the inferior surface of the biliary diverticulum, proximal to its enlarging terminal sacculations and lying quite close to the ventral wall of the gut, a third bud, the ventral pancreatic bud, has appeared.

The bud that gives rise to the liver and biliary tree, as it advances superiorly, is composed of a solid cord of entodermal cells and contains no lumen. The superior bud of the ventral sacculation finally reaches the septum transversum, the primitive mesodermal sheet that separates the thorax from the abdominal cavity. Just before it reaches the septum transversum, the advancing superior bud divides into a right and a left cellular column, each of which will form one of the lobes of the liver. The inferior head of the divided ventral sacculation is carried superiorly by the growth of the superior head to which it is attached. The advance of the inferior head stops just below the visceral surface of the liver, at which point it develops into the gallbladder and the cystic duct. On those rare occasions when the inferior head advances too far superiorly, an intrahepatic gallbladder will result, nearly always within the right lobe of the liver.

The growth superiorly of the superior bud of the biliary diverticulum is the mechanism by which the hepatic ducts, the common hepatic duct, and the common bile duct are formed. With the embryo at the 7 mm stage, the common bile duct is seen to be still attached to the ventral surface of the duodenum, with the ventral pancreatic bud attached to its inferior wall. The rotation of the ventral pancreatic bud is to the left and dorsalward and encompasses an arc of about 180 degrees. This rotation allows the ventral pancreatic bud to fuse with the dorsal pancreatic bud to form the complete pancreas. Since the most proximal segment of the com-

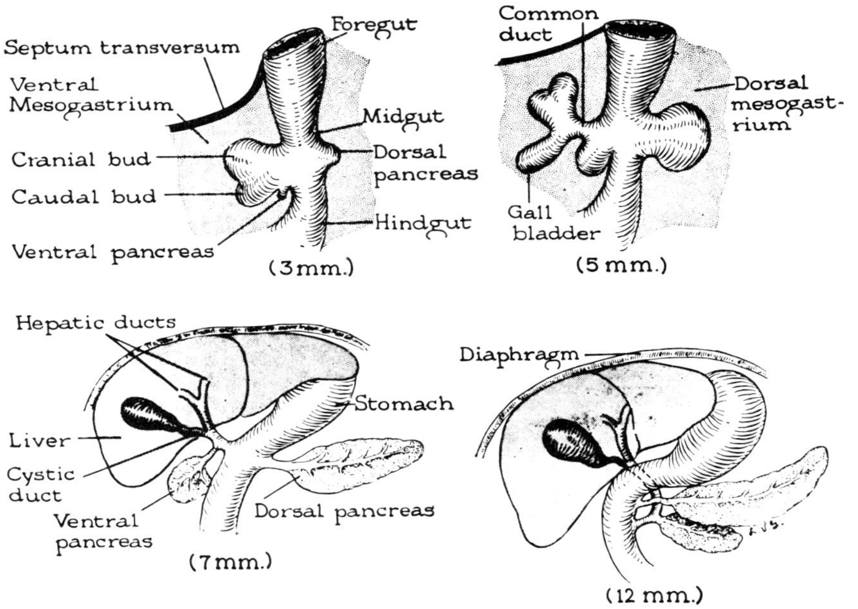

Figure 1–1. Development of extrahepatic biliary tract in the embryo from the 3 mm to the 12 mm stage.

mon bile duct is attached to the ventral pancreatic head, the combined rotation of the duodenum and the ventral pancreatic anlage serves finally to place the junction of the common bile duct and the duodenum on the posteromedial duodenal wall.

By the beginning of the seventh week of intrauterine life, vacuolization starts to take place within the future biliary tree. Within a week, a completely open lumen has formed within the gallbladder, the cystic duct, the hepatic ducts, and the common bile duct. By the end of the third month of fetal life, the liver begins to secrete bile, and it flows into the duodenum via the recently canalized extrahepatic biliary tree.

Embryologic Errors Resulting in Congenital Malformations of the Extrahepatic Biliary Tree[1]

Abnormalities of the Gallbladder (Table 1–1)

A double gallbladder probably results from the presence of an additional inferior bud on the superiorly advancing ventral biliary tract diverticulum. The extra bud usually presents at the site of junction of the common hepatic, cystic, and common bile ducts, and its failure to regress explains the origin of a double gallbladder (Fig. 1–2). If the duplication is drained by a single cystic duct the anomaly is known as a cleft, or bilobed, gallbladder. If the anomaly is drained by a separate cystic duct it is known as a true double gallbladder. Anomalous positions of the gallbladder are probably due to improper migration of the original inferior gallbladder sacculation or to the development of a second inferior gallbladder sacculation with coincidental failure of the primary sacculation to develop.

Table 1–1 CLASSIFICATION OF ABNORMALITIES OF THE GALLBLADDER

I. Anomalous forms
  1. Double gallbladder
    a. "Y" type
    b. "H" type
    c. Trabecular type
  2. Bilobed gallbladder
  3. Hourglass gallbladder
II. Diverticulum of the gallbladder
III. Congenital absence of the gallbladder
IV. Abnormal position of the gallbladder (it is important to remember that no matter where the gallbladder is located, the cystic duct always crosses to the right side of the abdomen and joins the common duct in a comparatively normal relationship).
  1. Abdominal wall
  2. Falciform ligament of the liver
  3. Intrahepatic gallbladder
  4. Retroperitoneal gallbladder
  5. Left-sided gallbladder
V. Abnormalities of the mesentery of the gallbladder (absent, too short, or too long)
VI. Miscellaneous abnormalities
  1. Aberrant gastrointestinal mucosa in the gallbladder wall
  2. Aberrant pancreatic tissue in the gallbladder wall

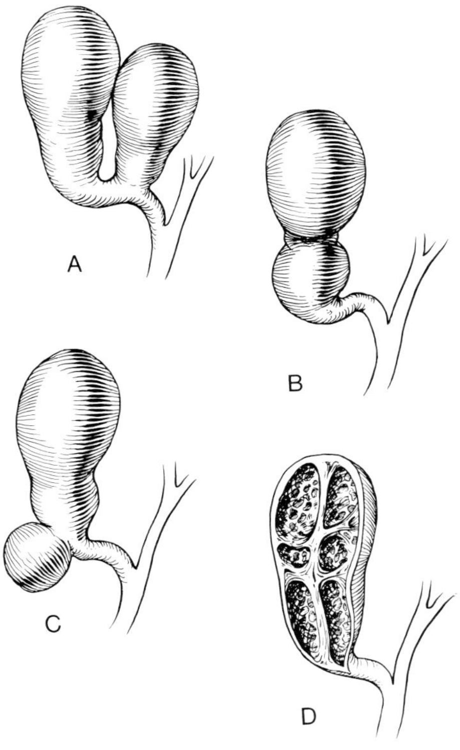

Figure 1–2. Anomalies of the gallbladder. *A*, Bilobed gallbladder. *B*, Hourglass gallbladder. *C*, Congenital enlargement of the infundibulum. *D*, Septate gallbladder.

The presence of a complete or an incomplete septum within the lumen of the gallbladder, abnormal valves of Heister in the cystic duct, a gallbladder diverticulum, or congenital stricture of the gallbladder or cystic duct is usually the result of incomplete vacuolization of the solid entodermal cord.

Congenital absence of the gallbladder is due either to failure of the inferior portion of the original biliary sacculation to develop or to failure of vacuolization during the seventh week of fetal life. Congenital absence of the gallbladder is frequently associated with atresia of one or more segments of the extrahepatic ductal system. Congenital absence of the gallbladder is usually not suspected until operation, and in such cases the possibility of a completely intrahepatic gallbladder must be considered if the gallbladder is not found elsewhere.

The so-called floating gallbladder is one in which the organ is completely covered by peritoneum; it is usually suspended from the liver by a mesentery (Fig. 1–3). If a mesentery is absent, the only connection of the gallbladder to the liver may be by a cystic duct mesentery. Both types of floating gallbladder predispose to gallbladder torsion.

An intrahepatic gallbladder is rare (Fig. 1–3). When present, it is usually close to the visceral surface of the right lobe of the liver. When inflamed, it may be mistaken for an intrahepatic abscess.

Abnormalities of the Extrahepatic Biliary Ducts[6]

Stenosis and Atresia (Fig. 1–4). Much confusion exists regarding the precise cause of stenosis and atresia of the biliary tract. Up until 1970, it was commonly held that all congenital stenoses and atresias of the biliary ducts were due to failure of the solid cord of entodermal cells to vacuolize during the seventh week of fetal life. Some investigations strongly suggest that congenital biliary stenosis and atresia are secondary to fetal hepatic or hepatoductal infection.[9] It has also been suggested that some cases of stenosis and atresia may result from abnormal vascular patterns supplying the ducts or that they might be due to pressure by abnormal bands upon vessels supplying specific sections of the ducts. Any segment of the extrahepatic ductal system may be congenitally stenotic or

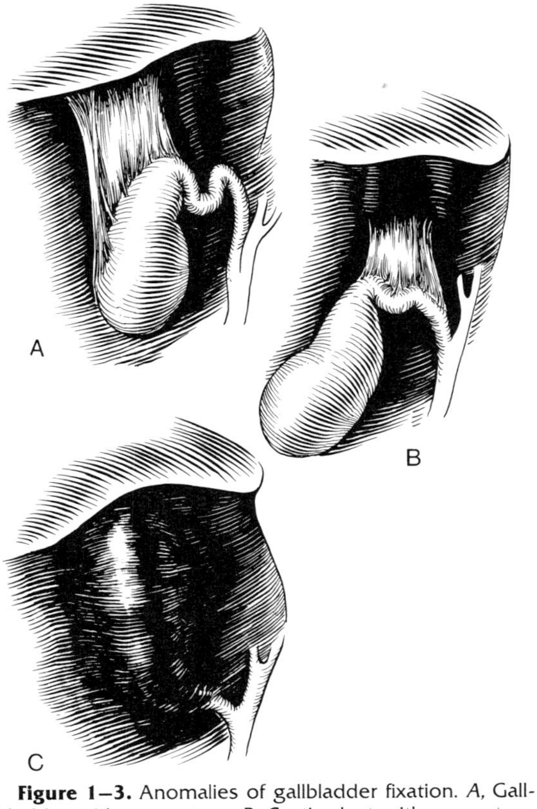

Figure 1–3. Anomalies of gallbladder fixation. *A*, Gallbladder with mesentery. *B*, Cystic duct with mesentery. *C*, Intrahepatic gallbladder.

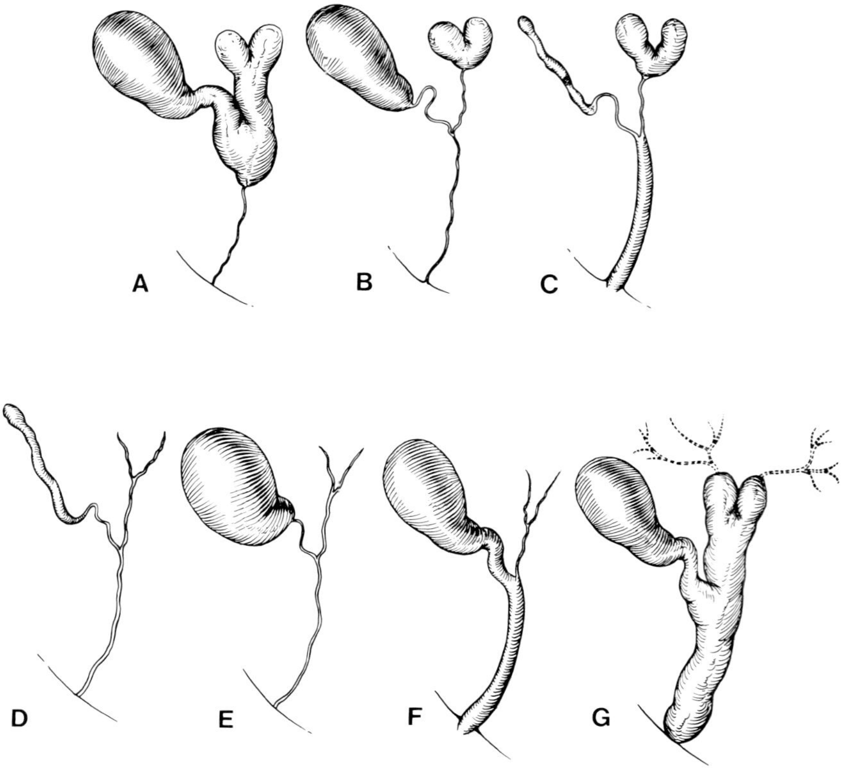

Figure 1–4. Types of stenosis and atresia of the extrahepatic biliary system.

completely obliterated. Multiple combinations of stenosis or atresia, or both, in multiple areas of the extrahepatic biliary tract may occur. Intrahepatic stenosis or atresia of the biliary ducts frequently accompanies extrahepatic anomalies.

True Accessory Extrahepatic Biliary Ducts. True accessory extrahepatic biliary ducts result from an extra bud being given off from the primary biliary anlage. Usually these extra buds disappear, but if they persist in the cephalic portion of the extrahepatic biliary tree and canalize, they form one or more true accessory biliary ducts. Accessory ducts are much more common on the right side of the biliary tree than on the left. They may run directly from the liver into the gallbladder, the right or left hepatic duct, the common hepatic duct, the common bile duct, or the cystic duct. In the performance of surgery upon the biliary tract, an accessory duct, particularly if it is small, may be inadvertently severed. The presence of an accessory bud growing from the biliary anlage close to its departure from the distal foregut may result in a duodenal diverticulum arising from the posteromedial aspect of the bowel and protruding into the head of the pancreas near the junction of the common bile duct and the duodenum.

Pseudo–Accessory Extrahepatic Biliary Ducts. Pseudo–accessory extrahepatic biliary ducts, unlike true anomalous ducts, which arise from an extra biliary bud, result from an extrahepatic course of a biliary duct that normally is contained within the liver substance. Such a duct joins the true right or left hepatic duct in an extrahepatic position rather than within the liver. These accessory ducts drain a liver segment, usually from the right lobe, and thus nearly always join the right hepatic duct. Even though they are not truly anomalous, they present the same surgical pitfalls as do true accessory ducts.

Cystic Disease of the Common Duct (Choledochal Cyst). Cystic disease of the common duct is a rare anomaly found three times more often in girls than in boys (see also Chapters 39 and 40). A large cyst is found in a supraduodenal position lying between the two layers of the hepatoduodenal ligament just superior to the pylorus of the stomach. The hepatic and cystic ducts usually open directly into the cystic area of the common bile duct, and the cystic duct joins the hepatic duct above or at the upper margin of the cyst. The etiology of the condition is not clear, but the most commonly held theory is that the cystic swelling is due to a valvelike obstruction of the common duct at the immediate supraduodenal level, the obstruction resulting from abnormal peritoneal fixation of the first and second portions of the duodenum. Some investigators believe that choledochal cysts develop secondary to repeated ascending infections of the lower common bile duct, with subsequent stenosis of the duct at the supraduodenal level.[14]

In nearly 95 per cent of cases of choledochal cyst, the pancreatic and common bile ducts join and form a common channel 1.5 to 2 cm superior to the ampulla of Vater but inferior to the cystic swelling. This unusual site of junction is a persistence of the embryonic hepaticopancreatic duct. It permits reflux of pancreatic juice into the biliary duct, a circumstance of probable etiologic importance in the development of the cystic change in the duct.

Patients with choledochal cysts experience episodes of cholangitis, but flow of bile from the common bile duct into the duodenum is never completely obstructed.

ANATOMY OF THE BILIARY TREE

The Gallbladder[5]

The gallbladder is a pear-shaped organ that lies in a depression on the inferior or visceral surface of the right lobe of the liver. The position of the gallbladder marks the boundary of the right and left hepatic lobes. The gallbladder is attached to the liver by areolar connective tissue that contains multiple small lymphatics and veins. These lymphatics and veins connect the venous and lymphatic systems of the gallbladder with those of the liver. Additionally, in rare cases one or more small accessory bile ducts pass through this tissue to enter the gallbladder directly.

Normally, only that portion of the gallbladder not in direct contact with the liver is covered with peritoneum. Some gallbladders, however, are suspended on a mesentery and thus are almost completely covered with peritoneum.

For purposes of gross description, the gallbladder is usually divided into a fundus, body, infundibulum, and neck. The fundus is the rounded blind end of the gallbladder, which usually projects 0.5 to 1 cm beyond the free edge of the right lobe of the liver. The top of the fundus is usually found lying in the angle formed by the right lateral border of the rectus abdominis muscle and the ninth costal cartilage. In this position it comes into contact with the anterior peritoneum of the abdominal wall. However, the positions of the gallbladder and the ninth costal cartilage vary enough that the gallbladder may be above or below this point. In hepatic and biliary tract disease, the relationship of the gallbladder to the anterior peritoneum may change considerably, depending on the size of the organ. It is the fundus that becomes palpable in the right upper abdominal quadrant when the gallbladder distends. Occasionally, the fundus is kinked upon itself, an anomaly referred to as a phrygian cap.

The fundus passes without a demonstrable transition into the body, which constitutes the largest segment of the organ. Unless a mesentery is present, the entire superior surface of the gallbladder body is closely attached to the visceral surface of the liver over the area of the gallbladder bed. It is this intimate relationship to the visceral surface of the liver that permits direct spread of gallbladder inflammation to the liver. It also enables early spread of carcinoma of the gallbladder into the liver. On occasion, rupture of a gallbladder containing stones will place the stones between the body of the gallbladder and the inferior liver surface.

The free surface of the body and the infundibulum of the gallbladder lie in close approximation to the first portion and the superior segment of the second portion of the duodenum (Fig. 1–5). In duodenal or biliary tract disease, inflammatory adhesions may form between the duodenum and the gallbladder. A fistula may develop at this spot, and gallstones may pass into the bowel. The body and infundibulum of the gallbladder are also in close relationship to the hepatic flexure and the right one third of the transverse colon. Adhesions between the gallbladder and colon are common, and fistulae may develop between these two structures. The serosal surfaces of the gallbladder may come into contact with loops of small bowel that reside in the right hypochondrium. In patients with a high-lying cecum and appendix, these organs may lie against the gallbladder.

The infundibulum of the gallbladder is the tapering transitional area between the body and neck of the organ. It usually appears as a shallow diverticulum, lying close to the

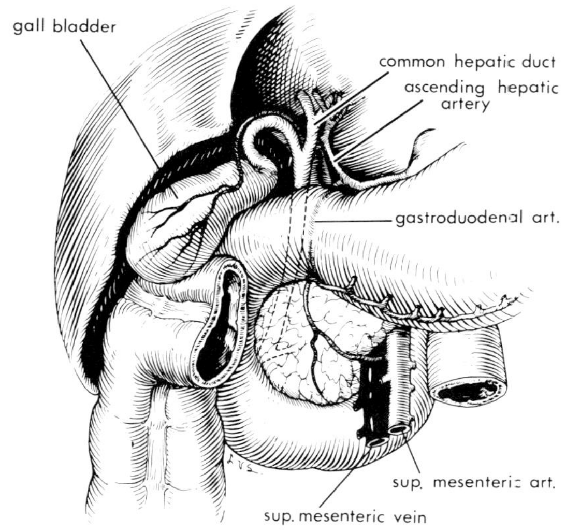

Figure 1–5. Relationship of structures in the gallbladder fossa.

undersurface of the cystic duct, and on occasion it completely hides the cystic duct from view. It is attached to the right lateral surface of the first part of the duodenum by a relatively avascular, double-layered peritoneal fold, which is derived from the inferior margin of the right free border of the hepatoduodenal ligament. This fold, called the cholecystoduodenal ligament, helps guide the surgeon to the major vascular and ductal structures lying in the biliary fossa.

Hartmann's pouch is an asymmetric bulge of the inferior surface of the gallbladder infundibulum. It lies close to the neck of the organ and is frequently a convenient area to put on traction to improve exposure of the neck of the gallbladder and the cystic duct. When particularly well developed, it may be so adherent to the cystic duct that the duct cannot be mobilized until Hartmann's pouch has been dissected free. Hartmann's pouch may also become adherent to the common bile duct, making cholecystectomy difficult and predisposing to common bile duct injury.

The infundibulum of the gallbladder rapidly tapers into the neck, which is narrow and curves upon itself in the form of an S. The neck is usually directed superiorly, dorsally, and to the left, but it may be directed transversely or inferiorly. It narrows into a well-marked constriction at its junction with the cystic duct. The transition between the neck of the gallbladder and the cystic duct may be abrupt or gradual. The neck is quite short (5 to 7 mm, for example). It occupies the deepest part of the "cystic fossa," situated close to the right lateral free border of the hepatoduodenal ligament (Fig. 1–5).

The *arterial supply to the gallbladder*[1, 7] is usually from a single cystic artery (Figs. 1–6 and 1–7). In a few cases (12 per cent), a double cystic artery is present. Normally the cystic artery arises from the proximal segment of the right hepatic artery, and it almost immediately divides into two branches—one running along the peritoneal surface of the gallbladder and the other usually lying between the gallbladder and the liver. The cystic artery usually lies superior to the cystic duct, but it may lie anterior to it, to the left of it, or dorsal to it (Fig. 1–7). If it arises to the left of the common bile duct, it may pass to the right, either dorsal or ventral to the common bile duct or the common hepatic duct.

The site of origin of the cystic artery varies greatly. It may arise from an aberrant right hepatic artery, from the left hepatic artery, from the common hepatic artery, or from one of the branches of the celiac artery other than the hepatic artery (Figs. 1–6 and 1–7). Rarely, it arises from the superior mesenteric artery.

After it departs from the right hepatic artery, the cystic artery may parallel the course of the parent artery for a varying distance. In such cases it may easily be confused with the right hepatic artery. In 7 to 10 per cent of cases, the cystic artery does not leave the right hepatic artery until just before that vessel enters the right lobe of the liver. In such cases the cystic artery is very short (a few millimeters), and it runs inferiorly from close to the visceral surface of the liver to the superior surface of the neck of the gallbladder. The cystic artery usually branches close to the neck of the gallbladder. If either the superficial or the deep branch of the cystic artery is not found at or near that point, one must always suspect the possibility of a double cystic artery.

The triangle of Calot is bounded on the left by the common hepatic duct, on the right by the cystic duct, and superiorly by the hilum of the liver. In and about this triangle are the majority of the structures of importance in cholecystectomy (Fig. 1–6). The apex of the triangle (the cystohepatic angle) is the most critical area, since in it are usually the cystic artery, the right hepatic artery, 95 per cent of accessory right hepatic arteries, and 90 per cent of accessory bile ducts. The size

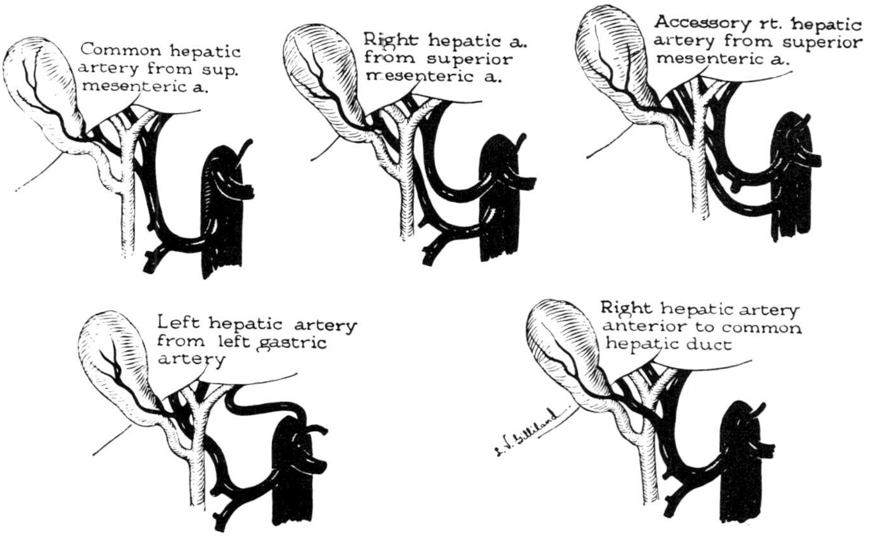

Figure 1–6. Variations in the relationship of the right hepatic artery to the right hepatic duct and the common hepatic duct.

of the triangle varies with both the length and the angle of union of the hepatic and cystic ducts.

There is no single major cystic vein per se. Venous return from the gallbladder leaves the organ via multiple small veins that run either from the hepatic surface of the gallbladder directly into the liver bed or toward the cystic duct, where they join with venous radicals from the common bile duct before eventually entering the portal venous system.

Lymphatic drainage from the gallbladder usually takes one or both of the following routes: (1) The lymph may run directly into the gallbladder bed of the liver via multiple small lymphatic channels. This may allow establishment of a localized hepatitis in the presence of inflammatory disease of the gall-

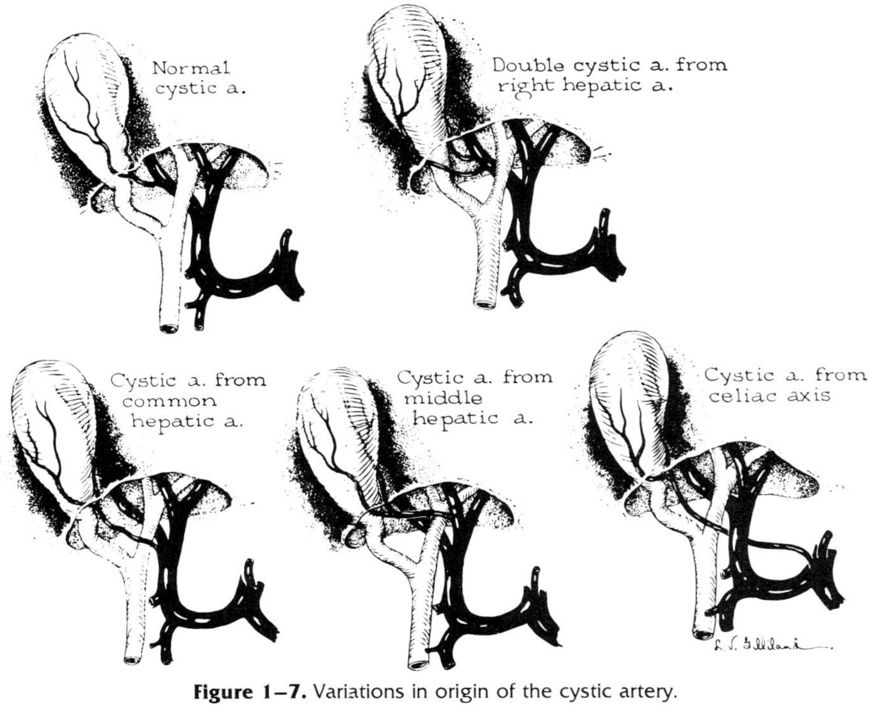

Figure 1–7. Variations in origin of the cystic artery.

bladder. (2) The lymph may drain toward the cystic duct and into a single node or a series of nodes overlying the cystic duct. From these nodes, lymph may pass superiorly via lymphatics in the hepatoduodenal ligament to nodes close to the hilum of the liver, or inferiorly into lymphatics in the inferior portion of the hepatoduodenal ligament. This inferior flow of lymph eventually enters the nodes about the celiac axis.

The gallbladder receives nerve fibers from both the sympathetic and the parasympathetic nervous systems. They travel via the hepatic plexus, beginning at the celiac plexus and extending superiorly toward the gallbladder along with the hepatic artery and the portal vein. The hepatic plexus contains afferent, sympathetic, and parasympathetic vagal fibers. The plexus is joined just inferior to the liver by branches from the left trunk of the vagus. The afferent fibers present in the hepatic plexus supplying the extrahepatic biliary system include some pain fibers. Consequently, pain from the extrahepatic biliary tree is usually referred to the epigastric or right hypochondrial areas and may be referred to the right scapular region. Conduction of pain from the biliary tract is transmitted entirely via fibers that run with the sympathetic nerves. The nerves supplying the gallbladder and the sphincter of Oddi facilitate, but are not essential for, gallbladder emptying.

Histologically the gallbladder wall comprises the following layers: (1) a mucous layer, composed of columnar epithelium and lamina propria; (2) a layer of smooth muscle; (3) a well-developed perimuscular connective tissue layer; and (4) an outer serous membrane.

The mucous layer has numerous folds that are particularly evident in the empty gallbladder. This increases the surface area of epithelium in contact with bile. The basal surface of the gallbladder epithelium is in contact with a lamina propria, which consists of loose connective tissue, elastic fibers, blood vessels, and lymphocytes. The epithelial cells contain a rich supply of mitochondria, and their nuclei are located in the basal third of the columnar cell. The apical region of the epithelial cells show abundant microvilli. Near the neck of the gallbladder the epithelium invaginates into the lamina propria and forms tubuloacinar glands, which possess a wide lumen. The cells lining these glands are similar to mucus-secreting cells and are responsible for the mucus in bile.

The muscular layer of the gallbladder consists of several layers of smooth muscle organized longitudinally and diagonally to the long axis of the gallbladder. A thick connective tissue layer connects the gallbladder to its liver bed. The visceral surface of the gallbladder is covered by a serous layer similar to the peritoneum.

At the *electron microscopic level*, the structure of the gallbladder epithelium is perfectly suited to its physiologic function of bile concentration. At the apical surface of the gallbladder epithelial cell, numerous microvilli are present. Immediately below the luminal surface of the epithelium, adjoining cells are tightly bound together by junctional complexes and associated tonofilaments (Fig. 1–8). These complexes (called tight junctions) separate the paracellular space from the gallbladder lumen. Lateral cell borders also contain numerous microvilli. During times of active bile concentration, the basolateral intercellular spaces are dilated from the presence of eletrolytes and water. In the resting stage, the lateral cellular spaces are collapsed and the microvilli are markedly interdigitated. Numerous small mitochondria are present, as is expected in any tissue involved in active ion transport. The Golgi complex is well developed and found in a supranuclear position.[12]

Right and Left Hepatic Ducts and Common Hepatic Duct

In each individual liver segment, the smaller bile ducts unite to form a single channel called the segmental bile duct. Rarely do two ducts drain one liver segment. The right and left hepatic ducts are formed by the confluence of the segmental ducts within the substance of the hepatic lobes. It is not unusual for as much as 1 to 3 cm of the lobar duct to lie within hepatic tissue. Generally the terminal intrahepatic segment of the left hepatic duct is easier to delineate than the similar segment of the right hepatic duct, because the tributary branches of the former join more proximally within the liver. This anatomic fact is of considerable importance in operative procedures in which an additional length of biliary duct is needed for an anastomosis to the gut. In about 95 per cent of cases, the right and left hepatic ducts unite in an extrahepatic position just inferior to the porta hepatis (Fig. 1–9). In the remainder, their union is intrahepatic. The usual extrahepatic length of each hepatic lobar duct varies from 0.5 to 1.5 cm. This portion of the duct can be seen only if the pylorus, the first portion of the duodenum, and the hepatoduodenal ligament are depressed inferiorly and the quadrate lobe of the liver is lifted anteriorly.

Depending partly upon their extrahepatic length, the right and left hepatic ducts may join at a wide angle or an acute angle, or they may descend parallel to each other for a variable distance before joining. Usually, however, the two ducts unite about 1 cm below the porta hepatis to form the common hepatic duct. However, they may remain separate until they reach the junction of the cystic duct with the common hepatic duct. Occasionally, the two hepatic ducts do not unite until after the cystic duct has joined the right hepatic duct. In this case, there is no common hepatic duct.

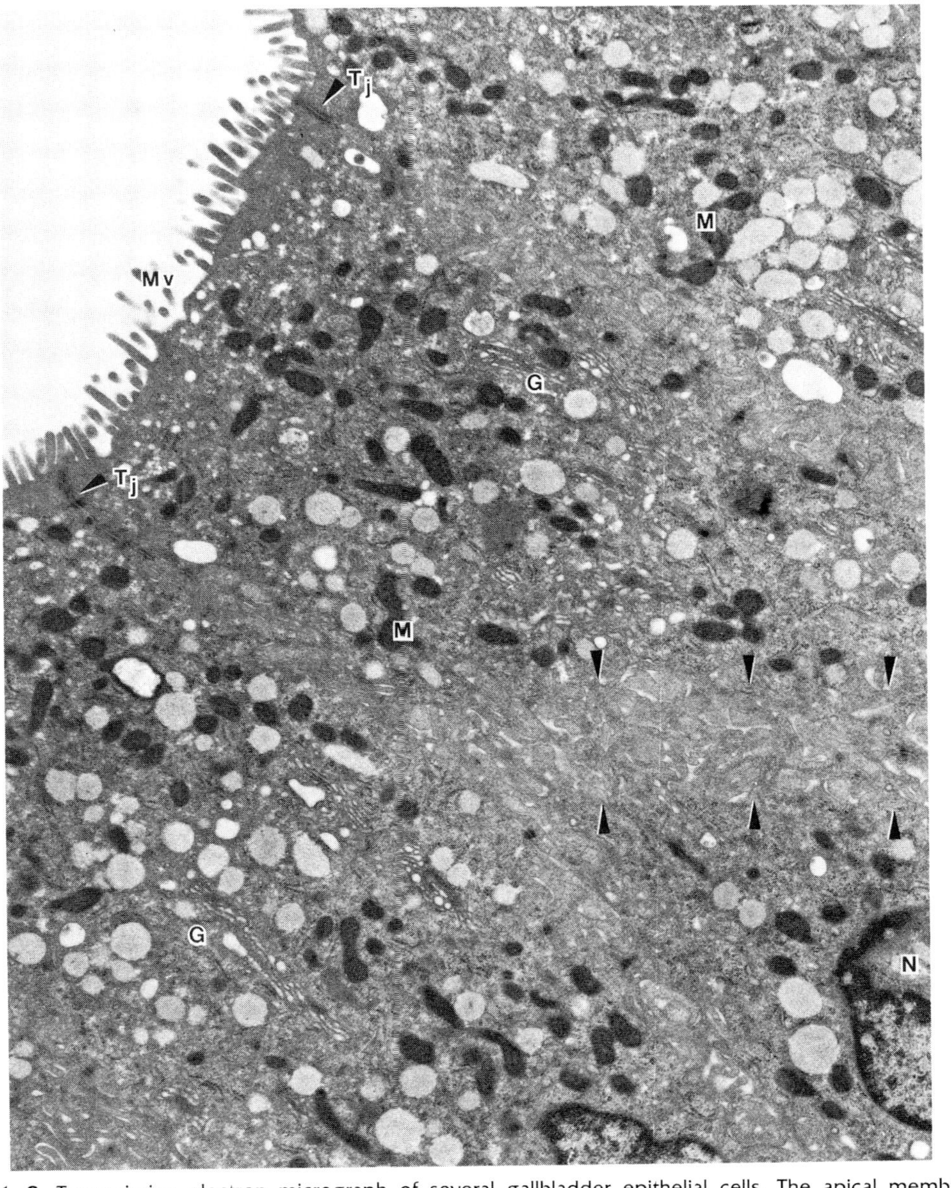

Figure 1–8. Transmission electron micrograph of several gallbladder epithelial cells. The apical membrane has abundant microvilli (Mv). The elaborate interdigitation of lateral cell membranes forms the intercellular space (*arrowheads*), sealed from the gallbladder lumen by the tight junctions (Tj) between the apical surfaces of two adjacent cells. Numerous mitochondria (M) and Golgi complexes (G) and the nucleus (N) are also seen (× 8300). (Courtesy of S. Raper and A. L. Jones.)

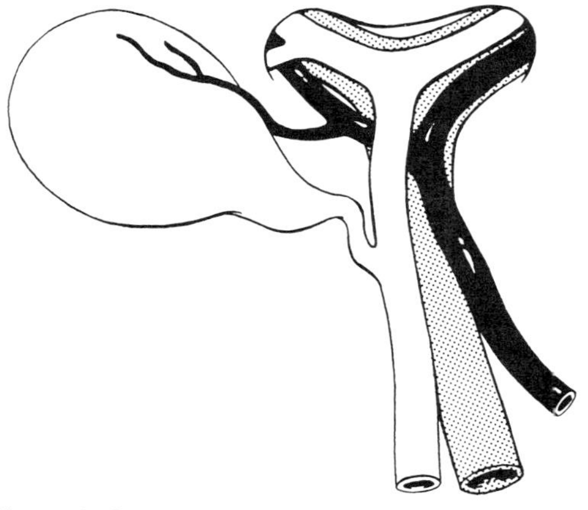

Figure 1–9. Most common type of relationship of the right, left, and common hepatic ducts and the branches of the hepatic artery and the portal vein at the hilum of the liver.

In about 20 per cent of cases, the right anterior and right posterior ducts do not join to form the right hepatic duct. Instead, the right posterior duct joins the left hepatic duct and the right anterior duct joins distally (Fig. 1–10). In these instances, there are three ducts emerging from the porta hepatis. In the past, the right anterior duct was called an accessory duct. This is a mistake, since this is the only duct that provides drainage to the right anterior segment of the liver, and division or damage of this duct may lead to jaundice, cholangitis, or biliary fistula. Because of its extrahepatic location the right anterior duct may also be confused with the cystic duct.

The left lobar segmental bile ducts join in one of two fashions. In 80 per cent of cases, the left medial and left lateral segmental bile ducts join to form the left hepatic duct. In 20 per cent of cases, two or three ducts may drain the left medial or the left lateral segment. However, no matter what the pattern of union of the segmental ducts, the left lobe is drained functionally by a single duct, the left hepatic duct.

The common hepatic duct varies in length from 2 to 6.5 cm. Its course is inferior and slightly to the right.

The hepatic duct and common bile duct lie between the serous layers of the hepatoduodenal ligament. The hepatic lobar ducts are separated from the adjacent right and left hepatic arteries and the subjacent portal vein (and its two superior branches) by a well-marked areolar tissue sheath.[1] This sheath normally compartmentalizes the structures in the upper portion of the hepatoduodenal ligament as far inferiorly as the junction of the cystic duct with the common hepatic duct. This condensation of fibrous areolar tissue about the most superior segment of the biliary ductal system begins intrahepatically, where it can be seen sheathing the segmental biliary ducts within the liver. The two hepatic ducts and their area of confluence are partially obscured by this fibrous tissue, which also extends to and fuses with the outermost layer of the common hepatic duct. This strong sheath of fibrous tissue binds the hepatic ducts to the adjacent vascular structures in such a way that the relationship of the upper segment of the biliary ductal system to the porta hepatis is not easily altered. As a result, even previous operative trauma or inflammation does little to change ductal relationships near their exit from the liver, a fact that is of importance when performing dissections in this area.

The relationship of the right hepatic duct and the common hepatic duct to the right hepatic artery is variable. Usually the right hepatic artery crosses from left to right dorsal to the right hepatic duct at a point just superior to the junction of the right and left hepatic ducts (see Figs. 1–6 and 1–9). However, the artery frequently passes ventral to the right hepatic duct. The right hepatic artery may cross the common hepatic duct either ventrally or dorsally at a level just superior to the transverse course of the cystic artery, in which case it may be difficult to distinguish these two vessels from each other. Finally, the right hepatic artery may not cross

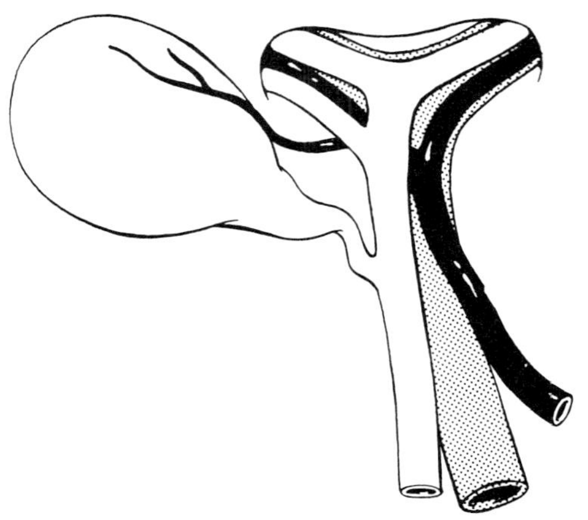

Figure 1–10. Relationship between biliary ducts and hepatic artery and portal vein at the liver hilum. On occasion, the right posterior and the right anterior ducts do not join to form the right hepatic duct. Instead, the right posterior duct joins the left hepatic duct. The right anterior duct may be confused with the cystic duct.

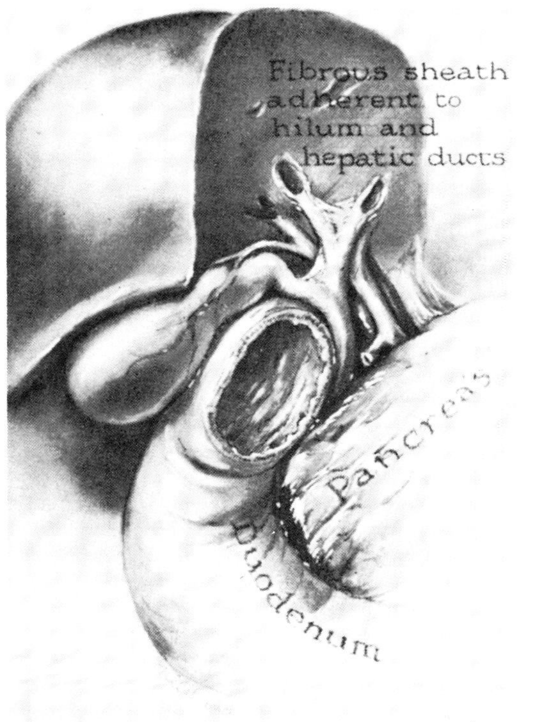

Figure 1–11. Note the fibrous sheath surrounding the junction of the hepatic ducts with the common bile duct extending both superiorly into the liver and inferiorly onto the common bile duct.

the right hepatic duct until just before the duct disappears into the porta hepatis. Because of its position, the right hepatic artery is especially susceptible to injury during biliary tract surgery; great care must be exercised to avoid mistaking it for the cystic artery (Fig. 1–11).

In about 80 per cent of cases, the left hepatic artery lies just ventral to the main trunk of the portal vein. In the remaining 20 per cent of cases, it lies slightly to the left of the portal vein (Fig. 1–9). It is seldom, if ever, dorsal or to the right of the portal vein. In almost 95 per cent of cases, the left hepatic artery lies to the left of the bile duct, but when there is a low union of the left and right hepatic ducts it has been found to run toward the liver between the two ducts. To summarize, the common hepatic duct is crossed by an artery, usually the right hepatic or the cystic artery, in about 30 per cent of cases. The right hepatic duct is close (ventral or dorsal) to the right hepatic artery in about 90 per cent of cases.

Like the gallbladder, the hepatic ducts receive their nerve supply from the anterior and posterior divisions of the hepatic plexus.

Both the hepatic ducts and the common bile duct are lined by a mucous membrane with a columnar epithelium whose cells contain an abundance of mitochondria. The lamina propria is thin and surrounded by a very thin layer of smooth muscle. As the common duct nears the duodenum the muscular layer becomes thicker; it is thickest in the pancreatic and intramural portions of the duct. There is a fibrous coat external to the thin muscular layer. The internal mucous layer contains numerous mucous glands that are markedly lobulated and that open via minute orifices.

The Cystic Duct

The cystic duct connects the neck of the gallbladder to the common hepatic duct. It is not too unusual, however, for the duct to join the right hepatic duct. Generally it is about 5 cm long, but its length may vary markedly (from 0.5 cm to 8 cm) depending upon its site and mode of junction with the hepatic duct. The circumference of the duct varies from 3 to 12 mm, and the larger ducts may allow gallbladder stones to enter the common bile duct. Congenital absence of the cystic duct has been reported, in which case the gallbladder is interposed between the hepatic and common bile ducts.

With the hepatoduodenal ligament placed on a stretch, the cystic duct usually runs dorsally, to the left, and inferiorly to join the common hepatic duct. On occasion its course may be quite tortuous. The cystic duct (1) may join the common hepatic duct at a right angle; (2) may parallel the right side of the common bile duct before entering it; (3) may run dorsal to the common duct and enter its dorsal surface; (4) may run dorsal to the common duct and enter it from its left side; (5) may enter the right hepatic duct; (6) may enter the common duct after passing behind the first portion of the duodenum; and (7) on rare occasions, may join the common duct just before the common duct enters the posteromedial duodenal wall.

The mode of entrance of the cystic duct into the common hepatic duct may be angular, parallel, or spiral (Fig. 1–12). The angular type is the most common, occurring in over 70 per cent of individuals. The angle of junction in the angular type may vary from a right angle to an acute angle (e.g., 10 degrees). In the parallel type of junction the two ducts run alongside each other for 1.5

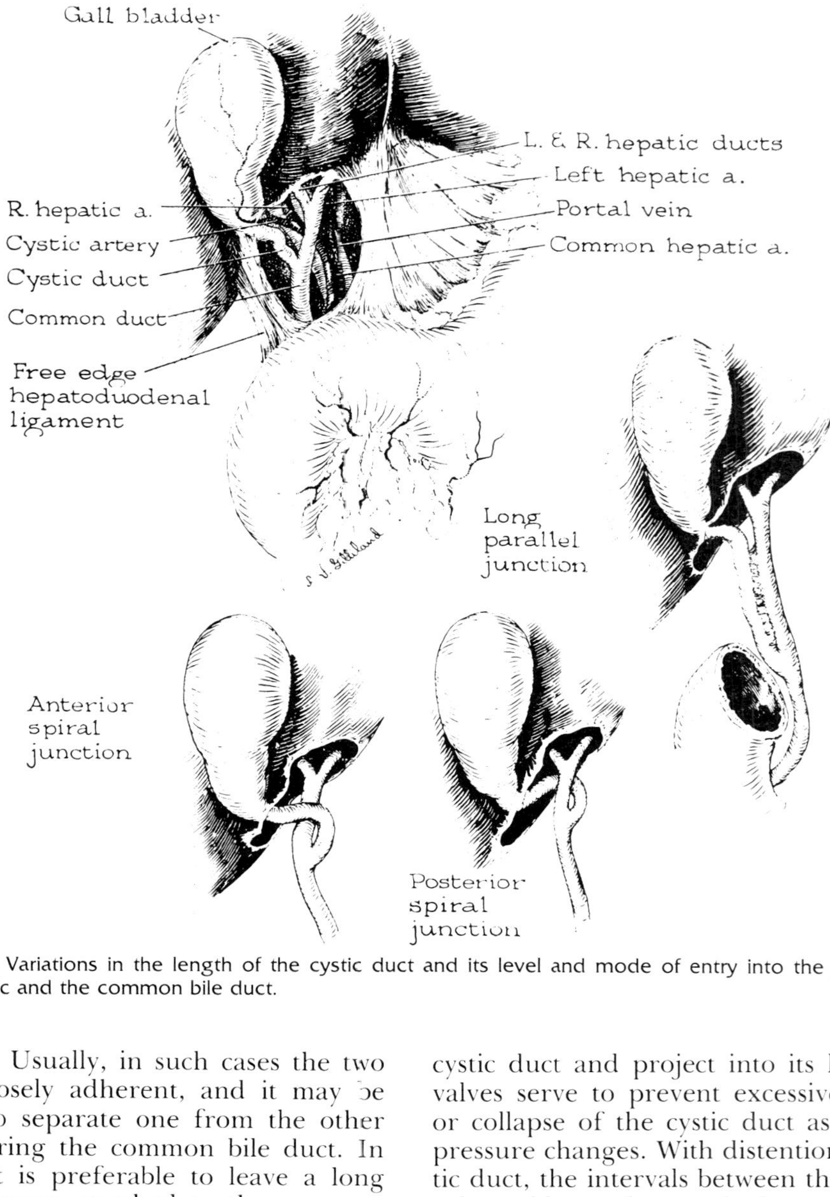

Figure 1–12. Variations in the length of the cystic duct and its level and mode of entry into the junction of the common hepatic and the common bile duct.

cm to 6 cm. Usually, in such cases the two ducts are closely adherent, and it may be impossible to separate one from the other without injuring the common bile duct. In such cases it is preferable to leave a long cystic duct stump attached to the common bile duct. In the spiral type of junction, the cystic duct may pass either ventral or dorsal to the common hepatic duct before joining it (Fig. 1–12). The spirals vary, so the cystic duct may lie anterior or anterolateral, or posterior or posterolateral, to the common bile duct. On occasion, a spiraling duct may even empty into the left lateral surface of the common hepatic duct.

The mucous membrane that lines the interior of the cystic duct has four to ten crescentic folds, referred to as the spiral valve of Heister. Similar folds are found in the terminal segment of the short gallbladder neck. They span the entire length of the cystic duct and project into its lumen. The valves serve to prevent excessive distention or collapse of the cystic duct as intraductal pressure changes. With distention of the cystic duct, the intervals between the individual valves widen and cause the lumen of the duct to appear twisted upon itself. The valves tend to block passage of a gallstone into the common bile duct.

The distal end of the cystic duct usually is found within the free right border of the hepatoduodenal ligament. This free border is known as the cholecystoduodenal ligament and is the key to the operative search for the cystic duct.

If the cystic artery comes off the right hepatic artery in a relatively low angular position close to the cystic duct, the artery usually runs transversely just superior to the cystic duct (see Fig. 1–6). Alternatively, it may lie dorsal to the cystic duct; in about 5 per cent of cases, it runs inferior to the cystic duct. If the cystic artery comes off the right hepatic artery in a high position, the cystic artery usually moves inferiorly to the neck or the body of the gallbladder, abandoning its usual close relationship to the cystic duct.

The right hepatic artery usually lies to the left of the cystic duct, but in 7 to 10 per cent of cases it passes behind the cystic duct, and on rare occasions it has been found to pass ventral to the cystic duct. The portal vein lies on a plane just dorsal and to the left of the cystic duct. The cystic duct and the cystic artery usually lie well superior to the epiploic foramen, the entrance to the lesser peritoneal sac. As a result, pressure exerted by one or two fingers inserted into the epiploic foramen will usually stop bleeding from the right hepatic artery or the cystic artery, or both.

The Common Bile Duct[2–4]

Short descriptions of the hepatoduodenal ligament, the ascending branch of the common hepatic artery, the portal vein, and the foramen of Winslow are needed in order to properly set the stage for an anatomic description of the common bile duct. These descriptions are of importance because the long supraduodenal portion of the common bile duct is intimately related to these structures.

The hepatoduodenal ligament is the name given to the right free border of the hepatogastric ligament (the lesser omentum). The hepatogastric ligament is derived from the posterior layer of the primitive ventral mesogastrium, which in fetal life suspends the foregut from the peritoneum of the ventrolateral abdominal wall. The hepatogastric ligament consists of two layers of peritoneum that run from the porta hepatis to the lesser curvature of the stomach, where they diverge to form the ventral and dorsal serosal coats of the stomach. Dorsal to the hepatogastric ligament lies the lesser sac, and consequently the hepatoduodenal ligament forms the right ventral border of the lesser sac. Between the two leaves of the hepatoduodenal ligament lie the common bile duct, the common hepatic duct, the right and left hepatic ducts, the ascending hepatic artery and its extrahepatic branches, and the portal vein and its right and left terminal branches. The inferior vena cava lies dorsal to the hepatoduodenal ligament and is separated from the ligament by the lesser peritoneal sac and the peritoneum of the posterior abdominal wall, the posterior boundary of the lesser sac.

The common hepatic artery is normally one of the three major branches of the celiac artery. It arises from the celiac artery dorsal to the posterior peritoneal wall of the lesser sac and proceeds to the right and slightly inferiorly, lying close to the right superior border of the head of the pancreas. It then turns ventrally and finally superiorly at about the level of the superior surface of the first portion of the duodenum and enters the hepatoduodenal ligament close to the inferior border of the foramen of Winslow. Just before its ascent in the hepatoduodenal ligament, the artery gives off its right gastric branch, which runs along the lesser curvature of the stomach, and its gastroduodenal branch, which runs inferiorly, dorsal to and closely attached to the first portion of the duodenum. The ascending hepatic artery (hepatica propria) in the hepatoduodenal ligament is of variable length. Normally the artery runs just to the left of the common bile duct and the common hepatic duct (see Figs. 1–6 and 1–7). Just after it enters the hepatoduodenal ligament it lies ventral to the foramen of Winslow, which allows the surgeon to occlude the artery with ventral finger pressure. In its course superiorly, the artery lies in a plane ventral to the portal vein and the inferior vena cava. An aberrant common hepatic artery has been noted on occasion to arise from the superior mesenteric artery, directly from the abdominal aorta, and, rarely, from a common celiac–superior mesenteric artery. Of these anomalies, the most frequent is the origin of the vessel from the superior mesenteric artery (about 15 per cent of cases).

The portal vein is formed dorsal to the neck of the pancreas by the junction of the splenic vein and the superior mesenteric vein. The inferior mesenteric vein enters the portal system by joining the splenic vein, the superior mesenteric vein, or the apex of the angle formed by the junction of the superior mesenteric and splenic veins. After its formation, the portal vein reaches the superior border of the pancreas and then turns ventrally to enter the hepatoduodenal ligament.

As it runs superiorly in the hepatoduodenal ligament, it receives blood from the coronary vein, from the superior pancreaticoduodenal vein, from the pyloric vein, and on occasion from the cystic vein. The portal vein lies dorsal to the common bile duct and the ascending hepatic artery and usually slightly to the left of the common bile duct. It should

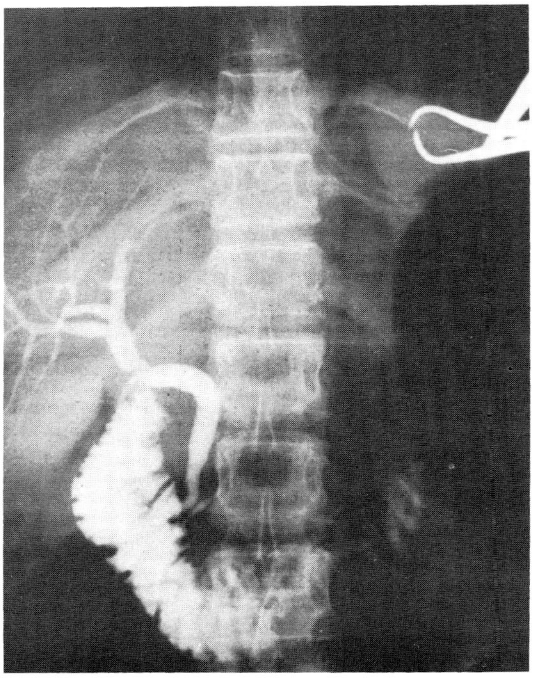

Figure 1–13. Normal operative cholangiogram. The common bile duct terminates into the posteromedial wall of the descending duodenum.

seldom be confused with the common bile duct. Since it lies between the two leaves of the hepatoduodenal ligament, the portal vein always lies ventral to the epiploic foramen.

The epiploic foramen connects the greater and lesser peritoneal cavities. It lies just superior to the upper border of the first portion of the duodenum and is bounded as follows: ventrally by the hepatoduodenal ligament containing the common bile duct, the ascending hepatic artery, and the portal vein; dorsally by the peritoneum of the posterior abdominal wall, which covers the ventral surface of the inferior vena cava; superiorly by the inferior layer of the coronary ligament of the liver as the ligament runs from the right ventral abdominal wall to the liver; and inferiorly by the superior border of the proximal portion of the first segment of the duodenum.

The common bile duct is formed by the junction of the common hepatic duct with the cystic duct. Its length varies with the length of the hepatic lobar ducts; it may be as short as 5 cm and as long as 17 cm. Its width varies from 3 to 15 mm but can become markedly distended as a result of obstructive biliary disease. Its normal diameter is 9 to 11 mm (Fig. 1–13).

Atresia, stenosis, and choledochal cyst, the principal anomalies of the common bile duct, are infrequent. In 20 per cent of individuals, the site of the opening of the common bile duct into the duodenum is other than at the usual point in the mid–descending duodenum. Duplication of the lower third of the common duct has been reported. A few cases have been seen in which the common bile duct has been double throughout its length, one of the ducts draining the right lobe, and the other, the left lobe of the liver. In cases of double common bile duct, the two ducts usually open separately into the duodenum.

The common bile duct has an outer coat of fibroareolar tissue, which contains only scanty amounts of smooth muscle fibers. The smooth muscle, when present, is usually arranged in circular fashion about the duct. The mucosal layer of the duct is continuous with the lining of the gallbladder, the other extrahepatic ducts, and the duodenum. The epithelium is of the columnar type and contains multiple mucous glands.

For purposes of description, the common bile duct is divided into four segments: supraduodenal, retroduodenal, pancreatic, and intraduodenal.

Supraduodenal Segment. The supraduodenal segment of the common bile duct is usually its longest segment, averaging about 2.5 cm in length. It lies within the right free border of the hepatoduodenal ligament (Fig. 1–12). The ascending hepatic artery lies on the same plane as the duct and slightly to the left of it. The portal vein lies dorsal to the duct, separated from it by a varying amount of loose areolar tissue. Just superior to the first portion of the duodenum, the common bile duct lies ventral to the epiploic foramen, separated from it by areolar tissue, the portal vein, and the posterior serosal layer of the hepatoduodenal ligament. This relationship allows the surgeon to palpate the supraduodenal portion of the duct between the index finger of the left hand placed in the epiploic foramen and the thumb placed on the ventral surface of the common bile duct. Consequently, a stone may be milked from the lower segment of the supraduodenal portion of the duct to its superior segment. Multiple lymph nodes lie close to the supraduodenal portion of the common bile duct, and, when enlarged, they may be mistaken for gallstones when the duct is palpated.

Retroduodenal Segment. The retroduodenal segment of the common bile duct varies in length from 2.5 to 4.5 cm. It lies dorsal to the midsegment of the first portion of the duodenum. As it runs inferiorly from the superior to the inferior surface of the duodenum, it slants obliquely from right to left. Lying just to the left of the retroduodenal portion of the duct is the gastroduodenal branch of the hepatic artery. The artery as it descends slants gradually to the right, which places the common bile duct closer to the artery at the inferior margin of the duodenum than at the superior margin. Because of its close relationship to the dorsal surface of the first portion of the duodenum, the common bile duct is sometimes involved in the inflammatory reaction associated with a posterior duodenal ulcer. Additionally, when transecting the proximal part of the first portion of the duodenum in order to perform a Billroth II gastrectomy, the surgeon must be careful not to sever the common bile duct or catch it in the suture closure of the duodenum. If there is difficulty in locating this portion of the common bile duct, a catheter or sound should be passed inferiorly from a choledochotomy in the supraduodenal portion of the duct; this will serve to demonstrate the duct's position. The superior 1 to 1.5 cm of the retroduodenal segment of the common duct is very loosely attached by a thin layer of areolar tissue to the posterior surface of the duodenum.

The retroduodenal segment of the duct may be surgically exposed by incising the ventral layer of the hepatoduodenal ligament just superior to the upper border of the duodenum and then drawing the duodenum inferiorly. In order to expose the entire retroduodenal portion of the common bile duct, one must mobilize the superior half of the descending duodenum using the Kocher maneuver. The avascular peritoneum on the lateral surface of the descending duodenum is incised, and the duodenum is bluntly dissected from the underlying retroperitoneal tissues and rolled to the left.

An often neglected relationship of the retroduodenal segment of the common bile duct is its close association with the middle colic artery. This vessel arises from the superior mesenteric artery just inferior to the sweep of the inferior surface of the pylorus and the first portion of the duodenum. The artery often lies in a fold of the transverse mesocolon that is loosely fused to the inferior surface of these segments of the bowel. During mobilization of the retroduodenal portion of the common bile duct, the fold containing the middle colic artery must be searched for, mobilized, and allowed to drop inferiorly. As the retroduodenal portion of the common bile duct descends behind the superior surface of the duodenum, it is on occasion crossed by the rather variable supraduodenal artery of Wilkie, the artery crossing ventral to the duct. A short distance farther inferiorly, the common bile duct is usually crossed anteriorly by the posterior superior pancreaticoduodenal artery. This is a relatively large vessel, which usually must be dealt with when mobilizing the second segment of the common duct.

Pancreatic Segment. The pancreatic portion of the common bile duct is usually from 2 to 3 cm in length except in those instances in which the duct empties distal to its normal point of entrance into the duodenum, in which case it may be as long as 6 cm. This segment of the duct is related to the head of the pancreas in one of two ways. It may be entirely retropancreatic, lying between the head of the pancreas and the areolar tissues of the retroperitoneum; or it may lie within the substance of the dorsal portion of the pancreatic head, being covered dorsally by a thin layer of pancreatic tissue. The third portion of the common bile duct describes a gentle convex curve to the left as it descends reltively close to the left border of the descending duodenum. Lying to the left lateral side of the duct is the vertebral column. About halfway along its pancreatic course, the third portion of the common duct starts to curve gently to the right; then quite abruptly it describes an almost 90 degree turn to the right to enter the posteromedial surface of the descending duodenum at about its midpoint, just superior to the crossing of the duodenum by the transverse colon. The inferior vena cava lies just dorsal to the third portion of the common duct, separated from it only by a thin layer of areolar tissue. As the portal vein runs obliquely, superiorly, and to the right, it has no close relationship to this portion of the common bile duct. Related to the superior half of the third portion of the common duct is the gastroduodenal artery, which lies just to the left of the duct. The superior pancreaticoduodenal branch of the gastroduodenal artery crosses the third portion of the common bile duct either ventrally or dorsally. It and its multiple duodenal and pancreatic branches make exposure of the third portion of the common duct hazardous. The large pancreaticoduodenal vein that runs on the posterior surface of the pancreatic head is related to the left border of the pancreatic portion of the bile duct just before the vessel joins the portal vein. It is easily torn during surgery on this portion of the duct or on the adjacent descending duodenum or pancreatic head.

Intraduodenal Segment.[8, 11, 15] Just before passing through the duodenal wall, the common bile duct lies dorsal and slightly superior to the major pancreatic duct. The common bile duct passes through the duodenal wall tangentially, similar in some respects to the passage of the ureters through the bladder wall. The course through the duodenal wall is almost 2 cm in length, passing at first through the smooth muscle layers and then, for most of its course, lying in a submucosal position. The classic anatomic description given for the site of penetration of the duodenum by the common duct is the posteromedial wall of the duodenum just superior to the crossing of the duodenum by the transverse colon. This site is generally about 7 cm distal to the pylorus. The passage of the common bile duct into the duodenum is complicated by the presence of the major pancreatic duct, which, like the common bile duct, empties into the duodenum at the summit of the major duodenal papilla.

The terminal portion of the common bile duct is related to the terminal portion of the major pancreatic duct in one of three ways. (1) There frequently is an extraduodenal junction of the two ducts just external to the posteromedial duodenal wall. In such instances, before the two ducts penetrate the duodenal wall they run parallel to one another for a distance of 2 mm to 10 mm. During this close extraduodenal association, the lumina of the two ducts may join, usually just external to the duodenal wall. (2) During the passage of the closely applied bile duct and pancreatic duct through the duodenal wall, the septum between their two lumina is lost, and together they form a true common channel that opens through a single ostium on the major duodenal papilla. (3) In some 20 per cent of cases, the septum between the lumina of the two ducts persists throughout the entire passage of the ducts through the thickness of the duodenal wall. In such cases there is no common channel just proximal to the major duodenal papilla, and the two ducts empty on the papilla by separate ostia. As the common bile duct proceeds through the duodenal wall it narrows markedly. Its normal extraduodenal diameter averages about 10 mm. Almost immediately upon entering the duodenal wall the diameter drops to about 6 mm. The narrowing is so pronounced and comes on so rapidly that it seems to form a ridge between the wide extraduodenal portion of the duct and the narrow intraduodenal portion. This fact is of great importance in common duct exploration, because unless care is taken when the area of the introduodenal junction is probed, a false passage may be formed.

The ampulla of Vater is formed within the intraduodenal portion of the common bile duct as a result of the junction of the lumina of the common bile duct and the major pancreatic duct. Depending upon whether there is an extraduodenal junction of the two ducts, an intraduodenal wall junction, or no junction at all, the length of the ampulla of Vater will vary markedly. The ampulla has been reported to be as long as 14 mm and as short as 3 mm. Obviously, if there is no ductal junction, there is no true ampulla of Vater. The ampulla extends from the point of confluence of the two ducts to just proximal to their exit through a single opening on the duodenal papilla. In over 50 per cent of cases, the common bile duct narrows just before it empties into the ampulla, and in all cases the ampulla narrows just before it empties via the major duodenal papilla. These two intraduodenal ductal areas of narrowing are favorite places for stone impaction in calculous disease of the biliary tract.

Rienhoff and Pickrell[13] described the anatomy of the pancreatic ductal system based on a study of 250 cases. They found no junction of the pancreatic and bile ducts in 29 per cent; two separate intraduodenal lumina separated by a septum reaching to within 2 mm of the apex of the duodenal papilla in 32 per cent (these individuals have a very short ampulla of Vater); and an ampulla longer than 2 mm in about 46 per cent of cases (the average diameter of the ampulla was about 3 mm).

The Muscular Apparatus at the Terminal End of the Common Duct (Sphincter of Oddi) (Fig. 1–14)

The intraduodenal portion of the common bile duct, including the ampulla of Vater, is surrounded by a sheath of smooth muscle fibers. The entire sphincteric system of the distal biliary tract is commonly referred to as the sphincter of Oddi. The smooth musculature of the sphincter is divided into several sections and contains both circular and longitudinal fibers. Thus, the term "sphincter of Oddi" is an extremely loose one, since it does not clearly denote the exact area of the biliary sphincter that is being referred to.

Early investigators felt that the sphincteric apparatus about the terminal segment of the common duct developed from the smooth muscular layers of the neighboring duodenum. However, Boyden and his coworkers showed that the sphincter develops much later in fetal life than does the duodenal muscle and that its genesis is via progressive differentiation of the primitive mesoderm surrounding the intramural portion of the biliary duct.[2, 3] Second, it has been demonstrated that if a manometer is placed in the common duct and a balloon in the duodenum, the biliary tract sphincter operates quite independently of the action of the duodenal musculature.

The placement of the smooth muscle surrounding the intraduodenal segments of the common bile duct is extremely complex (Fig. 1–14). The biliary and pancreatic ducts enter the posteromedial surface of the mid–descending duodenum through an elliptical slit in the circular muscle of the bowel. At their point of entrance, some smooth muscle fibers run to the angles of the opening; others connect the margins of the opening in both the longitudinal and the circular muscle of the duodenum with the major duodenal papilla and with the intraduodenal course of the ducts. These latter fibers serve both to erect the papilla and to anchor the duct securely to the aperture in the duodenal musculature. From the time it pierces the duodenal wall until its junction with the major pancreatic duct, the common bile duct is wrapped in a sheath of circular muscle, the sphincter choledochus (sphincter of Boyden). It is the action of this sphincter that is responsible for filling of the gallbladder during fasting. The sphincter choledochus is made up of two consecutive segments, a proximal one that surrounds the bile duct as it enters the duodenal wall and a distal segment that is completely intramural. When the common bile duct and the major pancreatic duct lie side by side within the duodenal wall, the choledochal sphincter usually interlaces with an inconstant sphincter pancreaticus in a figure-of-eight manner.

If the two ducts unite within the duodenal wall to form the ampulla, just before they do so a sheath of muscle fibers encircles both ducts. This marks the site of origin of the sphincter of the ampulla, which extends almost to the tip of the major duodenal papilla. If this sphincter becomes spastic, a common channel will be formed between the biliary and pancreatic ducts. If the two ducts do not join, but proceed distally to empty separately on the ampulla, the sphincter of the ampulla is replaced by the sphincter of the papilla.

Lindner and coworkers[11] studied 1000 operative cholangiograms and showed that the common bile duct entered the descending duodenum in 87 per cent of cases. The duct entered the angle formed by the junction of the descending and transverse duodenum or entered the proximal portion of the transverse duodenum in the remaining 13 per cent of cases (Figs. 1–15 and 1–16). This

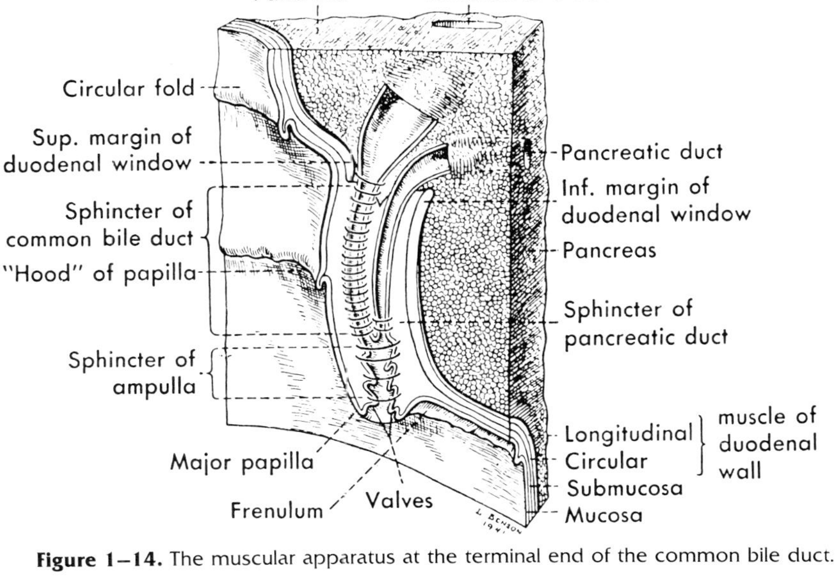

Figure 1–14. The muscular apparatus at the terminal end of the common bile duct.

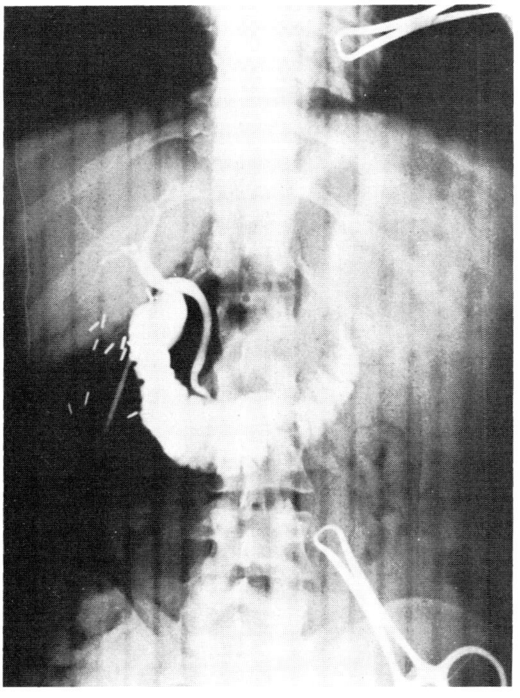

Figure 1–15. Example of the common bile duct terminating in the transverse duodenum. Note the distinct drop inferiorly (*left*) of the common duct in this case.

degree of variability was a sizable departure from previously accepted norms. There were no terminations of the common bile duct in the duodenal bulb or in the fourth portion of the duodenum, nor were there any terminations of the duct in extraduodenal sites. No relationship was found between the length of the descending duodenum and abnormalities of termination of the common bile duct. In those patients in whom the common bile duct entered the duodenum proximal to the junction of the desending and transverse duodenum, the length of the duct ranged from 2.5 cm to 6.9 cm. In those cases in which the entrance of the common bile duct was anomalous, the duct ranged in length from 3.8 to 10.1 cm. It was noted that the common bile ducts that terminated in the inferior duodenal angle or in the proximal transverse duodenum tended almost always to drop directly inferiorly from the inferior surface of the first portion of the duodenum, rather than curving first gently to the left and then compensating with a right curvature toward the descending duodenum (Fig. 1–15). Additionally, it was noted that during its descent inferiorly the common bile duct, in those cases in which it terminated anomalously, frequently lay close to the right lateral border of the vertebral column or, in some cases, actually ventral to the vertebra.

Nerve Supply to the Common Bile Duct (Fig. 1–17)

Whereas the anterior portion of the hepatic plexus gives fibers to the cystic and hepatic ducts, the posterior segment of the hepatic plexus sends nerve fibers to the common bile duct. The posterior hepatic plexus takes its origin from the right celiac plexus via two or three large nerve trunks that pass dorsal to the portal vein near its origin. The fibers then course superiorly along the right margin of the vein. The right side of the posterior hepatic plexus becomes the nerve of the common bile duct and lies upon the dorsal surface of the duct at the inferior border of the epiploic foramen (Fig. 1–17). The posterior hepatic plexus gives off several small descending branches that run on the dorsal aspect of the descending common duct. These nerves distribute several small branches to the pancreas and then penetrate the wall of the common bile duct, where they

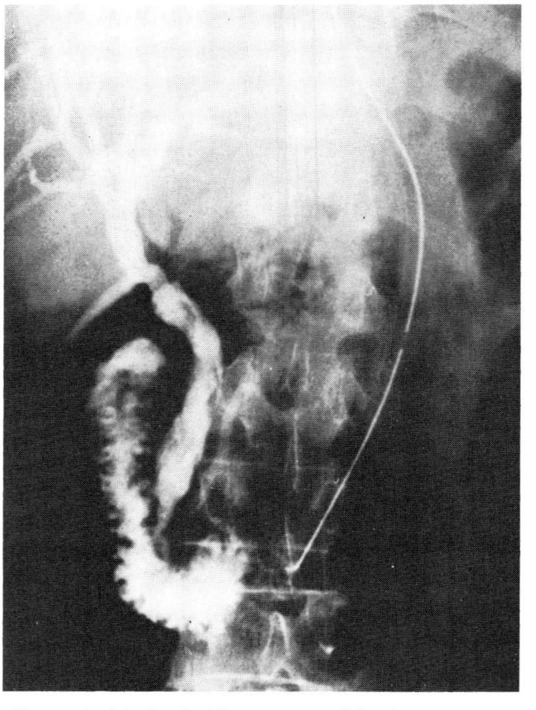

Figure 1–16. Angle: The common bile duct terminates at the junction between the descending and transverse duodenum.

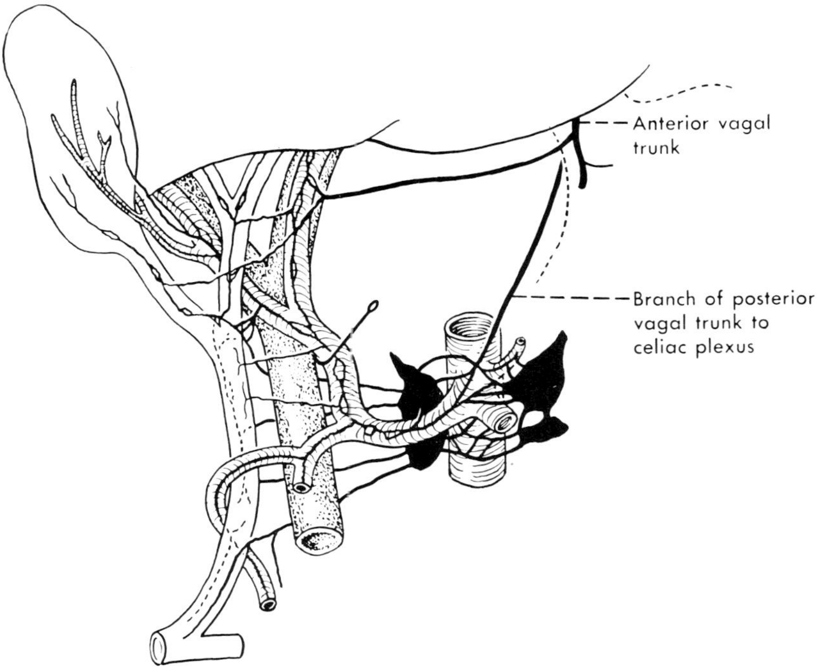

Figure 1–17. Nerve supply to the extrahepatic biliary tract.

can be followed in microscopic section right out to the apex of the duodenal papilla. There seems to be no connection between this nerve plexus and the duodenal wall.

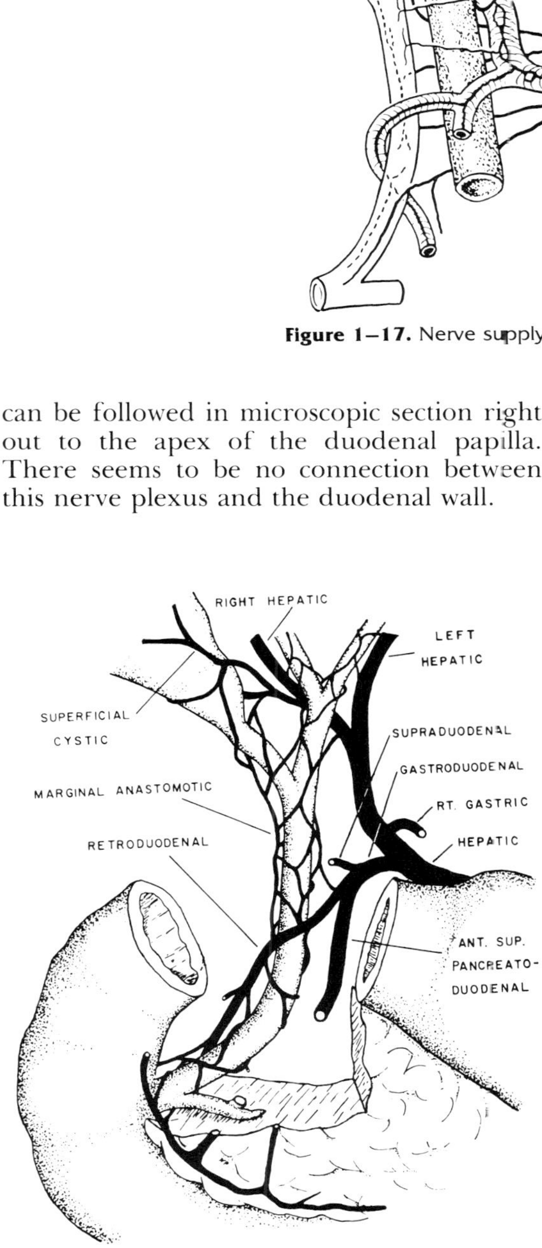

Figure 1–18. Arterial supply to the common bile duct.

Arterial Supply to the Common Bile Duct (Fig. 1–18)

The great variation in the distribution of the arterial supply to the common bile duct and the extremely inconstant anastomotic patterns of the vessels that supply the duct probably account for the postoperative ischemic sequelae that may follow mobilization of long segments of the duct.

Generally the arterial twigs supplying the common bile duct are quite small, easily disrupted, and most inconstant. The major arterial branches to the duct usually arise from the cystic artery or the posterior superior pancreaticoduodenal artery. The supraduodenal portion of the duct is usually nourished by small branches from the cystic artery. These vessels also supply the common hepatic duct and the lower part of the right hepatic duct. If ascending arterial branches from vessels supplying the lower segments of the common bile duct are not well developed, the cystic artery and, on occasion, the right hepatic artery will send off one or two descending branches to the first part of the duct (Fig. 1–18). The retroduodenal or second portion of the common bile duct is usually supplied by four to six branches from the posterior superior pancreaticoduodenal artery as this vessel loops around this segment of the common bile duct. On occasion, one of these branches will ascend to become an accessory cystic artery. The supraduodenal branch of the gastroduodenal artery occasionally will send a twig to the retroduodenal portion of the duct. This branch is usually ablated by the surgeon when he mobilizes the superior surface of the first part of the duodenum. The third and fourth portions of the common duct are supplied by both the anterior and the posterior superior pancreaticoduodenal arteries, and these portions of the duct seem to have a better anastomotic arterial pattern than do the first and second ductal segments.

Venous drainage from the superior portion of the common bile duct ascends along the surface of the common duct and the hepatic and cystic ducts. It enters the liver directly rather than by joining branches of the portal vein. The venous drainage from the inferior half of the common bile duct is into small radicals that directly enter the portal vein.

The ventral surface of the supraduodenal portion of the common bile duct is marked by a constant ascending vein. Bleeding from this vessel can become a nuisance during common duct surgery if it is not ligated above and below the site of the choledochotomy.

The lymphatic drainage from the common bile duct courses superiorly, first into nodes that lie along the course of the duct, and finally into a group of six to ten nodes adjacent to the structures entering and leaving the porta hepatis. Some lymphatic drainage from the common duct reaches the deep pancreatic group of nodes, which is situated near the origin of the superior mesenteric artery. The eventual final station for all common duct lymphatic drainage is into the deep celiac group of nodes lying close to the origin of the celiac artery.

REFERENCES

1. Anson BJ, McVay CB: Surgical Anatomy, 5th ed. Philadelphia, WB Saunders, 1971, pp 597–622.
2. Boyden EA: The sphincter of Oddi in man and certain representative mammals. Surgery 1937; *1*:25.
3. Boyden EA: Humoral vs. neural regulation of the extrahepatic biliary tract. Minn Med 1953;*36*:720.
4. Dowdy GS Jr, Waldron GW, Brown WG: Surgical anatomy of the pancreatico-biliary ductal system. Arch Surg 1962;*84*:229.
5. Goss CM (ed): Gray's Anatomy. 29th American ed. Philadelphia, Lea & Febiger, 1974.
6. Hicken NF, Coray QB, Franz B: Anatomic variations of the extrahepatic biliary system as seen by cholangiographic studies. Surg Gynecol Obstet 1949; *88*:577.
7. Hollinshead HW: The liver and the gall bladder. *In* Anatomy for Surgeons, 3rd ed. New York, Hoeber-Harper, 1982.
8. Keddie NC, Taylor AW, Sykes PA: The termination of the common bile duct. Br J Surg 1974;*61*:623.
9. Landing B: Considerations on the Pathogenesis of Neonatal Hepatitis, Biliary Atresia, Cholangiopathy, and Choledochal Cyst: The Concept of Infantile Obstructive Cholangiopathy. Baltimore, University Park Press, 1972.
10. Lindner HH, Green RB: Embryology and surgical anatomy of the extrahepatic biliary tract. Surg Clin North Am 1964;*44*:1273.
11. Lindner HH, Pena VA, Ruggieri RA: A clinical and anatomical study of anomalous termination of the common bile duct into the duodenum. Ann Surg 1976;*184*:626.
12. Mueller JC, Jones AL, Long JA: Topographic and subcellular anatomy of the guinea pig gallbladder. Gastroenterology 1972;*63*:856.
13. Rienhoff WF Jr, Pickrell KL: Pancreatitis: an anatomical study of the pancreatic and extrahepatic biliary systems. Arch Surg 1945;*51*:205.
14. Saito S, Ishida M: Congenital choledochal cyst. Prog Paediatr Surg 1974;*6*:63.
15. Schulenberg CAR: Anomalies of the biliary tract as demonstrated by operative cholangiography. Med Proc 1970;*16*:351.

*BRUCE F. SCHARSCHMIDT, M.D.**
RUDI SCHMID, M.D.

2

Bile Secretion, Intestinal Lipid Absorption, and the Enterohepatic Circulation of Bile Salts

INTRODUCTION

Hepatic bile formation serves two primary functions. First, it serves as a route of excretion for endogenous substances, such as bilirubin, as well as a variety of exogenous substances, including certain drugs and dyes. Second, bile plays an important role in the absorption of dietary lipids, including the fat-soluble vitamins. Hepatic bile consists of about 90 per cent water. The remaining 10 per cent is composed of electrolytes and organic solutes, such as bile acids, phospholipids, cholesterol, and conjugated bilirubin.

The bile secretory apparatus is illustrated schematically in Figure 2–1. Bile formation begins in the canaliculus; the first section of this chapter will be largely devoted to reviewing the microanatomy of the bile secretory apparatus and current concepts regarding the mechanisms by which the hepatocyte secretes organic and inorganic solutes and thus generates bile flow. Understanding of these basic mechanisms, although incomplete, is rapidly evolving and is an essential first step in characterizing the pathophysiology of cholestasis. Consideration of the relationship between hepatic secretion of bile acids, phospholipids, and cholesterol will serve as an important background for Chapter 4 on gallstone formation and dissolution. Attention will then be paid to the modifications that occur in the composition of canalicular bile as it passes through the intra- and extrahepatic biliary tree and gallbladder. The final areas covered in this chapter will be the role of bile acids in intestinal lipid absorption and the enterohepatic circulation of bile acids and other bile constituents under normal conditions and in certain disease states.

FUNCTIONAL ANATOMY OF THE BILE SECRETORY APPARATUS

The Primary Bile Secretory Unit: Hepatocyte and Canaliculus

Within the liver lobule, hepatocytes are arranged in one cell–thick plates bathed on either side by sinusoidal blood (Fig. 2–2).[1] Each hepatocyte is bounded by a cell membrane, which has three functionally and morphologically distinct areas: the sinusoidal face, which accounts for approximately 37 per cent of the cell surface; the lateral face, which contacts adjacent hepatocytes and accounts for about 50 per cent of the surface area; and the bile canalicular face, which accounts for the remaining 13 per cent of the cell surface.[2, 197]

Current evidence suggests that the membranes of all living cells, including hepatocytes, consist of a phospholipid bilayer in which the hydrophobic tails of the phospholipid fatty acids are oriented toward the center of the membrane and the polar phospholipid head groups are oriented toward the exterior (extracellular or cytoplasmic side) of the membrane.[3] Associated with this phospholipid bilayer are "peripheral" proteins that "float" on the surface of the membrane and are readily detached, and "integral" pro-

*Recipient of NIH Research Career Development and Award 5 KO4 AM-00323. This work was also supported in part by NIH Liver Center Grant PSO AM-26740, NIH Research Grant AM-26270, and The Walter C. Pew Fund.

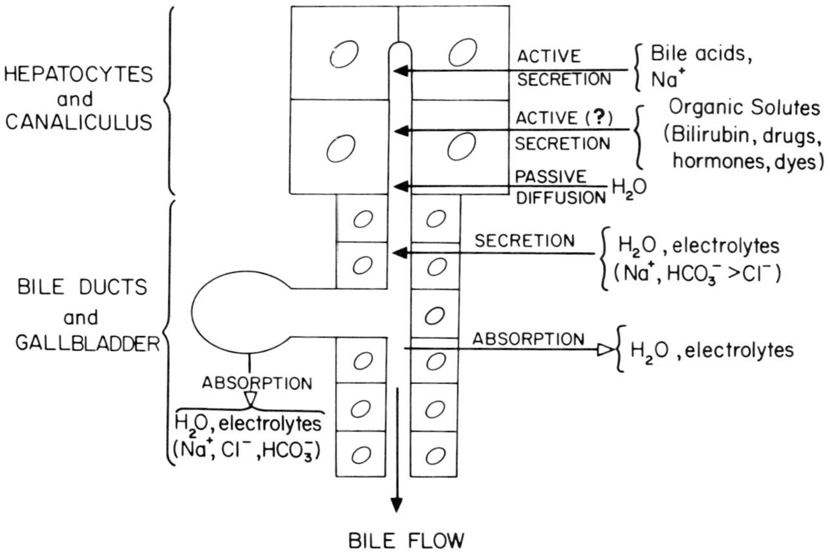

Figure 2–1. Schematic illustration of the mechanisms of bile formation. Bile secretion begins at the level of the bile canaliculus by active secretion of bile acids and possibly sodium and certain organic solutes. Active secretion of these substances is followed by passive water flow. Canalicular bile subsequently is modified in the bile ducts and gallbladder by secretion and reabsorption of water and electrolytes.

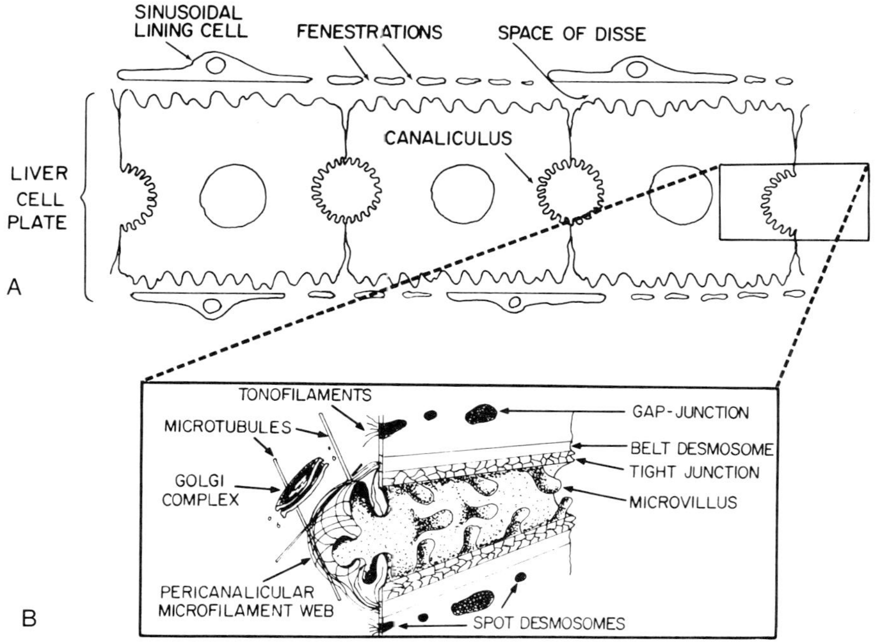

Figure 2–2. *A*, Schematic illustration of a liver cell plate. The single cell–thick liver plate is separated from the sinusoidal blood on either side by sinusoidal lining cells. These lining cells have large fenestrations in their cytoplasm that allow free access of plasma to the space of Disse. Each hepatocyte surface membrane consists of three distinct areas, the sinusoidal surface, the lateral surface, and the canalicular surface. *B*, An enlargement of the hemicanaliculus shown in *A*. The canalicular membranes of adjacent hepatocytes are joined by *tight junctions*, shown here en face, which seal the canalicular space from the lateral intercellular space and sinusoidal space. The *belt desmosomes* adjacent to the tight junction help hold the cells together and serve as the site of attachment of pericanalicular microfilaments. *Spot desmosomes* can be thought of as "spot welds" between adjacent liver cells. They also help hold cells together and are the sites of insertion of intracellular tonofilaments, which transmit passive forces to the membrane surface. *Gap junctions* allow direct passage of certain molecules between the cytoplasm of adjacent cells. The Golgi complex and microfilaments are characteristically concentrated in the pericanalicular area and may play a role in bile secretion.

teins that may actually span the entire width of the membrane. Such proteins serve structural purposes (as, for example, the creation of intercellular junctions), or they may function as receptors, carriers, or enzymes that play an active role in a variety of cellular processes. NaK-ATPase, alkaline phosphatase, 5′-nucleotidase, adenylate cyclase, leucine amino peptidase, and γ-glutamyltranspeptidase are all enzyme proteins known to be present in liver cell membranes.[2, 4, 5] These proteins are distributed unevenly among the three major membrane faces of the hepatocyte; their distribution as well as the distribution of phospholipids and other membrane proteins is largely responsible for the functional specialization exhibited by the three major regions of the hepatocyte membrane.

The liver cell membrane facing the sinusoid is actively involved in transport. Compounds such as bilirubin and sulfobromophthalein, which circulate in plasma tightly bound to albumin, as well as less tightly protein-bound substances, such as bile acids, are taken up by the hepatocyte across this membrane. On the other hand, substances such as lipoproteins and many plasma proteins synthesized in the liver are secreted across the membrane into the sinusoidal blood. This active bidirectional transport of large and frequently protein-bound substances is facilitated by the very large fenestrations present in the cytoplasmic extensions of the endothelial cells lining the sinusoid (Figs. 2–2*A* and 2–3). These gaps allow plasma proteins to enter the space of Disse and make direct contact with the sinusoidal membrane of the hepatocytes. Liver-blood exchange also is facilitated by the irregular microvilli covering the sinusoidal face, which greatly increase the surface of the cell (Fig. 2–2*A*) and sometimes protrude directly into the sinusoidal lumen through fenestrations in the endothelial lining cells.[2]

The lateral face of the hepatocyte extends from the sinusoid to the edge of the bile canaliculus and is relatively flat (Fig. 2–2*A*). This surface of the hepatocyte is specialized to allow attachment and communication between adjacent cells. The *tight junction* is an area immediately adjacent to the bile canaliculus, which joins adjacent hepatocytes and thus seals the bile canaliculus from the sinusoidal space (Fig. 2–2*B*). Structurally, the tight junction appears to consist of matching rows of integral membrane positions (one row contributed by each hepatocyte), which make head-to-head contact in a manner analogous to the teeth of a zipper and obliterate the intercellular space.[2, 6] Viewed en face, these rows of integral membrane proteins look like a random series of interconnecting lines (Fig. 2–2*B*). The number of rows and

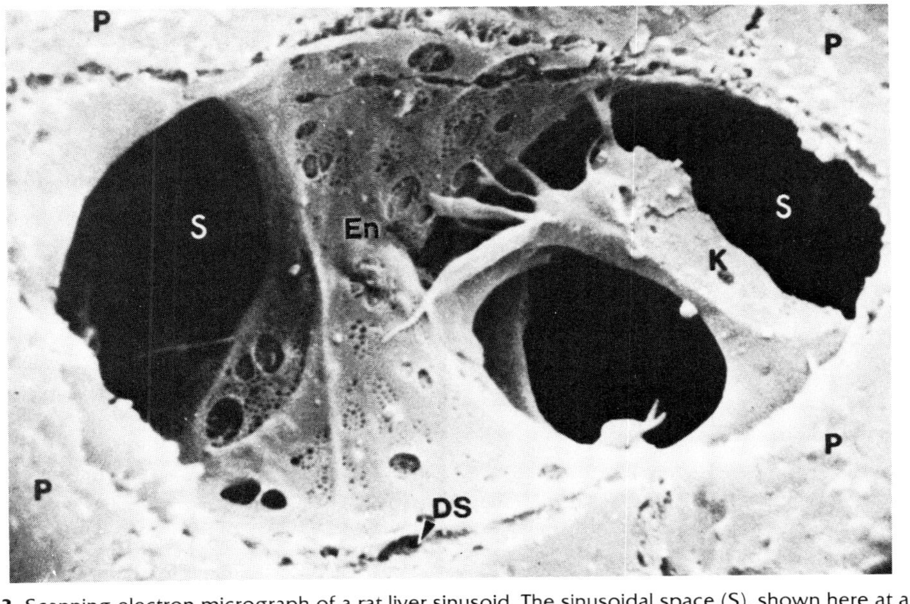

Figure 2–3. Scanning electron micrograph of a rat liver sinusoid. The sinusoidal space (S), shown here at a bifurcation point, is lined by endothelial cells (En) with many cytoplasmic fenestrations that allow blood proteins to enter the space of Disse (DS) and come into close contact with the sinusoidal membrane of hepatic parenchymal cells (P). A phagocytic Kupffer cell (K) is shown spanning the sinusoidal space (× 7500). (From Jones AL, Schmucker DL: Gastroenterology *73*:833, 1977. Used by permission.)

their spacing appear to correlate with the "tightness" of the tight junction.[6] Although it was originally believed that the tight junction was impermeable, subsequent studies have shown that tight junctions in some tissues, such as the proximal renal tubules, are actually rather leaky.[7] The tight junctions between liver cells show considerable regional heterogeneity[8] and are morphologically intermediate between "tight" tight junctions and "leaky" tight junctions,[2, 8] with respect to strand number and junction depth. Moreover, there is now considerable evidence that water, inorganic electrolytes such as sodium, and certain organic solutes too large to pass readily through cell membranes enter bile "paracellularly," i.e., by passing directly from sinusoid to canaliculus via the intercellular space through the tight junction.[9–11]

The next specialized area of the lateral cell surface as one proceeds outward from the bile canaliculus, past the tight junction toward the sinusoid, is the *zonula adherens* or *belt desmosome* (Fig. 2–2*B*).[2, 6] This is a continuous beltlike junction that serves the important function of holding adjacent liver cells together. The intercellular space is filled with filamentous material, and on each cytoplasmic side of the belt desmosome is a thick mat of intermeshed filaments. The *microfilaments* leading to this mat measure about 70 Å and appear to contain actin, a contractile protein.[12, 13] Thus, the belt desmosome not only serves an adhesive purpose but, because of the contractile actin fibers, may also transmit internally generated forces from cell to cell. As shown in Figure 2–2*B*, these actin fibers that insert in the belt desmosome form a weblike network around the canaliculus. Two other specialized structures are located on the lateral surface of the hepatocytes. *Spot desmosomes,* (maculae adherens), which can be thought of as "spot welds" between adjacent hepatocytes, serve as sites of attachment for cytoplasmic tonofilaments that presumably permit transmission of passive stresses between cells. *Gap junctions* (maculae communicans) are entirely different types of specialized membrane structures that directly connect the cytoplasm of adjacent cells via large molecular complexes. These complexes span the intercellular space and have in their center a hollow channel. Gap junctions thus allow direct transfer of substances from cell to cell.[2, 6]

The bile canaliculus is the third major portion of the surface membrane and represents the "business end" of the hepatocyte insofar as bile secretion is concerned. A substantial portion of this chapter will deal with the mechanisms by which the liver secretes bile acids, lipids, and inorganic solutes into the canaliculus and thus generates bile flow. The canaliculus actually consists of two (occasionally three) "hemicanaliculi"—specialized membrane areas of adjacent hepatocytes joined by tight junctions. The canalicular network is thus a more or less sealed intercellular space that lies in the middle of the liver cell plate.[2, 197] This is illustrated diagrammatically in Figure 2–2; Figure 2–4 is an actual scanning electron micrograph of a liver cell that has been "fractured" between the lateral cell membranes to expose the hemicanaliculus. The wall of the canaliculus consists of irregularly spaced microvilli and diverticulum-like structures, both of which serve to increase the total canalicular surface area, estimated to be about 10 m^2 in the whole human liver.[14] The *microfilaments* that surround the canaliculus also extend into the microvilli, where they insert on the inner leaflet of the microvillous membrane (Fig. 2–2*B*).[2] There is increasing evidence that microfilaments play a role in maintaining canalicular structure and perhaps in bile formation. Thus, experimental agents, such as cytochalasin B and phalloidin, that impair microfilamental function produce canalicular dilatation and loss of microvilli associated with a profound decrease in bile flow.[15–17] Canalicular dilatation, loss of microvilli, and alteration of the pericanalicular microfilamentous web also are seen in human cholestasis,[18] although it is not yet clear whether microfilament dysfunction is the cause of these nonspecific structural changes.

Microtubules are another component of the cytoskeleton that are also found in the pericanalicular web. As their name implies, they are long tubular structures, about 240 Å in diameter, composed of tubulin protein. Like microfilaments, microtubules are structural components that represent a dynamic equilibrium between cytoplasmic monomeric precursors and polymerized macromolecules; they probably play a role in the cellular mobility and movement of intracellular organelles. Microtubules also appear to be involved in bile secretion in that colchicine and vinca alkaloids, both of which depolymerize microtubules, have been reported to decrease bile flow and the biliary output of bile acids and perhaps lecithin.[19, 20]

The Bile Collecting System

Bile flows in the canalicular network from the pericentral area of the liver lobule toward the portal tract. This is opposite to the direction of blood flow in the sinusoids. After leaving the canaliculus, bile enters a slightly larger conduit often called the canal of Hering, which is bounded by a hepatocyte or two on one side and one or two ductular cells on the other.[21] Like canaliculi, the canals of Hering are difficult to identify by routine histologic examination of normal liver tissue. However, in extrahepatic obstruction and, less commonly, in prolonged intrahepatic cholestasis, bile plugs may be seen in dilated canals of Hering, which can then be recognized by their position outside the portal connective tissue.[22] The canals of Hering empty into ductules lined by poorly developed lining cells that rest on a basement membrane and have microvilli on the luminal surface.[21] These ductules, in turn, empty into interlobular bile ducts, which are lined by cuboidal or low columnar epithelium and are readily recognized by their position within the connective tissue stroma of the portal tracts. Proper identification of these structures is of major diagnostic importance, since the presence of bile plugs or polymorphonuclear leukocytes in the lumen of interlobular ducts, but not necessarily in the canaliculi or canals of Hering, is strongly suggestive of extrahepatic obstruction.[22]

Studies of the ductular system in rats and rabbits with scanning electron microscopy have revealed a complex of portal bile ductular channels. This richly anastomosing network of tubules 20 to 30 μm in diameter may play an important role in modifying canalicular bile secreted by hepatocytes because it provides an anatomic basis for exchange of water, electrolytes, and possibly other substances between ductules and sinusoids or ductules and venule branches of the portal system.[198] Interlobular bile ducts present in small portal tracts join to form large septal ducts, 100 μm or greater in diameter, which are lined by tall columnar cells with basal nuclei. Confluence of these septal ducts results in formation of the right and left lobular ducts, which continue outside the liver as the corresponding hepatic ducts. These join to form the common hepatic duct, which terminates as an intramural structure on the left side of the duodenum. The gallbladder is drained by the cystic duct, which usually joins the common hepatic duct 1 to 2 inches below the junction of the right and left hepatic ducts. However, variations in the length of the cystic duct and the site of its anastomosis to the common hepatic duct frequently occur. The anatomy of the extrahepatic biliary tree is discussed in more detail in Chapter 1.

FORMATION OF CANALICULAR BILE

In 1954, Brauer and coworkers demonstrated that bile secretory pressure is rela-

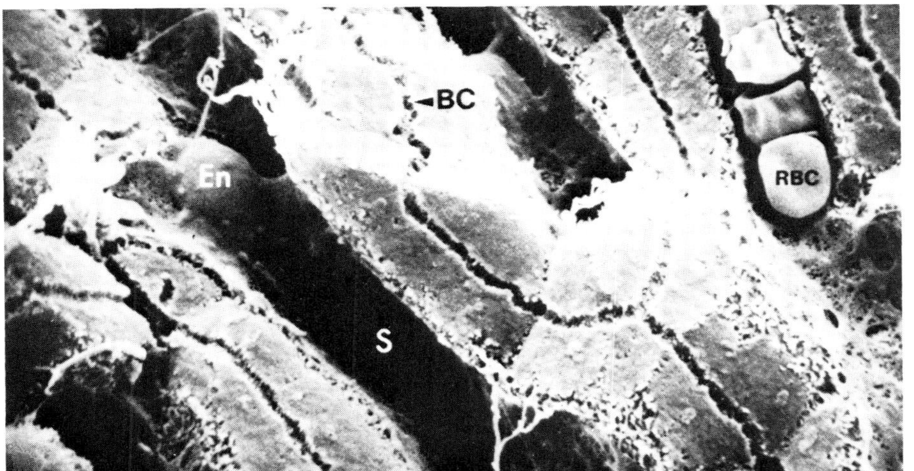

Figure 2–4. Scanning electron micrograph of rat liver. Adjacent hepatocytes in the liver cell plate have been separated along the lateral intercellular space, revealing a hemi-bile canaliculus (BC). The liver cell plates are bounded on either side by sinusoids (S) lined by endothelial cells (En). Red blood cells (RBC) are visible in one sinusoid (× 200). (From Jones AL, Schmucker DL: Gastroenterology *73*:833, 1977. Used by permission.)

tively independent of, and may even exceed, hepatic perfusion pressure.[23] These findings, which were subsequently confirmed and enlarged upon,[24] demonstrated a fundamental difference between the formation of primary urine and of canalicular bile. Whereas urine produced in the glomerulus represents an ultrafiltrate of plasma dependent for its formation on arterial perfusion pressure, canalicular bile is actively secreted by hepatocytes. Since active secretion of water per se is inherently inefficient and therefore unlikely, canalicular bile formation presumably is generated by active secretion of solute(s) into the canaliculus. This creates an osmotic gradient that results in a net flow of water into the canaliculus. Water may either diffuse from the hepatocyte across the canalicular membrane or enter via the paracellular pathway across "leaky" tight junctions.[199, 200] In either case, the active secretion of solute is the initiating event, and the years since Brauer's classic experiments have been devoted largely to identifying those solutes that are actively secreted as well as the factors controlling their rate of secretion.

The study of bile formation has been hampered by the fact that the bile canaliculus is too small (about 1 μm diameter) to be successfully micropunctured using currently available equipment. Thus, neither the electrical potential differences nor the unidirectional solute flux rates across the canalicular membrane can be measured directly. In addition, the free or effective concentration of biliary solutes on either side of the canalicular membrane is difficult to determine, because solutes in the hepatocyte may be compartmentalized or bound to cytoplasmic macromolecules and solutes in the bile may be associated with mixed micelles and other aggregates. For these and other reasons, information regarding the mechanisms of bile formation has to be derived by a variety of indirect techniques.

Measurement of Canalicular Bile Flow

Like the measurement of glomerular filtration rate with inulin, canalicular bile flow can be estimated by using one of several metabolically inert neutral solutes, such as erythritol or mannitol. These substances appear to enter bile predominantly or exclusively at the level of the canaliculus by diffusion and convection and are not appreciably secreted by the bile ducts and ductules.[25–28] Thus, infusion of bile acids or other substances that alter the rate of canalicular bile formation (see further on) causes parallel changes in erythritol clearance, whereas modification of the rate of ductular fluid secretion induced by secretin produces no change in erythritol clearance.[26] In the studies on the mechanisms of bile production (discussed later), canalicular bile flow has been estimated by using erythritol or some other suitable marker.

Bile Acid–Dependent Flow

Since bile acids are the predominant organic solute in bile, it is not surprising that the rate of canalicular bile flow is related to the rate of bile acid secretion. When canalicular bile flow is plotted versus bile acid output at varying rates of bile acid excretion, a linear relationship analogous to that shown in Figure 2–5 has been demonstrated in rats,[29, 30] dogs,[31, 32] humans,[33–35] and all other mammals thus far studied. The slope of the line, that is, the amount of water flow generated per molecule of bile acid secreted, is dependent both on the rate of total bile acid secretion[36] and on the type of bile acid.[34] This results, in part, from the fact that most bile acids aggregate to form *micelles* when present in solution above a certain concentration called the *critical micellar concentration.*

Micelles may be of several different types. For example, *pure bile acid micelles* contain two or more different species of bile acid. *Mixed micelles* of the type present in bile contain two or more different bile acids as well as cholesterol and phospholipid. Association of a particular bile acid with any type of micelle will decrease its concentration in free solution and thus decrease its osmotic effect. Hence, dehydrocholate, a bile acid that does not form micelles, has been found to be a more potent stimulator of canalicular bile flow than taurocholate, which does form micelles.[34] This probably reflects, in part, the fact that taurocholate presumably has a lesser free concentration in bile and hence a lesser osmotic effect than does dehydrocholate. Alterations in micelle size and aggregation number may also partially explain the observation that canalicular bile flow per unit of bile acid excreted is less at high rates of bile acid excretion than at low rates.[36]

The observations that canalicular bile flow is linearly related to bile acid output, and that bile acid concentration in hepatic bile (5 to 45 mM) normally exceeds that in plasma

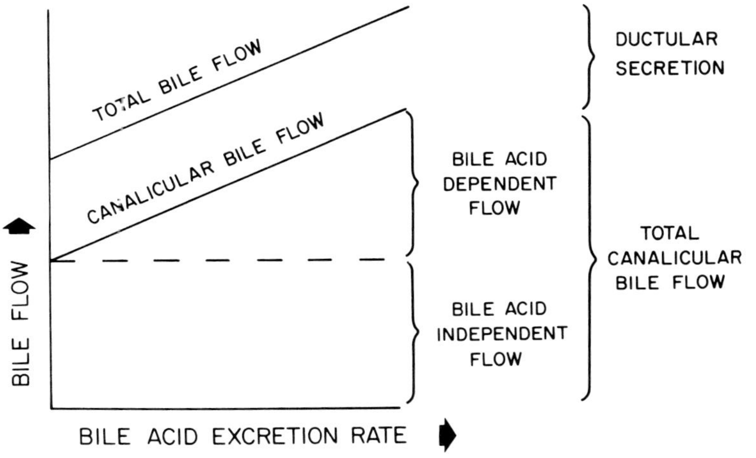

Figure 2–5. Schematic representation of the relationship between total bile flow, canalicular bile flow, and bile acid excretion. Total bile flow consists of a constant ductular secretion plus canalicular bile flow. Canalicular bile flow consists of a theoretically constant bile acid–independent fraction and a bile acid–dependent fraction, which, in turn, depend on total bile acid excretion and the slope of the line relating canalicular bile flow to bile acid excretion.

(1 to 5 μM) by three orders of magnitude, led to the concept that bile acids are actively secreted by the hepatocyte.[199, 201] Accordingly, that portion of bile flow resulting from the presumably active secretion of bile acids is generally termed *bile acid–dependent flow*. Operationally, this bile acid–dependent flow is determined from the slope of the line relating canalicular bile flow to bile acid output and the amount of bile acid secreted (Fig. 2–5). Under normal conditions, bile acids secreted by the liver are derived predominantly from portal blood, that is, from bile acids that have been reabsorbed from the intestine and have undergone enterohepatic circulation. Thus, the bile acid load reaching the liver, and hence bile acid–dependent flow, would be expected to decrease during periods of fasting but to increase following meal-stimulated gallbladder contraction. It has been estimated that in humans,[33, 34] bile acid–dependent flow accounts for about half of canalicular bile flow and for 35 to 40 per cent of total bile flow (Fig. 2–6).

The mechanism by which hepatocytes actively take up bile acids has recently been identified. A variety of studies using intact liver, freshly isolated hepatocytes, or cultured hepatocytes indicate that conjugated bile acids enter hepatocytes via a saturable, sodium-dependent, ouabain-suppressible mechanism presumably representing sodium-coupled transport.[37–39, 202] The driving force for bile acid uptake is believed to result from movement of sodium down its electrochemical gradient from sinusoidal blood into cytoplasm. The electrochemical sodium gradient is, in turn, attributable to NaK-ATPase in the liver cell plasma membrane. The sodium-coupled mechanism for hepatic bile acid uptake exhibits considerable substrate selectivity, preferring conjugated to unconjugated bile acids and trihydroxy to dihydroxy bile acids.[40] Unconjugated dihydroxy bile acids enter hepatocytes largely via a nonsaturable, non–sodium dependent process that may represent simple diffusion.[40]

In contrast to the comparatively well-characterized uptake step, relatively little is known regarding how bile acids are transported from inside the hepatocyte to the canaliculus. A bile acid receptor in liver plasma membranes has been identified and

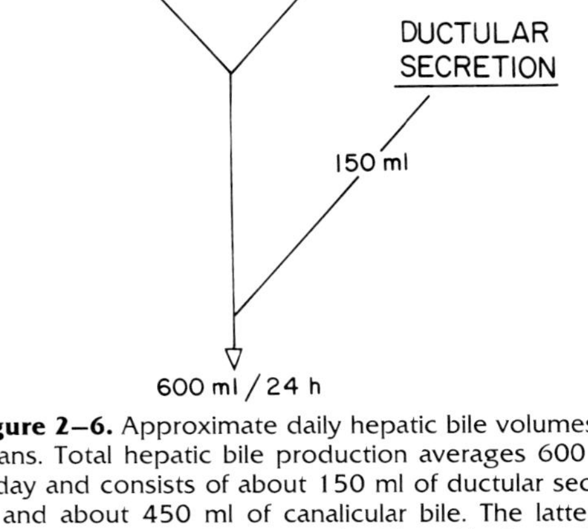

Figure 2–6. Approximate daily hepatic bile volumes in humans. Total hepatic bile production averages 600 ml per day and consists of about 150 ml of ductular secretion and about 450 ml of canalicular bile. The latter is nearly equally divided between the bile acid–dependent and bile acid–independent fractions. The reabsorptive role of the gallbladder is not shown.

partially characterized,[41] but it is unclear at present whether this receptor mediates uptake or excretion. The mechanisms that regulate bile acid transport and secretion are also unclear. Recent studies indicate that sympathetic neurotransmitters and peptide hormones may play a role by interacting with these membrane receptors.[203]

Finally, although bile acid–dependent flow is clearly related to bile acid excretion, bile acids per se account for only a minor portion of the osmolality of bile even during bile acid–induced choleresis. Rather, the most important biliary solutes in terms of osmolality are the inorganic electrolytes (sodium, chloride, and bicarbonate) that accompany the bile acids into the canaliculus. Thus, differences in the choleretic potency of various bile acids are at least in part attributable to the varying ability of different bile acids to stimulate inorganic electrolyte secretion and are not readily explainable on the basis of micelle-forming ability.

Bile Acid–Independent Flow

Within 10 years after the description and definition of bile acid–dependent flow, it became apparent that processes independent of bile acid secretion were responsible for a substantial portion of canalicular bile flow. Several major pieces of evidence led to this conclusion. First, the quantity of bile produced for a given bile acid output (that is, the slope of the line in Figure 2–5) differs markedly in different species,[41] and canalicular bile flow may change with temperature without accompanying changes in bile acid excretion. Second, in the isolated perfused rat liver, bile acid excretion may be reduced experimentally by 95 per cent, but this is accompanied by only a 31 per cent decrease in canalicular bile flow.[29] Finally, as shown in Figure 2–5, when the line relating canalicular bile flow to bile acid output is extrapolated to zero bile acid output, a positive "Y" intercept is obtained in dogs,[27] rabbits,[43] and humans.[33, 34] These findings would be difficult to explain if bile acid secretion were the sole determinant of canalicular bile flow; they indicate that there is a fraction of canalicular bile flow that is independent of bile acids—a so-called *bile acid–independent flow.*

In theory, this bile acid–independent flow should be determined by measuring bile flow in the complete absence of bile acid excretion. This, of course, is impossible in the intact animal because bile acids are being returned to the liver continuously via the enterohepatic circulation to be resecreted in bile. Even in the isolated perfused rat liver, ongoing hepatic bile acid synthesis and excretion make it impossible to reduce bile acid secretion to zero. Thus, bile acid–independent flow is generally defined as the extrapolated "Y" intercept of the line relating canalicular bile flow to bile acid excretion (Fig. 2–5). Using this operational definition, bile acid–independent flow accounts for about half of canalicular bile flow in guinea pigs, rats, rabbits, hamsters, and dogs. In humans, bile acid–independent flow also accounts for about half of canalicular bile flow and 35 to 40 per cent of total bile flow (Fig. 2–6).[33, 34] In practice, measurement of bile acid–independent flow by extrapolation may introduce some degree of error, because the line relating canalicular bile flow to bile acid output has been reported to be nonlinear at very low rates of bile acid secretion.[36] Moreover, the term "bile acid–independent flow" may not be strictly correct since, as discussed further on, there is evidence that bile acids may indirectly regulate bile acid–"independent" flow. Nonetheless, there is little doubt that a significant fraction of bile flow is not directly related to bile acid secretion, and the term "bile acid–independent flow" is widely used to designate this fraction.

Bile acid–independent formation of canalicular bile presumably results from secretion by the hepatocyte of inorganic electrolytes. However, the mechanism(s) of electrolyte secretion and, indeed, even the identity of electrolytes that are actively secreted have remained unclear.[204] Most investigation has focused on the roles of sodium and NaK-ATPase.[42, 205, 206] Sodium is quantitatively the most important inorganic electrolyte in bile, and biliary sodium output is linearly related to bile acid–independent flow. Both observations suggest a central role for sodium and hence for NaK-ATPase, which is an integral membrane protein found in the plasma membrane of hepatocytes and other cells. It catalyzes a complex reaction consisting of hydrolysis of one molecule of ATP to ADP and inorganic phosphate coupled with transport of three sodium ions out of the cell and two potassium ions into the cell. This combined hydrolysis-transport process is responsible for maintaining the low sodium and high potassium concentrations found in hepatocytes and most other living cells. This creates not only the proper intracellular conditions for normal cell metabolism but also a steep electrochemical gradient for sodium across the cell membrane, which is essential for such diverse processes as propagation of action potentials in nerve cells and concentrative sodium cotransport processes, such as the bile acid uptake mechanism described earlier.

It was originally postulated that sodium was pumped directly into the canaliculus by NaK-ATPase in the canalicular membrane.[42] This hypothesis was supported by a variety of observations, including: (1) cytochemical studies showing high ATPase activity in the canalicular membrane[45]; (2) apparently high NaK-ATPase activity in liver plasma membrane preparations believed to be enriched in canaliculi[46–50]; (3) an apparent parallelism between hepatic NaK-ATPase activity and bile acid–independent flow[48–54]; and (4) diminished bile flow by the isolated perfused liver following exposure to NaK-ATPase inhibitors.[43]

Each of these lines of evidence, however, has subsequently been refuted or questioned. Specifically, (1) cytochemical studies using newer techniques localized NaK-ATPase to the sinusoidal and lateral rather than to the canalicular membrane[5, 44]; (2) canaliculi-enriched liver plasma membrane fragments are frequently contaminated with NaK-ATPase–bearing sinusoidal and lateral membranes[58]; (3) several investigators reported a lack of parallelism between bile acid–independent bile flow and NaK-ATPase[55–59]; and (4) inhibitors of NaK-ATPase were reported to increase rather than decrease bile acid–independent bile flow. Although these observations rendered the original postulate untenable, they spawned a new hypothesis that NaK-ATPase might indirectly energize electrolyte transport via sodium-coupled transport. For example, sodium-coupled transport of chloride, in a fashion analogous to sodium-coupled transport of bile acids (see earlier), would tend to drive chloride into the cell against its electrochemical gradient. Subsequent movement of chloride into the canaliculus down its electrochemical gradient would create net solute and water movement. This mechanism has already been identified in a variety of other tissues, such as gallbladder, in which the basolateral localization of NaK-ATPase is analogous to its sinusoidal/lateral membrane location in the liver. Although this hypothesis is extremely attractive, evidence to support it has not yet been reported.[61] In contrast to the persistent uncertainty regarding the roles of sodium and NaK-ATPase in bile acid–independent bile flow, there is direct evidence that transport of bicarbonate may be important.[60, 62] The mechanism of bicarbonate transport is uncertain but has been speculated to involve sodium-coupled transport[63] or an ion pump separate from NaK-ATPase.[62]

Secretion of Biliary Lipids

The major lipids in bile are nonesterified cholesterol and the phospholipid phosphatidyl choline (lecithin). Lecithin is an amphipathic molecule, that is, it has both a water-insoluble (hydrophobic) portion and a water-soluble (hydrophilic) portion. In partially purified form, it is a thick greaselike substance that is minimally water-soluble. Pure cholesterol also is virtually insoluble in water, yet both cholesterol and lecithin are in solution in normal human bile. This results from the fact that bile acids, amphipathic molecules that are more water-soluble than either cholesterol or lecithin, function as detergents that solubilize cholesterol and lecithin by forming mixed micelles.[64] In these mixed micelles, the polar portion of both the phospholipid and the bile acid molecules is oriented toward the exterior. This allows interaction with surrounding water molecules and permits the micelles to remain in solution. The hydrophobic portion of the phospholipid and bile acid molecules is oriented toward the interior of the micelle, and the largely nonpolar cholesterol presumably is located in this hydrophobic interior. Although the exact size and shape of biliary mixed micelles are still uncertain, it is clear that a definable molar ratio of bile acid and phospholipid to cholesterol is necessary to prevent formation of insoluble cholesterol deposits. Thus, in theory, cholesterol cholelithiasis would be favored by an increase in biliary cholesterol or by a decrease in biliary phospholipid or bile acid.[64] Conversely, cholesterol stones may be dissolved by reversing these ratios. As discussed in Chapter 4, a combination of these processes is responsible for supersaturation of bile with cholesterol, which is a necessary condition for cholesterol cholelithiasis.

As shown in Figure 2–7, biliary excretion of both cholesterol and phospholipid in humans is curvilinearly related to bile acid output.[66] Excretion of both is close to zero at low bile acid excretion, increases rapidly with

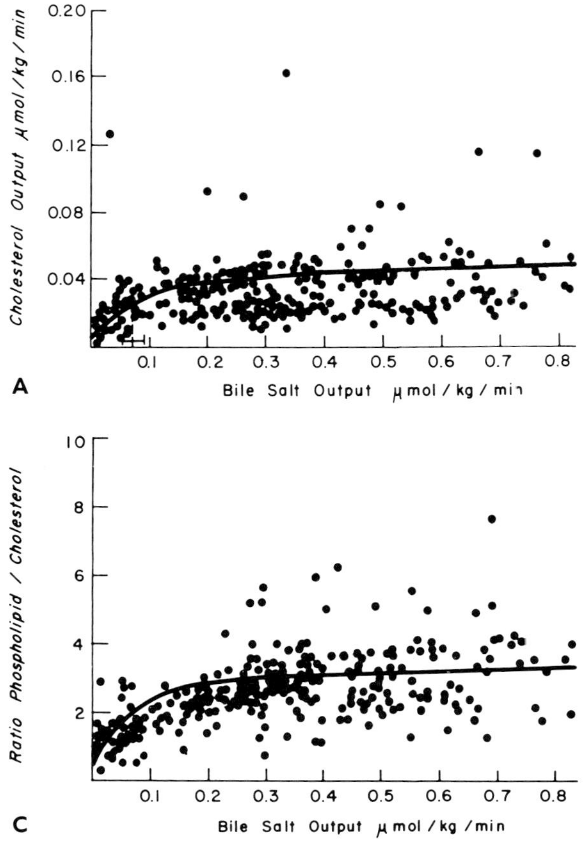

Figure 2–7. Relationship of cholesterol output (*A*), phospholipid output (*B*), and phospholipid/cholesterol molar ratio (*C*) to bile acid (here called bile salt) output in seven patients. Note that both cholesterol and phospholipid output are curvilinearly related to bile acid output, approaching limiting values at high rates of bile acid secretion. Note also that the molar ratio of phospholipid to cholesterol increases as bile acid output rises. Conversely, low rates of bile acid secretion are associated with a higher ratio of cholesterol to phospholipid and bile acid and hence greater cholesterol saturation. (From Wagner CI, Trolman BW, Soloway, RD: J Clin Invest *57*:473, 1976. Used by permission.)

increasing bile acid output, and approaches maximal values at high bile acid output. As is apparent from Figure 2–7, the curves relating output of cholesterol and phospholipid to that of bile acids are shaped differently. Thus, the ratio of phospholipid and bile acids to cholesterol increases with increasing rates of bile acid secretion. Conversely, low rates of bile acid secretion, as may occur during sleep[67] or following interruption of the enterohepatic circulation, are associated with a decreased ratio of bile acid and phospholipid to cholesterol, thereby enhancing the potential for cholesterol precipitation. Since dehydrocholate, a synthetic tri-keto bile acid unable to form micelles, does not increase lipid excretion, it appears to be the ability of natural bile acids to form micelles that underlies their regulatory effect on lipid excretion.

The source of biliary lipids has been intensively investigated.[65, 209–211] In experimental animals, cholesterol newly synthesized in the liver accounts for less than one third of biliary cholesterol; the remainder appears to be delivered to the liver by plasma lipoproteins. Furthermore, changes in hepatic cholesterol synthesis do not result in similar changes in biliary cholesterol output.[207, 208] In contrast, phospholipid is derived largely from the liver, and both the hepatic synthesis and the transcellular transport of phospholipid are closely linked to bile acid transport. While crucial to an understanding of cholesterol cholelithiasis, information regarding the mechanism of the link between bile acid transport and the excretion of cholesterol and phospholipid (Fig. 2–7) is not yet available.

It has not yet been established where micelle formation takes place. It has been suggested, however, that bile acids solubilize lipids from the canalicular membrane en route to the canaliculus. Alternatively, micelles may be prepackaged for export inside the hepatocyte, possibly in intracellular vesicles, and extruded intact into the canaliculus. The latter possibility is suggested by several observations, including the proximity of the Golgi apparatus and other vesicles to the biliary pole of the hepatocyte, the increased volume of this organelle in cells actively engaged in bile secretion,[68] the attachment of contractile microfilaments to the canalicular membrane,[2] and the fact that dysfunction of microfilaments and microtubules is associated with cholestasis and impaired lipid secretion.[15–17] Although these findings are consistent with the hypothesis that mixed micelles may be prepackaged in vesicles that are transported to the canaliculus via the microtubular-microfilament system, a role for these structures in bile secretion remains speculative.

Secretion of Other Organic Solutes

In addition to inorganic ions, bile acids, cholesterol, and phospholipid, the liver secretes a variety of organic solutes, including conjugated bilirubin and many drugs, dyes, and hormones. For a complete discussion of the hepatic metabolism of bilirubin and other organic anions the reader is referred to one of two reviews.[69, 70]

Bilirubin and other organic anions, such as sulfobromophthalein and indocyanine green, are transported across the sinusoidal membrane into the hepatocyte by a process that exhibits several features of carrier-mediated transport, including saturability with increasing dose; relatively selective, mutually competitive inhibition among substrates; and probably also countertransport and accelerative exchange diffusion.[71] The carrier system appears to be generally distinct from that for bile acids,[71–73] and preliminary evidence suggests that, unlike the carrier system for bile acids, it is not sodium-dependent.[73] Consistent with this hypothesis of carrier-mediated transport is the fact that proteins capable of binding bilirubin and other organic anions have been isolated from liver plasma membrane preparations.[74, 75] Together, these findings suggest that bilirubin tightly bound to albumin in the circulation enters the space of Disse in association with albumin through the large fenestrations in the endothelial lining cells. Bilirubin then presumably is stripped from its albumin carrier in the space of Disse by binding proteins on the liver cell membrane and is translocated by these putative carriers to the inside of the hepatocyte. Indeed, recent studies suggest that physical interaction of the bilirubin-albumin complex with the liver cell surface may be important in the uptake process.[196]

Once inside, bilirubin, which by itself is poorly water-soluble, appears to bind to one of two cytoplasmic protein fractions designated as "Y" protein, or ligandin, and "Z" protein.[76] Ligandin, which constitutes about 5 per cent of cytoplasmic protein in rat liver, originally was considered to be of importance in the transport process because of its ability to bind a variety of organic compounds, including steroids, aminoazodyes, and various organic anions.[77] It subsequently was found that ligandin is one of a family of glutathione S-transferases, which are enzymes that catalyze the conjugation of glutathione with many different electrophilic substrates.[78] Although there has been considerable controversy regarding the exact role of these intracellular binding proteins in bilirubin transport, the most recent evidence suggests that binding to "Y" protein (ligandin) facilitates net hepatic uptake of bilirubin and other organic anions by decreasing their free concentration in the hepatocyte and hence decreasing their availability for reflux back into plasma.[79]

In the hepatocyte, bilirubin is esterified with a variety of carbohydrate moieties, but bilirubin diglucuronide constitutes the major pigment fraction in human bile.[80] It is firmly established that esterification of bilirubin with the first molecule of glucuronic acid is mediated by a specific glucuronyltransferase located in the membranes of the smooth and rough endoplasmic reticulum. Despite extensive study, purification and characterization of this enzyme, like those of many other membrane-associated enzymes, have been only partially successful.[81] There is some evidence that conversion of mono- to diglucuronide may be catalyzed not by microsomal glucuronyltransferase but by an enzyme system with a different intracellular location, perhaps on the plasma membrane.[82, 83] In this proposed transglucuronidation mechanism, the glucuronic acid moiety of one bilirubin monoglucuronide molecule is said to be transferred to another monoglucuronide, resulting in equimolar formation of diglucuronide and unconjugated bilirubin.[82, 83] However, other studies have failed to demonstrate transglucuronidation in vivo[84] and are most compatible with the hypothesis that formation of both bilirubin mono- and diglucuronide is catalyzed by microsomal glucuronyltransferase.

Because it has not yet been possible to sample canalicular bile, the hepatic excretory mechanism for conjugated bilirubin and other organic anions has remained relatively obscure. Nonetheless, important inferences can be drawn from the available information. First, virtually every organic anion thus far studied, including bilirubin, has been found to have a definite maximal hepatic excretory rate (T_m). Since the observed T_m is less than the maximal uptake capacity for each of these anions[28] and since infusion rates exceeding the T_m result in reflux of conjugated bilirubin into plasma,[85] it is believed that transport across the canalicular membrane is a saturable process that may be rate-limiting in the overall transport of bilirubin and other organic anions from blood to bile. Intrahepatic sulfobromophthalein concentration has been shown to increase nonlinearly with increasing rates of sulfobromophthalein excretion, which also suggests a saturable excretory process.[86] Second, it appears that various organic anions compete for excretion into the bile.[87, 88] Together, these properties of saturation and competition suggest that canalicular excretion, like sinusoidal uptake, is a carrier-mediated process.

Normal human bile contains only a small amount of unconjugated bilirubin (1 per cent of total bilirubin in gallbladder bile), and the question of why bilirubin requires conjugation for excretion has long been a source of interest. It has been suggested that the conjugating moiety per se may allow bilirubin to "fit" with a specific carrier in the canalicular membrane. Alternatively, it has been postulated that conjugation serves simply to disrupt the internal hydrogen bonding responsible for the hydrophobic properties of unconjugated bilirubin IXα,[88, 89] thereby allowing transport by a carrier system(s) showing broad specificity for a variety of hydrophilic anions.[90] Several observations support this hypothesis. First, unlike bilirubin IXα, many hydrophilic organic anions are excreted into bile conjugated only in part (e.g., sulfobromophthalein), or they do not require conjugation for biliary excretion (e.g., indocyanine green, rose bengal, and i-urobilin). Second, bilirubin IXα isomers, which presumably are not internally hydrogen-bonded, are excreted largely in unconjugated form.[91, 92] This hypothesis also may help to explain why phototherapy results in enhanced hepatic excretion of unconjugated bilirubin IXα, causing reduction of plasma bilirubin concentration—namely, photoisomerization-like conjugation appears to disrupt the internal hydrogen bonds of bilirubin IXα, making it more suitable for secretion via the organic anion carrier system(s).[93, 94]

Studies on mutant Corriedale sheep, an animal model with many features of the Dubin-Johnson syndrome (see further on), have suggested that organic anions, including bilirubin and bile acids, are excreted via functionally distinct pathways.[95] This is consistent with the observation that the organic anions indocyanine green and probenecid do not compete with bile acids for binding to bile acid receptors in isolated liver surface membranes enriched in bile canaliculi, although sulfobromophthalein does show some competition.[96] Despite this apparent functional separation between bile acid and organic anion excretion, it has been observed that bile acid infusion increases the T_m for bilirubin,[97] sulfobromophthalein,[98–100] indocyanine green,[101] and iopanoic acid,[102] whereas compounds that increase canalicular bile flow without enhancing bile acid output fail to increase the T_m for most of the organic anions studied to date.[98, 102, 103] This relationship between excretion of bile acids and organic anions may help to explain the impaired excretion of biliary contrast materials and the poor opacification or nonopacification of the gallbladder or bile ducts that is characteristic of cholestasis. Decreased bile acid excretion also may account for the occasional inadequacy of these procedures in patients who have fasted before being studied.[104]

Whereas it is easy to understand why the excretion of hydrophobic substances, such as cholesterol and phospholipid, which are incorporated into mixed micelles, is dependent upon the rate of bile acid excretion, the link between excretion of bile acids and water-soluble substances, such as conjugated bilirubin, sulfobromophthalein, and biliary contrast media, is less obvious. Possible mechanisms are that bile acids directly stimulate organic anion excretion, or that the two membrane carrier systems are in some way coupled.[28, 98, 103] The observations that bile acid infusion also alters the appearance of bile canalicular membranes on scanning electron microscopy,[105] modifies bile canalicular membrane lipid composition and the activity of associated enzymes,[105] and reduces the K_m (as defined by standard transport kinetics) for sulfobromophthalein excretion[86] are all consistent with a direct membrane effect.

Another possibility is that bilirubin and other organic anions enter into a physicochemical self-association or association with bile salts or mixed micelles, or both. Such an arrangement would decrease the effective concentrations of conjugated bilirubin in bile, thereby reducing its availability for back-diffusion across the canalicular membrane, increasing its net excretion.[86, 97, 101, 103, 106] Although the functional importance of association of organic anions with various macromolecular aggregates in bile has yet to be established, this general hypothesis has been supported by ultracentrifugation and gel chromatography studies of normal bile or synthetic solutions, which indicated a physical association between sulfobromophthalein and taurocholate[106] and between bilirubin and mixed micelles or some other macromolecular complex of bile.[107, 108] Recent quantitative investigations have established that compounds excreted in bile in high concentration, including bilirubin and other organic anions for which T_m is increased by bile acid infusion, are associated with macromolecular aggregates, so that only a small percentage of these solutes (range 0 to 5 per cent) are present in bile in the form of monomers or complexes of low molecular weight.[109] These findings support the concept that the observed link between the biliary excretion of bile acids and organic anions may be related to physical association between these compounds.

The question of whether the excretory mechanism for organic anions is actively concentrative or equilibrative also remains to be resolved. Estimates of the bilirubin and sulfobromophthalein concentration ratios between bile and liver homogenate have ranged from 30:1 to 50:1.[88, 110, 111] Although measurement of whole liver homogenate ignores possible intracellular compartmentation, these findings have been taken as evidence that a steep concentration gradient exists across the canalicular membrane.[99, 112–114] Since binding to intracellular proteins presumably reduces the effective intracellular concentration and hence further increases the apparent concentration gradient, it is widely assumed that the excretory mechanism for organic anions is intrinsically concentrative, that is, active and energy-requiring.[99, 112–114] However, physical association of these anions with macromolecular aggregates [109] serves to reduce their free concentration. The effective concentration of these substances in bile thus may equal that inside the hepatocytes and thereby explain the apparent concentration gradient without necessarily invoking an intrinsically concentrative transport process.

Defects in the hepatic excretory mechanism for organic anions account for some types of hereditary hyperbilirubinemia simulating obstructive jaundice. Dubin-Johnson syndrome, inherited as an autosomal recessive disorder,[115] is characterized by variable conjugated hyperbilirubinemia that sometimes is not recognized until early adulthood.[116] Studies in such patients[117] and in an animal model closely resembling the Dubin-Johnson syndrome[118] indicated that the disorder results from a defective canalicular transport system for conjugated sulfobromophthalein and presumably other compounds secreted as conjugates, such as bilirubin and iodinated contrast media. Probably for this reason, oral cholecystography usually does not opacify the gallbladder, and sulfobromophthalein disappearance curves exhibit a characteristic secondary rise after 90 to 120 minutes, resulting from reflux of conjugated sulfobromophthalein into plasma. Rotor's syndrome, which probably also results from a defective excretory system, resembles Dubin-Johnson syndrome in inheritance and the presence of conjugated hyperbilirubinemia.[119] However, oral cholecystography in these patients usually opacifies the gallbladder, the sulfobromophthalein disappearance curve fails to show a secondary rise, and urinary coproporphyrin excretion does not exhibit the specific isomer abnormality seen in the Dubin-Johnson syndrome.[119] These disorders should be considered in the differential diagnosis of any apparently healthy child or young adult with chronic conjugated hyperbilirubinemia.

In addition to the excretory system for organic anions already discussed, the hepatocyte appears to have a separate excretory mechanism for organic cations, such as procainamide. Like the organic anion excretory system, it shows features, such as saturability and competitive inhibition between various cations, suggesting carrier-mediated transport.[120] Finally, the liver appears to have an excretory system for neutral organic compounds, including several cardiac glycosides.[121] However, these excretory processes have been less well characterized than the organic anion excretory system.

MODIFICATION OF CANALICULAR BILE BY THE BILE DUCTS AND GALLBLADDER

The Bile Ducts

After leaving the canaliculus, bile is altered by bile ductular secretion and reabsorption of water and electrolytes. Because the precise composition of canalicular bile is unknown, the modifications produced by the bile ducts can be assessed only indirectly. Moreover, there is marked species variation in bile ductular activity. Despite these complexities, certain general statements are possible regarding electrolyte and water transport by the bile ducts.

Net ductular secretion of fluid and electrolytes in response to secretin has been observed in many species, including humans, pigs, sheep, dogs, guinea pigs, and cats.[122, 212, 213] The magnitude of the secretin response varies in different species, but the general effect is to increase total bile flow without increasing the clearance of erythritol and other inert markers of canalicular bile flow and to decrease biliary concentration of bile acid, cholesterol, phospholipid, and bilirubin. This is exactly what one would expect if secretin augments bile flow by stimulating secretion of a ductular fluid containing inorganic electrolytes without altering canalicular bile secretion. Indirect measurements in vivo indicate that ductular fluid secreted in response to secretin, as is the case in the pancreas, has a bicarbonate concentration much greater than that of plasma (125 mEq/L in the pig) and contains considerable amounts of sodium and chloride.[123] These in vivo measurements have been confirmed by the direct in vitro observation that isolated bile ducts secrete fluid containing sodium, potassium, chloride, and bicarbonate.[124] Moreover, this secretion by isolated duct preparations continued in the face of opposing osmotic and electrochemical gradients but was inhibited by dinitrophenol. These findings confirm that bile ducts actively secrete a bicarbonate-rich fluid. This secretion is stimulated not only by secretin but also to a lesser extent by cholecystokinin, gastrin, cerulein, and bombesin.[125, 126, 212]

In addition to its secretory function, bile ductular epithelium can absorb water and electrolytes. Absorption is best demonstrated under conditions in which ductular secretion is suppressed, for example, by cholinergic blockage in dogs[27] or by resection of the gastric antrum and small bowel in monkeys.[127] Under these experimental conditions, bile-to-plasma erythritol concentration ratios may approach 2:1. Since eythritol, as discussed earlier, appears to enter bile by passive diffusion and convection at the level of the canaliculus, these findings demonstrate net ductular reabsorption of fluid. Bile-to-plasma erythritol ratios slightly greater than one also have been observed in the rat and rabbit. Intravenous infusion of somatostatin, a peptide present in the hypothalamus, gastric mucosa, and pancreas, causes a reduction in total bile flow and biliary bicarbonate output in the fasting dog.[214] Somatostatin also suppresses the choleresis produced by intravenous infusion of secretin[213] or by duodenal acidification.[212] The anticholeretic effect of somatostatin appears to be caused by either an enhancement of ductular reabsorption or an inhibition of the ductular secretion.[213] At present it is difficult to assess the functional significance of this reabsorption under physiologic conditions. It is possible, however, that following cholecystectomy, bile ducts may assume an absorptive function resembling that of the gallbladder.

Although most attention previously has been focused on absorption and secretion of water and inorganic electrolytes by the bile ducts, it has been reported that glucose entering the canaliculus also is reabsorbed by ductular epithelium in a manner analogous to that in the renal tubule.[128] Thus, bile ducts may participate in the bodily conservation of certain organic as well as inorganic solutes.

The Gallbladder

Hepatic bile enters the gallbladder, where it is stored and then released in response to a meal. The functional importance of a coordinated release of bile with a meal is debatable, since a number of mammals, including the rat, horse, deer, camel, elephant, whale, and rhinoceros, as well as many nonmammals appear to thrive without a gallbladder.[129] Since the capacity of the gallbladder in humans is only about 40 ml, it would quickly be filled with hepatic bile were it not for its truly remarkable absorptive capacity.

Absorption of fluid by the gallbladder proceeds rapidly. Within 3 to 4 hours,[130] up to 90 per cent of the water present in hepatic bile may be removed as an isotonic solution composed primarily of sodium chloride and sodium bicarbonate.[131] This results in the formation of gallbladder bile, which has very high concentrations of bile acids and sodium (both often above 200 mEq/L), potassium (10 mEq/L), and calcium (25 mEq/L) but low concentrations of chloride and bicarbonate (5 to 10 mEq/L). Given this resorptive capacity, the gallbladder theoretically is capable of storing the entire bile acid pool of the body.[129]

The mechanism of water absorption in the gallbladder has been the subject of much investigation. Perhaps the best characterized aspect of gallbladder transport is sodium-coupled transport of chloride by mucosal cells.[132–135] The existence of this mechanism was first suggested by the observation that substitution of either sulfate for chloride or choline for sodium reduced transport of both sodium and chloride in an equimolar fashion and reduced water absorption. Subsequent investigation of unidirectional ion fluxes has further suggested the presence of one-for-one coupling between sodium and chloride movements into mucosal cells. The presence of sodium-coupled chloride transport is most strongly supported by the observation that intracellular chloride activity, measured by using a chloride-sensitive electrode, is two to three times greater than would be expected for passive distribution and falls to that predicted for passive distribution on removal of sodium. Collectively, these findings indicate that movement of sodium into the mucosal cell down its electrochemical gradient is coupled to chloride movement so as to drive chloride into the cell.[215–218] The sodium gradient is presumably maintained by NaK-ATPase. The mechanism of chloride exit across the basolateral membrane is uncertain but presumably reflects differences in either permeability or transport systems between the luminal and basolateral membranes. The net result of this process is transcellular (i.e., transmucosal movement of chloride followed by sodium and water flow).

Morphologic studies during active gallbladder absorption have demonstrated dilatation of the intercellular space,[136, 137] suggesting that at least some of the water flow occurs paracellularly across the tight junction. This route of flow is supported indirectly by the observation that gallbladder tight junctions are, in fact, rather leaky and permeable to ionic lanthanum.

With respect to organic compounds, lipid solubility appears to be the major determinant of movement across the gallbladder wall. Conjugation of a variety of compounds, such as bilirubin, bile acids, steroid hormones, and biliary contrast media, therefore probably serves to alter their water solubility and pK_a and consequently to inhibit their absorption by the gallbladder.[129] For example, unconjugated bilirubin is readily absorbed,[140] whereas conjugated bilirubin is not. Conjugated bile acids, presumably because they are largely ionized at physiologic pH owing to their low pK_a (see Enterohepatic Circulation of Bile Acids), are absorbed only very slowly by the gallbladder.[141] By contrast, unconjugated bile acids, which have a higher pK_a, are absorbed more readily and furthermore damage the mucosa, causing a nonselective increase in absorption of other solutes.[141] Thus, increased absorption of bile acids, due either to bacterial deconjugation or to nonspecific mucosal change caused by inflammation, has been postulated to impair the ability of gallbladder bile to solubilize cholesterol and therefore to promote formation of cholesterol stones. Increased absorption of iopanoic acid by similar mechanisms may account for nonopacification of the gallbladder by oral cholecystography in patients with chronic cholecystitis.[141]

REGULATION OF BILE FLOW

The preceding discussion has emphasized the fact that bile entering the duodenum represents the end result of a complex array of interrelated functions. These include bile acid–dependent and –independent bile formation by the hepatocyte, modification and concentration of canalicular bile in the gallbladder, and ductular secretion. As outlined further on, these various processes appear to be orchestrated largely by events related to the ingestion and digestion of food.

In humans, bile acid–dependent canalicular bile formation is regulated primarily by the enterohepatic cycling of bile acids. In the fasting state, bile acids are largely sequestered in the gallbladder and bile acid–dependent flow is at its nadir. However, there is mounting evidence that the gallbladder contracts periodically during fasting, emptying 20 to 40 per cent of its contents.[219] With ingestion of food, the gallbladder is stimulated to contract by release of cholecystokinin and motilin[189] and possibly by cholinergic mechanisms.[190] The bolus of bile acids thus delivered to the gut may undergo enterohepatic cycling two to three times during the meal, thus stimulating bile acid–dependent flow. Infusion of certain peptide hormones, notably glucagon and insulin, has been reported to increase bile acid–independent canalicular bile flow in dogs and humans while decreasing biliary lipid output.[191] Although these findings suggest that bile acid–independent bile flow is subject to hormonal control, the importance of such an effect under physiologic conditions in humans is not yet clear. As previously discussed, meal-stimulated release of hormones such as secretin and cholecystokinin probably increases total bile flow by eliciting ductular secretion. Thus, all components of bile flow, i.e., bile acid–dependent and –independent canalicular bile flow and ductular secretion (see Fig. 2–6), are probably maximal in the immediate postprandial period.

MECHANISMS OF CHOLESTASIS

Definition of Cholestasis

Cholestasis is a term with different meanings in different settings. As used by the pathologist, it signifies plugging of canaliculi and ductules with bile. The physician uses it to denote the clinical manifestations of impaired bile secretion. Unfortunately, the presence of cholestasis as defined by the pathologist is not always accompanied by the typical clinical manifestations of cholestasis, and vice versa. Cholestasis can be defined more precisely in physiologic terms as a slowing or stoppage of bile flow. Since the clinician usually cannot measure bile flow directly, he must deduce from clinical and laboratory information that slowing has occurred. The most valuable findings for the diagnosis of cholestasis consist of evidence that substances normally excreted in bile are being retained in the plasma. Jaundice due to conjugated hyperbilirubinemia is probably used most frequently as an indicator of cholestasis. However, as noted earlier, conjugated hyperbilirubinemia occurs in certain hereditary disorders of bilirubin metabolism in the absence of true cholestasis. Serum bile acid levels, although not routinely measured, also are elevated with cholestasis and may be the earliest detectable abnormality. Accumulation of bile acids in the skin has generally been considered the cause of the pruritus that frequently accompanies cholestasis.[142, 143] However, recent studies have failed to demonstrate a correlation between pruritus and the quantity or type of bile acids in either plasma or skin, suggesting that bile acids, at least by themselves, may not be responsible for pruritus.[144] Hypercholesterolemia also is frequently associated with a prolonged cholestasis and is frequently accompanied by planar or tuberous xanthomata if the sterol level remains above 1500 mg/dl.[145] The presence of all three of these abnormalities—elevated blood levels of conjugated bilirubin, bile acids, and cholesterol—is unequivocal evidence of cholestasis.

Alkaline phosphatase and 5′-nucleotidase are enzymes located in the plasma membrane of hepatocytes.[4, 5, 45] Although increased activity of these enzymes in plasma frequently accompanies cholestasis and may be helpful diagnostically (see Chapter 13), the elevated plasma levels reflect enhanced hepatic synthesis or release of these enzymes into plasma, or both, rather than impaired biliary secretion.

Once the presence of cholestasis is established, the first and most important question facing the clinician is whether it is due to intrinsic liver dysfunction or to extrahepatic obstruction. This differentiation and the differential diagnosis of extrahepatic obstruction are discussed in detail in Chapters 9 through 13. In the past, when little was known about the mechanism of bile flow, all cases of cholestasis in which extrahepatic obstruction had been excluded were lumped together under the heading of "intrahepatic obstruction" or "intrahepatic cholestasis." Although our ability to identify functional abnormalities in patients with intrahepatic cholestasis is still in its infancy, some categorization is possible. It is clear that some cases of intrahepatic cholestasis result from multiple defects in the uptake, metabolism, or excretion of biliary solutes. One such example is acute viral hepatitis, which produces overt cellular injury throughout the liver lobule, obvious on histologic examination. Other forms of intrahepatic cholestasis may result from specific defects in the transport of biliary solutes that are not recognizable at the light microscopic level. It is from such defects, selectively summarized here, that we can learn the most about the pathophysiology of intrahepatic cholestasis.

Impaired Bile Acid Excretion

Two cholestatic syndromes have been described in infants that may be related to defective bile acid secretion, specifically Byler's disease, named after an Amish family in Pennsylvania and Ohio,[146] and a similar disorder described by Williams and associates.[147] Both disorders appear to be inherited as an autosomal recessive trait, make their appearance in early infancy with pruritus, and are characterized by severe and progressive cholestasis leading eventually to liver failure and death. In both, detailed studies of bile acid metabolism[147, 148] have suggested that hepatic uptake and conjugation of bile acids are only minimally impaired, but plasma bile acid levels are markedly elevated while duodenal bile acid concentration is reduced. These findings collectively suggest a primary defect in bile acid secretion.

Affected infants also have a markedly elevated plasma level of lithocholic acid, and it is possible that accumulation of this potentially hepatotoxic bile acid (see Enterohepatic Circulation of Bile Acids) may contribute to the progressive nature of the illness. Patients with Byler's disease have been reported to show defective excretion of sulfobromophthalein and bilirubin. This may reflect the above-mentioned interrelationship between excretion of bile acids and organic anions, or it may indicate that hepatic damage due to accumulation of toxic bile acids has progressed to the point of interfering with the transport of other biliary solutes.

Altered Physical and Functional Properties of Liver Plasma Membranes

The role of different portions of the hepatocyte membrane in generating bile flow has already been emphasized. Carriers in the sinusoidal membrane perform the essential first step of transporting substances such as bile acids and organic anions from sinusoidal blood into the hepatocyte, and it is possible that carriers in the canalicular membrane are responsible for their exit into bile.[96] Organic solutes, such as bilirubin, are conjugated by enzymes localized in membranes of the endoplasmic reticulum; NaK-ATPase, an enzyme present in liver plasma membranes, appears to be important in the transport of bile acids and possibly other solutes. Since the functioning of these carriers and enzymes may be dependent upon the proper membrane environment, any agent that alters the physical or functional characteristics of liver cell membranes could potentially alter bile flow in a variety of ways. For example, estrogens have been shown to modify the canalicular membrane permeability,[220] lipid composition,[149] fluidity (i.e., viscosity of the hydrophobic membrane interior),[58] and NaK-ATPase activity[58, 149] of liver plasma membranes. It is quite possible that the cholestatic effect of estrogens in humans (e.g., cholestasis related to pregnancy or the use of oral contraceptives) may result, at least in part, from these effects of estrogens on the plasma membrane and plasma membrane enzymes. Chlorpromazine, a well-recognized cause of cholestasis in humans, is a cationic detergent that is capable of physically interacting with biologic membranes. Administration of chlorpromazine to experimental animals decreases bile flow; produces ultrastructural changes in the sinusoidal, canalicular, and internal membranes of rat liver[150]; alters the physical properties of liver plasma membranes[151]; and decreases membrane-associated ATPase activity.[151] Chlorpromazine, like estrogens, may thus impair hepatic bile formation, at least in part, by its effect on hepatocyte membranes.

Impaired Microfilament Function

As previously discussed and illustrated in Figure 2–2, contractile microfilaments may play a role in maintaining the normal structure and function of the bile canaliculus. This hypothesis is supported by their strategic position surrounding the canaliculus and by the observation that agents such as cytochalasin B and phalloidin, which impair microfilament function, cause canalicular dilatation, loss of microvilli, and a profound decrease in bile flow.[15–17] Similar structural changes are seen in human cholestasis associated with a wide variety of causes[18] (e.g., anabolic steroid administration). Chlorpromazine, in addition to its effects on biologic membranes, has been shown in vitro to alter the polymerization of actin to its microfilamentous form.[152] While these observations certainly do not establish a role for microfilament dysfunction in human cholestasis, they provide tantalizing circumstantial evidence to support the hypothesis.

ROLE OF BILE ACIDS IN INTESTINAL LIPID ABSORPTION

Just as bile acids are essential in solubilizing biliary cholesterol and phospholipid, they also play an important role in the intestinal absorption of dietary lipids. Prolonged cholestasis of any cause, whether intrahepatic or extrahepatic, requires therapy directed specifically at the attendant abnormalities in the absorption of dietary lipids and lipid-soluble vitamins. Moreover, as discussed further on, abnormalities in the enterohepatic circulation of bile acids are characteristically accompanied by lipid malabsorption. For these reasons, an understanding of the role of bile acids in lipid absorption is of clinical importance. The intestinal absorption of lipids can be thought of as consisting of four interrelated, but more or less distinct, steps.[153, 154]

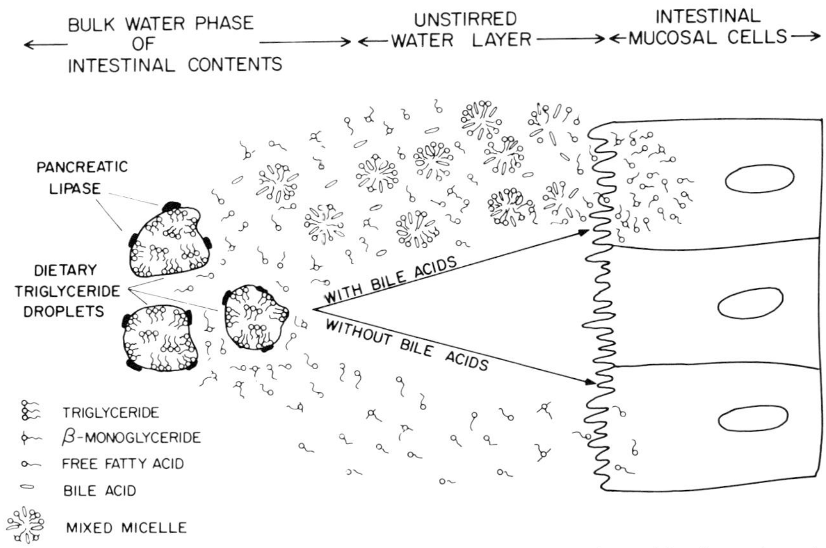

Figure 2–8. Intestinal fat absorption. β-Monoglyceride and free fatty acid released by the action of pancreatic lipase on triglyceride-containing lipid droplets are incorporated into mixed micelles in the presence of bile acids. Incorporation into mixed micelles greatly increases the aqueous solubility of these substances. The delivery of β-monoglycerides and fatty acids across the unstirred water layer to the absorptive surface of the mucosal cell is therefore increased more than 100 fold in the presence of bile acids (*top*) compared with simple diffusion in the absence of bile acids (*bottom*).

Lipolysis

Most dietary lipid is ingested in the form of triglycerides, which are neutral lipids consisting of three fatty acid molecules (in a normal diet, primarily long-chain fatty acids) bound in ester linkage to glycerol. Triglycerides are present in the gut lumen as water-insoluble oil droplets. The first stage of triglyceride digestion, lipolysis, is catalyzed by pancreatic lipase, an enzyme with two properties of prime physiologic importance. First, it is an interfacial enzyme, that is, it acts at the oil-water interface between triglyceride droplet and aqueous intestinal content.[155] The rate of triglyceride hydrolysis is dependent upon the available surface area of the droplets and hence on the particle size distribution of the emulsion. It is possible that bile acids, by virtue of their detergent property, act as emulsifying agents that increase the surface area and hence the rate of hydrolysis. Bile acids may also protect lipase from inactivation by irreversible adsorption to the triglyceride surface.[192] However, these potentially accelerating effects of bile acids require the presence of colipase,[156] a pancreatic polypeptide that binds to lipase and appears to prevent bile acids from inhibiting lipase activity at the oil-water interface.

The second important property of pancreatic lipase is that it catalyzes the stereospecific partial hydrolysis of triglyceride to β-monoglyceride and two molecules of fatty acid. Monoglycerides and fatty acids, but not di- or triglycerides, can be solubilized in the form of mixed micelles by bile acids. The specific partial hydrolysis of triglycerides to fatty acids and monoglycerides thus allows a redistribution of these products of digestion from the triglyceride oil droplets to a mixed bile acid–monoglyceride–fatty acid micelle (Fig. 2–8).[157] This redistribution may be important in absorption, as outlined further on, and also may facilitate ongoing hydrolysis by preventing accumulation of the more polar fatty acids and monoglycerides at oil-water interfaces.[153] Although lipases of pharyngeal[158] and intestinal[159] origin have been described, their role in triglyceride absorption has not yet been defined.

Luminal Solubilization

Before intraluminal digestion starts, nearly all dietary lipid is present in the oil phase. With continuing lipolysis, there is a gradual redistribution of monoglycerides and fatty acids from the oil droplet to mixed micelles stabilized by bile acids (Fig. 2–8). At the same time, the phospholipids initially present in mixed micelles are converted by pancreatic phospholipase to lysolecithin, some of which leaves the micelle and enters into free solution. Although characterization of the mixed lipid micelles present in the intestinal lumen is technically difficult, some measurements of their relative content of fatty acid, monoglyceride, lysolecithin, cholesterol, and bile acid have been reported.[160] Studies in which fat digestion occurring in vitro has been directly observed microscopically confirm the important role of bile acids but suggest that the traditional view of intraluminal digestion as a two-phase system (insoluble triglyceride and micelles) may be an oversimplification.[153]

Mucosal Uptake

Before fatty acids and monoglycerides present in mixed micelles can be absorbed, they must be transported to the surface of the intestinal mucosal cell. This is complicated by the fact that there is a layer of water adjacent to all biologic membanes, including the intestinal mucosal cell, through which solute molecules must move by simple diffusion.[161] Although the boundary between this unstirred water layer and the bulk water phase of the intestinal lumen is not sharply defined, the unstirred layer may be as thick as 0.5 mm. Fatty acids and monoglycerides, both of which are poorly water-soluble, would be expected to move only very slowly through such an unstirred water layer. A very important function of micelles is to facilitate diffusion of these products of digestion to the mucosal surface. It is estimated that micelle formation may accelerate this process 100 fold.[154] Micellarization is particularly important in the absorption of the fat-soluble vitamins D and K, which are minimally water-soluble.

Fatty acids incorporated into the micelle are not immobilized but are continuously exchanging with fatty acids in other micelles and also in free solution. Fatty acid molecules in solution that come in contact with the cell membrane may be absorbed. There is, in fact, evidence that the rate of fatty acid absorption by the mucosal cell is related directly to fatty acid concentration in molecular solution.[162] Thus, micelles may not participate directly in absorption, but they perform the important function of delivering poorly water-soluble lipid molecules across the unstirred water layer to the vicinity of the mucosal cell membrane, where absorption can occur (Fig. 2–8).

Intracellular Metabolism

Once inside the mucosal cell, triglycerides are resynthesized either by recombination of the absorbed β-monoglycerides with fatty acids[163] or by esterification of free glycerol derived from endogenous glucose with three molecules of fatty acid. Triglycerides are then packaged in the form of chylomicrons, which consist of an inner core of triglyceride and cholesterol esters surrounded by a layer of more polar lipids, including unesterified cholesterol and phospholipid, that, in turn, is coated with apoprotein. After extrusion from the mucosal cells, lipid packaged in the form of chylomicrons is transported from the intestine primarily via the lymphatics.

Fat Malabsorption in Cholestasis

Under normal circumstances, 96 per cent of the 60 to 100 gm of neutral fat ingested daily as a part of Western diet is absorbed. About 90 per cent of this absorption takes place in the proximal 100 cm of the jejunum. Although it is clear from the preceding discussion that bile acids participate in several steps of the overall process of lipid absorption, approximately 75 per cent of the ingested triglyceride can be absorbed in the complete absence of bile,[164] assuming, of course, that pancreatic and intestinal function is otherwise unimpaired. This is largely the result of the enormous intestinal reserve. For example, even though transit through the unstirred water layer is slowed markedly, recruitment of the normally "unused" mid- and distal jejunum and ileum for lipid absorption creates a vastly extended absorptive surface and partially compensates for the absence of bile acids. This does not apply to fat-soluble vitamins, which, because of their very limited solubility in water, are not detectably absorbed in the absence of micelles.[154] Patients with prolonged cholestasis therefore must be supplemented with parenteral or water-soluble preparations of vitamins A, D, and K to prevent deficiency states leading, respectively, to night blindness, osteoporosis, and osteomalacia and bleeding. At least in children, supplementation with vitamin E may also be advisable to prevent neurologic dysfunction.[194] Since malabsorption of dietary fat often causes flatulence, bloating, and diarrhea with bulky, greasy, foul-smelling stools, these patients also frequently require restriction of dietary fat and supplementation with medium-chain triglycerides. The latter are synthetic triglycerides in which the fatty acid is primarily C-8, octanoic acid. They are hydrolyzed more readily by lipase than are dietary long-chain triglycerides, and the liberated medium-chain fatty acids are relatively water-soluble and can therefore diffuse through the unstirred water layer to the intestinal surface even in the absence of bile acid.

ENTEROHEPATIC CIRCULATION OF BILIARY SOLUTES

Bile Acids

For a comprehensive review of the enterohepatic circulation of bile acids, the reader is referred to reference 165. In discussing the enterohepatic circulation of bile acids under physiologic and pathologic conditions, it is helpful to introduce some additional terminology and concepts. The first relates to the distinction between primary and secondary bile acids. *Primary bile acids* are those synthesized in the liver from cholesterol. The two primary bile acids in humans are *cholic acid* and *chenodeoxycholic acid*. Secondary bile acids are formed in the intestine by bacterial alteration of primary bile acids. The two secondary bile acids of importance in humans are deoxycholic acid and lithocholic acid, which are formed from cholic acid and chenodeoxycholic acid, respectively. Since patients with an ileostomy have relatively less deoxycholate than do healthy individuals,[166] it is likely that formation of secondary bile acids occurs primarily in the colon. However, there is also an increased proportion of secondary bile acids in patients who have undergone cholecystectomy,[167] that is, under conditions of continuous, uninterrupted enterohepatic circulation.

Although this may reflect a greater proportion of bile acids entering the colon, an alternative explanation is that bile acids dwell for a relatively longer time in the small intestine, which would suggest that some formation of secondary bile acids occurs in the small bowel as well as in the colon. Since both primary and secondary bile acids undergo enterohepatic circulation, both are found in normal bile. Primary bile acids usually account for about 60 to 90 per cent of the total bile pool, and secondary bile acids, primarily deoxycholate, make up the remaining 10 to 30 per cent. Lithocholate, which is present in normal bile in only trace amounts,[168] produces cholestasis in experimental animals[105] and liver injury in subhuman primates. The ability to form 3-ester sulfate derivatives of glyco- and taurolithocholic acid appears to protect humans from the potentially toxic effect of this bile acid by decreasing its absorption in the bowel.[165] This is an important consideration with respect to the therapeutic use of chenodeoxycholic or ursodeoxycholic[221] acid for dissolution of gallstones (see Chapter 4). The enterohepatic circulation of primary and secondary bile acids is schematically illustrated in Figure 2–9.

The second item of terminology relates to the difference between conjugated and unconjugated bile acids. Bile acids in humans are conjugated in the liver with either taurine or glycine by an amide linkage. This conjugation markedly lowers the pK_a of bile acids from about 6 to 4 for glycine conjugates and to 2 for taurine conjugates. This low pK_a

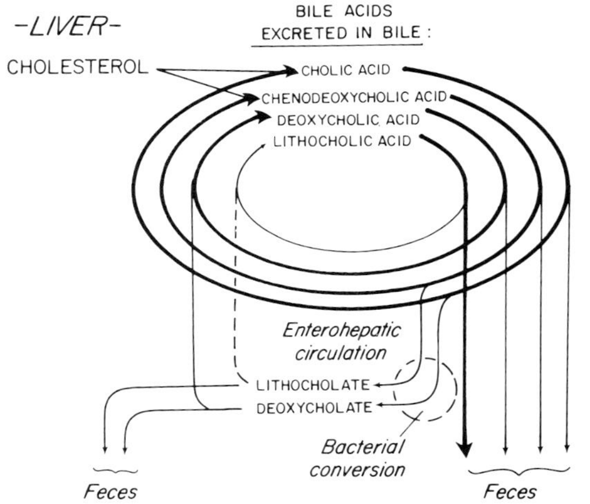

Figure 2–9. Enterohepatic circulation of bile acids. The primary bile acids, cholic acid and chenodeoxycholic acid, are formed in the liver from cholesterol. The secondary bile acids, deoxycholic acid and lithocholic acid, are formed in the bowel by the action of bacterial enzymes on cholic acid and chenodeoxycholic acid respectively. All four bile acids are secreted in bile conjugated with either glycine or taurine, making a total of eight different principal bile acid species in human bile. Bile acids are absorbed either by an active transport mechanism in the terminal ileum or by non-ionic diffusion. Non-ionic diffusion is operative primarily for bile acids that have been deconjugated by intestinal bacteria, and it occurs in the colon and probably also in the small intestine. Lithocholic acid, in addition to being conjugated with glycine or taurine, is sulfated. Sulfation decreases both active and passive absorption of this bile acid in the bowel, and lithocholate therefore is present in human bile in only small amounts (<5% of total bile acids).

ensures that conjugated bile acids are largely ionized at the pH range normally encountered in the intestinal lumen. The ionized form of the acid is less lipid-soluble than the protonated form and is therefore less likely to move passively through the intestinal wall by nonionic diffusion. Virtually all primary and secondary bile acids secreted by the liver are conjugated, and the ratio of glycine to taurine conjugates normally ranges from 3:1 to 4:1 but may be reduced by taurine feeding.[169] No disease states have thus far been described in which significant amounts of unconjugated bile acids are secreted by the liver. A variety of intestinal bacteria, including enterococci, bacteroides, and clostridia, are capable of hydrolyzing this amide linkage,[170] i.e., deconjugating bile acids. Unconjugated bile acids that are returned from the intestine to the liver are subsequently reconjugated with either glycine or taurine before re-excretion in bile.

Bile acids enter the duodenum following meal-stimulated gallbladder contraction and participate in dietary lipid absorption primarily in the proximal 100 cm of jejunum. Farther downstream, in the distal 100 to 150 cm of ileum, bile acids are reabsorbed by an active sodium-dependent transport process. This process appears analogous to hepatic sodium-coupled bile acid transport and, in fact, closely resembles the hepatic transport process in its substrate selectivity.[171] About 70 to 80 per cent of the total enterohepatic circulation occurs via this route. The remaining enterohepatic circulation takes place via an absorptive mechanism operative primarily for unconjugated bile acids. Because of their higher pK_a, a significant proportion of unconjugated bile acids are not dissociated at the pH of the intestinal lumen and therefore may be absorbed via nonionic diffusion. Since nonionic diffusion does not require a specialized transport system, it is potentially operative throughout the entire length of the small and large intestine. One would anticipate that most nonionic diffusion would occur in the colon, where bile acids that have escaped the ileal transport mechanism would be deconjugated by the abundant colonic flora. However, hydrolysis of taurine and glycine conjugates appears to proceed at rates in excess of those predicted for the colon alone,[172] which suggests that limited absorption of unconjugated bile acids, and perhaps even of glycine-conjugated bile acids,[173] may occur via nonionic diffusion in the small bowel.

The liver synthesizes 300 to 600 mg of primary bile acids per day, and the total bile acid pool is approximately 3 to 4 gm. It is estimated that this bile acid pool undergoes enterohepatic circulation four to eight times per day depending on dietary habits,[174, 224] with total daily fecal losses[175] equaling the hepatic synthetic rate. The hepatic uptake system for bile acids is very efficient and cannot be saturated by endogenous bile acids in healthy individuals. Measurement of peripheral serum bile acids can, therefore, provide information as to the status of the enterohepatic circulation.[223] It is thus evident that the enterohepatic circulation of bile acids functions very efficiently and allows the liver to deliver 10 to 15 times more bile acids to the intestine than would be possible on the basis of synthesis alone. This helps to ensure that the biliary concentration of bile acids is adequate to solubilize the excreted cholesterol and that the luminal concentration of bile acids in the proximal small bowel is sufficient to allow efficient lipid absorption.

Although a detailed description of abnormalities of the enterohepatic circulation of bile acids is beyond the scope of this chapter, many of the causes and sequelae of such disorders are predictable on the basis of the preceding discussion. For example, patients with ileal resection or intrinsic ileal disease due to granulomatous enteritis, amyloid infiltration, or radiation damage have been found to have bile acid malabsorption.[171] Although such patients may partially compensate by increasing bile acid synthesis in the liver and nonionic resorption of unconjugated bile acids in the colon, they frequently have a relative bile acid deficiency that produces characteristic clinical problems. For example, they may exhibit malabsorption of dietary fat and fat-soluble vitamins as a direct result of decreased concentrations of bile acids in the intestinal lumen. They also have an increased incidence of gallstones,[176] which presumably results from inadequate cholesterol-solubilizing capacity of hepatic bile. This may be partially explained by findings of the type shown in Figure 2–7, which illustrate that the molar ratio of cholesterol to phospholipid and bile acid increases at low rates of bile acid excretion.[66] Ileal resection or disease also causes excessive delivery of bile acids to the colon, where they have been found to inhibit colonic water absorption[177]; this may explain the syndrome of watery diarrhea termed choleretic enteropathy that frequently is associated with ileal dysfunction.[178] An isolated defect of the ileal active bile acid transport has been described. This defect resulted in an interruption of the enterohepatic circulation leading to chronic diarrhea, steatorrhea, and growth failure.[222]

An understanding of normal bile salt metabolism also helps to explain the clinical manifestations frequently encountered in patients with disordered small bowel motility, partial small bowel obstruction, or anatomic "blind loops." Once bacterial proliferation in the affected segment(s) of small bowel enhances deconjugation of bile acids, which are less water-soluble than conjugated bile acids and therefore are reabsorbed by nonionic diffusion, the intraluminal concentration of bile acids may fall below that required for adequate micelle formation.[179] This appears to be the principal cause of fat malabsorption in these conditions, although it is possible that mucosal toxicity of unconjugated bile acids and bacterial overgrowth may be contributing factors.

Urobilinogen

Conjugated bilirubin is not absorbed in the small intestine and probably remains largely intact en route to the distal small bowel and colon.[180, 181] Thus there is no appreciable enterohepatic circulation of conjugated bilirubin in humans. In the terminal ileum and large bowel, bilirubin glucuronide is hydrolyzed to unconjugated bilirubin by bacterial β-glucuronidases, and the unconjugated bilirubin is reduced to a complex series of tetrapyrroles collectively referred to as urobilinogens.[182] These colorless chromogens, or their oxidized orange derivatives called urobilin, appear in the stool. A small fraction of these compounds is absorbed in the terminal ileum or colon, and they are re-excreted primarily by the liver, with a much smaller amount appearing in the urine.[183] Quantitative measurement of urinary or fecal urobilinogen is of limited usefulness in the diagnosis of hepatobiliary disorders. For example, increased urinary urobilinogen excretion may occur with either intrinsic liver disease or excessive bile pigment production, but in neither case is it a constant or reliable laboratory finding.[184] Similarly, fecal urobilinogen excretion is a poor measure of increased bilirubin production, as occurs, for example, in hemolysis. In complete biliary tract obstruction, urinary and fecal urobilinogen are absent, but this provides little more information than noting that the stool is clay-colored.

With respect to stool color, it frequently is assumed that urobilinogen and urobilin are responsible for the normal brown appearance of feces. This is unlikely, however, since these compounds are either colorless or orange. There is evidence to suggest that stool color is derived largely from dietary pigments, presumably plant pigments such as chlorophylls, which readily undergo enterohepatic circulation and chemical modification in the liver.[185] Thus the acholic stool characteristic of biliary tract obstruction does not result from absence of bilirubin degradation products but rather from interruption of the enterohepatic circulation of dietary pigments. Definition of the term "bile pigment" therefore should be broadened to include bilirubinoid as well as nonbilirubinoid pigments appearing in the bile.

Exogenous Substances

In addition to endogenous substances, such as bile acids and urobilinogen, a variety of exogenous substances of clinical importance are secreted in bile and undergo enterohepatic circulation. The role of dietary pigments in conferring to stool its normal brown color already has been mentioned.

Digitoxin is an example of a drug that undergoes enterohepatic circulation.[186] Indeed, the extensive enterohepatic circulation is responsible for digitoxin's relatively long biologic half-life of 11 days. It has been demonstrated that interruption of this enterohepatic circulation by use of the anion exchange resin cholestyramine markedly shortens the half-life of digitoxin,[187] a maneuver that may be useful in patients with digitalis toxicity.

One interesting report has illustrated in dramatic fashion the importance of enterohepatic circulation of exogenous substances.[188] A group of factory workers were exposed over many months to high concentrations of chlordecone, an organochlorine pesticide. This lipophilic substance accumulated in many tissues and produced a variety of toxic manifestations, including tremor, stuttering speech, neuropsychiatric disturbances, hepatomegaly with altered liver histology, and oligospermia. Studies in affected workers and experimental animals indicated that chlordecone is excreted in bile (as well as perhaps directly across the bowel wall) but that less than 10 per cent of the amount excreted in bile appeared in feces. This extensive enterohepatic circulation undoubtedly contributes to the long half-life of chlordecone, reported to be approximately 5 and 1/2 months. In a controlled clinical trial, interruption of the enterohepatic circulation by oral administration of cholestyramine shortened chlordecone's half-life by 50 per cent and accelerated the disappearance of its toxic manifestations. These studies illustrate how manipulation of the enterohepatic circulation can be turned to therapeutic advantage.

SUMMARY

This chapter has reviewed current concepts regarding the mechanisms of hepatic bile formation and cholestasis, the role of bile acids in lipid absorption, and the enterohepatic circulation of bile acids, urobilinogen, and other biliary solutes. Hemodynamic considerations make it clear that bile secretion is an active process, and bile acid–dependent canalicular bile formation is closely related to the active secretion of bile acids. The biliary secretion of cholesterol and phospholipid is curvilinearly related to bile acid excretion, and the molar ratio of cholesterol to phospholipid and bile acid is an important determinant of cholesterol gallstone formation. Bilirubin and other organic solutes appear to enter bile by a secretory pathway distinct from that of bile acids, although there is evidence of some relationship between the two processes. Bile acids play a crucial role in several stages of lipid absorption and are subsequently reabsorbed in the distal small bowel and colon and returned to the liver. Disorders of this enterohepatic circulation of bile acids are associated with alterations in bile secretion rate, biliary lipid composition, and intestinal fat absorption. Urobilinogen and some exogenous substances also undergo enterohepatic circulation; an understanding of this process is clinically useful in such diverse ways as interpreting stool color and treating drug toxicity.

REFERENCES

1. Grisham JW, Nopanitaya W, Compagno J: Scanning electron microscopy of the liver: A review of the methods and results. *In* Popper H, Schaffner F (eds): Progress in Liver Diseases. Vol 5. New York, Grune & Stratton, 1976.
2. Desmet VJ: Anatomy 1: Hepatocyte-canaliculus. *In* Bianchi L, Gerok W, Sickinger K (eds): Liver and Bile. Lancaster, MTP Press Ltd, 1977.
3. Capaldi RA: A dynamic model of cell membranes. Sci Am 1974;*230*:26.
4. Ma MH, Biempica L: The normal human liver cell. Cytochemical and ultrastructural studies. Am J Pathol 1971;*62*:353.
5. Blitzer BL, Boyer JL: Cytochemical localization of Na^+, K^+-ATPase in the rat hepatocyte. J Clin Invest 1978;*62*:1104.
6. Staehelin LA, Hull BE: Junctions between living cells. Sci Am 1978;*238*:140.
7. Claude P, Goodenough DA: Fracture faces of zonulae occludentes from "tight" and "leaky" epithelia. J Cell Biol 1973;*45*:272.
8. Lagarde S, Elias E, Wade JB, et al: Structural heterogeneity of hepatocyte "tight" junctions: a quantitative analysis. Hepatology 1981;*1*:193.
9. Graff J, Peterlik M: Mechanism of transport of inorganic ions into bile. *In* Taylor W (ed): The Hepatobiliary System—Fundamental and Pathological Mehanisms. New York, Plenum Press, 1975.
10. Bradley SE, Merz R: Permselectivity of biliary canalicular membrane in rats: clearance probe analysis. Am J Physiol 1978;*235*:E570.
11. Layden TJ, Elias E, Boyer JL: Bile formation in the rat. The role of the paracellular shunt pathway. J Clin Invest 1978;*62*:1375.
12. Govindan VM, Wieland TH: Isolation and identification of actin from rat liver. FEBS Lett 1975;*59*:117.
13. Phillips MJ, Oda M: The bile canalicular web. Fed Proc 1974;*33*:626.
14. Wheeler HO: Principles of bliary secretion. *In* Hepatology—Research and Clinical Issues. 2. Jaundice. New York, Plenum Press, 1975.
15. Gabbiani G, Montesano R, Tuchweber B, et al: Phalloidin-induced hyperplasia of actin filaments in rat hepatocytes. Lab Invest 1975;*33*:562.
16. Dubin M, Maurice M, Feldman G, et al: Phalloidin-induced cholestasis in the rat: relation to changes in microfilaments. Gastroenterology 1978;*75*:450.
17. Phillips MJ, Oda M, Mak E, et al: Microfilament dysfunction as a possible cause of intrahepatic cholestasis. Gastroenterology 1975;*69*:48.
18. Adler M, Chung KW, Schaffner F: Pericanalicular hepatocyte and bile ductular microfilaments in cholestasis in man. Am J Pathol 1980;*98*:603.
19. Dubin M, Maurice M, Feldman G, et al: Influence of colchicine and phalloidin on bile secretion and hepatic ultrastructure in the rat. Gastroenterology 1980;*79*:646.
20. Gregory DH, Vlahcevic ZR, Prugh MF, et al: Mechanism of secretion of biliary lipids: role of a microtubular system in hepatocellular transport of lipids in the rat. Gastroenterology 1978;*74*:93.
21. Schaffner F: The ultrastructure of bile secretion. *In* Gerok W, Sickinger K (eds): Drugs and the Liver. New York, FS Schattauer Verlag, 1973.
22. Ishak KG: Liver biopsy: special techniques. *In* Race GJ (ed): Laboratory Medicine. New York, Harper & Row, 1973.
23. Brauer RW, Leong SF, Holloway RJ: Mechanics of bile secretion. Effect of perfusion pressure and temperature on bile flow and bile secretion pressure. Am J Physiol 1954;*177*:103.
24. Tavoloni N, Reed JS, Boyer JL: Hemodynamic effects of determinants of bile secretion in isolated rat liver. Am J Physiol 1978;*234*:E584.
25. Barnhart JL, Combes B: Erythritol and mannitol

clearances with taurocholate and secretin-induced choleresis. Am J Physiol 1978;*234*:E146.

26. Forker EL: Two sites of bile formation as determined by mannitol and erythritol clearance in the guinea pig. J Clin Invest 1967;*46*:1189.
27. Wheeler HO, Ross ED, Bradley SE: Canalicular bile production in dogs. Am J Physiol 1968; *214*:866.
28. Forker EL: Mechanisms of hepatic bile formation. Ann Rev Physiol 1977;*39*:323.
29. Boyer JL, Klatskin G: Canalicular bile flow and bile secretory pressure. Evidence for a non–bile salt dependent fraction in the isolated perfused rat liver. Gastroenterology 1970;*59*:853.
30. Paumgartner G, Herz R, Sauter K, et al: Taurocholate excretion and bile formation in the isolated perfused rat liver. An *in vitro–in vivo* comparison. Naunyn-Schmiedebergs Arch Pharmacol 1974; *285*:165.
31. Wheeler HO, Ramos OL: Determinants of the flow and composition of bile in the unanesthetized dog during constant infusions of sodium taurocholate. J Clin Invest 1960;*39*:161.
32. Preisig R, Cooper HL, Wheeler HO: The relationship between taurocholate secretion rate and bile production in the unanesthetized dog during cholinergic blockage and during secretin administration. J Clin Invest 1962;*41*:1152.
33. Prandi D, Erlinger S, Glasinovic JC, et al: Canalicular bile production in man. Eur J Clin Invest 1975;*5*:1.
34. Boyer JL, Bloomer JR: Canalicular bile secretion in man: studies utilizing the biliary clearance of [^{14}C] mannitol. J Clin Invest 1974;*54*:773.
35. Linblad L, Schersten T: Influence of cholic and chenodeoxycholic acid on canalicular bile flow in man. Gastroenterology 1976;*70*:1121.
36. Balabaud C, Kron K, Gumucio JJ: The assessment of the bile salt–nondependent fraction of canalicular bile water in the rat. J Lab Clin Med 1977;*89*:393.
37. Reichen J, Paumgartner G: Uptake of bile acids by perfused rat liver. Am J Physiol 1976;*231*:734.
38. Dietmaier A, Gasser R, Graf J, et al: Investigations on the sodium dependence of bile acid fluxes in the isolated perfused rat liver. Biochim Biophys Acta 1976;*443*:81.
39. Scharschmidt BF, Stephens JE: Transport of sodium, chloride and taurocholate by cultured rat hepatocytes. Proc Natl Acad Sci USA 1981;*78*:986.
40. Van Dyke RW, Stephens JE, Jones AL, et al: Bile acid uptake by cultured rat hepatocytes. Gastroenterology 1981;*80*:1352.
41. Gonzales MC, Sutherland E, Simon FR: Regulation of hepatic transport of bile salts: effect of protein synthesis inhibition on excretion of bile salts and their binding to liver surface membrane fractions. J Clin Invest 1979;*63*:684.
42. Erlinger S: Bile acid–independent secretion. *In* Bianchi L, Gerok W, Sickinger K (eds): Liver and Bile. Lancaster, MTP Press, 1976.
43. Erlinger S, Dhumeaux D, Berthelot P, et al: Effects of inhibition of sodium transport on bile formation in the rabbit. Am J Physiol 1970;*219*:416.
44. Latham PS, Kashgarian M: The ultrastructural localization of transport ATPase in the rat liver at nonbile canalicular plasma membranes. Gastroenterology 1979;*76*:988.
45. Essner E, Novikoff AB, Masek B: Adenosin-triphosphate and 5′-nucleotidase activities in plasma membrane of liver cells as revealed by electron microscopy. J Biophys Biochem Cytol 1958;*4*:711.
46. Boyer JL, Reno D: Properties of (Na^+-K^+)–activated ATPase in rat liver plasma membranes enriched with bile canaliculi. Biochim Biophys Acta 1975;*401*:59.
47. Reichen J, Paumgartner G: Relationship between bile flow and Na^+, K^+ adenosinetriphosphatase in liver plasma membranes enriched in bile canaliculi. J Clin Invest 1977;*60*:429.
48. Simon FR, Sutherland E, Accatino L: Stimulation of hepatic sodium and potassium–activated adenosine triphosphatase activity by phenobarbital. J Clin Invest 1977;*59*:849.
49. Wannagat F-J, Adler RD, Ockner RK: Bile acid–induced increase in bile acid–independent flow and plasma membrane NaK-ATPase activity in rat liver. J Clin Invest 1978;*61*:297.
50. Layden TJ, Boyer JL: The effect of thyroid hormone on bile salt–independent bile flow and Na^+K^+-ATPase activity in liver plasma membranes enriched in bile canaliculi. J Clin Invest 1976;*57*:1009.
51. Samuels AM, Carey MC: Effects of chlorpromazine hydrochloride and its metabolites on Mg^{2+}- and Na^+, K^+-ATPase activities of canalicular-enriched rat liver plasma membranes. Gastroenterology 1978;*74*:1183.
52. Ros ER, Small DM, Carey MC: The effects of chlorpromazine hydrochloride (CPZ) on bile formation and biliary lipid secretion in the primate. Gastroenterology 1975;*68*:975.
53. Laperche Y, Launay A, Oudea P: Effects of phenobarbital and rose bengal on the ATPase of plasma membranes of rat and rabbit liver. Gut 1972;*13*:920.
54. Dhumeaux D, Erlinger S, Benhamou J-P, et al: Effects of rose bengal on bile secretion in the rabbit: inhibition of a bile salt independent fraction. Gut 1976;*11*:134.
55. Riely CA, Dobbins JW, Binder HJ: The effect of phenobarbital on canalicular enriched liver plasma membranes (LPM). (Abstract.) Gastroenterology 1976;*71*:A-33/926.
56. Gumucio JJ, Balabaud C, Gray RH, et al: Study of the stimulation of the bile salt non-dependent fraction of canalicular bile water (BSNDF) by phenobarbital. Gastroenterology 1975;*68*:1077.
57. Boyer JL, Reno D, Layden TJ: Bile canalicular membrane Na^+K^+-ATPase. *In* Leevy CM (ed): Diseases of the Liver and Biliary Tract. Basel, S. Karger, 1976.
58. Keeffe EB, Scharschmidt BF, Blankenship NM, et al: Studies of relationships among bile flow, liver plasma membrane NaK-ATPase, and membrane microviscosity in the rat. J Clin Invest 1979; *64*:1590.
59. Leffell D, Dobbins J, Riely CA, et al: Evidence against stimulation of bile flow by Na-K ATPase. (Abstract.) Clin Res 1977;*25*:315.
60. Hardison WGM, Wood CA: Importance of bicarbonate in bile salt independent fraction of bile flow. Am J Physiol 1978;*235*:E158.
61. Scharschmidt BF, Van Dyke RW, Stephens JE: Chloride transport by intact rat liver and cultured rat hepatocytes. Am J Physiol 1982;*242*:G628.
62. Van Dyke RW, Stephens JE, Scharschmidt BF: Effect of ion substitution on bile acid–dependent and bile acid–independent bile formation by rat liver. J Clin Invest 1982;*70*:505.

63. Blitzer BL, Boyer JL: Cellular mechanisms of bile formation. Gastroenterology 1982;*82*:345.
64. Carey MC, Small DM: The physical chemistry of cholesterol solubility in bile. Relationship to gallstone formation and dissolution in man. J Clin Invest 1978;*61*:998.
65. Grundy SM, Kern F Jr: Workshop on regulation of hepatic cholesterol and bile acid metabolism. J Lipid Res 1980;*21*:496.
66. Wagner CI, Trolman BW, Soloway RD: Kinetic analysis of biliary lipid excretion in man and dog. J Clin Invest 1976;*57*:473.
67. Northfield TC, Hofmann AF: Biliary lipid output during three meals and an overnight fast. I. Relationship to bile acid pool size and cholesterol saturation of bile in gallstone and control subjects. Gut 1975;*16*:1.
68. Jones AL, Schmucker DL, Mooney JS, et al: Alteration in hepatic pericanalicular cytoplasm during enhanced bile secretory activity. Lab Invest 1979;*40*:512.
69. Schmid R, McDonagh AF: Hyperbilirubinemia. *In* Stanbury JB, Wyngaarden JB, Fredrickson DS (eds): The Metabolic Basis of Inherited Disease. New York, McGraw-Hill, 1978.
70. Scharschmidt BF, Gollan JL: Current concepts of bilirubin metabolism and hereditary hyperbilirubinemia. *In* Popper H, Schaffner F (eds): Progress in Liver Diseases. Vol VI. New York, Grune & Stratton, 1979.
71. Scharschmidt BF, Waggoner JG, Berk PD: Hepatic organic anion uptake in the rat. J Clin Invest 1975;*56*:1280.
72. Paumgartner G, Reichen J: Kinetics of hepatic uptake of unconjugated bilirubin. Clin Sci Molec Med 1976;*51*:169.
73. Mender E, Paumgartner G: Disparate Na^+-requirement of bile acids and indocyanine green uptake by isolated hepatocytes. (Abstract.) Gastroenterology 1977;*73*:A37/1235.
74. Wolkoff AW, Chung CT: Identification, purification, and partial characterization of an organic anion binding protein from rat liver cell plasma membranes. J Clin Invest 1980;*65*:1152.
75. Reichen J, Blitzer BL, Berk PD: Binding of unconjugated and conjugated sulfobromophthalein to rat liver plasma membrane fractions in vitro. Biochim Biophys Acta 1981;*640*:298.
76. Levi AJ, Gatmaitan Z, Arias IM: Two hepatic cytoplasmic protein fractions, Y and Z, and their role in the hepatic uptake of bilirubin, sulfobromophthalein, and other anions. J Clin Invest 1969;*48*:2156.
77. Litwack G, Ketterer B, Arias IM: Ligandin: an abundant protein which binds steroids, bilirubin, carcinogens, and a number of exogenous organic anions. Nature 1971;*234*:466.
78. Habit WH, Pabst MJ, Fleischner G, et al: The identity of glutathione S-transferase B with ligandin, a major binding protein of rat liver. Proc Natl Acad Sci USA 1974;*71*:3879.
79. Wolkoff AW, Goresky Sellin J, Gatmaitan Z, et al: Role of ligandin in the transfer of bilirubin from plasma from liver. Am J Physiol 1979;*236*:E638.
80. Gordon ER, Goresky CA, Chang T-H, et al: The isolation and characterization of bilirubin diglucuronide, the major bilirubin conjugate in dog and human bile. Biochem J 1976;*155*:477.
81. Burchell B: Studies on the purification of rat liver uridine diphosphate glucuronyl-transferase. Biochem J 1977;*161*:543.
82. Jansen PLM, Chowdhury JR, Fischberg EG, et al: Enzymatic conversion of bilirubin monoglucuronide to diglucuronide by rat liver plasma membranes. J Biol Chem 1977;*252*:2710.
83. Chowdhury JR, Jansen PLM, Fischberg EB, et al: Hepatic conversion of bilirubin monoglucuronide to diglucuronide in uridine diphosphate glucuronyltransferase deficient man and rat by bilirubin glucuronoside glucuronosyltransferase. J Clin Invest 1978;*62*:191.
84. Blanckaert N, Gollan J, Schmid R: Mechanism of bilirubin formation in intact rats. J Clin Invest 1980;*65*:1332.
85. Schalm L, Weber APH: Jaundice with conjugated bilirubin in hyperhaemolysis. Acta Med Scand 1964;*176*:549.
86. Forker EL: Canalicular anion transport. *In* Berk PD, Berlin NI (eds): Chemistry and Physiology of Bile Pigments. DHEW Publication No. (NIH) 77-1100, Washington, DC, Government Printing Office, 1977.
87. Clarenberg R, Kao CC: Shared and separate pathways for biliary excretion of bilirubin and BSP in rats. Am J Physiol 1973;*225*:192.
88. Whelan G, Combes B: Competition of unconjugated and conjugated sulfobromophthalein sodium (BSP) for a single excretory system. J Lab Clin Med 1971;*78*:230.
89. Bonnett R, Davies JE, Hursthouse MB: Structure of bilirubin. Nature 1976;*262*:326.
90. Schmid R: Bilirubin metabolism: state of the art. Gastroenterology 1978;*74*:1307.
91. Blanckaert N, Fevery J, Heirwegh KPM, et al: Characterization of the major diazo-positive pigments in bile of homozygous Gunn rats. Biochem J 1977;*164*:237.
92. Blanckaert N, Heirwegh KPM, Zaman A: Comparison of the biliary excretion of the four isomers of bilirubin IX in Wistar and homozygous Gunn rats. Biochem J 1977;*164*:229.
93. McDonagh AF, Palma LA, Lightner DA: Blue light and bilirubin excretion. Science 1980;*208*:145.
94. McDonagh AF, Palma LA: Hepatic excretion of circulating bilirubin photoproducts in the Gunn rat. J Clin Invest 1980;*66*:1182.
95. Arias IM: The excretion of conjugated bilirubin by the liver cell. Medicine 1966;*45*:513.
96. Accatino L, Simon FR: Identification and characterization of a bile acid receptor in isolated liver surface membranes. J Clin Invest 1976;*57*:496.
97. Goresky CA, Haddad HH, Kluger WS, et al: The enhancement of maximal bilirubin excretion with taurocholate-induced increments in bile flow. Can J Physiol Pharmacol 1974;*52*:389.
98. Barnhart J, Ritt D, Ware A, et al: A comparison of the effects of taurocholate and theophylline on BSP excretion in dogs. *In* The Liver: Quantitative Aspects of Structure and Function. Basel, S Karger, 1973.
99. O'Maille ERL, Richards TG, Short AH: Factors determining the maximal rate of organic anion excretion by the liver and further evidence of the hepatic site of action of the hormone secretin. J Physiol (London) 1966;*186*:424.
100. Boyer JL, Scheig RL, Klatskin G: The effect of sodium taurocholate on the hepatic metabolism of sulfobromophthalein sodium (BSP). The role of bile flow. J Clin Invest 1970;*49*:206.
101. Vonk RJ, Veen HVD, Prop G, et al: The influence of taurocholate and dehydrocholate choleresis on plasma disappearance and biliary excretion of in-

docyanine green in the rat. Naunyn-Schmiedebergs Arch Pharmacol 1974;*282*:401.
102. Berk RN, Goldberger LE, Loeb P: The role of bile salts in the hepatic excretion of iopanoic acid. Invest Radiol 1974;*9*:7.
103. Gibson GE, Forker EL: Canalicular bile flow and bromsulphthalein transport maximum: the effect of a bile salt–independent choleretic, SC-2644. Gastroenterology 1974;*66*:1046.
104. Dunn CR, Berk RN: The pharmacokinetics of Telepaque metabolism: the relation of blood concentration and bile flow to the rate of hepatic excretion. Am J Roentgenol 1972;*114*:758.
105. Nemchausky BA, Layden TJ, Boyer JL: Effects of chronic choleretic infusions of bile acids on the membrane of the bile canaliculus. Lab Invest 1977;*36*:259.
106. Ware AJ, Carey MC, Combes B: Solution properties of sulfobromophthalein sodium (BSP) compounds alone and in association with sodium taurocholate (TC). J Lab Clin Med 1976;*87*:443.
107. Juniper K: Physicochemical characteristics of bile and their relation to gallstone formation. Am J Med 1965;*39*:98.
108. Nakayama F: Nature of cholesterol complexing macromolecular fractions in bile. Clin Chim Acta 1966;*13*:212.
109. Scharschmidt BF, Schmid R: The "micellar sink": A quantitative assessment of the association of various organic anions with mixed micelles and other aggregates in rat bile. J Clin Invest 1978;*62*:1122.
110. Bloomer JR, Zaccaria J: Effect of graded bilirubin loads on bilirubin transport by perfused rat liver. Am J Physiol 1976;*230*:736.
111. Billing BH, Maggiore Q, Cartter MA: Hepatic transport of bilirubin. Ann NY Acad Sci 1963;*111*:319.
112. Goresky CA: The hepatic uptake and excretion of sulfobromophthalein and bilirubin. Can Med Assoc J 1965;*92*:851.
113. Sperber I: Biliary secretion of organic anions and its influence on bile flow. *In* Taylor W (ed): The Biliary System. Oxford, Blackwell Scientific Publications, 1965.
114. Fleischner G, Arias IM: Recent advances in bilirubin formation, transport, metabolism, and excretion. Am J Med 1970;*49*:576.
115. Wolkoff AW, Cohen LE, Arias IM: The inheritance of the Dubin-Johnson syndrome. N Engl J Med 1973;*288*:113.
116. Dubin IN, Johnson FB: Chronic idiopathic jaundice with unidentified pigment in liver cells: new clinicopathologic entity with report of 12 cases. Medicine 1954;*33*:155.
117. Abe H, Okuda K: Biliary excretion of conjugated sulfobromophthalein (BSP) in constitutional hyperbilirubinemias. Digestion 1975;*13*:272.
118. Barnhart JL, Gronwall RR, Combes B: Selective defect in biliary excretion of conjugated BSP compounds in mutant Corriedale sheep: evidence for a second canalicular carrier. (Abstract.) Gastroenterology 1977;*73*:A-59/1257.
119. Wolkoff AW, Wolpert E, Pascasio FN, et al: Rotor's syndrome. A distinct inheritable pathophysiologic entity. Am J Med 1976;*60*:173.
120. Schanker LS: Hepatic transport of organic cations. *In* Taylor, W (ed): The Biliary System. Oxford, Blackwell Scientific Publications, 1965.
121. Kupferberg HJ, Schanker LS: Biliary secretion of ouabain-H^3 and its uptake by liver slices in the rat. Am J Physiol 1968;*214*:1048.
122. Wheeler HO: Secretion of bile. *In* Schiff L (ed): Diseases of the Liver. Ed 4. Philadelphia, JB Lippincott, 1975.
123. Hardison WGM, Norman JC: Electrolyte composition of the secretin fraction of bile from the perfused pig liver. Am J Physiol 1968;*214*:758.
124. Chenderovitch J: Secretory function of the rabbit common bile duct. Am J Physiol 1973;*223*:695.
125. Jones RS, Grossman MI: Choleretic effect of cholecystokinin, gastrin II and caerulin in the dog. Am J Physiol 1970;*219*:1014.
126. Gardiner BN, Small DM: Simultaneous measurement of the pancreatic and biliary response to CCK and secretin. Primate biliary physiology. XIII. Gastroenterology 1976;*70*:403.
127. Strasberg SM, Ilson RG, Siminovitch KA, et al: Analysis of the components of bile flow in the rhesus monkey. Am J Physiol 1975;*228*:115.
128. Guzelian P, Boyer JL: Glucose reabsorption from bile. Evidence for a biliohepatic circulation. J Clin Invest 1974;*53*:526.
129. Wheeler HO: Concentrating function of the gallbladder. Am J Med 1971;*51*:588.
130. Dietschy JM: Water and solute movement across the wall of the everted rabbit gallbladder. Gastroenterology 1964;*47*:395.
131. Frizzell RA, Heintze K: Transport functions of the gallbladder. Int Rev Physiol 1980;*21*:221.
132. Frizzell RA, Field M, Schultz SG: Sodium-coupled chloride transport by epithelial tissues. Am J Physiol 1979;*236*:F1.
133. Frizzell RA, Dugas M, Schultz SG: Sodium chloride transport by rabbit gallbladder: direct evidence for a coupled NaCl influx process. J Gen Physiol 1975;*65*:769.
134. Whitlock RT, Wheeler HO: Coupled transport of solute and water across rabbit gallbladder epithelium. J Clin Invest 1964;*43*:2249.
135. Duffy ME, Turnheim K, Frizzell RA, et al: Intracellular chloride activities in rabbit gallbladder: direct evidence for the role of the sodium-gradient in energizing "uphill" chloride transport. J Membr Biol 1978;*42*:229.
136. Kaye GI, Wheeler HO, Whitlock RT, et al: Fluid transport in the rabbit gallbladder. A combined physiological and electron microscopic study. J Cell Biol 1966;*30*:237.
137. Tourmey JM, Diamond JM: Studies on the structural basis of water transport across epithelial membranes. Fed Proc 1966;*25*:1458.
138. Diamond JM: Channels in epithelial cell membranes and junctions. Fed Proc 1978;*37*:2639.
139. Macken TE, Erlis D, Wooding FBP: Permeable junction complexes. The movement of lanthanum across rabbit gallbladder and intestine. J Cell Biol 1972;*54*:302.
140. Ostrow JD: Absorption of bile pigments by the gallbladder. J Clin Invest 1967;*46*:2035.
141. Ostrow JD: Absorption by the gallbladder of bile salts, sulfobromophthalein and iodipamide. J Lab Clin Med 1969;*74*:482.
142. Javitt NB: Bile acids and hepatobiliary disease. *In* Schiff L (ed): Diseases of the Liver. Vol 4. Philadelphia, JB Lippincott, 1975.
143. Schoenfield LJ, Sjovall J, Perman E: Bile acids on the skin of patients with pruritic hepatobiliary disease. Nature 1967;*213*:93.
144. Ghent CN, Bloomer JR, Klatskin G: Elevations in

skin tissue levels of bile acids in human cholestasis: relation to serum levels and to pruritus. Gastroenterology 1977;*73*:1125.
145. Ahrens EH Jr: Primary biliary cirrhosis. Medicine 1950;*29*:299.
146. Clayton RJ, Iber FL, Ruebner BH, et al: Byler disease: fatal intrahepatic cholestasis in an Amish kindred. Am J Dis Child 1969;*117*:112.
147. Williams CN, Kaye R, Baker L, et al: Progressive familial cholestatic cirrhosis and bile acid metabolism. J Pediatr 1972;*81*:493.
148. Linarelli LG, Williams CN, Phillips MJ: Byler's disease: fatal intrahepatic cholestasis. J Pediatr 1972; *81*:484.
149. Simon FR, Gonzalez M, Sutherland E, et al: Reversal of ethinyl estradiol–induced bile secretory failure with Triton WR-1339. J Clin Invest 1980;*65*:851.
150. Hruban Z, Tavoloni N, Reed JS, et al: Ultrastructural changes during cholestasis induced by chlorpromazine in the isolated perfused rat liver. Virchows Arch (Zellpathol) 1978;*26*:289.
151. Keeffe EB, Blankenship NM, Scharschmidt BF: Alteration of rat liver plasma membrane fluidity and ATPase activity by chlorpromazine hydrochloride and its metabolites. Gastroenterology 1980;*79*:222.
152. Elias E, Boyer JL: Chlorpromazine and its metabolites alter polymerization and gelation of actin. Science 1979;*206*:1402.
153. Borgstrom B: Digestion and absorption of lipids. *In* Young DB (ed): Gastrointestinal Physiology. II. International Review of Physiology. Vol 12. Baltimore, University Park Press, 1977.
154. Hofmann AF: Fat absorption and malabsorption: Physiology, diagnosis and treatment. View Dig Dis 1977;*9*(4):1.
155. Sarda L, Desmielle P: Action de la lipase pancréatique sur les ésters en émulsion. Biochim Biophys Acta 1958;*30*:513.
156. Borgstrom B, Erlanson C: Pancreatic juice colipase: physiological importance. Biochim Biophys Acta 1971;*242*:509.
157. Hofmann AF, Borgstrom B: The intraluminal phase of fat digestion in man. The lipid content of the micellar and oil phases of intestinal content obtained during fat digestion and absorption. J Clin Invest 1964;*43*:247.
158. Cohen M, Morgan RGH, Hofman AF: Lipolytic activity of human gastric and duodenal juice against medium and long chain triglycerides. Gastroenterology 1974;*60*:1.
159. Serrero G, Negrel R, Ailhaud G: Characterization and partial purification of an intestinal lipase. Biochem Biophys Res Comm 1975;*65*:89.
160. Mansbach CM, Cohen RS, Leff PB: Isolation and properties of the mixed lipid micelles present in intestinal content during fat absorption in man. J Clin Invest 1975;*56*:781.
161. Dietschy JM, Westergaard H: The effect of unstirred water layers on various transport processes in the intestine. *In* Csaky TZ (ed): Intestinal Absorption and Malabsorption. New York, Raven Press, 1975.
162. Simmonds WJ: Absorption of lipids. *In* Young DB (ed): Gastrointestinal Physiology. MTP International Review of Science. Physiology Series I. Baltimore, University Park Press, 1974.
163. Johnston JM: Mechanism of fat absorption. *In* Code CF (ed): Handbook of Physiology. Vol 3. 1968.
164. Knodel LK: Intestinal absorption in vivo of micellar and nonmicellar lipid. Am J Physiol 1972;*223*:255.
165. Hofmann AF: The enterohepatic circulation of bile acids in man. Adv Intern Med 1976;*21*:501.
166. Miettinen TA, Deltohallo P: Bile salt, fat, water, and vitamin B_{12} excretion after ileostomy. Scand J Gastroenterol 1971;*6*:543.
167. Sjovall J: Bile acids in man under normal and pathological conditions. Bile acids and steroids 73. Clin Chim Acta 1966;*13*:207.
168. Vlahcevic ZR, Meller JR, Farrar JT, et al: Kinetics and pool size of primary bile acids in man. Gastroenterology 1971;*61*:85.
169. Garbutt JT, Kenney TJ: Effect of cholestyramine on bile acid metabolism in normal man. J Clin Invest 1972;*51*:2781.
170. Donaldson RM: Small bowel bacterial overgrowth. Adv Intern Med 1965;*16*:191.
171. Lack L: Properties and biologic significance of the ileal bile salt transport system. Environ Health Perspect 1979;*33*:79.
172. Hepner GW, Sturman JA, Hofmann AF, et al: Metabolism of steroid and amino acid moieties of conjugated bile acids in man. III. Cholyl taurine (taurocholic acid). J Clin Invest 1973;*52*:433.
173. Hislop IG, Hofmann AF, Schoenfield LJ: Determinants of the rate and site of bile acid absorption in man. J Clin Invest 1967;*46*:1070.
174. Sorensen TIA: Jejunum and bile acid synthesis. Comparison of effects of jejunoileal bypass with 3:1 and 1:3 jejunoileal ratio. Scand J Gastroenterol 1982;*17*:557.
175. Moore RB, Anderson JT, Taylor HL, et al: Effect of dietary fat on the fecal excretion of cholesterol and its degradation products in man. J Clin Invest 1968;*47*:1517.
176. Heaton KW, Read AE: Gallstones in patients with disorders of the terminal ileum and disturbed bile salt metabolism. Br Med J 1969;*3*:494.
177. Mekhjian HS, Phillips SF, Hofmann AF: Specific bile acids provoke secretion of electrolytes and water in the human colon. (Abstract.) Clin Res 1969;*17*:307.
178. Hofmann AF: The syndrome of ileal disease and the broken enterohepatic circulation: choleretic enteropathy. Gastroenterology 1967;*52*:752.
179. Isaacs PET, Kim YS: The contaminated small bowel syndrome. Am J Med 1979;*67*:1049.
180. Lester R, Schmid R: Intestinal absorption of bile pigments. I. The enterohepatic circulation of bilirubin in the rat. J Clin Invest 1963;*42*:736.
181. Lester R, Schmid R: Intestinal absorption of bile pigments. II. Bilirubin absorption in man. N Engl J Med 1963;*269*:178.
182. Watson CJ: Gold from dross: the first century of the urobilinoids. Ann Intern Med 1969;*70*:839.
183. Bourke E: Mechanisms of renal excretion of urobilinogen. Br Med J 1965;*2*:1510.
184. Bloomer JR: Comparison of fecal urobilinogen excretion with bilirubin production in normal volunteers and patients with increased bilirubin production. Clin Chim Acta 1970;*29*:643.
185. Lester R, Sachdev A, Van Thiel DH: What makes stool brown? Gastroenterology 1978;*74*:1055.
186. Okita GT, Talso PJ, Curry JH, et al: Metabolic fate of radioactive digitoxin in human subjects. J Pharmacol Exp Ther 1955;*115*:371.
187. Caldwell JH, Bush CA, Greenberger NJ: Interruption of the enterohepatic circulation of digitoxin by cholestyramine. II. Effect on metabolic dispo-

sition of tritium-labeled digitoxin and cardiac systolic intervals in man. J Clin Invest 1971;*50*:2638.

188. Cohn WJ, Boylan JJ, Blaschke RV, et al: Treatment of chlordecone (Kepone) toxicity with cholestyramine. Results of a controlled clinical trial. N Engl J Med 1978;*298*:243.
189. Takayashi J, Suzuki T, Aizawa I, et al: Comparison of gallbladder contractions induced by motilin and cholecystokinin in the dog. Gastroenterology 1982;*82*:419.
190. Hansen WE, Haberland MH: The effect of sham feeding on gallbladder volume and circulation of bile acids. Hepatogastroenterology 1982;*29*:100.
191. Meyers WC, Jones RS: Glucagon or insulin suppressed biliary lipid excretion in dogs and man. Ann Surg 1979;*190*:710.
192. Borgstrom B, Erlanson C: Interactions of serum albumin and other proteins with porcine pancreatic lipase. Gastroenterology 1978;*75*:382.
193. Patton JC, Carey MC: Watching fat digestion. Science 1979;*204*:145.
194. Rosenbaum JL, Keating JP, Prensky AL, et al: A progressive neurologic syndrome in children with chronic liver disease. N Engl J Med 1981;*304*:503.
195. Dumont M, Erlinger S, Uchman S: Hypercholeresis induced by ursodeoxycholic acid and 7-ketolithocholic acid in the rat: possible role of bicarbonate transport. Gastroenterology 1980;*79*:82.
196. Weisiger RA, Gollan JL, Ockner RK: Receptor for albumin on the liver cell surface may mediate uptake of fatty acids and other albumin-bound substances. Science 1981;*211*:1048.
197. Jones AL, Schmucker DL, Renston RH, et al: The architecture of bile secretion. A morphological perspective of physiology. Dig Dis Sci 1980;*25*:609.
198. Yamamoto K, Phillips MJ: A hitherto unrecognized bile ductular plexus in normal rat liver. Hepatology 1984;*4*:381.
199. Klaassen CD, Watkins JB III: Mechanisms of bile formation, hepatic uptake, and biliary excretion. Pharmacol Rev 1984;*36*:1.
200. Scharschmidt BF, Van Dyke RW: Mechanisms of hepatic electrolyte transport. Gastroenterology 1983;*85*:1199.
201. Anwer MS, Hegner D: Importance of solvent drag and diffusion in bile acid–dependent bile formation: ion substitution studies in isolated perfused rat liver. Hepatology 1982;2:580.
202. Inoue M, Kinne R, Tran T, et al: Taurocholate transport by rat liver sinusoidal membrane vesicles: evidence of sodium cotransport. Hepatology 1982;2:572.
203. Gewirtz DA, Randolph JK, Goldman ID: Induction of taurocholate release from isolated rat hepatocytes in suspension by γ-adrenergic agents and vasopressin: implications for control of bile salt secretion. Hepatology 1984;*4*:205.
204. Graff G: Canalicular bile salt–independent bile formation: concepts and clues from electrolyte transport in rat liver. Am J Physiol 1983;*244*:G233.
205. Erlinger S: Does Na^+-K^+-ATPase have any role in bile secretion? Am J Physiol 1982;*243*:G243.
206. Erlinger S: Hepatocyte bile secretion: current views and controversies. Hepatology 1981;*1*:352.
207. Maton PN, Reuben A, Dowling RH: Relationship between hepatic cholesterol synthesis and biliary cholesterol secretion in man: hepatic cholesterol synthesis is not a major regulator of biliary lipid secretion. Clin Sci 1982;*62*:515.
208. Turley SD, Spady DK, Dietschy JM: Alteration of the degree of biliary cholesterol saturation in the hamster and rat by manipulation of the pools of preformed and newly synthesized cholesterol. Gastroenterology 1983;*84*:253.
209. Kortz WJ, Meyers WC, Schirmer BD, et al: Effects of dibutyryl cyclic AMP and theophylline on biliary cholesterol secretion. J Surg Res 1984;*36*:62.
210. Bickerstaff KI, Garberoglio CA, Baker AL, et al: Hormonal control of biliary lipid secretion in dogs. Ann Surg 1983;*198*:168.
211. Lin DS, Connor WE, Phillipson BE: Sterol composition of normal human bile. Effects of feeding shellfish (marine) sterols. Gastroenterology 1984; *86*:611.
212. Kaminski DL, Deshpande YG: Effect of somatostatin and bombesin on secretin-stimulated ductular bile flow in dogs. Gastroenterology 1983; *85*:1239.
213. Rene E, Danzinger RG, Hofmann AF, et al: Pharmacologic effect of somatostatin on bile formation in the dog. Enhanced ductular reabsorption as the major mechanism of anticholeresis. Gastroenterology 1983;*84*:120.
214. Hanks JB, Kortz WJ, Andersen DK, et al: Somatostatin suppression of canine fasting bile secretion. Gastroenterology 1983;*84*:130.
215. Spring KR: Fluid transport by gallbladder epithelium. J Exp Biol 1983;*106*:181.
216. Kottra G, Fromter E: Functional properties of the paracellular pathway in some leaky epithelia. J Exp Biol 1983;*106*:217.
217. Corcia A, Armstrong WMcD: A mechanism for basolateral chloride exit in Necturus gallbladder. J Membr Biol 1983;*76*:173.
218. Zeuthen T: Ion activities in the lateral intercellular spaces of gallbladder epithelium transporting at low external osmolarities. J Membr Biol 1983; *76*:113.
219. Itoh Z, Takahashi J, Nakaya M, et al: Interdigestive gallbladder bile concentration in relation to periodic contraction of gallbladder in the dog. Gastroenterology 1982;*83*:645.
220. Adinolfi LE, Utili R, Gaeta GB, et al: Cholestasis induced by estradiol-17β-D-glucuronide: mechanisms and prevention by sodium taurocholate. Hepatology 1984;*4*:30.
221. Nilsell K, Angelin B, Leijd B, et al: Comparative effects of ursodeoxycholic acid and chenodeoxycholic acid on bile acid kinetics and biliary lipid secretion in humans. Evidence for different modes of action on bile acid synthesis. Gastroenterology 1983;*85*:1248.
222. Heubi JE, Balistreri WF, Fondacaro JD, et al: Primary bile acid malabsorption: defective in vitro ileal active bile acid transport. Gastroenterology 1982;*83*:804.
223. Angelin B, Bjorkhem I, Einarsson K, et al: Hepatic uptake of bile acids in man. Fasting and postprandial concentrations of individual bile acids in portal venous and systemic blood serum. J Clin Invest 1982;*70*:724.
224. Kupfer RM, Northfield TC: Diurnal variation in cholesterol saturation of gall-bladder bile. Gut 1983;*24*:950.

CARLOS A. PELLEGRINI, M.D.
MARCO G. PATTI, M.D.

3

Motility of the Gallbladder and Bile Ducts and the Kinetics of Bile Flow

Progress in the understanding of biliary motility and its role in the pathogenesis of gallstones and other gallbladder diseases was remarkably slow for many years. The lack of reliable noninvasive methods precluded direct studies in humans, and after Admirand and Small described the chemical basis of cholesterol solubility in bile[1] the attention of most biliary physiologists focused primarily on the role of supersaturated bile in gallstone formation.

Over the last decade our understanding of biliary motility has improved substantially. Classic concepts regarding the motor function of the biliary tract have been challenged and the kinetics of bile flow have been redefined. Bile stasis has been identified as a major factor in gallstone formation and growth. The clinical application of these new concepts is just beginning to surface. For example, in patients on total parenteral nutrition, in whom gallstone formation is primarily due to gallbladder stasis, cholelithiasis may be prevented by inducing periodic gallbladder emptying. Characterization of the biliary motility disorder associated with biliary dyskinesia may provide a rational therapeutic approach to this problem.

This chapter is divided into three sections. The first is a discussion of the motor function of each portion of the biliary tract: the gallbladder, the sphincter of Oddi, the cystic duct, the common bile duct, and the bile canaliculus. The second deals with the integrated motor function of these organs and the kinetics of bile flow in the digestive and interdigestive periods. The third covers specific disorders of biliary motility, such as those associated with cholelithiasis, diabetes mellitus, vagotomy, and biliary dyskinesia.

NORMAL BILIARY MOTILITY

Gallbladder Motor Function

The motor function of the gallbladder includes two different phases: gallbladder emptying and gallbladder filling. Gallbladder emptying is a brief, predominantly active phase, during which most of the gallbladder contents are evacuated. Gallbladder filling is a long, predominantly passive phase, during which hepatic bile flows preferentially into the gallbladder.

Gallbladder Emptying

Gallbladder emptying is caused by contraction of the gallbladder muscle layer, a result of active stimulation by cholecystokinin, motilin, and other factors.

Cholecystokinin (CCK) is probably the major hormonal regulator of gallbladder contraction. CCK, first isolated by Ivy in 1928, is a linear polypeptide, normally produced by the mucosa of the proximal intestine. CCK circulates in at least three different molecular forms:[2] a 39–amino acid polypeptide (CCK-39); a 33–amino acid polypeptide (CCK-33), which consists of the carboxy-terminal 33–amino acid chain of CCK-39; and an octapepide (CCK-8), also a carboxy-terminal fragment of CCK-39.

CCK is released in response to fat, peptones, and other substances. As the levels of CCK in plasma rise, the gallbladder contracts. Indeed, using a CCK radioimmunoassay, several studies have found that rising plasma levels of CCK correlate with gallbladder emptying; falling plasma levels of CCK correlate with gallbladder filling.[3–5]

In normal subjects an intravenous injection of CCK (0.020 U/kg/min) initiates gallbladder contraction within a few minutes.[6] Gallbladder contraction in response to CCK is smooth and continuous (i.e., there is no peristalsis).[7] Within 15 minutes of stimulation about 50 per cent of gallbladder bile is evacuated, and the degree of emptying plateaus at 75 per cent by 30 minutes. This response is dose-related.[7]

The rate of gallbladder emptying postprandially varies in relation to the character (e.g., osmolality, caloric density, solid or liquid) of the meal. An average meal of solid food results in 30 per cent emptying of the gallbladder within 30 minutes and a maximum of 80 per cent emptying by 120 minutes.[8] Sham feeding also induces emptying, which in the first 60 minutes closely matches the rate induced by a meal, but maximum emptying after sham feeding (about 65 per cent) falls short of the maximum in response to food.[9]

Steigerwalt et al. demonstrated the presence of CCK receptors in the smooth muscle layer of the gallbladder.[10] It is believed that CCK, acting through these receptors, induces changes in cyclic nucleotides. For example, intracellular 3′-5′ adenosine monophosphate (cAMP) is decreased by CCK.[11] Agents that decrease intracellular cAMP produce contraction of an in vitro preparation of rabbit gallbladder muscle, whereas agents that increase intracellular cAMP cause the preparation to relax.[11] In addition, CCK causes a rise in intracellular 3′-5′ guanosine monophosphate (cGMP) levels and activation of intracellular phosphodiesterase—possible mediators of gallbladder contraction.[12]

The effects of CCK on gallbladder smooth muscle in vitro are not blocked by anticholinergics or by alpha- or beta-blocking agents. Experiments in vivo have yielded different results. For example, Takahashi et al. demonstrated that CCK-8–induced contraction of the gallbladder was inhibited by atropine. This inhibition was dose-related, probably reflecting competitive antagonism.[13] Similarly, Behar and Biancani found that, in vivo, parasympathetic blockade by hexamethonium and atropine or tetrodotoxin decreased CCK-induced gallbladder contraction in the cat. They concluded that the gallbladder muscle has two kinds of CCK receptors, one on muscle cells and one on intramural postganglionic cholinergic neurons,[14] and that loss of vagal innervation may decrease the gallbladder response to CCK.

Motilin may play a major role in gallbladder motor function, especially during fasting.[15] Motilin is a 22–amino acid polypeptide isolated by Brown in 1971.[16] In the conscious dog, motilin-induced gallbladder contractions differ from CCK-induced contractions in two aspects: they are not dose-related, and they have a limited duration despite continued infusion of motilin.[13] Since plasma motilin levels vary in a cyclic manner during the interdigestive state and peak plasma levels coincide with phase III of the duodenal interdigestive migrating motor complex,[17, 18] motilin may be the humoral factor responsible for initiating interdigestive gallbladder contractions.[15] The site of action of motilin in the gallbladder has not been identified. In vivo, motilin causes gallbladder contraction in the pig,[19] in the dog,[15] and in humans.[20] In vitro, it has no effect on human gallbladder muscle strips.[20] This may indicate that its action is indirect and may be mediated by another agent. Lee et al. found that vagal stimulation produces substantial motilin release and proposed that motilin is responsible for some of the actions previously thought to be due to a direct vagal stimulation of the biliary tree.[21] Takahashi et al. showed that motilin-induced gallbladder contractions were abolished by atropine.[13] However, Yoshiya et al. found that truncal vagotomy did not influence the concentration of plasma motilin in the fasting state or motilin secretion after the ingestion of food.[22] Therefore, the exact mechanism of action of motilin on the gallbladder remains unknown.

Gastrin, with a C-terminal tetrapeptide identical to that of CCK, has some cholecystokinetic effect, but its potency is low. Physiological levels of gastrin are not likely to influence biliary motor function.[23]

Secretin does not alter gallbladder pressure at doses that stimulate pancreatic secretion, but when administered with CCK, secretin potentiates the effect of CCK on gallbladder contraction.[24]

Histamine increases pressure in the gallbladder by stimulating receptors on the smooth muscle cells.[25] Studies with receptor agonists and antagonists[26] indicate that histamine contractile effects are mediated via H_1 receptors. H_2 stimulation relaxes the body of the gallbladder but has no effect on the gallbladder neck and cystic duct. The effects of histamine on the motility of the diseased human gallbladder decrease as the inflammation becomes more severe.[26]

Prostaglandins contract the gallbladder

muscle in vitro and in vivo and can increase intraluminal gallbladder pressure.[27] In strips from gallbladders with chronic cholecystitis, PGF_2, PGB_2, and PGD_2 caused concentration-dependent contractions. PGE_1 and PGE_2 also contracted the strips, although the response was variable.[28] Thornell and coworkers found that intravenously administered indomethacin abolished the abdominal pain and tenderness associated with cholecystitis.[29] They postulated that by inhibiting the synthesis of prostaglandins, indomethacin reduced the intraluminal pressure in the gallbladder, relieving biliary pain. Prostaglandins also play a role in the control of intestinal motility and may, indirectly, participate in the genesis of the interdigestive gallbladder contractions.[30]

Various studies have shown that *cholinergic stimulation* causes contraction of the gallbladder muscle and gallbladder emptying. Yau and Youther studied the effect of cholinergic stimulation using an isolated guinea pig gallbladder preparation subjected to transmural field stimulation. They showed that contraction of the gallbladder is associated with release of acetylcholine from intrinsic cholinergic neurons.[31] Fisher and coworkers studied the effect of cholinergic stimulation and cholinergic blockade on normal subjects using cholescintigraphy.[32] They demonstrated that cholinergic stimulation by bethanecol produced 40 per cent gallbladder emptying, whereas cholinergic blockade with atropine sulfate decreased gallbladder emptying in response to a liquid and a solid meal. (The effects of vagotomy on the motor function of the gallbladder are discussed elsewhere in this chapter.)

Adrenergic control of gallbladder contraction is less important than cholinergic stimulation. Alpha-receptor stimulation produces only a weak contraction, and beta-receptor stimulation produces weak relaxation of gallbladder strips in vitro.[33]

Gallbladder Filling

Gallbladder filling occurs when pressure within the gallbladder is lower than pressure in the common bile duct. Intraluminal resting gallbladder pressure is approximately 5 mm Hg,[34] and pressure in the common bile duct is about 10 mm Hg; therefore, bile flows into the gallbladder continuously. Gallbladder filling during fasting is interrupted periodically by gallbladder contraction.

Intraluminal pressure in the gallbladder is determined, for the most part, by smooth muscle tone. Muscular tone of the gallbladder wall does not increase with increasing volume,[35] for if it did, gallbladder filling would not be possible within the pressure range normally present in the common duct. Instead, when the muscle is stretched, its fibers rearrange internally by sliding filaments in such a manner that tension development is minimal. As gallbladder volume increases, the wall becomes thinner and the number of muscle cells per cross-sectional area of gallbladder wall decreases. Thus, compliance of the gallbladder wall is high, and pressure-volume curves show that relatively large changes in volume occur with little change in pressure.[36] For example, when the gallbladder of the opossum is slowly filled with saline and the cystic duct is occluded, 50 per cent of the maximal gallbladder pressure is not attained until about two thirds of the gallbladder volume has been filled. With scarring (as in chronic cholecystitis), compliance may be impaired, affecting gallbladder filling.

The endogenous factors that influence gallbladder filling have not yet been completely identified. It was once thought that gallbladder filling occurred passively, reflecting decreased circulating CCK. Increasing evidence, however, suggests that gallbladder filling is an active process involving specific neural and/or hormonal intermediates that stimulate gallbladder relaxation or sphincter of Oddi contraction. Progressive relaxation of the muscle layer would be responsible for the high compliance of the gallbladder, and increased resistance to flow through the sphincter of Oddi would divert hepatic bile to the gallbladder.

Pancreatic polypeptide (PP) probably plays a key role in the regulation of postprandial gallbladder filling, causing relaxation of the gallbladder muscle. PP is a 36–amino acid peptide, found almost exclusively in the pancreas. Plasma levels of PP rise shortly after a meal and stay elevated for up to 6 hours.[37] Release of PP occurs in a biphasic manner.[37] The first release occurs as a result of vagal stimulation; the second, more prolonged rise occurs in response to hormonal stimulation, predominantly cholecystokinin. In addition, the vagal action may also modulate PP release through its effects on CCK release.[38] Studies on prairie dogs,[39] pigs,[40] and humans[41] suggest that PP reduces bile delivery to the duodenum directly through induction of gallbladder relaxation, so that bile preferentially flows into the gallbladder. The relaxant effects of PP are not seen on isolated gallbladder muscle strips;[20] thus, it seems likely that PP does not exert its action directly on the gallbladder muscle.

Vasointestinal polypeptide (VIP) also causes relaxation of the gallbladder muscle.[42] The presence of VIP in nerve fibers and cell bodies in the gallbladder wall suggests that VIP plays a physiologic role in gallbladder motility or in the secretory behavior of the gallbladder epithelium. VIP nerve fibers reach the gallbladder via vagal branches.

There is some evidence to suggest that *adrenergic* pathways may be involved in gallbladder relaxation and may participate in the regulation of overall gallbladder compliance. For example, beta-receptor stimulation produces weak relaxation of gallbladder strips in vitro.[33] Also, there is evidence of inhibitory innervation of the gallbladder musculature mediated by nonadrenergic transmitters. Candidates for this inhibitory neurotransmitter include ATP[43] and VIP.[44]

Sphincter of Oddi Motor Function

The resting pressure in the common bile duct, about 10 mm Hg, results from the combined effects of the rate of bile secretion by the liver and the resistance imposed by the sphincter of Oddi. Sphincter of Oddi motility has been studied in many species,[45–48] but the American opossum has been most commonly used. In this animal the sphincter of Oddi is 2 to 3 cm long and is mostly extraduodenal. Thus, manometry and electromyography can be carried out with negligible interference from duodenal motor activity.[49, 50]

The sphincter of Oddi has phasic activity, with contraction waves that originate near the cephalic margin and propagate distally along its entire length. These contractions, which generate pressures up to 200 mm Hg, occur at a rate of 2 to 8 per minute, and last about 5 seconds. They are not abolished by tetrodotoxin, which suggests a myogenic origin. Concurrent myoelectric and manometric recordings show that each phasic contraction is immediately preceded by an electrical spike burst, which also propagates in a caudal direction.

In the conscious opossum[50–52] and in the dog[53] the frequency of phasic sphincter activity exhibits a cyclic pattern related in time to the intermittent myoelectric migratory complex (IMMC). The frequency of sphincter of Oddi spike potentials increases from phase I to phase III of the IMMC and then decreases rapidly during phase IV to start a new cycle. Delivery of bile from the common bile duct into the duodenum is higher in phases I and II but decreases in phase III.[53] Basal sphincter of Oddi pressure in humans is about 3 mm Hg higher than the pressure in the common bile duct and the pancreatic duct.[45, 54] Studies in humans have also demonstrated peristaltic phasic contractions of the sphincter.[45, 54] The majority of peristaltic waves propagate in a caudal direction; only 15 per cent of the contractions are retrograde.

The sphincter of Oddi segment appears to fill between contractions, a phase called "diastole." The rhythmic peristaltic contractions ("systolic phase") actively empty the sphincter into the duodenum. The degree of diastolic filling depends on the magnitude of the common bile duct pressure, the rate of common bile duct flow, and the duration of sphincter of Oddi diastole.

CCK is probably the most important hormonal regulator of sphincter of Oddi activity in the immediate postprandial period. In man, CCK reduces the frequency and amplitude of the phasic motor activity and the basal pressure, thus decreasing resistance to flow.[45] However, in the opossum, CCK increases the frequency and amplitude of the sphincter's contractions and increases the resistance to flow across the sphincter.[46, 47, 55] The action of CCK is unaffected by adrenergic or cholinergic blockade but is reversed by tetrodotoxin.[14] This suggests that CCK has two sites of action: the first, an inhibitory effect via noncholinergic nonadrenergic fibers; the second, a direct excitatory effect on the smooth muscle. CCK activates adenyl cyclase, which increases the level of intracellular cyclic AMP and produces muscle relaxation. It also activates phosphodiesterase in sphincteric smooth muscle.[56]

Motilin is thought to regulate sphincter of Oddi activity during fasting. The increase in the frequency of sphincter phasic contractions that precedes phase III of the duodenal IMMC has been thought to be caused by motilin.[51] Takahashi et al. showed that plasma levels of motilin in the conscious opossum peak coincident with phase III activity and that motilin has an excitatory effect on the sphincter of Oddi.[55] This effect is abolished by atropine, suggesting that the excitatory effect of motilin on the sphincter of Oddi and upper gastrointestinal tract of the opossum is mediated by cholinergic nerves.

Studies in the opossum[47, 57] have shown that *glucagon* decreases the frequency of sphincter of Oddi and duodenum spike potentials. A reduction in sphincter of Oddi pressure was also observed in humans.[58] The effect of *secretin* on the myoelectric activity of the sphincter of Oddi is controversial. Geenen et al. showed that in humans secretin has a biphasic activity, causing an initial increase in the frequency and amplitude of the sphincter of Oddi activity, followed by a decrease.[58] However, Coelho et al. showed that, in the conscious opossum, secretin decreases the sphincter of Oddi and duodenal spike burst frequencies and often delays the onset of the IMMC.[57] Selective relaxation of the pancreatic duct sphincter was also observed in humans.[59] *Pentagastrin* increases the frequency and amplitude of sphincter of Oddi contractions.[46]

Behar and Biancani proposed the presence of two opposing neural pathways in the cat sphincter of Oddi: one excitatory and one inhibitory.[60] *Enkephalins* are thought to play an important role in activating opioid receptors present on intramural serotoninergic neurons that stimulate postganglionic cholinergic neurons and the circular muscle. This causes an increment in basal sphincter of Oddi activity. The inhibitory pathway consists of intramural neurons that utilize an unidentified nonadrenergic, noncholinergic neurotransmitter, and it is activated by CCK.[14] Leucine-enkephalin may play a role in this pathway too.[60] Sphincter of Oddi contraction induced by enkephalins is partially blocked by atropine, methysergide, and naloxone. The effect of naloxone has been confirmed by clinical studies in subjects with a normal sphincter of Oddi,[61] but not in cases of very high frequency of contractions (tachyrhythmia).[62]

Vagal stimulation produces relaxation of the sphincter of Oddi and decreases resistance to flow.[14] Truncal vagotomy increases the frequency and amplitude of the phasic activity of the sphincter of Oddi[48] and increases resistance to flow.[63] Alpha-adrenergic stimulation increases resistance to flow through the sphincter of Oddi, whereas beta-adrenergic stimulation decreases resistance.[64]

Cystic Duct, Common Bile Duct, and Biliary Canaliculus Motor Function

The cystic duct is the narrowest portion of the extrahepatic biliary tract and, in primates, is convoluted by a system of prominent mucosal folds called the valves of Heister. These folds do not seem to constitute a valve, as was once thought; there is some debate, nevertheless, as to whether the cystic duct possesses a sphincter-like function as a result of activity of the muscle in its wall.[65, 66] Resting pressure within the cystic duct has been measured at about 35 mm Hg, substantially higher than simultaneously measured gallbladder or common duct pressure. Some investigators have found that resistance to flow through the cystic duct increased following the administration of CCK, epinephrine, or morphine.[67, 68] Other observers have concluded, however, that any resistance imposed by the cystic duct is more likely to result from passive mechanical factors than from muscular contractions.[34, 69]

The wall of the common duct contains sparse muscle fibers in only 20 per cent of humans, and any active role for the duct in biliary dynamics is unlikely. The duct never exhibits anything resembling peristaltic activity, and pressures within the duct remain steady following various stimuli that might be expected to affect a responsive organ.[49, 65, 69–71]

Although the extrahepatic ducts behave as passive conduits, actin filaments are present within the hepatocytes and may endow the canaliculi with contractile properties and a weak ability to pump bile toward the larger system.[72] Observations in freshly prepared liver cell monolayers show that contractions occur in the bile canaliculus. The contractions last 60 seconds and appear forceful, emptying the canaliculus. Relaxation appears to be passive and occurs over 5 to 6 minutes. Canalicular contractions show periods of regular activity interspersed with sequences in which definite regular intervals are present. The control mechanism of these contractions and the role they play in bile flow or in different diseases are not yet understood.[73, 74]

BILE FLOW*

Bile is produced continuously by the liver and flows through the hepatic radicles to the common bile duct. The flow of bile through

*Bile flow as used in this chapter refers to the actual movement of bile through the biliary tract. Bile secretion, commonly referred to as "bile flow," is discussed in detail in Chapter 2.

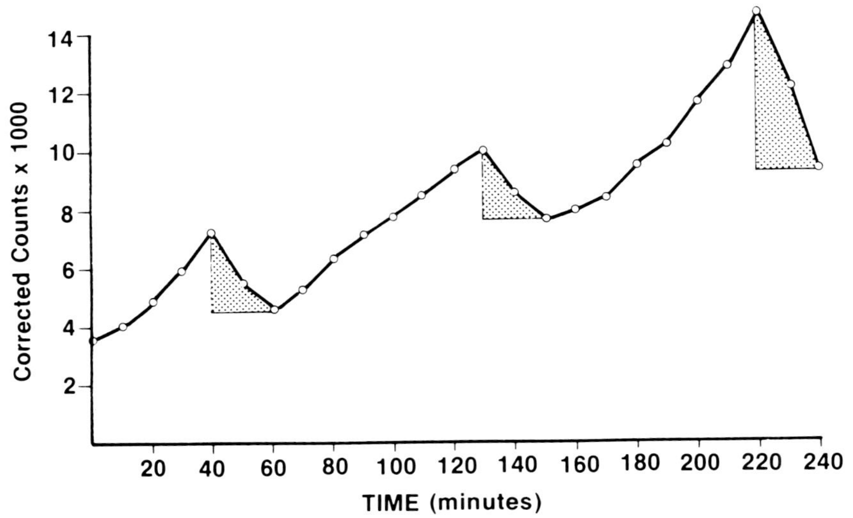

Figure 3–1. Time-activity curve of the gallbladder area during continuous infusion of ^{99m}Tc-DIDIDA in a dog. Note that progressive gallbladder filling is periodically interrupted by gallbladder emptying. The periods of gallbladder emptying are regular, and the ejection fraction of these contractions is approximately 35 per cent.

the extrahepatic biliary tract follows two distinct patterns depending on whether the subject is in a fasted or a fed state.

Fasting (or Interdigestive) Bile Kinetics

Classic physiology regarded the fasting state as a relatively uneventful period in gastrointestinal motility. However, Szurszewski in 1969[75] reintroduced Boldyreff's observation that the small intestine demonstrated a cyclic pattern of motility during the fasting period.[76] The electrical and mechanical characteristics of this motility pattern conform to the interdigestive migratory myoelectric complex.[77–79] The biliary tract exhibits a similar cyclic pattern of motility during fasting. Fasting biliary motility maintains a close temporal relationship to the fasting motility of the duodenum.[15, 51] For example, the output of bile and pancreatic juice increase during phase II of the IMMC.[18, 80, 81]

During phase II of the IMMC, the gallbladder contracts. These contractions are associated with a rise in the plasma level of motilin and are thought to be caused by it.[13, 15, 19] Traynor et al., using a transducer implanted in the gallbladder, first showed that in the fasted conscious dog, gallbladder filling was interrupted, during duodenal phase II of the IMMC, by a period of increased gallbladder pressure and an associated ejection of up to 15 per cent of gallbladder contents.[82] They suggested that increased gallbladder pressure was caused initially by contraction of the gallbladder against a closed sphincter of Oddi. Subsequent sphincter relaxation was associated with partial gallbladder emptying and flow of bile into the duodenum.

We have studied gallbladder bile flow in conscious dogs using a continuous infusion of ^{99m}Tc-diethyl-HIDA and have confirmed these observations. During fasting, bile flow exhibited a cyclic pattern that consisted of a period of gallbladder filling (when more than 90 per cent of the bile entered the gallbladder) lasting approximately 80 minutes, and a period of gallbladder emptying (during which hepatic bile completely bypassed the gallbladder) lasting approximately 20 minutes. About 35 per cent of the gallbladder contents were evacuated during the emptying period. The total duration of the cycle was close to 100 minutes, the time that it takes for a complete cycle of the IMMC in the dog (Fig. 3–1).[83] We have also found that in the prairie dog gallbladder filling during fasting is periodically interrupted by gallbladder contraction.[84] During these contractions, the sphincter of Oddi relaxes and bile flows into the duodenum.

There is evidence that a similar cyclic pattern, with periodic gallbladder emptying, occurs in humans. For example, Peeters et al. found an increased output of bile acids into the duodenum prior to duodenal phase III activity,[85] and Bloom et al., using cholescintigraphy, found periodic gallbladder emptying, of approximately 20 per cent of its con-

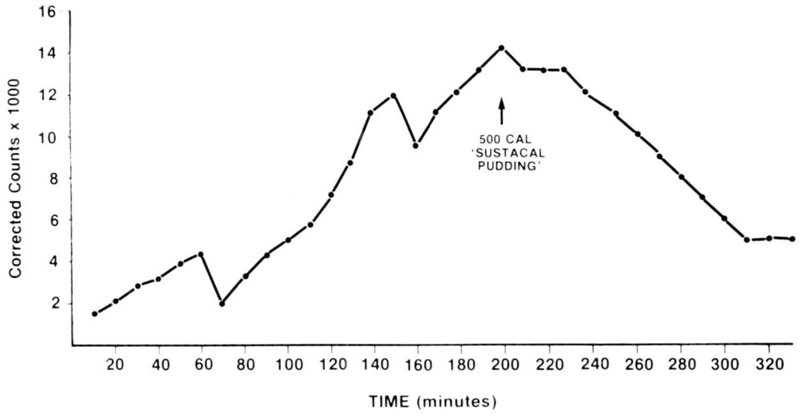

Figure 3–2. Time-activity curve of the gallbladder area during continuous infusion of ^{99m}Tc-DIDIDA in a human subject. Note that the progressive gallbladder filling is periodically interrupted by gallbladder emptying. The periods of gallbladder emptying are regular, and the ejection fraction of these contractions is approximately 30 per cent. Following ingestion of 500 cal of a fat-containing pudding (Sustacal) 70 per cent of the gallbladder bile was evacuated over 120 min.

tents, 20 minutes prior to peak plasma motilin levels.[86] We have also observed periodic gallbladder contractions during fasting in normal subjects (Fig. 3–2).[84]

Postprandial Bile Kinetics

The evidence suggests that postprandial bile kinetics follow the ensuing pattern. Gallbladder emptying in response to a meal may be initiated by a "cephalic" phase presumably mediated by the vagus, either directly or through the release of motilin. The substantial gallbladder contraction observed in response to sham feeding lends support to this theory. The second phase of gallbladder emptying is probably triggered by the release of CCK as a result of entry of food into the duodenum.[8] Using cholescintigraphy we have shown that in the conscious dog gallbladder emptying following the ingestion of food can be divided into three phases: prompt gallbladder emptying (ejection fraction of 30 per cent) for the first 7 to 8 minutes, followed by a period of gallbladder filling for about 12 to 15 minutes, and then by a sustained gallbladder contraction (ejection fraction of 60 to 70 per cent) for the next 60 minutes (Fig. 3–3).[83] The sphincter of Oddi also exhibits a cyclic pattern of electrical and mechanical activity; maximal action potential rate (the electrical counterpart of a peristaltic wave of contraction) occurs during late duodenal phase II of the IMMC.[51]

Several studies have shown that CCK plasma levels increase after a meal, and that this increase is responsible for the smooth,

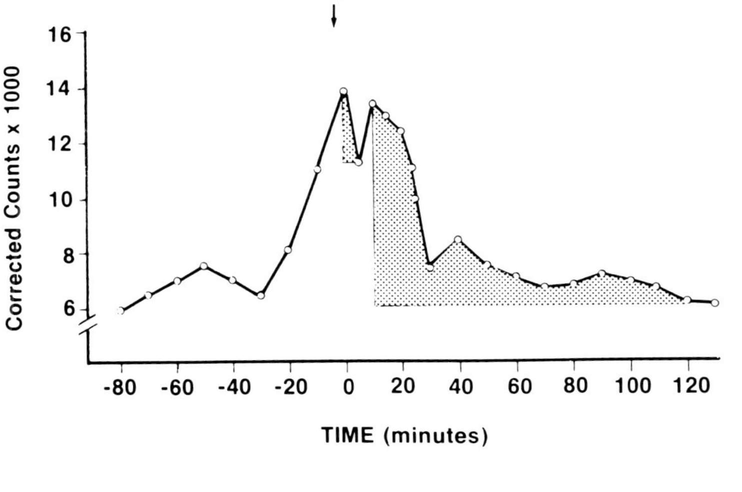

Figure 3–3. Time-activity curve of the gallbladder area during continuous infusion of ^{99m}Tc-DIDIDA in a dog. The picture depicts the last 80 minutes of the fasting period. The dog was fed at time "0." Immediately following the meal there was a 30 per cent emptying of the gallbladder, followed by progressive filling, and finally by a sustained contraction that emptied over 70 per cent of gallbladder contents.

continuous, tonic contraction of the gallbladder that leads to evacuation of about 65 to 80 per cent of gallbladder bile.[3, 5, 82] In association with this gallbladder contraction, CCK decreases the resistance to flow through the sphincter of Oddi[45] and bile enters the intestine. The amount of bile that enters the intestine varies in relation to the character of the meal. Bile enters the duodenum in spurts because of the phasic activity of the sphincter of Oddi.

Although gallbladder emptying is maximal at 120 minutes (ejection fraction of 80 to 90 per cent),[9] gallbladder filling and the cyclic pattern of gallbladder activity that characterize the fasting state do not return for the next few hours. Similarly, intestinal interdigestive motility patterns do not return for 3 to 10 hours.[83] Takahashi[87] et al. reported that gallbladder motor function in the postprandial period can be divided into three stages. The first is a gallbladder contraction of short duration associated with feeding, with gallbladder tone rapidly returning to basal levels. Bile concentration in the gallbladder continues to rise, indicating minimal ejection of bile during this period. Second, approximately 30 minutes after feeding, there is a period of rhythmic contractions and sustained rise in tone, which lasts approximately 4 hours. This period is associated with a substantial fall in gallbladder bile concentration. A final period is characterized by irregular tonic contractions with a return to basal values between contractions. Interestingly, gallbladder bile concentration initially increases but then falls toward the end of this period, which terminates with the return of the characteristic interdigestive motility pattern.

Traynor et al. on the other hand, noted a sustained isotonic gallbladder contraction, which started approximately 4 minutes after the ingestion of the meal, lasted 85 minutes, and was followed by a period of 5.5 hours of large-amplitude rhythmic contractions.[81] In our cholescintigraphic study in dogs we also found that after a postprandial contraction and for the ensuing 4 to 6 hours, nearly 90 per cent of the hepatic bile entered the intestine, and gallbladder filling was erratic and sporadic (Fig. 3–4).[83] It seems reasonable to assume that the immediate postprandial period may represent vagally mediated activity with a minimal ejection of gallbladder bile. The rhythmic contraction period may represent a CCK-induced contraction with ejection of most of the gallbladder bile. Finally, the irregular contraction period seems to represent intermittent gallbladder filling and partial emptying.

The Influence of Sex Hormones on Biliary Motility

Since cholelithiasis is more prevalent in women than in men, hormones have been thought to play a role, affecting either gallbladder motility or bile composition. Biliary motility has been studied in this context to determine the influence of: (1) menstrual cycle,[88–90] (2) the use of contraceptives,[91–99] and (3) pregnancy.[91, 92, 101, 102]

Fried and coworkers[89] compared CCK release and gallbladder emptying in men and

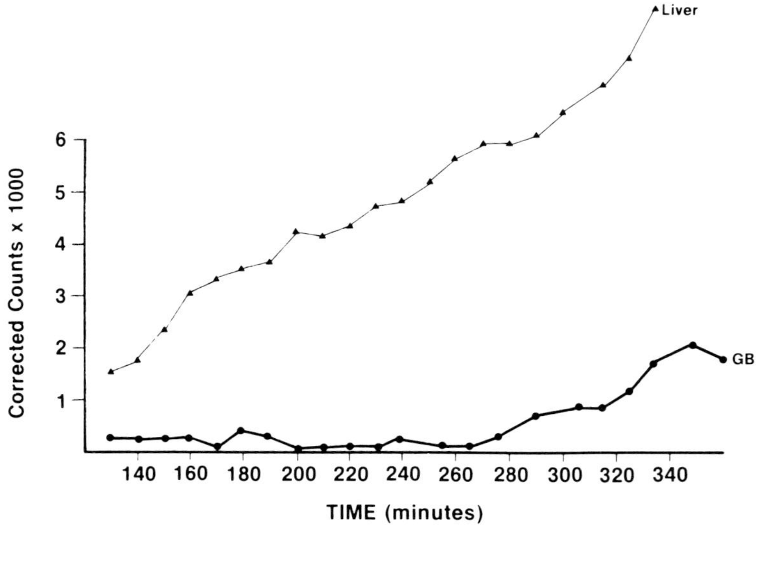

Figure 3–4. Time-activity curve of the gallbladder area and the liver during continuous infusion of ^{99m}Tc-DIDIDA in a dog 2 to 6 hours after feeding. During this period, gallbladder filling is minimal.

in women. Each woman was studied on days 14 and 21 of her menstrual cycle, corresponding to the presumed estrogen and progesterone peaks. Data from their study showed no difference in the release of CCK or in gallbladder contraction in women at different times of their menstrual cycle. Furthermore, they found no difference between sexes in release of CCK or gallbladder contraction.

Women taking *oral contraceptives* have an increased risk of cholesterol gallstone disease. The risk is higher only in younger women (i.e., less than 29 years)[98, 99] and during the first 4 years of contraceptive use. Paradoxically, the risk of developing gallstones declines after 4 years of oral contraceptive use to a rate below that of controls.[98] These women have cholesterol supersaturation of bile. The changes in biliary lipid secretion are thought to be caused by estrogens[94] or by a combination of estrogens and a progestin[95, 96] and may be prevented by the administration of S-adenosyl-L-methionine.[97] Gallbladder motor function is unaffected by contraceptive steroids.[91, 92]

During *pregnancy*, emptying of the gallbladder is sluggish.[91, 92] After the first trimester the resting gallbladder volume doubles; in response to stimulation by a liquid meal, the rate of emptying is decreased by 30 per cent and the residual volume is twice normal.[91, 92] In the guinea pig, pregnancy decreases the magnitude of the contractile response of the gallbladder to acetylcholine and CCK-8.[100] It is thought that the decreased contractility of the gallbladder smooth muscle is mediated by progesterone.[101]

DISORDERED BILIARY MOTILITY

Cholelithiasis

Biliary motility relates to cholelithiasis in two different ways: disordered biliary motility may lead to the development of gallstones, and gallstones, once present, produce additional changes in biliary motility. It is not always possible to differentiate, especially in studies involving humans with cholelithiasis, whether motility changes are the result or the cause of gallstones. However, a considerable body of experimental evidence suggests that abnormal biliary motility plays a major role in the development and growth of cholesterol and pigment stones[102–115] In both types of stones, gallbladder bile stasis is the most obvious abnormality, and in both, gallbladder stasis seems to develop before gallstones form.[102–104, 116–119]

Motility Changes Associated with the Formation of Gallstones

Cholesterol Gallstones. In the case of cholesterol gallstones, gallbladder stasis produces changes in the size of the bile acid pool that lead to cholesterol supersaturation of bile and the formation of crystals.[11] Once crystals have formed, bile stasis enhances crystal nucleation and the growth of stones.[120, 121]

The size of the bile acid pool is influenced by fasting and postprandial gallbladder motility. During fasting, about two thirds of the bile acid pool is contained in the gallbladder. Periodic gallbladder contractions (every 90 to 120 minutes; ejection fraction 15 to 30 per cent) maintain the rest of the bile acid pool in circulation.[81, 86] Thus, during this period, the physiologic storage of bile in the gallbladder reduces, but does not interrupt, the enterohepatic circulation. This decreases hepatic secretion of bile acids and produces lithogenic bile.[122] The amount of bile acids sequestered in the gallbladder during fasting is determined by the frequency and the ejection fraction of fasting gallbladder contractions.[123] Following a meal, the gallbladder delivers bile with a high concentration of bile acids in the intestine, which then contains most of the bile acid pool. Thus, changes in gallbladder dynamics during fasting or postprandially affect bile salt recycling and may change bile composition, bile flow, rate of bile acid synthesis, and size of the bile acid pool.

If gallbladder filling is increased owing to decreased gallbladder tone or increased sphincteric resistance, or if gallbladder emptying is slowed (e.g., during pregnancy), an increasing fraction of the bile acid pool is sequestered within the gallbladder, lowering the rate of bile acid secretion. This increases the cholesterol saturation of bile because the rate of cholesterol secretion remains about the same. Conversely, increased gallbladder emptying decreases the size of the bile acid pool, probably because of increased cycling. Since gallbladder contraction is in part determined by CCK stimulation, a diet rich in sucrose and low in fat, common in some North American Indian tribes, may decrease the cycling frequency of the bile acid pool.

Several studies in the prairie dog suggest that gallbladder stasis develops during gall-

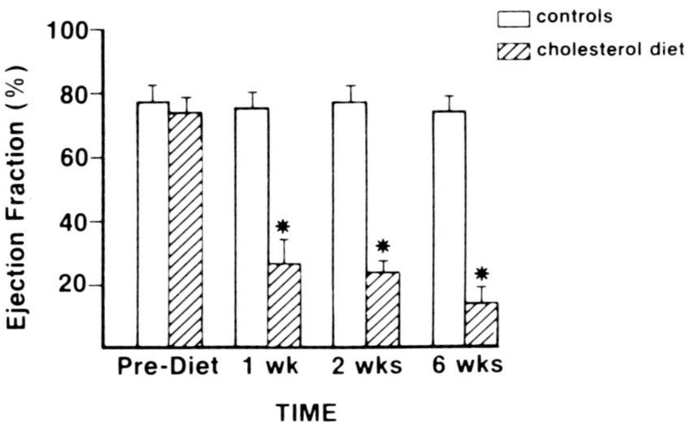

Figure 3–5. Gallbladder ejection fraction in response to CCK before, and 1, 2, and 6 weeks after, placing prairie dogs on a 0.4 per cent cholesterol diet (crossed bars) compared with that of control animals. Gallbladder emptying in response to intravenous CCK was significantly affected 1 week after initiation of the lithogenic diet, and decreased further at 6 weeks.

stone formation. For example, the development of lithogenic bile is associated with an increased resistance to flow through the cystic duct,[106, 124, 125] and gallstone formation can be prevented by promoting gallbladder contraction.[42] The changes in biliary motility appear shortly after initiation of a lithogenic diet and before gallstones form. For example, 8 days into the cholesterol diet, the ratio of the bile salt concentration in the gallbladder relative to hepatic bile doubles, reflecting impaired gallbladder motility.[102] We examined the relationship between biliary motility and early events in gallstone formation in this animal model, using cholescintigraphy, and found that within 1 week of starting cholesterol feeding the response of the gallbladder to intravenous CCK decreased markedly: ejection fraction fell from 75 per cent to about 25 per cent (Fig. 3–5). These animals had developed supersaturation of bile but had not yet developed cholesterol crystals or gallstones, suggesting that the motility changes preceded the formation of stones and were probably induced by the presence of lithogenic bile.[126] Indeed, in vitro studies suggest that the decreased gallbladder motility observed during gallstone formation is due to a direct effect of lithogenic bile on the gallbladder smooth muscle.[105]

As the process of gallstone formation progresses, gallbladder motility is affected even more. For example, gallbladders from prairie dogs with cholesterol crystals generate less isometric tension in vitro in response to CCK-8 than do those from animals with supersaturated bile only.[127]

The effects of lithogenic bile in other areas of the biliary tract and their relationship to the process of gallstone formation are less clear. In the prairie dog, sphincterotomy prevents gallstone formation[104] and atropine reverses the effect of sphincterotomy.[128] Whether these changes enhance gallstone formation and growth directly or through alterations in gallbladder filling is unclear.

As pointed out earlier, studies in humans who have already developed gallstones are more difficult to interpret, but indirect evidence suggests that cholesterol gallstone formation is associated with gallbladder stasis, at least in certain groups. For example, long-term parenteral nutrition,[129–132] treatment with contraceptive steroids,[91] pregnancy,[92] and other conditions that lead to gallbladder stasis[116] increase the risk of developing gallstones. Likewise, diabetics[108] and postvagotomy patients[109] are thought to have altered gallbladder motility, and both these groups have an increased incidence of gallstones.[110, 111] Prolonged opacification of the gallbladder following oral cholecystogram has been reported in subjects with gallstone disease, diabetes mellitus, and after truncal vagotomy.[112]

Pigment Gallstones. Biliary stasis has also been shown to play a role in the formation of pigment stones.[117, 118, 133] For example, pigment stones are found more commonly than cholesterol stones in patients with strictures[119] and other conditions that lead to common bile duct stasis.[134] We have found pigment stones as early as 3 days after cystic duct ligation in the dog.[116] The mechanism whereby gallbladder or common bile duct stasis (which appears to play a greater role in pigment stone formation than it does in cholesterol stone formation) leads to the formation of pigment gallstones is not as clear as in the case of cholesterol stones. In animals that form pigment stones, bile is nonlithogenic with regard to cholesterol, is sterile, and does not contain any apparent impetus to stone formation other than a high concentration of mucin.[116]

Mucin may indeed play a major role in the development of pigment stones. For example, pigment stone formation is almost always preceded by the formation of sludge, and sludge is associated with a marked increase in total content and concentration of mucin.[116] It appears that accumulation of mucin, which is not adequately flowing down the biliary tract because of stasis, serves as a nidus on which bilirubin, calcium-bilirubinate complexes, and other particles are trapped and precipitated, initiating the formation of stones.[116] In fact, Womack and others have suggested that gallstones form by heterogeneous nucleation of bile solids (cholesterol, bilirubin, or calcium salts) on a macroscopic lattice of mucin.[135, 136] It is also possible that bilirubin precipitation may be enhanced by biliary infection, commonly associated with biliary stasis. For example, infection with *E. coli* leads to increases in biliary glucuronidase activity, which may lead to deconjugation of bilirubin. Since unconjugated and monoconjugated bilirubins are less water-soluble than conjugated bilirubin, their precipitation is more likely. This mechanism has been proposed as the main explanation for the high incidence of pigment gallstones in Japanese patients.[137, 138]

Motility Changes Induced by Gallstones

The presence of gallstones can also lead to changes in the dynamics of the extrahepatic biliary tract. For example, gallstones in the gallbladder cause chronic cholecystitis, which frequently leads to mural fibrosis and decreased compliance. Decreased gallbladder compliance leads to decreased filling. Chronic inflammation of the gallbladder wall may also lead to decreased response to CCK and other stimulants. The end result is a functional exclusion of the gallbladder from the biliary tract. For example, in a study of gallbladder bile flow during gallstone formation in the prairie dog, we found no alteration in the process of gallbladder filling during the formation of gallstones; however, gallbladder filling was substantially impaired after stones had formed.[126]

Cholescintigraphic studies of gallbladder bile flow in humans with cholelithiasis have also shown profound changes in gallbladder motility. Shaffer et al., for example, found that subjects with radiolucent stones and functioning gallbladder had normal gallbladder filling but decreased gallbladder emptying in response to CCK.[6] Northfield et al., on the other hand, found that patients with gallstones had an increased sensitivity to CCK.[113] More recently, Thompson et al. reported that stone-forming patients can be divided into "contractors" (normal gallbladder emptying in response to decreased CCK release) and "noncontractors" (poor gallbladder emptying in response to normal CCK release).[114] Finally, Fisher et al., in a controlled study, found that patients with gallstones had decreased gallbladder emptying in response to ingestion of a standard liquid meal when compared with control subjects.[115] These apparently different results may reflect various degrees of cholecystitis and various stages of gallbladder disease among the patients studied, which would be expected to produce different alterations in biliary motility.

Choledocholithiasis may lead to common bile duct obstruction. In the presence of sudden complete ductal obstruction, bile pressure rises to about 25 to 35 mm Hg, reflecting the activity of the bile secretory apparatus within the liver. With time, however, ductal pressure falls to normal.[47] In the absence of a gallbladder, the pressure of the duct must reach 12 to 15 cm H_2O for bile to flow through the normal sphincter.[139] Passage pressure may be increased in patients with choledocholithiasis as a result of mechanical obstruction to flow by the stones, but usually the pressure is normal.[47] Common duct pressure is also normal in patients with cholelithiasis confined to the gallbladder.[47, 140]

Vagotomy

Several clinical and experimental observations suggest that vagotomy leads to gallstone formation,[107, 141–143] but the mechanism is not clear. Although vagotomy increases lithogenicity of bile in some species,[144, 145] it appears to have an opposite effect in humans.[146, 147] Therefore, changes in bile composition alone do not explain the development of cholelithiasis after vagotomy. Indirect evidence suggests that biliary motility becomes abnormal after vagotomy and may be related to gallstone formation. For example, truncal vagotomy has been reported to increase the resting volume of the gallbladder.[109, 148, 149] Rudick and Hutchison[149] found that vagotomy impaired gallbladder emptying after a fatty meal, and Ihasz and Griffith[143] reported a high incidence of gallstones in patients whose gallbladders dilated after vagotomy and failed to contract in response to a fatty meal.

Attempts to define the exact nature of these motility changes have led to conflicting results. Some workers have found that vagotomy causes hypotonia of the gallbladder and biliary stasis,[143, 148, 149] whereas others have reported that it increases intragallbladder pressure and sensitivity of the gallbladder to CCK stimulation.[150, 151] These changes may reflect altered gallbladder function[150, 151] or altered sphincter of Oddi motility.[48] Using cholescintigraphy, a method that yields more accurate information regarding bile flow,[146, 152] we found that neither gallbladder filling nor the response to exogenous CCK was affected by vagotomy in the prairie dog and in humans.[84] Contrary to what we expected, neither the frequency nor the ejection fraction of fasting gallbladder contractions was altered by vagotomy.[84] Our study, therefore, did not show any changes in the motility of the biliary tract secondary to vagotomy. We did not study the effect of meals on gallbladder contraction after vagotomy, but Fisher and coworkers, who did, showed that cholinergic blockade with atropine sulfate decreased gallbladder emptying responses to a liquid and a solid meal. In their study, patients with vagotomies had 60 per cent gallbladder emptying in response to a liquid meal at 120 minutes compared with 80 per cent in control subjects.[32] It is possible, therefore, that vagotomy leads to more subtle changes in biliary motor function than we expected. Further studies in the field are needed to characterize biliary motility after vagotomy.

Total Parenteral Nutrition

Several investigators have reported that a substantial number of infants, children, and adults on total parenteral nutrition (TPN) develop intrahepatic cholestasis and gallbladder disease.[131, 153–157] Complications from cholelithiasis in these patients are not uncommon, and the possibility of cholelithiasis must be kept in mind in the differential diagnosis of patients with abdominal pain on TPN. This is especially true in children who have a particular tendency to develop complications of cholelithiasis while on TPN.[157]

Gallbladder stasis, caused by the lack of periodic gallbladder contractions in response to meals, is thought to cause sludge[130] and, eventually, pigment stones. The longer the patient has been on TPN, the higher the chances of finding sludge in the gallbladder. For example, Messing et al. found that whereas only 6 per cent of patients on TPN had sludge at 3 weeks, 50 per cent developed sludge between the fourth and sixth weeks, and 100 per cent had it after 6 weeks.[131] Progression of sludge to gallstones was demonstrated in 6 of 14 patients in one study, and none of the patients without sludge developed gallstones.Three of the patients who developed gallstones required cholecystectomy while on TPN because of biliary colic, cholecystitis, or cholangitis. Gallbladders from these patients were filled with sludge, and in two patients stones between 3 and 5 mm were also discovered.[131] On the other hand, the evidence indicates that sludge disappears when intravenous nutrition is replaced by oral feedings. Indeed, of eight patients who developed sludge during TPN in one study, none had sludge after the fourth week off hyperalimentation and on oral feedings.[131]

Since gallbladder stasis appears to be a critical factor in the pathogenesis of TPN-induced gallbladder disease, stimulation of gallbladder emptying by oral administration of fat or intravenous CCK may prevent the development of gallbladder disease in these patients. Doty and coworkers[158] have demonstrated that daily administration of intravenous CCK-8 prevented gallbladder stasis and reduced the incidence of gallstone formation in prairie dogs on TPN. The majority of TPN-induced gallstones are of the pigment variety,[133] and thus, bile acid dissolution is not applicable. Because of the relatively high incidence of complications, some have advocated early cholecystectomy.[132]

Diabetes Mellitus

Patients with diabetes mellitus have a higher prevalence of gallstones, although the exact frequency varies among studies.[159–161] Alterations of gallbladder motility caused by peripheral or autonomic neuropathy or alterations in bile constituents caused by the disease have been proposed as etiologies.

Diabetic cholecystopathy was first reported by Gitelson et al.,[108, 162] who noted large, poorly contracting and slow-filling gallbladders among diabetic patients, especially those with evidence of either peripheral or autonomic neuropathy. In related work, Grodski[163] and others[164] have found that diabetics had decreased gallbladder emptying when compared with controls. Gallbladder atony may play a role in gallstone formation in diabetics, but these patients also have supersaturated bile and a reduced bile acid pool.[161] Under these conditions the propensity for cholesterol to precipitate and form stones is enhanced. Paradoxically, it has been found that bile lithogenicity is greater during insulin treatment than during uncontrolled hyperglycemia.[165, 166]

Although Gracie and Ransohoff[167] have proposed that routine prophylactic operation for silent gallstones is not necessary in the general population, the general advice has been to remove the gallbladder in asymptomatic diabetics who have gallstones.[168–170] This approach is based on the belief that the risk of developing cholecystitis and cholangitis is greater among diabetics, and that when these complications occur, the outcome is worse than among nondiabetics. However, since it is not known whether such complications occur more frequently in diabetics, and whether the outcome of emergency operations is any different in these patients, the traditional advice of early operation has been recently challenged.[171, 172] Well-controlled studies are needed to determine whether routine ultrasonographic screening for gallstones and prophylactic surgery are worthwhile and cost-effective in diabetics.

Biliary Dyskinesia

Biliary dyskinesia is a term that defines a form of motor incoordination of the biliary tract that is responsible for symptoms in patients in whom a complete diagnostic workup of the biliary tract does not show any organic abnormality. Although the very existence of biliary dyskinesia was challenged for some time, as our ability to study biliary motor function improves it is becoming an established clinical entity. There are two areas of the biliary tract where abnormal motility is thought to cause symptoms: the gallbladder and the sphincter of Oddi. In clinical practice, gallbladder motor function is studied primarily by cholescintigraphy or by CCK cholecystography, and sphincter of Oddi motor function by direct manometry.

Intravenous CCK given during the course of an oral cholecystogram may be used to relate biliary motor activity to symptoms. For example, Griffen has found that patients whose gallbladders failed to empty normally and who experienced right upper quadrant pain following CCK stimulation of the gallbladder usually had histologic evidence of chronic cholecystitis and were relieved of their symptoms by cholecystectomy.[173] This experience has been confirmed by other studies.[174, 175] For further details on the use of cholecystography and cholescintigraphy in patients with biliary dyskinesia, refer to Chapters 7 and 12.

Following cholecystectomy some patients complain of episodic right upper quadrant pain, have transient abnormalities of liver function tests or serum amylase, and have normal ultrasound, computerized tomography, endoscopic retrograde cholangiopancreatography, and transhepatic cholangiography. In these patients, direct evaluation of the sphincter of Oddi function is advised. In 1973 Nardi[176] introduced the morphine-neostigmine provocation test as an aid in the diagnosis of biliary dyskinesia. A positive study consisted of a twofold increase in serum amylase concentration and reproduction of the patient's pain after intramuscular injection of these drugs. Other studies have shown, however, that this test is not as specific as was initially thought.[177, 178]

An important step in identifying the nature of these postcholecystectomy symptoms has been the development of peroral transendoscopic sphincter of Oddi manometry. This is done following endoscopic retrograde cholangiopancreatography. A catheter with one or multiple holes is passed through the biopsy channel of the endoscope and positioned in the common bile duct or pancreatic duct, flushed with water, and connected at its proximal end to a pneumohydraulic capillary infusion system for manometric measurements. Pressures are transmitted to transducers, converted to electrical signals, and transcribed on a polygraph recorder. Ductal pressure, basal sphincter of Oddi pressure, amplitude of the phasic contractions of the sphincter of Oddi, and the direction of propagation of these contractions can be studied.[62, 179–184]

The most consistent manometric finding in patients with biliary dyskinesia is elevated resting sphincter of Oddi pressure. This is thought to be caused by muscle spasm or fibrotic stenosis of the sphincter,[179–184] but excess retrograde contraction,[179, 182] high contraction frequency,[62, 179] and paradoxical response to CCK (increase in frequency of phasic contractions and in basal pressure of the sphincter of Oddi)[179] may also be involved. A high frequency of retrograde phasic contractions has been described also in patients with common bile duct stones,[54] probably caused by the irritative action of the stone. An abnormally high frequency of contractions, which shortens the diastolic phase and decreases filling of the sphincter of Oddi, may impair bile flow and cause pain.

Endoscopic sphincterotomy has been used

with encouraging results in patients with suspected sphincter of Oddi dysfunction in whom presphincterotomy manometry showed an elevated basal pressure.[180, 181, 184] Geenen and associates[183] examined the effects of endoscopic sphincterotomy (performed to remove common bile duct stones) on the sphincter of Oddi. Follow-up studies at 12 and 24 months showed that the common bile duct to duodenal pressure gradient and the sphincter of Oddi basal pressure were eliminated. The amplitude of sphincter of Oddi phasic contractions was lower at 12 months but returned to presphincterotomy levels by 2 years. Endoscopic sphincterotomy carries significant morbidity (5 to 10 per cent) and mortality (1 per cent), and despite initial encouraging results,[187–189] longer follow-up of these patients is needed before the procedure can be recommended.

Pharmacologic agents that relax the sphincter of Oddi have been tried. Gregg and Antal showed that administration of naloxone to patients with high frequency of contractions did not have significant effect on either the frequency or the symptoms.[62] In an isolated case report, isosorbide dinitrate (10 mg tid) was described as decreasing basal and phasic sphincter activity, with disappearance of the pain, in a patient with papillary dysfunction demonstrated by endoscopic manometry.[185]

In a randomized placebo-controlled double-blind trial, Basso and coworkers showed that 9 of 12 patients with biliary colic treated with cerulein experienced significant pain relief. This effect is probably due to a reduction of the pressure within the biliary tree, secondary to relaxation of the sphincter of Oddi.[186] Such treatment may be useful in patients with high sphincter of Oddi pressure and biliary pain.

REFERENCES

1. Admirand WH, Small DM: The physiochemical basis of cholesterol gallstone formation in man. J Clin Invest 1968;*47*:1043.
2. Rehfeld JF: Four basic characteristics of the gastrin-cholecystokinin system. Am J Physiol 1981; *240*:G255.
3. Byrnes DJ, Borody T, Daskalopoulos G, et al: Cholecystokinin and gallbladder contraction: Effect of CCK infusion. Peptides 1981;2:259.
4. Lilta P, Fagan C, Weiner I, et al: Infusion of pure cholecystokinin in humans. Gastroenterology 1982; *83*:256.
5. Weiner I, Inoue K, Fagan C, et al: Release of cholecystokinin in man. Ann Surg 1981; *194*:321.
6. Shaffer EA, McOrmond P, Duggan H: Quantitative cholescintigraphy. Assessment of gallbladder filling and emptying and duodenogastric reflux. Gastroenterology 1980;*79*:899.
7. Spellman SJ, Shaffer EA, Rosenthall L: Gallbladder emptying in response to cholecystokinin. Gastroenterology 1979;*77*:115.
8. Rock E, Malmud L, Fisher RS: Gallbladder emptying after meals of different composition. Gastroenterology 1981;*80*:1263 (Abstr).
9. Rock E, Malmud L, Fisher RS: Gallbladder emptying in response to sham feeding. Gastroenterology 1981;*80*:1263 (Abstr).
10. Steigerwalt RW, Goldfine ID, Williams JA, et al: Characterization of cholecystokinin receptors on bovine gallbladder membranes. Am J Physiol 1984;*247*:G709.
11. Amer MS: Studies with cholecystokinin *in vitro* III. Mechanism of the effect on the isolated rabbit gallbladder strips. J Pharmacol Exp Ther 1972;*183*:535.
12. Amer MS, McKinnery GR: Studies with cholecystokinin *in vitro* IV. Effect of CCK and related peptide on phosphodiesterase. J Pharmacol Exp Ther 1972;*183*:535.
13. Takahashi I, Suzuki T, Aizawa I, et al: Comparison of gallbladder contractions induced by motilin and cholecystokinin in dogs. Gastroenterology 1982; *82*:419.
14. Behar J, Biancani P: Effect of cholecystokinin and the octapeptide of cholecystokinin on the feline sphincter of Oddi and gallbladder: mechanisms of action. J Clin Invest 1980:*66*:1231.
15. Itoh Z, Takahashi I: Periodic contractions of the canine gallbladder during the interdigestive state. Am J Physiol 1981;*140*:183.
16. Brown JC, Mutt V, Dryburgh JR: The further purification of motilin, a gastric motor activity stimulating polypeptide from the mucosa of the small intestine of dogs. Can J Physiol 1971;*49*:399.
17. Lee KY, Chey WY, Tai HH, et al: Radioimmunoassay of motilin: validation of studies on the relationship between plasma motilin and interdigestive myoelectric activity of the duodenum of dog. Am J Dig Dis 1978;*23*:789.
18. Keane FB, DiMagno EP, Dozois RR, et al: Relationships among canine interdigestive exocrine pancreatic and biliary flow, duodenal motor activity, plasma pancreatic polypeptide and motilin. Gastroenterology 1980;*78*:310.
19. Adrian TE, Michenere P, Sagor GR, et al: Effect of motilin and other gut hormones on gallbladder pressure. Regul Pept 1980;*1*(Suppl 1):51 (Abstr).
20. Pomeranz IS, Davison JS, Shaffer EA: In vitro effects of pancreatic polypeptide and motilin on contractility of human gallbladder. Dig Dis Sci 1983;*28*:539.
21. Lee KY, Chey WY, Chang TM: Cholinergic influence on release and action of motilin in dogs. Gastroenterology 1981;*80*:1206 (Abstr).
22. Yoshiya K, Yamamura T, Ishikawa Y, et al: The failure of truncal vagotomy to affect motilin release in dogs. J Surg Res 1985;*38*:263.
23. Lin T: Actions of gastrointestinal hormones and related peptides on the motor function of the biliary tract. Gastroenterology 1975;*69*:1006.
24. Stening GF, Grossman MI: Potentiation of action of cholecystokinin by secretin. Clin Res 1969; *17*:528.
25. Shoetz DJ, Wise WE, La Morte WW, et al: Hista-

mine receptors in the primate gallbladder. Gastroenterology 1978;*74*:1090.
26. Lennon F, Feeley TM, Clanachan AS, et al: Effects of histamine receptors stimulation on diseased gallbladder and cystic duct. Gastroenterology 1984;*87*:257.
27. Thornell E, Jansson R, Kral JG, et al: Inhibition of prostaglandin synthesis as a treatment for biliary pain. Lancet 1979;*1*:584.
28. Kotwall CA, Clanachan AS, Boer HP, et al: Effects of prostaglandins on motility of gallbladders removed from patients with gallstones. Arch Surg 1984;*119*:709.
29. Thornell E, Jansson R, Svanvik J: Indomethacin intravenously: A new way for effective relief of biliary pain. A double blind study in man. Surgery 1981;*90*:468.
30. Bueon L, Fargeas MJ, Fioramonti J, et al: Central control of intestinal motility by prostaglandins: A mediator of the actions of several peptides in rats and dogs. Gastroenterology 1985;*88*:1888.
31. Yau WM, Youther ML: Modulation of gallbladder motility by intrinsic cholinergic neurons. Am J Physiol 1984;*247*:G662.
32. Fisher RS, Rock E, Malmud LS: Cholinergic effects on gallbladder emptying in humans. Gastroenterology 1985:*89*:716.
33. Persson CGA: Dual effects on the sphincter of Oddi and gallbladder induced by stimulation of the right great splanchnic nerve. Acta Physiol Scand 1973;*87*:334.
34. Oster MJ, Csendes A, Funch-Jensen P, et al: Intraoperative pressure measurements of the choledochoduodenal junction, common bile duct, cysticocholedochal junction and gallbladder in humans. Surg Gynecol Obstet 1980;*150*:385.
35. Schoetz DJ, LaMorte WW, Birkett DH, et al: Gallbladder tone in the primate: Dynamic description by a new method. Gastroenterology 1978;*74*:1090.
36. Ryan J, Cohen S: Gallbladder pressure-volume reponse to gastrointestinal hormone. Am J Physiol 1976;*238*:1461.
37. Lanovics J, Devitt P, Watson LC, et al: Pancreatic polypeptide: A review. Arch Surg 1981; *116*:1256.
38. Greenberg GR, Chan B, Nordgren SR, et al: Effect of vagal blockade on food- and hormone-stimulated release of pancreatic polypeptide and motilin in dogs. Dig Dis Sci 1985;*30*:946.
39. Conter R, Roslyn JJ, Muller EL, et al: Effect of pancreatic polypeptide on gallbladder filling. J Surg Res 1985;*38*:461.
40. Adrian TE, Mitchenere P, Sagor G, et al: The effect of pancreatic polypeptide on gallbladder pressure and hepatic bile secretion. Am J Physiol 1982;*243*:G204.
41. Greeberg GR, McCloy RF, Chadwick VS, et al: Effect of bovine pancreatic polypeptide on basal pancreatic and biliary outputs in man. Dig Dis Sci 1979;*24*:11.
42. Jansson R: Effects of gastrointestinal hormones on concentrating function and motility in the gallbladder. An experimental study in the cat. Acta Physiol Scand (Suppl) 1978;*456*:1.
43. Davison JS, Al-Hassani M, Crowe R: The nonadrenergic, inhibitory innervation of the guineapig gallbladder. Pflugers Arch 1978;*377*:43.
44. Sundler F, Alumets J, Hakanson R: VIP innervation of the gallbladder. Gastroenterology 1977; *72*:1375.
45. Toouli J, Hogan WJ, Geenen JE, et al: Action of cholecystokinin-octapeptide on sphincter of Oddi basal pressure and phasic wave activity in humans. Surgery 1982;*92*:497.
46. Becker JM, Moody FG, Zinsmeister AR: Effect of gastrointestinal hormones on the biliary sphincter of the opossum. Gastroenterology 1982;*82*:1300.
47. Honda R, Toouli J, Dodds WJ, et al: Effect of enteric hormones on sphincter of Oddi and gastrointestinal myoelectric activity in fasted conscious opossums. Gastroenterology 1983;*84*:1.
48. Pitt HA, Doty JE, DenBesten L, et al: Altered sphincter of Oddi phasic activity following truncal vagotomy. J Surg Res 1982;*32*:598.
49. Toouli J, Dodds WJ, Honda R, et al: Motor function of the opossum sphincter of Oddi. J Clin Invest 1983;*71*:208.
50. Coelho JCU, Moody FG, Senninger N: A new method for correlating pancreatic and biliary duct pressures and sphincter of Oddi electromyography. Surgery 1985;*97*:342.
51. Honda R, Toouli J, Dodds WJ, et al: Relationship of sphincter of Oddi spike bursts to gastrointestinal myoelectric activity in conscious opossums. J Clin Invest 1982;*69*:770.
52. Takahaski I, Dodds WJ, Itoh Z, et al: Influence of transsphincteric fluid flow on spike burst rate of the opossum sphincter of Oddi. Gastroenterology 1984;*87*:1292.
53. Scott RB, Strasberg SM, El-Sharkawy TY, et al: Fasting canine biliary secretion and the sphincter of Oddi. Gastroenterology 1984;*87*:793.
54. Toouli J, Geenen JE, Hogan WJ, et al: Sphincter of Oddi motor activity: A comparison between patients with common bile duct stones and controls. Gastroenterology 1982;*82*:111.
55. Takahashi I, Honda R, Dodds WJ, et al: Effect of motilin on the upper gastrointestinal tract and sphincter of Oddi in the conscious opossum. Am J Physiol 1983;*245*:G476.
56. Andersson KD, Andersson R, Hedner P, et al: Effect of cholecystokinin on the level of cyclic AMP and on mechanical activity in the isolated sphincter of Oddi. Life Sci 1972;*11*:723.
57. Coelho JCU, Moody FG, Senninger N, et al: Effects of gastrointestinal hormones on Oddi's sphincter and duodenal myoelectric activity and pancreatobiliary pressure. Arch Surg 1985;*120*:1060.
58. Geenen JE, Hogan WJ, Dodds WJ, et al: Intraluminal pressure recording from the human sphincter of Oddi. Gastroenterology 1980;*78*:317.
59. Carr-Locke DL, Gregg JA, Chey WY: Effects of exogenous secretin on pancreatic and biliary ductal and sphincteric pressure in man demonstrated by endoscopic manometry and correlation with plasma secretin levels. Dig Dis Sci 1985;*30*:909.
60. Behar J, Biancani P: Neural control of the sphincter of Oddi. Gastroenterology 1984;*86*:134.
61. Gregg JA: Endoscopic manometry of the pancreatic and bile duct sphincters after naloxone administration. Gastroenterology 1981;*80*:1163 (Abstr).
62. Gregg JA, Antal RD: Rhythm abnormalities of the biliary and pancreatic sphincters: Diagnosis by endoscopic manometry. Am J Surg 1984;*148*:602.
63. Pitt HA, Doty JE, Roslyn JJ, et al: The role of extrahepatic biliary function in the pathogenesis of gallstones after vagotomy. Surgery 1981;*90*:418.
64. Persson CGA: Adrenergic, cholecystokinetic and morphine induced effects on extrahepatic biliary motility. Acta Physiol Scand (Suppl) 1972;*383*:4.

65. Csendes A, Kruse A, Funch-Jensen P, et al: Pressure measurements in the biliary and pancreatic duct systems in controls and in patients with gallstones, previous cholecystectomy, or common bile duct stones. Gastroenterology 1979;*77*:1203.
66. Scott GW, Wlodzimierz JO: Resistance and sphincter-like properties of the cystic duct. Surg Gynecol Obstet 1979;*149*:177.
67. Courtney DF, Clanachan AS, Scott GW: Cholecystokinin constricts the canine cystic duct. Gastroenterology 1983;*85*:1154.
68. Scott GW: Resistance and sphincter-like properties of the cystic duct. Surg Gynecol Obstet 1979; *149*:177.
69. Miranda M, Espinoza M, Csendes A: Manometric characteristics of the extrahepatic biliary tract in dogs. Dig Dis Sci 1981;*26*:417.
70. Ludwick JR, Bass P: Contractile and electric activity of the extrahepatic biliary tract and duodenum. Surg Gynecol Obstet 1967;*124*:536.
71. Shaffer EA: Gallbladder function and bile composition after vagotomy and gastric surgery. Gastroenterology 1981;*80*:1348.
72. Oshio C, Phillips MJ: Contractility of bile canaliculi: implications for liver function. Science 1981; *212*:1041.
73. Phillips MJ, Oshio C, Miyairi M, et al: A study of bile canalicular contractions in isolated hepatocytes. Hepatology 1982;*2*:763.
74. Phillips MJ, Oda M, Mak E, et al: Microfilament dysfunctions as a possible cause of intrahepatic cholestasis. Gastroenterology 1975;*69*:48.
75. Szurszewski JH: A migrating electric complex of the canine small intestine. Am J Physiol 1969; *217*:1757.
76. Boldyreff W: Einige neue seiten der latigkeit des pankreas: der uberstritt des pankreassaftes und anderer darmsekrete in den magen; die physiologische and klinische bedeutung deiser ekscheinung. Ergeb Physiol 1911;*11*:185.
77. Code CF, Marlett JA: The interdigestive myoelectric complex of the stomach and small bowel of dogs. J Physiol 1975;*246*:289.
78. Itoh Z, Takeuchi S, Aizawa I, et al: Characteristic motor activity of the gastrointestinal tract in fasted conscious dogs measured by implanted force transducers. Dig Dis 1978;*23*:229.
79. Sarna SK: Cyclic motor activity; Migrating motor complex: 1985. Gastroenterology 1985;*89*:894.
80. Owyang C, Achem-Karam SR, Vink AI: Pancreatic polypeptide and intestinal migrating motor complex in humans. Effects of pancreatico-biliary secretions. Gastroenterology 1983;*84*:10.
81. Traynor OJ, Dozois RR, DiMagno EP: Relationship of interdigestive and postprandial gallbladder motility and emptying to bile flow into the duodenum. Gastroenterology 1982;*82*:1198 (Abstr).
82. Traynor OJ, Dozois RR, DiMagno EP: Canine interdigestive and postprandial gallbladder motility and emptying. Am J Physiol 1984;*246*:G432.
83. Ryan TD, Pellegrini CA, Way LW: Bile kinetics in the conscious dog. Surg Forum 1983;*35*:234.
84. Pellegrini CA, Lewin M, Patti MG, et al: Gallbladder filling and response to cholecystokinin are not affected by vagotomy. Surgery 1985;*98*:452.
85. Peeters TL, Vantrappen G, Janssens J: Bile acid output and the interdigestive migrating motor complex in normals and in cholecystectomy patients. Gastroenterology 1980; *79*:678.
86. Bloom SR, Adrian TE, Mitchenere P: Motilin-induced gallbladder contraction—a new mechanism. Gastroenterology 1977;*112*:750.
87. Takahashi I, Nakaya M, Suzuki T, et al: Postprandial changes in contractile activity and bile concentration in the gallbladder of the dog. Am J Physiol 1982;*243*:G365.
88. Shaffer, EA, Taylor PJ, Logan K, et al.: The effect of progestin on gallbladder function in young women. Am J Obstet Gynecol 1984;*148*:504.
89. Fried GM, Ogden WD, Fagan CJ, et al: Comparison of cholecystokinin release and gallbladder emptying in men and women at estrogen and progesterone phases of the menstrual cycle. Surgery 1984;*95*:284.
90. Bennion LJ, Knowler WC, Mott DM, et al: Development of lithogenic bile during puberty in Pima Indians. N Engl J Med 1979;*300*:873.
91. Everson GT, McKinley C, Lawson M, et al.: Gallbladder function in the human female: effect of the ovulatory cycle, pregnancy, and contraceptive steroids. Gastroenterology 1982;*82*:711.
92. Braverman DZ, Johnson ML, Kern F Jr.: Effects of pregnancy and contraceptive steroids on gallbladder function. N Engl J Med 1980;*302*:362.
93. Down RHL, Whiting MJ, Watts J, et al: Effects of synthetic oestrogens and progestagens in oral contraceptives on bile lipid composition. Gut 1983;*24*:253.
94. Tritapepe R, DiPadova C, Zuin M, et al: Lithogenic bile after conjugated estrogens. N Engl J Med 1976;*295*:961.
95. Bennion J, Ronald MD, Ginsberg L, et al: Effects of oral contraceptives on the gallbladder bile of normal women. N Engl J Med 1976;*294*:189.
96. Kern F Jr, Everson GT, DeMark B, et al: Biliary lipids, bile acids, and gallbladder function in the human female: Effects of contraceptive steroids. J Lab Clin Med 1982;*99*:798.
97. DiPadova C, Tritapepe R, DiPadova F, et al: S-Adenosyl-L-Methionine antagonizes oral contraceptive–induced bile cholesterol supersaturation in healthy women: Preliminary report of a controlled randomized trial. Am J Gastroenterol 1984;*79*:941.
98. Scragg RKR, McMichael AJ, Seamark RF: Oral contraceptives, pregnancy, and endogenous oestrogen in gallstone disease: A case control study. Br Med J 1984;*288*:1795.
99. Royal College of General Practitioners' Oral Contraception Study: Oral contraceptives and gallbladder disease. Lancet 1982;*2*:957.
100. Ryan JP: The effect of pregnancy on gallbladder contractility in the guinea pig. Gastroenterology 1984;*87*:674.
101. Ryan JP, Pellecchia D: Effect of progesterone pretreatment on guinea pig gallbladder motility in vitro. Gastroenterology 1982;*83*:81.
102. Meyer PD, DenBesten L, Gurll NJ: Effects of cholesterol gallstone induction on gallbladder function and bile salt pool size in the prairie dog model. Surgery 1978;*83*:599.
103. Roslyn JJ, DenBensten L: Effects of CCK on gallbladder stasis and cholesterol gallstone formation. J Surg Res 1981;*30*:200.
104. Hutton SW, Sievert CE, Vennes JA, et al: The effect of sphincterotomy on gallstone formation in the prairie dog. Gastroenterology 1981;*81*:663.
105. Fridhandler, T, Davidson J, Pomeranz I, et al: Progressive defect in gallbladder contractility during the early stages of cholesterol gallstone formation. Clin Res 1983;*31*:31A.

106. Pitt HA, Roslyn JJ, Kuckenbecker SL, et al.: The role of cystic duct resistance in the pathogenesis of cholesterol gallstones. J Surg Res 1981;*30*:508.
107. Thomas MJ, Pellegrini CA, Broderick WC, et al: Vagotomy enhances cholesterol precipitation in the gallbladder of the prairie dog. Surg Forum 1981;*32*:145.
108. Gitelson S, Schwartz A, Fraenkel M, et al: Gallbladder dysfunction in diabetes mellitus. Diabetes 1963;*12*:308.
109. Johnson FE, Boyden EA: The effect of double vagotomy on the motor activity of the human gallbladder. Surgery 1952;*32*:591.
110. Lieber MM: The incidence of gallstones and their correlation with other diseases. Ann Surg 1952;*135*:394.
111. Clave RH, Caspar MR: Incidence of gallbladder disease after vagotomy. Am J Surg 1969;*118*:169.
112. Jacob CO, Modon M, Hzchak Y, et al: Prolonged opacification of the gallbladder after oral cholecystography: a reevaluation of its clinical significance. Gastroenterology 1981;*81*:936.
113. Northfield TC, Kupfer, RM, Maudgal DP, et al: Gallbladder sensitivity to cholecystokinin in patients with gallstones. Br Med J 1980;*1*:143.
114. Thompson JC, Fried GM, Ogden DW, et al: Correlation between release of cholecystokinin and contraction of the gallbladder in patients with gallstones. Ann Surg 1982;*195*:670.
115. Fisher RS, Stelzer F, Rock E, et al: Abnormal gallbladder emptying in patients with gallstones. Dig Dis Sci 1982;*27*:1019.
116. Bernhoft RA, Pellegrini CA, Broderick WC, et al: Pigment sludge and stone formation in the acutely ligated dog gallbladder. Gastroenterology 1983; *85*:1166.
117. Pikula JV, Dunphy JE: Some effects of stenosis of the terminal common bile duct on the biliary tract and liver. N Engl J Med 1959;*260*:315.
118. Imamoglu K, Perry JF Jr., Wangensteen OH: Experimental production of gallstones by incomplete stricture of the terminal common bile duct. Surgery 1957;*42*:623.
119. Soloway RD, Trotman BW, Ostrow JD: Pigment gallstones. Gastroenterology 1977;*72*:167.
120. Sedaghat A, Grundy SM: Cholesterol crystals and the formation of cholesterol gallstones. N Engl J Med 1980;*302*:1274.
121. Small D: Cholesterol nucleation and growth in gallstone formation. N Engl J Med 1980;*302*:1305.
122. Mok HYI, Von Bergmann K, Grundy SM: Kinetics of the enterohepatic circulation during fasting: Biliary lipid secretion and gallbladder storage. Gastroenterology 1980;*78*:1033.
123. Northfield TC, Hofmann AF: Biliary lipid output during three meals and an overnight fast. Gut 1975;*16*:1.
124. Doty JE, Pitt HA, Kuchendecker SL, et al: Impaired gallbladder emptying before gallstone formation in the prairie dog. Gastroenterology 1983;*85*:168.
125. Pitt HA, Doty JE, DenBesten L: Stasis before gallstone formation: altered gallbladder compliance or cystic duct resistance? Am J Surg 1982;*143*:144.
126. Pellegrini CA, Ryan T, Broderick W, Way LW: Gallbladder filling and emptying during cholesterol formation in the prairie dog: A cholescintigraphic study. Gastroenterology 1986;*90*:143.
127. Fridhandler TM, Davison JS, Shaffer EA: Defective gallbladder contractility in the ground squirrel and prairie dog during the early stages of cholesterol gallstone formation. Gastroenterology 1983; *85*:830.
128. Hutton SW, Sievert CE, Vennes JA, et al: Inhibition of gallstone formation by sphincterotomy in the prairie dog: reversal by atropine. Gastroenterology 1982;*82*:1308.
129. Holzbach RT: Gallbladder stasis: Consequence of long-term parenteral hyperalimentation and risk factor for cholelithiasis. Gastroenterology 1983; *84*:1055.
130. Allen B, Bernhoft R, Blanckaert N, et al: Sludge is calcium bilirubinate associated with bile stasis. Am J Surg 1981;*141*:51.
131. Messing B, Bories C, Kunstlinger F, et al: Does total parenteral nutrition induce gallbladder sludge formation and lithiasis? Gastroenterology 1983; *84*:1012.
132. Roslyn JJ, Pitt HA, Mann L, et al: Parenteral nutrition–induced gallbladder disease: A reason for early cholecystectomy. Am J Surg 1984;*148*:58.
133. Pitt HA, Berquist WE, Mann L, et al: Parenteral nutrition induces calcium bilirubinate gallstones. Gastroenterology 1983;*84*:1274.
134. Bernhoft R, Pellegrini CA, Motson RW, Way LW: Composition, morphology and clinical features of common bile duct stones. Am J Surg 1984;*148*:77.
135. Womach NA, Zeppa R, Irvin GL III: The anatomy of gallstones. Ann Surg 1963;*157*:670.
136. Maki T, Matsushiro T, Suzuki N, et al: Role of sulfated glycoprotein in gallstone formation. Surg Gynecol Obstet 1971;*132*:846.
137. Masuda H, Nakayama F: Composition of bile pigment in gallstones and bile and their etiological significance. J Lab Clin Med 1979;*93*:353.
138. Maki T: Pathogenesis of calcium bilirubinate gallstone: Role of E coli, beta-glucuronidase and coagulation by inorganic ions, polyelectrolytes and agitation. Ann Surg 164;*90*:1966.
139. Schein CJ, Gliedman ML: Vagotogenic cholecystitis. Am J Gastroenterol 1978;*69*:708.
140. Wong HN, Frey CF, Gacic MN: Intraoperative common duct pressure and flow measurements. Am J Surg 1980;*139*:691.
141. Sapala MA, Sapala JA, Resto Soto AD, et al: Cholelithiasis following subtotal gastric resection with truncal vagotomy. Surg Gynecol Obstet 1970;*148*:36.
142. Tompkins RK, Kraft AR, Zimmerman E, et al: Clinical and biochemical evidence of increased gallstone formation after complete vagotomy. Surgery 1972;*71*:196.
143. Ihasz M, Griffith CA: Gallstone after vagotomy. Am J Surg 1981;*141*:48.
144. Deveney CCW, Gardiner BN, Way LW: Effect of truncal vagotomy on bile kinetics in rhesus monkey. Surg Forum 1974;*25*:402.
145. Cowie AGA, Clark CG: The lithogenic effect of vagotomy. Br J Surg 1972;*59*:365.
146. Shaffer EA: The effect of vagotomy on gallbladder function and bile composition in man. Ann Surg 1982;*195*:413.
147. Stempel JM, Duane WC: Biliary lipids and bile acid pool size after vagotomy in man. Evidence against a predisposition to gallstones. Gastroenterology 1978;*75*:608.
148. Parkin GJS, Smith RB, Johnston D: Gallbladder volume and contractility after truncal, selective, and highly selective vagotomy in man. Ann Surg 1973;*178*:581.
149. Rudick J, Hutchison JSF: Evaluation of vagotomy

and biliary function by combined oral cholecystography and intravenous cholangiography. Gastroenterology 1974;*66*:22.
150. Malagelada JR, Go VLW, Summerskill WHJ: Altered pancreatic and biliary function after vagotomy and pyloroplasty. Gastroenterology 1974; *66*:22.
151. Tinker J, Cox G: Gallbladder function after vagotomy. Br J Surg 1960;*56*:779.
152. Krishnamurthy GT, Bobba VR, Kinstone E: Radionuclide ejection fraction: A technique for quantitative analysis of motor function of the human gallbladder. Gastroenterology 1981;*80*:482.
153. Klein GL, Rivera D: Adverse metabolic consequences of total parenteral nutrition. Cancer 1985;*55*:305.
154. Whitington PF: Cholestasis associated with total parenteral nutrition in infants. Hepatology 1985;*4*:693.
155. Roslyn JJ, Berquist WE, Pitt HA, et al: Increased risk of gallstones in children receiving total parental nutrition. Pediatrics 1983;*71*:784.
156. Roslyn JJ, Pitt HA, Mann L, et al: Gallbladder disease in patients on long term parenteral nutrition. Gastroenterology 1983;*84*:148.
157. Andrassy RJ, Treadwell TA, Rather IA, et al: Gallbladder disease in children and adolescents. Am J Surg 1976;*132*:19.
158. Doty JE, Pitt HA, Porter-Fink V, et al: Cholecystokinin prophylaxis of parenteral nutrition–induced gallbladder disease. Clin Res 1984;*32*:24.
159. Lieber MM: The incidence of gallstones and their correlation with other diseases. Ann Surg 1952;*135*:394.
160. Foster KJ, Griffith AH, Dewbury K, et al: Liver disease in patients with diabetes mellitus. Postgrad Med J 1980;*56*:767.
161. Ponz De Leon M, Ferenderes R, Carulli N: Bile lipid composition and bile acid pool size in diabetes. Dig Dis 1978;*23*:710.
162. Gitelson S, Oppenheim D, Schwartz A: Size of the gallbladder in patients with diabetes mellitus. Diabetes 1969;*18*:493.
163. Grodski M, Rozynska E, Cayayk A: Diabetic cholecystopathy. Diabetologia 1968;*4*:345.
164. Onodera H, Sugawara H, Hirata T, et al: Diurnal profile of gallbladder size in diabetic patients: Ultrasonographic evaluation of diabetic neurogenic gallbladder. Tohoku J Exp Med 1983;*139*:179.
165. Bennion LJ, Scott MG: Effects of diabetes mellitus on cholesterol metabolism in man. N Engl J Med 1977;*296*:1355.
166. The metabolic disorder in cholesterol gallstone disease. Nutr Rev 1978;*36*:45.
167. Gracie WA, Ransohoff DF: The natural history of silent gallstones. N Engl J Med 1982;*307*:798.
168. Mundth ED: Cholecystitis and diabetes mellitus. N Engl J Med 1962;*267*:642.
169. Turrill FL, McCarron MM, Mikkelsen WP: Gallstones and diabetes: An ominous association. Am J Surg 1961;*102*:184.
170. Walsh DB, Eckhauser FE, Ramsburg SR, et al: Risk associated with diabetes mellitus in patients undergoing gallbladder surgery. Surgery 1982; *91*:254.
171. Sandler RS, Maule WF, Baltus ME: Factors associated with postoperative complications in diabetics following biliary tract surgery. Gastroenterology 1986;*91*:157.
172. Pellegrini CA: Asymptomatic gallstones. Does diabetes mellitus make a difference? Gastroenterology 1986;*91*:245.
173. Griffen WO, Bivins BA, Rogers EL, et al: Cholecystokinin cholecystography in the diagnosis of gallbladder disease. Ann Surg 1980;*191*:636.
174. Valdberg LS, Jabbari M, Kerr JW, et al: Biliary pain in young women in the absence of gallstones. Gastroenterology 1971;*60*:1020.
175. Goldstein F, Grunt R, Margulies M: Cholecystokinin cholecystography in the differential diagnosis of acalculous gallbladder disease. Am J Dig Dis 1974;*19*:835.
176. Nardi GL: Papillitis and stenosis of the sphincter of Oddi. Surgery Clin North Am 1973;*53*:1149.
177. Lo Giudice JA, Geenen JE, Hogan WJ, et al: Efficacy of the morphine-neostigmine test for evaluating patients with suspected papillary stenosis. Dig Dis Sci 1979;*24*:455.
178. Steinberg WM, Salvato RF, Toskes PP: The morphine-prostigmin provocative test: Is it useful for making clinical decisions? Gastroenterology 1980;*78*:728.
179. Toouli J, Roberts-Thomson IC, Dent J, et al: Manometric disorders in suspected sphincter of Oddi dysfunction. Gastroenterology 1985;*88*:1243.
180. Bar-Meir S, Geenen JE, Hogan WJ, et al: Biliary and pancreatic duct pressure measured by ERCP manometry in patients with suspected papillary stenosis. Dig Dis Sci 1979;*24*:209.
181. Funch-Jensen P, Kruse A, Csendes A, et al: Biliary manometry in patients with post-cholecystectomy syndrome. Acta Chir Scand 1982;*148*:267.
182. Meshkinpour H, Mollot M, Gordon B, et al: Bile duct dyskinesia: Clinical and manometric study. Gastroenterology 1984;*87*:759.
183. Geenen JE, Toouli J, Hogan WJ, et al: Endoscopic sphincterotomy: Follow-up evaluation of effects on the sphincter of Oddi. Gastroenterology 1984;*87*:754.
184. Geenen JE, Hogan W, Toouli J, et al: A prospective randomized study of the efficacy of endoscopic sphincterotomy for patients with presumptive sphincter of Oddi dysfunction. Gastroenterology 1984;*86*:1086 (Abstr).
185. Bar-meir S, Halpern Z, Bardan E: Nitrate therapy in a patient with papillary dysfunction. Am J Gastroenterol 1983;*78*:94.
186. Basso N, Bagarani M, Materia A, et al: Effect of caerulein in patients with biliary colic. Gastroenterology 1985;*89*:605.
187. Tanaka M, Ikeda S, Matsumoto S, et al: Manometric diagnosis of sphincter of Oddi spasm as a cause of postcholecystectomy pain and treatment by endoscopic sphincterotomy. Ann Surg 1985; *202*:712.
188. Roberts-Thomson IC, Toouli J: Is endoscopic sphincterotomy for disabling biliary-type pain after cholecystectomy effective? Gastrointest Endosc 1985;*31*:370.
189. Shaffer EA, Hershfield NB, Logan K et al: Cholescintigraphic detection of functional obstruction of the sphincter of Oddi. Effect of papillotomy. Gastroenterology 1986;*90*:728.

JAMES McK. WATTS, M.B., B.S., F.R.A.C.S.
JAMES TOOULI, Ph.D.
MALCOLM J. WHITING, Ph.D.

4

The Formation and Dissolution of Gallstones

Gallstones have been observed in man throughout recorded history, but their importance in human disease was not realized until about the seventeenth century.[1] Human and animal gallstones were once used as charms, as artist's pigment, or as a ground powder in the potions and draughts of apothecaries and alchemists.

Early attempts at the treatment of gallstones were highly empirical, since there was no certain method of diagnosis. Many attempts were made to dissolve the stones or to stimulate their expulsion from the gallbladder. Preventive measures were aimed at elimination of bile stagnation. In the nineteenth century, patients with liver disorders and colic were sent to the great European spas "to take the waters," which were rich in mineral salts, especially magnesium.

Surgical treatment for gallstones started sporadically in the mid-nineteenth century, and Langenbach is credited with the first cholecystectomy in 1882. The real impetus to surgical treatment was the introduction of cholecystography by Graham and Cole in 1924.[2] This permitted accurate diagnosis for the first time. A further impetus was the control of the bleeding tendency that accompanied obstructive jaundice, with the discovery and therapeutic use of vitamin K.

Charlatans had for many years claimed that they were able to dissolve gallstones by oral medication, but their methods were arbitrary, as the chemical mechanisms of gallstone formation were unknown. Commonly used agents were purgatives, olive oil, and mixed bile salts, usually given in large doses over short periods. There is certainly no evidence that these methods were successful, and it is likely that many patients in whom success was claimed did not have gallstones in the first place. The first record of successful dissolution of human gallstones was that of Rewbridge[3] in 1937, who was successful in dissolving gallstones in two of five patients using prolonged administration of mixed bile salts and olive oil. The modern era of gallstone dissolution was heralded by the study of Danzinger and his colleagues,[4] who reported successful dissolution of gallstones in man by the oral administration of the primary bile acid, chenodeoxycholic acid.

PREVALENCE OF GALLSTONES

Because the majority of people with gallstones do not have any symptoms, the true prevalence of gallstone disease in any given population is unknown. We do know that gallstones are exceedingly rare in some populations, such as the African Masai and the Eskimos, and exceedingly common in others, such as the Pima Indians of North America. In these Indians, 70 per cent of the women have gallstones by the age of 30, and 70 per cent of the men by the age of 60. If the results of the Framingham study[5] are extrapolated to the United States population, 12 million women and 4 million men have (or have had) gallstones and 800,000 new cases are presented for treatment each year. A study in South Wales,[6] where oral cholecystography was carried out on a weighted random sample of the population between 45 and 69 years of age, showed that the overall gallstone prevalence rate for males was 6.2 per cent and for females 12.1 per cent. Within the age limits investigated there was no marked increase of prevalence with age shown in either sex in this study.

Autopsy studies have provided some evidence about gallstone disease in a number of populations. These studies, which give suggestive information about prevalence, show that after the American Indian, the prevalence of gallstones is probably highest in Sweden and a little less common in the white populations of the United States, Western Europe, South Africa, Australia, and Israel.[7]

Autopsy data generally confirm that there are large differences in gallstone prevalence between developed and developing countries. They have also provided evidence to suggest that there has been an increase in prevalence of gallstones in Europe, North America, and Australia. In many areas of the world, such as Asia, the USSR, the Middle East, and South America, little is known about the prevalence of gallstone disease.

CHEMICAL COMPOSITION OF GALLSTONES

Human gallstones vary in composition from individual to individual and contain the same range of constituents, but in different proportions. Human gallstones are usually classified as either cholesterol or pigment depending on their major constituent. Pure cholesterol stones are uncommon: Gallstones usually contain some calcium salts and varying amounts of pigment.

Pigment Gallstones

Pigment stones are usually red-brown to black, irregular in shape and between 2 mm and 5 mm in diameter. About half are radiopaque to x-rays because of a high calcium content. By definition, pigment stones contain less than 25 per cent cholesterol.[8] They are composed of varying amounts of unidentified pigment and calcium salts of bilirubin, phosphate, carbonate, and other anions. Pigment stones vary in appearance from small, glassy, black stones to large, soft, chocolate-brown stones. The solids are predominately calcium bilirubinate complexed with glycoprotein.[9–11] The pigment in the small black stones is mainly polymerized bilirubin,[12, 13] which is invulnerable to known solvents. The soft, brown, earthy stones that form as the result of stasis are composed of calcium bilirubinate, which can be dissolved by EDTA solutions.

Pigment stones often occur in diseases involving rapid hemoglobin breakdown, such as chronic hemolytic anemia and prosthetic heart valve–induced hemolysis. However, most patients with pigment stones have no evidence of hemolysis, and total bilirubin concentration in bile is the same as that found in patients with cholesterol gallstones, although the level of unconjugated bilirubin may be increased.[14]

Patients with pigment stones have a different gallbladder bile composition from those with cholesterol stones, but there is a large overlap between the two groups. The bile from patients with pigment stones usually contains less cholesterol than the bile from patients with cholesterol stones. Their bile is also less likely to become supersaturated during periods of low bile salt output.[15]

Pigment stones result from precipitation and agglomeration of unconjugated bilirubin.[9] The proportion of unconjugated bilirubin in gallbladder bile from subjects with pigment stones exceeds the 2 per cent upper limit of unconjugated bilirubin found in normal bile, but the cause of the excess unconjugated bilirubin has not been clearly elucidated.

It has been proposed that the increased concentration of unconjugated bilirubin is derived from hydrolysis of conjugated bilirubin by β-glucuronidase derived from bacteria-infected bile (particularly *Escherichia coli*).[16] The unconjugated bilirubin then combines with calcium to form the water-insoluble calcium bilirubinate (Fig. 4–1).

The infection theory of pigment stone formation may be true for many patients in the Orient and Asia, where pigment stones predominate and infected bile is so common. *E. coli* is commonly cultured from bile in patients with recurrent pyogenic cholangitis,[17] a disease principally seen in the Chinese. In this disorder, pigment stones characteristically occur in the intrahepatic bile ducts. Similar gram-negative organisms commonly infect the biliary tract of Japanese patients with pigment stones. Eggs or cuticle fragments from *Ascaris lumbricoides* have also been observed in the calcium bilirubinate stones of Japanese patients.[16]

While this mechanism may apply to patients in Asia and the Orient, it cannot be the explanation in Western countries, where pigment stones commonly occur in the absence of biliary infection.[14] The explanation for the precipitation of bile pigment in such patients

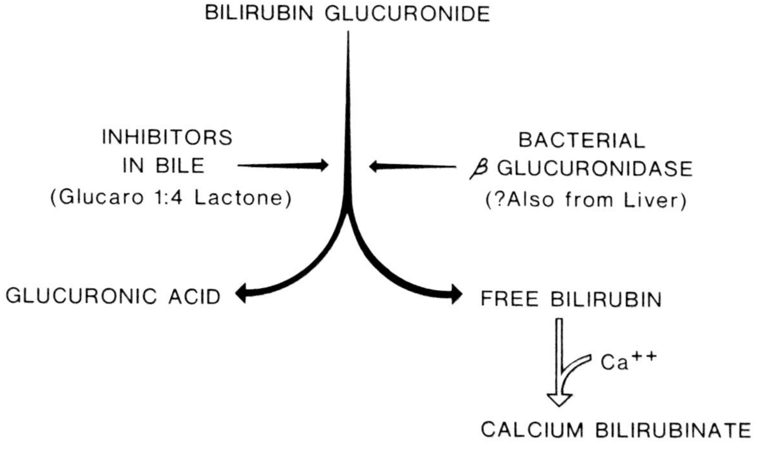

Figure 4–1. One possible mechanism of pigment stone formation, in which β-glucuronidase from bacteria deconjugates bilirubin glucuronide to produce free bilirubin. Free bilirubin is insoluble and combines with calcium to form calcium bilirubinate stones.

is unknown. However, the solubility of unconjugated bilirubin is influenced by pH and ionized calcium, both of which may be altered in the presence of stasis. Stasis is known to cause calcium excretion from the biliary mucous membrane. Pigment may also precipitate with sulfated glycoproteins, which bind calcium salts tightly and are present in increased amounts in patients with pigment gallstones.[8]

Epidemiology of Pigment Stones

Pigment stones are far more common than cholesterol stones in the Orient and Asia, although there is some evidence that the prevalence of cholesterol stones is increasing, at least in some of these countries. In Japan, pigment stones were found in 70 per cent of gallstone patients in the 1940s,[16] but by 1966 the proportion was only 30 to 40 per cent, a difference believed to be due to a change in diet and living conditions and a reduction of infestation with intestinal parasites.[18] In the United States, a study of gallstones from 92 consecutive patients undergoing cholecystectomy in Philadelphia showed that 27 of these patients had pigment stones.[19] A report from Japan[20] indicates that young Japanese adults predominantly have cholesterol gallstones but that elderly Japanese usually have pigment stones, both in their gallbladders and in their bile ducts. In Adelaide, Australia, only 41 of 356 patients undergoing cholecystectomy had pigment stones in the gallbladder, a proportion of 12 per cent. However, 21 of 61 stones (34 per cent) in this study[21] and 50 of 115 stones (43 per cent) in another report[22] surgically removed from the common bile duct were pigment stones, a finding that may indicate that stasis and infection are more important in the etiology of common bile duct stones.[21]

Clinical Correlates of Pigment Stones

The proportion of patients with pigment stones increases with advancing age. In contrast to cholesterol stones, sex, parity, and obesity appear to have no influence on the prevalence. Apart from their association with hemolytic disorders, pigment stones are found more frequently in patients with hepatic cirrhosis.[23]

Cholesterol Gallstones

Cholesterol is the major constituent of gallstones in people having a Western style of life and diet, but regional differences exist between the urban and rural populations in some countries, such as Japan.[16, 20] Sutor and Wooley[24] studied gallstones from eight countries. Cholesterol accounted for 71 per cent of the crystalline material in these stones, calcium carbonate 15 per cent, and calcium palmitate 6 per cent. Small amounts of calcium phosphate and α-palmitic acid were also found. Stones from different countries varied greatly in composition; for example, cholesterol accounted for 89 per cent of the weight of stones from Sweden but only 41 per cent of the weight of stones from South Africa.

These geographic differences in stone composition may indicate different processes of stone formation or differences in the composition of bile, which may, in turn, be related to be a different environment or a different diet. The composition of the gallstone nucleus may give a clue to the initial events in cholesterol gallstone formation. Some studies[25, 26] suggest that the stone nucleus is either predominantly pigment or composed of glycoprotein. Minor chemical differences have been shown between the nucleus and the rest of the stone; Sutor and Wooley[24] found more calcium phosphate and amorphous material in the center of gallstones. Calcium carbonate, on the other hand, is more frequently found on the surface of cholesterol gallstones than in the interior.[27] After the lipids of a cholesterol gallstone have been dissolved, the matrix of the stone is found to consist of a mucin-bilirubin complex, which constitutes 12.5 per cent of the weight of large stones.[28]

Cholesterol gallstones have no single characteristic appearance. The stones are usually hard, are often yellow, and may vary in size from a speck to so large that they occupy the whole lumen of the gallbladder. They may be single and spherical or multiple and faceted. Probably their most characteristic appearance is observed after the stone is bisected, when radiating sheets of cholesterol are seen, particularly in large and pure cholesterol stones.

Cholesterol Solubility in Bile

There are three major lipids in bile—cholesterol, phospholipids, and bile acids. Cholesterol is insoluble in water but is kept in solution in bile by the presence of the bile acids and phospholipids. The bile acids are synthesized in the liver from cholesterol (Fig. 4–2). During this synthetic process, the bile acids acquire polar hydroxyl groups on one side of the molecule and become amphipathic (Fig. 4–3). In aqueous solution, these amphipathic molecules aggregate at a critical concentration to form micelles, which can incorporate both phospholipid and cholesterol molecules within them (Fig. 4–4). The capacity for these mixed micelles to keep cholesterol in solution is related to the relative concentrations of cholesterol, phospholipids, and bile acids.

Although it was known in 1862 that bile acids could dissolve cholesterol and the micelle was described in 1913 by McBain,[29] it was not until the classic work of Admirand and Small[30] in 1968 that the important relationship between the biliary lipids in bile was understood. The relative molar proportions of these lipids can be plotted on triangular coordinates (Fig. 4–5). By estimation of the relative lipid composition of any bile sample (of between 5 and 25 per cent solid content), it is possible to represent the bile sample as a point within the triangle. Admirand and Small defined a line at the base of the triangle that represented the maximum relative mole concentrations of cholesterol that remain in micellar solution at various relative concentrations of phospholipids and bile acids. At points above that line, the bile is supersaturated and cholesterol is likely to come out of solution, either as free cholesterol crystals or, more likely, by deposition of cholesterol on an existing gallstone or other nidus.

Further studies on human bile[31, 32] defined a lower equilibrium line (Fig. 4–5), the area between the two lines being a metastable zone within which cholesterol may come out of solution when certain nucleating factors are present. Carey and Small have defined a family of cholesterol solubility curves for different lipid concentrations.[33]

Another method by which cholesterol is transported in bile is in relatively large (500 to 1000 A) phospholipid vesicles.[34] The phospholipid:cholesterol ratio in these spherical structures is about 1:1, making them much more efficient than bile salt micelles as cholesterol carriers. It seems likely that a sizable portion (10 to 60 per cent) of biliary cholesterol is solubilized in this way. The stability of these vesicles needs to be determined under a variety of circumstances, and their

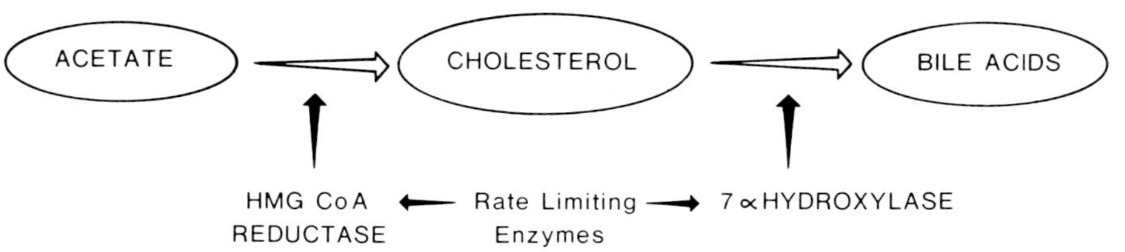

Figure 4–2. Both cholesterol and the primary bile acids are synthesized in the liver. The synthetic rate of cholesterol is controlled by the rate-limiting enzyme 3-hydroxyl-3-methyl glutaryl CoA (HMGCoA) reductase and the synthetic rate of bile acids by the rate-limiting enzyme cholesterol 7α-hydroxylase.

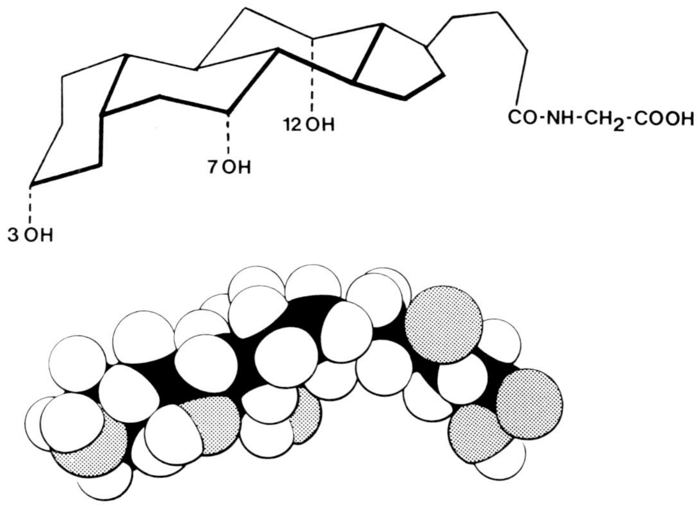

Figure 4–3. The molecular configuration of cholic acid. The hydrophilic polar groups (stippled in the lower diagram) are oriented on one side of the molecule. The molecule is therefore amphipathic and has detergent properties. In an aqueous solution at the critical micellar concentration, the molecules aggregate to form micelles.

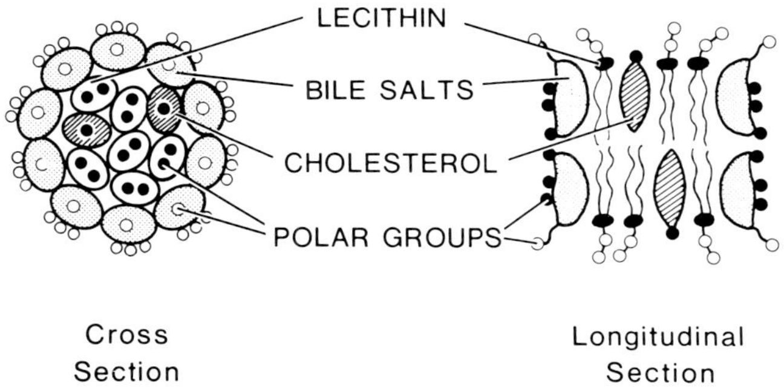

Figure 4–4. A diagrammatic representation of a mixed micelle found in bile. Bile acid molecules aggregate with hydrophilic polar groups externally and with hydrophobic surfaces internally. They incorporate the water-insoluble phospholipid and cholesterol molecules within the micelle. Note that the polar groups of all molecules lie externally.

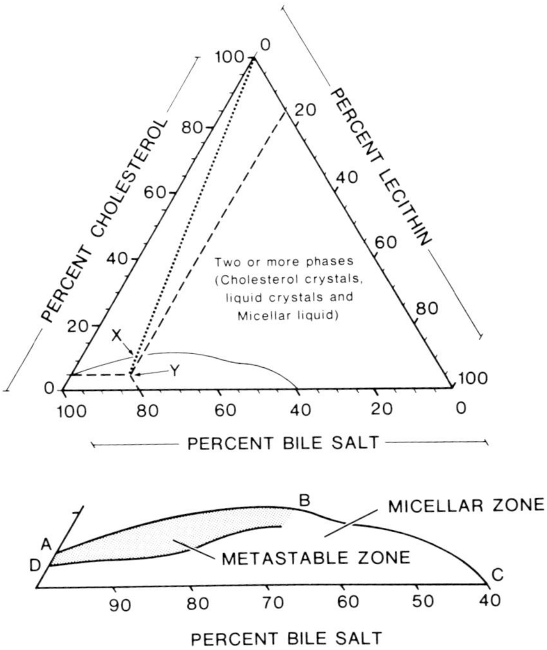

Figure 4–5. The three biliary lipids plotted as mole percentages on triangular coordinates. On the upper diagram, point Y represents a bile with 15 per cent phospholipid (lecithin), 80 per cent bile salt, and 5 per cent cholesterol and is within the micellar zone. The dotted line connecting Y to the apex of the triangle intersects at point X the line of maximum solubility of cholesterol as defined by Admirand and Small.[30] To calculate the saturation index of the bile represented by Y, the actual mole per cent cholesterol (5) is divided by the mole per cent cholesterol at point X (9), to give a value of 0.56. The expanded lower diagram shows a line DBC that indicates the true equilibrium solubility line of bile (Hegardt and Dam, 1971[31]; Holzbach et al., 1971[32]). Bile with a lipid composition, represented by a point between ABC and DBC, lies within a metastable zone where cholesterol may require nucleating factors to precipitate from solution. It is usual to calculate the saturation index using the line DBC and not ABC. (Redrawn from Small, 1975.[50])

physiology needs to be related to cholesterol precipitation and gallstone formation.[35]

The Saturation Index

The cholesterol saturation of bile is expressed as the saturation or lithogenic index.[36] This is the ratio of the actual amount of cholesterol in any bile sample to the maximum amount of cholesterol that can be dissolved in that sample (Fig. 4–5). Therefore, bile samples that have a composition represented by a point that lies below the equilibrium line have a saturation index of less than 1, a sample lying on the line has an index of 1, and a sample lying above the line has an index of greater than 1. The equilibrium line has been defined by a mathematical equation,[37] which simplifies the determination of the saturation index. Further refinements in this equation depend on the total solid content of bile, which influences the saturation index.[33]

Mechanisms of Cholesterol Supersaturation in Bile

A normal person weighing 70 kg has a total bile acid pool of between 2.5 and 4.0 gm, synthesizes 350 to 550 mg of bile acid a day, and secretes 15 to 35 gm of bile acid and about 0.75 gm of cholesterol a day. The bile acid pool circulates between 5 and 15 times a day. The mean hepatic return of bile acids is slightly less than the secretion rate because a small proportion of the bile acid pool is lost in the feces; in the steady state, this fecal loss equals the synthesis rate (Fig. 4–6). Supersaturated bile may occur when any of the normal mechanisms are disturbed (Table 4–1).

Increased Biliary Cholesterol Secretion. Cholesterol gallstones occur commonly in the very obese. Bile secretion studies in obese people indicate an excessive biliary cholesterol secretion but a normal bile salt and phospholipid secretion.[38] The size of their bile acid pool is normal or higher than normal.

Excessive biliary cholesterol secretion may also occur in association with high-calorie diets,[39] high-cholesterol diets,[40] and diets rich in polyunsaturated fats.[41, 42] Administration of clofibrate in hypercholesterolemic states may also produce an increase in biliary cholesterol, but there is also a decrease in the biliary concentration, pool size, and synthesis

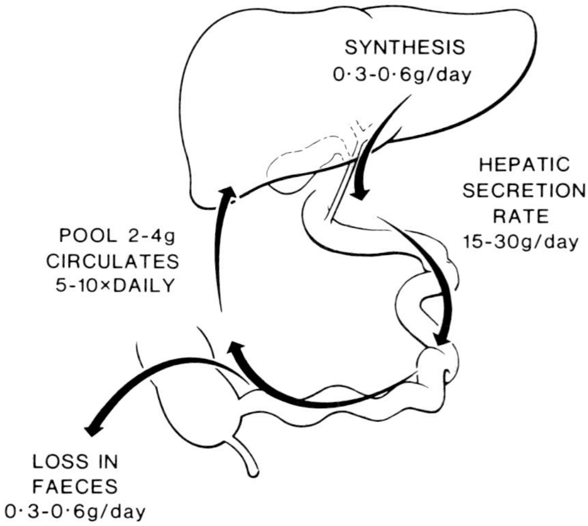

Figure 4–6. The enterohepatic circulation of bile acids. The bile acid pool size is maintained by hepatic synthesis, which in the steady state equals fecal losses.

of bile acids.[43] Estrogen or progesterone administration, as in oral contraceptives, may also lead to an increase in biliary cholesterol secretion.[44]

The mechanism for increased biliary cholesterol secretion is excessive cholesterol input or deficient cholesterol conversion into bile acids, or a combination of both.[45] Increased hepatic cholesterol synthesis appears to be responsible for the increased cholesterol secretion,[46] since there is no evidence that patients with gallstones absorb more cholesterol than those without stones.[47]

Decreased Biliary Bile Acid Secretion. When the biliary bile acid secretion is decreased, the bile acid pool is smaller than normal. Low rates of bile acid secretion are also accompanied by a reduction in biliary phospholipid secretion. Although biliary cholesterol secretion is also decreased, the decrease in cholesterol secretion is proportionally less than for the other lipids, so that bile saturation increases. There are three disorders that may lead to decreased biliary bile acid secretion.

Excessive Bile Acid Loss. This is seen clinically in patients with disease of the ileum (as in Crohn's disease) or in patients who have had a resection or a bypass of the ileum.[48, 49] There is a high incidence of gallstones under these conditions. The reason for the excessive bile acid loss is that the area of active bile acid transport in the terminal ileum does not function and unabsorbed bile acids are excreted in the feces. If this excess loss of bile

Table 4–1 DISORDERS ASSOCIATED WITH CHOLESTEROL SUPERSATURATION OF BILE

Defect	Possible Mechanism	Associated Clinical States
Increased biliary cholesterol secretion	Increased HMGCoA reductase activity and/or decreased 7α-hydroxylase activity[46]	Obesity[38] High-calorie diets[39] High-cholesterol diets[40] High–polyunsaturated fat diets[41, 42] Estrogen/progesterone administration[43] Clofibrate administration[43]
Decreased biliary bile acid secretion—with reduction of bile acid pool size	Excessive bile acid loss in feces from defective active absorption in ileum Decreased bile acid synthesis (decreased 7α-hydroxylase activity)[46] Rapid enterohepatic cycling of bile acid pool and oversensitive feedback inhibition of bile acid synthesis	Patients with ileal disease or ileal resection Nonobese cholesterol stone-formers[38] People with low bile acid pool[51]
Disorders of the extrahepatic biliary tract	Defect in gallbladder contraction → sequestering of bile salt pool and layering of supersaturated bile in the gallbladder Increased cystic duct resistance → diminished gallbladder emptying[64] Gallbladder mucus hypersecretion→ nucleation of biliary cholesterol[65] Abnormal intraluminal pressures or inflammation → bile acid absorption from damaged mucosa (?)	Pregnancy[57, 58] Vagotomy (?)[61] Estrogen/progesterone[57] Biliary dyskinesia Cholecystitis

acids is greater than the synthetic rate in the liver, a new equilibrium is set up, with a decreased hepatic bile acid secretion and a decreased bile acid pool size. Supersaturated bile is produced, and cholesterol is likely to come out of solution.

Decreased Bile Acid Secretion. This is thought to be the explanation for cholesterol supersaturation of bile in the majority of nonobese cholesterol gallstone patients.[38] The bile acid pool is smaller than normal, and both the bile acid and the phospholipid secretion rates are reduced, leading to supersaturated bile. Whether this occurs because of an oversensitive bile acid feedback mechanism that is genetically determined is uncertain.[50] However, a decrease in activity of the rate-limiting liver enzyme responsible for the conversion of cholesterol to bile acids—cholesterol 7 α-hydroxylase—has been demonstrated in people with cholesterol gallstones.[46]

Rapid Enterohepatic Cycling of the Bile Acid Pool (See also Chapter 2). In the economy of the enterohepatic circulation, there should be an inverse relationship between the bile acid pool size and the enterohepatic cycling rate.[51] Some people with normal bile composition and a smaller than normal bile acid pool must have increased frequency of pool cycling in order to prevent supersaturation. An increase in cycling rate is seen after cholecystectomy,[38] and this more than offsets the reduction in pool size, so that bile cholesterol saturation improves.[52, 53] A similar improvement in bile cholesterol saturation is seen in patients with nonfunctioning gallbladders.[54–56] Rapid enterohepatic cycling and a small bile salt pool size may not normally lead to supersaturated bile, but under conditions such as prolonged fasting, when the bile acids are sequestered in the gallbladder, insufficient bile acid may be present to prevent cholesterol precipitation. This explanation for supersaturation is speculative.

Disorders of the Extrahepatic Biliary Ducts. The search for biochemical mechanisms for the production of cholesterol gallstones has dominated research into their etiology in recent years. The role of the gallbladder is not so well defined, but it is obviously important for two reasons. First, it is the site of the occurrence of most gallstones, and second, the cholesterol saturation of bile improves after the gallbladder is removed. The gallbladder could influence gallstone formation in the following ways.

Deficient Motor Function. Defects in gallbladder concentration have been demonstrated in pregnancy.[57, 58] In patients with celiac disease, the gallbladder fails to contract normally after a meal because there is a decreased release of cholecystokinin from the damaged duodenal mucosa.[59, 60] The gallbladder may dilate after vagus nerve division.[61] There is also evidence that gallbladder emptying is abnormally slow in at least some patients with gallstone disease.[62, 63]

The result of this postulated defect in motor function of the gallbladder would be to sequester the bile acid pool, leading to increased synthesis and an increased total bile acid pool size with a decreased pool cycling rate. Whether this mechanism would lead to supersaturated bile is unproved, but if the pool size did not expand, this would be expected. A further effect of decreased gallbladder motor function is that layering of supersaturated bile may occur in the gallbladder. This may allow time for nucleation and aggregation of cholesterol crystals.

Experimental studies on resistance to flow through the cystic duct and sphincter of Oddi have been carried out in the prairie dog fed a high-cholesterol diet.[64] Increased resistance to flow through the cystic duct occurred before gallstone formation and continued to increase during stone formation. This increased cystic duct resistance provides a mechanism for diminished gallbladder emptying and suggests an etiologic role for increased cystic duct resistance in the pathogenesis of cholesterol gallstones.[64]

Other studies have shown that the cholesterol-fed prairie dog develops gallbladder mucus hypersecretion.[65] Increased mucus production may explain increased cystic duct resistance. Mucus is also a nucleating agent for biliary cholesterol in the gallbladder.[65] For further details on the relationship of gallbladder motility to cholesterol gallstone formation see Chapter 3.

Mucosal Damage Leading to Bile Acid Absorption or Change in Biliary Lipids. Gallbladder or bile duct mucous membrane may be damaged from infection or abnormal increases in intraluminal pressure from motility disorders (dyskinesia). Inflamed mucosa may absorb bile acids, or bacterial enzymes may cause changes in biliary lipids leading to supersaturated bile. The theory that alterations occur in human bile as a result of abnormalities of biliary tract motility is pure speculation, but it is certainly possible that increases in intraluminal pressure in the gallbladder lead to mucosal damage. Intermittent biliary obstruction in primates can readily produce decreased bile acid synthesis and secretion, accompanied by increased cholesterol secretion and supersaturated bile.[66]

Stages of Cholesterol Gallstone Formation

There are three stages in cholesterol gallstone formation: saturation, crystallization, and growth.

Saturation. Supersaturation with cholesterol is a prerequisite for cholesterol precipitation in bile. Even normal people secrete supersaturated bile on occasion, especially after overnight fasting, when presumably a large amount of the bile acid pool is sequestered within the gallbladder.[67, 68] However, as fasting continues beyond 20 hours, the cholesterol saturation of bile appears to decline.[69, 70] Conversely, patients who form cholesterol gallstones may have normal bile, especially following a meal, when the biliary bile acid secretion rate is high. The difference between normal patients and gallstone formers may be in the duration of supersaturation. In any 24-hour period, patients with cholesterol gallstones secrete a bile containing excess cholesterol relative to the bile acids and phospholipids that keep it in solution.[71]

Crystallization. In this stage, supersaturated bile changes to a liquid phase of bile saturated with cholesterol and a solid phase of cholesterol crystals. These cholesterol crystals can be seen microscopically in bile and may aggregate around a nidus of, for example, bile pigment, mucoproteins, or bacteria.

Supersaturated bile may not necessarily lead to cholesterol crystal formation; many otherwise normal persons have supersaturated bile at times. This is particularly evident in obese patients without cholesterol gallstones, whose gallbladder bile may be highly supersaturated but not contain crystals, even after incubation at 37° C for periods of up to 3 weeks.[72, 73] In contrast, patients with cholesterol gallstones almost always have crystals.[73]

The explanation for these differences seems to be that supersaturated bile from subjects without gallstones contains either antinucleating[164] or pronucleating[74] agents that, respectively, prevent or foster the formation of cholesterol crystals. Holzbach and his colleagues[75, 76] have shown that some bile proteins (apolipoproteins) exert a stabilizing influence, which accounts for the slow nucleation time of normal bile. One pronucleating agent is gallbladder mucus, which has been shown to promote cholesterol crystallization from supersaturated bile.[65, 77] Other experiments, however, have demonstrated the presence of a heat-labile protein other than mucus, which appears to be the most important initiating factor.[78] This substance is absent from normal bile but present in bile from patients with gallstones. When it is added to bile with a slow nucleation time, the nucleation time is greatly accelerated.

Growth. Pure cholesterol stones are found rarely. Presumably, these stones grow by simple surface accretion of cholesterol. In most stones, cholesterol is deposited in an organic matrix along with calcium-containing mineral salts. The rate of stone growth is determined by the balance between the rate of precipitation and the rate of dissolution. "Families" or "crops" of gallstones are often found, presumably as a result of periodic episodes during which conditions in the bile and gallbladder are favorable to nucleation and the growth of stones.[164]

Clinical Correlates of Cholesterol Gallstone Disease

The important clinical correlates of cholesterol gallstone disease are shown in Table 4–2.

Table 4–2 CLINICAL STATES ASSOCIATED WITH AN INCREASED INCIDENCE OF CHOLESTEROL GALLSTONES

Some racial groups (e.g., Pima Indians)
Family history of gallstones
Female sex
Obesity
Parity and female sex hormones
Clofibrate administration
Disease or resection of the ileum

BILE ACIDS

The major acids found in human bile are illustrated in Figure 4–7. There are two primary bile acids, cholic and chenodeoxycholic acid. They are conjugated by the liver with the amino acids glycine and taurine. Both these primary bile acids are dehydroxylated in the 7α position by the action of bacterial dehydroxylases in the intestine. The secondary bile acids formed in this way are deoxycholic acid from cholic acid and lithocholic acid from chenodeoxycholic acid. Most deoxycholic acid is absorbed and enters the enterohepatic circulation, but only traces of lithocholic acid are reabsorbed and secreted into the bile. Lithocholic acid undergoes further modification by the liver during enterohe-

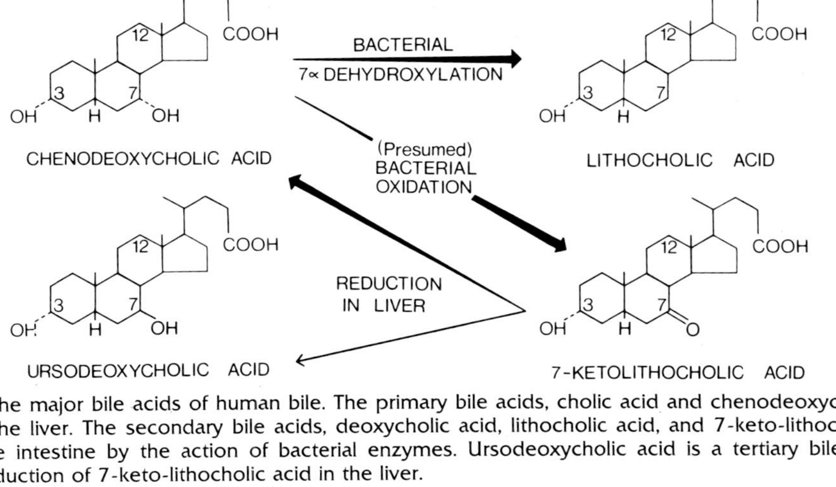

Figure 4–7. The major bile acids of human bile. The primary bile acids, cholic acid and chenodeoxycholic acid, are synthesized in the liver. The secondary bile acids, deoxycholic acid, lithocholic acid, and 7-keto-lithocholic acid, are produced in the intestine by the action of bacterial enzymes. Ursodeoxycholic acid is a tertiary bile acid, as it is produced by reduction of 7-keto-lithocholic acid in the liver.

patic circulation. A large proportion undergoes sulfate esterification at the 3-hydroxyl group, making it water-soluble. The approximate ratio of bile acids in normal bile is cholic acid 40 per cent, chenodeoxycholic acid 40 per cent, deoxycholic acid 20 per cent, and lithocholic acid 1 to 3 per cent. All other bile acids are found only in trace amounts in human bile. One of these bile acids is 7-ketolithocholic acid, which is formed from chenodeoxycholic acid by bacterial oxidation in the intestine and is readily absorbed. It is reduced in the liver to chenodeoxycholic acid and, in varying proportion, to ursodeoxycholic acid, the 7β epimer of chenodeoxycholic acid. Ursodeoxycholic acid is sometimes found in large quantities (up to 20 per cent of the total) in the bile of patients on long-term therapy with chenodeoxycholic acid.

GALLSTONE DISSOLUTION BY ORAL AGENTS

Most gallstones in people from developed countries are composed principally of cholesterol. Most patients with cholesterol gallstones have both fasting gallbladder and fasting hepatic bile that is supersaturated with cholesterol. Alterations in bile composition that reduce the relative molar proportion of cholesterol should therefore lead to cholesterol stone dissolution.

Rewbridge[3] in 1937 was the first to report the disappearance of gallstone shadows on x-ray. This occurred in two of five patients with gallstones who were fed bile salts in a dose of 600 mg a day for 9 months. In 1971, the primary bile acid, chenodeoxycholic acid, when fed orally, was found to increase the cholesterol-solubilizing capacity of bile.[79] In 1972, the first report of gallstone dissolution in man by oral chenodeoxycholic acid was made by Danzinger and his colleagues from the Mayo Clinic.[4]

THERAPEUTIC METHODS TO ALTER BILIARY LIPID COMPOSITION AND PROMOTE GALLSTONE DISSOLUTION

Chenodeoxycholic Acid

Chenodeoxycholic acid (CDCA) is an effective and safe agent for gallstone dissolution. Its ability to desaturate bile was first reported in 1971,[79] and its efficacy in gallstone dissolution in man was then reported in 1972.[4, 80] It is now an established agent for medical treatment of gallstones and is available on prescription.

Mechanism of Action

Patients with cholesterol gallstones have smaller bile acid pools than do normal people.[81] The effect of CDCA was at first thought to be an expansion of the pool of this bile acid and a relative increase in the biliary secretion of bile acids and phospholipids over cholesterol, which desaturated bile and led to conditions in which dissolution could occur. Although this theory has now been shown to be incorrect, the exact mechanism of action of CDCA in desaturating bile is still unclear.[82] One explanation is that CDCA suppresses the activity of 3-hydroxyl-3-methyl glutaryl CoA (HMGCoA) reductase, the rate-limiting enzyme of hepatic cholesterol synthesis. Liver biopsies taken from patients with gallstones show reduced activity of this enzyme after CDCA treatment.[83, 84] However, it is doubtful whether secretion of cholesterol into bile is closely linked to the rate of hepatic synthesis;[82] the cholesterol in bile comes from a preformed pool of cholesterol, not newly synthesized cholesterol. Other mechanisms of action of CDCA, such as alterations in cholesterol absorption from the intestine,[85] are still plausible.

Effective Dose of CDCA

Changes in bile composition leading to desaturation occur with doses of CDCA as low as 250 mg/day.[86] However, the effect is dose-dependent, and high doses promote a greater relative decrease in biliary cholesterol concentration and a reduction in the saturation index. Although gallstone dissolution has been observed with a dose as low as 250 mg/day,[87] this is exceptional; it is now clear that the dose given should be based on the body weight,[88, 89] 15 mg/kg/day being an optimal dose. At this dose, all except some obese patients will have unsaturated bile.[90] Desaturation of the bile obtained by duodenal intubation is believed to be a prerequisite for gallstone dissolution, but dissolution has been observed in patients in whom the duodenal bile remained supersaturated.[88] However, infrequent sampling may not give a true representation of the duration of bile supersaturation throughout the day,[91] and in any case, measurement of the cholesterol saturation index in duodenal bile at the same time on different days shows considerable biologic variation.[92]

The pharmacokinetics and bioavailability of CDCA have been studied by Ponz de Leon et al.,[93] and most of the ingested dose is absorbed. The bile acid is usually given in gelatin capsules as a single dose at night.[94]

Results of Therapy with CDCA

For dissolution to occur, gallbladder stones must be exposed to unsaturated bile; therefore, patients with poor or absent gallbladder opacification on oral cholecystography are unsuitable. The stones must also be composed principally of cholesterol and must contain insufficient calcium to make them radiopaque on x-ray. The results of gallstone dissolution may be different from one country to another because of differences in stone composition. Reports are also difficult to compare because of differences in patient selection, dosage schedules, and patient compliance.

Radiologic assessment of a decrease in gallstone size or disappearance is often difficult. However, when stones are seen to decrease in size, prolonged administration of CDCA will lead to complete dissolution in about two thirds of cases. Assessment of complete dissolution by oral cholecystography is insufficient by itself and must be supplemented by ultrasonic examination before treatment is stopped.

Gallbladder Stones. Chenodeoxycholic acid has now been administered to many thousands of patients. The results have been variable and often disappointing.[88, 89, 95–102]

Three studies from England, Australia, and the United States will be used to illustrate the results of treatment, the optimal dose, and the influence of gallstone size and other factors on the outcome of treatment.

English Study (Table 4–3).[97] One hundred and twenty-five patients with radiolucent stones were treated with CDCA (13 to 15 mg/kg/day in most cases). Most patients had stones with a diameter of less than 15 mm. Complete dissolution was observed in 47 (38 per cent). If the 21 patients who withdrew from the study before completing 6 months of treatment are excluded from the analysis, the complete dissolution rate was 45 per cent.

Table 4–3 RESULTS OF TREATMENT WITH CHENODEOXYCHOLIC ACID IN 125 PATIENTS WITH RADIOLUCENT STONES*

Results of Treatment	Patients *Number*	*Per Cent of Total*
Complete dissolution	47	37.6
Partial dissolution	7	5.6
Unchanged	50	40.0
Withdrawal or dropout (> 6 months treatment)	21	16.8
Total	125	100

*Most patients received 13 to 15 mg/kg/day.
From Maton et al., Medicine 1982;*61*:86.[97]

Also, if patients with stones less than 15 mm in diameter were treated with CDCA (≥ 13 mg/kg/day) for not less than 1 year and their bile became unsaturated during treatment, the complete dissolution rate was 78 per cent. The median duration of treatment for complete dissolution was 7.5 months for stones ≤ 5 mm in diameter, 12 months for stones 5 to 10 mm in diameter, and 22 months for stones 10 to 15 mm in diameter.

Australian Study. (Table 4–4).[102] Ninety-four patients with radiolucent gallstones were treated with CDCA (15 mg/kg/day) for at least 6 months. The complete dissolution rate was only 32 per cent, but it was 42 per cent in patients with stones less than 15 mm in diameter and 66 per cent in patients with stones less than 5 mm in diameter. Therefore, the results of this study were similar to those of the English study.[97]

American National Cooperative Gallstone Study. (Table 4–5).[100] This multicenter study involved 916 patients with radiolucent stones. Patients were allocated randomly to three

Table 4–4 RESULTS OF TREATMENT WITH CHENODEOXYCHOLIC ACID IN 94 PATIENTS WITH RADIOLUCENT STONES IN A FUNCTIONING GALLBLADDER*

Result of Treatment	Diameter of Largest Stone *< 5 mm*	*5–15 mm*	*> 15 mm*	All Stones
Complete dissolution	19 (66%)	10 (25%)	1 (4%)	30 (32%)
Partial dissolution	4	6	3	13
Unchanged	6	24	21	51
Total	29	40	25	94

*Dosage was ≃ 15 mg/kg/day. All patients completed at least 6 months of therapy.
Unpublished data from Flinders Medical Centre, Adelaide, and Austin Hospital, Melbourne.[102]

Table 4–5 RESULTS OF A DOUBLE-MASKED STUDY IN 916 PATIENTS WITH RADIOLUCENT GALLSTONES TO DETERMINE THE EFFICACY OF CHENODEOXYCHOLIC ACID*

	Treatment Group					
	Placebo		*350 mg/day*		*750 mg/day*	
Result of Treatment	Number	%	Number	%	Number	%
Complete dissolution	2	0.8	16	5.2	41	13.5
Partial dissolution	31	10.2	56	18.4	83	27.3
Unchanged	227	74.4	184	60.1	133	43.6
Withdrawals and dropouts	47	14.7	50	16.3	48	15.7
Total	307	100	306	100	305	100

*At doses of 350 mg/day or 750 mg/day for 2 years.
Modified from Schoenfield LJ et al: Ann Intern Med 1981; *95*:257.

CDCA treatment groups: 750 mg/day, 375 mg/day, and placebo.

After 2 years' treatment, complete dissolution occurred in 13.5 per cent (750 mg/day group), 5.2 per cent (375 mg/day group), and 0.8 per cent (placebo group). All patients who started treatment were included; 15 per cent of the total group failed to complete the course of treatment. Dissolution occurred more frequently in female patients, thin patients, patients with small or floating gallstones, and patients with serum cholesterol levels ≥ 227 mg/dl. The daily dose of CDCA was fixed in this study, so that most patients did not receive the 13 to 15 mg/kg/day employed in the English and Australian studies, which may partly explain the lower efficacy in this study. Another possible reason for the poor results in the American study was the exclusion of females under the age of 40 years. Younger women have a high prevalence of small radiolucent stones, which are particularly susceptible to dissolution treatment.

The results of these studies indicate that even in carefully selected patients, prolonged therapy with CDCA is often unsuccessful in achieving complete gallstone dissolution. Nevertheless, with careful selection of patients, an acceptable rate of dissolution can be attained.

Common Duct Stones. There is little information about the efficacy of CDCA for the treatment of radiolucent stones in the common bile duct, presumably because most patients are symptomatic or have bile duct obstruction and require surgical or endoscopic intervention. Nevertheless, common duct stones occasionally dissolve during therapy with CDCA,[103] although the results are less predictable than with gallbladder stones. CDCA may be useful in patients with recurrent intrahepatic cholesterol stones as an alternative to multiple and hazardous surgical procedures.

Factors Influencing Response to CDCA

Chemical Composition of Stones. As expected from the mechanism of action of CDCA, stones low in cholesterol content are not suitable for dissolution therapy with this agent. However, there is potential error in assuming that all radiolucent stones are rich in cholesterol. This error, estimated to be between 14 and 20 per cent,[104, 105] must account for some treatment failures. In a study of the gallstones of 14 patients who had been unsuccessfully treated with CDCA for at least 6 months, it was found that the stones of two patients were pigment in type.[27] Although there is at present no completely accurate way of distinguishing patients with cholesterol stones from those with pigment stones, careful analysis of radiographic features[106] and microscopic examination of duodenal bile for cholesterol crystals or pigment granules[73, 107] may help.

Apart from pigment stones, it is also possible that some radiolucent gallstones of high cholesterol content will not respond to treatment owing to the presence of calcium salts on their surface.[27]

Size of the Stones. It would be expected that stone size influences the dissolution rate, because the larger the stone, the smaller the surface available for dissolution in relation to stone volume. This proposition has been confirmed in all reported studies.

The efficacy of CDCA in stones greater than 15 mm in diameter is so poor and the time taken for dissolution so long that, except in unusual circumstances, dissolution therapy should not be contemplated. Large stones are older than small stones, are more likely to contain calcium-rich rings inhibiting dissolution, and also contain more tightly packed cholesterol.[108]

Floating Stones. Small stones that float in the gallbladder (as seen on oral cholecystography) are composed of cholesterol and dissolve more readily than other radiolucent stones.[100]

Dose of CDCA. Although there may be individual variations in response to CDCA, the overall response is dose-related.[100] A dose of 13 to 15 mg/kg/day is believed to be optimal.[88, 89] At this dose, a small proportion of patients have troublesome diarrhea.

Duration of Therapy. Provided that the stones are capable of being dissolved, a response to therapy is almost always observed after 6 to 9 months of treatment.[97, 100, 102] Treatment should not be continued unless there is a definite reduction in stone volume after 9 months.

Obesity. Obesity may lead to difficulty with bile desaturation and dissolution of stones. Dosage schedules that are based on body weight have recognized this "resistance" to chenodeoxycholic acid therapy in the overweight patient. Some patients greater than 130 per cent of ideal body weight had supersaturated bile even if chenodeoxycholic acid were given at 15 mg/kg/day.[97] Higher doses may be necessary in these individuals.[90]

Hypertriglyceridemia. There may be a relationship between systemic triglyceride metabolism and biliary lipids that influences the response to CDCA therapy. The ability of CDCA to lower bile cholesterol saturation correlated with the presence of hypertriglyceridemia in one study.[109] However, this finding was not confirmed in the United States National Cooperative Gallstone Study.[100]

Recurrence of Gallstones After Dissolution and its Prevention

It is predictable that gallstones should recur after cessation of CDCA, as nothing has been done to influence the abnormal mechanisms leading to their formation. Reported recurrence rates are presented in Table 4–6. These recurrent stones may be redissolved by further treatment of CDCA in full therapeutic doses, as intermittent or low-dose therapy appears to be ineffective in maintaining unsaturated bile.[110] Dietary modification, including decreased caloric intake or addition of bran to the diet,[111, 112] may be useful to prevent recurrence, but the effect of these measures is unproven. It is impossible to justify lifelong chenodeoxycholic acid treatment on economic grounds, and unless simpler measures, such as dietary manipulation, can be shown to be effective in preventing recurrence, this will seriously limit the usefulness of oral dissolution therapy. In the future, it may be possible to identify those patients in whom stones will recur, either by bile analysis or by some form of assessment of gallbladder function.

Table 4–6 RECURRENCE OF GALLSTONES AFTER DISSOLUTION WITH CDCA

Series	Duration of Follow-up	Number of Patients Studied	Number of Patients With Recurrence
Thistle et al[88] (1978)	6–48 months	15	3
Iser et al[89] (1975)	12 months	10	5
Beker[95] (1977)	6 months	9	2
Ruppin and Dowling[101] (1982)	7½ years	54	25
Collected series		98	35

Side Effects of CDCA

Diarrhea. This is by far the most common side effect of oral CDCA treatment and occurs in more than half the treated patients. It is dose-related and always responds to temporary cessation of treatment. The severity of diarrhea is rarely sufficient to stop treatment, but some patients need constant encouragement to persist, particularly during the first few weeks. Ultimately, adaptation usually occurs, and diarrhea may cease altogether or occur episodically for a few hours every 10 to 14 days.

The cause of diarrhea is unabsorbed bile acid in the colon; this occurs when the ability of the small intestine to absorb bile acid is exceeded. Presumably, lessening of diarrhea after a time is related to more efficient bile acid absorption in the terminal ileum.

Abnormal Liver Function Tests. When chenodeoxycholic acid therapy was introduced, there was considerable anxiety that this bile acid or its bacterial metabolite, lithocholic acid, might cause liver damage in man. Lithocholic acid is very toxic to the liver in many animal species,[113] but in man it undergoes sulfation,[114, 115] which is probably responsible for its lack of toxicity.

Up to one third of patients undergoing CDCA treatment show transient rises in the serum levels of hepatic transaminases. In the United States National Cooperative Gallstone Study,[100] clinically significant hepatotoxicity occurred in 3 per cent of patients on 750 mg/day CDCA. The mechanisms for these abnormalities are unknown, and histologic and electron microscopic studies have not revealed specific CDCA-related disease.[115–119] In vitro studies have demonstrated direct toxic effects of CDCA on hepatocytes. Another possibility is the ability of CDCA to deplete canalicular membranes of cholesterol.

It is usual for hepatic enzyme elevations to return toward normal despite continuation of the drug. Occasionally the elevated levels persist, and the drug should then be discontinued. Under these circumstances, it is important to remember that biliary obstruction may be responsible for these biochemical abnormalities.

The effect of CDCA on the liver of the human fetus is unknown, and CDCA is therefore contraindicated in women capable of becoming pregnant. Studies in pregnant rhesus monkeys receiving high doses of CDCA demonstrated that this bile acid, or lithocholic acid, may cross the placenta and produce severe damage to the fetal monkey liver.[120]

Changes in Fasting Serum Lipids. Since CDCA suppresses the catabolism of cholesterol to bile acids, it was predicted that prolonged administration might lead to hypercholesterolemia and increased atherosclerosis.[121] A 10 per cent increase in serum LDL cholesterol levels was detected in the large multi-institutional United States trial, but other studies have failed to show changes.[100, 122] Fasting levels of serum triglyceride are lowered during CDCA therapy.[123–125]

Other Effects. Many patients undergoing dissolution treatment with CDCA are agreeably surprised at the improvement in their symptoms. Not only is there a reduction in the frequency of biliary pain, but also a reduction in the frequency of the common minor gastrointestinal symptoms (for example, bloating, flatulence, and intolerance of fatty foods), which are commonly ascribed by the patient to gallstones. However, the United States National Cooperative Gallstone Study[100] revealed no difference in the frequency of biliary pain, dyspepsia, or nausea between patients treated with CDCA and placebo. It is therefore likely that the symptomatic improvement during CDCA treatment is simply a placebo effect.

CDCA has now been used in man for more than 10 years, and no serious long-term side effects have been encountered. There is no evidence that the frequency of gastrointestinal or hepatobiliary cancer is increased in patients who have had prolonged treatment with CDCA.

Supervision During CDCA Therapy

Minimal patient supervision is necessary during therapy. It is usually sufficient to see the patient only 1 month after starting treatment and then at approximately 2-month intervals.

An investigation plan for patients undergoing gallstone dissolution is shown in Table 4–7. Before treatment is started, liver function tests are performed, and the patient is instructed to increase the dose gradually to the prescribed level over several days. If diarrhea occurs, one or more doses of the drug are omitted. At 1 month, liver function tests are repeated. If transaminase levels are raised to more than twice normal, they are measured again after another 2 weeks, and treatment is discontinued if elevated levels persist.

It would be valuable to be able to monitor the effectiveness of therapy by obtaining pre- and post-treatment samples of fasting gallbladder bile by duodenal intubation and stimulation of the gallbladder by intravenous cholecystokinin. However, this test is not tolerated by most patients, and the dose of CDCA selected is usually based on body weight.

Table 4–7 INVESTIGATION PLAN FOR PATIENTS UNDERGOING DISSOLUTION THERAPY WITH ORAL CDCA OR UDCA

Investigation	Before Treatment	4–6 Weeks	6 Months	12 Months
Oral cholegram	+	–	+	*
Ultrasound study of gallbladder	+	–	+	+
Liver function tests	+	+	+	+
Bile sampling (microscopy and saturation index)	*	*	–	–

* = the investigation is optional.

It can be useful to obtain a pretreatment sample of fasting gallbladder bile for analysis in order to exclude some patients who are likely to have pigment stones. If pigment granules are found on microscopy and the bile saturation index is less than unity, the chances of the stones being composed of cholesterol are less than 50 per cent.[107, 126] Conversely, the finding of cholesterol crystals in the bile indicates a 99 per cent probability that the stones are cholesterol in type.[107] The finding of a saturation index of less than unity in the presence of multiple small radiolucent stones indicates that these stones are more likely to be composed of pigment.[126] Estimation of the saturation index of fasting duodenal bile after several weeks of CDCA treatment may indicate an inadequate dose of bile acid, especially in an obese patient.[90] However, the saturation index is subject to considerable biologic variation,[92] and this must be borne in mind in interpreting changes in saturation index values.

Patient compliance during CDCA treatment can be monitored by analyzing serum for its CDCA content relative to the other bile acids and predicting the percentage of CDCA present in gallbladder bile.[127] When bile contains greater than 70 per cent CDCA, it is usually unsaturated with cholesterol. This method has the advantage of avoiding duodenal intubation, but it does require a specialized laboratory to perform the bile acid analysis.

Ursodeoxycholic Acid

Ursodeoxycholic acid (L., ursus = bear) was first isolated in the bile of polar bears in 1902.[128] Bear bile has been given for many gastrointestinal and hepatic ailments in Japan and has been credited with making gallstones disappear.

Ursodeoxycholic acid (UDCA), the 7β epimer of CDCA, normally occurs in low concentrations in human bile. The proportion of UDCA in human bile increases in some patients during CDCA therapy, sometimes up to 51 per cent of the bile acid pool.[129–131] UDCA becomes the major bile acid in human bile after its oral administration, and the concentration reached is dose-related.[130–133]

The first therapeutic trial of UDCA in man was carried out by Makino in 1975.[134] He reported success in dissolving radiolucent gallstones in five of nine patients who were treated for 4 to 12 months.

Mechanism of Action

Experimental studies with UDCA in the rhesus monkey indicated that its mechanism of action on bile cholesterol saturation may be similar to that of CDCA.[135] There was a similar suppression of hepatic HMGCoA reductase after both UDCA and CDCA, which was thought to indicate reduction in cholesterol synthesis and excretion into bile. UDCA, unlike CDCA, was not hepatotoxic in this species and produced no rise in biliary lithocholic acid.

Administration of UDCA in man was also found to suppress HMGCoA reductase in some experiments[84, 133] but to have no such effect in others.[136] UDCA produced a rise in biliary and plasma UDCA without an increase in biliary or plasma lithocholic acid.[137, 138] UDCA does not suppress bile acid synthesis from cholesterol as does CDCA, so absolute biliary output of cholic and chenodeoxycholate acids remains about the same after starting UDCA as during the pretreatment control period.[139, 140]

UDCA is a poor detergent in terms of cholesterol solubility capacity,[141] and the dissolution rate of cholesterol in vitro is significantly faster in CDCA solutions than in UDCA solution.[142] However, the results of clinical trials with UDCA indicate this bile acid to be comparable to CDCA with respect to cholesterol gallstone dissolution in vivo.[143] This paradox has been explained by in vitro studies[144] comparing cholesterol gallstone dissolution in bile acid–lecithin solutions. Cholesterol release from the gallstones into a lecithin-UDCA–containing medium continued far beyond the apparent equilibrium solubility in the isotropic phase by formation of a turbid liquid crystalline phase (mesophase). Ultimately the saturation index reaches about 140 per cent in UDCA solutions.[145, 146] In comparison, cholesterol release from stones in the lecithin-CDCA medium stopped once the micellar equilibrium solubility was reached.

Effective Dose

The dose of UDCA at which bile is consistently desaturated with cholesterol is approximately 5 mg/kg/day,[133, 143] although desaturation may occur with a dose as low as 1.9 mg/kg/day.[147] The optimal dose for gallstone dissolution is 8 to 10 mg/kg/day. However, definite dissolution responses have been observed at a dose as low as 150 mg/day (2.8 mg/kg/day).[147]

Results of Therapy with UDCA

Reports on clinical experience with UDCA to treat radiolucent gallstones are limited (Table 4–8). Ashizawa and his colleagues[132] treated 55 patients with radiolucent gallstones in a multicenter double-blind trial for an average of 5 months. Complete gallstone dissolution was observed in 29 per cent of 24 patients on 600 mg a day, 13 per cent of 16 patients on 150 mg a day, and 7 per cent of 15 patients on placebo. The combined Japanese experience with UDCA at varying doses was summarized by Nakayama.[148] A total of 287 patients were treated with UDCA for varying lengths of time. There was complete dissolution of the stones in 53 patients and partial dissolution in 63 patients, an overall response rate of 40 per cent. The results are similar to those obtained with CDCA.

In a double-blind controlled trial comparing CDCA and UDCA,[149] the latter drug produced better results after 12 months of therapy (UDCA, 30 per cent complete and 30 per cent partial dissolution; CDCA, 7 per cent complete and 40 per cent partial dissolution). Erlinger and coworkers[150] reported a 29 per cent rate of gallstone dissolution after 1 year of UDCA therapy (8.4 mg/kg/day), similar to the experience of Neligan and coworkers.[151] There is some evidence that a combination of CDCA and UDCA may be more effective than equivalent doses of either drug alone.[152]

Side Effects of UDCA

Side effects of UDCA are uncommon. Diarrhea occurs rarely, even with high doses, possibly because UDCA has a much lower water solubility than does CDCA.[153]

Abnormalities in liver transaminases, serum cholesterol, or serum triglyceride have not been observed during UDCA therapy.[132–134, 147, 154, 168] The explanation may be related to the lower micellar capacity for cholesterol of UDCA, with resultant decreased effects on canalicular membranes.

UDCA in Gallstone Dissolution Therapy

UDCA is about as effective as CDCA in dissolving gallstones, but without any of the major side effects of CDCA. It is more expensive at equivalent doses than CDCA, because it is synthesized from this bile acid.

Other Possible Oral Dissolution Agents

Rowachol

Rowachol is a proprietary choleretic consisting of a mixture of monoterpene compounds. It has been advocated for gallstone dissolution by Bell and his colleagues, who reported a response rate of 7 of 24 patients (29 per cent) in 6 months when the preparation was given alone,[155] and 13 of 22 patients (59 per cent) when it was given in combination with CDCA at 375 mg/day for 12 months.[156] Common duct stones have also disappeared following treatment with Rowachol for up to 12 months.[156, 157] These results need to be confirmed by other studies to fully assess the potential of this agent.

Dietary Manipulation

The role of the diet in the cause and prevention of gallstones is unclear, because it is so difficult to carry out experiments

Table 4–8 RESULTS OF TREATMENT WITH UDCA FROM PUBLISHED CLINICAL TRIALS

Author	Number of Patients	Dose (mg/day)	Complete Dissolution	Partial Dissolution	Total Response
Makino et al.[134] (1975)	9	450–2000	5	0	5
Ashizawa et al.[132] (1977)	24	600	7 (29%)	3 (13%)	10 (42%)
	16	150	2 (13%)	1 (6%)	3 (19%)
	15	Placebo	1 (7%)	0	1 (7%)
Nakagawa et al.[147] (1977)	15	600	2 (13%)	0	2 (13%)
	16	150	3 (19%)	3 (19%)	6 (38%)
	13	Placebo	0	0	0
Nakayama[148] (1980) Combined Japanese Trial	287	150–2000	53 (19%)	63 (22%)	116 (40%)
Tint et al.[154] (1981)	18	1000	—	—	15 (85%)
	18	500	—	—	12 (69%)
	17	250	—	—	11 (62%)

involving dietary manipulations for long periods in large groups of people. No therapeutic trials on gallstone dissolution have been carried out using dietary manipulation alone. However, fiber-enriched diets[111, 112] reduce the cholesterol saturation of supersaturated bile and may therefore be usefully combined with therapeutic agents such as chenodeoxycholic acid or used to prevent recurrent stones after successful dissolution. Maudgal and colleagues claim that a low-cholesterol diet enhances the effect of CDCA in patients with gallstones.[158]

Glycerophosphate

This substance, which is a phospholipid precursor, was reported to improve cholesterol solubility in bile when fed orally to patients with supersaturated bile,[159] but this was not confirmed in a later study.[160] There is no evidence that this substance can lead to gallstone dissolution.

Phospholipids

Although large doses of lecithin may improve cholesterol solubility,[161] there is no evidence that oral lecithin alone can lead to gallstone dissolution. The combination of essential phospholipids with cholic acid has been reported to reduce cholesterol saturation and possibly to dissolve gallstones,[162] but this combination is unlikely to be as effective as chenodeoxycholic acid alone.

Phenobarbitone

Phenobarbitone induces microsomal enzymes and affects bile acid synthesis by inducing cholesterol 7α-hydroxylase. Phenobarbitone was found to increase the cholesterol-holding ability of human bile but was ineffective in dissolving gallstones.

Phenobarbitone has also been used in combination with chenodeoxycholic acid, but there is no evidence that this combination accelerates either the unsaturating effect or the dissolution rate over that observed with chenodeoxycholic acid alone.[88]

Choline

Choline is a component of the biliary lecithin molecule. Oral administration of choline alone did not induce desaturation of bile, nor did choline in combination with chenodeoxycholic acid enhance the unsaturating effect of CDCA alone.[88]

β-Sitosterol

β-Sitosterol competes for cholesterol-binding sites in the intestine. It may desaturate bile by reducing cholesterol absorption and therefore biliary cholesterol excretion. Administration of large doses of this substance to patients with gallstones did not produce unsaturated bile.[88] In combination with chenodeoxycholic acid, however, β-sitosterol appeared to enhance the effect of the former.[163] Whether this finding is of clinical importance is as yet unknown.

Clofibrate

This compound inhibits cholesterol synthesis, but in man it increases the saturation of bile[43, 79] and is therefore unsuitable for gallstone dissolution.

Thyroid Hormones

Thyroid hormones increase primary bile acid synthesis and increase the amount of chenodeoxycholic acid in bile.[165] Their effect on bile cholesterol saturation is unknown.

Cholic Acid

On theoretical grounds, cholic acid feeding should increase the bile acid pool, increase both biliary bile acid and phospholipid output more than biliary cholesterol output, and therefore desaturate bile. However, feeding cholic acid increases the proportion of cholic acid in the bile acid pool, inhibits bile acid synthesis, and leaves the saturation index of bile unchanged. No evidence of gallstone dissolution was found in 17 patients with radiolucent stones who were treated with cholic acid for 1 year.[88]

Without doubt, many other agents will be investigated for gallstone dissolution in the future. The most promising approach, however, appears to be the investigation of adjuvant accelerators to cholesterol dissolution that are absorbed orally and excreted in the bile. Compounds such as steroidal amines and the bile acid derivatives containing the amine nitrogen or the quaternary nitrogen functional groups require investigation.[166]

FACTORS INFLUENCING RESPONSE TO DISSOLUTION AGENTS

The factors influencing cholesterol gallstone dissolution with CDCA or UDCA in man are shown in Figure 4–8.[88] The biologic factors leading to unsaturated bile depend on patient compliance and intestinal absorption of an adequate dose of bile acid. Desaturation is usually not difficult to achieve except in obese patients.[90]

The physical factors involved in dissolution depend on the stone type and composition and on the ability of the unsaturated bile to obtain access to the stone. The factors involved in stone dissolution in unsaturated bile are the surface-volume ratio of the stones and the interfacial barriers.

SELECTION OF PATIENTS FOR DISSOLUTION THERAPY

It is probably unnecessary to treat all patients found to have gallstones, but a patient found to have radiolucent stones at cholecystography usually has had enough symptoms to justify the investigation and therefore requires treatment. The alternative to dissolution treatment for symptomatic gallstones is surgery, which today can be carried out with minimal mortality and morbidity and with only temporary inconvenience to the patient.

For gallstone dissolution to be contemplated, the following conditions should apply.

1. Patients of any age or sex can be treated, but females capable of becoming pregnant must have adequate contraception. Obvious candidates for dissolution therapy are patients with radiolucent stones who have cardiac or pulmonary disease severe enough to make surgery hazardous. Information about recurrence rates and prevention of recurrence after successful dissolution in the young patient is not available. However, many young patients, especially females, have small cholesterol stones that dissolve readily, so further studies on this group are justified.

2. The patient must not have severe and persistent symptoms. This requirement is not absolute, as symptoms often improve after taking CDCA.

3. The patient must comply with treatment and be prepared to take tablets for a minimum of 6 to 9 months, at which point response to treatment is first assessed.

4. The stones must be radiolucent, and the largest stone must not exceed 1.5 cm. The gallbladder must opacify on oral cholecystectomy, indicating a patent cystic duct and the ability of the gallbladder mucosa to concentrate bile.

5. There must be a reasonable expectation that the stones are cholesterol in type. The most reliable indicators are floating stones on oral cholecystography and the presence of cholesterol crystals in a fasting sample of gallbladder bile obtained after duodenal intubation.

WHAT IS THE IMPACT OF DISSOLUTION THERAPY ON GALLSTONE DISEASE?

Gallstone dissolution therapy has a limited place in the management of patients with gallstone disease. The proportion of individuals suitable for dissolution treatment is illustrated by an analysis of 406 symptomatic patients who presented with gallbladder stones over a 30-month period to Flinders Medical Centre, a community general hospital in South Australia.[167]

Cholecystectomy was performed in 387, and 19 were treated by oral chenodeoxycholic acid. Only 43 out of 406 gallstone patients (11 per cent) had functioning gallbladders that contained radiolucent stones 1 cm or less in diameter. The stones of 33 of these patients were analyzed, and 25 (76 per cent) had a cholesterol content greater than 80 per cent. Therefore, only between 5 and 10 per cent of all symptomatic gallstone patients presenting to the hospital had functioning gallbladders containing stones with

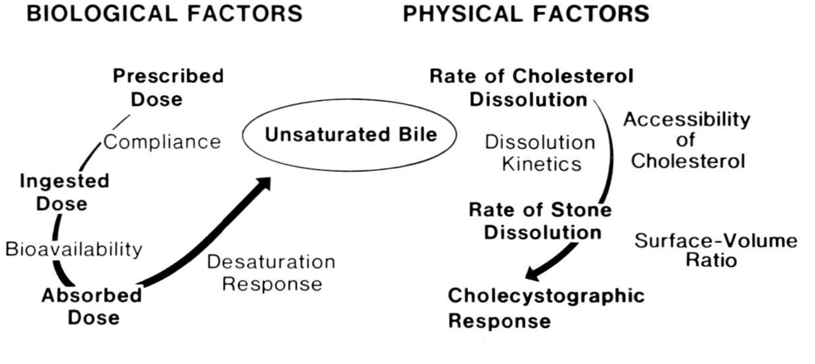

Figure 4–8. The biologic and physical factors involved in gallstone dissolution by chenodeoxycholic acid or ursodeoxycholic acid.

the physical and chemical characteristics required for successful dissolution.

THE FUTURE OF GALLSTONE DISSOLUTION

Most research effort should be directed at the detection of those patients at high risk for developing gallstones and the development of effective methods of prevention. It seems unlikely that the economics of bile acid therapy will allow it to be used for preventive treatment. Elective biliary tract surgery is now so safe that for any method of prevention to be justified it must be cheap and effective, and this is simply not the case with CDCA or UDCA.

Dissolution therapy will be much more attractive if it can be made to work faster. Additives to bile acid therapy are of interest and the most promising approach is the use of accelerating substances that decrease the interfacial resistance to dissolution.[166] Recently, dissolution of gallstones has been achieved in a few hours by direct infusion of an ether solvent into the gallbladder and aspiration of the dissolved cholesterol via a percutaneous catheter.[169] This direct approach is under further investigation to establish its safety. There are no known dissolving agents for black pigment stones, but this is not surprising, since very little is known about their chemical composition or why they occur.

REFERENCES

1. Rains AJH: Gallstones: Causes and Treatment. London, Heinemann Medical, 1964.
2. Graham EA, Cole WH: Roentgenologic examination of the gallbladder: preliminary report of a new method utilizing the injection of tetrabromphenolthalein. JAMA 1924;*82:*613.
3. Rewbridge AG: Disappearance of gallstone shadows following prolonged administration of bile salts. Surgery 1937;*1:*395.
4. Danzinger RG, Hofmann AF, Schoenfield LJ, et al: Dissolution of cholesterol gallstones by chenodeoxycholic acid. N Engl J Med 1972;*286:*1.
5. Friedman GD, Kannel WB, Dawber TR: The epidemiology of gallbladder disease: observations in the Framingham study. J Chronic Dis 1966;*19:*273.
6. Bainton D, Davies GT, Evans KT, et al: Gallbladder disease. Prevalence in a South Wales industrial town. N Engl J Med 1976;*294:*1147.
7. Brett M, Barker DJ: The world distribution of gallstones. Int J Epidemiol 1976;*5:*335.
8. Soloway RD, Trotman BW, Ostrow JD: Pigment gallstones. Gastroenterology 1977;*72:*167.
9. Ostrow JD: The etiology of pigment gallstones. Hepatology 1984;*4:*215s.
10. Soloway RD, Fayusal EB, Trotman BW, Weston NE, Ficca JF: Water content of gallstones: Location and contribution to a hypothesis concerning stone structure. Hepatology 1982;*2:*223.
11. Lamont JT, Ventola AS, Trotman BW, Soloway RD: Mucin glycoprotein content of human pigment gallstones. Hepatology 1983;*3:*377.
12. Wosiewitz U, Schroebler S: On the chemistry of "black' pigment stones from the gallbladder. Clin Chim Acta 1978;*89:*1.
13. Ohkubo H, Ostrow JD, Carr SH, Rege RV: Polymer networks in pigment and cholesterol gallstones assessed by equilibrium swelling and infrared spectroscopy. Gastroenterology 1984;*87:*805.
14. Boonyapisit ST, Trotman BW, Ostrow JD: Unconjugated bilirubin, and the hydrolysis of conjugated bilirubin, in gallbladder bile of patients with cholelithiasis. Gastroenterology 1978;*74:*70.
15. Wagner CI, Trotman BW, Soloway RD: Biliary lipid excretion in patients with pigment gallstones. Am J Dig Dis 1978;*23:*85.
16. Maki T: Pathogenesis of calcium bilirubinate gallstones: role of *E. coli*, beta-glucuronidase and coagulation by inorganic ions, polyelectrolytes and agitation. Ann Surg 1966;*164:*90.
17. Ong GB: A study of recurrent pyogenic cholangitis. Arch Surg 1962;*84:*199.
18. Matsushiro T, Suzuki N, Sato T, et al: Effects of diet on glucaric acid concentration in bile and the formation of calcium bilirubinate gallstones. Gastroenterology 1977;*72:*630.
19. Trotman BW, Soloway RD: Pigment vs cholesterol cholelithiasis: clinical and epidemiological aspects. Am J Dig Dis 1975;*20:*735.
20. Nagase M, Tanimura H, Setoyama M, Hikasa Y: Present features of gallstones in Japan. Am J Surg 1978;*135:*788.
21. Watts JMcK, Whiting MJ, Bradley B, et al: The chemical composition of common bile duct stones. Int Biliary Assoc Meeting, New York, 1981 (Abstract).
22. Bernhoft RA, Pellegrini CA, Motson RW, Way LW: Composition and morphologic and clinical features of common duct stones. Am J Surg 1984;*148:*77.
23. Nicholas P, Rinaudo PA, Conn HO: Increased incidence of cholelithiasis in Laennec's cirrhosis. Gastroenterology 1972;*63:*112.
24. Sutor DJ, Wooley SE: A statistical survey of the composition of gallstones in eight countries. Gut 1971;*12:*55.
25. Bogren H: The composition and structure of human gallstones. Acta Radiol (Diagn) (Stockh) Suppl 1964;*266:*1.
26. Womack NA, Zeppa R, Irvin GL 3d: The anatomy of gallstones. Ann Surg 1963;*157:*670.
27. Whiting MJ, Jarvinen V, Watts JMcK: Chemical composition of gallstones resistant to dissolution therapy with chenodeoxycholic acid. Gut 1980;*21:*1077.
28. Smith BF, LaMont JT: Identification of gallbladder mucin-bilirubin complex in human cholesterol gallstone matrix. J Clin Invest 1985;*76:*439.
29. McBain JW: Mobility of highly charged micelles. Trans Faraday Soc 1913;*9:*99.
30. Admirand WH, Small DM: The physiochemical basis of cholesterol gallstone formation in man. J Clin Invest 1968;*47:*1043.

31. Hegardt FG, Dam H: The solubility of cholesterol in aqueous solutions of bile salts and lecithin. Z Ernahrungswiss 1971;*10:*223.
32. Holzbach RE, Marsh M, Holan K: Cholesterol solubilizing capacity: A direct assessment of lithogenic potential in bile. Gastroenterology 1971; *60:*777 (Abstract).
33. Carey MC, Small DM: The physical chemistry of cholesterol solubility in bile. J Clin Invest 1978;*61:*998.
34. Somjen GJ, Gilat T: Contribution of vesicular and micellar carriers to cholesterol transport in human bile. J Lipid Res 1985;*26:*699.
35. Gilat T, Somjen GJ: Why does cholesterol ever precipitate out of human bile? J Clin Gastroenterol 1985;*7:*197.
36. Metzger AL, Heymsfield S, Grundy SM: The lithogenic index—a numerical expression for the relative lithogenicity of bile. Gastroenterology 1972;*62:*449.
37. Thomas PJ, Hofman AF: A simple calculation of the lithogenic index of bile: expressing biliary lipid composition on rectangular coordinates. Gastroenterology 1973;*65:*698 (Letter).
38. Shaffer EA, Small DM: Biliary lipid secretion in cholesterol gallstone disease. The effect of cholecystectomy and obesity. J Clin Invest 1977;*59:*828.
39. Sarles H, Gerolami A, Cros RC: Diet and cholesterol gallstones. A multicentre study. Digestion 1978;*17:*121.
40. DenBesten L, Connor WE, Bell S: The effect of dietary cholesterol on the composition of human bile. Surgery 1973;*73:*266.
41. Watanabe N, Gimbel NS, Johnston CG: Effect of polyunsaturated and saturated fatty acids on the cholesterol holding capacity of human bile. Arch Surg 1962;*85:*136.
42. Sturdevant RA, Pearce ML, Dayton S: Increased prevalence of cholelithiasis in man ingesting a serum-cholesterol–lowering diet. N Engl J Med 1973;*288:*24.
43. Pertsemlidis D, Panvelwalla D, Ahrens EH Jr: Effects of clofibrate and of an estrogen-progestin combination on fasting biliary lipids and cholic acid kinetics in man. Gastroenterology 1974;*66:*565.
44. Bennion LJ, Mott DM, Howard BV: Oral contraceptives raise the cholesterol saturation of bile by increasing biliary cholesterol secretion. Metabolism 1980;*29:*18.
45. Grundy SM, Metzger AL, Adler RD: Mechanisms of lithogenic bile formation in American Indian women with cholesterol gallstones. J Clin Invest 1972;*51:*3026.
46. Salen G, Nicolau G, Shefer S, Mosbach EH: Hepatic cholesterol metabolism in patients with gallstones. Gastroenterology 1975;*69:*676.
47. Goldstein LI, Schoenfield LJ: Gallstones: pathogenesis and medical treatment. Adv Intern Med 1975;*20:*89.
48. Cohen S, Kaplan M, Gottlieb L, et al: Liver disease and gallstones in regional enteritis. Gastroenterology 1971;*60:*237.
49. Heaton KW, Read AE: Gallstones in patients with disorders of the terminal ileum and disturbed bile salt metabolism. Br Med J 1969;*3:*494.
50. Small DM: The formation and treatment of gallstones. *In* Schiff L (ed): Diseases of the Liver, 4th ed. Philadelphia, JB Lippincott 1975.
51. Mok HY, Von Bergmann K, Grundy SM: Regulation of pool size of bile acids in man. Gastroenterology 1977;*73:*684.
52. Simmons F, Ross AP, Bouchier IA: Alterations in hepatic bile composition after cholecystectomy. Gastroenterology 1972;*63:*466.
53. Nakayama F, van der Linden W: Role of gallbladder in gallstone formation. Acta Chir Scand 1974;*140:*45.
54. van der Linden W, Nakayama F: Occurrence of cholesterol crystals in human bile. Gut 1974; *15:*630.
55. Antsaklis G, Lewin MR, Sutor DJ, et al: Gallbladder function, cholesterol stones, and bile composition. Gut 1975;*16:*937.
56. Redinger RN: The effect of loss of gallbladder function on biliary lipid composition in subjects with cholesterol gallstones. Gastroenterology 1976;*71:*470.
57. Braverman DZ, Johnson ML, Kern F: Effects of pregnancy and contraceptive steroids on gallbladder function. N Engl J Med 1980;*302:*362.
58. Gerdes MM, Boyden EA: Rate of emptying of human gallbladder in pregnancy. Surg Gynecol Obstet 1938;*66:*145.
59. DiMagno EP, Go WL, Summerskill WH: Impaired cholecystokinin-pancreozymin secretion, intraluminal dilution and maldigestion of fat in sprue. Gastroenterology 1972;*63:*25.
60. Low-Beer TS, Heaton KW, Heaton ST, et al: Gallbladder inertia and sluggish enterohepatic circulation of bile salts in coeliac disease. Lancet 1971;*1:*991.
61. Rudick J, Hutchinson JSF: Effects of vagal nerve section on the biliary system. Lancet 1964;*1:*579.
62. Holzbach RT: Factors influencing cholesterol nucleation in bile. Hepatology 1984;*4:*173S.
63. Pomeranz IS, Shaffer EA: Abnormal gallbladder emptying in a subgroup of patients with gallstones. Gastroenterology 1985;*88:*787.
64. Pitt HA, Roslyn JJ, Kuchenbecker SL, Doty JE, DenBesten L: The role of cystic duct resistance in the pathogenesis of cholesterol gallstones. J Surg Res 1981;*30:*508.
65. Lee SP, Lamont T, Carey MC: Role of gallbladder mucus hypersecretion in the evolution of cholesterol gallstones. J Clin Invest 1981;*67:*1712.
66. Redinger RN, Strasberg SM, Small DM: Primate biliary physiology. IX. Effects of obstruction on biliary lipid metabolism in the monkey. Am J Physiol 1974;*226:*776.
67. Holzbach RT, Marsh M, Olszewski M, et al: Cholesterol solubility in bile. Evidence that supersaturated bile in frequent in healthy man. J Clin Invest 1973;*52:*1467.
68. Metzger AL, Adler R, Heymsfield S, Grundy SM: Diurnal variation in biliary lipid composition. N Engl J Med 1973;*288:*333.
69. Duane WC, Ginsberg RL, Bennion LJ: Effects of fasting on bile acid metabolism and biliary lipid composition in man. J Lipid Res 1976;*17:*211.
70. Bloch HM, Thornton JR, Heaton KW: Effects of fasting on the composition of gallbladder bile. Gut 1980;*21:*1087.
71. Small DM, Rapo S: Source of abnormal bile in patients with cholesterol gallstones. N Engl J Med 1970;*283:*53.
72. Holan KR, Holzbach RT, Hermann RE, et al: Nucleation time: a key factor in the pathogenesis of cholesterol gallstone disease. Gastroenterology 1979;*77:*611.
73. Sedaghat A, Grundy SM: Cholesterol crystals and the formation of cholesterol gallstones. N Engl J Med 1980;*302:*1274.

74. Burnstein MJ, Ilson RG, Petrunka CN, Taylor RD, Strasbert SM: Evidence for a potent nucleating factor in the gallbladder bile of patients with cholesterol gallstones. Gastroenterology 1983;*85*:801.
75. Holzbach RT: Metastability behavior of supersaturated bile. Hepatology 1984;*4*:155S.
76. Holzbach RT, Kibe A, Thiel E, Howell JH, Marsh M, Hermann RE: Biliary protein: Unique inhibitors of cholesterol crystal nucleation in human gallbladder bile. J Clin Invest 1984;*73*:35.
77. Levy PF, Smith BF, LaMont JT: Human gallbladder mucin accelerates nucleation of cholesterol in artificial bile. Gastroenterology 1984;*87*.270.
78. Gallinger S, Taylor RD, Harvey PRC, Petrunka CN, Strasberg SM: Effect of mucous glycoprotein on nucleation time of human bile. Gastroenterology 1985;*89*:648.
79. Thistle JL, Schoenfield LJ: Induced alterations in composition of bile of persons having cholelithiasis. Gastroenterology 1971;*61*:488.
80. Bell GD, Whitney B, Dowling RH: Gallstone dissolution in man using chenodeoxycholic acid. Lancet 1972;*2*:1213.
81. Vlahcevic ZR, Bell CC Jr, Buhac I, et al: Diminished bile acid pool size in patients with gallstones. Gastroenterology 1970;*59*:165.
82. Andersen JM: Chenodeoxycholic acid desaturates bile—but how? Gastroenterology 1979;*77*:1146.
83. Coyne MJ, Bonorris GG, Godstein LI, et al: Effect of chenodeoxycholic acid and phenobarbital on the rate-limiting enzymes of hepatic cholesterol and bile acid synthesis in patients with gallstones. J Lab Clin Med 1976;*87*:281.
84. Maton PN, Ellis HJ, Higgins MJ, et al: Hepatic HMGCoA reductase in human cholelithiasis: effects of chenodeoxycholic and ursodeoxycholic acids. Eur J Clin Invest 1980;*10*:325.
85. Ponz de Leon M, Carulli N, Loric P, et al: The effect of chenodeoxycholic acid on cholesterol absorption in man. Gastroenterology 1979;*77*:223.
86. Marks JW, Bonorris GG, Chung A, Coyne MJ, Okun R, Lachin MJ, Schoenfield LJ: Feasibility of low-dose and intermittent chenodeoxycholic acid therapy of gallstones. Am J Dig Dis 1977;*22*:856.
87. Danzinger RG, Kurlas TK, Torchia MG: Low-dose chenodeoxycholic acid for gallstone dissolution: a randomised trial in poor operative risk patients. Dig Dis Sci 1980;*25*:785.
88. Thistle JL, Hofmann AF, Ott BJ, et al: Chenotherapy for gallstone dissolution. I. Efficacy and safety. JAMA 1978;*239*:1041.
89. Iser JH, Dowling RH, Mok HY, et al: Chenodeoxycholic acid treatment of gallstones. A follow-up report and analysis of factors influencing response to therapy. N Engl J Med 1975;*293*:378.
90. Iser JH, Maton PN, Murphy GM, Dowling RH: Resistance to chenodeoxycholic acid (CDCA) treatment in obese patients with gallstones. Br Med J 1978;*1*:1509.
91. LaRusso NF, Hoffman NE, Hofmann AF, et al: Effect of primary bile acid ingestion on bile acid metabolism and biliary lipid secretion in gallstone patients. Gastroenterology 1975;*69*:1301.
92. Whiting MJ, Down RH, Watts JMcK: Precision and accuracy in the measurement of the cholesterol saturation index of duodenal bile. Gastroenterology 1981;*80*:533.
93. Ponz de Leon M, Loria P, Carulli N, et al: Intestinal solubilisation, absorption, pharmacokinetics and bioavailability of chenodeoxycholic acid. Eur J Clin Invest 1980;*10*:261.
94. Maudgal DP, Bird R, Northfield TC: Optimal timing of doses of chenic acid in patients with gallstones. Br Med J 1979;*1*:922.
95. Beker S: Treatment of cholesterol gallstones with chenic acid. A follow-up study of 25 patients. Am J Gastroenterol 1977;*68*:456.
96. Bateson MC, Ross PE, Murison J, Bouchier IAD: Comparison of fixed doses of chenodeoxycholic acid for gallstone dissolution. Lancet 1978;*1*:111.
97. Maton PN, Iser JH, Reuben A, et al: Outcome of chenodeoxycholic acid treatment in 125 patients with radiolucent gallstones. Medicine 1982;*61*:86.
98. Barbara L, Roda E, Road A, et al: The medical treatment of cholesterol gallstones: experience with chenodeoxycholic acid. Digestion 1976;*14*:209.
99. Toouli J, Jablonski P, Watts JMcK: Treatment of gallstones by chenodeoxycholic acid. Med J Aust 1980;*1*:478.
100. Schoenfield LJ, Lachin JM, et al: Chenodiol (chenodeoxycholic acid) for dissolution of gallstones: the National Cooperative Gallstone Study. Ann Intern Med 1981;*95*:257.
101. Ruppin DC, Dowling RH: Is recurrence inevitable after gallstone dissolution by bile acid treatment? Lancet 1982;*1*:181.
102. Watts JMcK, Iser JH: Personal communication, 1982.
103. Sue SO, Taub M, Pearlman BJ, Marks JW, Bonorris GG, Schoenfield LJ: Treatment of choledocholelithiasis with oral chenodeoxycholic acid. Surgery 1981;*90*:32.
104. Bell GD, Dowling RH, Whitney B, et al: The value of radiology in predicting gallstone type when selecting patients for medical treatment. Gut 1975;*16*:359.
105. Trotman BW, Petrella EJ, Soloway RD, et al: Evaluation of radiographic lucency or opaqueness of gallstones as a means of identifying cholesterol or pigment stones. Correlation of lucency or opaqueness with calcium and mineral. Gastroenterology 1975;*68*:1563.
106. Dolgin SM, Schwartz JS, Kressel HY, et al: Identification of patients with cholesterol or pigment gallstones by discriminant analysis of radiographic features. N Engl J Med 1981;*304*:808.
107. Whiting MJ, Down RHL, Watts JMcK: Biliary crystals and granules, the cholesterol saturation index, and the prediction of gallstone type. Surg Gastroenterol 1982;*1*:17.
108. Wolpers C: Morphologie der Gallensteine. Leber Magen Darm 1974;*4*:43.
109. Bateson MC, Ross PE, Murison J, et al: Effect of prolonged feeding with chenodeoxycholic acid on bile in patients with and without gallstones. Gut 1977;*18*:599.
110. Iser JH, Murphy GM, Dowling RH: Speed of change in biliary lipids and bile acids with chenodeoxycholic acid—is intermittent therapy feasible? Gut 1977;*18*:7.
111. Pomare EW, Heaton KW, Low-Beer TS, et al: Effect of wheat bran on bile salt metabolism and bile composition. Gut 1974;*15*:824.
112. Watts JMcK, Jablonski P, Toouli J: The effect of added bran to the diet on the saturation of bile in people without gallstones. Am J Surg 1978; *135*:321.
113. Hunt RD, Leveille GA, Sauberlich HE: Dietary bile acids and lipid metabolism. II. Effects of lithocholic acid in mammalian species. Proc Soc Exp Biol Med 1964;*115*:277.
114. Palmer RH, Bolt MG: Bile acid sulphates. I. Syn-

thesis of lithocholic acid sulphates and their identification in human bile. J Lipid Res 1971;*12:*671.
115. Cowen AE, Korman MG, Hofmann AF, et al: Metabolism of lithocholate in healthy man. I. Biotransformation and biliary excretion of intravenously administered lithocholate, lithocholylglycine and their sulphates. Gasteroenterolgy 1975;*69:*59.
116. Coyne MJ, Bonorris GG, Chung A, et al: Treatment of gallstones with chenodeoxycholic acid and phenobarbital. N Engl J Med 1975;*292:*604.
117. Bouma ME, Levy VG, Infante R: Liver ultrastructure in cholesterolic gallstone patients before and after treatment with chenodeoxycholic acid. Gastroenterol Clin Biol 1980;*4:*569.
118. Hartmann W, Paulini K, Goebell H: Light and electron microscopy of human liver before and during chenodeoxycholic acid therapy. Hepatogastroenterology 1980;*27:*91.
119. Koch MM, Giampieri MP, Lorenzini K, Jezequel AM, Orlandi F: Effect of chenodeoxycholic acid on liver structure and function in man: a stereological and biochemical study. Digestion 1980;*20:*8.
120. Palmer AK, Heywood R: Pathological changes in the rhesus fetus associated with the oral administration of chenodeoxycholic acid. Toxicology 1974;*2:*239.
121. Small DM: Prestone gallstone disease—is therapy safe? N Engl J Med 1971;*284:*214.
122. Hoffman NE, Hofmann AF, Thistle J: Effects of bile acid feeding on cholesterol metabolism in gallstone patients. Mayo Clin Proc 1974;*49:*236.
123. Miller NE, Nestel PJ: Triglyceride-lowering effect of chenodeoxycholic acid in patients with endogenous hypertriglyceridemia. Lancet 1974;*2:*929.
124. Angelin B, Einarsson K, Leijd B: Effect of chenodeoxycholic acid on serum and biliary lipids in patients with hyperlipoproteinaemia. Clin Sci 1978;*54:*451.
125. Camarri E, Fici F, Marcolongo R: Influence of chenodeoxycholic acid on serum triglycerides in patients with primary hypertriglyceridemia. Int J Clin Pharmacol Biopharm 978;*16:*523.1
126. Bruusgaard A, Malver E, Pedersen LR, et al: Criteria for selection of patients for medical treatment (chenodeoxycholic acid therapy) of gallstones. Scand J Gastroenterol 1977;*12:*97.
127. Whiting MJ, Watts JMcK: Prediction of the bile acid composition of bile from serum bile acid analysis during gallstone dissolution therapy. Gastroenterology 1980;*78:*220.
128. Hammarsten O: Untersuchungen uber die Galle einiger Polar-thiere. I. Ueber die Galle des Eisbaren. Physiol Chem 1902;*36:*525.
129. Fromm H, Erbler HC, Eschler A, Schmidt FW: Alterations of bile acid metabolism during treatment with chenodeoxycholic acid. Studies of the role of the appearance of ursodeoxycholic acid in the dissolution of gallstones. Klin Wochenschr 1976;*54:*1125.
130. Stiehl A, Raedsch R, Rudolph G, Walker S: Effect of ursodeoxycholic acid on biliary bile acid and bile lipid composition in gallstone patients. Hepatology 1984;*4:*107.
131. von Bergmann K, Epple-Gutsfeld M, Leiss O: Differences in the effects of chenodeoxycholic and ursodeoxycheolic acid on biliary lipid secretion and bile acid synthesis in patients with gallstones. Gastroenterology 1984;*87:*136.
132. Ashizawa S, Ishii N, Ishihara F, Ito Y, Ueno Y, Osawa H, Osuga T, et al: A clinical study of gallstone dissolution with ursodeoxycholic acid. A controlled double blind trial. Igaku No Ayumi 1977;*101:*922.
133. Maton PN, Murphy GM, Dowling RH: Ursodeoxycholic acid treatment of gallstones. Dose-response study and possible mechanism of action. Lancet 1977;*2:*1297.
134. Makino I, Shinozaki K, Yoshinok, Nakagawa SS: Dissolution of cholesterol gallstones by ursodeoxycholic acid. Jpn J Gastroenterol 1975;*72:*690.
135. Fedorowski T, Salen G, Zaki FG, et al: Comparative effects of ursodeoxycholic acid and chenodeoxycholic acid in the Rhesus monkey: Biochemical and ultrastructural studies. Gastroenterology 1978;*74:*75.
136. Angelin B, Ewerth S, Einarsson K: Ursodeoxycholic acid treatment in cholesterol gallstone disease: effects on hepatic 3-hydroxy-3-methylglautaryl coenzyme A reductase activity, biliary lipid composition, and plasma lipid levels. J Lipid Res 1983;*24:*461.
137. Stiehl A, Raedsch R, Czygan P, et al: Effects of biliary bile acid composition on biliary cholesterol saturation in gallstone patients treated with chenodeoxycholic acid and/or ursodeoxycholic acid. Gastroenterology 1980;*79:*1192.
138. Makino I, Nakgawa S: Changes in biliary lipid and biliary bile acid composition in patients after administration of ursodeoxycholic acid. J Lipid Res 1978;*19:*723.
139. Fromm H: Gallstone dissolution and the cholesterol–bile acid–lipoprotein axis. Propitious effects of ursodeoxycholic acid. Gastroenterology 1984; *87:*229.
140. Hardison WGM, Grundy SM: Effect of ursodeoxycholate and its taurine conjugate on bile acid synthesis and cholesterol absorption. Gastroenterology 1984;*87:*130.
141. Carey MC: Critical tables for calculating the cholesterol saturation of native bile. J Lipid Res 1978;*19:*945.
142. Igimi H, Carey MC: Cholesterol gallstone dissolution in bile: dissolution kinetics of crystalline (anhydrate and monohydrate) cholesterol with chenodeoxycholate, ursodeoxycholate and their glycine and taurine conjugates. J Lipid Res 1981;*22:*254.
143. Thistle JL, Carlson GL, LaRusso NF, Hofmann AF: Comparison of the effects of 5 to 10 mg./kg./day of ursodeoxycholic acid and chenodeoxycholic acid on cholesterol saturation of bile in patients with gallstones. *In* Proceedings of V. Bile Acid Meeting, Falk Symposium Nr 1978;*26:*14 (Abstract).
144. Corrigan OL, Su CC, Higuchi WI, et al: Mesophase formation during cholesterol dissolution in ursodeoxycholate-lecithin solution: a new mechanism for gallstone dissolution in humans. J Pharm Sci 1980;*69:*869.
145. Park Y-H, Igimi H, Carey MC: Dissolution of human cholesterol gallstones in simulated chenodeoxycholate-rich and ursodeoxycholate-rich biles: an in vitro study of dissolution rates and mechanisms. Gastroenterology 1984;*87:*150.
146. Su CC, Higuchi WI, Gilmore IT, Danzinger RG, Hofmann AF: Mesophase formation during cholesterol gallstone dissolution in human bile: effect of bile acid composition. J Pharm Sci 1984;*73:*1160.
147. Nakagawa S, Makino I, Ishizaki T, et al: Dissolution of cholesterol gallstones by ursodeoxycholic acid. Lancet 1977;*2:*367.

148. Nakayama F: Oral cholelitholysis—Cheno versus urso. Japanese experience. Dig Dis Sci 1980; *25*:129.
149. Fromm H, Roat JW, Gonzalez V, Sarva RP, Farivar S: Comparative efficacy and side effects of ursodeoxycholic and chenodeoxycholic acids in dissolving gallstones: A double-blind controlled study. Gastroenterology 1983;*85*:1257.
150. Erlinger S, Le Go A, Husson JM, Feverty J: Franco-Belgian cooperative study of ursodeoxycholic acid in the medical dissolution of gallstones: a double-blind, randomized, dose-response study, and comparision with chenodeoxycholic acid. Hepatology 1984;*4*:308.
151. Neligan P, Bateson MC, Trash DB, Ross PE, Bouchief IAD: Ursodeoxycholic acid for the dissolution of radiolucent gallbladder stones. Digestion 1983;*28*:227.
152. Podd M, Zuin M, Dioguardi ML, Festorazzi S, Dioguardi N: A combination of chenodeoxycholic acid and ursodeoxycholic acid is more effective than either alone in reducing biliary cholesterol saturation. Hepatology 1982;*2*:334.
153. Debongnie JC, Phillips SF: Colonic function and diarrhoea. Gastroenterology 1977;*72*:1046 (Abstract).
154. Tint GS, Colallilo A, Salen G, Graber D, Shefer S: Ursodeoxycholic acid is a safe and effective gallstone dissolving agent in humans. Gastroenterology 1981;*80*:1304 (Abstract).
155. Bell GD, Doran J: Gallstone dissolution in man using an essential oil preparation, Rowachol. Br Med J 1979;*1*:24.
156. Ellis WR, Bell GD, Middleton B, et al: Adjunct to bile acid treatment for gallstone dissolution: low-dose chenodeoxycholic acid combined with a terpene preparation. Br Med J 1981;*1*:611.
157. Ellis WR, Bell GD: Treatment of biliary duct stones with a terpene preparation. Br Med J 1981;*1*:611.
158. Maudgal DP, Bird R, Blackwood WS, et al: Low-cholesterol diet: enhancement of effect of CDCA in patients with gallstones. Br Med J 1978;*2*:851.
159. Linscheer WG, Raheja KL: Effect of glycerophosphate on lithogenic bile. A new approach to treatment of cholelithiasis. Lancet 1974;*2*:551.
160. Holan KR, Holzbach RT, Hsieh JY, et al: Effect of administration of "essential' phospholipid, β-glycerophosphate and linoleic acid on biliary lipids in patients with cholelithiasis. Digestion 1979; *19*:251.
161. Tompkins RK, Burke LG, Zollinger RM, et al: Relationship of biliary phospholipid and cholesterol concentrations to the occurrence and dissolution of human gallstones. Ann Surg 1970; *172*:936.
162. Toouli J, Jablonski P, Watts JMcK: Gallstone dissolution in man using cholic acid and lecithin. Lancet 1975;*2*:1124.
163. Tangedahl TN, Matseshe JW, Thistle JL, Hofmann AF: Plant sterols increase effectiveness of chenodeoxycholic acid therapy in lowering cholesterol saturation of fasting state bile in patients with radiolucent gallstones. Gastroenterology 1977; *72*:A-115 (Abstract).
164. Whiting MJ, Watts JMck: Supersaturated bile from obese patients without gallstones supports cholesterol crystal growth but not nucleation. Gastroenterology 1984;*86*:243.
165. Faloon WW: Gallstone prophylaxis and therapy. Am J Dig Dis 1974;*19*:81.
166. Kwan KH, Higuchi WI, Molokhia AM, et al: Cholesterol gallstone dissolution rate accelerators. I. Exploratory investigations. J Pharm Sci 1977; *66*:1106.
167. Whiting MJ, Bradley BM, Watts JMcK: Chemical and physical properties of gallstones in South Australia: implications for dissolution treatment. Gut 1983;*24*:11.
168. Roda E, Bazzoli F, Labate AMM, Mazella G, Roda A, Sama C, Festi D, Aldini R, Taroni F, Barbara L: Ursodeoxycholic acid vs chenodeoxycholic randomized study. Hepatology 1982;*2*:804.
169. Allen MJ, Borody TJ, Bugliosi TF, et al: Rapid dissolution of gallstones by methyl tert-butyl ether. N Engl J Med 1985;*312*:317.

JOHN ALEXANDER-WILLIAMS, M.D.

5

Bacteriology of Biliary Disease

PREVALENCE OF BACTERIA IN NORMAL BILE

It is not known how common bacterobilia is in the normal subject or how often bacteria appear in the bile in the absence of disease. There have been few studies of the bacteriology of the bile in normal people, presumably because of ethical considerations. In one study,[1] gallbladder bile was aspirated and cultured in patients undergoing laparotomy who were known to have none of the normally accepted criteria of biliary disease. In none of these patients were any organisms cultured from the bile. In another study,[2] bile samples were aspirated at operation from 46 patients who were considered to have no biliary or pancreatic disease. All samples of gallbladder bile were sterile on culture. However, anaerobic intestinal bacteria were recovered from the liver in 14 per cent of cases. Taken at face value, these observations suggest that although the liver may act as a bacteriologic filter of the portal tract, it does not normally excrete these bacteria into the biliary system. However, these observations are on a small number of patients, studied only during the course of an abdominal operation.

It is well known that pathogenic microorganisms are often found in the bile of patients with biliary disease, that certain biliary disorders are much more likely than others to be associated with bacteria in the bile, and that the presence of bacteria in the bile predisposes to the development of septic complications of biliary operations.

Infective complications of biliary tract surgery include potentially fatal conditions, such as suppurative cholangitis, infected biliary peritonitis, and local subhepatic or subphrenic abscesses with septicemia. Less severe but more common infections include infection of the wound or of the wound drainage site. Although wound infection and drainage site infection may be the result of organisms introduced from the hospital environment or from the patient's skin (exogenous infection), in the majority of cases the infection after biliary operations is due to organisms identical to those found in the bile (endogenous infection).

The least that postoperative infection can do to a patient is to cause discomfort and malaise and to retard complete recovery. At worst, it lengthens hospital stay, predisposes to postoperative wound herniation, and occasionally causes loss of life. The economic consequences of these serious complications are severe.

The prevention of sepsis after biliary operations by preventing infected bile from successfully colonizing the wound or tissue spaces is a commendable goal for all who practice biliary surgery.

PREVALENCE OF BACTERIA IN THE BILE OF PATIENTS WITH BILIARY DISEASE BEFORE AND AFTER BILIARY TRACT OPERATIONS

The incidence of bacterobilia in patients with biliary disease varies in different series from 20 to 50 per cent (Table 5–1).[2–12] The incidence rises to nearly 50 per cent in most patients with common duct stones or with obstruction of the cystic duct.[7, 9] Emergency operations, or operations on patients with acute biliary disease, show an even higher incidence of bacterobilia from 40 to 100 per cent.[1, 13] Sianesi found that the incidence of bacterobilia in patients with acute cholecystitis changes with time and the patient's condition. For example, although only 20 per cent of patients operated on within 24 hours of admission had positive bile cultures, 70 per cent of those operated on after 48 hours

Table 5–1 INCIDENCE OF BACTEROBILIA AT OPERATION

Authors	Year	Center	Incidence of Bacterobilia (%)
In Patients Having Elective Biliary Surgery			
Keighley et al	1974	Leeds, England	33
Keighley et al.	1977	Birmingham, England	42
Csendes et al.	1975	Santiago, Chile	30 (33% in gallbladder wall)
McLeish et al.	1977	Birmingham, England	32
Truedson et al.	1982	Umea, Sweden	16
Kaufman et al.	1984	Tel Aviv, Israel	24.5
Glen and Joffe	1985	Columbus, Ohio, USA	21
In Patients With Acute Biliary Disease or Emergency Operation			
Csendes et al.	1975	Santiago, Chile	43 (47% in gallbladder wall)
Keighley et al.	1974	Leeds, England	100
Glen and Joffe	1985	Columbus, Ohio, USA	52

for failure of medical therapy had positive cultures. The incidence of positive cultures was only 15 per cent in those patients operated on more than 8 weeks after the attack.

Although the overall incidence of bacterobilia is 20 to 30 per cent, the chances of an individual patient having infected bile are related to the etiology of the biliary tract disease. It can frequently be predicted from the symptoms. For example, Suzuki, in a study of 295 patients from whom bile was obtained by transhepatic aspiration, found that 89 per cent of the specimens were positive when the patients had high fever and were on antibiotics at the time of the study. By contrast, positive cultures were obtained in 39 per cent of the patients who were not so ill as to require antibiotics. The overall incidence of biliary infection was 90 per cent in patients with bile duct stones.[11] This is a higher incidence than most other reports of patients with ductal stones, but this study includes several patients with intrahepatic stones, in which the incidence of bacterobilia is almost always 100 per cent. Bacterobilia in these patients may play an etiologic role. *Escherichia coli, Bacteroides,* and *Clostridium* may contribute to the formation of bile pigment calcium stones by producing β-glucuronidase and thus deconjugating bilirubin diglucuronide to form free unconjugated bilirubin; this, in turn, combines with calcium, leading to stone formation.[25]

In a study that included only patients considered at high risk for bacterobilia, Pitt et al. found that 66 per cent had at least one organism isolated from the biliary tract.[10] Although 30 per cent of the patients had sterile bile at the time of operation, 85 per cent of bile samples collected from biliary drainage catheters postoperatively were infected.[10] It is important to recognize that colonization of the biliary tract occurs commonly when drainage tubes are left in place,[10, 19] when the biliary tract is anastomosed to the intestine, and after sphincterotomy and sphincteroplasty.[20] For example, Gregg et al. have shown that of 45 patients with sterile bile at the time of sphincterotomy, 70 per cent had bile colonized by enteric organisms 6 to 36 months later. Growth was heavy to moderate in most of the patients. Despite bacterobilia, no patient had symptomatic cholangitis, presumably owing to excellent drainage of bile. These investigators thought that the most likely source of the bacterobilia was direct extension of duodenal organisms into the common bile duct.[20] Even though it has been suggested that the presence of contaminated bile for long periods may produce favorable conditions for precipitation of calcium bilirubinate, triggering new pigment stone formation,[19] antibiotics are not useful. Indeed, these patients have no clinical signs of infection unless obstruction supervenes, and they do not require treatment. It is important to recognize this, since antibiotics are ineffective and may be detrimental.[10]

Types of Microorganisms Found in the Bile of Patients With Biliary Disease

Most reports of the bacteriology of biliary organisms show a predominance of alimentary organisms such as coliforms, fecal streptococci, and *Klebsiella,* with a lower incidence of streptococci, staphylococci, and anaerobic organisms such as clostridia.[2, 10–12, 14–18] The morphology of the organisms cultured from the bile in patients undergoing biliary operations in our institution is shown in Table 5–2. The most common organisms found are aerobic, gram-negative species; however, 13 per cent of the bile samples had anaerobic bacteria.

The presence of anaerobic bacteria in bile was thought to be rare until the mid-1970s. In 1977, England and Rosenblatt from the Mayo Clinic noted that, of 371 patients whose bile was cultured for aerobic and anaerobic bacteria, 69 per cent had bacterobilia and 41 per cent of these grew anaerobes. Anaerobes were found to be associated with aerobic organisms in most instances, and in only two patients were they found to be the only infecting organisms.[21] The incidence of anaerobic infection and the rarity of pure cultures of anaerobes have been confirmed by other reports.[22] *Bacteroides fragilis* was the most common organism isolated and ranked fourth behind *E. coli,* Group D streptococci, and *Klebsiella* in terms of overall isolates in the Mayo Clinic series.[21] In that study, *Bacteroides fragilis* accounted for 7 per cent of the total aerobic and anerobic isolates and was present in 21 per cent of all positive cultures.[21] In Kaufman's series, anaerobes were found in 6 per cent of bile cultures.[7] The clinical significance of anaerobic bacteria in bile is not completely clear. Anaerobic infection has been associated with (1) a history of complex, multiple, biliary tract operations often involving biliary-intestinal anastomoses and common bile duct manipulation; (2) severe symptoms; and (3) a high incidence of postoperative infectious complications, especially wound infection.[23] Roberts et al. found that the incidence of anaerobic infection was 37 per cent in patients with common duct obstruction, whereas the overall incidence in their study was 7 per cent. The wound infection rate in patients with anaerobic bacterobilia was 27 per cent, but anaerobic organisms rarely grew from the infected wound.[22] By the same token, although *B. fragilis,* fusobacteria, clostridia other than *C. perfringens,* non–spore-forming gram-positive bacilli, and anaerobic streptococci have been found in bile collected from a large number of patients, these organisms were not generally responsible for sepsis among these patients.[21, 24]

Table 5–2 BACTERIA IN THE BILE: MORPHOLOGY OF 199 ORGANISMS

Organism	Number
Aerobic: 174 (87%)	
Gram-positive: 42 (21%)	
Streptococcus faecalis	30
Beta-hemolytic streptococci	4
Streptococcus viridans	1
Staphylococcus aureus	3
Staphylococcus albus	4
Gram-negative: 132 (66%)	
Escherichia coli	77
Klebsiella aerogenes	22
Enterobacter spp.	8
Proteus spp.	13
Pseudomonas aeruginosa	4
Actinobacter spp.	4
Serratia spp.	2
Aeromonas spp.	2
Anaerobic: 25 (13%)	
Gram-positive: 23 (12%)	
Clostridium welchii	16
Anaerobic streptococci	7
Gram-negative: (1%)	
Bacteroides spp.	2

Incidence of Wound Infection After Biliary Operations

In two reported series, the incidence of wound infection after biliary surgery was no more than 5 per cent.[26, 27] However, both these studies are retrospective analyses of case notes and therefore probably grossly underestimate the true incidence of infected wounds. Several series in which a prospective analysis was made are listed in Table 5–3. The true incidence of wound infection after elective operations in patients without prophylactic antibiotic coverage appears to be between 15 and 30 per cent.[1, 3, 4, 7, 13, 28, 29] The wide variation in the incidence is the result of many factors, including technical ones such as operative technique and wound hematoma. However, other factors, such as the type of biliary pathology found, contribute heavily to the risk of infection. The incidence of wound sepsis and septicemia in different groups of our patients having biliary surgery is shown in Table 5–4, which demonstrates how high the risk of infection is in patients having emergency operations and in those with stones in the common bile duct. Subsequent studies have reported similar results.[7, 28, 29]

In our experience, most wound sepsis is due to organisms identical to those isolated from the bile, and the presence of bacteria in the bile significantly increases the risk of infection. The relationship between biliary organisms and wound sepsis organisms was

Table 5–3 INCIDENCE OF WOUND INFECTION AFTER BILIARY OPERATIONS

Authors	Year	Center	Incidence of Infected Wounds (%)*
Keighley et al.	1974	Leeds, England	22
Keighley et al.	1977	Birmingham, England	21
Papachristodoulou	1978	Southampton, England	16
Morran et al.	1978	Glasgow, Scotland	21
Kaufman et al.	1984	Tel Aviv, Israel	24.5
Lewis et al.	1984	Montreal, Canada	20
Cainzos et al.	1985	Galicia, Spain	28

*Patients not given prophylactic antibiotics.

investigated in 282 patients. When organisms were found in the bile at operation, the incidence of wound sepsis was 38 per cent and the incidence of septicemia was 16 per cent. This was significantly greater than that found in patients with sterile bile, in whom the wound sepsis rate was 10 per cent and the septicemia rate 5 per cent. Infections were caused by organisms that had previously been isolated from the bile in 64 per cent of the patients who had wound sepsis and in 90 per cent of those who had septicemia. The fact that septic complications are related to the presence of bacteria in bile has been supported by several other investigators. For example, Kaufman found that the overall wound sepsis after biliary operations was 24 per cent. It was 45 per cent, however, among those patients with positive bile cultures.[7] Pitt found that wound sepsis and renal failure after surgery in patients undergoing urgent and complex biliary operations was significantly higher among those with positive bile cultures.[10]

As most infections after biliary operations are due to microorganisms from the bile being implanted in the tissues, there are three principal ways in which we can attempt to minimize the risk: (1) reducing the size of the inoculum, (2) using meticulous surgical technique, and (3) providing adequate antibiotic cover.

Most of the variables in the first two groups have not been studied in a scientific manner because of the difficulty in providing a control series. However, some worthwhile studies have been made.

Size of the Inoculum. The size of the inoculum can be reduced by (a) trying to sterilize the bile before operation, (b) decreasing spillage or carefully packing the wound to prevent contamination, (c) washing out the peritoneal cavity at the end of the operation to dilute the inoculum, or (d) using topical antiseptics, such as chlorhexidine, around the wound edge.

Chetlin and Elliott[30] have shown that the administration of the antibiotic cephaloridine, to which 90 per cent of biliary organisms are sensitive, did not reduce the incidence of positive bile cultures in high-risk patients, that is, those with acute cholecystitis, common duct stones, jaundice, and so forth. However, they found that in low-risk patients, those under the age of 70 years with chronic cholecystitis, the incidence of positive bile cultures was reduced from 13.6 per cent in controls to 5.8 per cent in those receiving cephaloridine. Therefore, it seems that giving preoperative antibiotics in the hope of reducing the concentration of bacteria in the bile is of little value in those patients at greatest risk. In one of our prospective controlled trials we found no significant differ-

Table 5–4 INCIDENCE OF WOUND SEPSIS AND SEPTICEMIA IN PATIENTS NOT RECEIVING PROPHYLACTIC ANTIBIOTICS

	Number of Patients			Wound Sepsis				Septicemia			
Emergency operation			17			7	(41%)			3	(18%)
Elective operation			164			29	(18%)			9	(6%)
Cholecystectomy alone		101			10		(10%)		1		(1%)
Choledochotomy		63			19		(31%)		8		(12%)
Stones	23			8			(35%)	5			(22%)
Carcinoma	13			4			(31%)	1			(8%)
No stones	27			7			(26%)	2			(7%)
Total			181			36	(20%)			12	(7%)

After Keighley, 1977.

ence in the incidence of bacteria in the bile between control patients (38 per cent) and patients who received preoperative rifamide (30 per cent) or gentamicin (24 per cent).[3]

If the bacteria found in wound infections come from infected bile, then clearly the quantity of bile spilled at operation must influence the risk. It seems obvious that a gallbladder that is ruptured during the course of cholecystectomy and spills infected bile into the wound will be much more likely to lead to infection than a gallbladder that is removed cleanly with only the minimal quantity of bile lost from the cystic duct stump. Although there are no reliable data to support this statement, it seems sensible to use particular care when a large bile spillage has occurred. Some surgeons believe that operative cholangiography increases the risk of wound infection because of the inevitable spillage of a small quantity of common bile duct bile. This may be true, but there is no reliable supportive evidence.

If the risk of infection is related to the size of the inoculum, it would seem logical to dilute the inoculum by thorough lavage of the wound or peritoneal cavity as a means of preventing infection. Serial dilution with volumes of up to 5 liters of normal saline should theoretically reduce the size of an inoculum to insignificant proportions. However, there are few, if any, data published to substantiate this belief. Preliminary work in our department so far indicates that the actual reduction in the concentration of the bacteria inoculum by serial dilution is very much less than would be expected. A 4 liter serial dilution reduces the concentration of inoculum only from 10^4 to 10^2. However, such a reduction may be critical in preventing wound infection.

Wheeler[31] has shown that plastic wound drapes do not decrease the risk of wound infection unless the wound is surrounded by a chlorhexidine-soaked towel.

Surgical Technique. Meticulous surgical technique is needed to ensure minimal damage to the tissues of the wound and minimal collection of blood or serum postoperatively.

Some surgeons always seem to have much less wound infection than others. The surgeons with the lower infection rate tend to attribute this to better surgical technique with less tissue damage. Controlled clinical studies have failed to show any advantage from diathermy over suture or ligation of blood vessels in the prevention of wound infection. Nevertheless, I still harbor the belief that a careful, meticulous surgeon who damages tissue very little is less likely to have a wound infection than one who is rough with the tissues.

Antibiotic Cover. The provision of an adequate quantity of antimicrobial antibiotic or chemotherapeutic agents in the tissues at the time of contamination should reduce the risk of infection.

There are many reports about the results of prophylactic antibiotics.[7, 16, 17, 28, 29, 32, 33] A large number of prospective controlled studies have all shown that appropriate prophylaxis is effective in reducing the incidence of wound infection after biliary operations. The critical factor is the provision of the appropriate antimicrobial agent in the right concentration, in the right place, at the time of contamination. We have found that a wound infection rate of 22 per cent and a bacteremia rate of 14 per cent after biliary operations in patients receiving no antibiotics could be reduced to 6 per cent with prophylactic gentamicin (Table 5–5).

Chetlin and Elliott[30] reduced the infective complications after biliary operations from 27 per cent in the control series to 4 per cent in patients receiving prophylactic cephaloridine. Stone and his colleagues[34] reduced the incidence of wound infection from 11 per cent in the control series to 3 per cent in those patients treated with cefazolin. Kaufman reported that wound sepsis in patients undergoing biliary surgery was 43 per cent and could be reduced to 7 per cent by the use of gentamicin.[7] If the analysis was limited to patients who had positive bile cultures, the infection rate was 43 per cent and was reduced to 7 per cent by gentamicin.[7] Cainzos et al., in another prospective randomized study of 52 high-risk patients, found that

Table 5–5 RESULTS OF PROPHYLACTIC ANTIBIOTIC THERAPY IN BILIARY OPERATIONS

	Gentamicin (50)	Controls (50)	Rifamide (50)
Biliary infection	12 (24%)	19 (38%)	10 (20%)
Wound sepsis	3 (6%)*	11 (22%)	5 (10%)
Bacteremia	1 (2%)*	7 (14%)	4 (8%)

*P <0.05 compared with controls.
After Keighley, 1977.

whereas the wound infection rate was 28 per cent among the control patients, it was nil among those who received 2 gm of cefamandole IM 30 minutes before operation and 2 gm every eight hours for 2 days postoperatively.[29] This may be excessive treatment, as Lewis et al., in a prospective randomized study, found that a single preoperative dose of cefazolin (2 gm) significantly reduced postoperative sepsis in high-risk biliary surgery.[28]

DETERMINING WHICH PROPHYLACTIC ANTIBIOTICS TO GIVE

Which antibiotic? The choice can be based on selecting the "best bet" antibiotic obtained from the table of antibiotic sensitivities derived from bile cultures of patients undergoing cholecystectomy. The distribution of the antibiotic sensitivity pattern of different organisms isolated from the bile in our patients is shown in Table 5–6. However, it must be stressed that this distribution of antibiotic sensitivities will not necessarily be the same for other biliary patients in other parts of the world or even within the same country. Nor does it mean that the antibiotic sensitivity pattern in 1978 will be the same as that in 1988. However, it seems that, in general, organisms found in the bile of patients with biliary disease are more likely to be sensitive to aminoglycosides such as gentamicin or cephalosporins such as cephaloridine, cefamandole, or cefazolin than they are to other commonly employed antibiotics.

Clearly, it is best to give appropriate antibiotics depending on the culture of the bile in the biliary tract at the time of operation. However, this is usually impractical if the bile is aspirated at the time of operation, because by the time the sensitivity pattern of the organisms is known the optimum time for antibiotic prophylaxis will have long passed. It seems apparent that each hospital needs to keep a running audit of the types of organisms isolated from its patients with biliary disease, to monitor the antibiotic sensitivity pattern, and to update accordingly its antibiotic policy for biliary disease.

In general, it is better to reserve for prophylaxis those antibiotics that will have the fewest side effects and not to use antibiotics that may be required later in therapy. Prophylactic antibiotic administration has been criticized by some on the grounds that it will promote the emergence of resistant strains of organisms. This objection is valid in theory, but there is no evidence to show that short courses of prophylactic antibiotics in one, two, or three doses promote the emergence of resistant strains. It is much more likely that prolonged antibiotic therapy will be responsible for allowing resistant strains to flourish and spread.

Some manufacturers of antibiotics will encourage us to use drugs that are secreted in high concentrations in the bile rather than those that reach high concentration in the tissues. To investigate this question we conducted a randomized control trial of 150 patients undergoing biliary surgery to determine whether an antibiotic that is excreted almost entirely in the bile (rifamide) is preferable to one having satisfactory serum levels only (gentamicin). Patients were allocated to one of three groups: 50 received gentamicin, 50 received rifamide, and 50 controls received no antibiotic cover. In the absence of duct obstruction, rifamide achieved high bile levels but low serum concentrations. However, in jaundiced patients, both the bile and the serum concentrations of rifamide were too low to be of therapeutic value. In contrast, gentamicin achieved adequate serum concentration in 88 per cent of patients.

The incidence of postoperative sepsis was not reduced by rifamide compared with con-

Table 5–6 SENSITIVITY TO FIVE ANTIBIOTICS OF 170 ORGANISMS ISOLATED FROM BILE (310 PATIENTS)

Antibiotic	All Organisms (%)	Aerobic: Gram-Positive (24) (%)	Aerobic: Gram-Negative (131) (%)	Anaerobic (%)
Gentamicin	85	56	100	0
Cephaloridine	76	58	71	66
Tetracycline	54	58	51	74
Rifampicin	50	67	46	66
Ampicillin	43	93	27	100

After Keighley, 1977.

trols. However, despite poor bile levels, gentamicin was associated with a significant reduction of wound infection, from 22 per cent to 6 per cent, and septicemia, from 14 per cent to 2 per cent, compared with controls. Therefore, it seems that to reduce the septic complications of biliary operations, adequate serum levels of an effective antimicrobial agent are more important than high bile levels of an antibiotic that does not achieve high serum levels.[3]

Thomas has emphasized the importance of attaining adequate serum and tissue levels of antibiotics. Prevention of septic complications is probably related to bactericidal levels of antibiotic in the wall of the bile ducts and the gallbladder (not necessarily in the bile) and in the surrounding tissue—the gallbladder bed, the liver, and the wound.[18]

Thus, as described previously, there is now plenty of evidence to support the concept that systemic prophylactic antibiotics significantly reduce the sepsis rate after biliary tract surgery. There is also some evidence to indicate that topical antibiotics may yield the same results. For example, in a prospective, randomized study of patients undergoing "high-risk" biliary surgery, Pitt et al. found that the incidence of infectious complications after surgery was the same whether the patients received parenteral antibiotics (gentamicin and penicillin) or wound irrigation with neomycin and polymyxin.[35] Similarly, Freischlag et al., in another prospective randomized study, showed that cefamandole nafate 0.4 per cent solution used to irrigate the wound and the subhepatic space in patients undergoing biliary surgery was as effective as cefamandole nafate given parenterally 2 hours before and 6, 12, and 18 hours after the operation.[36]

Because we realized that the wide variety of organisms that can be found in a diseased biliary tract would make it difficult to find one antibiotic that covered all possibilities, we set out to try to increase the chances of picking the most appropriate antibiotic by attempting to achieve instantaneous recognition of organisms in the bile. As has already been said, it is not possible to wait 24 to 48 hours for sensitivity patterns to be available before prescribing a prophylactic antibiotic. However, if the particular type of organism could be identified immediately, it might make possible a more informed guess as to the right antibiotic to use. In an attempt to study this question we took aspiration samples from the gallbladder or common duct at the beginning of the biliary operation and sent them immediately to the bacteriology department, where they had instant Gram stains and were cultured. The results of the Gram stains were telephoned to the operating room within 20 minutes of collection. Accuracy of the Gram stains was checked against the subsequent culture of organisms from the bile. The overall accuracy rate of the immediate Gram stain reports compared with the subsequent bile cultures was 77 per cent. The incidence of false positive results was 12 per cent, and of false negative results 7 per cent. The organism was identified incorrectly by the Gram stain in 4 per cent of patients.[4]

Logically, the next step was to put our hypothesis to the test by basing our antibiotic policy on the result of immediate Gram stains. In a nonrandomized prospective study we compared two groups of patients: 119 consecutive patients in whom the antibiotics were administered during operation according to the results of the immediate Gram stain of the bile, and a group of 101 patients, none of whom received prophylactic antibiotics. Those having antibiotics were given gentamicin if gram-negative bacteria were seen, ampicillin if gram-positive organisms were seen, and no antibiotics if no bacteria were seen on the Gram stains. The control group had an incidence of wound sepsis of 22 per cent and a septicemia rate of 8 per cent. In the group receiving antibiotics, if organisms were located on the Gram stain, there was a significant reduction of sepsis to 7 per cent ($p \leq 0.005$) and a septicemia rate of only 2 per cent. Seventy-six of the 119 patients having Gram stains had no organisms identified on the stain. In 70 of these the subsequent culture was also sterile, and only 2 of these (3 per cent) developed wound infection. However, in six, although the Gram stain was negative, the subsequent culture grew organisms. These patients received no antibiotics, and two of them (33 per cent) were infected—a false negative result for the antibiotic policy. Fourteen patients had organisms identified on a Gram stain, but the subsequent culture was sterile. Those patients may have received an unnecessary antibiotic cover, but none of them developed infection. In two patients the organism was incorrectly identified, and the inappropriate antibiotic was given in one; these patients became infected. It seems, therefore, that the policy of obtaining immediate Gram stain on aspirated bile at the time of operation produces a satisfactory lowering of the incidence of sepsis in high-risk patients and avoids the necessity of giving antibiotics to those patients who do not need it because they do not have infected bile. Gallagher et al., however, found a poor correlation between the results of microscopic examination of bile at the time of operation and the results of bile culture and did not find this procedure useful.[37] Despite the theoretical attraction of this policy, we have now abandoned this method of giving appropriate antibiotic cover because, in terms of laboratory time, it is not cost-effective.[5]

If one wishes to detect infective bile before operation and make accurate assessment of the organisms and their sensitivity pattern, it is possible to make a reliable estimation of bacteriology of the bile by performing duodenal aspiration and culture. A series of 47 patients had preoperative duodenal aspirates examined by culture and viable count. These results were later compared with operative bile cultures. Small numbers of oral commensals were isolated frequently from the duodenum, even in patients with sterile bile. However, if concentrations of organisms of more than 10^5 per ml are considered significant, 75 per cent of those patients with bacteria in the bile were correctly identified from duodenal aspiration, with a 6 per cent incidence of false positive and an 11 per cent incidence of false negative findings. Suzuki et al. also found that 85 per cent of specimens from duodenal aspirates grew the same organism as a simultaneously obtained bile sample.[11] Although this method of preoperative investigation is possible with a reasonable degree of accuracy, it is technically too cumbersome to make it of much practical value.[4]

When to Give the Antibiotic

Animal experimental work suggests that the optimum time for antibiotic prophylaxis is one that achieves the highest level of tissue antibiotic concentration at the time of contamination.[38] Stone and his coworkers[34] showed that the incidence of wound infection in biliary surgery was 11 per cent if no antibiotics were given, 9 per cent if cefazolin was given 4 hours postoperatively, and zero if cefazolin was given 1 hour preoperatively. It has been shown that the optimum tissue levels of gentamicin are maintained for 1 to 2 hours after an intramuscular injection.[39] Therefore, it seems that the optimum time to give prophylactic antibiotics is either with the premedication or at the beginning of induction of anesthesia. However, we found that antibiotics given 20 minutes after the aspiration of bile from the gallbladder at the beginning of the operation were just as effective as antibiotics given 1 hour preoperatively.

The question of how long to continue prophylactic antibiotic therapy has been the subject of much investigation and controversy. In many of our early studies we gave prophylactic antibiotics for as long as 5 days but later reduced this to 3 days and then to 1 day without finding any lessening of its efficacy in sepsis prevention. Single-dose prophylaxis appears to be as effective as multiple-dose prophylaxis and has much to recommend it on grounds of ecology, economy, safety, and convenience.

In a study by Morran and colleagues it was shown that prophylactic co-trimoxazole (equivalent to 160 mg of trimethoprim and 800 mg of sulfamethoxazole) infused intravenously for 80 minutes before operation reduced wound sepsis from 21 per cent in controls to 4 per cent in the treated group.[6]

Several studies have shown the efficacy of cephalosporins. In one study, a single dose of 2 gm intramuscular cefazolin given at the time of premedication reduced the wound infection rate in biliary surgery from 16 per cent in a control group to 0.5 per cent in the treated group.[32] In another study, Cainzos et al. showed that cefamandole 2 gm IM 30 minutes before surgery and 2 gm every 8 hours for 2 days brought the infection rate from 28 per cent to zero.[29] Similarly, Lewis et al. have shown that a single preoperative dose of 2 gm cefazolin prevented postoperative sepsis.[28]

One must remember that some of the most severe biliary tract infections have associated common bile duct obstruction, a factor that prevents the entry of most antibiotics into bile.[40] In addition, several antibiotics, such as ampicillin, erythromycin, and penicillin G, are excreted into the bile at a much lower rate when there is any evidence of hepatocellular disease.[33] The choice of an antimicrobial agent for either prophylaxis or therapy of biliary tract infections is difficult only because of the wide variety of available agents with a broad spectrum against the pathogens causing disease and readily found in high levels in both serum and bile. No single agent, however, will be effective against all the likely pathogens, and the choice of the appropriate drug or drugs will depend on the patient's renal function, history of drug allergy, and probable infecting pathogen. However, most importantly, if obstruction of the biliary tree is present, it must be removed before the infection can be controlled and antimicrobial agents can reach the site of that infection.

To Whom Should Prophylaxis Be Given?

This question has already been answered in part. Prophylaxis should be given to those at risk of developing endogenous infection. These are, by definition, patients with bacteria in the bile that can inoculate the peritoneal cavity and the wound at the time of operation. It seems unnecessary to give prophylactic antibiotics to patients with sterile bile as, in them, no significant reduction in wound infection results from doing so. It has been shown to be possible, but impractical, to determine the organisms in the bile by sampling from the duodenum before operation. It is possible but impractical to determine whether there are organisms in the bile by performing the immediate Gram stains during operation, and we have now abandoned this policy.

How then can we determine to whom we should give antibiotics? We attempted to answer this question by performing a multivariate analysis of 17 clinical and 10 operative variables to correlate with the presence or absence of bacteria in the bile aspirated at operation. The study was performed on 181 patients; 136 patients were classified as low risk, and in them the incidence of infected bile was 19 per cent. Forty-five patients were classified as high risk, and in them the incidence of infected bile was 67 per cent ($p \leq 0.001$). Eight variables were more common in the high-risk than in the low-risk group; these included jaundice at the time of operation, recent rigors, emergency operations or operations within 4 weeks of emergency admission, age over 70 years, previous biliary operation, common duct obstruction, and stones in the common duct. In 67 patients in whom one or more "high-risk factors" were present, the bile contained organisms in 37 (53 per cent); when four "high-risk factors" occurred in the same patient (16 cases), biliary organisms were isolated from 14 (87 per cent). Several subsequent studies by other investigators have confirmed these findings.[7, 28, 29, 35]

We believe that the presence of one or more "high-risk factors" indicates a patient in whom prophylactic antibiotics should be advised during an operation on the biliary tract. In this study, no patient received prophylactic antibiotics. The incidence of wound infection in the high-risk group was 38 per cent, and in the low-risk group 14 per cent.[3]

CONCLUSIONS

Patients undergoing biliary operations who have bacteria in their bile have a very high risk of developing septic complications due to contamination of the abdomen or the wound with infected bile. Patients at high risk are the elderly; those with common duct obstruction, particularly due to stones; and those with recent acute septic cholecystitis. The organisms responsible for the infected bile and septic operative complications are usually gram-positive *Streptococcus faecalis* or gram-negative *Escherichia coli, Klebsiella,* or *Proteus;* clostridia are occasionally present. Most organisms, particularly the gram-negative ones, are sensitive to gentamicin and cephalosporins. The latter are suitable for prophylaxis because they are unlikely to be needed in therapy if serious septic complications do supervene. Antibiotics such as gentamicin and chloramphenicol are probably best reserved for therapy rather than prophylaxis.

Appropriate antibiotic prophylaxis given at the time of induction of anesthesia by the intravenous or intramuscular route gives effective protection against the risk of septic complications, with great savings of time and money to the patient and the hospital service. It does not seem necessary or advisable to give prophylactic antibiotics to those patients who do not have infected bile. However, many surgeons and many hospitals believe that the risks of "one-shot prophylaxis" are so small that it is expedient to give such prophylaxis to all patients undergoing biliary surgery.

REFERENCES

1. Csendes A, Fernandez M, Uribe P: Bacteriology of the gallbladder bile in normal subjects. Am J Surg 1975;*129*:629.

2. Edlund YA, Mollstedt BO, Ouchterlony O: Bacteriological investigation of the biliary system and liver in biliary tract disease correlated to clinical data and microstructure of the gallbladder and liver. Acta Chir Scand 1959;*116*:461.
3. Keighley MRB, Flinn R, Alexander-Williams J: Multivariate analysis of clinical and operative findings associated with biliary sepsis. Br J Surg 1976;*63*:528.
4. Keighley MRB, McLeish AR, Bishop HM, et al: Identification of the presence and type of biliary microflora by immediate gram stains. Surgery 1977;*81*:469.
5. McLeish AR, Keighley MRB, Bishop HM, et al: Selecting patients requiring antibiotics in biliary surgery by immediate gram stains of bile at operation. Surgery 1977;*81*:473.
6. Morran C, NcNaught W, McArdle CS: Prophylactic co-trimoxazole in biliary surgery. Br Med J 1978;*2*:462.
7. Kaufman Z, Engelberg M, Eliashiv A, Reiss R: Systemic prophylactic antibiotics in elective biliary surgery. Arch Surg 1984;*119*:1002.
8. Reiss R, Eliashiv A, Deutsch A: Septic complication and bile culture in 800 consecutive cholecystectomies. World J Surg 1982;*6*:195.
9. Glen P, Joffe SN: Bacteria in the biliary tract. Contemp Surg 1985;*27*(1):25.
10. Pitt HA, Postier RG, Cameron JL: Biliary bacteria. Significance and alterations after antibiotic therapy. Arch Surg 1982;*117*:445.
11. Suzuki Y, Kobayashi A, Ohto M, Tsuchiya Y, et al: Bacteriological study of transhepatically aspirated bile. Relation to cholangiographic findings in 295 patients. Dig Dis Sci 1984;*29*:109.
12. Truedson H, Elmros T, Holm S: The incidence of bacteria in gallbladder bile at acute and elective cholecystectomy. Acta Chir Scand 1982;*194*:308.
13. Keighley MRB, Lister DM, Jacobs SJ, Giles GR: Hazards of surgical treatment due to micro-organisms in the bile. Surgery 1974;*75*:578.
14. Sianesi M, Ghirarduzzi A, Percudani M, Dell'Ana B: Cholecystectomy for acute cholecystitis: Timing of operation, bacteriologic aspects and postoperative course. Am J Surg 1984;*148*:609.
15. Keighley MRB: Micro-organisms in the bile. Ann R Coll Surg Engl 1977;*59*:328.
16. Stone HH, Haney BE, Klob LD, et al: Prophylactic and preventive antibiotic therapy: Timing duration and economics. Ann Surg 1979;*189*:691.
17. Kahng KU, Beaton JL: Infectious complications of biliary surgery in the antibiotic era. Infect Surg 1985;*4*:455.
18. Thomas M: Antibiotics in bile. J Antimicrob Chemother 1983;*12*:419.
19. Feretis CB, Contou CT, Manouras AJ, et al: Long term consequences of bacterial colonization of the biliary tract after choledochostomy. Surg Gynecol Obstet 1984;*159*:363.
20. Gregg JA, De Girolami P, Carr-Locke DL: Effects of sphincteroplasty and endoscopic sphincterotomy on the bacteriologic characteristics of the common bile duct. Am J Surg 1985;*149*:668.
21. England DM, Rosenblatt JE: Anaerobes in human biliary tracts. J Clin Microbiol 1977;*6*:494.
22. Roberts AB, Finlay-Jones JJ, Watts JM: Infection in biliary surgery: Anaerobic organisms and acute cholecystitis. Surg Gastroenterol 1982;*1*:183
23. Bourgault AM, England DM, Rosenblatt JE, et al: Clinical characteristics of anaerobic bactibilia. Arch Intern Med 1979;*139*:1346.
24. Finegold SM: Anaerobes in biliary tract infection. Arch Intern Med 1979;*139*:1338.
25. Tabata M, Nakayama F: Bacteria and gallstones. Etiological significance. Dig Dis Sci 1981;*26*:218.
26. Raine PAM, Gunn AA: Acute cholecystitis. Br J Surg 1975;*62*:697.
27. Todd GJ, Reemtsma K: Cholecystectomy with drainage. Am J Surg 1978;*135*:622.
28. Lewis RT, Allan CM, Goodall RG, et al: A single preoperative dose of cefazolin prevents postoperative sepsis in high-risk biliary surgery. Can J Surg 1984;*27*:44.
29. Cainzos M, Potel J, Puente JL: Prospective randomized controlled study of prophylaxis with cefamandole in high risk patients undergoing operations upon the biliary tract. Surg Gynecol Obstet 1985;*160*:27.
30. Chetlin SH, Elliott DW: Preoperative antibiotics in biliary surgery. Arch Surg 1973;*107*:319.
31. Wheeler MH: Abdominal wound protection by means of plastic drapes. *In* Strachan CJL (ed): Surgical Sepsis. London, Academic Press, 1979, pp 3–13.
32. Papachristodoulou AJ, Mackenzie A, Norman J, et al: Single-dose cephalosporin prophylaxis in major abdominal surgery. *In* Siegenthaler W, Luethy R (eds): Current Chemotherapy. Zurich, 1978, pp 856–885.
33. Nagar H, Berger SA: Collective review. The excretion of antibiotics by the biliary tract. Surg Gynecol Obstet 1984;*158*:601.
34. Stone HH, Hooper CA, Kolb LD, et al: Antibiotic prophylaxis in gastric, biliary and colonic surgery. Ann Surg 1976;*184*:443.
35. Pitt HA, Postier RG, Gadacz TR, Cameron JL: The role of topical antibiotics in "high-risk" biliary surgery. Surgery 1982;*91*:518.
36. Freischlag J, McGrattan M, Busuttil RW: Topical vs systemic cephalosporin administration in elective biliary operations. Surgery 1984;*96*:686.
37. Gallagher P, Ostick G, Jones D, et al: Intraoperative microscopy of bile—is it useful? Br J Surg 1982; *69*:473.
38. Burke JK: The effective period of preventing antibiotic action in experimental incisions and dermal lesions. Surgery 1961;*50*:161.
39. Winters RE, Litwack KD, Hewitt WL: Relation between dose and levels of gentamicin in blood. J Infect Dis 1971;*124*:S90.
40. Weinstein L, Dalton AC: Host determinants of response to antimicrobial agents. N Engl J Med 1968; *279*:580.

CARLOS A. PELLEGRINI, M.D.

6

Pathophysiology of Biliary Obstruction

Biliary obstruction is caused by gallstones, tumors, and benign strictures in over 90 per cent of cases. Parasites and inflammatory and neoplastic processes occasionally cause biliary obstruction (see Chapters 36, 37, and 43).

Gallstones in the common bile duct produce variable degrees of biliary obstruction depending on their number and size. Biliary obstruction caused by choledocholithiasis is typically a partial obstruction. Periodically the obstruction is aggravated by the temporary impaction of a gallstone in the distal (and narrower) portion of the bile duct. Mucus, debris, and associated cholangitis contribute to these periodic exacerbations. As the pressure builds up in the proximal ducts, and aided by duodenal peristalsis, the stone eventually passes through the ampulla of Vater or, more commonly, is dislodged and moves back to larger areas of the bile duct, where it has less effect on bile flow.

Biliary obstruction caused by *tumors* is usually progressive, until all bile flow stops. Since the biliary tract in these patients has not been previously colonized by bacteria (as opposed to that of patients with cholelithiasis) and since the tumor eventually produces a complete obstruction that separates the stagnant bile from the intestinal environment, this form of biliary obstruction is rarely associated with cholangitis.

Benign biliary strictures frequently cause a more or less fixed and relatively high-grade obstruction. Thus, the effects of sustained biliary obstruction on liver morphology and function are more commonly seen in these patients than in those with gallstones or tumors. Periodically, edema, mucus, biliary sludge, or gallstones (secondary to proximal bile stasis) aggravate the biliary obstruction, which may lead to a complete cessation of bile flow with or without associated cholangitis.

Regardless of cause, obstruction of the bile duct produces structural and functional changes in the canalicular system and the liver parenchyma, the extent and severity of which depend on the degree, duration, and site of obstruction. Connective tissue proliferation with permanent functional damage to the liver is the end result of sustained and prolonged biliary tract obstruction. Abnormalities in liver function and accumulation of substances normally cleared by the liver produce alterations in several other organ systems. This chapter deals with the local (i.e., liver and bile ducts) and systemic effects of biliary obstruction, the recovery of liver function following relief of obstruction, and the risks of surgery in patients with biliary obstruction.

LOCAL EFFECTS OF BILIARY OBSTRUCTION

Morphologic Changes in the Liver and Bile Ducts

Increases in biliary pressure produce dilatation of the common bile duct up to two and one-half times the normal diameter.[1, 2] When high intrabiliary pressure is sustained for a prolonged period, the final extent of dilatation is related to the cause of the obstruction. Dilatation is more marked in patients with neoplastic obstruction. In these patients the obstruction affects an otherwise normal bile duct, which becomes progressively distended until, eventually, bile flow ceases. In patients with choledocholithiasis or biliary strictures, dilatation is rarely as marked. This is because the obstruction is not complete, and the inflammatory process that affects the wall of the ducts usually prevents marked dilatation.

If the point of obstruction is below the junction of cystic duct and common duct, the gallbladder may dilate enough so that it can be felt on examination of the abdomen.

Courvoisier's law states that a palable nontender gallbladder in a jaundiced patient indicates that the obstruction is from a neoplasm rather than from a gallstone or some benign lesion. This is usually true because the obstruction in neoplastic disease is more complete and continuous, and the gallbladder is usually unscarred. With gallstone disease, common duct obstruction is both less complete and intermittent, and gallbladder dilatation is inhibited by the effects of chronic inflammation in its wall. An exception to this rule may be seen in patients with Mirizzi's syndrome.[3] Mirizzi's syndrome is a rare form of common hepatic duct obstruction that results from an inflammatory response secondary to a gallstone impacted in the cystic duct or neck of the gallbladder. Most individuals with this syndrome have a cystic duct that runs parallel to the common hepatic duct and inserts unusually low into the bile duct.[4] These patients have acute cholecystitis and may have a palable, *tender* gallbladder associated with biliary obstruction.[3–5]

A number of investigators have studied the relationship between the structural changes in the bile ducts and liver and the duration and degree of obstruction.[6–10] In rats, total obstruction produces marked dilatation of the common bile duct, with the appearance of focal necrosis around small ducts within 48 hours. Early signs of bile duct proliferation, such as syncytial buds from the bile ducts, appear after 48 to 72 hours of total obstruction. If obstruction persists and the animal survives, the dilatation of the extrahepatic biliary tree becomes saccular, the liver parenchyma is compressed, and cirrhosis develops in 5 to 6 weeks.[8, 9] Extrapolation of these changes to humans is difficult, and the extent of dilatation of the human common bile duct is never as great as in the rat.

In most other animals[7] and in man,[9, 10] long-standing obstruction leads to changes in the microvascular anatomy of the liver. This may decrease blood flow through the sinusoids and explain the decreased clearance of organic anions.

Both intrahepatic and extrahepatic cholestasis produce canalicular bile plugging. In extrahepatic biliary obstruction in humans the most specific histologic feature is plugging of interlobular biliary canaliculi. Centrilobular bile stasis and dilatation of biliary radicles result in periductular extravasation of bile, which causes reactive edema and infiltration of polymorphonuclear leukocytes. With progressive dilatation of the canalicular system the liver cells become flattened, and degenerative changes occasionally occur. The inflammatory reaction appears to stimulate proliferation of bile ducts and may lead to periportal and intralobular fibrosis, which gives the picture of biliary cirrhosis.[10, 11] Infection may lead to pericholangitis and occasionally to liver abscess formation.

Ultrastructural studies of the liver in patients with obstructive jaundice show subcellular changes in the bile canalicular membrane and the adjacent hepatocyte cytoplasm. In the early stage, the microfilaments located within the pericanalicular cytoplasm increase, while intracellular membranes (i.e., endoplasmic reticulum and Golgi complex) and the volume density of mitochondria and lysosomes decrease.[12] After a longer period (i.e., 3 weeks) the bile canaliculus becomes very dilated and the microvilli of the canalicular membrane flatten and become fewer (Fig. 6–1). Complete bile duct obstruction leads to loosening of the tight junction network, increasing the depth of the fibril texture and producing marked irregularities of its pattern.[13–15]

Changes in Hepatocytic Function, Bile Secretion, and Bile Flow

The normal pressure of bile in the common duct, 10 to 15 cm of water, results from the resistance of the sphincter of Oddi and the rate of bile flow produced by the bile secretory apparatus. Obstruction results in increased common bile duct pressure proportional to the degree and duration of obstruction.[16] Complete obstruction gives a pressure of 25 to 35 cm H_2O. If the gallbladder is present, the rate at which common duct pressure climbs is slowed owing to absorption of water in the gallbladder.

Elevated biliary pressure leads to changes in bile flow and the secretion of bile constituents.[17–20] When pressure in the common duct of dogs exceeds 15 cm of water, bile flow decreases. At bile pressures in excess of 30 cm of water, net bile secretion stops.[21] Experiments in monkeys show that at pressures up to 14 cm H_2O there is no change in bile flow. Pressures between 17 and 22 cm H_2O decrease bile flow and bile acid secretion to approximately half normal, suggesting that the effect is principally on the bile salt–dependent fraction of flow.[22, 23] Partial ob-

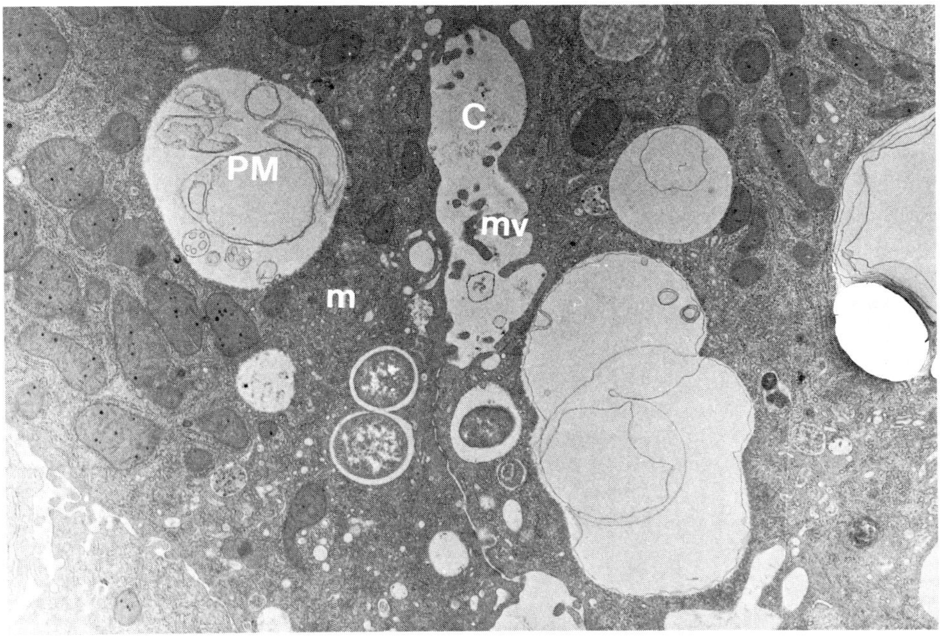

Figure 6–1. Electron micrograph of the biliary canaliculus of a rat 5 days after ligation of the common bile duct. The canaliculus (C) is dilated; microvilli (mv) are sparse and microfilaments (m) are increased in the pericanalicular cytoplasm. Fragments of the plasma membrane (PM) (which presumably give rise to the high molecular-weight fraction of the serum alkaline phosphatase) are seen inside the cell. (Courtesy of S. Raper and A. Jones.)

struction of the common bile duct in the dog results in inspissation of bile[24, 25] and occasionally in sludge and pigment stone formation.[26]

In rats, the flow of bile ceases when bile duct pressure reaches approximally 20 cm of water.[18, 19] At pressures of 16 to 17 cm of water, bile flow is 65 per cent of normal in these animals. A similar decrease in erythritol clearance suggests that the decreased bile flow is secondary to decreased canalicular secretion of bile rather than to increased absorption. Cholesterol output is decreased to the same extent as bile flow, and thus its concentration in bile does not change. Bile salt concentration and phospholipid secretory rates are not altered. Inulin excretion is increased in rats with partial common bile duct obstruction.[18, 19] Since the biliary excretion of inert solutes with large molecular radius, such as inulin, is dependent more on diffusion than on solvent drag, this increased inulin clearance suggests that biliary obstruction increases canalicular permeability.

When the ducts are partially obstructed, bile continues to be secreted into the canaliculus. Increased hydrostatic pressure in the biliary canaliculi distorts the tight junctions. Desmet and De Vos[15] suggest that tight junctions remain functionally intact even with extreme dilatation of the canaliculus. However, morphologic and physiologic studies show increased permeability of hepatocytic tight junctions in cholestasis.[27, 28] It is likely that discontinuities in the texture of the tight junctions and the higher number of free-ending loops interfere with the barrier function of the tight junctions.[29] Therefore, the liver has two main pathways for reflux of bile during cholestasis: transjunctional reflux into the paracellular space (and from there to the lymphatics and portal sinusoids) and transcellular reflux back into the portal sinusoids. For example, Jones et al. have shown that during times of elevated biliary pressure, hepatocytes can readily transport macromolecules from the biliary canaliculus to the portal sinusoids via non–receptor mediated, membrane-limited vesicles.[30]

Experiments in the dog show that about 10 per cent of canalicular bile enters the systemic circulation via the lymphatics. Indeed, after complete common bile duct obstruction, bile acid and bilirubin concentrations in the hepatic lymphatics increase for 6 hours, plateau for a short period, and then drop slightly to reach a new plateau at a level higher than normal. The eventual decrease in bilirubin concentration in the lymphatics is due in part to a decreased capacity of the hepatocyte to secrete organic anions.[31]

The maximal biliary excretion of bilirubin

(bilirubin Tm = 0.65 ± 0.24 mg/min in normal subjects) decreases during biliary tract obstruction. Excretion of sulfobromophthalein (i.e., anion transport) and the capacity of the liver to store anionic compounds also decrease.[32] Bilirubin metabolism by the hepatocyte may be increased by the administration of phenobarbital and spironolactone, presumably owing to the ability of these drugs to induce microsomal enzymes.[33, 34] Pretreatment with phenobarbital or spironolactone does not decrease serum bilirubin levels in rats with bile duct obstruction.[35]

Decreased anion excretion is aggravated in late obstruction by decreased uptake of bilirubin by liver cells and by alterations in the conjugate pattern of bilirubin in bile.[36] This suggests that, in addition to canalicular transport, uptake and conjugation of bilirubin are altered by obstruction.

The clearance of IgA immune complexes from the circulation is also reduced after acute bile duct obstruction.[37] By contrast, clearance rates for IgG and beta-glucuronidase, both of which are supposed to be removed from the circulation predominantly by the liver, are not affected.

Whether the decrease in bile salt secretion that follows increases in intraductal pressure results from decreased secretion by the hepatocyte (due to impaired canalicular membrane transport) or from reabsorption of bile salts from canalicular bile is not clear. Bile salt concentrations in the hepatocyte and in the systemic circulation increase, which inhibits bile salt synthesis and decreases the size of the bile salt pool. Phospholipid and cholesterol secretion also decline. When biliary tract pressure is restored to normal, the cholesterol secretion returns to normal faster than does phospholipid or bile acid secretion, and the lithogenic index transiently increases.[22, 23]

SYSTEMIC EFFECTS OF BILIARY OBSTRUCTION

Serum Bilirubin and Alkaline Phosphatase

Complete obstruction of the common bile duct causes the serum bilirubin, alkaline phosphatase, 5′ nucleotidase, and leucine aminopeptidase levels to rise. The serum glutamic oxalacetic and glutamic pyruvic transaminase levels also climb, but marked elevations of these enzymes in extrahepatic biliary obstruction have only rarely been observed.[38] The plasma concentration of bile acids and salts increases several fold, from less than 0.01 mg/dl to 2 to 6 mg/dl.[39, 40]

The serum bilirubin level starts to rise within 1 hour after total occlusion of the common bile duct.[41] In complete obstruction in humans, the serum bilirubin concentration rises for days to weeks and then plateaus. Accumulation of bilirubin in plasma and tissues causes jaundice, and excretion of conjugated bilirubin by the kidney is responsible for choluria—cardinal signs of biliary obstruction. The average final height of the bilirubin concentration with complete obstruction ranges from 20 to 30 mg/dl. At this point, the daily bilirubin load is excreted by the kidneys. Higher bilirubin values suggest concomitant hemolysis or renal dysfunction.[39]

Differential determination of serum bilirubins by assaying direct bilirubin (bilirubin conjugated with one or two glucuronic acid moieties) and indirect (unconjugated) bilirubin is useful to distinguish hepatobiliary disease (associated with an increase of direct bilirubin) from unconjugated hyperbilirubinemias, usually the result of overproduction or deficient hepatic conjugation of bilirubin. Traditionally this has been done using the method introduced by van den Bergh; however, alkaline methanolysis[42] combined with high-performance liquid chromatography[43] is a much more sensitive and specific method to measure serum bilirubin. This method can accurately determine the amount of unconjugated bilirubin and that of esterified (mono- or diconjugated) bilirubin. Using this technique, esterified bilirubin is not measurable in normal subjects; thus, even very small amounts of esterified bilirubin in the serum imply some degree of cholestasis (see also Chapter 13).

In addition to unconjugated bilirubin and its ester conjugates, patients with biliary obstruction have bilirubins covalently linked to serum protein, predominantly albumin.[45] Since only esterified (conjugated) bilirubin links itself to serum protein,[44] these bilirubin-protein complexes are seen only in patients with cholestasis.

In general, neoplastic obstruction produces the highest bilirubin values, and those caused by benign (e.g., post-traumatic) strictures and choledocholithiasis are substantially lower (Fig. 6–2).[46] The cause of the jaundice is

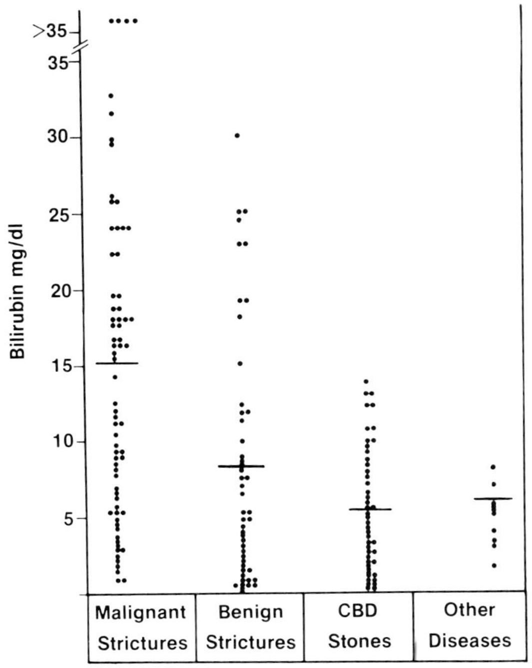

Figure 6–2. Serum bilirubin values in 178 patients with obstructive jaundice grouped according to the cause of the biliary obstruction. Although there is considerable overlap, the mean serum bilirubin in patients with malignant strictures was substantially higher than that of patients with choledocholithiasis. None of the latter had serum bilirubin values higher than 14 mg/dl.

often obvious from the history in patients with bile duct stricture due to a ductal injury. Most of the remaining patients with obstructive jaundice will have either neoplastic obstruction or gallstone obstruction. One is usually correct in assuming that the diagnosis is neoplasm if the bilibrubin value is greater than about 13 mg/dl, and that it is choledocholithiasis if the bilirubin value is below 10 mg/dl and the syndrome also includes short-term fluctuations in the bilirubin level, cholangitis, or episodes of colic. Of course, additional tests are usually needed before the evaluation can be considered complete, but these simple guidelines allow one to make a fairly accurate initial estimate of the cause of obstructive jaundice in the average patient. (See Chapter 13 for further details.)

The *alkaline phosphatase* concentration is a more sensitive indicator of the presence of biliary obstruction than the bilirubin concentration is (Fig. 6–3).[46] Its rise is rapid, precedes that of bilirubin, and occurs in almost every case of bile duct obstruction. In dogs, the serum alkaline phosphatase concentration begins to increase when the common bile duct pressure reaches 15 cm of water, but the serum bilirubin concentration does not change until the pressure exceeds 15 cm, and the bilirubin remains normal in some animals with pressures above 18 cm of water.[47] The absolute height of the alkaline phosphatase level does not correlate closely with the degree of obstruction.

In the rat, ligation of the common bile duct causes a progressive elevation of alkaline phosphatase, which reaches a maximum about 36 hours after the obstruction and then plateaus.[48, 49] Rats also have a transient increase of the intestinal alkaline phosphatase, which peaks at about 12 hours. Interestingly, intraperitoneal injection of bile from bile duct–ligated animals into normal rats causes the same increases in serum alkaline phosphatase activity.[50] Addition of bile from bile duct–ligated animals to organ explants of liver and intestine also causes a threefold increase of alkaline phosphatase activity.[50]

Although it was thought for some time that the elevation of alkaline phosphatase activity was the result of the lack of excretion of alkaline phosphatase from extrahepatic sources, it is now well accepted that this increased activity is the result of *de novo*

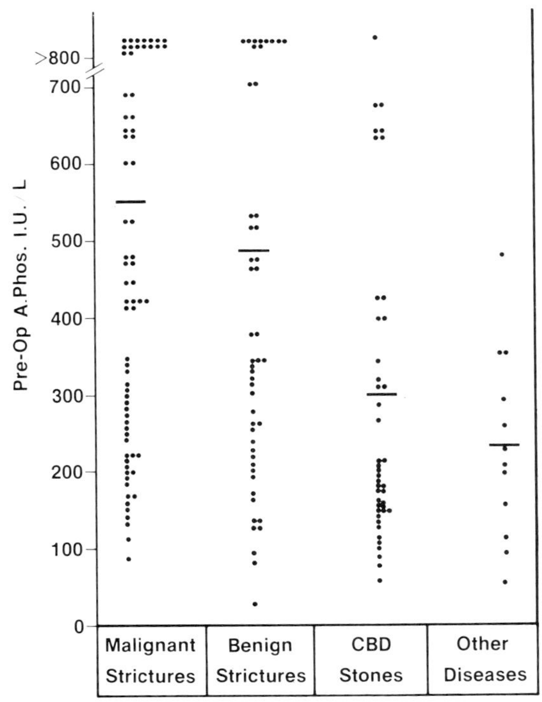

Figure 6–3. Serum alkaline phosphatase values in 178 patients with biliary obstruction grouped according to the cause of the obstruction. Although there is considerable overlap, the highest values are observed in patients with malignant strictures.

enzyme synthesis by the plasma membrane of the hepatocytes in the obstructed liver.[48–51] Indeed, the increase of alkaline phosphatase caused by biliary obstruction can be prevented by inhibitors of protein synthesis.[50, 52]

There is evidence that the serum of patients with intrahepatic cholestasis or focal extrahepatic obstruction contains at least two different forms of alkaline phosphatase: liver alkaline phosphatase and a high molecular weight isoenzyme.[53] The latter is the result of a release of fragments of hepatocytic plasma membrane into the blood stream. These fragments are caused by ruptured membranes as a result of high degrees of biliary obstruction or tumoral invasion of the liver cells (see Fig. 6–1).

The alkaline phosphatase level usually increases with segmental obstruction (e.g., solitary parenchymal metastasis, solitary hepatic abscess, and so forth), a situation in which the bilirubin level (measured with the van den Bergh reaction) is often normal. The reason is as follows. The serum bilirubin concentration rises during obstruction because excretion is blocked, and bilirubin is regurgitated into the hepatic sinusoids and lymphatics. Hepatocyte uptake and excretion are impaired with prolonged obstruction.[32] Bilirubin excretion is not impaired, however, until about half of the biliary tree is blocked. On the other hand, the serum alkaline phosphatase value rises because of increased synthesis of alkaline phosphatase by hepatocytes proximal to the point of obstruction and regurgitation into the sinusoids.[48, 54, 55]

Within a few days of the onset of bile duct obstruction, the *cholesterol* concentration in plasma rises. This is the result of increased cholesterol synthesis, not decreased excretion as was once thought, but the mechanism is unknown.[56]

Cardiovascular Changes

Patients with obstructive jaundice have a tendency to hypotension and an increased susceptibility to hemorrhagic shock.[39, 57] These effects are thought to be due to a combination of the following: (1) decreased peripheral vascular resistance,[59, 60] (2) impaired left ventricular function,[61, 62] and (3) hypovolemia secondary to the diuretic effect of bile.[63]

The decreased peripheral resistance observed in association with obstructive jaundice is probably secondary to an altered response of the smooth muscle of the blood vessels to the normal regulatory mechanisms. For example, several animal experiments suggest that cholemia leads to blunting or refractoriness to the pressor action of angiotensin, norepinephrine, and other sympathomimetic amines.[39, 64] In vitro studies of vascular and extravascular smooth muscle from animals who have bile duct ligation have shown that the contractile response to norepinephrine is reduced.[65] Similarly, exposure of normal smooth muscle of rats to bile salts causes a reduction in contractility to tyramine and norepinephrine. This reduction is different for each bile salt and for each concentration. The site of this loss of contractile response appears to be postjunctional, since bile or bile salts do not affect neuronal amine uptake.[65]

The changes in the response to regulatory mechanisms described previously lead to vasodilatation and decreased peripheral resistance. The kidney and the brain respond differently, both with vasoconstriction.[66, 67] The vasconstriction observed in the kidney results in part from a normal response to the relative hypoperfusion caused by the generalized decrease of peripheral vascular resistance. In addition, biliary obstruction alters the sensitivity of the renal vasculature to endogenous vasoactive agents differently than it does in other vascular beds.[39, 60, 68] For example, there is an enhancement of the action of norepinephrine and angiotensin in the circulation of the kidney in animals with bile duct ligation,[60, 61, 63] and there is blunting of response to dopamine (normally a kidney vasodilator) and complete refractoriness to glucagon, glycine, and bradykinin, all of which normally produce renal vasodilatation.[69]

The effects of cholemia on cardiac performance are less clear. Older studies suggested that hyperbilirubinemia was associated with marked bradycardia.[70] This chronotropic effect of cholemia has been substantiated by several experimental studies,[62, 71] but it is unlikely that ventricular performance is significantly affected by bradycardia, and most studies in conscious animals with biliary obstruction suggest that cardiac output is unchanged.[39, 60]

There are still other mechanisms that may contribute to the development of postoperative hypotension in patients with jaundice. For example, endotoxemia, found in half of patients with biliary obstruction,[72] causes vasodilatation and decreased peripheral resistance.[72, 73]

Changes in Renal Function

Patients with biliary obstruction have a high risk of developing renal failure, particularly after operations or manipulations of the biliary tract. For example, in one report, postoperative renal failure was 60 times more common after emergency operations in patients with biliary obstruction than after operations for perforated peptic ulcer[74]; it was responsible for over 50 per cent of the deaths following surgery to treat obstructive jaundice in another.[75] Similarly, one third of jaundiced patients had some evidence of impaired renal function preoperatively, and 36 per cent developed oliguria and increased serum creatinine levels after surgery, according to another report.[76]

In jaundiced patients, postoperative creatinine clearance is decreased to a greater degree than in nonjaundiced patients, and the decrease is proportional to the degree of hyperbilirubinemia.[74] The mechanism whereby renal failure develops in the presence of obstructive jaundice involves several factors. For example, cholemia has diuretic effects, and, as discussed earlier, jaundiced patients have a tendency to hypotension; therefore, it is likely that, at least in the initial stages, renal failure in these patients may be prerenal. However, there is ample evidence that cholemia has a nephrotoxicity of its own, probably mediated by its action on the renal vasculature. For example, as early as 4 hours after bile duct ligation in the dog, although tubular function is preserved (assessed by the diuretic response to furosemide), there is marked attenuation of the vasodilatory effects of dopamine and lack of response to other vasodilators.[69] Interestingly, intravenous infusion of small amounts of whole bile, but not bilirubin or bile salts alone, has the same effects, and relief of obstruction results in immediate recovery of the response to vasodilators in these animals.[59] Prostaglandins are thought to play a compensatory role under these circumstances. Renal prostaglandin synthesis is markedly increased after common bile duct ligation in the dog.[58, 77] This increase in vasodilatory prostaglandins may contrarest the negative effects of renal vasoconstriction by redistributing renal blood flow toward the inner cortex, which leads to increased glomerular filtration rate. In fact, inhibition of prostaglandin synthesis (with return to normal levels) in animals with biliary obstruction results in a marked decrease of renal blood flow through the inner cortex and decreased urine output.[77]

Endotoxemia in patients with obstructive jaundice is commonly associated with impaired renal function, although the mechanism of this association remains unknown.[72]

In summary, the high incidence of renal dysfunction associated with biliary obstruction is caused initially by renal hypoperfusion, resulting from relative hypovolemia secondary to the diuretic effects of bile salts, and the generalized vasodilation associated with biliary obstruction. It is later aggravated by the vasoconstriction of the renal vascular bed due to altered responses to regulatory mechanisms, and finally it may be worsened by endotoxemia, so common in these patients.

Changes in the Host-Defense Mechanism

Sepsis is a major cause of morbidity and mortality in patients with biliary obstruction.[78–80, 125–127] Gram-negative septicemia often complicates manipulation of the obstructed biliary tract and may progress to septic shock with multiple organ failure. Endotoxemia occurs preoperatively in 20 to 65 per cent of patients with obstructive jaundice[76, 81] and postoperatively in 50 to 85 per cent.[72, 76, 81–84] For example, in a study that compared 27 jaundiced patients with 13 patients with biliary tract disorders but no jaundice, endotoxins were found in 68 per cent of jaundiced patients, but in only one of the nonjaundiced patients before surgery. Following operation, the incidence of endoxemia increased to 80 per cent in the jaundiced patients. The incidence of endotoxemia did not correlate with the serum bilirubin value and was not changed by the use of the antitoxin polymyxin B.[76] Ingoldby et al. found an association between preoperative endotoxemia and postoperative mortality.[76] Portal endotoxemia is found in over half of patients with obstructive jaundice.[72, 76]

There is evidence that biliary obstruction causes a partial inhibition of the phagocytic function of the reticuloendothelial system,[80, 83, 85, 124, 125] and, therefore, bacteria, endotoxin, and immune complexes are not cleared as efficiently from the plasma. For example, biliary obstruction of 21 days in the rat decreases the ability of the reticuloendothelial system to clear colloidal carbon from the plasma, and these animals have a higher mortality following an intravenous administration of endotoxin.[80, 85] Indeed, one study showed that whereas 90 per cent of rats with 3 days of complete biliary obstruction died following an endotoxin injection, mortality was only 20 per cent among the control animals.[85] Injection of viable *E. coli* in rats with common bile duct ligation is cleared from the blood, at least initially, at the same rate as that of control animals. However, while bacteria accumulate predominantly in the Kupffer cells of the liver in normal rats, they are trapped in the lung in the animals with common duct ligation. This leads to thickening of the lung interstitium and may explain the tendency to pulmonary failure in patients with biliary obstruction.[86] In addition to depessing RES phagocytic capacity, prolonged biliary obstruction results in splenomegaly.

Depression of Kupffer cell activity is probably secondary to increased biliary intraductal pressure and to the accumulation of compounds toxic to the reticuloendothelial system in the systemic circulation. Alternatively, this could represent a decreased number of Kupffer cells or depletion of serum opsonins.

Extrahepatic Cellular Damage

Cholemia may lead to direct cellular damage. Although it is clear that in very high concentrations, bile constituents lead to alterations of key cellular functions, which of the bile constituents is responsible for the effects is not known. It is possible that different constituents of bile may have different effects on different tissues. For example, kernicterus and renal medullary damage in jaundiced infants are thought to represent direct cellular injury caused by hyperbilirubinemia.[39] High bilirubin levels inhibit oxidative phosphorylation in the brain cells.[87] High serum bilirubin may also cause hemolysis by direct cellular injury. Likewise, high concentrations of bile acids inhibit lymphocyte function[128] and can also produce tissue injury. They inhibit ATPase activity, oxygen uptake, and protein synthesis in the small intestine of the rat,[88] they are capable of disrupting lysosomes,[58] and they may lead to the destruction of cellular membranes.[39]

RELIEF OF BILIARY OBSTRUCTION AND RECOVERY OF LIVER FUNCTION

Relief of biliary obstruction is accompanied by an immediate choleresis,[89, 91] consisting of increases in both the bile acid–dependent and the bile acid–independent fractions of bile flow. Bile acid excretion initially is lower than normal, but it recovers in about 4 days in humans.[90] In rats, 5 days after bile duct ligation, relief of the obstruction is followed by a high bile flow for the first few minutes. Bile flow, however, falls to relatively normal levels within 1 hour.[92] This choleretic state is associated with increased erythritol and inulin clearances and augmented Na^+, K^+, and ATPase activity, and thus it is most probably caused by increased canalicular permeability.[18, 19] Support of this hypothesis comes from the observation that the estimate of bile acid–independent bile flow during the initial choleretic period that follows bile duct ligation in the rat is three times higher than that of controls.[92] Following relief of bile duct obstruction the excretion rate of bile acids is initially very high, coinciding with the marked choleresis. The excretion rate falls sharply over the first hour, just as the bile flow does, and becomes significantly lower than that of controls for the next 3 to 4 hours.[92] Infusion of sodium taurocholate in the immediate postobstructive period induces choleresis by increasing bile acid–dependent flow.

Bilirubin transport is more sensitive than bile acid transport to the effects of biliary tract obstruction. For example, the maximal rate of bilirubin excretion is decreased when bile flow is obstructed, but, contrary to what happens to bile acid secretion, it is not improved by infusions of bile salts that increase bile flow.[91] Indeed, after a brief period of biliary obstruction in dogs (less than a week), the bilirubin returns to normal in 4 to 7 days. There is no correlation between the duration of obstruction and the rate of return of serum bilirubin or serum alkaline phosphatase values to normal.[89] In humans, as the preoperative serum bilirubin level becomes

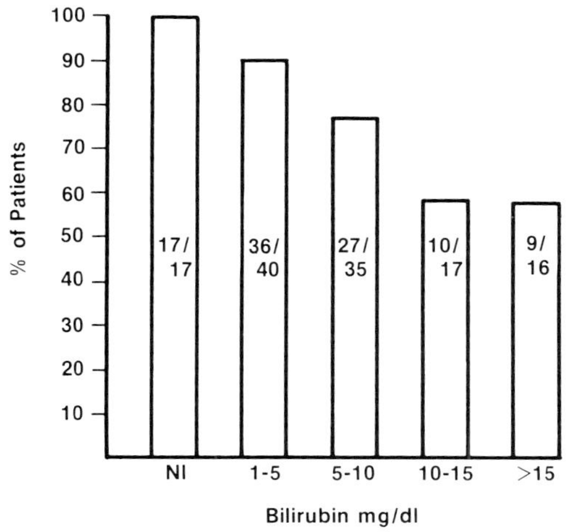

Figure 6–4. Relationship between postoperative normalization of serum bilirubin and preoperative serum bilirubin values in 125 patients operated on for biliary obstruction. About 40 per cent of patients whose preoperative bilirubin value was greater than 10 mg/dl did not achieve normal serum bilirubin postoperatively. However, a considerable number of these patients had malignant biliary obstruction.

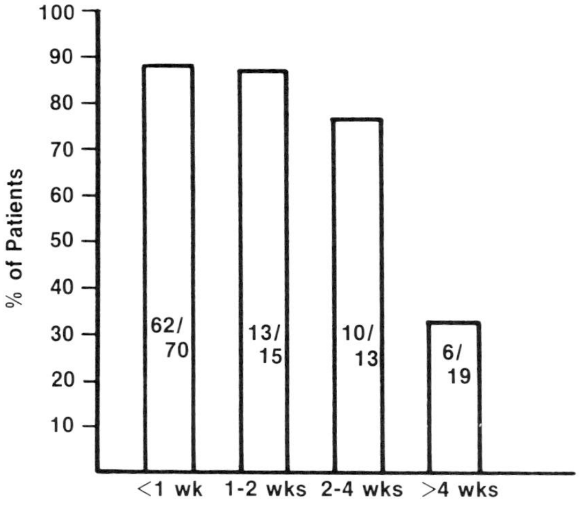

Figure 6–5. Relationship between postoperative normalization of serum bilirubin values and preoperative duration of jaundice in 117 patients followed for at least 3 months after decompression of the bile duct. Note that less than 40 per cent of those who were jaundiced for over 4 weeks before operation eventually achieved a normal serum bilirubin postoperatively.

higher, the chances of postoperative return to normal decrease. For example, in a study of 278 patients with biliary obstruction, we found that 45 per cent of those whose preoperative serum bilirubin value was higher than 10 mg/dl never reached normal values postoperatively (Fig. 6–4).[46] Similarly, the duration of biliary obstruction preoperatively may play a role, as we found a normal serum bilirubin value postoperatively in only one third of patients who had been jaundiced for over 4 weeks preoperatively (Fig. 6–5).[46]

In humans the serum bilirubin value decreases exponentially at an average rate of 8 per cent per day (Fig. 6–6); this is not affected by the duration of obstruction, the height of the preoperative bilirubin value, or the cause of the obstruction.[46] The rate is slower than the 14.5 per cent per day disposal of an additional bilirubin load in normal subjects.[93] This difference may reflect persistent impairment of the excretory mechanism following relief of the obstruction. Support for this view is based on the fact that both humans and dogs exhibit abnormal sulfobromophthalein excretion for a while following relief of bile duct obstruction, even after the serum bilirubin level has become normal.[89, 94] Decreased clearance of organic anions may also be the result of decreased sinusoidal blood flow induced by long-standing biliary obstruction.[7, 10] Nevertheless, it is of interest that while there is a precipitous fall of serum bilirubin values in the first day or two following relief of biliary obstruction, the rate of descent of serum bilirubin becomes much slower after the first 72 to 96 hours.

Van Hootegem et al. have suggested that this apparently slower decline in the value of serum bilirubin is due to the presence of bilirubin covalently linked to serum proteins and thus not available for the hepatocytes for

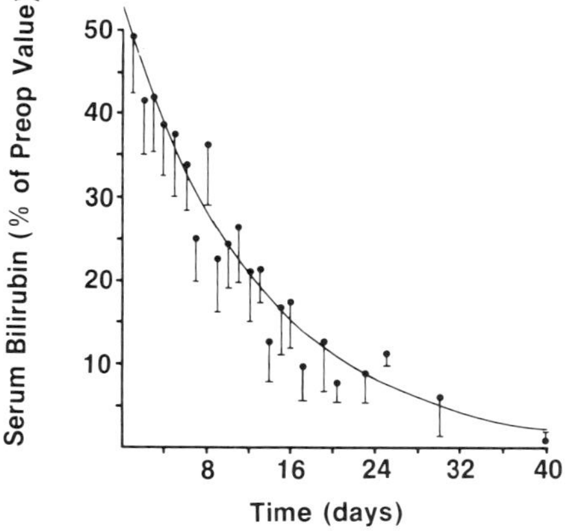

Figure 6–6. Mean serum bilirubin values in 98 patients operated on for biliary obstruction who eventually achieved a normal serum bilirubin level. Serum bilirubin was about 25 per cent of the preoperative value by day 10 and was about 10 per cent of the preoperative value 3 weeks after operation.

clearance from the plasma. In their study they found that 10 days after relief of obstruction, although total bilirubin values had declined to about 20 per cent of the preoperative value, the fraction of bilirubin linked to protein had declined only to about 70 per cent of its preoperative value.[44] This concept is supported by a study of the plasma clearance of injected albumin-linked bilirubin in rats with intact hepatobiliary function. The study showed that, unlike esterified bilirubins, bilirubin-albumin conjugates cannot be excreted in bile at an appreciable rate.[95] The plasma level of this assumed protein-conjugated bilirubin decreases slowly from day 7 onward with a plasma half-life of approximately 17 days, comparable to that of plasma albumin.[44, 96] Therefore, it is possible that this slower clearance of bilirubin from the serum of patients who had relief of biliary obstruction may not be totally due to hepatocytic dysfunction, but rather to the accumulation of other bilirubin compounds not available to the hepatocytes for excretion.

After release of obstruction in rats and dogs, the bilirubin concentration returns to normal earlier than the alkaline phosphatase concentration does.[41] In humans the decline in alkaline phosphatase values after release of obstruction is sluggish compared with that of bilirubin values (Fig. 6–7), and a transient rebound elevation often occurs after the initial decline.[46, 97, 98] These differences reflect the different pathways of elimination of bilirubin and alkaline phosphatase. In general, the liver does not excrete alkaline phosphatase from serum to bile but catabolizes it like other plasma proteins. This is due in part to the size and high molecular weight of a considerable portion of the alkaline phosphatase present in the serum of patients with biliary obstruction.[53, 99] Thus, the disappearance of alkaline phosphatase from serum is largely independent of hepatocytic secretory function or patency of the biliary tract.[49] In fact, 8 days after surgery for biliary obstruction, and while the plasma concentration of alkaline phosphatase was in excess of 500 units, De Broe et al. found alkaline phosphatase activity barely detectable in the bile.[53] Because the catabolic pathway for alkaline phosphatase is not dependent on biliary excretion and its half-life in the circulation is long (7 days), the serum concentration changes slowly in response to the decreased production that follows release of obstruction.

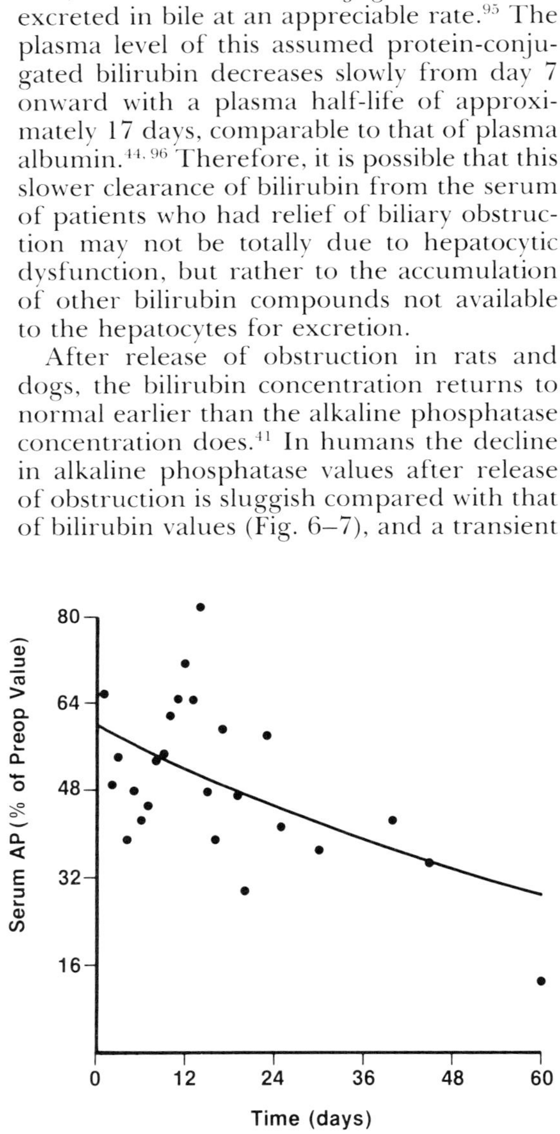

Figure 6–7. Mean serum alkaline phosphatase values in 98 patients operated on for biliary obstruction who eventually achieved a normal serum bilirubin. The decline of serum alkaline phosphatase was sluggish when compared with that of serum bilirubin. There was a rebound about 2 weeks after operation.

RISK OF OPERATION IN PATIENTS WITH BILIARY OBSTRUCTION

The effects of biliary obstruction in the function of the liver, the kidneys, the cardiovascular system, and the immune defense mechanisms described earlier lead to an increased risk of complications and death in these patients. It is important to determine preoperatively the risks of biliary surgery in patients with biliary obstruction and perhaps identify those groups who, because of prohibitive mortality rates, might benefit from less invasive procedures. Several studies have identified risk factors associated with poor outcome in patients with obstructive jaundice.[100–103]

Pitt et al. analyzed 15 clinical and laboratory parameters taken on admission in 155 consecutive patients undergoing biliary tract surgery and found that 10 factors correlated with hospital mortality. They were malignancy, age greater than 60 years, temperature higher than 38 C°, hematocrit value less than 30 per cent, white blood cell count more than 10,000/mm^3, blood urea nitrogen level more than 20 mg/dl, serum creatinine level more than 1.3 mg/dl, serum albumin level less than 3 gm/dl, bilirubin level more than

10 mg/dl, and alkaline phosphatase level more than 100 IU/L.[101] Most of these factors were also found by Blamey et al. to correlate significantly with mortality after surgery for biliary obstruction.[102] Dixon, et al. in a similar retrospective study, identified only three risk factors that were associated with increased postoperative mortality and morbidity: an initial bilirubin level more than 100 μmol/L, a hematocrit value of 30 per cent or less, and a diagnosis of malignant obstruction.[103]

Other authors have attempted to measure the degree of hepatocellular function by different tests and have correlated the test results with the outcome after operations in the biliary tract. McPherson et al. have suggested that measurement of antipyrine clearance is useful to predict the outcome of surgery. Antipyrine is normally cleared by the hepatocytes and thus may give a dynamic measure of hepatic function. The antipyrine test is performed by taking blood samples immediately before, and 4 and 24 hours after, the administration of 600 mg of antipyrine, a minor analgesic. In normal volunteers the half-life of antipyrine is less than 15 hours. McPherson et al. found that among patients with biliary obstruction the chance of postoperative death was significantly higher in those with antipyrine half-life of over 15 hours. In fact, 10 of 25 patients with an abnormal test died, as opposed to 2 of 21 patients with a normal test.[100] This is relatively safe test, which can be repeated to assess changes in liver function over time. Gill et al. have proposed the use of the C-14-aminopyrine breath test, which measures hepatic microsomal function.[104] This test successfully quantitates liver dysfunction in patients with liver disease undergoing surgery but has the disadvantage that it cannot be readily repeated because it involves the use of C-14. Prothrombin time, a reflection of hepatocytic synthetic function, has prognostic value in patients with cirrhosis, but it is not helpful in patients with biliary obstruction. Similarly, measurements of other blood coagulation parameters, such as antithrombin III, plasminogen, and alpha-2 antiplasmin, have been looked at in prospective studies and found to be of very little value to assess risks in patients with biliary obstruction.[105]

At present there is no single test of hepatic function that can accurately predict the outcome of surgery. Knowledge of all the risk factors, and measurement of liver secretory or synthetic function in some patients, help determine the general risk category in which to place the patient but should not be used individually to decide who should or should not get an operation. It appears clear from all the studies that, aside from the general risk factors of all major operations, the absolute level of serum bilirubin and the presence of associated biliary infection are the most important factors that determine the immediate outcome of surgery in patients with biliary obstruction.

The wide availability and relatively low risk of percutaneous transhepatic biliary drainage, and the recognition of biliary obstruction as a major risk factor, fueled the enthusiasm for preoperative percutaneous decompression of the biliary tract in the last decade. Moreover, several retrospective studies[106–108] and a nonrandomized analysis[109] suggested that routine preoperative percutaneous biliary drainage might be helpful. Many clinicians accepted this technique, and its use became routine in several centers during the early 1980s. Since then, several authors have found that percutaneous biliary drainage had a relatively high complication rate[110–118] and failed to reduce the number of complications or the mortality in patients with biliary obstruction.[119, 120] Three prospective randomized trials have also shown that, when applied indiscriminately to all patients with biliary obstruction, preoperative percutaneous drainage does not reduce the operative risk.[121–123] A fourth prospective controlled trial showed that although preoperative percutaneous drainage improved renal function and decreased the number of surgical complications, when the complications of drainage itself were included, the clinical impact of percutaneous drainage was minimal.[129] This technique, however, may be useful in patients who require preoperative nutritional support and in whom the operation has to be delayed, in those whose serum bilirubin levels exceed 20 to 22 mg/dl,[117] and in those who have associated cholangitis.

REFERENCES

1. Beneventano TC, Jacobson HG, Hurwitt ES, Schein CJ: Cine-cholangiomanometry: physiologic observations. Am J Roentgenol 1967;*100*:673.
2. Schein CJ, Beneventano TC: Choledochal dynamics in man. Surg Gynecol Obstet 1968;*126*:591.
3. Mirizzi PL: Sindrome del conducto hepatico. J Int Chir 1948;*8*:731.

4. Montefusco P, Spier N, Geiss AC: Another facet of Mirizzi's syndrome. Arch Surg 1983;*118*:1221.
5. McSherry CK, Ferstenberg H, Virshup M: The Mirizzi's syndrome classification and surgical therapy. Surg Gastroenterol 1983;*1*:219.
6. Cantarow A, Stewart HL: Alteration in serum bilirubin and bromsulphalein retention in relation to morphological changes in the liver and bile passages in cats with total biliary stasis. Am J Pathol 1935;*11*:561.
7. Hunt DR: Changes in liver blood flow with development of biliary obstruction in the rat. Aust NZ J Surg 1979;*49*:733.
8. Cameron GR, Oakley CL: Ligation of the common bile duct. J Pathol 1932;*35*:769.
9. Cameron GR, Hasan SM: Disturbances of structure and function in the liver as the result of biliary obstruction. J Pathol Bacteriol 1958;*75*:333.
10. Gall EA, Dobrogorski O: Hepatic alterations in obstructive jaundice. Am J Clin Pathol 1964; *41*:126.
11. Shorter RG, Baggenstoss AH: Extrahepatic cholestasis: I. Histologic changes in hepatic interlobular bile ducts and ductules in extrahepatic cholestasis. Am J Clin Pathol 1959;*32*:1.
12. Adler M, Chung KW, Schaffner F: Pericanalicular hepatocytic and bile ductular microfilaments in cholestasis in man. Am J Pathol 1980;*98*:603.
13. DeVos R, Desmet VJ: Morphologic changes of the junctional complex of the hepatocytes in the rat liver after bile duct ligation. Br J Exp Pathol 1978;*59*:220.
14. Koga A, Todo S: Morphological and functional changes in the tight junctions of the bile canaliculi induced by bile duct ligation. Cell Tissue Res 1978;*195*:267.
15. Desmet VJ, De Vos R: Tight junctions in the liver. *In* Popper H, Schaffner F (eds.): Progress in Liver Disease, Vol III. New York, Grune & Stratton, 1982, pp 31–50.
16. Williams RD, Fish JC, Williams DD: The significance of biliary pressure. Arch Surg 1967;*95*:374.
17. Strasberg SM, Redinger RN, Small DN, Egdahl RH: The effect of elevated biliary tract pressure on biliary lipid metabolism and bile flow in nonhuman primates. J Lab Clin Med 1982;*99*:342.
18. Accatino, L, Contreras A, Fernandez S, et al: The effect of complete biliary obstruction on bile flow and bile acid excretion: post-cholestatic choleresis in the rat. J Lab Clin Med 1979;*93*:706.
19. Accatino L, Contreras A, Berdichevsky E, et al: The effect of complete biliary obstruction on bile secretion. Studies on the mechanisms of post-cholestatic choleresis in the rat. J Lab Clin Med 1981;*97*:525.
20. Accatino L, Gavilan P, Contreras A, Quintana C: Effects of increased biliary resistance on bile secretion in the rat. J Lab Clin Med 1984;*104*:51.
21. Jonson, G. Sundman L: Bile and dry matter output at elevated liver secretion pressure. Acta Chir Scand 1964;*128*:153.
22. Strasberg SM, Dorn BC, Redinger RN, Small DM, Egdahl RH: Effects of alteration of biliary pressure on bile composition—A method for study: Primate biliary physiology V. Gastroenterology 1971;*61*: 357.
23. Strasberg SM, Dorn BC, Small DM, Egdahl RH: The effect of biliary tract pressure on bile flow, bile salt secretion, and bile salt synthesis in the primate. Surgery 1971;*70*:140.
24. Imamoglu K, Perry JF, Wangensteen OH: Experimental production of gallstones by incomplete stricture of the terminal common bile duct. Surgery, 1957;*42*:623.
25. Pikula JV, Dunphy JE: Some effects of stenosis of the terminal common bile duct on the biliary tract and liver. N Engl J Med 1959;*260*:315.
26. Bernhoft RA, Pellegrini CA, Broderick WC, Way LW: Biliary sludge and stone foundation in the acutely ligated dog gallbladder. Gastroenterology 1983;*85*:1166.
27. Peterson RE, Fujimoto JM: Increased biliary tree permeability produced in rats by hepatoactive agents. J Pharmacol Exp Ther 1977;*202*:732.
28. Boyer JL: Tight junctions in normal and cholestatic liver: does the paracellular pathway have functional significance? Hepatology 1983;*3*:614.
29. Metz J, Aoki A, Merlo M, et al: Morphological alterations and functional changes of interhepatocellular junctions induced by bile duct ligation. Cell Tissue Res 1977;*182*:299.
30. Jones AL, Hradek GT, Schmucker DL, Underdown BJ: The fate of polymeric and secretory immunoglobulin A after retrograde infusion into the common bile duct in rats. Hepatology 1984;*4*:1173.
31. Szabo G, Magyar Z, Szentirmai A, et al: Bile constituents in blood and lymph during biliary obstruction. II. The absorption and transport of bile acids and bilirubin. Lymphology 1975;*8*:36.
32. Wheeler HO, Meltzer JI, Bradley SE: Biliary transport and hepatic storage of sulfobromophthalein sodium in the unanesthetized dog, in normal man and in patients with hepatic disease. J Clin Invest 1960;*39*:1131.
33. Simon FR, Sutherland E, Accatino LA: Stimulation of hepatic sodium and potassium activated adenosine triphosphate activity by phenobarbital—its possible role in regulation of bile flow. J Clin Invest 1977;*59*:849.
34. Zsigmond G, Solymoss B: Increased canalicular bile production induced by pregnenolone-16 alfacarbonitrile, spironolactone and cortisol in rats. Proc Soc Exp Biol Med 1974;*145*:631.
35. Solymoss B, Zsigmond G: Effect of microsomal enzyme inducers on the liver changes produced by common bile duct ligature. Proc Soc Exp Biol Med 1974;*147*:430.
36. Van Damme BV, Fevery J, Heirwegh K: Altered composition of bilirubin conjugates in rat bile after obstruction of the common bile duct. Experientia 1971;*27*:27.
37. Harmatz PR, Kleinman RE, Bunnell BW, McClenathan DT, Walker WA, Bloch KJ: The effect of bile duct obstruction on the clearance of circulating IgA immune complexes. Hepatology 1984;*4*:96.
38. Ginsberg AL: Very high levels of SGOT and LDH in patients with extrahepatic biliary tract obstruction. Am J Dig Dis 1970;*15*:803.
39. Green J, Beyar R, Bomzon L, Finberg JPM: Jaundice, the circulation and the kidney. Nephron 1984;*37*:145.
40. Rickers H, Christensen M, Arnfred T, et al: The diagnostic value of fasting serum total bile acid concentration in patients with suspected liver disease. Scand J Gastroenterol 1982;*17*:565.
41. Corlette MB, Mendes-Monteiro AC, Bismuth H, Morin J: Transient bile duct obstruction. Arch Surg 1976;*111*:1017.

42. Blanckaert N: Analysis of bilirubin and bilirubin mono- and diconjugates. Determination of their relative amounts in biological samples. Biochem J 1980;*185*:115.
43. Blanckaert N, Kabra P, Farina F, et al: Measurement of bilirubin and its monoconjugates and diconjugates in human serum by alkaline methanolysis and high-performance liquid chromatography. J Lab Clin Med 1980;*96*:198.
44. Van Hootegem P, Fevery J, Blanckaert N: Serum bilirubins in hepatobiliary disease: Comparison with other liver function tests and changes in the postobstructive period. Hepatology 1985;*5*:112.
45. Blanckaert N, D'Argenio G: Presence of bilirubins linked covalently to albumin in serum of patients with cholestasis (Abstr). Gastroenterology 1982; *82*:1222.
46. Pellegrini CA, Thomas MJ, Way LW: Bilirubin and alkaline phosphatase values before and after surgery for biliary obstruction. Am J Surg 1982;*143*:167.
47. Aronsen KF: Liver function studies during and after complete extra-hepatic biliary obstruction in the dog. II. Complete biliary stasis. Acta Chir Scand (Suppl) 1961;*275*:16.
48. Kaplan MM, Righetti A: Induction of rat liver alkaline phosphatase: the mechanism of the serum elevation in bile duct obstruction. J Clin Invest 1970;*49*:508.
49. Kaplan MM: Alkaline phosphatase. N Engl J Med 1972;*286*:200.
50. Komoda T, Kumegawa M, Yajima T, Tamura G, Alpers DH: Induction of rat hepatic and intestinal alkaline phosphatase activity produced by bile from bile duct–ligated animals. Am J Physiol 1984; *246*:G393.
51. Moss DW: Clinical biochemistry of alkaline phosphatase. Cell Biochem Funct 1983;*1*:70.
52. Kaplan MM, Ohkubo A, Zuaroni GE, Sze-Tu D: Increased synthesis of rat liver alkaline phosphatase by bile duct ligation. Hepatology 1983;*3*:368.
53. De Broe ME, Roels F, Nouwen EJ, Claeys L, Wieme RJ: Liver plasma membrane: The source of high molecular weight alkaline phosphatase in human serum. Hepatology 1985;*5*:118.
54. Price CP, Sammons HG: An interpretation of the serum alkaline phosphatase isoenzyme patterns in patients with obstructive liver disease. J Clin Pathol 1976;*29*:976.
55. Righetti AB, Marshall MK: Disparate responses of serum and hepatic alkaline phosphatase and 5′ nucleotidase to bile duct obstruction in the rat. Gastroenterology 1972;*62*:1034.
56. McIntyre N, Harry DS, Pearson AJG: The hypercholesterolaemia of obstructive jaundice. Gut 1975;*16*:379.
57. Bismuth H, Kuntziger H, Corlette MB: Cholangitis in acute renal failure: Priorities in therapeutics. Ann Surg 1975;*181*:881.
58. Fletcher J, Weswick J, Kakkar VV: Endotoxin, prostaglandins and renal fibrin deposition in obstructive jaundice. Br J Surg 1982;*69*:625.
59. Melman A: Effect of angiotensin II inhibition on the bile duct ligated dog. J Surg Res 1978;*24*:277.
60. Alon U, Berant M, Mordechovitz D, Hashmonai M, Better OS: Effect of isolated cholaemia on systemic haemodynamics and kidney function in conscious dogs. Clin Sci 1982;*63*:59.
61. Hishida A, Honda N, Sudo M Nagase M: Mechanisms of altered renal perfusion in the early stage of obstructive jaundice. Kidney Int 1980;*17*:223.
62. Lunzer MR, Manghani KK, Newman SP, Sherlock SPV, Bernard AE, Ginsburg J: Impaired cardiovascular responsiveness in liver disease. Lancet 1975;*2*:382.
63. Alon U, Berant M, Mordechovitz D, Better OS: The effect of intrarenal infusion of bile on kidney function in the dog. Clin Sci 1982;*62*:431.
64. Finberg JPM, Syrop HA, Better OS: Blunted pressor response to angiotensin and sympathomimetic amines in bile duct ligated dogs. Clin Sci 1981;*61*:535.
65. Bomzon A, Finberg JPM, Tovbin D, Naidu SG, Better OS: Bile salts, hypotension and obstructive jaundice. Clin Sci 1984;*67*:177.
66. Bloom DS, Eidelman BH, McCalden TA: Modification of the cerebrovascular response to noradrenaline by bile duct ligation. Gut 1975;*16*:732.
67. Bomzon L, Rosendorff C, Scriven DRL, Farr J: The effect of noradrenaline, adrenergic blocking agents and tyramine on the intrarenal distribution of blood flow in the baboon. Cardiovasc Res 1975;*9*:314.
68. Bomzon L, Kew MC: Renal blood flow in experimental obstructive jaundice. *In* Epstein ME (ed.): The Kidney in Liver Disease, 2nd ed. New York, Elsevier Science Publishing Company, 1983; pp 313–326.
69. Levy M, Finestone H, Fechner C: Action of renal vasodilators in dogs following acute biliary obstruction. J Surg Res 1984;*36*:163.
70. Wakim KG, Essex HE, Mann FC: The effects of whole bile and bile salts on the perfused heart. Am Heart J 1939;*18*:171.
71. Wakim KG, Essex HE, Mann FC: The effects of whole bile and bile salts on the innervated and denervated heart. Am Heart J 1940;*20*:486.
72. Bailey ME: Endotoxin, bile salts and renal function in obstructive jaundice. Br J Surg 1976;*63*:774.
73. Liehr H, Grun M, Thiel H, Brunswig D, Rasenack U: Endotoxin-induced liver necrosis and intravascular coagulation in rats enhanced by portacaval collateral circulation. Gut 1975;*16*:429.
74. Dawson JL: Acute postoperative renal failure in obstructive jaundice. Ann R Coll Surg 1968; *42*:163.
75. Zollinger RM, Williams RD: Surgical aspects of jaundice. Surgery 1956;*39*:1016.
76. Ingoldby CJ, McPherson GAD, Blumgart LH: Endotoxemia in human obstructive jaundice. Effect of Polmyxin B. Am J Surg 1984;*147*:766.
77. Zambraski EJ, Dunn MJ: Importance of renal prostaglandins in control of renal function after chronic ligation of the common bile duct in dogs. J Lab Clin Med 1984;*103*:549.
78. Freedman LR, Goldenberg IS: The relationship between bacterial infection of the hepato-biliary system and common bile duct obstruction in man. Yale J Biol Med 1963;*35*:318.
79. Drivas G, James O, Wardle N: Study of reticuloendothelial phagocytic capacity in patients with cholestasis. Br Med J 1976;*1*:1568.
80. Holman JM Jr, Rikkers LF: Biliary obstruction and host defense failure. J Surg Res 1982;*32*:208.
81. Wardle EN: Renal failure in obstructive jaundice—pathogenic factors. Postgrad Med J 1975;*51*:512.
82. Wilkinson SP, Moodie H, Stamatakis JD, Kakkar WV, Williams R: Endotoxaemia and renal failure in cirrhosis and obstructive jaundice. Br Med J 1976;*2*:1415.
83. Tanaka N, Ryden S, Bergqvist L, Christensen P,

Bengmark S: Reticulo-endothelial function in rats with obstructive jaundice. Br J Surg 1985;*72*:946.

84. Allison MEM, Prentice CRM, Kennedy AC, Blumgart LH: Renal function and other factors in obstructive jaundice. Br J Surg 1979;*66*:392.
85. Wardle EN, Wright NA: Endotoxin and acute renal failure associated with obstructive jaundice. Br Med J 1970;*4*:472.
86. Katz S, Grosfeld JL, Gross K, Plager DA, Ross D, Rosenthal RS, Hull M, Weber TR: Impaired bacterial clearance and trappings in obstructive jaundice. Ann Surg 1984;*199*:14.
87. Zetterstrom R, Ernster L: Bilirubin, an uncoupler of oxidative phosphorylation in isolated mitochondria. Nature 1956;*178*:1335.
88. Parkinson TM, Olson JA: Inhibitory effects of bile acids on adenosine triphosphatase oxygen consumption, and the transport and the diffusion of water soluble substances in the small intestine of the rat. Life Sci 1964;*3*:107.
89. Aronsen KF: Liver function studies during and after complete extrahepatic biliary obstruction in the dog. VII. Results of examinations performed after release of complete biliary obstruction. Acta Chir Scand (Suppl) 1961;*275*:71.
90. Preisig R, Bucher H, Stirneman H, Tauber J: Postoperative choleresis following bile duct obstruction in man. Rev Franc Etud Clin Biol 1969;*14*:151.
91. Zsigmond G, Bernhoft RA, Way LW: Bilirubin transport or segmental biliary obstruction. Surg Forum 1982;*32*:155.
92. Cleland DP, Bartholomew TC, Billing BH: Hepatic transport of sulfated and nonsulfated bile acids in the rat following relief of bile duct obstruction. Hepatology 1984;*4*:477.
93. Berk PD, Bloomer J, Howe R, Berlin N: Constitutional hepatic dysfunction (Gilbert's Syndrome). A new definition based on kinetic studies with unconjugated radiobilirubin. Am J Med 1970;*49*:296.
94. Zsigmond G, Alant O, Flautner L, et al: Indirect methods for evaluation of canalicular, mitochondrial and microsomal function of liver cells in patients with obstructive jaundice before and after surgery. I. Canalicular function. Proc XX Biennial World Congress of the International College of Surgeons, Vol 3. Lourus NC (ed). Amsterdam, Excerpta Medica, 1977, pp 1073–1075.
95. Blanckaert N, Servaes R: Formation and excretability in bile of the bilirubin covalently linked to albumin present in serum of rats with conjugated hyperbilirubinemia (Abstr). Gastroenterology 1983;*84*:1364.
96. Rothschild M, Gratz M, Schreiber S: Albumin metabolism. Prog Liver Disease 1972; *4*:9.
97. Mori K, Misumi A, Sugiyama A, et al: Percutaneous transhepatic bile drainage. Ann Surg 1977; *185*:111.
98. Wiechel KL: Percutaneous transhepatic cholangiography. Acta Chir Scand (Suppl) 1964;*330*:1.
99. De Broe ME, Borgers M, Wieme RJ: The separation and characterization of liver plasma membrane fragments circulating in the blood of patients with cholestasis. Clin Chim Acta 1975;*59*:369.
100. McPherson GAD, Benjamin IS, Boobis AR, Blumgart LH: Antipyrine elimination in patients with obstructive jaundice: a predictor of outcome. Am J Surg 1985;*149*:140.
101. Pitt HA, Cameron JL, Postier RG, Gadacz TR: Factors affecting mortality in biliary tract surgery. Am J Surg 1981;*141*:66.
102. Blamey SL, Fearon KCH, Gilmour WH, Osborne DH, Carter DC: Predictors of risk in biliary surgery. Br J Surg 1983;*70*:535.
103. Dixon JM, Armstrong CP, Duffy SW, Davies GC: Factors affecting morbidity and mortality after surgery for obstructive jaundice. A review of 373 patients. Gut 1983;*24*:845.
104. Gill RA, Goodman MW, Gene GR, Onstad FG, Bubnick MP: Aminopyrine breath test predicts surgical risk for patients with liver disease. Ann Surg 1983;*198*:701.
105. Rodzynek JJ, Urbain D, Leautaud P, Wettendorff P, Delcourt A: Antithrombin III, plasminogen and alpha-2 antiplasmin in jaundice. Clinical usefulness and prognostic significance. Gut 1984;*25*:1050.
106. Koyama K, Takagi Y, Kenji I, Sato T: Experimental and clinical studies on the effect of biliary drainage in obstructive jaundice. Am J Surg 1981;*142*:293.
107. Gundry SR, Strodel WE, Knol JA, Eckhauser FE, Thompson NW: Efficacy of preoperative biliary tract decompression in patients with obstructive jaundice. Arch Surg 1984;*119*:703.
108. Ellison EC, Van Aman ME, Carey LC: Preoperative transhepatic biliary decompression in pancreatic and periampullary cancer. World J Surg 1984;*8*:862.
109. Denning DA, Ellison EC, Carey LC: Preoperative percutaneous transhepatic biliary decompression lowers operative morbidity in patients with obstructive jaundice. Am J Surg 1981;*141*:61.
110. Blenkharn JI, McPherson GAD, Blumgart LH: Septic complications of percutaneous transhepatic biliary drainage. Am J Surg 1984;*147*:318.
111. Mueller PR, vanSonnenberg E, Ferrucci JT Jr: Percutaneous biliary drainage: Technical and catheter-related problems in 200 procedures. AJR 1982;*138*:17.
112. McPherson GAD, Benjamin IS, Habib NA, Bowley NG, Blumgart LH: Percutaneous transhepatic drainage in obstructive jaundice: advantages and problems. Br J Surg 1982;*69*:261.
113. Wong JH, Krippaehne WW, Fletcher WS: Percutaneous transhepatic biliary decompression. Results and complications in 30 patients. Am J Surg 1984;*147*:615.
114. Clouse ME, Evans D, Costello P, Miguel A, Edwards SA, McDermott WV Jr: Percutaneous transhepatic biliary drainage. Ann Surg 1983;*198*:25.
115. Dooley JS, Dick R, George P, Kirk RM, Hobbs KEF, Sherlock S: Percutaneous transhepatic endoprosthesis for bile duct obstruction. Gastroenterology 1984;*86*:905.
116. Clark RA, Mitchell SE, Colley DP, Alexander E: Percutaneous catheter biliary decompression. AJR 1981;*137*:503.
117. Stambuk EC, Pitt HA, Pais SO, Mann LL, Lois JF, Gomes AS: Percutaneous transhepatic drainage. Risks and benefits. Arch Surg 1983;*118*:1388.
118. Gobien RP, Stanley JH, Soucek CD, Anderson MC, Vujic I, Gobien BS: Routine preoperative biliary drainage: effect on management of obstructive jaundice. Radiology 1984;*152*:353.
119. Norlander A, Kalin B, Sundblad R: Effect of percutaneous transhepatic drainage upon liver function and postoperative mortality. Surg Gynecol Obstet 1982;*155*:161.
120. Thomas JH, Connor CS, Pierce GE, MacArthur

RI, Iliopoulos JI, Hermreck AS: Effect of biliary decompression on morbidity and mortality of pancreatoduodenectomy. Am J Surg 1984;*148*:727.

121. Hatfield ARW, Terblanche J, Fataar S, Kernoff L, Tobias R, Girdwood AH, Harries-Jones R, Marks IN: Preoperative external biliary drainage in obstructive jaundice. A prospective controlled clinical trial. Lancet 1982;*2*:896.

122. McPherson GAD, Benjamin IS, Hodgson HJF, Bowley NB, Allison DJ, Blumgart LH: Pre-operative percutaneous transhepatic biliary drainage: The results of a controlled trial. Br J Surg 1984;*71*:371.

123. Pitt HA, Gomes AS, Lois JF, et al: Does preoperative percutaneous biliary drainage reduce operative risk or increase hospital cost? Ann Surg 1985;*201*:545.

124. Tanaka N, Christensen P, Ryden S, Klofyer-Stahl B, Bengmark S: Impaired liver clearance of bacteria in rats with chronic biliary obstruction. Res Exp Med 1985;*185*:173.

125. Pain JA, Cahill CJ, Bailey ME: Perioperative complications in obstructive jaundice: therapeutic considerations. Br J Surg 1985;*72*:942.

126. Malchow-Moller A, Thomsen C, Hilden J, Matzen P, Mindeholm L, Juhl E, The Copenhagen Computer Icterus Group: Survival after jaundice: a prospective study of 1000 consecutive cases. Scand Gastroenterol 1985;*20*:155.

127. Armstrong CP, Dixon JM, Taylor TV, Davies GC: Surgical experience of deeply jaundiced patients with bile duct obstruction. Br J Surg 1984;*71*:234.

128. Keane RM, Gadacz TR, Munster AM, Birmingham W, Winchurch RA: Impairment of human lymphocyte by bile salts. Surgery 1984;*95*:439.

129. Smith RC, Pooley M, George CRP, Faithful GR: Preoperative percutaneous transhepatic internal drainage in obstructive jaundice: A randomized, controlled trial examining renal function. Surgery 1985;*97*:641.

SECTION II

DIAGNOSTIC PROCEDURES

ROBERT N. BERK, M.D.

7

Oral Cholecystography, IV Cholangiography

ORAL CHOLECYSTOGRAPHY

Most physicians consider oral cholecystography to be an uncomplicated radiologic procedure that is simple to perform and easy to interpret. However, in reality, few examinations in radiology require more expertise. The proper performance of oral cholecystography demands sound judgment based on knowledge of the pathophysiology of diseases of the hepatobiliary system, familiarity with the clinical manifestations of these diseases, and an understanding of the pharmacology of biliary contrast materials. Radiographs of excellent technical quality are a prerequisite. Only with this background can oral cholecystography be conducted with sufficient competence to ensure maximum accuracy, efficiency, and safety.

Oral cholecystography was introduced in 1924 by Graham and Cole.[1] The technique is based on two physiologic principles: Halogenated dyes are excreted into the bile and the gallbladder concentrates bile eight to ten times. Thus, the halogen appears in bile and is sufficiently concentrated to permit radiographic visualization of the gallbladder. The most frequently used dye is iopanoic acid (Telepaque). Iopanoic acid is fat-soluble. When the patient takes 6 gm (12 tablets) of Telepaque by mouth, the contrast material is absorbed by passive diffusion in the jejunum and ileum; it is then bound to albumin and taken up by the liver. Iopanoic acid is conjugated with glucuronide by the hepatocytes and excreted into the bile as a water-soluble compound in a process that resembles bilirubin transport. Once in the gallbladder, the contrast material is concentrated by absorption of water. A concentration of 0.5 to 1 per cent iodine is required for proper opacification.[2] In the normal gallbladder, this concentration usually is reached 14 to 17 hours after ingestion of Telepaque. Water-soluble compounds are more rapidly absorbed than is Telepaque. For example, with the use of tyropanoate sodium (Bilopaque) or ipodate (Orografin) the gallbladder opacifies in 10 to 12 hours.[41] Oral cholecystography is done primarily for the diagnosis of cholelithiasis. Gallstones are usually seen as radiolucent defects in the opacified gallbladder. When cystic duct obstruction prevents the contrast material from reaching the gallbladder or when chronic cholecystitis impairs gallbladder absorption and iodine concentration in bile is less than 0.25 per cent, the gallbladder does not opacify.

Considering that nearly 20 million people in the United States have gallstones, and that more than one-half million require hospitalization each year for problems related to that disease,[3] it is not surprising that 2 million oral cholecystograms are performed each year in this country.[4] However, the use of oral cholecystography is decreasing as cholecystosonography has become the preferred diagnostic test for cholelithiasis. For example, data from the Massachusetts General Hospital show that the number of oral cholecystograms performed decreased approximately 80 per cent between 1976 and 1985.[5]

At present, oral cholecystography is done only when clinical findings suggest the presence of cholelithiasis. It is not customary to perform the study to detect gallstones in asymptomatic individuals, although this may be worthwhile in exceptionally high-risk groups, such as diabetics, American Indians, and patients with hemolytic anemia, Crohn's disease, and cirrhosis.[12] Oral cholecystography should not be attempted in patients with impaired liver function or biliary obstruction in whom the serum bilirubin is 2 mg/dl or higher, because with this degree of cholestasis the possibility of opacification of the gallbladder is negligible.

Burhenne summarized the major problems related to oral cholecystography as follows[4]: (1) overrated accuracy in the diagnosis of gallstones; (2) problems associated with nonopacification and impaired opacification of the gallbladder after a single dose of contrast material; (3) misunderstanding concerning the indications for oral cholecystography compared with those for intravenous cholangiography; (4) uncertainty regarding the value of cholecystokinin cholecystography in the diagnosis of acalculous cholecystitis, biliary dyskinesia, and the cystic duct syndrome; and (5) the practice of obtaining oral cholecystograms without preliminary plain abdominal radiographs.

Accuracy of Oral Cholecystography

Numerous reports indicate accuracy rates for oral cholecystography in the range of 97 to 99 per cent.[13–20] However, these studies involved only patients in whom a positive oral cholecystogram was correlated with the pathologic findings at surgery. These data showed that the interpretation of an oral cholecystogram is nearly 100 per cent correct when gallstones are visible in the opacified gallbladder, or when there is nonopacification of the gallbladder on two consecutive studies and extrabiliary causes of nonopacification have been excluded. Hence, these studies show that false positive cholecystograms are exceedingly rare; however, they give no indication concerning the number of patients who have gallstones but in whom the cholecystogram is interpreted as normal (false negative). Since cholecystectomy is rarely justified in patients who have an apparently normal oral cholecystogram, until recently there were only a few reports concerning the incidence of false negative results on oral cholecystography. For example, Dunn et al. found small gallstones at surgery in 2 of 29 patients who had a cholecystectomy despite having a normal cholecystogram—a 7 per cent incidence of false negative examinations.[21] Kolodny et al. reported three examples of patients who had normal cholecystograms but who had gallstones at cholecystectomy.[24] These small stones may be obscured by contrast material, even on upright spot views. Some are missed even by ultrasonography. Because small stones have the potential to develop serious complications, other diagnostic tests, such as ERCP, may be needed in these patients.

With the advent of cholecystosonography and computerized tomography of the gallbladder, it has been possible to evaluate the false negative rate of oral cholecystography with accuracy. Based on comparative studies with ultrasound evaluation of the gallbladder, the accuracy of oral cholecystography in detecting gallstones is probably closer to 90 per cent than 98 per cent.[4, 6–11] Even with ideal radiographic technique and good opacification of the gallbladder, gallstones that are 2 to 3 mm or less in diameter occasionally may be missed.[4, 25] Consequently, when a patient's symptoms are highly suggestive of gallbladder disease, a normal oral cholecystogram should not be taken as conclusive evidence against the presence of gallstones.

Technique of Oral Cholecystography

Preparation of Patient

Experimental data in dogs indicate that the enterohepatic circulation of bile salts plays a major role in facilitating both the intestinal absorption and the hepatic excretion of Telepaque.[26, 27] Therefore, it is important to ensure that fat is given in the diet at the same time as Telepaque is administered. Fat stimulates the release of cholecystokinin, which causes the gallbladder to contract and to empty bile salts stored in the gallbladder into the intestine.

Data reported by Stanley et al. provide clinical evidence that fat in the diet is important in the adequate opacification of the gallbladder with Telepaque.[28] In their study, 47 per cent of patients given Telepaque with a nonfat supper had satisfactory first-day examinations, compared with 70 per cent when Telepaque was given with a high-fat meal. Opacification with Cholebrine and Bilopaque was unaffected by the presence or absence of fat in the diet. Nonopacification of the gallbladder with Telepaque in volunteers on a low-fat diet, reported by Zboralske and Amberg,[29] may be due to poor absorption and excretion of Telepaque rather than to stasis of nonopaque bile in the gallbladder as suggested by the authors.

On the contrary, Mauthe failed to show any difference in the incidence of poor first-dose gallbladder opacification in patients given Telepaque with a fatty meal compared with those in whom Telepaque was given with a low-fat supper.[30] He used a dosage schedule for the contrast material based on body weight (0.5 gm/20 lb), so that, in general, his patients were given more Telepaque than the usual 3 gm dose. The higher dose may have overcome the difficulties with intestinal absorption and hepatic excretion that otherwise might have occurred in the absence of circulating bile salts.

Consequently, data concerning the value of a high-fat diet administered with contrast material are conflicting.[30–33] Whether a regular or a high-fat diet should be recommended depends on which contrast agent is used, and this remains to be clarified. Nevertheless, the present routine of giving a low-fat supper is not warranted and may be counterproductive.

The optimal dose of Telepaque and the other oral cholecystographic contrast agents has not been studied sufficiently. Most authors recommend a single 3 gm dose,[6, 9] but some use 2 gm in order to avoid producing opacification of the gallbladder so dense that gallstones may be obscured.[34] This is not a problem if compression spot films are made. Administering more than 3 gm of Telepaque may be necessary in obese patients, but the routine use of large doses should be avoided because the degree of toxicity produced by the contrast agent is probably proportional to the amount of the compound given. The routine use of a double dose (6 gm) is not warranted, because most reported cases of renal failure due to oral cholecystographic contrast materials have been in patients who received high doses of the compound.[35]

Patients should be adequately hydrated following the administration of the contrast agent because of the potent uricosuric effects of the compounds.[35] Water should be allowed ad lib. If the patient is known to have gout, fluids should be encouraged and the urine should be alkalinized to avoid precipitation of urate crystals in the urine. A small dose of aspirin may be given to reduce the uricosuria associated with Telepaque.[36] When 600 mg (2 tablets) of aspirin are given with 3 gm of Telepaque, followed by an additional dose of 600 mg of aspirin 2 hours later, the uricosuric effect of the Telepaque is reduced by a factor of 10.

Fecal material in the colon may interfere with optimal visualization of the gallbladder. However, because Telepaque frequently has a cathartic effect, it is not necessary to routinely administer a laxative. Conversely, it has been shown that castor oil does not interfere with opacification of the gallbladder when it is given with Telepaque.[37, 38] Since castor oil stimulates the gallbladder to contract, there is experimental evidence, at least, to suggest that it may improve the absorption and excretion of Telepaque.[35]

Patients should be evaluated for a history of previous allergic reaction to any of the radiographic contrast materials before oral cholecystography is undertaken. Crossover reactions with the urographic and angiographic contrast materials may occur. Adverse reactions in a patient with known allergy to contrast material can be avoided by treatment with corticosteroids and antihistaminics prior to administration of the cholecystographic contrast agent.

Radiographic Technique

Ideally, a preliminary plain abdominal radiograph should be made before the administration of contrast material in order to detect calcification of the wall of the gallbladder or radiopaque gallstones that might be obscured by contrast material in the gallbladder, and to recognize milk of calcium bile that could be confused with a normally opacified gallbladder. This is in keeping with the basic radiologic tenet that a preliminary radiograph should be made before any contrast agent is used. However, it is impractical in most cases to require patients to make an additional trip to the radiology department for the preliminary examination. Consequently, one must weigh the inconvenience and expense of the preliminary radiograph against the number of times gallbladder disease will be overlooked without it. Despite the lack of precise data concerning the latter, it is not customary to make a preliminary film.[4] If upright spot films of the gallbladder are made with graded compression, it is exceedingly unlikely that radiopaque gallstones will not be identified in the fundus of the opacified gallbladder. However, two such cases were reported by Moadel and Bryk,[39] and undoubtedly others occur. One must keep in mind that such false negative cholecystograms may happen if the preliminary radiograph is omitted. In special cases (e.g., in patients with apparently normal cholecystograms who have characteristic symptoms of biliary colic or in whom significant symptoms persist), a plain abdominal radiograph should be made at some point in the radiologic work-up.

Care must be taken to make the radiographs of the gallbladder at the appropriate time following the administration of the contrast material. Poor gallbladder opacification will occur if the radiographs are taken prematurely or if they are delayed. Peak opacification of the gallbladder with Telepaque occurs between 14 and 19 hours after ingestion of the contrast material.[40] With the use of Bilopaque, a water-soluble agent, optimal gallbladder opacification occurs at 10 hours.[41] Consequently, the timing of the radiograph depends upon which contrast material is used.

The actual number and type of radiographs that are made as a part of a cholecystogram vary depending upon the preference of the radiologist, but in all cases the following principles must be observed: (1) Upright spot films made with fluoroscopy or right lateral decubitus radiographs should be included if gallstones are not evident on prone or supine radiographs (Figs. 7–1 and 7–2)[42–45]; (2) at least one radiograph should include the entire abdomen; (3) the radiograph should be of excellent technical quality and made using low-kilovoltage technique; and (4) the radiograph should be viewed before the patient leaves the department so that additional films can be obtained if necessary.

The Fatty Meal. The routine use of a fatty meal in oral cholecystography has been recommended by various authors[46–55] in order to (1) free the gallbladder from overlying gas and fecal material in the colon; (2) evaluate gallbladder function; (3) detect small gallstones, especially those that lie in the neck of the gallbladder; (4) opacify the cystic and common ducts; (5) diagnose cholesterolosis and adenomyomatosis; and (6) differentiate a gallstone from a fixed filling defect in the gallbladder wall.

It is generally agreed that the response of the gallbladder to a fatty meal is too variable to permit valid conclusions regarding its ability to empty normally.[4, 48] Cholecystokinin has replaced the fatty meal for this purpose.

Miller et al. emphasized the importance of giving a fatty meal routinely to opacify the neck of the gallbladder, where they believe

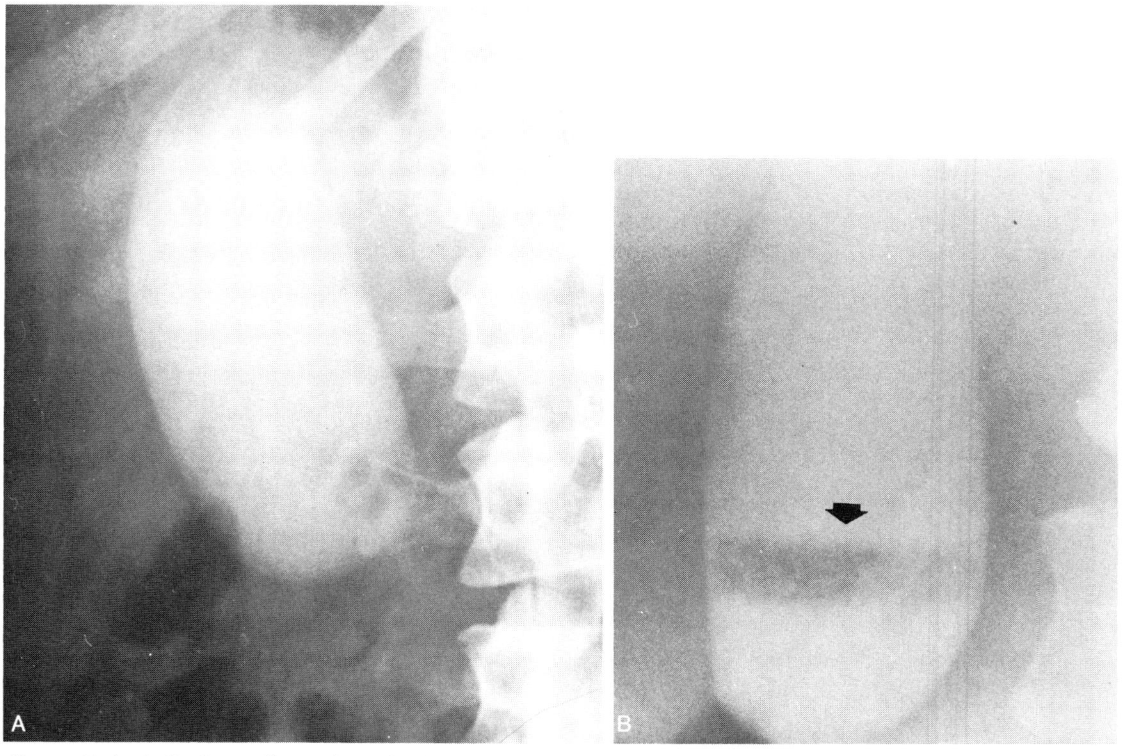

Figure 7–1. *A*, Supine radiograph made during oral cholecystography, showing no gallstones in the gallbladder. *B*, Upright spot films of the gallbladder in the same patient, made with the use of fluoroscopy. A layer of small gallstones is visible, which was not evident on supine or prone radiographs (*arrow*).

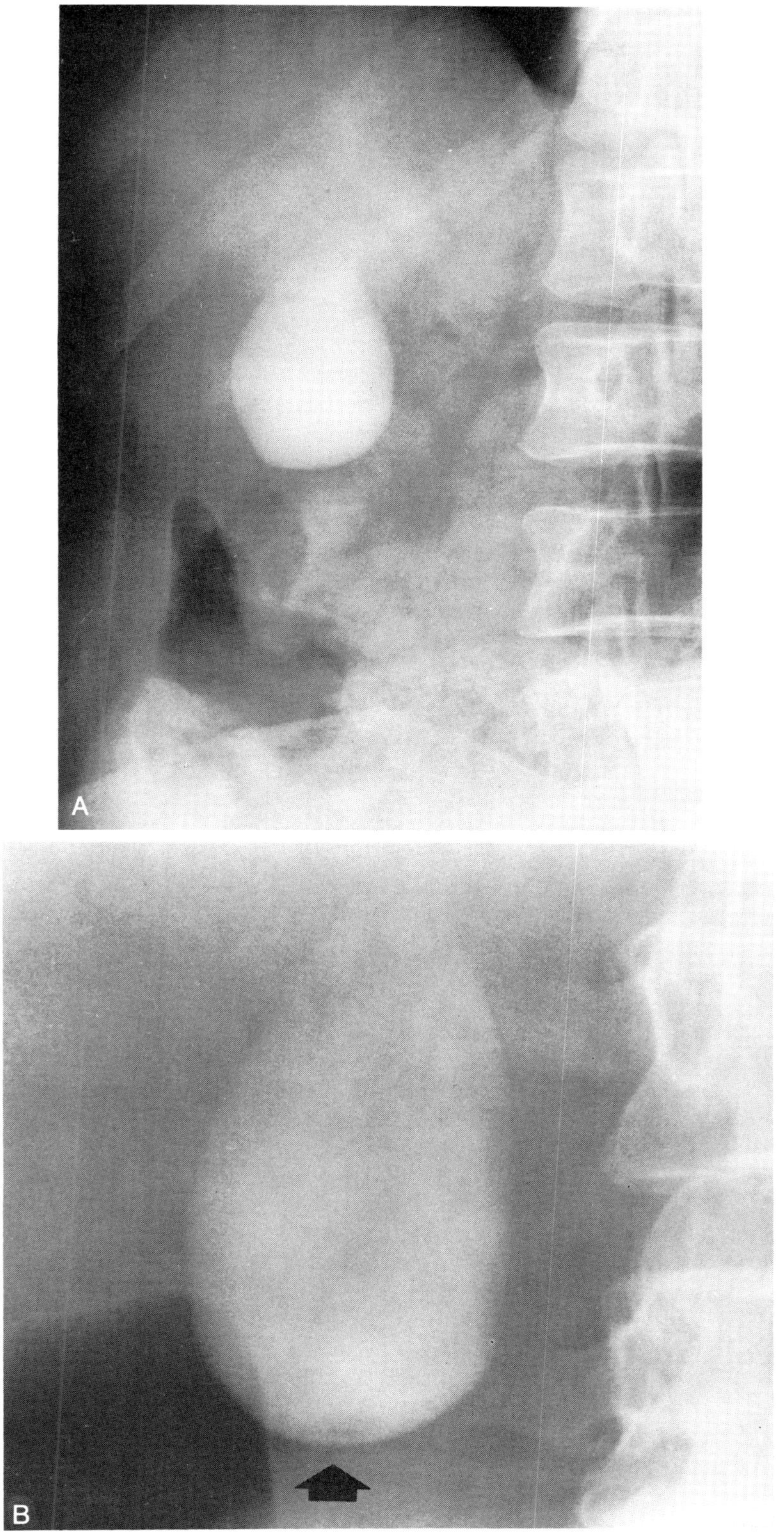

Figure 7–2. *A*, Supine radiograph made during oral cholecystography, showing a well-opacified gallbladder with no evidence of cholelithiasis. *B*, A gallstone is visible only on an upright spot film of the gallbladder made at fluoroscopy (*arrow*).

stones are often missed.[46] However, Laufer and Gledhill compared the diagnosis before and after a fatty meal in 231 patients undergoing cholecystography and found only one patient in whom a stone was detected only on the post–fatty meal radiograph.[56] In this case, the stone was missed on the original film because of overlying gas and not because it was hidden in the neck of the gallbladder.

Opacification of the cystic and common ducts does not justify the routine use of a fatty meal. If the gallbladder is opacified on the oral cholecystogram, it is reasonable to assume that there are no calculi in the cystic duct. Furthermore, it can be assumed that there are no gallstones in the common duct if there are none in the gallbladder. Choledocholithiasis is uncommon in the absence of gallstones in the gallbladder.

Another putative indication for giving a fatty meal is the detection of cholesterolosis and adenomyomatosis on the post–fatty meal radiograph, when these abnormalities are not evident on the initial films. In Laufer and Gledhill's series of 231 patients, this occurred only three times.[56] In addition, since the clinical significance of cholesterolosis and adenomyomatosis is uncertain, one might question the importance of establishing the diagnosis of these diseases, especially in patients in whom the changes are so mild that they are not apparent on pre–fatty meal radiographs of the gallbladder. However, a fatty meal is useful to evaluate a compartmentalized gallbladder for circumscribed adenomyomatosis.

In view of the considerable inconvenience, expense, and additional exposure involved in the use of a fatty meal, there are few objective data to justify its routine use in cholecystography.[9, 57] A fatty meal may be useful in specific circumstances, such as when the fundus of the gallbladder cannot otherwise be separated from fecal material in the colon, and when the initial radiograph suggests the presence of adenomyomatosis or cholesterolosis.

The Problem of Impaired First-Dose Opacification of the Gallbladder. Repeat examination in cases of impaired opacification of the gallbladder on a single-dose oral cholecystogram is required with disturbing regularity and is an important practical problem.[58–60] The incidence varies depending on the degree of gallbladder opacification that individual radiologists are willing to accept as adequate for diagnosis on the first-dose examination. Mujahed et al.[17] found a second-dose examination necessary in 25 per cent of their patients, whereas approximately 50 per cent of Stanley's patients required a second study.[28]

The difficulty arises from the fact that gallbladder opacification is not always maximal on the first study and sometimes can be improved by a second dose of contrast material.[58] As a result, initial nonopacification of the gallbladder is not a definite indication of the presence of gallbladder disease, and a second study is required before the diagnosis can be made. Poor opacification of the gallbladder after a single dose of contrast material not only occurs in a significant percentage of apparently normal patients but also occurs regularly in patients with acute pancreatitis[61–64] or acute peritonitis;[65] after trauma,[66, 67] surgery,[65] and fasting;[29] in patients with pernicious anemia;[68] in infants under 6 months of age;[69] and in women in the late stage of pregnancy.[70] Kaden et al. showed that two thirds of 25 patients with acute pancreatitis had nonopacification or poor opacification of the gallbladder with Telepaque when the examination was performed during the first week of an acute exacerbation of the disease.[61] Subsequent cholecystograms performed after recovery showed that the gallbladders in these patients were normal. Nonopacification of the gallbladder with Telepaque in patients with acute pancreatitis cannot be attributed to common bile duct obstruction secondary to inflammation of the pancreas, since there is no correlation between failure of the gallbladder to opacify and the serum bilirubin or alkaline phosphatase concentration.

The reason for inadequate opacification of the gallbladder in the absence of gallbladder disease and other causes, such as biliary obstruction, liver disease, failure to take the contrast material, vomiting, and so forth, has not been clearly defined. Impaired first-dose opacification in apparently normal patients may be due to inadequate intestinal absorption or deficient hepatic excretion of Telepaque in the absence of circulating bile salts.[35] This occurs in patients who are fasting or who are on low-fat diets, in whom bile salts are sequestered in the gallbladder. Poor absorption of the contrast material also may be related to diminished secretion of pancreatic juice, with an associated decrease in intestinal pH.[35] Poor opacification in patients with acute pancreatitis may be related to the fact that these individuals usually are fasting, because of abdominal pain and as part of their therapy. This would explain the persistent failure of the gallbladder to opacify after patients have resumed a normal diet, as described by Sanchez-Ubeda et al.[65] However, these data may be in error in light of the more current report of Roller et al.,[71] who were able to obtain satisfactory gallbladder opacification in 90 per cent of patients with acute pancreatitis before discharge from the hospital, when the examination was performed after intake of solid food was resumed.

Techniques to Eliminate the Need for A Second-Dose Cholecystogram. Burhenne and Obata[72] recommend avoiding a second cholecystogram in patients with initial nonvisualization or poor visualization of the gallbladder by administering two consecutive 3 gm doses of Telepaque each evening before the day the radiographs are made. Their data from over 600 single-visit oral cholecystograms indicate that failure of the gallbladder to opacify under these circumstances is reliable evidence of gallbladder disease, when extrabiliary causes of nonopacification, such as liver disease, are excluded. Their technique requires that the patient be relied upon to take the contrast material as directed but is a clever solution to the problem of having to perform second-dose cholecystograms.

Administering Oragrafin calcium to patients with first-dose nonopacification or poor opacification of the gallbladder is a useful alternative to performing a second-day cholecystogram (reinforcement cholecystography).[73, 74] Radiographs made 4 hours after administering 6 gm of Oragrafin calcium showed sufficient improvement in opacification to allow a diagnosis in 80 per cent of Beseman's patients with initial poor opacification.[73] When the original cholecystogram showed nonopacification of the gallbladder, the chance of increased opacification with Oragrafin was only 13 per cent. In a series of 115 patients with initial nonopacification, Crummy showed that persistent failure of the gallbladder to opacify on radiographs made 5 hours after a second dose of 3 gm of Oragrafin calcium is conclusive evidence of gallbladder disease, when extrabiliary causes of nonopacification are excluded.[74]

Opacification of the common duct is accurate evidence that there has been adequate intestinal absorption and hepatic excretion of the contrast material to opacify the gallbladder. Nonopacification of the gallbladder in this circumstance indicates the presence of cystic duct obstruction. Tomography of the right upper quadrant of the abdomen can reduce the need for a second cholecystogram by demonstrating opacification of the common bile duct in the absence of gallbladder opacification in 70 to 80 per cent of patients with nonopacification of the gallbladder on cholecystography.[75, 76] Tomography may reveal calcification in the obstructing cystic duct calculus that is not visible on the conventional cholecystogram, or it may identify the gallstone as a crescentic filling defect in the cystic duct. Frequently, tomography of the nonopacified gallbladder will permit identification of faintly calcified stones that are not visible or definite on the initial films. Tomography sometimes reveals nonopaque stones in faintly opacified gallbladders that were believed to be nonopacified on the initial films. Often the gallbladder can be identified on retrospective review of the conventional films. When tomography does not reveal a stone or opacification of the gallbladder or bile ducts, an extrinsic cause for the lack of gallbladder opacification should be considered. The use of tomography is unnecessary in patients who have nonopacification of the gallbladder after two doses of contrast material, because this is, in itself, an accurate indication of gallbladder disease when other causes of nonopacification are excluded.[17]

Another alternative to a second-day cholecystogram in patients with initial nonopacification of the gallbladder is an intravenous cholangiogram with Cholografin on the same day as the first examination. This is more hazardous for the patient than the oral study, since Cholografin is more toxic than Telepaque[35]; the examination also is more time-consuming for the radiology department. However, if the common bile duct opacifies without opacification of the gallbladder after 4 hours, the intravenous cholangiogram provides accurate direct evidence of gallbladder disease.[77] Opacification of the gallbladder without evidence of gallstones during an intravenous cholangiogram does not exclude the presence of gallstones. In one series of patients with consecutive nonopacification of the gallbladder following Telepaque administration, and in whom gallbladder disease was proved at surgery, 17 per cent had a normal intravenous cholangiogram.[17] Consequently, a normal intravenous cholangiogram in a patient with nonopacification of the gallbladder on oral studies does not exclude gallbladder disease. In these patients, the oral cholecystogram should be repeated at a later date. With the ready availability of cholecystosonography in most hospitals, the easiest way to approach patients who have nonopacification following a single dose of Telepaque is to perform an ultrasound examination of the gallbladder.

The Cause and Significance of Nonopacification of the Gallbladder After a Second-Dose Cholecystogram. Failure of the gallbladder to opacify after the administration of two consecutive doses of cholecystographic contrast material is reliable evidence of gallbladder disease, if other causes of nonopacification can be excluded. Most commonly, it represents either failure of the contrast agent to reach the lumen of the gallbladder owing to cystic duct obstruction or failure of the mucosa of the gallbladder to absorb water and concentrate the dye owing to chronic cholecystitis. Cholelithiasis is likely to be present in either case.

In a series of 5000 patients having cholecystography reported by Mujahed et al.,[17] 14 per cent of the group that had persistent nonopacification of the gallbladder on consecutive studies had an extrabiliary cause. Two thirds of these patients had liver disease. The others had a previous cholecystectomy, had pyloric obstruction, or had received no contrast material. All patients who had consecutive nonopacifications with no extrabiliary reason for it had gallbladder disease at surgery—nearly always chronic cholecystitis and cholelithiasis. Hence, failure of the gallbladder to opacify after a second dose of contrast material is highly reliable evidence for the presence of gallbladder disease. Further evaluation by intravenous cholangiography, tomography, or ultrasound is unnecessary.

There are many extrabiliary causes for nonopacification of the gallbladder. Low-Beer et al. presented evidence that small bowel disease is rarely a cause of nonopacification of the gallbladder on oral cholecystography with Oragrafin.[78] They reported 84 patients with diseases that produce malabsorption (celiac disease, Crohn's disease, ileal resections, small intestinal diverticulosis, and so forth), 95 per cent of whom had satisfactory gallbladder opacification. Goldberg noted that, in his experience, patients with Crohn's disease or ileal resection may have nonopacification of the gallbladder on oral cholecystography with Telepaque owing to impaired intestinal absorption of the contrast materials, perhaps related to a deficiency of bile salts.[79]

Cholecystokinin (CCK) Cholecystography

Fatty food intolerance, heartburn, flatulence, epigastric fullness, and upper abdominal discomfort are considered to be classic symptoms of cholelithiasis. However, patients with a normal cholecystogram have these dyspeptic complaints as frequently as do those with gallstones.[80] Consequently, although these symptoms may originate in the gallbladder, they are not always the result of cholelithiasis.

Patients who have undiagnosed abdominal pain related to the ingestion of fatty foods, but who have a normal cholecystogram, often are considered to have psychosomatic disease, no matter how much the pain resembles biliary colic. Some of these patients have gallstones that have been missed on cholecystography or diseases such as peptic ulcer and pancreatitis that have been overlooked. However, most suffer from one of a number of marginal organic diseases and questionable physiologic disorders of the biliary tract that present an enigma in terms of their actual existence, diagnosis, and treatment. These symptoms have been variously termed biliary dyskinesia, acalculous chronic cholecystitis, and the cystic duct syndrome. The clinical manifestations, pathologic changes, and results of surgery are so variable in these putative disorders that most surgeons are reluctant to perform a cholecystectomy in these patients. However, this inflexible approach to cholecystectomy for patients complaining of biliary tract pain has probably led to the underdiagnosis of biliary tract disease.[81] A reliable radiographic procedure for the diagnosis of these abnormalities and a technique to determine which patients would benefit from surgery would be exceedingly valuable.

Diagnosis of Biliary Dyskinesia on Oral Cholecystography

The fatty meal has been used since the inception of oral cholecystography in an effort to recognize abnormalities of gallbladder evacuation in patients with symptoms of biliary tract disease but a normal cholecystogram. Unfortunately, the degree that the normal gallbladder empties following a fatty meal varies widely and thus has little diagnostic significance.[4, 53–55] The difficulty arises from the fact that a fatty meal leaves the stomach at different rates, and when it reaches the duodenum it has a variable effect on stimulating the release of cholecystokinin by the duodenal mucosa.

It has been suggested that persistent opacification of the gallbladder 36 hours after administration of Telepaque is diagnostic of biliary dyskinesia.[82–84] However, it is not certain how many normal patients have persistent opacification of the gallbladder at 36 hours, nor has it been established that all those with prolonged opacification have biliary tract disease. It may be that persistent opacification of the gallbladder at 36 hours is due to the enterohepatic recirculation of conjugated Telepaque.[35] It also seems likely that prolonged opacification is closely related to diet. Patients would be expected not to empty their gallbladders if they had little or no fat in their diet following the cholecystogram.

Technique of Cholecystokinin (CCK) Cholecystography

CCK cholecystography is performed by giving 1.0 Ivy dog unit of CCK or equidoses of the octapeptide of CCK intravenously, after first opacifying the gallbladder by oral cholecystography performed in the usual manner.[85–93] Four or five serial radiographs of the gallbladder are then made in the prone oblique projection during the 15- to 20-minute interval after the injection. The optimal rate of the injection has not been defined, but the CCK usually is given over 1 to 3 minutes. No change in the patient's position is allowed during this study, since this might affect gallbladder size and configuration. A positive examination, although defined differently by various investigators, is one in which (1) the CCK induces the patient's symptoms (usually upper abdominal pain)[88, 89] or (2) the radiographs show incomplete emptying or spasm of the gallbladder (Fig. 7–3).[86–89] Incomplete emptying implies reduction in volume of less than 20 to 50 per cent in the 15- to 20-minute interval.[86–88, 91–96]

Accuracy of CCK Cholecystography

Goldstein et al. were enthusiastic about their experience with CCK cholecystography performed between 1959 and 1972, in which the diagnosis of cystic duct syndrome was apparently made correctly on the basis of a positive test in 28 patients.[86, 91, 93] The response to CCK was considered abnormal if the gallbladder emptied less than 50 per cent. In many of these cases the gallbladder assumed a globular configuration (fighting gall-

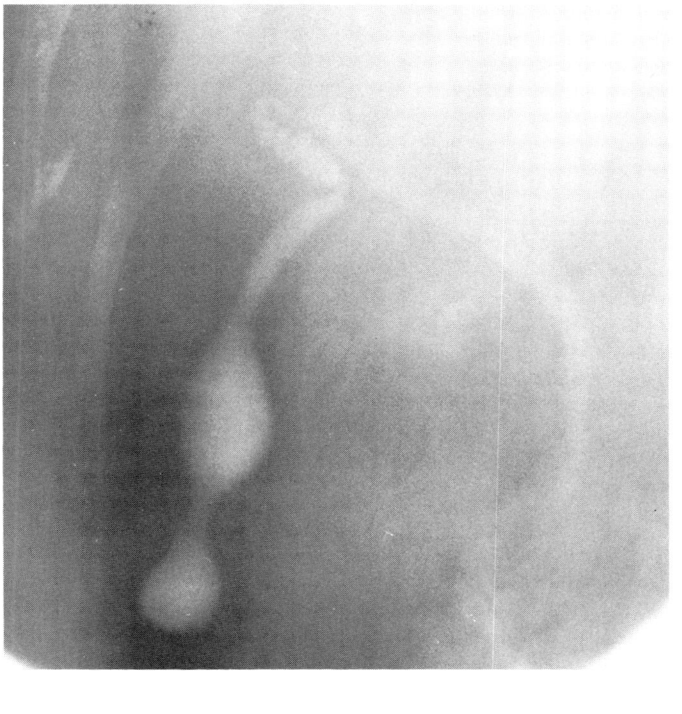

Figure 7–3. Cholecystokinin cholecystogram showing spasm of the body of the gallbladder. The patient underwent a cholecystectomy and was relieved of his symptoms. The pathologic diagnosis was mild chronic cholecystitis.

bladder), as if it were attempting to empty against increased resistance. All patients with deficient gallbladder contraction developed upper abdominal pain after the CCK injection. Cholecystectomy was performed in 25 of the 28 patients. All but three were relieved of their symptoms during follow-up periods ranging from 6 months to 11 years. Histologic examination of the gallbladder showed varying degrees of chronic cholecystitis with kinks or narrowing of the cystic duct in 18 of the 25 patients. The gallbladder was normal in five, and histologic data were not available in two. CCK cholecystography was performed in 17 control subjects. In every instance the gallbladder contracted 50 per cent or more, and no patient had upper abdominal pain.

Valberg et al.[90] had an equally good experience with cholecystokinin in 13 patients with typical attacks of biliary-like pain who had normal conventional cholecystograms. CCK, injected in 1 minute, produced typical attacks of pain in each patient. Changes in size or shape of the gallbladder were not taken into consideration. Twelve of the 13 patients underwent cholecystectomy and had complete relief of their symptoms. None of the 30 control subjects developed pain after the cholecystokinin.

In a third optimistic report, Nathan et al.[89] compared the results of CCK cholecystography in 141 patients with the results in 142 normal controls. Nathan et al.[89] differed from Goldstein et al.[93] in that they did not concern themselves with the degree of gallbladder emptying but considered only spasm of the gallbladder to be significant (Fig. 7–3). Transient spasm of the cystic duct was evident in both the patient group and the controls. However, prolonged spasm of the cystic duct or spasm of the body, fundus, or neck of the gallbladder occurred more frequently in the patients than in the control group. Nausea and upper abdominal cramps (not defined) occurred with approximately equal frequency in the control group and in the patients.

Nathan et al.[89] defined a positive response to CCK as spasm of the neck, body, or fundus of the gallbladder on the radiographs or the production of upper abdominal pain, or both. Subsequently, 79 patients in their series with a positive examination had a cholecystectomy. The gallbladders in 77 of these had histologic evidence of mild or minimal chronic cholecystitis, and in 2 the gallbladders were normal. Marked relief of the patient's symptoms occurred in 94 per cent of those having surgery in follow-up periods ranging from 3 months to 4 years.

Goldberg was equally sanguine about the value of CCK cholecystography in detecting patients with disease of the biliary tract in the presence of a normal conventional cholecystogram.[92] He defined a positive test more stringently than did Goldstein et al.[93] or Nathan et al.[89] by requiring that, for the gallbladder to be considered abnormal, it must contract less than 20 per cent on the radiographs and the patient must have reproduction of pain. Goldberg reported that 14 of 15 patients with a positive response to CCK who had a cholecystectomy either were completely cured or had marked improvement during the follow-up period of 6 months to 4 years. Others have reported similar experiences.[94–96]

Consequently, despite the facts that (1) differing criteria were used to define a "positive" response to CCK, (2) the CCK was injected at different rates, (3) the control subjects were evaluated by varying standards according to the investigator, and (4) the patients were followed for different lengths of time postoperatively, all the above-named authors were able to reach the same conclusion. This is that nearly all patients with biliary type pain who had a cholecystectomy based on a "positive" response to CCK are cured, despite having a normal conventional cholecystogram. This indicates that no matter which of the various criteria is used to define a "positive" examination or how the CCK is injected, there are few false positive CCK cholecystograms. The incidence of false negative tests has not been determined by these studies because none of the patients with a negative response to CCK had a cholecystectomy.

Despite these favorable reports,[86–96] CCK cholecystography has not been accepted enthusiastically as an accurate diagnostic modality in this enigmatic group of patients. Some radiologists are skeptical because of their own unsatisfactory experience with a fatty meal during cholecystography, in which the response of the gallbladder is variable and the production of symptoms is difficult to evaluate. In addition, there is lack of confidence in CCK cholecystography because investigators do not agree on what constitutes a "positive" response to CCK. Is it the degree of emptying of the gallbladder that is significant, or is it the presence of spasm in various portions of the gallbladder? If the former, what degree of contraction should be considered abnormal? Is it a gallbladder that contracts less than 50 per cent, 30 per cent, or 20 per cent? Many clinicians are doubtful about the reliability of putative successful results in patients who have had a cholecystectomy after positive CCK cholecystography. They recognize that the clinical symptoms in this group of patients are difficult to evaluate because the symptoms vacillate, are often poorly defined, and are sometimes associated with a potpourri of complaints in other organ systems.

In most cases, surgeons are still reluctant to operate when the conventional cholecystogram is normal, despite a positive response to CCK, because the pathologic findings in the gallbladder often are marginal and subject to differing interpretations. The histologic criteria for the diagnosis of cholecystitis are ambiguous. Inflammatory cellular infiltrates can be identified in the wall of the gallbladder in many asymptomatic subjects. The importance of the potential placebo effect of surgery per se in relieving or altering the complaints in these patients cannot be underestimated. Finally, some skeptics are fearful that the duration of follow-up of the patients in many of the reports is too short; they believe that those with initial successful results after cholecystectomy may have an exacerbation of their symptoms when they are observed for longer periods.

A study by Dunn et al. emphasizes some of these considerations. These investigators performed CCK cholecystography in 44 control subjects and in 74 patients who had a history suggestive of gallbladder disease but in whom routine cholecystography was normal.[21] The patients were assigned to one of two categories: "possible biliary colic" or "dyspepsia," depending on their symptoms. In order to be placed in the "possible biliary colic" group the patient must have had distinct attacks of abdominal pain. Patients assigned to the "dyspepsia" group had pain day after day and generally had epigastric or right upper quadrant discomfort or pain after meals and a feeling of fullness in the epigastrium, with or without food intolerance, belching, and flatulence. These patients had more persistent abdominal discomfort or pain than those in the "possible biliary colic" group. Some pain was required for inclusion in either category. Those with heartburn, food intolerance, belching, and flatulence were not included in the study unless they also had pain.

The radiographs were evaluated by three radiologists who had no knowledge of the patient's history. They were interpreted as "normal," "probably normal," "probably abnormal," or "definitely abnormal." The decision was based on changes in gallbladder shape; spasm of the fundus, body, or neck; cystic duct spasm; or abnormal patterns of emptying.

The clinical and radiographic responses are shown in Table 7–1. If the interpretations of the three radiologists are averaged, 28 per cent of the controls, 31 per cent of those with "possible biliary colic," and 43 per cent of those with "dyspepsia" had an abnormal or probably abnormal response to CCK. The differences are not significant. In approximately 28 per cent of the cases the radiologists differed in major ways in their interpretation of the radiographs. There was poor

Table 7–1 CCK CHOLECYSTOGRAPHY INTERPRETATION OF RADIOGRAPHS BY THREE RADIOLOGISTS*

	Average Age, Yr (Range)	Radiologist	X-ray Film Results				Gallbladder-like Pain After CCK
			Normal	*Probably Normal*	*Probably Abnormal*	*Abnormal*	*% of Patients*
Controls	33.8	1	48	16	16	20	27
n = 44	(20–58)	2	68	18	5	9	
		3	52	14	16	18	
Biliary	37.6	1	47	21	10	22	66
colic	(22–61)	2	62	12	12	14	
n = 49		3	33	31	12	24	
Dyspepsia	40.5	1	36	16	0	48	44
	(17–64)	2	52	8	12	28	
		3	32	28	12	28	

*Values given are percentages.
From Dunn FH, Christensen ED, Reynolds J, et al: JAMA 1974;*228*:997. Used by permission.

TABLE 7–2 RESPONSE TO CHOLECYSTECTOMY RELATED TO CLINICAL RESPONSE TO CHOLECYSTOKININ*

	Number of Patients	Number Cured	Number Improved	Number Same	Number of Follow-up
Pain or discomfort reproduced	20	14	3	2	1
Roentgenogram					
Abnormal†	9	7	2	—	—
Normal‡	11	7	1	2	1
Pain or discomfort not reproduced	9	4	2	3	—
Roentgenogram					
Abnormal	3	0	1	2	—
Normal	6	4	1	1	—

*No one's condition deteriorated as a result of therapy.
†Abnormal indicates roentgenogram read as abnormal or probably abnormal by at least two of the three radiologists.
‡Normal indicates roentgenogram read as normal or probably normal by at least two of the three radiologists.
From Dunn FH, Christensen ED, Reynolds J, et al: JAMA 1974;*228*:997. Used by permission.

correlation not only when three interpretations were compared but also when a second interpretation by an individual radiologist was compared with his initial reading.

Biliary-like pain or discomfort was produced in 27 per cent of the controls, 65 per cent of the patients with "possible biliary colic," and 44 per cent of the patients with dyspepsia. This was gallbladder-like pain and was carefully differentiated from the abdominal symptoms that can be produced by CCK, such as lower abdominal cramping, abdominal fullness, and nausea.

Twenty-nine of the patients were subjected to cholecystectomy because of severe and recurrent abdominal distress. The decision to operate was made without knowledge of the results of the CCK cholecystogram. Forty-one per cent of this group were in the "possible biliary colic" group, and 35 per cent were in the "dyspepsia" category. Eighty per cent considered themselves cured or definitely improved by cholecystectomy, regardless of the results of CCK cholecystography.

Table 7–2 shows the results of cholecystectomy related to the clinical response to CCK. Eighty-five per cent of the patients with pain reproduced by CCK who had a cholecystectomy were cured or improved, whereas 66 per cent of those with a negative symptomatic response to CCK were improved. Follow-up data on patients who did not have a cholecystectomy are given in Table 7–3. Of the patients who were contacted, 65 per cent of those in the "biliary colic" group were cured or improved, whereas 50 per cent of the "dyspepsia" group were cured or improved.

Dunn et al. concluded that CCK cholecystography, as currently performed and interpreted, is of little or no value in the diagnosis and management of patients with possible acalculous biliary tract disease. They give four reasons for their assertions: (1) The incidence of "abnormal" gallbladder contraction in normal subjects is high (14 to 36 per cent). (2) CCK cholecystography does not help predict which patients will be cured by cholecystectomy. Their results show that

Table 7–3 FOLLOW-UP IN PATIENTS WHO DID NOT HAVE GALLBLADDER SURGERY

	Number Cured	Number Improved	Number Same	Number Worse	Average Length of Follow-up (Months)	Range of Follow-up (Months)
Biliary colic (26 of 29 contacted)	6	11	6	3	20.1	6–32
Roentgenogram						
Abnormal*	0	3	1	1	19.6	6–28
Normal†	6	8	5	2	20.2	7–32
Dyspepsia (14 of 16 contacted)	2	5	4	3	21.7	6–34
Roentgenogram						
Abnormal*	1	1	1	1	19.8	11–32
Normal†	1	4	3	2	22.7	6–34

*Abnormal indicates roentgenogram read as abnormal or probably abnormal by at least two of the three radiologists.
†Normal indicates roentgenogram read as normal or probably normal by at least two of the three radiologists.
From Dunn FH, Christensen ED, Reynolds J, et al: JAMA 1974;*228*:997. Used by permission.

patients with both normal and abnormal responses to CCK usually are cured or improved by cholecystectomy. (3) CCK cholecystography does not help predict histologic findings in the gallbladder. Patients with normal and abnormal CCK responses without a cholecystectomy had similar histologic findings in their gallbladders. (4) There is a high degree of observer disagreement (approximately 28 per cent) in the interpretation of radiographs.

Davis et al. studied a smaller group of patients and normal subjects with cholecystokinin cholecystography, sonography, and scintigraphy and showed that the percentage of emptying of the gallbladder varies markedly and cannot be reliably used to determine the presence of acalculous cholecystitis.[22] In order to improve the diagnostic accuracy of cholecystokinin cholecystography, Burnstein has used it in combination with biliary drainage tests to evaluate patients with biliary colic–like pain and normal conventional cholecystograms. Patients with negative and positive tests were operated upon and followed. Although the pathologic findings were fewer in patients with negative tests, the symptomatic outcome was no different.[23]

Hyperplastic Cholecystoses

"Hyperplastic cholecystoses" is a generic term introduced by Jutras in 1960 for a group of abnormalities of the gallbladder that appear to be separate from inflammatory diseases.[97] Hyperplasia implies a benign proliferation of normal tissue elements, whereas cholecystoses indicates a pathologic process that is distinct from inflammation. The two main categories of hyperplastic cholecystoses are cholesterolosis and adenomyomatosis. According to Jutras, both types cause functional abnormalities of the gallbladder consisting of hyperconcentration, hypercontraction, and hyperexcretion. These can be detected on radiographs made during cholecystography and are clues to the diagnosis.

Cholesterolosis

Cholesterolosis, or "strawberry gallbladder," is characterized by abnormal deposits of cholesterol esters in fat-laden macrophages in the lamina propria of the gallbladder. The lipid creates coarse, yellow, speckled excrescences on the surface of the reddened hyperemic gallbladder mucosa and gives the latter a "strawberry" appearance. The cause of the cholesterol deposition is unknown, although it has been attributed to excess cholesterol absorption across the gallbladder mucosa. Cholesterolosis is not related to the serum cholesterol concentration, but cholesterol gallstones develop in 50 to 70 per cent of patients with the abnormality.

When the cholesterol deposits are big enough, the cholecystogram may show fixed radiolucencies, either localized or generalized, in the opacified gallbladder (Fig. 7–4). The lipid protrusions into the gallbladder lumen may be single or multiple, usually vary in size, are of uneven distribution, and may involve any portion of the gallbladder. The lesions are often best seen after partial evacuation of the gallbladder and on radiographs made with compression. Indirect radiographic findings include hyperconcentration and hyperexcretion, which are general features of all of the hyperplastic cholecystoses.[97] Cholesterolosis can be differentiated from cholelithiasis by determining that the radiolucent defects are fixed in position within the gallbladder on radiographs made in different positions; gallstones are usually free to move about and to collect by gravity in the dependent portion of the gallbladder or to form a layer in the bile.

The management of patients with cholesterolosis is uncertain. Some surgeons reserve cholecystectomy for those patients who also have cholelithiasis. However, in 269 cases of cholesterolosis without gallstones reported by Salmenkivi, about 90 per cent of patients had complete or partial relief of symptoms following surgery.[98]

Adenomyomatosis

Adenomyomatosis consists of proliferation of mucosa, increased thickness of the muscle coat, and formation of outpouches of mucosa into or through the muscularis.[97] These diverticula, which are termed Rokitansky-Aschoff sinuses, may be segmental or diffuse throughout the gallbladder.

Radiographically, the sinuses are seen as multiple or single oval collections of contrast material of various sizes adjacent to the lumen of the gallbladder (Fig. 7–5). Any portion of the gallbladder may be involved. At times, calcified concretions are present within the diverticula. Adenomyomatosis often is associated with compartmentalization of the

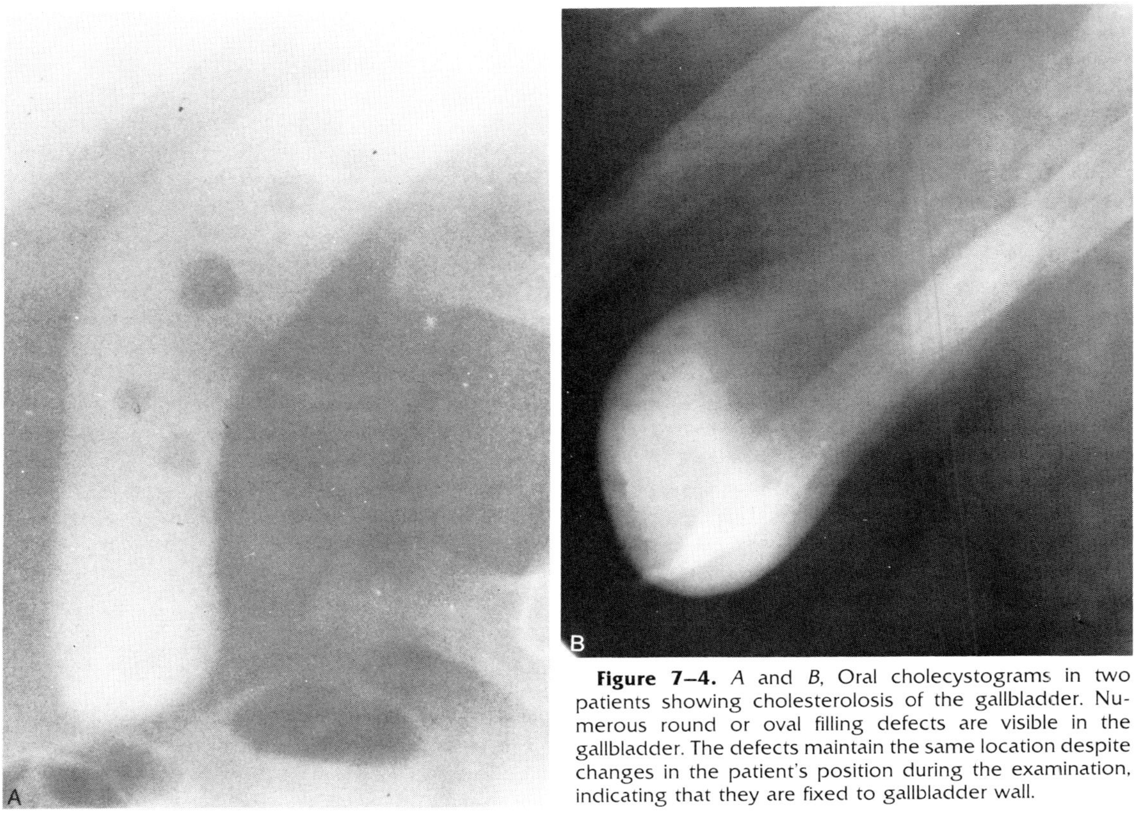

Figure 7–4. *A* and *B*, Oral cholecystograms in two patients showing cholesterolosis of the gallbladder. Numerous round or oval filling defects are visible in the gallbladder. The defects maintain the same location despite changes in the patient's position during the examination, indicating that they are fixed to gallbladder wall.

gallbladder caused by septal folds or annular thickening of the gallbladder wall. Whether compartmentalization is the cause or the effect of adenomyomatosis is not certain. Compartmentalization may be due to circumferential adenomyomatosis, a congenital septum, or adenomyomatosis superimposed on a congenital septum. Aguirre et al. believe that the circumferential form of adenomyomatosis producing compartmentalization originates in a congenital septum.[99] It often is difficult to determine by cholecystography whether the stenosis is a simple septum or whether the adenomyomatosis is already present.

The combination of adenomyomatosis and cholesterolosis is not unusual, and gallstones are often present. Like cholesterolosis, adenomyomatosis is often more easily identified and appears more marked on radiographs made after partial emptying of the gallbladder. Fundal adenomyomatosis has various radiologic patterns, ranging from a filling defect or mass in the fundus due to focal hyperplasia of the gallbladder wall to multiple diverticular outpouches filled with contrast material or small calculi localized to the fundus (Fig. 7–6).

Adenomyomatosis is observed much more commonly pathologically than radiographically. In one series, 50 per cent of patients having cholecystectomy for gallstones had associated adenomyomatosis found by the pathologist that was not apparent on cholecystography.[100] Whether a cholecystectomy should be performed on a patient with adenomyomatosis depends on the severity and duration of the symptoms and the presence of cholelithiasis.

INTRAVENOUS CHOLANGIOGRAPHY

The introduction of sodium iodipamide (Biligrafin) in Germany in 1953 and the United States shortly thereafter provided a unique radiologic modality for the diagnosis of diseases of the bile ducts. Because iodipamide has six iodine atoms per molecule, the concentration of iodine that is achieved when iodipamide is excreted in bile is greater than that of the oral contrast agents (excreted at the same rate but with only three iodine atoms per molecule). Since radiographic opacification depends on the number of iodine atoms in the path of the x-ray beam,

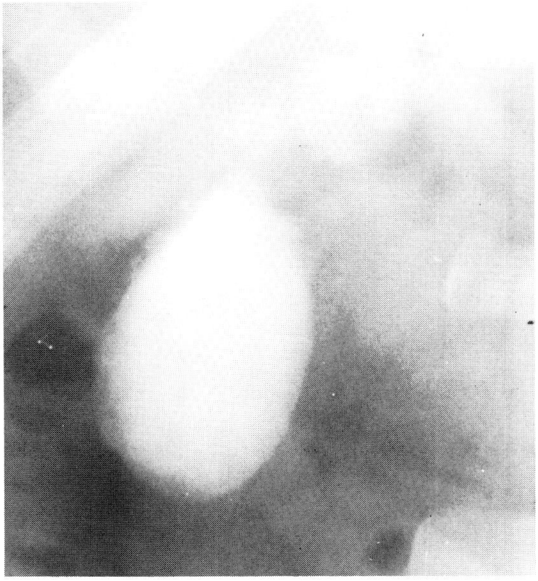

Figure 7–5. Oral cholecystogram showing diffuse adenomyomatosis of the gallbladder. Small outpouches of the gallbladder wall filled with contrast material are visible.

the concentration of iodine with iodipamide is adequate for opacification of the bile ducts directly, and further concentration of the contrast material in the gallbladder is unnecessary.

It is regrettable that the biliary excretion of these agents is inexorably associated with the simultaneous flow of relatively large volumes of water into the bile (choleresis). This automatically dilutes the contrast agents and establishes an unavoidable maximum concentration of the contrast material that can be achieved in bile. Therefore, there is an inherent limitation to the degree of radiographic opacification of the bile ducts that is possible with this contrast agent. For example, the radiographic density of the bile ducts during intravenous cholangiography with Cholografin (meglumine iodipamide) is at most only one half of that achieved in the kidney during intravenous pyelography[113] and 10 to 20 per cent of that which can be achieved by direct cholangiography. Consequently, opacification of the biliary tree with the intravenous cholangiographic agents is relatively poor.

It will be a momentous occasion in radiology when a new contrast material is developed that can achieve iodine concentrations in bile that are 10- or 100-fold greater than those now possible with Cholografin. Until then, intravenous cholangiography will be of limited value. The biliary tree is opacified so much better by endoscopic retrograde cholangiography and transhepatic cholangiography that, as these procedures are refined and simplified, they inevitably will tend to replace intravenous cholangiography as it is currently performed. In addition, excellent opacification of the biliary tree can be achieved with the direct-injection procedures despite the presence of jaundice, which would make opacification with intravenous cholangiography impossible.

Indications for Intravenous Cholangiography

In most radiology departments the use of intravenous cholangiography has decreased by as much as 80 per cent over the last decade.[5, 9] Until recently, intravenous cholangiography was indicated primarily in the evaluation of postcholecystectomy patients with right upper quadrant abdominal symptoms to evaluate the common bile duct, and in patients suspected of having acute cholecystitis to determine cystic duct obstruction. Direct cholangiography via ERCP or percutaneously has largely replaced intravenous cholangiography in the evaluation of the postcholecystectomy syndrome. Hepatobiliary scintigraphy, a noninvasive method that yields useful information regarding cystic duct obstruction, has replaced intravenous

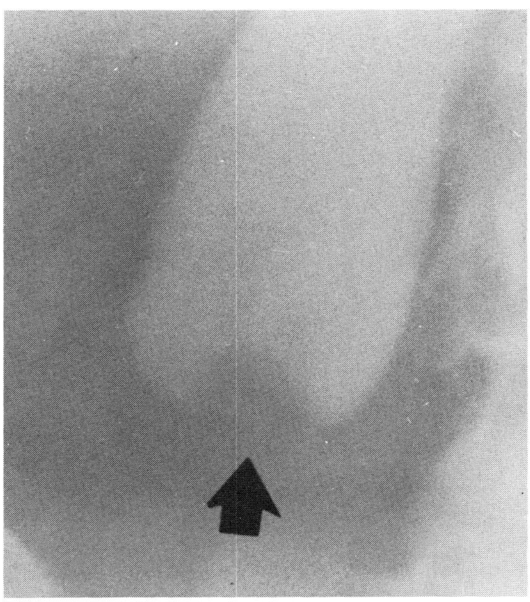

Figure 7–6. Oral cholecystogram showing fundal adenomyomatosis. A typical radiolucency is visible (*arrow*).

cholangiography in the diagnosis of acute cholecystitis.

Therefore, while intravenous cholangiography was once the only method to opacify the bile ducts nonoperatively, the advent of newer diagnostic procedures sharply reduced its indications. At present, intravenous cholangiography is reserved for (1) evaluation of patients suspected of having acute cholecystitis, when ultrasound is either not possible or technically inadequate and cholescintigraphy is unavailable; and (2) evaluation of the common bile duct after cholecystectomy, when endoscopic retrograde cholangiography and transhepatic cholangiography cannot be performed.

Intravenous Cholangiography in the Diagnosis of Acute Cholecystitis

Intravenous cholangiography may be useful to establish or exclude the diagnosis of acute cholecystitis in patients with acute abdominal pain, when cholescintigraphy is unavailable.[121] The premise is that the gallbladder will not fill with contrast material in patients with acute cholecystitis, because the cystic duct is obstructed. Consequently, the diagnosis can be established on intravenous cholangiography when the common duct, but not the gallbladder, is opacified. If both the common duct and the gallbladder are opacified, the diagnosis of acute cholecystitis can be excluded. Numerous reports found no false positive or false negative examinations.[101–106] All patients in whom there was common duct opacification without opacification of the gallbladder had acute cholecystitis at surgery. Similarly, 100 per cent of patients in whom both the common duct and the gallbladder opacified were shown not to have acute gallbladder disease. These investigators emphasized that false positive examination can be avoided only if radiographs

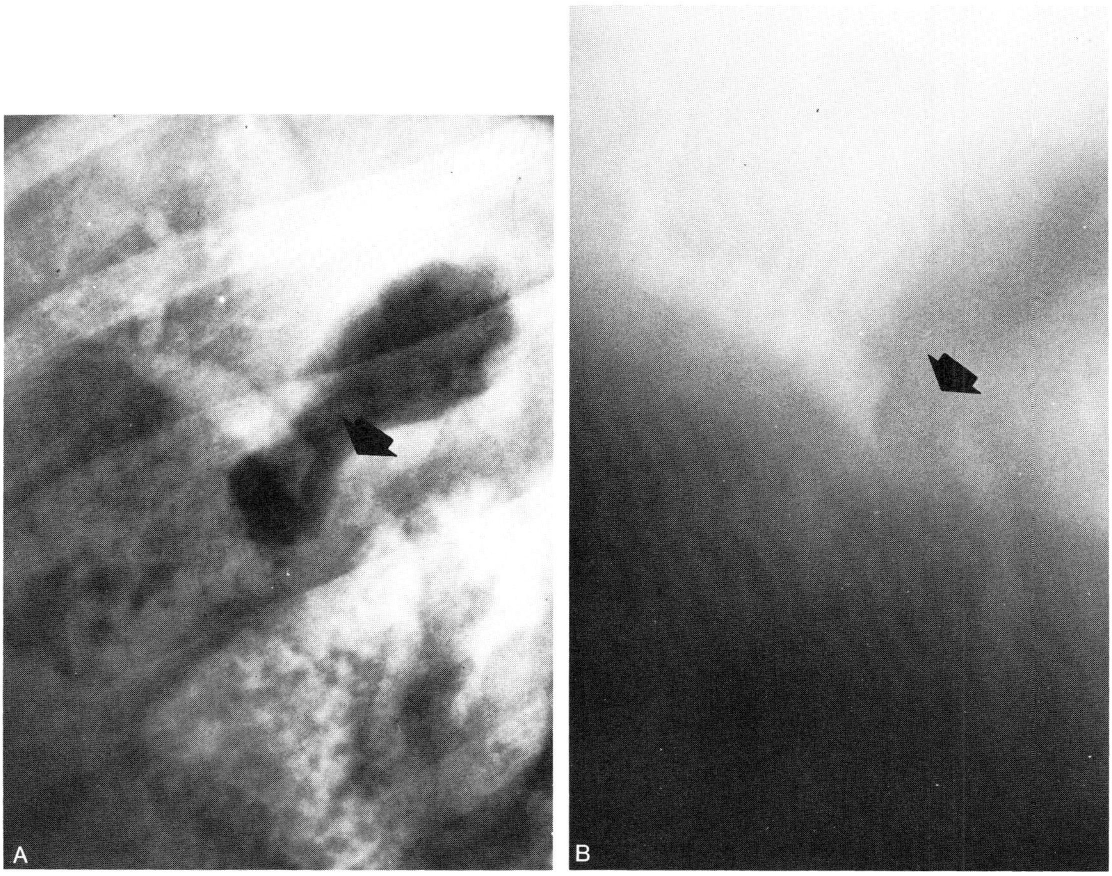

Figure 7–7. Conventional radiograph (*A*) and tomogram (*B*) made during an intravenous cholangiogram in a postcholecystectomy patient, showing a stone in the common bile duct (*arrows*). Note dilatation of the duct proximal to the calculus.

are made up to 4 hours after the injection of contrast material. Most authors emphasize the importance of obtaining 4-hour and 24-hour radiographs during intravenous cholangiography if the gallbladder fails to opacify earlier.[106, 107] There is delayed opacification of some apparently normal gallbladders for reasons that are obscure.[108, 109] This requirement rules out the use of intravenous cholangiography as an emergency procedure, since 1 day is required before the gallbladder can be assumed to be obstructed. However, the *absence* of acute cholecystitis can be demonstrated promptly when the gallbladder is opacified on early radiographs.

Intravenous cholangiography is principally warranted in patients with suspected acute cholecystitis when the diagnosis cannot be established with reasonable certainty on the basis of clinical and laboratory findings and cholescintigraphy is unavailable. The surgeon caring for the patient must decide how firm the clinical diagnosis of acute cholecystitis is and whether confirmation on cholangiography is necessary. Intravenous cholangiography is not indicated if the patient has had previous verified radiographic evidence of biliary disease, if gallstones can be seen on the plain abdominal radiograph, if a tender mass is palpable in the right upper quadrant of the abdomen, or if the patient is jaundiced. Patients with an established diagnosis of acute cholecystitis should not have intravenous cholangiography merely to evaluate the common duct before surgery. This can best be accomplished by operative cholangiography, which most surgeons believe should be performed routinely during cholecystectomy.

Examination in the Postoperative Patient

The most valuable role of intravenous cholangiography was the detection of common duct stones in patients with recurrent symptoms after cholecystectomy. However, direct injection of contrast material via the endoscopic or percutaneous route has largely replaced intravenous cholangiography in the work-up of patients suspected of having choledocholithiasis after cholecystectomy.[9] When these techniques are not available or cannot be performed, intravenous cholangiography may demonstrate the presence of stones in the bile ducts. The radiographic findings of gallstones in the common duct on intravenous cholangiography include identification of the gallstones directly as radiolucent defects in the opacified duct and the detection of partial obstruction of the common duct (Figs. 7–7 and 7–8). Rarely, gas bubbles in the duct may simulate gallstones in patients who have a biliary-enteric anastomosis or fistula.[116] In these cases, the correct diagnosis is usually obvious from the history and from the preliminary radiograph.

Evidence of partial obstruction of the common duct, such as loss of the normal tapered configuration of the common duct, delayed drainage, and dilatation (hydrohepatosis), provide indirect evidence of choledocholithiasis.[107] Because of the wide variation in the normal diameter of the common duct (2 to 15 mm), duct size is of certain value only in extreme cases. For example, the likelihood of common bile duct pathology is greater when the size of the common duct is greater than 10 mm and is almost certain when it exceeds 15 mm.[117, 118, 122]

A cystic duct remnant is a frequent occurrence after cholecystectomy and, in the absence of stones, should not be considered to be of clinical importance (Fig. 7–9).

The main problem with intravenous cholangiography to detect common or bile duct pathology remains the poor or very marginal

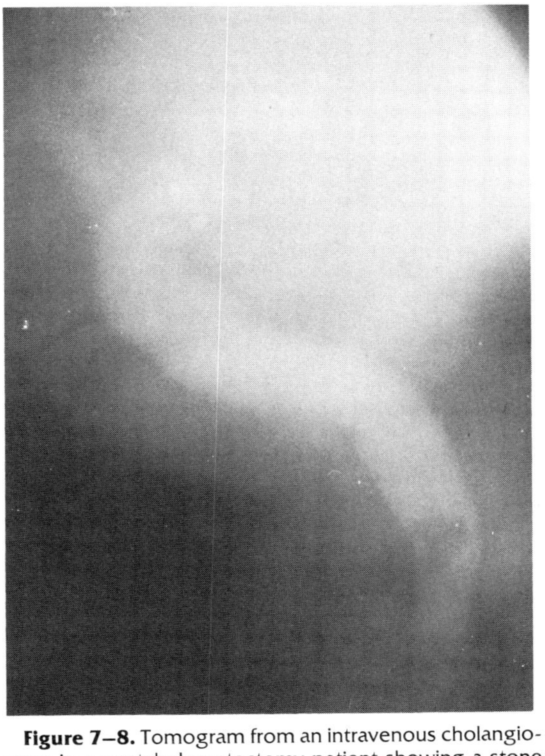

Figure 7–8. Tomogram from an intravenous cholangiogram in a postcholecystectomy patient showing a stone in the common duct. Dilatation of the duct is apparent.

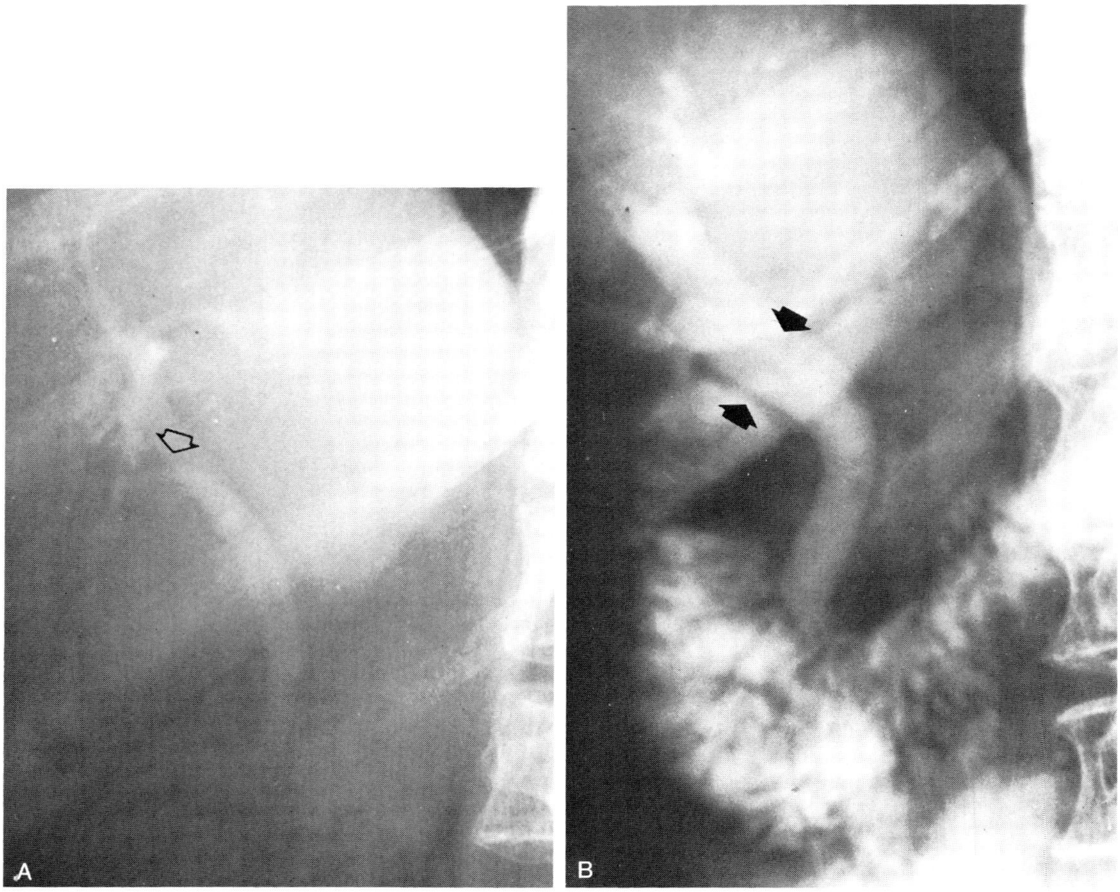

Figure 7–9. *A* and *B*, Intravenous cholangiogram in two postcholecystectomy patients showing cystic duct remnants (*arrows*).

opacification of the ducts obtained by this technique. Indeed, in nearly half the studies, opacification of the duct is so poor that no interpretation at all is possible. In the remainder, the margin of error is far greater than with direct cholangiography.[119, 120]

Other Indications and Contraindications of Intravenous Cholangiography

An intravenous cholangiogram is indicated for the evaluation of the biliary tree in patients in whom opacification of the gallbladder cannot be expected on oral cholecystography (Fig. 7–10). However, examination by ultrasound is also an excellent alternative in this group of patients.

Technical Aspects

Because of the uricosuric effect of Cholografin and the associated hazard of precipitating uric acid crystals in the renal tubules,[110] it is important that liquids be allowed freely before intravenous cholangiography. Johnson and Wise showed that the incidence of minor reactions is significantly reduced when patients are examined in a well-hydrated, nonfasting state.[111] A cathartic given the night before the examination is useful to eliminate fecal material in the colon that might otherwise obscure the biliary tree.

Wise gives a 1-ml test injection of Cholografin and waits 3 minutes before administering the remainder of the dose.[107] Until better data are available it appears that the optimal method for performing intravenous cholangiography is to limit the amount of Cholografin used to 20 ml in most patients. An infusion given over 10 to 15 minutes is most convenient and facilitates control of toxicity, if it should occur. Wise and Martinez et al.[112] recommend the use of an antihistamine given intramuscularly before the examination in an effort to reduce the inci-

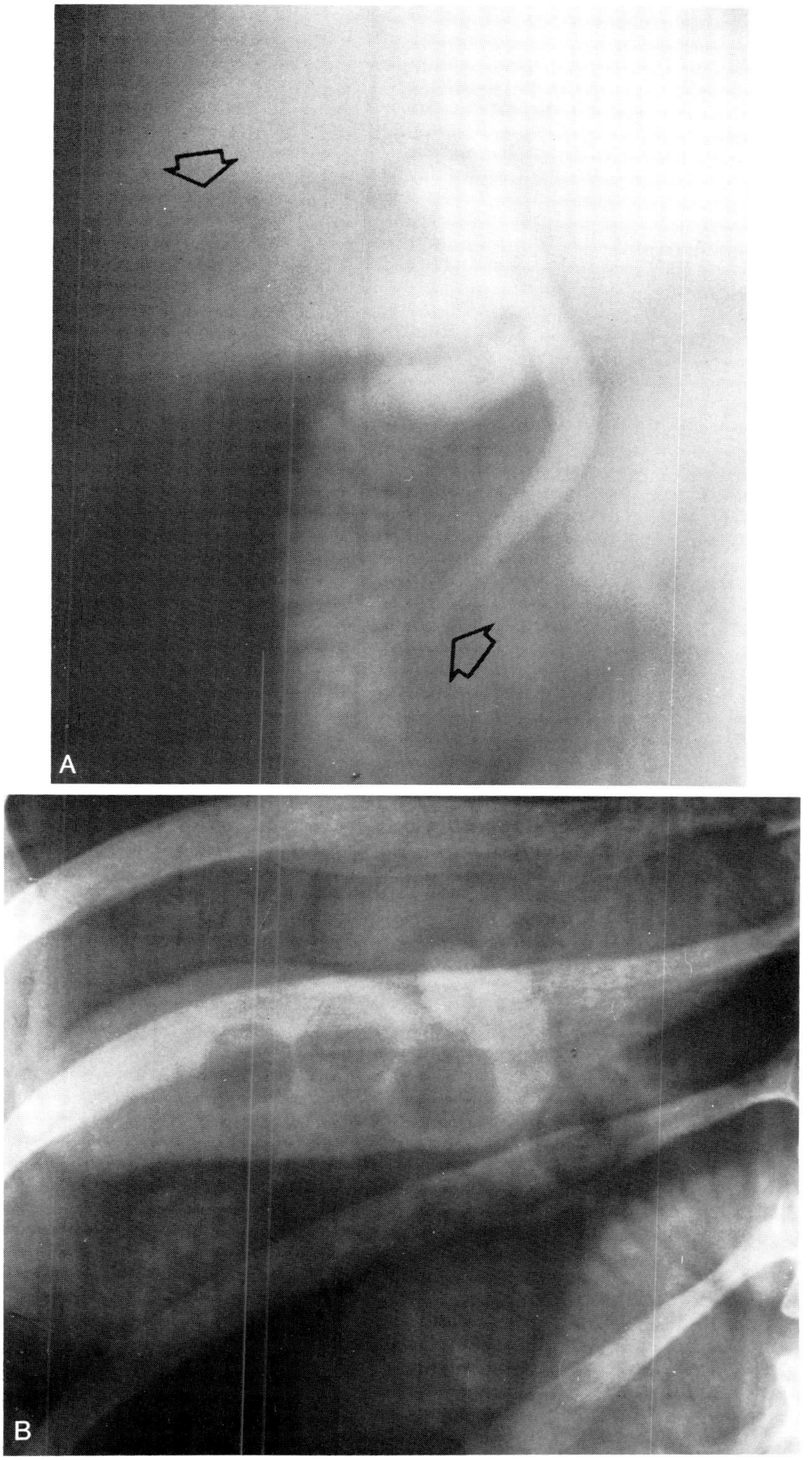

Figure 7–10. Intravenous cholangiogram in two patients with nonopacification of the gallbladder on second-day oral cholecystography. *A*, Gallstones are visible in the gallbladder and common duct *(arrows)*. Note contrast material in the duodenum. *B*, Gallstones in the gallbladder.

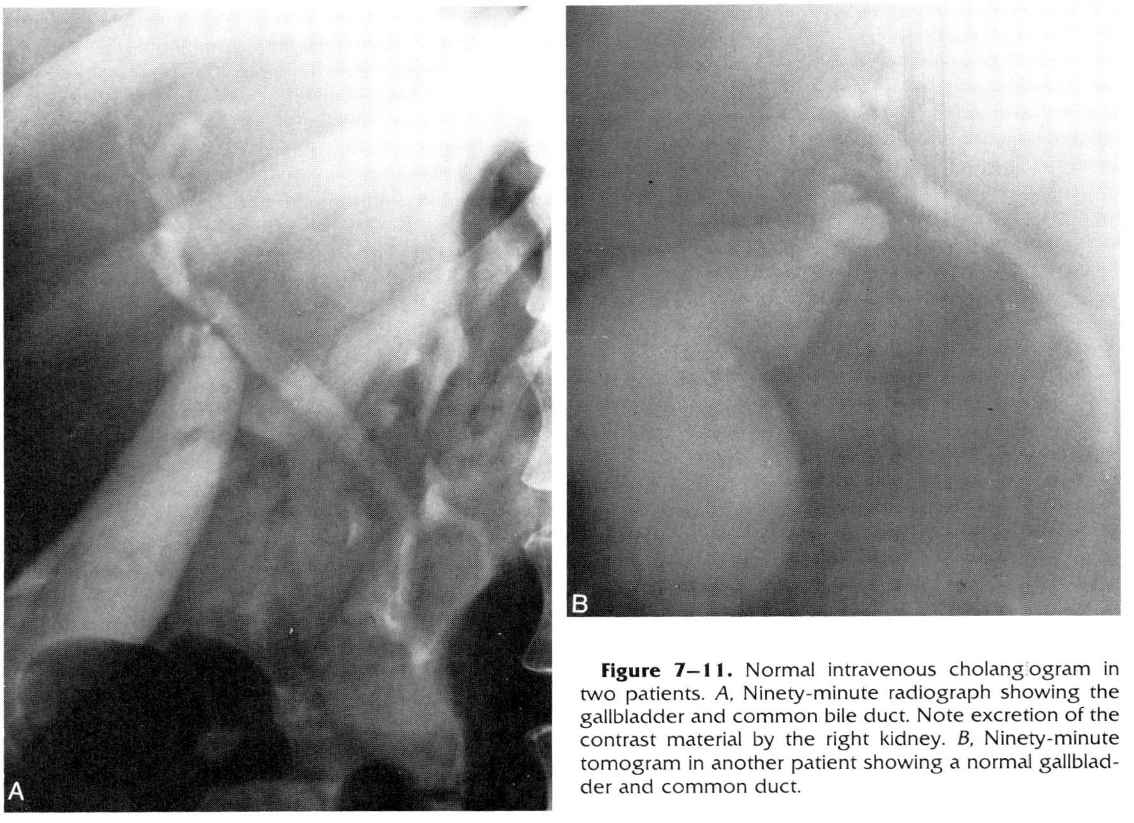

Figure 7–11. Normal intravenous cholangiogram in two patients. *A,* Ninety-minute radiograph showing the gallbladder and common bile duct. Note excretion of the contrast material by the right kidney. *B,* Ninety-minute tomogram in another patient showing a normal gallbladder and common duct.

dence of side effects. Wise recommends the use of morphine when it is necessary to increase the radiographic density of bile ducts.[107] Morphine causes contraction of the sphincter of Oddi, thereby increasing the amount of contrast material retained in the duct. According to Wise, the drug should not be given routinely, because the delayed emptying and dilatation of the common duct associated with its use cannot be distinguished from partial obstruction of the duct due to an anatomic abnormality.[107] Tomography of the bile duct after intravenous administration of contrast medium enhances diagnostic accuracy.[9]

The Normal Intravenous Cholangiogram

The average normal diameter of the bile duct at the level of the insertion of the cystic duct is about 5.5 mm, with a range of 2 to 15 mm (Fig. 7–11).[107] Maximal opacification of the common bile duct during intravenous cholangiography occurs 45 to 60 minutes after the injection of the contrast material.[107] This normal time-density relationship indicates proper drainage of the duct. The gallbladder usually begins to fill at 1 hour, although opacification occasionally is delayed until 4 hours or even 24 hours in apparently normal patients.

A round collection of contrast material lateral to the common bile duct, due to reflux of contrast material into the duodenal bulb, may simulate opacification of the gallbladder (Fig. 7–12).[113] Differentiation from contrast material in the gallbladder is based on the variability of the contrast material in the duodenum compared with that in the gallbladder. Opacification of the gallbladder persists and becomes progressively denser on serial radiographs; on the other hand, contrast material in the duodenum is transient, does not progressively increase in density, and sometimes can be seen to be continuous with contrast material in the second portion of the duodenum. Contrast material in the duodenal cap usually disappears when the patient's position is changed.

Another potential pitfall is mistaking incomplete mixing of radiopaque and nonopaque bile in the gallbladder for cholelithiasis

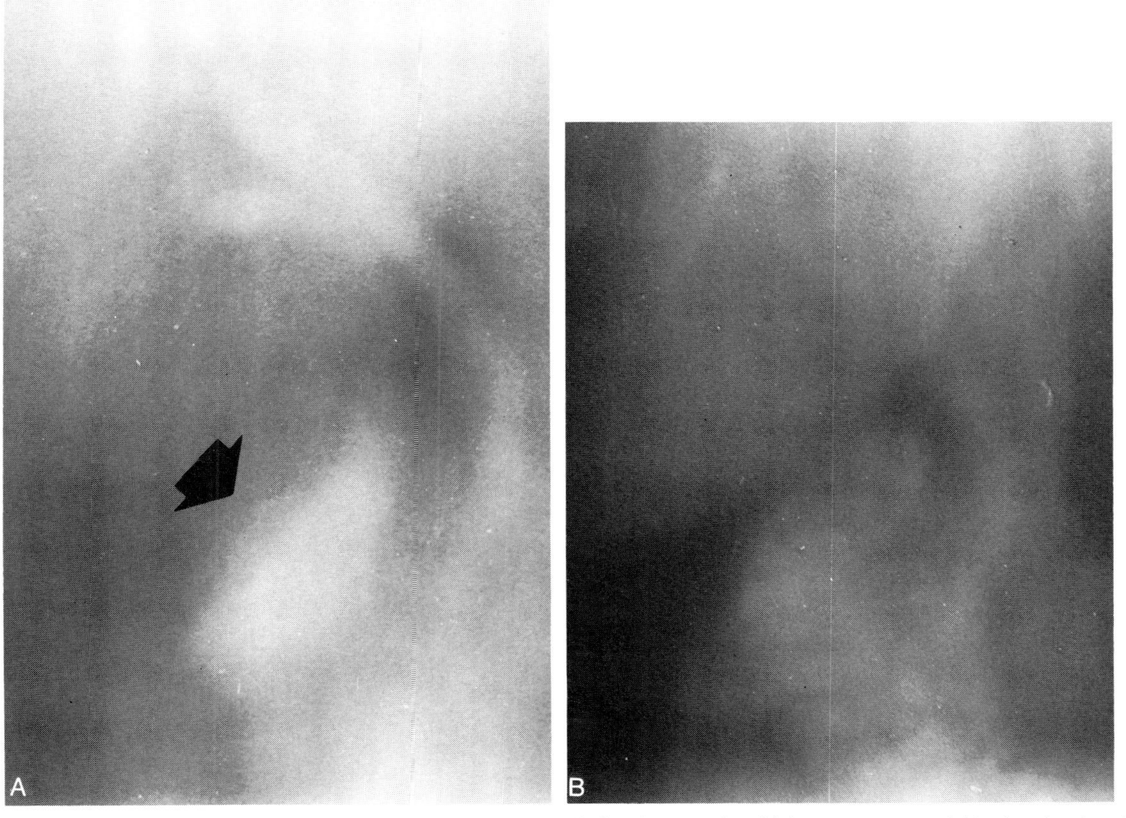

Figure 7–12. *A*, Tomogram made during an intravenous cholangiogram, in which contrast material in the duodenal bulb (*arrow*) simulated opacification of the gallbladder. *B*, Radiograph made later in the examination, in which it is apparent that the contrast material is in the duodenum and not the gallbladder.

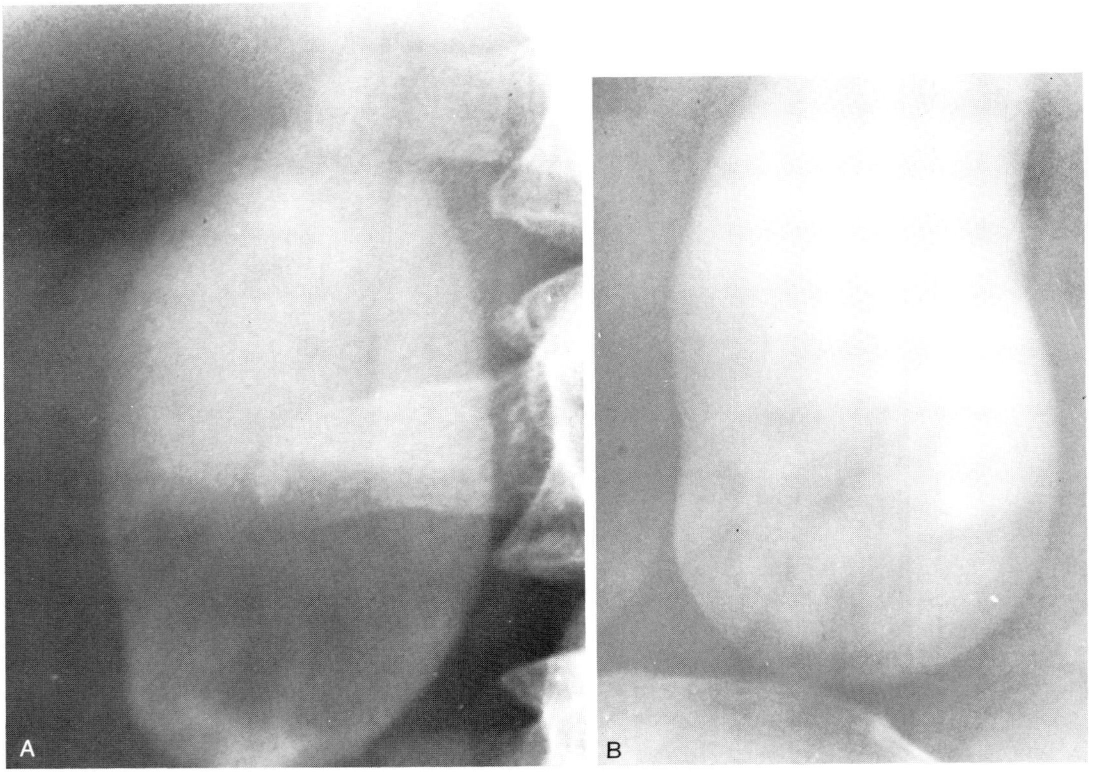

Figure 7–13. *A* and *B*, Upright spot films made at 120 minutes after the injection of Cholografin for intravenous cholangiography in two patients. There is incomplete mixing of bile containing contrast material and nonopaque bile in the gallbladder.

(Fig. 7–13).[114] Rapid filling of the gallbladder with contrast-laden bile during intravenous cholangiography does not allow time for thorough mixing with the nonopaque bile already in the gallbladder. Consequently, the latter appears as a radiolucency in the gallbladder. On upright or decubitus radiographs, incomplete mixing produces stratification of the bile with opaque layers of bile interspersed with the nonopaque bile. Radiolucent bile is variable in size and shape compared with gallstones and does not persist on delayed radiographs.

A final area of difficulty concerns the sphincter of Oddi. When the sphincter contracts, it may produce an abrupt termination in the distal portion of the common duct, with a concave defect on the cholangiogram that is indistinguishable from a gallstone (pseudocalculus sign).[115] This appearance is more common during operative and postoperative cholangiography, but it may also be visible during intravenous studies. When the defect is due to contraction of the sphincter, it is transient; however, a defect due to a gallstone persists and is associated with dilatation and poor drainage of the common duct. If the defect persists, glucagon can be used to relax the sphincter, so that a gallstone in the duct can be identified or excluded on subsequent radiographs.

In summary, intravenous cholangiography, once the only method to opacify the biliary ducts nonoperatively, has given way to newer techniques. Because its ability to opacify the ducts is marginal, the technique should be used only as a second or third test of choice in most instances. Indeed, unless a new contrast agent capable of producing adequate opacification of the biliary ducts is discovered, it is unlikely that intravenous cholangiography will survive as a useful diagnostic tool.

REFERENCES

1. Graham E, Cole W: Roentgenologic examination of the gallbladder. Preliminary report of a new method utilizing the intravenous injection of tetrabromphenolphthalein. JAMA 1924;82:613.
2. Joffe H, Wachowski RJ: Relationship of density of

cholecystographic shadows of the gallbladder to the iodine content. Radiology 1942;*38*:43.
3. Ingelfinger FJ: Digestive disease as a national problem. Gastroenterology 1968;*55*:102.
4. Burhenne HJ: Problem areas in the biliary tract. Curr Probl Radiol 1975;*5*:1.
5. Ferrucci JT Jr, Fordtran JS, Cooperberg PL, et al: The radiological diagnosis of gallbladder disease. Radiology 1981;*141*:49.
6. Rabinowitz JG, Yeh H-C, Cohen BA: Gallstone update—radiology. Semin Liver Dis 1983;*3*:120.
7. Yeh HC: Update on the gallbladder. *In* Sanders RC (ed): Ultrasound Annual. New York, Raven Press, 1982, pp 135–172.
8. Raghavendra BN, Redmond PE: Ultrasonography in the false normal oral cholecystogram. Am J Gastroenterol 1980;*73*:146.
9. Frommhold W, Wolf F: Radiological and radionuclide methods for the diagnosis of biliary disorders. Clin Gastroenterol 1983;*12*:65.
10. Krook PM, Allen FH, Bush WH Jr, et al: Comparison of real-time cholecystosonography and oral cholecystography. Radiology 1980;*135*:145.
11. Cooperberg PL, Burhenne HJ: Real-time ultrasonography. Diagnostic technique of choice in calculous gallbladder disease. N Engl J Med 1980; *302*:1277.
12. Amberg J: Radiography of the biliary tract. *In* Sleisenger MH, Fordtran JS (eds): Gastrointestinal Disease. Philadelphia, WB Saunders, 1973, p 1101.
13. Alderson DA: The reliability of Telepaque cholecystography. Br J Surg 1960;*47*:655.
14. Baker HI, Hodgson JR: Oral cholecystography: an evaluation of its accuracy. Gastroenterology 1958;*34*:1137.
15. Baker HI, Hodgson JR: Further studies on the accuracy of oral cholecystography. Radiology 1960;*74*:239.
16. Ferguson AN, Palmer WL: Cholecystography: its clinical evaluation. JAMA 1933;*100*:809.
17. Mujahed Z, Evans JA, Whalen JP: The nonopacified gallbladder on oral cholecystography. Radiology 1974;*112*:1.
18. Ochsner SF: Performance and reliability of cholecystography. South Med J 1970;*63*:1268.
19. Whitehouse WM: Correlation of surgical pathology with Telepaque cholecystography in doses of two grams. Surg Gynecol Obstet 1950;*100*:211.
20. Wickbom IG, Rentzhog U: The reliability of cholecystography. Acta Radiol 1955;*44*:185.
21. Dunn FH, Christensen ED, Reynolds J, et al: Cholecystokinin cholecystography. JAMA 1974;*228*:997.
22. Davis GB, Berk RN, Scheible FW, et al: Cholecystokinin cholecystography, sonography, and scintigraphy: detection of chronic acalculous cholecystitis. AJR 1982;*139*:1117.
23. Burnstein MJ, Vassal KP, Strasberg SM: Results of combined biliary drainage and cholecystokinin cholecystography in 81 patients with normal oral cholecystograms. Ann Surg 1982;*196*:627.
24. Kolodny M, Colker JL, Callahan EW, et al: Falsely negative cholecystography and cholangiography. Am J Dig Dis (New Series) 1968;*13*:669.
25. Ashmore JD, Kane JJ, Pettie HS, et al: Experimental evaluation of operative cholangiography in relation to calculus size. Surgery 1956;*40*:191.
26. Berk RN, Goldburger RE, Loeb PM: The role of bile salts in the hepatic excretion of iopanoic acid. Invest Radiol 1974;*9*:7.
27. Goldberger LE, Berk RN, Loeb PM: Biopharmaceutical factors influencing intestinal absorption of iopanoic acid. Invest Radiol 1974;*9*:16.
28. Stanley RJ, Melson GL, Cubillo E, et al: A comparison of three cholecystographic agents: a double blind study with and without a fatty meal. Radiology 1974;*112*:513.
29. Zboralske FF, Amberg JR: Cholecystocholestasis: a cause of cholecystographic error. Am J Dig Dis (New Series) 1962;*7*:339.
30. Mauthe H: The low-fat meal in gallbladder examinations. Radiology 1974;*112*:5.
31. Brewer AA: Physiological stasis: a cause of cholecystographic error. AJR 1974;*58*:106.
32. Curl H: High fat diet preceding cholecystography. JAMA 1942;*119*:607.
33. Whitehouse WM: Re-evaluation of fat-free preparatory meal in Telepaque cholecystography. AJR 1956;*76*:21.
34. Hodgson JR, Baker HL: New concepts in cholecystography and cholangiography. Postgrad Med 1959;*26*:283.
35. Berk RN, Loeb PM: Pharmacology and physiology of the biliary radiographic contrast materials. Semin Roentgenol 1976;*11*:147.
36. Postlethwaite AE, Kelly WN: Radiocontrast agents and aspirin. JAMA 1972;*219*:1479.
37. Sengpiel GW: The compatibility of castor oil and Priodax in concurrent examination of the colon and gallbladder. Radiology 1947;*53*:75.
38. McConnell RW, Rice RP: Effect of Neoloid on Telepaque cholecystography. AJR 1967;*101*:617.
39. Moadel E, Bryk D: Obscuration of opaque gallstones in oral cholecystography. J Can Assoc Radiol 1974;*25*:55.
40. Whalen JP, Rizzuti RJ, Evans JA: Time of optimal gallbladder opacification with Telepaque (iopanoic acid). Radiology 1972;*105*:523.
41. Oliphant M, Whalen HP, Evans JA: Times of optimal gallbladder opacification with Bilopaque (tyropanoate sodium). Radiology 1974;*112*:531.
42. Ettinger A: The value of the upright position in gallbladder examinations. Radiology 1940;*34*:481.
43. Greenwood F, Samuel E: The pathological gallbladder. Br J Radiol 1948;*21*:438.
44. Lubert M, Krause GR: Upright cholecystography using the fluoroscopic spotfilmer with graded compression. Radiology 1953;*61*:879.
45. Jensen R, Kaude J: Oral cholecystography. Acta Radiol 1970;*10*:499.
46. Miller RE, Chernish SM, Rodda BE: Cholecystography: a cost reduction study. Radiology 1974;*110*:61.
47. Hodgson JR: The technical aspects of cholecystography. Radiol Clin North Am 1970;*8*:85.
48. Harvey IC, Thwe M, Low-Beer TS: The value of the fatty meal in oral cholecystography. Clin Radiol 1976;*27*:117.
49. Sachs MD, Partington PF: The distended gallbladder. AJR 1960;*83*:835.
50. Heaton KW, Gibson MJ: The use of fatty meals in oral cholecystography: report of a postal survey in England and Wales. Clin Radiol 1973;*24*:90.
51. Lorman HG, Rosenbaum HD: How to do an oral cholecystogram. Semin Roentgenol 1976;*11*:165.
52. Wise RE: Pitfalls in roentgenographic diagnosis of gallbladder disease. Lahey Clin Found Bull 1966;*15*:109.
53. Miller RE: Simple apparatus for decubitus films with horizontal beam. Radiology 1970;*97*:682.

54. Amberg JR, Zboralske FF, Johnson ER: The inclined lateral decubitus position for cholecystography. AJR 1964;*92*:1128.
55. Etter LE: Left-sided gallbladder. AJR 1953;*70*:987.
56. Laufer I, Gledhill L: The value of the fatty meal in oral cholecystography. Radiology 1975;*114*:525.
57. Hoeffel J-C, Burger G, Senot P, et al: Oral cholecystography: Is the fatty meal always necessary? Radiology 1980;*20*:24.
58. Berk RN: The problem of impaired first-dose visualization of the gallbladder. AJR 1971;*113*:186.
59. Rosenbaum HD: The value of re-examination in patients with inadequate visualization of the gallbladder following a single dose of Telepaque. AJR 1959;*82*:1011.
60. Berk RN: The consecutive dose phenomenon in oral cholecystography. AJR 1970;*110*:230.
61. Kaden VG, Howard JM, Doubleday LC: Cholecystographic studies during and immediately following acute pancreatitis. Surgery 1955;*38*:1082.
62. Radakovich M, Greenlaw RH, Strain WH: Iodinated organic compounds as contrast media for radiographic diagnoses. X. Interrelationship of gallbladder and pancreas. Soc Exp Biol Med 1951;*77*:156.
63. Radakovich M, Greenlaw RH, Strain W: Iodinated organic compounds as contrast media for radiographic diagnoses. XIV. The influence of pancreatic function on cholecystography. NY State J Med 1951;*51*:2880.
64. Silvani HL, McCorkle HJ: Temporary failure of gallbladder visualization by cholecystography in acute pancreatitis. Am Surg 1948;*127*:1207.
65. Sanchez-Ubeda R, Ruzicka FF, Rousselot LM: Effect of peritonitis of nonbiliary origin on the function of the gallbladder as measured by cholecystography, its frequency and its duration. N Engl J Med 1957;*257*:389.
66. Howard JM: Gallbladder function (cholecystographic studies) following non-specific trauma. Surgery 1954;*36*:1051.
67. Sparkman RS, Jernigan R: Visualization of gallbladder and bile ducts following trauma. Surgery 1957;*41*:595.
68. Lindqvist T, Sohrne G: X-ray investigation of the gallbladder in pernicious anemia. Acta Med Scand 1944;*116*:117.
69. Harris RC, Caffey J: Cholecystography in infants. JAMA 1953;*153*:1333.
70. Levyn L, Beck EC, Aaron AH: Further cholecystographic studies in the late months of pregnancy. AJR 1933;*30*:774.
71. Roller R, Mallory A, Caruthers SB, et al: Oral cholecystography after alcoholic pancreatitis. Gastroenterology 1977;*73*:218.
72. Burhenne HJ, Obata WG: Single-visit oral cholecystography. N Engl J Med 1975;*292*:627.
73. Beseman EF: Can ipodate calcium save the patient one day in hospitalization? AJR 1970;*110*:226.
74. Crummy AB: Five-hour reinforcement cholecystography. Gastrointest Radiol 1976;*1*:91.
75. Stephens DH, Carlson HC, Gisvold JJ: Tomography in problem cholecystograms. Radiol Clin North Am 1976;*14*:15.
76. Stephens DH, Gisvold JJ, Carlson HC: Tomography of the gallbladder in oral cholecystography. Gastrointest Radiol 1976;*1*:93.
77. Berk RN: Radiology of the gallbladder and bile ducts. Surg Clin North Am 1973;*53*:973.
78. Low-Beer TS, Heaton KW, Roylance J: Oral cholecystography in patients with small bowel disease. Br J Radiol 1972;*45*:427.
79. Goldberg JI: Small bowel disease and oral cholecystography. Gastroenterology 1976;*71*:529.
80. Price WH: Gallbladder dyspepsia. Br Med J 1963;*2*:138.
81. Farrar ZT: Underdiagnosis of biliary tract disorders. Gastroenterology 1966:6051:1074.
82. Adams TW, Foxley EG: A diagnostic technique for acalculous cholecystitis. Surg Gynecol Obstet 1976:*142*:168.
83. Jacob CO, Modan M, Itzchak Y, et al: Prolonged opacification of the gallbladder after oral cholecystography: a reevaluation of its clinical significance. Gastroenterology 1981;*81*:938.
84. Hoffmann TH, Glanges E: Cholecystitis and delayed emptying of the gallbladder. Surg Gynecol Obstet 1980;*151*:70.
85. Goldberg HE: Cholecystokinin cholecystography. Semin Roentgenol 1976;*11*:175.
86. Goldstein F, Ginsberg DK, Johnson RG: Biliary dyskinesia—report of two cases with physiologic studies. Am J Gastroenterol 1961;*36*:268.
87. Cozzolino HJ, Goldstein F, Greening RR, et al: The cystic duct syndrome. JAMA 1963;*185*:920.
88. Camishion RC, Goldstein F: Partial, noncalculous cystic duct obstruction (cystic duct syndrome). Surg Clin North Am 1967:*47*:1107.
89. Nathan MH, Newman A, Murray DJ, et al: Cholecystokinin cholecystography. AJR 1970;*110*:240.
90. Valberg LS, Jabbari M, Kerr JW, et al: Biliary pain in young women in the absence of gallstones. Gastroenterology 1971;*60*:1020.
91. Goldstein F, Grunt R, Margulies M: Cholecystokinin cholecystography in differential diagnosis of acalculous gallbladder disease. Gastroenterology 1972;*62*:756.
92. Goldberg HI, Moss AA, Montgomery CK, et al: Contractility of the inflamed gallbladder: an experimental study using the technique of cholecystokinin cholecystography. Invest Radiol 1972; *7*:447.
93. Goldstein F, Grunt R, Margulies M: Cholecystokinin cholecystography in the differential diagnosis of acalculous gallbladder disease. Am J Dig Dis 1974;*19*:835.
94. Rajagoplan AE, Pickleman J: Biliary colic and functional gallbladder disease. Arch Surg 1982; *117*:1005.
95. Lennard TWJ, Farndon JR, Taylor RMR: Acalculous biliary pain: diagnosis and selection for cholecystectomy using the cholecystokinin test for pain reproduction. Br J Surg 1984;*71*:368.
96. Griffen WO Jr, Bivins BA, Rogers EL, et al: Cholecystokinin cholecystography in the diagnosis of gallbladder disease. Ann Surg 1980;*191*:636.
97. Jutras JA: Hyperplastic cholecystoses. AJR 1960;*83*:795.
98. Salmenkivi K: Cholesterolosis of the gallbladder, a clinical study based on 269 cholecystectomies. Acta Chir Scand (Suppl) 1964:*324*:1.
99. Aguirre JR, Boher RO, Guraieb S: Hyperplastic cholecystoses: a new contribution to the unitarian theory. AJR 1969;*107*:1.
100. Lubera RJ, Clinie ARW, Kling GE: Cholecystitis and the hyperplastic cholecystoses. A clinical, radiologic and pathologic study. Am J Dig Dis 1967;*12*:696.
101. Glenn F, et al: Intravenous cholangiography. Ann Surg 1954:*140*:600.

102. Johnson HC, McLaren JR, Weens HW: Intravenous cholangiography in the differential diagnosis of acute cholecystitis. Radiology 1960;*74*:790.
103. Sparkman RS, Ellis PR: Intravenous cholecyst-cholangiography in emergency abdominal diagnosis. Ann Surg 1956;*143*:416.
104. Harrington OB, Beall AC Jr, Noon G, et al: Intravenous cholangiography in acute cholecystitis. Arch Surg 1964:*88*:585.
105. Ehrlich EW, Debras J, Howard JM: Intravenous cholecystography as an immediate aid in differential diagnosis of acute pancreatitis and acute cholecystitis. Ann Surg 1962:*156*:287.
106. Thorpe CD, Olsen WR, Fischer H, et al: Emergency intravenous cholangiography in patients with acute abdominal pain. Am J Surg 1973;*125*:46.
107. Wise RE: Intravenous Cholangiography. Springfield, IL, CC Thomas, 1962.
108. Eckelberg ME, Carlson HC, McIlrath DC: Intravenous cholangiography with intact gallbladder. AJR 1970;*110*:235.
109. Halasz NA: Counterfeit cholecystitis. Am J Surg 1975;*130*:189.
110. Postlethwaite AE, Kelley WN: Uricosuric effect of radiocontrast agents. A study in man of four commonly used preparations. Ann Intern Med 1971;*74*:845.
111. Johnson JH, Wise RE: Intravenous cholangiography: a study of reactions to iodipamide methylglucamine. Lahey Clin Found Bull 1964:*13*:245.
112. Martinez LO, Viamonte M Jr, Gassman P, et al: Present status of intravenous cholangiography. AJR 1971;*113*:10.
113. Berk RN: Radiology of the Gallbladder and Bile Ducts. Ed 1. Philadelphia, WB Saunders, 1983.
114. Twiggs HI, Zelna A: Stratification in intravenous cholangiography. Radiology 1963:*80*:774.
115. Martinex LO, Cohen G: The pseudocalculus sign in intravenous cholangiography. South Med J 1972:*65*:1066.
116. Scholz FJ, Larsen CR, Wise RE: Intravenous cholangiography: recurring concepts. Semin Roentgenol 1976;*11*:197.
117. Edmunds R, Katz S, Garciano V, et al: The common duct after cholecystectomy. Arch Surg 1971;*103*:79.
118. Reiss R, Pikielny S: The clinical significance of the diameter of the common bile duct in cholecystectomized patients. Isr J Med Sci 1971;7:1070.
119. Goodman MW, Ansel HJ, Vennes JA, et al: Is intravenous cholangiography still useful? Gastroenterology 1980;*79*:642.
120. Eubanks B, Martinez CR, Mehigan D, et al: Current role of intravenous cholangiography. Am J Surg 1982;*143*:731.
121. Pedersen JH, Hancke S, Christensen B, et al: Ultrasonography ^{99m}Tc-DIDA cholescintigraphy and infusion tomography in the diagnosis of acute cholecystitis. Scand J Gastroenterol 1982;*17*:77.
122. Graham MF, Cooperberg PL, Cohen MM, et al: The size of the normal common bile duct following cholecystectomy: an ultrasonographic study. Radiology 1980;*135*:137.

ROY A FILLY, M. D.
PETER W. CALLEN, M. D.

8

Ultrasonography of the Gallbladder and Bile Ducts

In the last decade, ultrasonography has changed from a procedure with limited applications in the biliary tract to a major diagnostic modality for detection of gallbladder and bile duct pathology. This is due, in part, to the improvement in image quality that resulted from the development of gray-scale image processing. With this display, abnormal morphologic changes can be demonstrated accurately. Recent advances in the quality of the receivers employed on ultrasonographic systems have encouraged the use of higher frequency transducers, which yield improved resolution. In addition, real-time ultrasonography, tantamount to ultrasound "fluoroscopy," has become widely available. This is an important advancement with regard to gallbladder ultrasonography. Since static gray-scale ultrasonograms are tomograms, the ultrasonographer has always been faced with the problem of determining how many ultrasonic tomograms are necessary to adequately study the gallbladder. This is especially true when searching for stones. Real-time ultrasonography solves the problem by enabling the ultrasonographer to obtain a very large number of contiguous tomograms in a very short time.

This chapter includes the ultrasonographic assessment of the gallbladder, the detection of dilated bile ducts, and the use of ultrasound in the evaluation of patients following biliary tract surgery.

THE GALLBLADDER

Technique

The utility of ultrasonography for visualization of the gallbladder is, in large part, secondary to its high degree of resolution to identify fluid-containing viscera. If possible, the patient should be fasting for 8 to 12 hours preceding the examination in order to maximally distend the gallbladder. Ultrasonographic examination of a distended gallbladder yields more accurate results. Parasagittal scans are obtained at 1 to 2 cm intervals from the lateral right upper abdomen medially until the gallbladder is identified (Fig. 8–1). Then, very closely spaced longitudinal scans are performed, preferably through the long axis of the gallbladder. It is most important to visualize all segments of the gallbladder. The segments most commonly missed by inexperienced sonographers are the tip of the fundus and the neck. In order to be certain that the neck is properly imaged the ultrasonographer must bear in mind the virtually constant relationship of the gallbladder neck to the portal venous system.[15] Thus, when the gallbladder is noted to come into close proximity with either the right or the main portal vein, the ultrasonographer may feel confident that he has visualized the gallbladder neck adequately (Fig. 8–2).

Unless an unusual technical problem is encountered, the gallbladder can be visualized in essentially all normal fasting individuals. This has caused some ultrasonographers to ascribe a pathologic etiology if the gallbladder is not demonstrated in fasting individuals.[2, 30, 35, 39] In general, we subscribe to this concept although, clearly, with advanced imaging technology, very few patients should fall into this category.

Cross-sectional scans are less valuable than longitudinal scans but should be performed in all cases. Any gallbladder that appears normal on routine supine, transverse, and longitudinal scans requires additional scans in the left decubitus position.[21] Occasionally, by so doing, a small, solitary stone that was

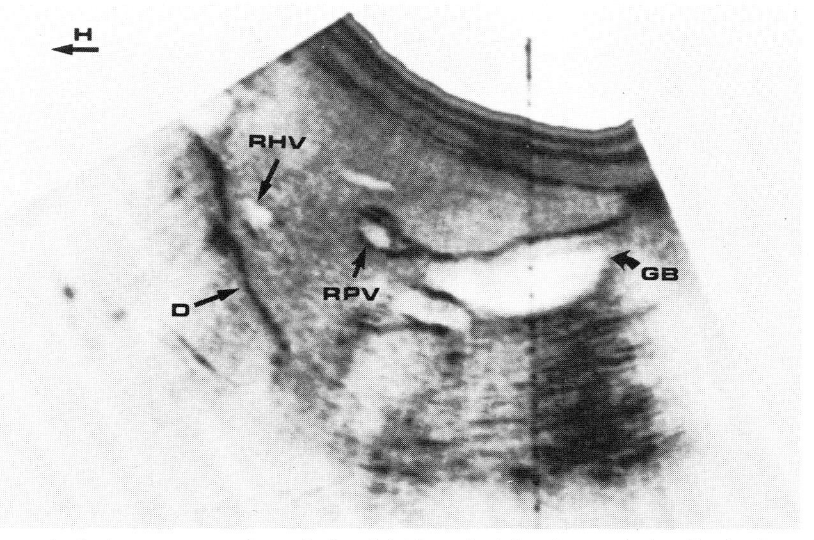

Figure 8–1. Parasagittal ultrasonogram through the right hepatic lobe demonstrates the body and fundus of the gallbladder (GB). (H = head; D = diaphragm; RPV = right portal vein; RHV = right hepatic vein.)

not previously seen gravitates to a position in the gallbladder in which it is easily identified. Additionally, real-time ultrasonography should be considered a virtually mandatory part of gallbladder examination.

Diagnosis of Cholelithiasis

In the late 1970s it became clear that ultrasonography could be used to complement oral cholecystography in the diagnosis of cholelithiasis,[4–6, 15] although accuracy in the detection of gallstones was less than ideal.[2, 3, 37, 38] The use of ultrasound tomography in the diagnosis of cholelithiasis has evolved as improvements in the equipment and identification of diagnostic features led to increased accuracy.[2–5, 15, 37, 38] It is now clear that the ultrasonographic diagnosis surpasses oral cholecystography,[31, 34, 44] and most agree that ultrasonography is the initial study of choice in the diagnosis of cholelithiasis.[6, 11, 26, 50, 54]

There are a number of features by which

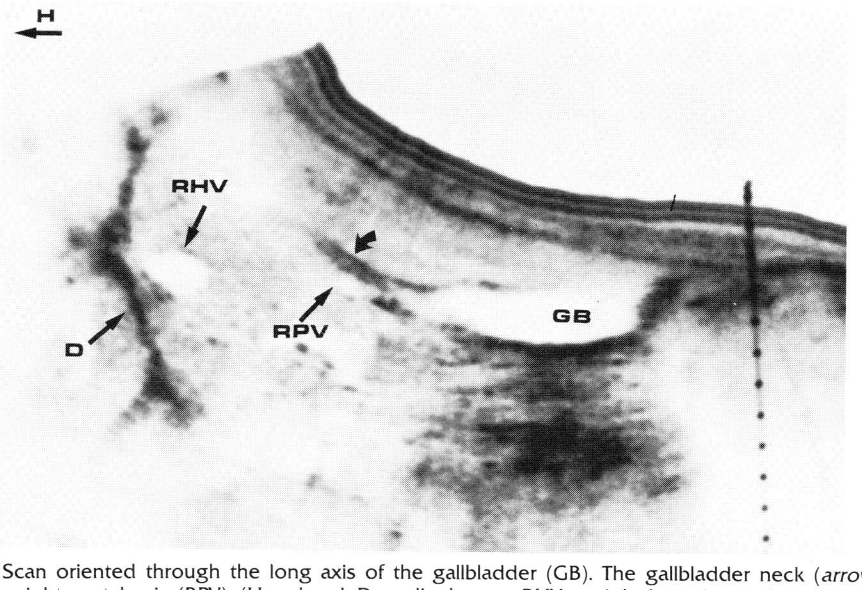

Figure 8–2. Scan oriented through the long axis of the gallbladder (GB). The gallbladder neck (*arrow*) is seen in contact with the right portal vein (RPV). (H = head; D = diaphragm; RHV = right hepatic vein.)

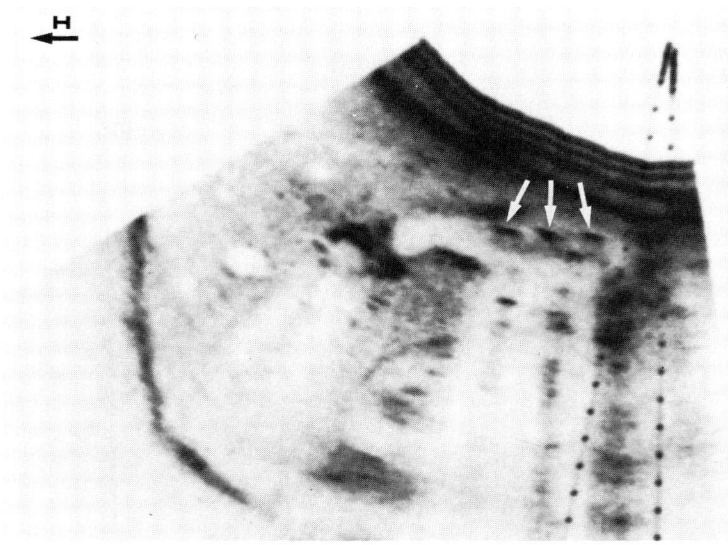

Figure 8–3. Parasagittal ultrasonogram demonstrating typical high-amplitude echoes (*arrows*) originating from stones in the gallbladder. Acoustic shadows are generated by the stones. (H = head.)

the ultrasonographer may diagnose gallstones.[2, 12, 15, 28, 48, 54] Some of these features are very reliable, whereas others are only moderately so.

The most reliable findings of gallstone disease on an ultrasonogram are: (1) demonstration of one or more high-amplitude reflections *within the gallbladder lumen*, which (2) cast well-defined acoustic shadows and (3) gravitate to the dependent portion of the gallbladder when the patient is placed in the decubitus or upright position (Fig. 8–3). The demonstration of these features is virtually, if not absolutely, diagnostic of cholelithiasis.

If it is not possible to demonstrate one or more of these findings, the degree of confidence in the diagnosis of cholelithiasis decreases. Nonetheless, demonstration of a high-amplitude echo within the gallbladder that gravitates dependently when the patient's position is altered is excellent evidence that gallstones are present, even though an acoustic shadow is not demonstrated. By contrast, a high-amplitude echo within the gallbladder that does not cast an acoustic shadow and that cannot be seen in all planes of section or demonstrated to gravitate dependently is inconclusive evidence for cholelithiasis. It may be secondary to another type of gallbladder pathology, such as a polyp, or it may be entirely spurious.

There are frequent instances in which the gallbladder is small and largely filled with stones. In such cases, the bile, which serves as an acoustic contrast agent, is absent. Thus, the gallbladder itself is not seen.[35, 54] The major diagnostic findings are (1) inability to demonstrate the gallbladder in a fasting individual and (2) the presence of an acoustic shadow emanating from the anatomic location in which one anticipates finding the gallbladder (Fig. 8–4). Since bowel gas in the duodenum or hepatic flexure of the colon also casts an acoustic shadow, caution must be exercised in the interpretation of ultrasonograms that fall in this category. The acoustic

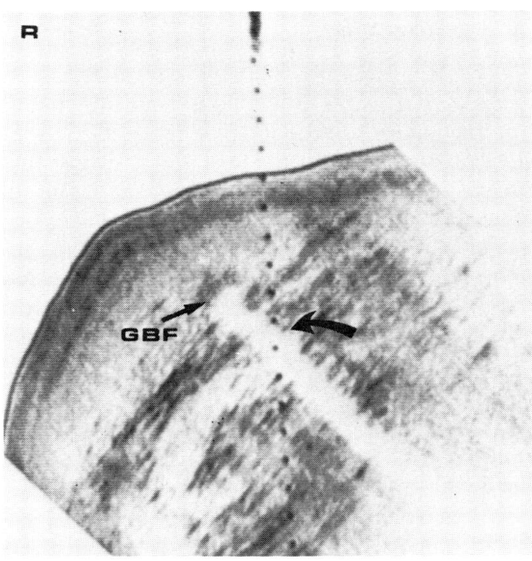

Figure 8–4. Limited transverse scan demonstrating the gallbladder fossa (GBF). While the gallbladder itself is not seen, characteristic shadowing is noted (*arrows*). (R = right.)

shadow cast by gallstones is generally an abrupt and complete cessation of sound transmission. It is a "clean" acoustic shadow. Conversely, shadows caused by bowel gas generally display multiple reverberative echo artifacts (Fig. 8–4). This distinction, however, is not absolute.[55]

The position of the acoustic shadow is critical in such cases. The best evidence that the shadow is caused by cholelithiasis is demonstration on limited transverse scans that the shadow originates in the gallbladder fossa. Since the gallbladder is the only viscus with a true fossa on the inferomedial edge of the liver, an acoustic shadow emanating from this depression may be confidently diagnosed as originating within the gallbladder. However, the origin of the shadow may be from gas in the gallbladder (emphysematous cholecystitis) or wall calcification (porcelain gallbladder). Thus, this finding is not definite for cholelithiasis, even though both these conditions are usually associated with cholelithiasis and are managed surgically.

If one is unable to demonstrate the aforementioned finding, the next most reliable approach is to analyze the relationship of the shadow to the proximal right portal vein on longitudinal sections. If the cephalic edge of the shadow lies very close to the right portal vein, the likelihood is high that the shadow originates in the gallbladder and thus is due to gallstones.

Relationship of Ultrasonography to Oral Cholecystography

Although the oral cholecystogram (OCG) is an excellent diagnostic test, our confidence in it has been somewhat overstated.[6] Ultrasonography is assuming an increasingly important role in the evaluation of patients suspected of harboring gallstones. In experienced hands, ultrasonography is probably the preferred technique for identification of cholelithiasis.[11, 26, 31, 33, 44, 50] Whether one subscribes to this view or not, there are several clearly defined areas where ultrasonography is preferred to the OCG. Patients who are allergic to iodinated contrast agents, particularly the oral biliary contrast agents, ought to be examined ultrasonically. Since ultrasound is a mechanical rather than an ionizing radiation method, it is preferable in pregnant patients. Obviously, the OCG cannot be performed adequately in patients with abnormal hepatocellular function or jaundice of any cause. Ultrasonography is a function-independent imaging technique. Thus, it can be used in patients with abnormal liver function and in normal individuals with equal success. Known malabsorption, gastric outlet obstruction, or pancreatitis as well as other problems not related to biliary dysfunction may result in nonopacification of the gallbladder with oral contrast agents. Such problems do not degrade the ultrasonic image.

Ultrasonography is indicated when the OCG is poorly opacified, unless gallstones are obvious. Patients with well-opacified "normal" OCGs in whom the weight of clinical evidence favors gallbladder disease should also be considered for ultrasonography, since false negative (well-opacified) OCGs may occur. In general, the clinician should remember that the false diagnoses of these two modalities are different. Whenever the interpretation of the OCG causes doubt, the ultrasonogram may be employed, and vice versa. Unfortunately, the quality of ultrasonography varies greatly from one institution to another.

Acute Cholecystitis. Sonographic demonstration of gallbladder stones in a patient with right upper quadrant pain, fever, and leukocytosis is inferential evidence of acute cholecystitis. A positive Murphy sign may be elicited using the ultrasound probe, which allows for precise determination of the location of the gallbladder fundus.[43] Ultrasonography, however, offers no information regarding gallbladder function and cystic duct patency, both of which can be determined much more accurately by cholescintigraphy (see Chapter 12). Some have proposed that increased gallbladder wall thickness or a rim of echolucency is diagnostic of acute cholecystitis;[32, 42, 43, 57, 59] however, others dispute this claim.[13, 46] The presence of intramural gas in the gallbladder wall is suggestive of emphysematous cholecystitis.[8]

The sensitivity of ultrasonography in patients with acalculous cholecystitis is much less than in patients with cholecystitis and cholelithiasis.[52] The most reliable sign of acalculous cholecystitis appears to be the demonstration of gallbladder wall thickening.[17, 41, 48] However, the sensitivity and reliability of this finding are still in question.[16] Several pitfalls in the interpretation of diffuse gallbladder wall thickening have already been described. When the normal gallbladder is distended by fasting, the wall is imperceptible ultrasonographically; however, when the gallbladder is not distended, the wall is visible and may be erroneously perceived as pathologically thickened.

Similarly, a variety of pathologic events not directly related to the gallbladder may result in wall thickening, including hypoalbuminemia and infectious hepatitis.[21, 52] However, in a dilated gallbladder (lumen greater than 4 cm), the finding of a thick wall appears to be a reliable sign of acute cholecystitis.[14, 17, 49] In very high-risk patients with acute cholecystitis, it is possible to use ultrasonography to place a catheter percutaneously. The technique of percutaneous cholecystostomy is relatively safe and can be performed at the patient's bedside.[19] Moreover, in some patients with neoplastic biliary obstruction this technique can be used to provide biliary drainage when the transhepatic approach is not possible.

Dilatation of the Gallbladder. Gallbladder dilatation may occur in the absence of signs or symptoms of acute cholecystitis. When the gallbladder is prominently dilated it is readily imaged. In patients with hydropic gallbladder or extrahepatic obstruction, the gallbladder is seen as a large fluid-filled structure in the right upper quadrant. The problem is determining a measurement above which the gallbladder may be confidently said to be pathologically dilated. In our experience, the length of the gallbladder is too highly variable to be of use. The diameter of the gallbladder is more applicable, but definitive criteria for pathologic enlargement have not been established. Our impression is that a diameter exceeding 4.5 to 5.0 cm indicates pathologic dilatation, although, rarely, a patient undergoing prolonged fasting will demonstrate a gallbladder diameter of this dimension (Fig. 8–5). The major problem with this limit is a false negative diagnosis. Many patients with common bile duct obstruction or an acute hydrops will have a gallbladder diameter within this limit.

Sludge. Sludge refers to the ultrasonic finding in which an echogenic layer of sediment is seen within the gallbladder (Fig. 8–6).[4] While this constitutes a pathologic finding, it is well known to be readily reversible. This finding is usually noted in patients who have extrahepatic biliary obstruction or who have undergone a prolonged fast and have been confined to bed. The obvious common denominator in these patients is bile stasis.[1, 58]

Patients on nasogastric suction or hyperalimentation commonly demonstrate prominent gallbladders that contain sludge.[1, 45] However, sludge is also seen in patients with hydrops, acute and chronic cholecystitis, and gallbladder neoplasms (Fig. 8–7). Thus, this finding should never be simply ignored as a "normal variant." In addition, there is increasing evidence of a relationship between sludge and the development of gallstones[7, 45] and acute acalculous cholecystitis. The identification of sludge on the ultrasonogram slightly complicates the demonstration of gallstones that may also be present within the gallbladder.

The precise etiology of this finding and the explanation of the mechanism by which

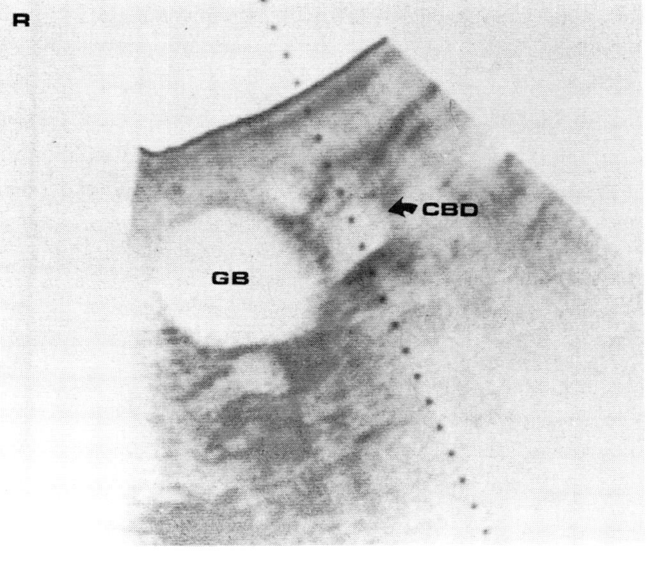

Figure 8–5. Limited transverse scan demonstrating a grossly dilated gallbladder (GB). The common bile duct (CBD) is also dilated (R = right.)

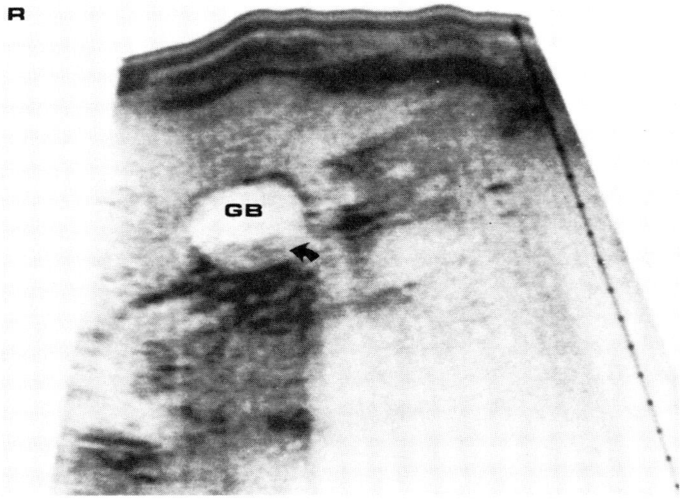

Figure 8–6. Limited transverse scan demonstrating "sludge" (*arrow*) within the gallbladder (GB). (R = right.)

sludge generates echoes are not known. This type of bile is viscous, but high viscosity per se does not cause echoes. Recent evidence indicates that calcium bilirubinate granules and, to a lesser degree, cholesterol crystals are the source of these echoes in biliary sludge.[1]

Polyps and Gallbladder Carcinoma. Polyps are occasionally identified on ultrasonic studies of the gallbladder.[34] Polyps generate medium- to high-amplitude echoes along the mucosal lining of the gallbladder, which fail to cast an acoustic shadow and do not gravitate with changes in patient position (Fig. 8–8). The sensitivity and accuracy of ultrasonography for demonstrating polyps are unknown. Gallbladder cancer may be seen as a focal mass within the gallbladder or as a complete disruption of the gallbladder appearance by a mass.

THE BILE DUCTS

Ultrasonography is a superb technique for the detection of extrahepatic and intrahepatic biliary dilatation, and it should be the procedure of choice in the initial evaluation of patients suspected of obstructive jaundice.[26, 27, 36, 41, 47] The accuracy of ultrasound diagnosis compares favorably with that of computed tomography and is considerably less expensive.[27, 56] Transhepatic cholangiography has a high diagnostic accuracy, but as an invasive procedure it entails both discomfort and risk.[33] Similar problems apply to endoscopic retrograde cholangiography.

The problem of diagnosing bile duct dilatation is an interesting one for the ultrasonographer, who possesses no specific contrast agents for either the biliary or the vascular system. In normal individuals the intra- and extrahepatic portal venous system and the hepatic veins are seen in virtually all technically satisfactory scans.[9] In general, the intrahepatic components of the biliary and arterial tree, which travel very close to the portal veins, are not seen. However, the extrahepatic components are visible in many individuals. When the intrahepatic bile ducts dilate,

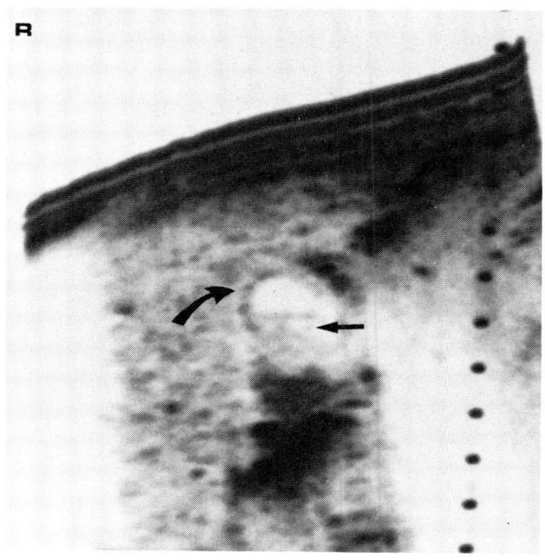

Figure 8–7. Limited transverse scan in a patient with acute acalculous cholecystitis. The gallbladder wall (*curved arrow*) is thickened. Sludge (*arrow*) is also present. (R = right.)

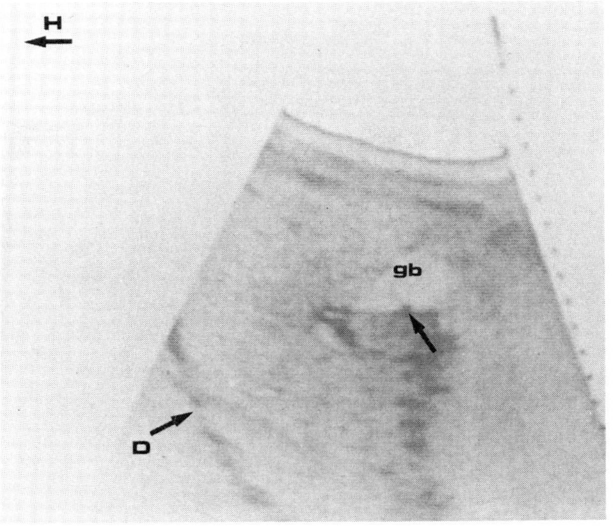

Figure 8–8. Parasagittal ultrasonogram demonstrating a polyp (*arrow*) within the gallbladder (GB). Note the absence of acoustic shadowing. (H = head; D = diaphragm.)

they cross the threshold of visibility. Thus, in order to recognize dilated bile ducts, the ultrasonographer must (1) be able to distinguish between hepatic and portal veins; (2) be aware of the normal portal anatomy and its few variations;[23] and (3) when the bile ducts are dilated, be able to recognize that a normally unseen set of tubular, fluid-filled structures is now coursing in association with the portal venous system. Fortunately, these tasks are reasonably straightforward. The methods have been clearly outlined in the literature.[26, 36]

Five features assist in differentiating dilated bile ducts from portal veins.[36] The most important is a typical alteration in the anatomic appearance of the portal venous region caused by dilated bile ducts (Fig. 8–9). Basically, the right portal vein is invariably seen as a solitary tubular vascular structure along its proximal segment. Any other tubular structures coursing with the portal vein in this region may be inferentially diagnosed as dilated bile ducts. This inference is highly accurate.

The second feature is the result of the

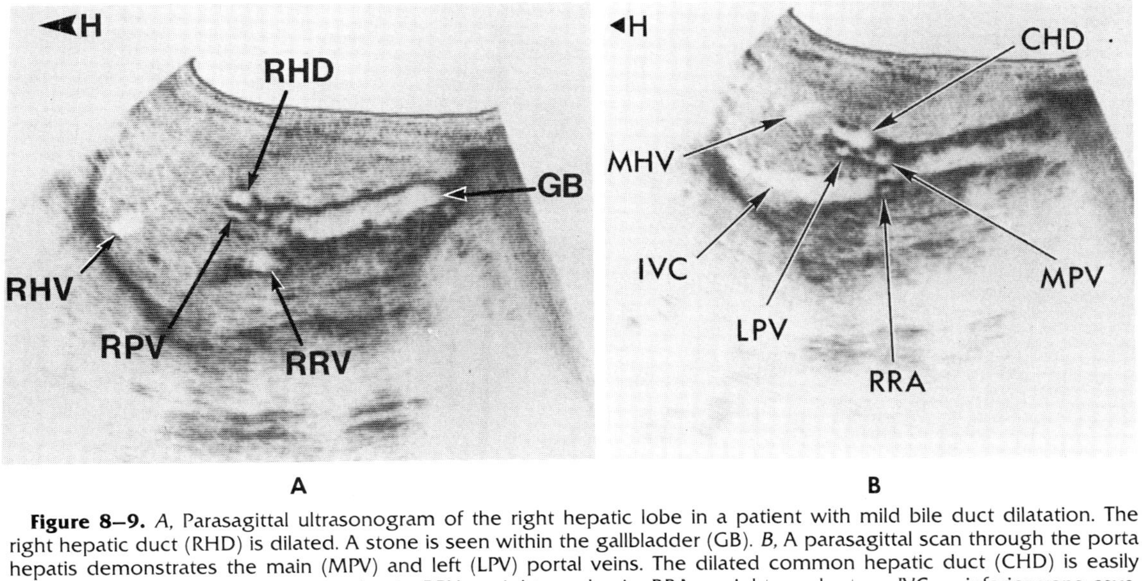

Figure 8–9. *A*, Parasagittal ultrasonogram of the right hepatic lobe in a patient with mild bile duct dilatation. The right hepatic duct (RHD) is dilated. A stone is seen within the gallbladder (GB). *B*, A parasagittal scan through the porta hepatis demonstrates the main (MPV) and left (LPV) portal veins. The dilated common hepatic duct (CHD) is easily seen. (H = head; RPV = right portal vein; RRV = right renal vein; RRA = right renal artery; IVC = inferior vena cava; MHV = middle hepatic vein.) (Reproduced from J Clin Ultrasound with permission.)

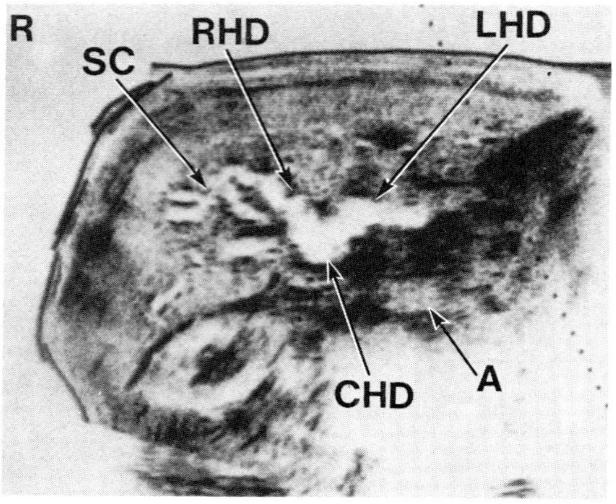

Figure 8–10. Limited transverse scan in a patient with severe bile duct dilatation. Note the irregular undulating course of the right (RHD) and left (LHD) hepatic ducts. A "stellate" or "spoke wheel" confluence (SC) is also seen. (R = right; CHD = common hepatic duct; A = aorta.) (Reproduced from J Clin Ultrasound with permission.)

irregular margins and serpiginous course of dilated ducts. Portal veins have smooth walls and taper gradually toward the periphery of the liver. Dilated bile ducts, particularly when the dilatation is severe, have lobulated margins and a serpiginous course (Fig. 8–10). The third feature is enhanced sound transmission. Blood attenuates sound more than bile, in most instances. Thus, acoustic enhancement is rarely seen in association with portal veins but is commonly identified in association with dilated bile ducts (Fig. 8–11).

The final two features are a "stellate" confluence of dilated ducts (Fig. 8–10) and a peripheral location of dilated ducts (Fig. 8–12). They are difficult to explain on an anatomic basis. Nonetheless, they are quite reliable for distinguishing a portal vein from a dilated bile duct.

The ability of ultrasonography to identify dilated bile ducts must be clearly distinguished from its ability to determine the cause of the obstruction. Although ultrasonography is an excellent modality for imaging stones in the gallbladder, it is a poor one for demonstrating stones in the bile ducts. Occasionally, a stone in the bile duct can be seen. Stones identified in the gallbladder of a patient with bile duct dilatation occasionally bear no relationship to the cause of the obstruction. Similarly, biliary strictures, small pancreatic and ampullary carcinomas, and many cholangiocarcinomas escape detection. Pseudocysts and larger carcinomas of the pancreas are usually seen. Sclerosing cholangitis is, in general, difficult to diagnose ultrasonographically.

Dilatation of the extrahepatic ducts without associated intrahepatic dilatation is not uncommon. Fortunately, the common hepatic

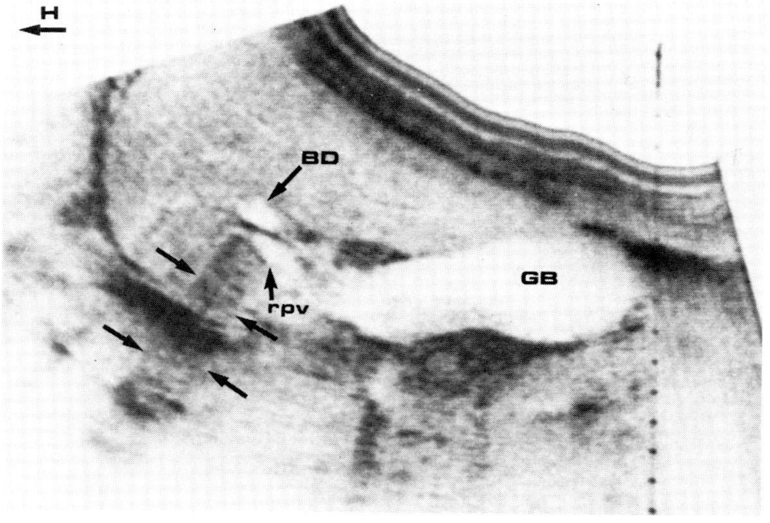

Figure 8–11. Parasagittal decubitus scan in a patient with dilated ducts. Acoustic enhancement (*arrows*) is seen posterior to the dilated right hepatic duct (BD). (H = head; rpv = right portal vein; GB = gallbladder.)

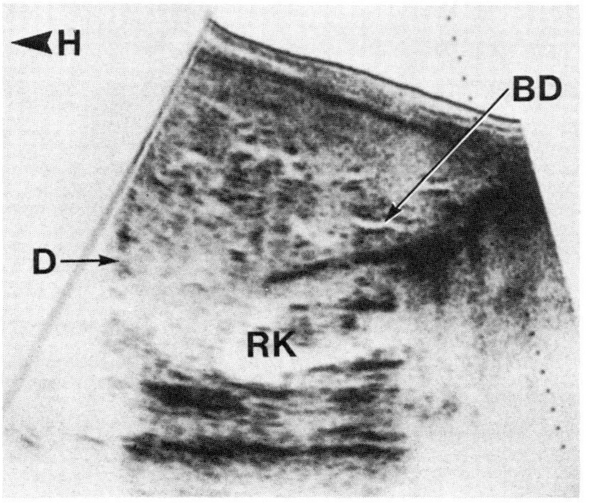

Figure 8–12. Parasagittal ultrasonogram in a patient with severe ductal dilatation. The bile duct designated by the arrow extends nearly to the liver edge. (H = head; D = diaphragm; RD = right kidney.) (Reproduced from J Clin Ultrasound with permission.)

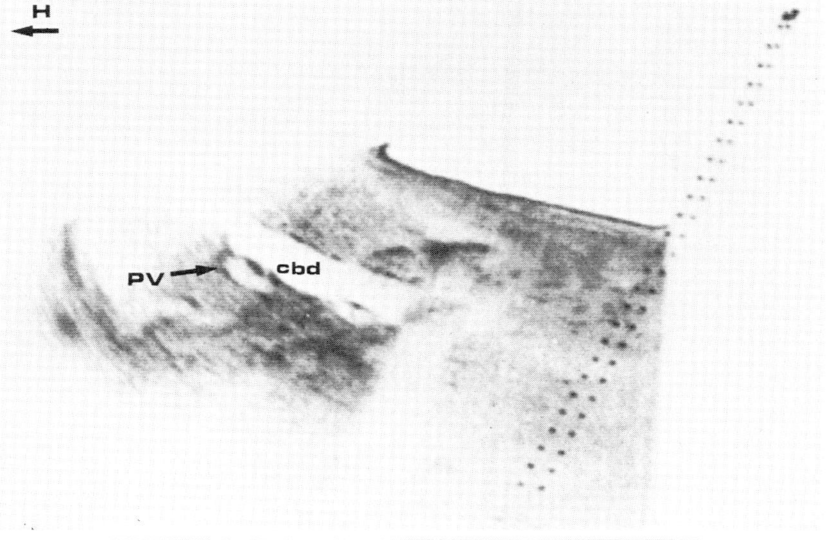

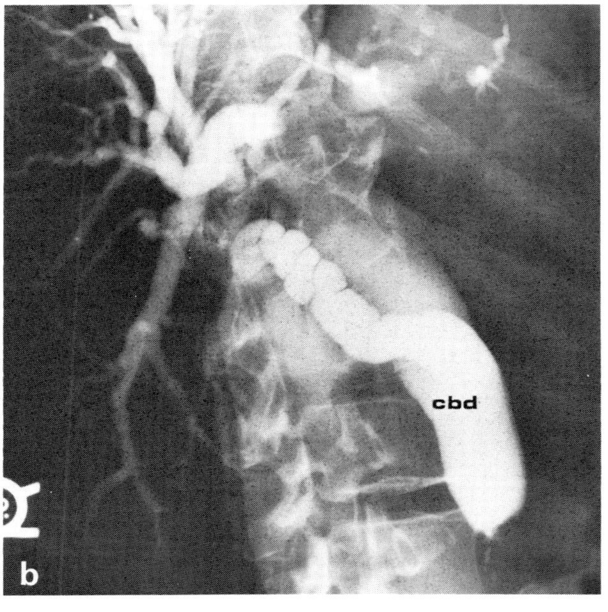

Figure 8–13. *A*, Parasagittal scan of the porta hepatis demonstrates a severely dilated common bile duct (cbd). (H = head; PV = portal vein.) *B*, Transhepatic cholangiogram correlates well with the ultrasonogram.

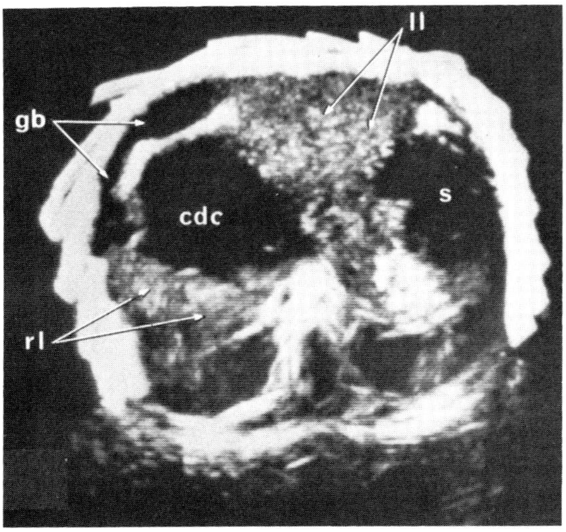

Figure 8–14. Transverse scan (reversed polarity—white on black) of a child with jaundice and a palpable mass. The gallbladder (gb) is draped over a large choledochal cyst (cdc). (ll = left lobe of liver; rl = right lobe of liver; s = spine.) (Reproduced from J Clin Ultrasound with permission.)

and common bile ducts, especially if dilated, are reliably detected by ultrasound (Fig. 8–13*A*).[10, 29, 38]

In jaundiced patients, ultrasonography is a useful screening procedure, and not infrequently it provides sufficient information to proceed with surgery. However, computed tomography, transhepatic cholangiography, or endoscopic cholangiography is frequently employed in conjunction with the ultrasonogram. Technically poor studies, equivocal results, or unanswered questions can usually be resolved by these additional tests. A situation that frequently results in unsatisfactory ultrasonograms is the evaluation of patients with choledocho- or cholecystoenterostomies. Intrabiliary gas and the anatomic changes engendered by these procedures generally decrease the quality of the examination and make interpretation of the ultrasound scan more difficult.

Choledochal Cyst. Ultrasound is extraordinarily sensitive for the detection of fluid. Renal, pancreatic, and ovarian cysts are among the most common indications for ultrasound diagnosis. Choledochal cysts would appear to be no exception to this rule. Although uncommon, choledochal cysts are an anatomic biliary deformity for which ultrasonography may be diagnostic (Fig. 8–14).[22] Since jaundice is commonly present in individuals with choledochal cysts, oral cholecys-

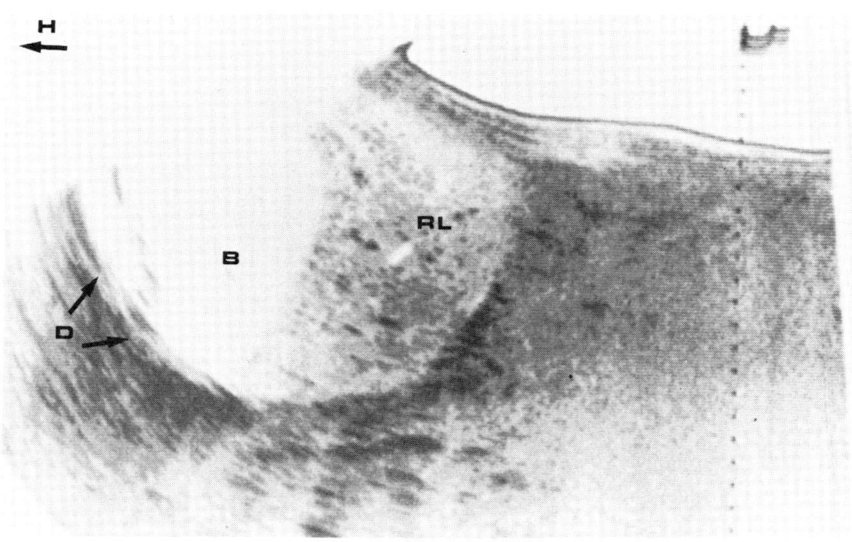

Figure 8–15. Parasagittal scan of the right abdomen in a patient who had had a recent cholecystectomy. A large bile collection (B) is seen indenting the right hepatic lobe (RL) and separating it from the diaphragm (D). (H = head.)

tography and intravenous cholangiography are frequently ineffective. Ultrasonography can provide a specific diagnosis of choledochal cyst if either the common hepatic or the cystic ducts are seen to join the lesion.

Ultrasonography in the Detection of Complications of Biliary Tract Surgery. Because of its sensitivity for the detection of fluid collections, ultrasonography is of considerable usefulness in the detection of postoperative bile leaks or abscesses. Such collections are usually identified in the subhepatic or subdiaphragmatic spaces (Fig. 8–15). In the examination of the right upper quadrant, ultrasonograms are usually not encumbered by gas-containing bowel, since the liver serves to displace bowel out of this region. In the left upper quadrant, image degradation from bowel gas is common. While ultrasonography is sensitive for detecting fluid collections, it is nonspecific regarding the type of fluid contained in the lesion (i.e., blood, pus, or bile).

SUMMARY

Ultrasonography has become an important diagnostic tool in the evaluation of the biliary tract. The two major areas of contribution are the detection of cholelithiasis and extrahepatic biliary obstruction. In the detection of cholelithiasis, ultrasonography, when performed by an experienced examiner, may be considered superior to oral cholecystography. Ultrasound should be considered as the first diagnostic imaging procedure in the majority of patients suspected of bile duct obstruction, and it should be considered in the evaluation of almost all patients suspected of pathology of the biliary system.

REFERENCES

1. Allen B, Bernhoft R, Blanckaert N, et al: Sludge is calcium bilirubinate associated with bile stasis. Am J Surg 1981;*141*:51.
2. Anderson JC, Harned RK: Gray scale ultrasonography of the gallbladder: an evaluation of accuracy and report of additional ultrasound signs. AJR 1977;*129*:975.
3. Arnon S, Resenquist CJ: Gray scale cholecystosonography: An evaluation of accuracy. AJR 1976; *127*:817.
4. Azimi F, Marangola JP, Bryan PJ: Ultrasound evaluation of the nonvisualized gallbladder. Gastrointest Radiol 1977;*1*:293.
5. Bartrum RJ, Crow HC, Foote SR: Ultrasound examination of the gallbladder—an alternative to "double-dose" oral cholecystography. JAMA 1976; *236*:1147.
6. Berk RN, Ferrucci JT, Fordtram JS, et al: The radiologic diagnosis of gallbladder disease. Radiology 1981;*141*:49.
7. Bernhoft RA, et al: Pigment sludge and stone formation in the acutely ligated dog gallbladder. Gastroenterology 1983;*85*:1166.
8. Bloom RA, et al: Shifting intramural gas—A new ultrasound sign of emphysematous cholecystitis. J Clin Ultrasound 1984;*12*:40.
9. Carlsen EN, Filly RA: Newer ultrasonographic anatomy in the upper abdomen: the portal and hepatic venous anatomy. J Clin Ultrasound 1976;*4*:85.
10. Cooperberg PL: Accuracy of common hepatic duct size in the evaluation of extrahepatic biliary obstruction. Radiology 1980;*135*:141.
11. Cooperberg PL, Burhenne HJ: Real-time ultrasonography. Diagnostic technique of choice in calculous gallbladder disease. N Engl J Med 1980;*302*:1277.
12. Crade M: Surgical and pathologic correlation of cholecystosonography and cholecystography. AJR 1978;*131*:227.
13. Crade M, Taylor KJW, Visconu GN: Need for care in assessing gallbladder wall thickening. AJR 1980;*135*:423.
14. Croce F et al: Ultrasonography in acute cholecystitis. Br J Radiol 1981;*54*:927.
15. Crow HC, Bartrum RJ, Foote SR: Expanded criteria for the ultrasonic diagnosis of gallstones. J Clin Ultrasound 1976;*4*:289.
16. Davis GB, Berk RN, Scheible FW, et al: Cholecystokinin cholecystography, sonography and scintigraphy: detection of chronic acalculous cholecystitis. AJR 1982;*139*:1117.
17. Deitch EA, Engel JM: Acute acalculous cholecystitis. Ultrasonic diagnosis. Am J Surg 1981;*142*:290.
18. Dillon E, Parkin GJS: The role of upper abdominal ultrasonography in suspected acute cholecystitis. Clin Radiol 1980;*31*:175.
19. Elyaderani MK, McDowell DE, Gabriele OF: A preliminary report of percutaneous cholecystostomy under ultrasonography and fluoroscopy guidance. J Clin Gastroenterol 1983;*5*:277.
20. Engel JM: Gallbladder wall thickness: sonographic accuracy and relation to disease. AJR 1980;*134*:907.
21. Filly RA, Allen B, Minton MJ, et al: In vitro investigation of the origin of echoes within biliary sludge. J Clin Ultrasound 1980;*8*:193.
22. Filly RA, Carlsen EN: Choledochal cyst: report of a case with specific ultrasonographic findings. J Clin Ultrasound 1976;*4*:7.
23. Filly RA, Laing FC: Anatomic variation of portal venous anatomy in the porta hepatis: ultrasonic evaluation. J Clin Ultrasound 1978;*6*:94.
24. Fiske CE: Ultrasonographic evidence of gallbladder wall thickening in association with hypoalbuminemia. Radiology 1980;*135*:713.
25. Foster SC, McLaughlin SM: Improvement in the ultrasonic evaluation of the gallbladder by using the left lateral decubitus position. J Clin Ultrasound 1977;*5*:253.
26. Frommhold W, Wolff J: Radiologic and radionuclide methods for the diagnosis of biliary disorders. Clin Gastroenterol 1983;*12*:65.
27. Goldberg HI, Filly RA, Korobkin M, et al: Capability of CT body scanning and ultrasonography to demonstrate the status of the biliary ductal system in patients with jaundice. Radiology 1978;*129*:731.
28. Good LI, Edell SL, Soloway RD, et al: Ultrasonic properties of gallstones. Effects of stone size and composition. Gastroenterology 1979;*77*:258.

29. Graham MF, Cooperberg PL: Ultrasonographic screening of the common hepatic duct in symptomatic patients after cholecystectomy. Radiology 1981;*138*:137.
30. Harbin WP, Ferrucci JT: Nonvisualized gallbladder by cholecystosonography. AJR 1979;*132*:727.
31. Hessler PC: High accuracy sonographic recognition of gallstones. AJR 1981;*136*:517.
32. Kene RA: Ultrasonographic diagnosis of gangrenous cholecystitis and empyema of the gallbladder. Radiology 1980;*134*:191.
33. Koenigsberg M, Wiener SN: The accuracy of sonography in the differential diagnosis of obstructive jaundice: a comparison with cholangiography. Radiology 1979;*133*:157.
34. Krook PM, Allen FH: Comparison of real-time cholecystosonography and oral cholecystography. Radiology 1980;*135*:145.
35. Laing FC, Gooding GAW, Herzog KA: Gallstones preventing ultrasonographic visualization of the gallbladder. Gastrointest Radiol 1977;*1*:301.
36. Laing FC, London LA, Filly RA: Ultrasonographic identification of dilated intrahepatic bile ducts and their differentiation from portal venous structures. J Clin Ultrasound 1978;*6*:90.
37. Lawson TL: Gray scale cholecystosonography: diagnostic criteria and accuracy. Radiology 1977; *122*:247.
38. Lee TG, Henderson SC, Ehrlich R: Ultrasound diagnosis of common bile duct dilatation. Radiology 1977;*124*:793.
39. Leopold GR, et al: Gray scale ultrasonic cholecystography: a comparision with conventional radiographic techniques. Radiology 1976;*121*:445.
40. Malini S, Sabel J: Ultrasonography in obstructive jaundice. Radiology 1977;*123*:429.
41. Marchal G, Crolla D, Baert AL, et al: Gallbladder wall thickening: a new sign of gallbladder disease visualized by gray scale cholecystosonography. J Clin Ultrasound 1978;*6*:177.
42. Marchal GJF, Casaer M, Baert AL, et al: Gallbladder wall sonolucency in acute cholecystitis. Radiology 1979;*133*:429.
43. Matolo NM, Stadalnik RC, McGahan JP: Comparison of ultrasonography, computerized tomography, and radionuclide imaging in the diagnosis of acute and chronic cholecystitis. Am J Surg 1982;*144*:676.
44. McIntosh DMF, Penney HF: Gray-scale ultrasonography as a screening procedure in the detection of gallbladder disease. Radiology 1980;*136*:725.
45. Messing B, Bories C, Kunstlinger F, et al: Does total parenteral nutrition induce gallbladder sludge formation and lithiasis? Gastroenterology 1983; *84*:1012.
46. Mindell HJ, Ring A: Gallbladder wall thickening: ultrasonic findings. Radiology 1979;*133*:699.
47. Neiman HL, Mintzer RA: Accuracy of biliary duct ultrasound: comparison with cholangiography. AJR 1977;*129*:979.
48. Okuda K, Tsuchiya Y: Ultrasonic anatomy of the biliary system. Clin Gastroenterol 1983;*12*:50.
49. Orlando R, Gleason E, Drezner AD: Acute acalculous cholecystitis in the critically ill patient. Am J Surg 1983;*145*:472.
50. Rabinowitz JC, Yeh HC, Cohen BA: Gallstone update—Radiology. Semin Liver Dis 1983;*3*:120.
51. Sample WF: Techniques for improved delineation of normal anatomy of the upper abdomen and high retroperitoneum with gray scale ultrasound. Radiology 1977;*124*:197.
52. Sanders RC: The significance of sonographic gallbladder wall thickening. J Clin Ultrasound 1980; *8*:143.
53. Shuman WP, Rogers JV, Rudd TG, et al: Low sensitivity of sonography and cholescintigraphy in acalculous cholecystitis. AJR 1984;*142*:531.
54. Simeone JF, Ferrucci JT Jr: New trends in gallbladder imaging. JAMA 1981;*246*:380.
55. Sommer FG, Taylor KJW: Differentiation of acoustic shadowing due to calculi and gas collections. Radiology 1980;*135*:399.
56. Thomas MJ, Pellegrini CA, Way LW: Usefulness of diagnostic tests for biliary obstruction. Am J Surg 1982;*144*:102.
57. Ulreich S, Foster KW, Stier SA, et al: Acute cholecystitis. Comparison of ultrasound and intravenous cholangiography. Arch Surg 1980;*115*:158.
58. Van der Linden W, Kempi V, Edlund G: Function of liver, gallbladder and sphincter of Oddi after major surgery studied by computer-assisted cholescintigraphy and real-time ultrasonography. Br J Surg 1983;*70*:497.
59. Worthen NJ, Uszler JM, Funamura JL: Cholecystitis: prospective evaluation of sonography and ^{99m}TC-HIDA cholescintigraphy. AJR 1981;*137*:973.

H. GOLDBERG, M.D.

9

Computed Tomography and Magnetic Resonance Imaging of the Gallbladder and Bile Ducts

INTRODUCTION

Computed tomography (CT) provides information about biliary tract pathology by direct imaging of the biliary ducts, by identification of extrahepatic masses (porta hepatis, head of the pancreas, periduodenal region), and by detection of intrahepatic masses secondary to biliary tract or gallbladder disease. In most instances, ultrasonography is the imaging method of choice for the biliary system, but when ultrasonography of the extrahepatic ductal system is unsuccessful, CT may act as a substitute in the anatomic delineation of the extrahepatic biliary tract and gallbladder.

In this chapter, the contribution of computed tomography (CT) to the detection of both benign and malignant mechanical obstruction of the extrahepatic biliary tree will be discussed, including biliary strictures and common bile duct stones, primary malignancy of the bile ducts and gallbladder, and extrinsic masses compressing the extrahepatic ducts. The use of magnetic resonance imaging (MRI) of the gallbladder, bile ducts, and porta hepatis, although much less well defined because of the lack of experience, will also be discussed.

GENERAL ROLE OF CT IN IMAGING THE BILIARY TRACT

While ultrasound remains the primary method of noninvasive evaluation of the biliary ductal system and gallbladder, CT may be used in cases in which ultrasound is unsuccessful. Therefore, in the extremely obese patient or one with extensive ascites or massive abdominal ileus, CT is effective in determining whether intrahepatic ducts are dilated, whether the extrahepatic common hepatic duct and common bile duct are dilated, and whether there are masses extrinsic to the ductal system affecting the duct.[1]

The porta hepatis can be evaluated best by CT if a bolus of 50 to 100 ml of iodinated contrast agent is given intravenously and if a rapid-sequence technique is used to detect selective opacification of the portal vein and hepatic artery (Fig. 9–1). The bolus technique provides information about any other nonenhancing structure in the porta hepatis, such as common bile duct, lymph nodes, or metastatic masses.[2] However, in some patients, particularly those with very little periportal fat, detection of metastasis in the porta hepatis and the gastrohepatic ligament may be difficult. Currently, there are no specific data on the accuracy of CT in detecting lesions of the porta hepatis.

Detection of Biliary Obstruction

In suspected extrahepatic biliary obstruction, the role of CT is to detect the presence of dilated intra- or extrahepatic ducts. Normal intrahepatic ducts are not usually seen on CT, although occasionally the main right and left duct may be seen near their confluence. Dilated intrahepatic ducts appear as low-density branching structures adjacent to portal veins (Fig. 9–2). When intravenous contrast material is given, the portal veins enhance to the same degree as the liver parenchyma, or to an even greater degree.

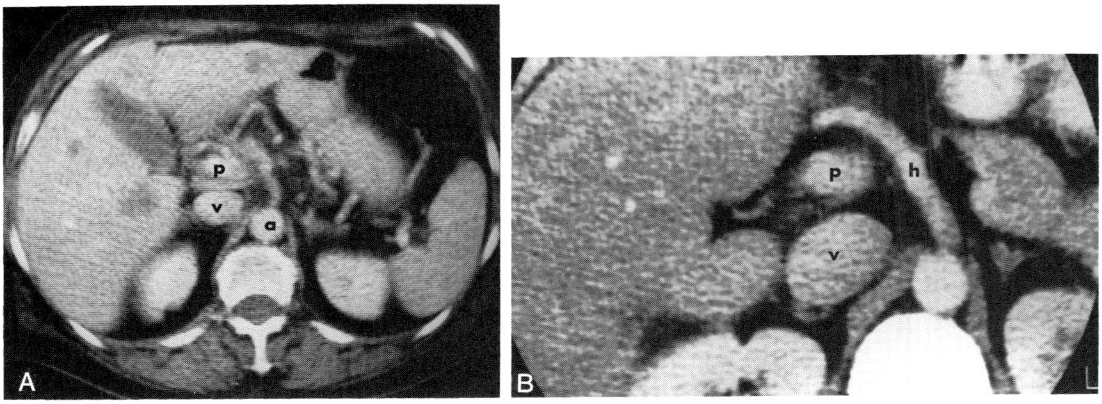

Figure 9–1. *A,* CT scan showing the normal porta hepatis region. The patient has received 100 ml of 30 per cent iodinated contrast material intravenously over 100 seconds so that the aorta (a), vena cava (v), and portal vein (p) are all opacified. In addition, the celiac artery is seen in the midline arising from the aorta. The hepatic artery courses on top of the portal vein, and a replaced right hepatic artery is seen between the portal vein and the vena cava. No additional strictures are seen in a normal porta hepatis. The patient had three low-density lesions in the liver, representing metastasis from colon carcinoma. *B,* A close-up of a CT scan in the porta hepatis in a patient with normal anatomy of the region. The hepatic artery (h), portal vein (p), and vena cava (v) are all easily identified because they are enhanced by the use of a bolus of iodinated contrast agent delivered intravenously.

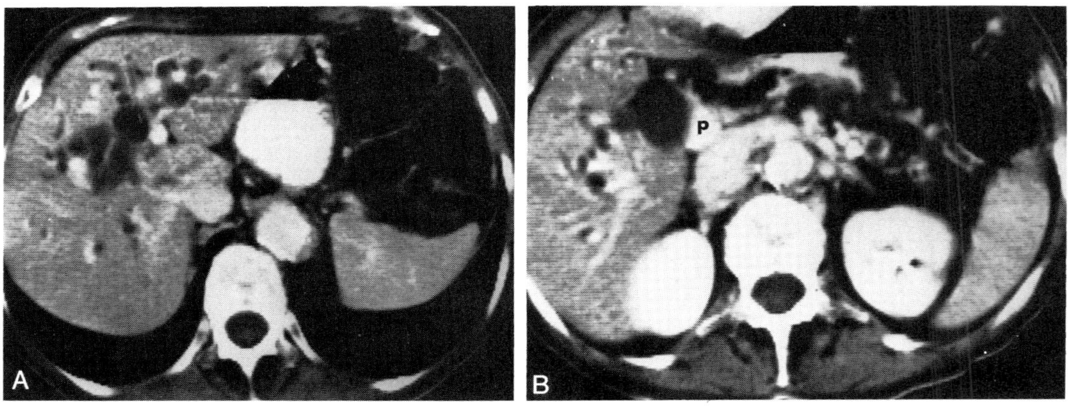

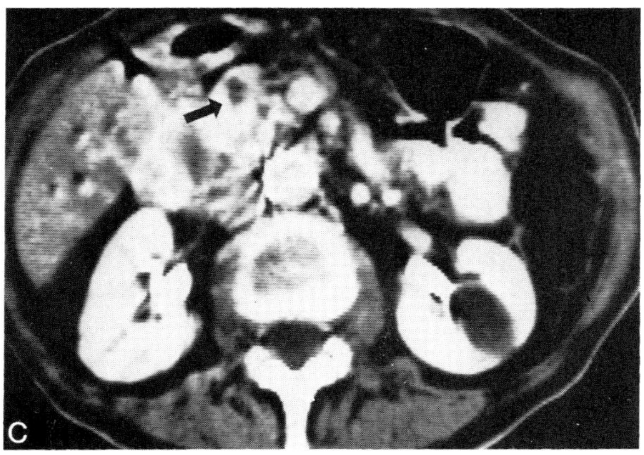

Figure 9–2. *A,* In this patient with extensive calcific pancreatitis obstructing the distal common bile duct, the CT scan demonstrates massively dilated intrahepatic bile ducts (low-density tubular structures). The portal veins appear as high-density tubular structures adjacent to the dilated ducts. *B,* The dilated common hepatic duct is adjacent to the contrast-enhanced portal vein (p). *C,* In the head of the pancreas, where extensive calcification is present, the common bile duct narrows (*arrow*).

The remaining low-density structures are the bile ducts. The accuracy of CT in the diagnosis of biliary obstruction appears to be greater than 90 per cent.[1, 3, 4] This level of accuracy in detecting dilated ducts is similar to that of ultrasound.

Not only can generalized ductal dilatation be seen, but also segmental dilatation of the intrahepatic biliary tree may be demonstrated on CT (Fig. 9–3).[5, 6] This may occur in patients without elevated serum bilirubin values, in whom the only clue to biliary disease is an elevation of the serum alkaline phosphatase value.

While there is general agreement that the normal common bile duct should not exceed 8 mm in diameter as measured on CT,[1] or less on ultrasound,[7, 8] there is only a loose relationship between the caliber of the bile duct and the presence or absence of obstruction. Although it is possible to detect the dilated duct, it is not always possible, using CT, to determine whether the duct is dilated because it is obstructed. Some patients have a dilated common bile duct owing to the recent passage of gallstones. Following cholecystectomy the common bile duct may dilate slightly, in the absence of obstruction. Therefore, the isolated finding of a dilated common duct in the absence of intrahepatic ductal dilatation, and in the absence of history or biochemical evidence of biliary obstruction, should be considered an isolated finding, not necessarily indicating the presence of obstruction. On the other hand, the absence of intrahepatic duct dilatation, particularly in cirrhotic patients, does not necessarily rule out mechanical obstruction of the biliary tract, as in some conditions (e.g., cirrhosis, sclerosing cholangitis) periductal fibrosis may prevent ductal dilatation even in the case of obstruction.[9] It is possible that cirrhotic patients with mechanical obstruction will demonstrate only common duct dilatation on CT. Therefore, careful evaluation of clinical history, in addition to the CT findings, is required to assess the isolated common duct dilatation detected by CT.

CT Detection of Choledocholithiasis

Gallstones in the gallbladder may be detected by CT when they have enough calcium to be radiopaque. Because the CT density of pure cholesterol stones blends with that of the bile, gallstones may not always be detected, however.

In biliary obstruction suspected to be due to choledocholithiasis, particularly in the postcholecystectomy patient, ERCP is recognized as the primary diagnostic modality. If ERCP fails, ultrasound or CT may be indicated to delineate the presence of stones in the biliary ducts (Fig. 9–4). The success of ultrasound in detecting common duct stones ranges from 20 to 40 per cent,[1, 10] except in one report[22] in which an overall sensitivity of 75 per cent for detecting choledocholithiasis was noted. The success rate in detecting these stones on CT is considerably higher.[11, 15] However, in the absence of a definitive diagnosis of biliary duct stones by CT, an invasive technique, such as percutaneous transhepatic cholangiography (PTC), must be used as the alternative to a failed ERCP.

CT plays no major role in the evaluation of benign strictures. Stricture detection and characterization require direct opacification of the ducts via ERCP or PTC. The role of CT is to detect the dilatation that may occur proximal to the stricture and to define the

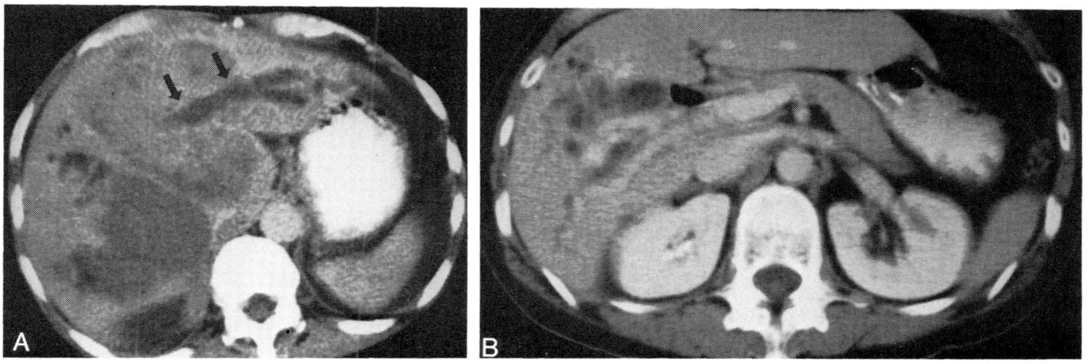

Figure 9–3. *A,* Segmental dilatation of the left hepatic duct is present (*arrows*), owing to a large hepatocellular carcinoma obstructing the duct near its confluence with the right duct. *B,* Selective dilatation of the right hepatic duct system is due to cholangiocarcinoma. The site of obstruction is at the origin of the right hepatic duct.

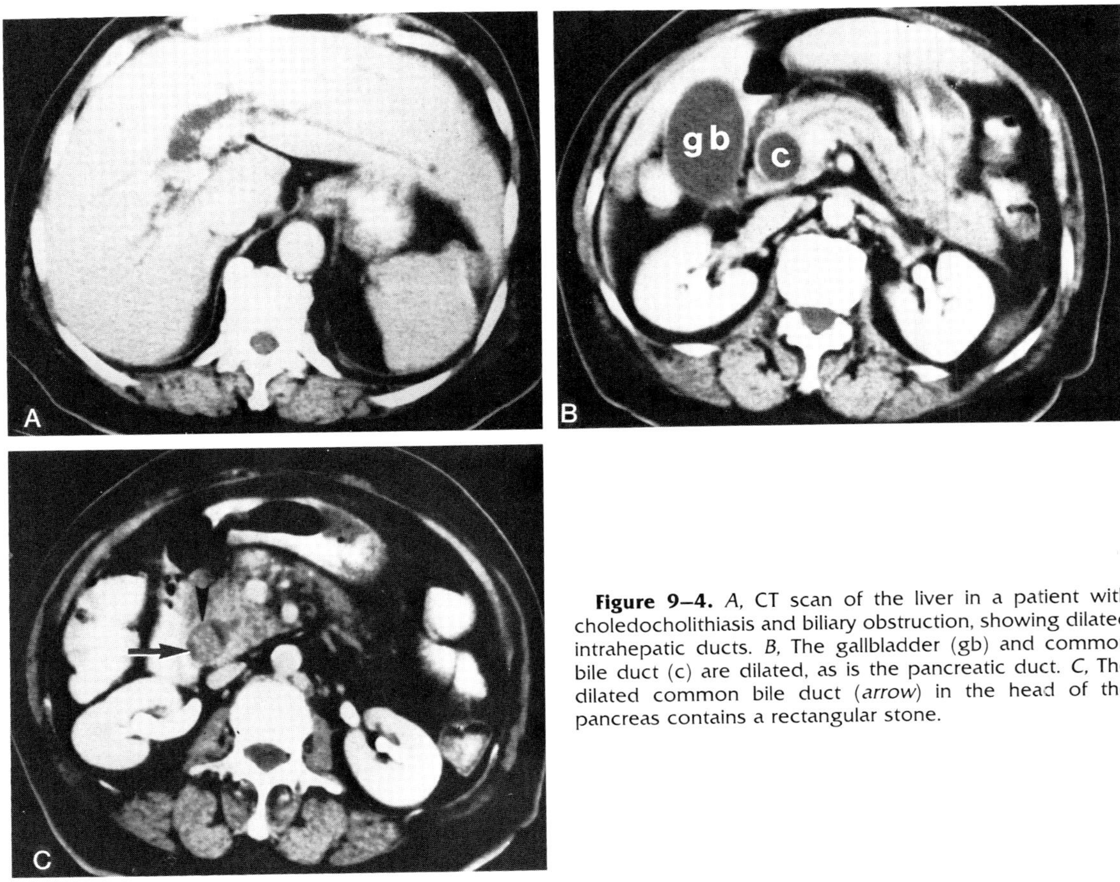

Figure 9–4. *A,* CT scan of the liver in a patient with choledocholithiasis and biliary obstruction, showing dilated intrahepatic ducts. *B,* The gallbladder (gb) and common bile duct (c) are dilated, as is the pancreatic duct. *C,* The dilated common bile duct (*arrow*) in the head of the pancreas contains a rectangular stone.

level of the stricture.[4] Occasionally, the smooth narrowing caused by a benign stricture may be detected as progressive decrease in the diameter of the common duct on several consecutive scans (Fig. 9–5).[12]

Primary Malignancy of the Biliary Ductal System

Because most ductal carcinomas expand along the ductal system to narrow and obstruct it, CT does not always contribute greatly to the detection or characterization of this disease. However, the CT scan will frequently indicate the presence of dilated intrahepatic ducts in the absence of extrahepatic ductal dilatation when lesions of the porta hepatis are present. In addition, some cholangiocarcinomas infiltrate into the liver hilum. These may be seen on CT as fan-shaped areas of increased enhancement after a bolus injection (Fig. 9–6). In some cases, cholangiocarcinoma may spread diffusely throughout the liver, producing multiple low-density areas.[13] Segmental dilatation due to involvement of one major ductal system may also be seen (See Fig. 9–3*B*).[5, 6] Therefore, in the overall staging of cholangiocarcinoma, CT is of considerable value because of its ability to detect extraductal nodal involvement in the peripancreatic, celiac, and perigastric nodes as well as direct spread of tumor into the liver parenchyma and distant liver metastasis.

CT-guided percutaneous fine needle biopsy of the porta hepatis is of limited use because the tumors are usually small and the exact site of tumor in relation to the common duct cannot always be determined on CT. Furthermore, the pathologic process is such that infiltration of the ductal system occurs along with considerable fibroblastic response, so that the cell yield of fine needle aspiration is low. When the tumor bulk is large, however, and spreads widely along the course of the intrahepatic bile ducts, percutaneous biopsy is often successful.[13]

Gallbladder Carcinoma

Carcinoma of the gallbladder can be detected and characterized by CT scans.[13, 14] In gallbladder cancer, the gallbladder is often

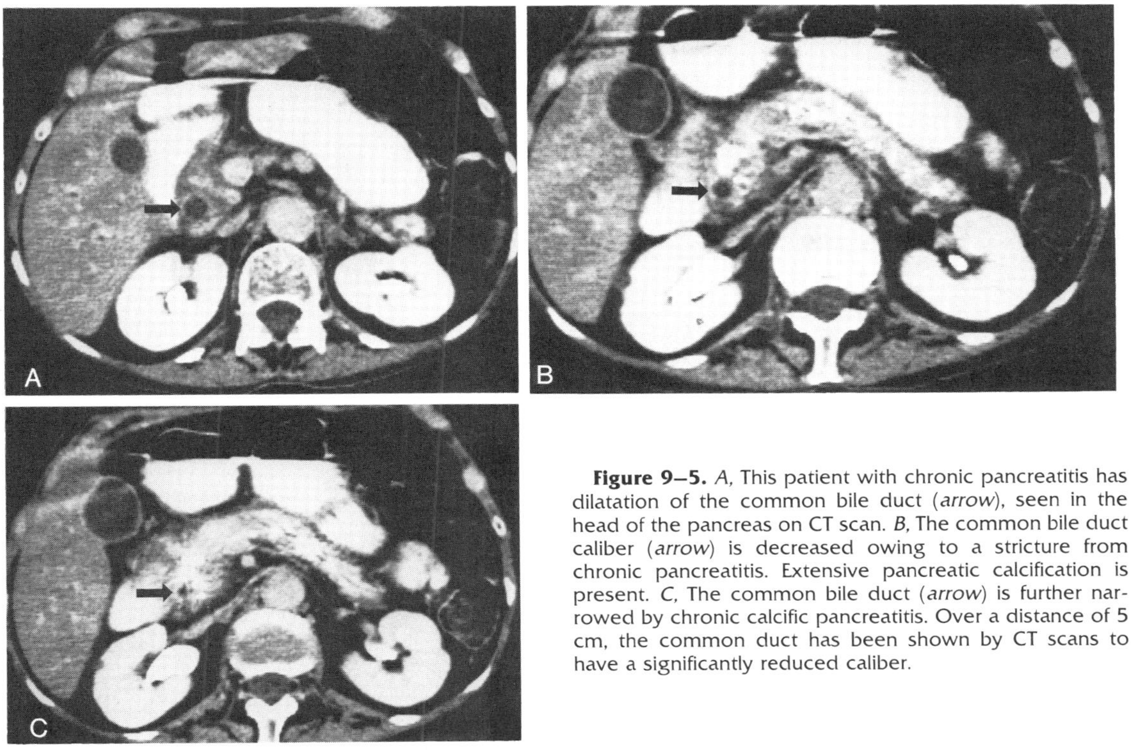

Figure 9–5. *A*, This patient with chronic pancreatitis has dilatation of the common bile duct (*arrow*), seen in the head of the pancreas on CT scan. *B*, The common bile duct caliber (*arrow*) is decreased owing to a stricture from chronic pancreatitis. Extensive pancreatic calcification is present. *C*, The common bile duct (*arrow*) is further narrowed by chronic calcific pancreatitis. Over a distance of 5 cm, the common duct has been shown by CT scans to have a significantly reduced caliber.

enlarged and the wall thickened. A soft tissue mass can be seen on CT projecting into the lumen of the gallbladder or extending external to the wall in some cases (70 per cent), indicating the presence of a primary tumor (Fig. 9–7). The level of biliary obstruction and the spread of gallbladder cancer by direct extension into the liver, to the porta hepatis, or to the regional lymph nodes as well as distant liver metastasis can all be defined by CT scans. The simultaneous occurrence of chronic cholecystitis and a primary liver tumor may be confused with primary gallbladder cancer associated with liver metastasis.[14] In general, the CT scan is the best method for evaluating the extent of gallbladder cancer.

Metastasis Involving the Biliary Ductal System

Metastasis to the porta hepatis occurs frequently with carcinoma of the pancreas and other abdominal neoplasms as well as with carcinoma of the lung and breast. The major challenge for CT is to identify the normal structures in the porta hepatis so that abnormal ones can be easily distinguished. This

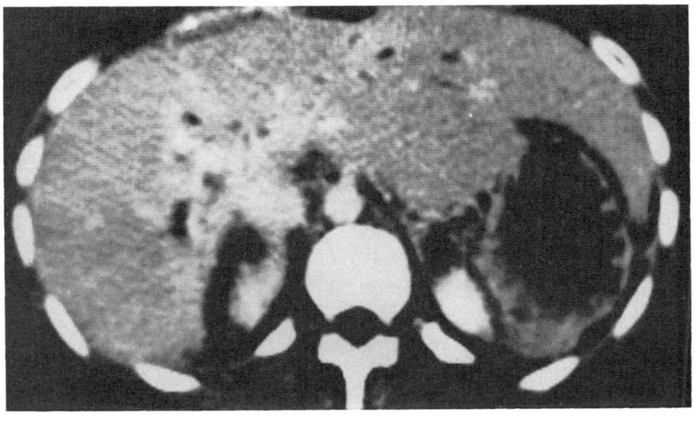

Figure 9–6. This CT scan of a patient with cholangiocarcinoma of the common hepatic duct demonstrates dilated intrahepatic bile ducts and a diffuse periductal infiltration by tumor, seen here as a fan-shaped area of increased density in the medial portion of the liver with extensions along the bile ducts. This appearance is seen after intravenous bolus injection of iodinated contrast material.

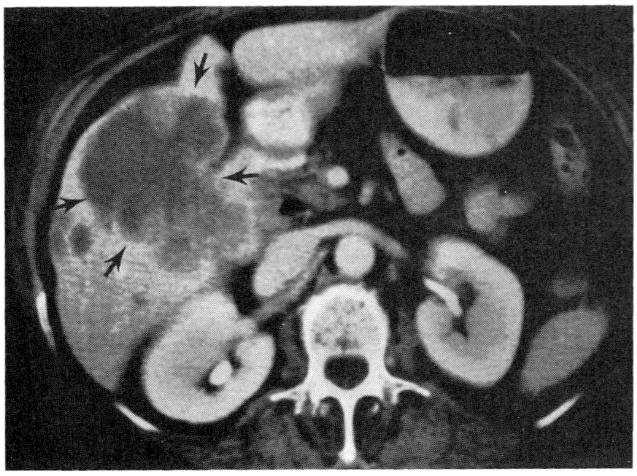

Figure 9–7. A large gallbladder carcinoma is present (*arrows*), with a tumor nodule projecting into the gallbladder lumen from the anterior wall. In addition, there are infiltration of the right lobe of the liver medially and three small metastatic lesions on the lateral surface of the right lobe.

requires excellent intravenous selective opacification of the portal vein and hepatic artery using high-volume bolus injection technique with rapid sequence scanning (See Fig. 9–1). When the portal vein, hepatic artery, and common duct are identified, any extra tissue can be considered abnormal and should be considered suspect for metastatic neoplasm (Fig. 9–8).

Metastasis may appear as a single round soft tissue density in the porta hepatis or gastrohepatic ligament, or as multiple separate densities 1 cm or greater in size (Fig. 9–9), or as a sheet of tissue obliterating the normal fat planes between the medial segment of the left lobe of the liver and the stomach and obscuring the boundaries between normal structures. In some instances, carcinoma of the pancreas will extend directly into the porta hepatis. Solitary metastasis and involvement by lymphoma may produce focal soft tissue densities compressing the common hepatic duct in the porta hepatis and displacing it along with the portal vein.

Pancreatic Carcinoma and Biliary Ductal Obstruction

CT scanning is an excellent method to evaluate carcinoma of the pancreas and its involvement of the common bile duct.[12] Because of the ability of CT to delineate the fat planes, the vasculature, the liver, and the adjacent lymph node areas, CT is the recommended noninvasive diagnostic study for this disease.[16] While ultrasonography is the method of choice for evaluating dilated intrahepatic ducts, technical factors usually

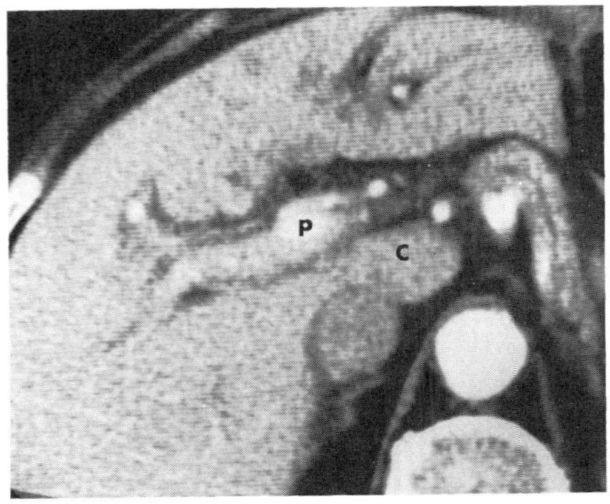

Figure 9–8. Metastasis to the porta hepatis from colon cancer is seen on this CT scan. The portal vein (p) is opacified by a bolus of iodinated contrast material, and the hepatic artery lying above the portal vein is also opacified. The caudate lobe (c) defines the posterior border of the porta hepatis on this section, and a portion of the tortuous hepatic artery is present at the tip of the caudate lobe. The remaining soft tissue density between all of these vascular structures represents metastatic tumor.

prevent an adequate sonogram of the pancreatic region.

A primary tumor of the head of the pancreas obstructing the bile duct can be detected by CT, either as a soft tissue mass extending beyond the normal confines of the pancreas, or as a lesion producing low density within the head of the pancreas without enlarging it (Fig. 9–10). Often the dilated common bile duct can be traced by CT in its course from the porta hepatis into the head of the pancreas and may be seen to abruptly change in caliber as the obstructing mass

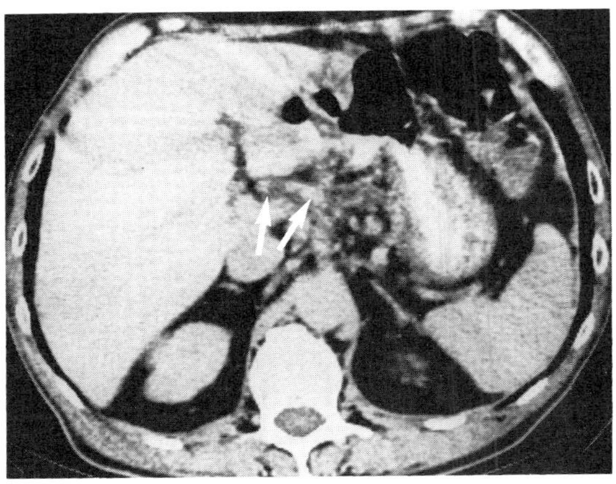

Figure 9–9. Multiple soft tissue densities, representing metastasis greater than 1 cm, occupy the space adjacent to the celiac artery and the hepatic artery as it branches into the porta hepatis (*arrows*). These can best be appreciated by comparing this scan with the normal appearance in Figure 9–1.

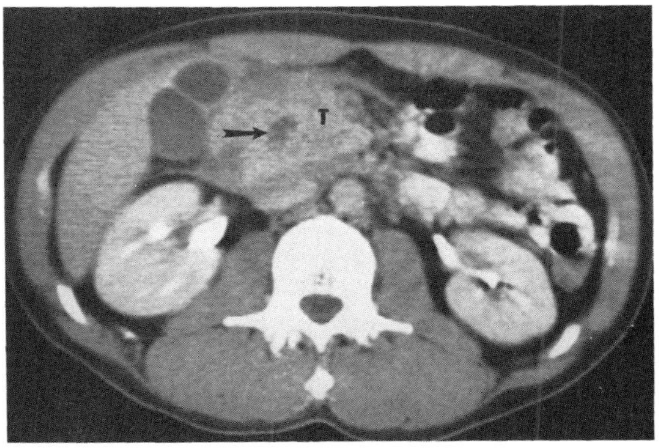

Figure 9–10. A carcinoma of the head of the pancreas (T) has produced obstruction of the distal common bile duct. The dilated duct appears as a low-density, oval structure (*arrow*).

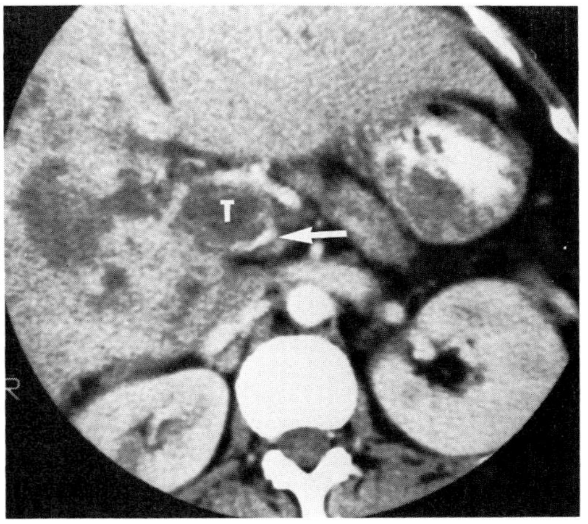

Figure 9–11. Tumor thrombus (T) is present in the portal vein of this patient with a primary hepatocellular carcinoma. The hepatic artery is arched over the enlarged portal vein. A small amount of contrast material is seen in the portal vein proximal to the tumor thrombus (*arrow*).

compresses or invades it. The CT scan of the patient with biliary obstruction due to carcinoma of the pancreas may also reveal metastasis to the liver, direct invasion of the celiac or superior mesenteric lymph nodes, and encasement of vessels such as splenic artery, superior mesenteric artery, or portal vein. In this setting, should a tissue diagnosis be necessary, a fine needle percutaneous CT-guided biopsy can be performed at the same time as the diagnostic study. Success rate in confirming the presence of carcinoma of the pancreas by aspiration biopsy is greater than 90 per cent, and the complication rate is about 1 per cent.[17]

Distal common bile duct obstruction may also be due to chronic pancreatitis, and the CT findings will frequently aid in differentiating this disease from carcinoma. In the patient with distal common duct obstruction and enlargement of the head of the pancreas, the finding of calcifications in the head of the pancreas provides strong evidence for the presence of pancreatitis (See Fig. 9–5). When this information is added to that obtained from the ERCP or PTC appearance of the distal duct, the diagnosis frequently can be made.

Occasionally, CT will demonstrate abnormalities relating to primary liver tumors that may affect the biliary ductal system and portal vein. Hepatocellular carcinoma may invade both the portal vein and the bile ducts as it grows into the porta hepatis.[6] An enlarged common hepatic duct and portal vein with tumor thrombus in it may be detected by CT (Fig. 9–11).

In summary, CT scanning is a useful and accurate method of detecting biliary ductal dilatation due to obstruction, defining the level of obstruction, and occasionally determining the cause of biliary obstruction. It is less useful in patients with benign biliary strictures. Most often, the CT detection of masses affecting the porta hepatis or extrahepatic biliary ducts should be followed by direct imaging of the biliary tract, either by ERCP or by PTC. The determination of dilated intrahepatic ducts in the absence of extrahepatic dilatation on CT should likewise be studied by PTC, or by ERCP in most patients.

MAGNETIC RESONANCE IMAGING (MRI) OF THE GALLBLADDER AND BILIARY DUCTS

Because of the lack of experience in evaluating diseases of the biliary tract and gallbladder by magnetic resonance imaging (MRI), little can be said definitively about this technique when compared with CT scanning or sonography. However, it appears that there are certain situations in which MRI may be useful.

MRI can detect both the shrunken and the distended gallbladder. The gallbladder is seen mainly because of its internal contents. Fresh hepatic bile in the gallbladder has a very low signal intensity and appears dark on the MRI scans obtained using spin-echo techniques with short repetition rates (TR = 0.5 to 1 sec).[18] This is typical of biologic fluid that has a high water content. It is only when the repetition rates are lengthened to 2 sec that the fresh hepatic bile provides a more

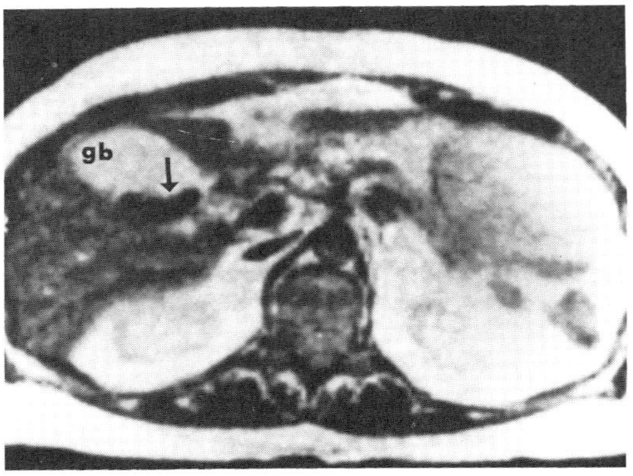

Figure 9–12. The gallbladder, imaged here by spin-echo magnetic resonance with a TR (repetition rate) of 2 sec and a TE (echo delay) of 56 msec, appears as a pear-shaped structure (gb) with a bright signal due to bile. The gallstones appear as a black sausage-shaped line at the base of the gallbladder (*arrow*). Gallstones characteristically provide no detectable signal.

intense signal. On the other hand, concentrated bile, containing less water, has a much more intense signal on the short repetition rates. Therefore, frequently one sees layering of fresh bile as a dark area on top of a more intense bright area within the gallbladder, indicating old bile. Some cases have been demonstrated that on oral cholecystography have had nonopacification of the gallbladder and on MRI have shown small thick-walled gallbladders with appearance of fresh bile, suggesting bile that has not been concentrated. Thus, MRI may have a role in the evaluation of gallbladder function, although this still must be proved by more extensive experimentation.

Gallstones are easily detectable on MRI because they provide almost no signal, always appearing black.[18–20] They may be hidden against fresh bile, which also has a very low intensity signal on the short repetition rate, but when the repetition rate is extended to 2 sec, the gallstones still remain without a signal, whereas the fresh bile will show an intense signal (Fig. 9–12).

Although there are no reports on the use of MRI to evaluate patients with gallbladder carcinoma, spread of gallbladder cancer after surgery has been seen in the liver and is easily differentiated from normal liver (Fig. 9–13).

Experience with imaging cholangiocarcinoma by magnetic resonance is limited. However, spread of tumor along the course of bile ducts has been noted. This may become a useful technique for staging the intrahepatic, extraductal extent of tumors (Fig. 9–14).

Dilated bile ducts may be seen within the liver in patients with obstruction at the porta hepatis or the distal common bile duct. Bile ducts can be differentiated from portal veins by manipulating the various spin-echo sequences. In the short repetition rates and the first echoes (TR = 0.5, TE = 28) both the portal veins and the bile ducts appear as black holes when seen transaxially or, occasionally, as branching structures. However, on the longer repetition rate the portal veins still appear as black holes because no signal emanates from flowing blood, whereas the dilated bile ducts have an increasing signal intensity owing to the fresh bile within them.[18] Therefore, using MRI, multiple se-

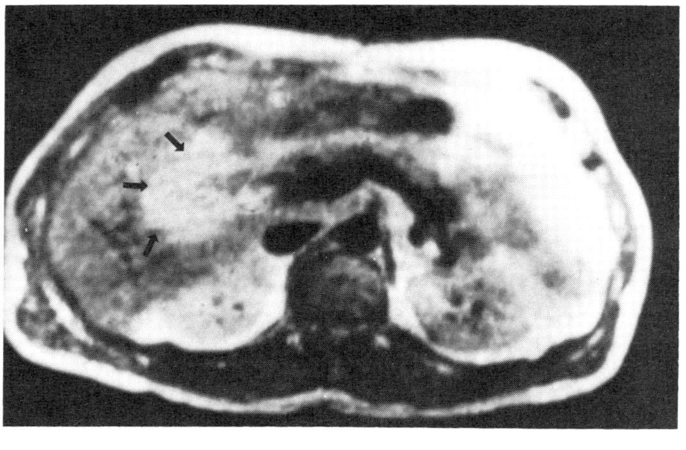

Figure 9–13. In this patient, who is 3 months status postcholecystectomy for focal gallbladder cancer, this MRI scan was performed to search for hepatic involvement. The spin-echo scan (TR = 2.0, TE = 28) demonstrates an area of bright signal from the medial portion of the liver adjacent to the gallbladder bed (*arrows*). Ultrasound-guided fine needle aspiration biopsy showed this to be recurrent tumor.

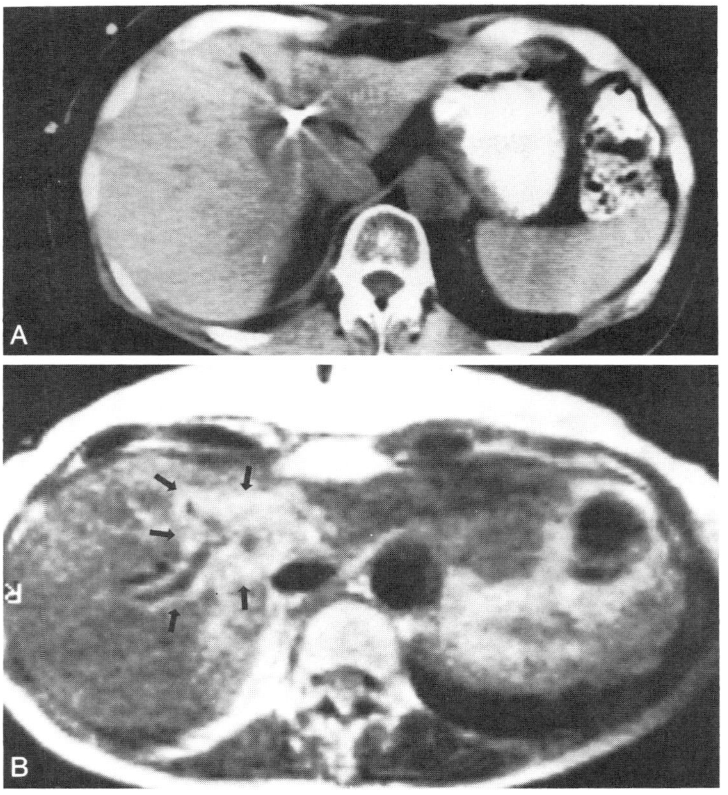

Figure 9–14. *A*, CT scan of a patient with cholangiocarcinoma occurring at the bifurcation of the major ducts. A biliary stent is present, causing streak artifacts that degrade the image and render interpretation of the medial part of the liver and porta hepatis difficult. *B*, The MRI scan clearly demonstrates the extent of the cholangiocarcinoma, shown here as an area of bright signal intensity in the liver hilum and extending along the portal veins (*arrows*). Note that because no signal is detected from the biliary stent, no artifacts due to the stent are present.

quences may be used to evaluate the problem of dilated bile ducts in obstructed jaundice.

The common bile duct, when dilated, may be seen on MRI and distinguished from portal veins by the use of multiple spin-echo sequences just as with the intrahepatic bile duct.

Obstructive jaundice caused by tumors of the head of the pancreas can be detected by MRI both on the basis of change in size and shape and on the change in signal intensity from the tumor itself. Metastasis from cholangiocarcinoma and pancreatic tumors may also be detected by MRI.[21] It is too early at this time to predict whether MRI will be useful in evaluating the jaundiced patient.

REFERENCES

1. Baron RL, Stanley RJ, Lee JKT, et al: A prospective comparison of the valuation of biliary obstruction using computed tomography and ultrasonography. Radiology 1982;*145*:91.
2. Foley WD, Wilson CR, Quiroz FA, et al: Demonstration of the normal extrahepatic biliary tract with computed tomography. J Comput Assist Tomogr 1980;*4*:48.
3. Goldberg HI, Filly RA, Korobkin M, et al: Capability of CT body scanning and ultrasonography to demonstrate the status of the biliary ductal system in patients with jaundice. Radiology 1978;*129*:731.
4. Pedrosa CS, Casanova R, Rodriguez R: CT in obstructive jaundice. Part I. The level of obstruction. Radiology 1981;*139*:627.
5. Thomas JL, Bernardino ME: Segmental biliary obstruction: its detection and significance. J Comput Assist Tomogr 1980;*4*:48.
6. Araki T, Itai Y, Tasaka A: Computed tomography of localized dilatation of the intrahepatic bile ducts. Radiology 1981;*141*:733.
7. Niederau C, Sonnenberg A, Mueller J: Comparison of the extrahepatic bile duct size measured by ultrasound and by different radiographic methods. Gastroenterology 1984;*87*:615.
8. Berk RN, Cooperberg PL, Gold RP, et al: Radiography of the bile ducts. Radiology 1982;*145*:1.
9. Shanser JD, Korobkin M, Goldberg HI, et al: Computed tomographic diagnosis of obstructive jaundice in the absence of intrahepatic ductal dilatation. AJR 1978;*131*:389.
10. Gross BH, Harter LP, Gore RM, et al: Ultrasonic evaluation of common bile duct stones: prospective comparison with endoscopic retrograde cholangiopancreatography. Radiology 1983;*146*:471.
11. Baron RL, Stanley RJ, Lee JKT, et al: Computed tomographic features of biliary obstruction. AJR 1983;*140*:1173.
12. Pedrosa CS, Casanova R, Lezana AH, et al: CT in obstructive jaundice. Part II. The cause of obstruction. Radiology 1981;*139*:635.
13. Thorsen MK, Quoroz F, Lawson TL, et al: Primary biliary carcinoma: CT evaluation. Radiology 1984;*152*:479.

14. Itai Y, Araki T, Yoshikawa K, et al: Computed tomography of gallbladder carcinoma. Radiology 1980;*137*:713.
15. Jeffrey RB, Federle MP, Laing FC, et al: Computed tomography of choledocholithiasis. AJR 1983; *140*:1179.
16. Federle MP, Goldberg HI: Computed tomography of the pancreas. *In* Moss AA, Gamsu G, Genant HK (eds): Computed Tomography of the Body. Philadelphia, W. B. Saunders 1983.
17. Harter LP, Moss AA, Goldberg HI, et al: CT-guided fine-needle aspirations for diagnosis of benign and malignant disease. AJR 1983;*140*:363.
18. Moss AA, et al: Liver, gallbladder, spleen, pancreas, peritoneal cavity and alimentary tube. *In* Margulis AR, Higgins CE, Kaufman L, et al (eds): Clinical Magnetic Resonance Imaging. Radiology Research and Education Foundation. San Francisco, University of California Printing Department, 1983.
19. Moon KL, Hricak H, Margulis AR, et al: Nuclear magnetic resonance imaging characteristics of gallstones in vitro. Radiology 1983;*148*:753.
20. Hricak H, Filly RA, Margulis AR, et al: Nuclear magnetic resonance imaging of the gallbladder. A preliminary report. Radiology 1983;*147*:481.
21. Moss AA, Goldberg HI, Stark DD, et al: Hepatic tumors: magnetic resonance and CT appearance. Radiology 1983;*150*:141.
22. Laing F, Jeffrey RB, Wing VW: Improved visualization of choledocholithiasis by sonography. AJR 1984;*143*:949.

ROBERT K. KERLAN, JR., M.D.
ERNEST J. RING, M.D.

10

Percutaneous Transhepatic Cholangiography and Interventional Radiology of the Gallbladder and Bile Ducts

INTRODUCTION

Direct cholangiography performed through needles placed percutaneously provides an excellent outline of biliary anatomy. Using fluoroscopy, catheters for temporary or permanent biliary drainage can be inserted above or through obstructed segments of the biliary tract. In addition, balloon dilating catheters can be inserted, and calculi can be removed with basket retrieval systems. In most situations, these techniques are not competitive with surgical therapy; rather, they are adjuncts to aid surgeons in the management of patients with biliary disease.

Access for fluoroscopically guided catheter manipulations of the biliary system can be obtained through surgically created tracts, percutaneous transhepatic puncture, and peroral retrograde catheterization. This chapter discusses the indications, therapeutic effectiveness, and limitations of catheter manipulations in the management of biliary tract disease.

PROCEDURES PERFORMED THROUGH SURGICALLY CREATED TRACTS

Removal of Retained Biliary Calculi

History

Removal of retained calculi was the first interventional radiologic procedure performed in the bile ducts. During the late 1960s and early 1970s, various instruments were passed through T-tube tracts to remove retained stones within the biliary tree, including Fogarty catheters, forceps, and Dormia baskets.[1] Widespread acceptance of the technique awaited the series of 220 cases reported by Mazzariello of Argentina in 1973.[2] Further technical modifications were subsequently reported by Burhenne from the United States,[3,4] who popularized the use of steerable catheters to position retrieval basket systems more precisely. With the advent of ultrasonic and electrohydraulic lithotripsy in the early 1980s, another technique has become available to fragment large retained calculi.[5]

Technique

Retained common duct calculi nearly always follow a common duct exploration that has resulted in the detection and removal of other stones. Because it is impossible to exclude completely the possibility that a stone has been left behind, the surgeon should take steps to facilitate instrumentation of the duct through the T-tube tract postoperatively, if that becomes necessary. A 14 F or larger T-tube should be used, and the stem should be brought out through a *lateral* subcostal stab wound. Whelan-Moss T-tubes are identical to the standard tubes, except that they have been made with thicker stems than horizontal limbs. For example, the tube with a 14 F limb for inserting in the duct has an 18 F stem, which creates a tract that better accommodates instruments for extracting retained stones. Since Whelan-Moss tubes have no drawbacks, they should be used routinely after common duct explorations for calculous disease. A lateral position for the T-tube site facilitates fluoroscopic manipulations and reduces radiation exposure to the radiologist's hands. Before stone extraction is attempted, the T-tube tract should be allowed to mature for 4 to 6 weeks from the time of operation. The mature (i.e., thick-walled) tract enables instrumentation within the biliary tree and minimizes the risk of making a false passage.

In the majority of patients, stone extraction can be performed as an outpatient procedure. However, elderly or debilitated individuals should be observed following the procedure and may require a brief hospitalization. Prophylactic use of a broad-spectrum antibiotic is initiated 24 hours before the procedure and is continued for 2 days. On the day of the examination, the patient is given a liquid diet. Although the procedure usually is not painful, most patients benefit from a mild sedative.

The patient is placed supine on a tilting fluoroscopy table, and the T-tube is removed by gentle traction. The skin surrounding the tube entry site is cleansed with antiseptic solution and is sterilely draped.

To avoid creation of false passages, the tract is catheterized with a soft red-rubber catheter or a blunt-tipped, steerable catheter.* If a red-rubber catheter is placed through the tract first, it is exchanged over a guide wire for a curved angiographic catheter. The tip of this catheter is positioned just beyond the stone and exchanged for a Dormia basket sheath over a guide wire. When the steerable catheter is used, it is directed to a point adjacent to the stone. The basket sheath is then passed through the catheter beyond the stone.

The diameter of the retrieval basket should be selected to match the size of the duct in which the stone is located. The basket is advanced to the tip of the sheath and positioned so that the midportion of the basket is adjacent to the stone. The sheath is then withdrawn while the basket is held in place, which allows the basket to open in an appropriate position (Fig. 10–1). The basket is rotated, trapping the stone within the wire mesh. The sheath is then gently advanced, locking the stone within the basket, and the stone is removed through the tract (Fig. 10–2). Conventional baskets are constructed with

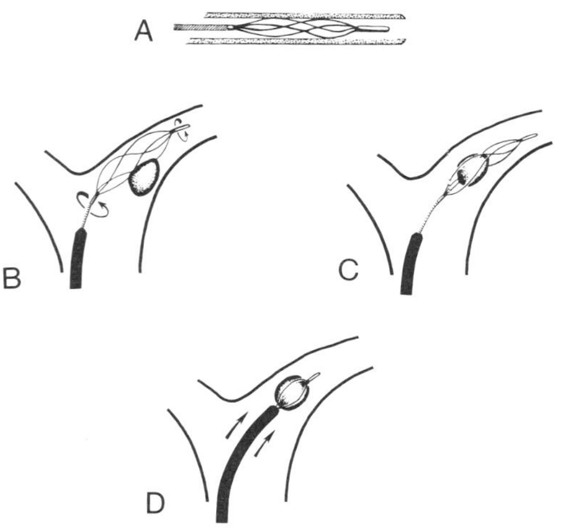

Figure 10–1. Technique of trapping biliary calculus with Dormia basket. *A,* Helical wires of Dormia basket fold together to fit into a sheathed catheter. *B,* The sheath is positioned beyond the stone, and the basket is introduced. The basket is opened adjacent to the stone and rotated (*arrows*). *C,* The basket is rotated until the stone is shown fluoroscopically to project within its wires. *D,* The basket is then closed around the stone by advancing the sheath (*arrows*). The basket and sheath are held together tightly and forcefully withdrawn through the T-tube tract.

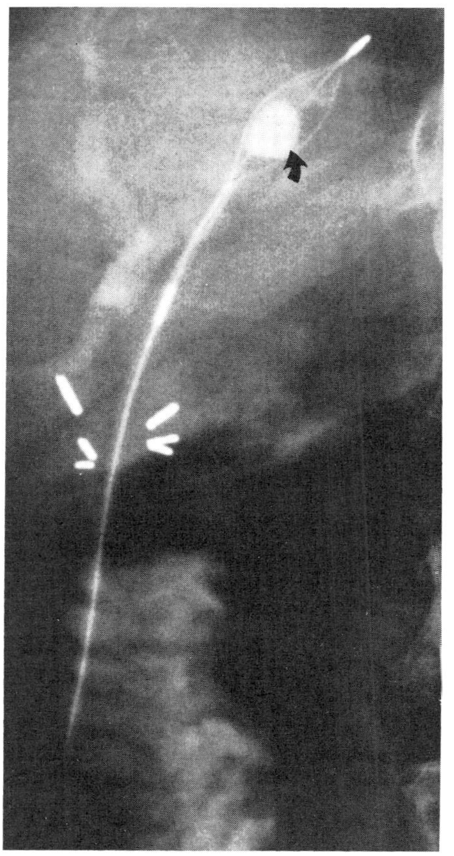

Figure 10–2. Radiopaque stone (*arrow*) trapped in the wires of a Dormia basket.

*Meditech, Watertown, MA.

four wires arranged in a helical configuration. Baskets made with three to six wires may be helpful to trap small stones when there is a marked discrepancy between stone size and ductal diameter.

Occasionally, resistance is encountered when the stone is extracted through the choledochotomy site. However, if continuous traction is applied under moderate tension, most stones can be extracted through 14 F or larger tracts, even though the stone may be slightly larger than the tract. Damage to the ductal system is very rare.

Following removal of all stones, the cholangiogram is repeated to ensure that no additional stones are present. Owing to the introduction of small amounts of air and the formation of blood clots, the postextraction cholangiogram may be difficult to interpret. It is therefore advisable to reinsert a drainage tube through the tract and perform another cholangiogram 24 to 48 hours later. Only when the cholangiogram is unequivocally normal should the drainage tube be removed and the tract allowed to heal.

Indications

Any patient with a retained common duct stone and an indwelling T-tube is a candidate for the procedure. It is also possible to remove retained stones via an endoscopic sphincterotomy, but in the majority of cases, removal through the T-tube tract is the procedure of choice.

Contraindications

There are no absolute contraindications to stone removal through a mature T-tube tract. Even very large stones can be removed with this technique, although in selected cases electrohydraulic or ultrasonic lithotripsy may be required to fragment them.

Stones lodged in cystic duct remnants or in diverticular outpouchings of the bile duct may be impossible to retrieve. When a stone is in one of these locations, it should be left undisturbed. Then, after a week or two of normal activity, the stone usually migrates into another position from which it can be more easily removed.

Results

Combining the two largest reported series of Mazzariello[2] and Burhenne[3] of over 850 patients, the overall success rate of stone removal through a T-tube tract is about 95 per cent. Removal of multiple stones often necessitates more than one procedure.

Complications

The complication rate is less than 5 per cent,[6] and only one patient has been reported to have died from the procedure.[7] Transient low-grade fevers are common, but clinical sepsis is unusual.

T-Tube Replacement

History

Before the 1970s, replacement or repositioning of indwelling T-tubes required a laparotomy. During the early 1970s, techniques were developed to disimpact T-tubes occluded by debris, but malpositioned tubes continued to require surgical replacement. In 1977, Crummy[8] described a technique whereby T-tubes could be replaced percutaneously under fluoroscopic control.

Technique

The indwelling T-tube is removed by gentle traction over a guide wire. The removed T-tube serves as a model for fashioning the limb length of the new tube. Limb length adjustments can be made easily on the basis of the cholangiogram.

Because there is so much friction between the rubber tube and the stainless steel guide wire, replacement is greatly facilitated by coating the T-tube generously with sterile water-soluble lubricant. The proximal limb of the T-tube is threaded over the guide wire, and the end of the wire is directed through the long external limb. The T-tube is passed over the wire with the distal limb trailing alongside the external limb. The tube is advanced until the tip of the trailing limb springs entirely into the lumen of the duct. The long external limb is retracted, seating the internal limbs into appropriate position (Fig. 10–3). The T-tube also may be inserted with the distal limb leading if the biliary anatomy is more suitable for this approach.

Indications

Although durable and comfortable, T-tubes sometimes become occluded with debris after 6 to 12 months. Simple flushing

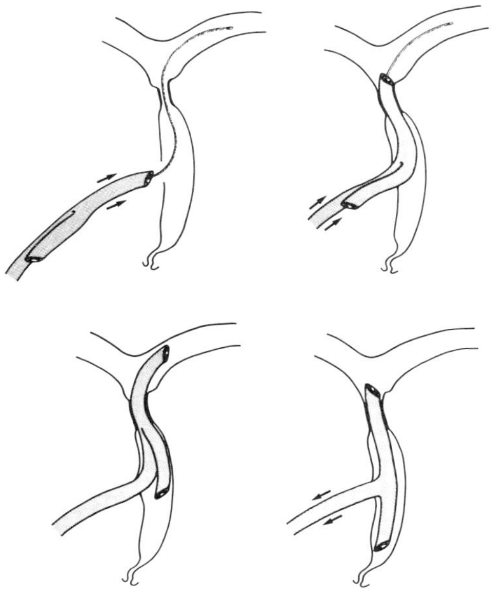

Figure 10–3. Technique of replacing T-tube. After the guide wire has been positioned in intrahepatic duct, the T-tube is placed on the guidewire. The lead limb of the "T" is placed on the guide first, followed by the external limb. The distal limb trails behind. As it passes completely through the choledochotomy site, the trailing limb springs into position into the distal duct. In general, traction is applied externally, and the lower vertical limb will descend into the common duct, positioning the T-tube.

with saline rarely is sufficient to disimpact the tube because the solution just escapes through the unobstructed limb. This is an indication for T-tube replacement.

When T-tubes are used to stent obstructing malignancies of the extrahepatic bile duct, growth of the lesion may eventually occlude a previously functioning system. This most commonly occurs cephalad to the proximal limb as a result of metastases or direct tumor extension. In this situation, a new tube with a longer proximal limb can be placed to re-establish bile flow (Fig. 10–4).

T-tubes may be malpositioned surgically in two ways: (1) the tube fails to stent an obstructing lesion, or (2) one limb is not placed into, or slips out of, the extrahepatic bile duct. Repositioning a recently placed T-tube is extremely difficult because there is no well-formed tract, but it is usually possible to pass an angiographic catheter into the duct. This preserves access to the duct and provides temporary bile drainage. If indicated, the catheter may be replaced with a T-tube 4 to 5 weeks later.

Finally, patients are occasionally encountered who have uncontrolled fistulae from the extrahepatic bile duct. Insertion of a T-tube is an ideal way to control the leak. Percutaneously placed sump catheters also may be required to evacuate associated abscesses.

Complications

As with any manipulation of the biliary tract, sepsis may occur if excessive amounts of contrast media are injected in the presence of infected bile. Therefore, broad-spectrum antibiotics should be given before manipulations of this kind are performed.

In addition, if the T-tube tract has not matured, access to the biliary tree may be lost during the procedure. Although this is infrequent, reoperation or percutaneous transhepatic catheterization may be necessary if biliary obstruction is present.

PROCEDURES PERFORMED THROUGH A DIRECT PERCUTANEOUS APPROACH

Percutaneous Transhepatic Cholangiography and Biliary Drainage

History

Percutaneous transhepatic cholangiography (PTC) was first attempted in Southeast Asia during the late 1930s.[9] However, the technique was rarely used in the United States and Europe until the 1960s.[10, 11] Even with technical modifications, at that time most centers considered PTC too dangerous unless it was followed immediately by laparotomy. In the early 1970s, it was shown that when PTC was performed with a fine needle (22- or 23-gauge), there were few risks even in the presence of complete ductal obstruction. Opacification of the biliary tree with the fine needle technique approaches 100 per cent when the ducts are dilated and over 80 per cent when the ducts are of normal caliber.[12] The ease of performance of PTC encouraged its rapid dissemination, and thin needle transhepatic cholangiography became the procedure of choice for routine preoperative depiction of biliary anatomy.

Endoscopic cannulation of the bile ducts was introduced at about the same time, but it did not become popular for several years because it requires greater skill. Now that both methods are available at most institutions, the techniques have become complementary. Endoscopic retrograde cholangiog-

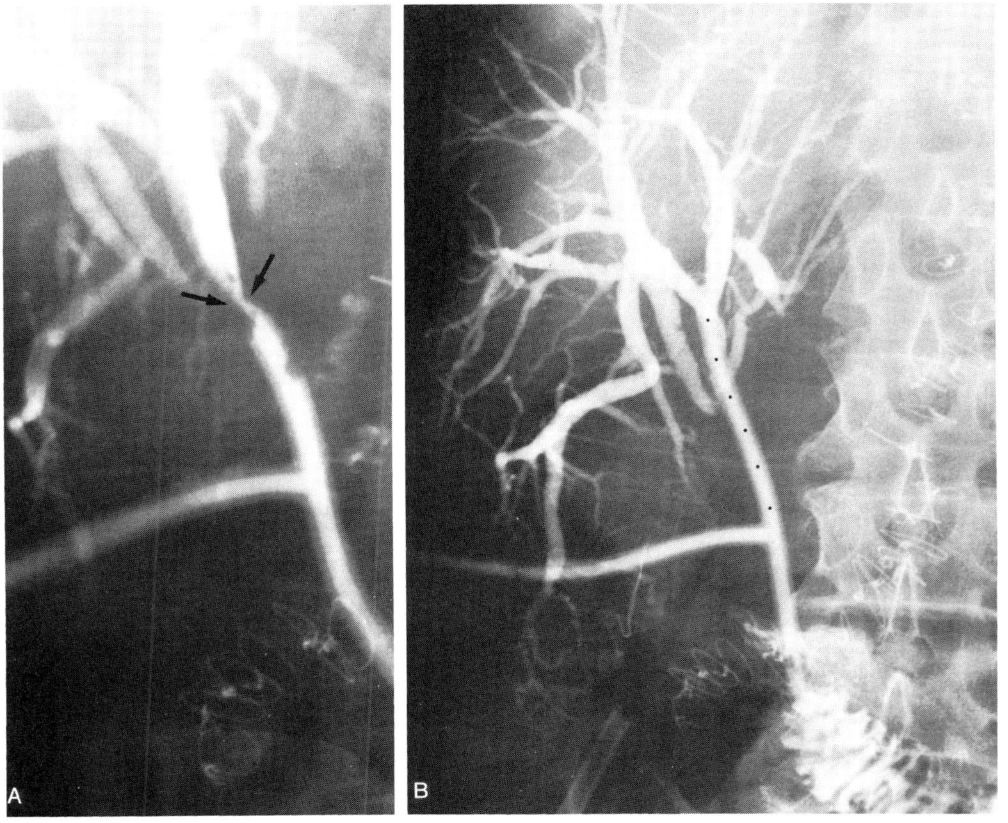

Figure 10–4. Exchanging T-tube for longer limb T-tube to stent a recurrent tumor. *A,* Six months after stenting T-tube had been placed, the patient developed recurrent cholangitis. T-tube cholangiogram shows irregular obstruction of the duct immediately proximal to the upper limb of the tube (*arrows*). *B,* The T-tube was removed and replaced. The new tube was fashioned with a longer proximal limb to extend into the intrahepatic ducts above the tumor.

raphy is used when a distal obstruction or gallstone disease is suspected or when the pancreatic duct must be outlined. PTC is the method of choice for demonstrating more proximal lesions and is especially important to delineate the ducts when the obstructing lesion is at the level of the porta hepatis. If the ducts cannot be opacified by THC, ERCP can be used, and vice versa.[13]

Percutaneous Biliary Drainage

Before the advent of the thin needle technique, attempts were made to enhance the safety of PTC by leaving a small catheter within the biliary tree and allowing temporary decompression of the bile ducts. This decreased the chance of bile leakage after the procedure. However, it was difficult to keep the catheter in position, and complications were frequent. In the mid-1970s, the feasibility of manipulating modified angiographic catheters through the biliary system and across obstructing lesions was demonstrated.[14] Transhepatic catheters could be securely anchored beyond the obstruction, and side holes positioned on either side of the obstruction permitted bile to drain internally into the duodenum. This procedure gained considerable popularity in the late 1970s as technical refinements were made and large series of patients were reported.[15, 16]

Technique

The patient is placed on broad-spectrum antibiotics immediately before the procedure. If there is evidence of cholangitis, parenteral antibiotics should be given. A sedative hypnotic and narcotic analgesic are administered. Additional analgesics may be given intravenously during the procedure as needed, but general anesthesia is rarely necessary.

The skin over the right upper quadrant, the right flank, and the right chest wall is cleansed with an antiseptic solution and is sterilely draped. The diaphragmatic border is identified fluoroscopically, and an entry point for the needle is selected in the midaxillary line, usually immediately above the tenth or eleventh rib.

The transhepatic cholangiogram is performed with a thin-walled, 22-gauge needle passed slightly cephalad through the liver parenchyma to a point just to the right of the vertebral body. Contrast medium is injected through the needle as it is slowly withdrawn through the parenchyma. When the tip of the needle enters the ductal system, contrast agent begins to outline the biliary tree. If no contact is made with a duct, the needle is withdrawn to a point just beneath the liver capsule and another pass is made more anteriorly or posteriorly. Caution should be used to avoid overdistention of the biliary system with contrast medium, as this may precipitate septicemia. The transhepatic cholangiogram is reviewed to determine the feasibility of percutaneous drainage.

When percutaneous drainage is deemed appropriate, a needle puncture site is selected in the midaxillary line that provides an almost horizontal approach to a branch of the right hepatic duct (Fig. 10–5). After the administration of local anesthesia, a 16-gauge sheathed needle is advanced into the duct, and the stylet is removed. Bile returns freely through the sheath when its tip lies within a bile duct. The sheath is then directed through the duct and the obstruction, using specially designed steerable guide wires.

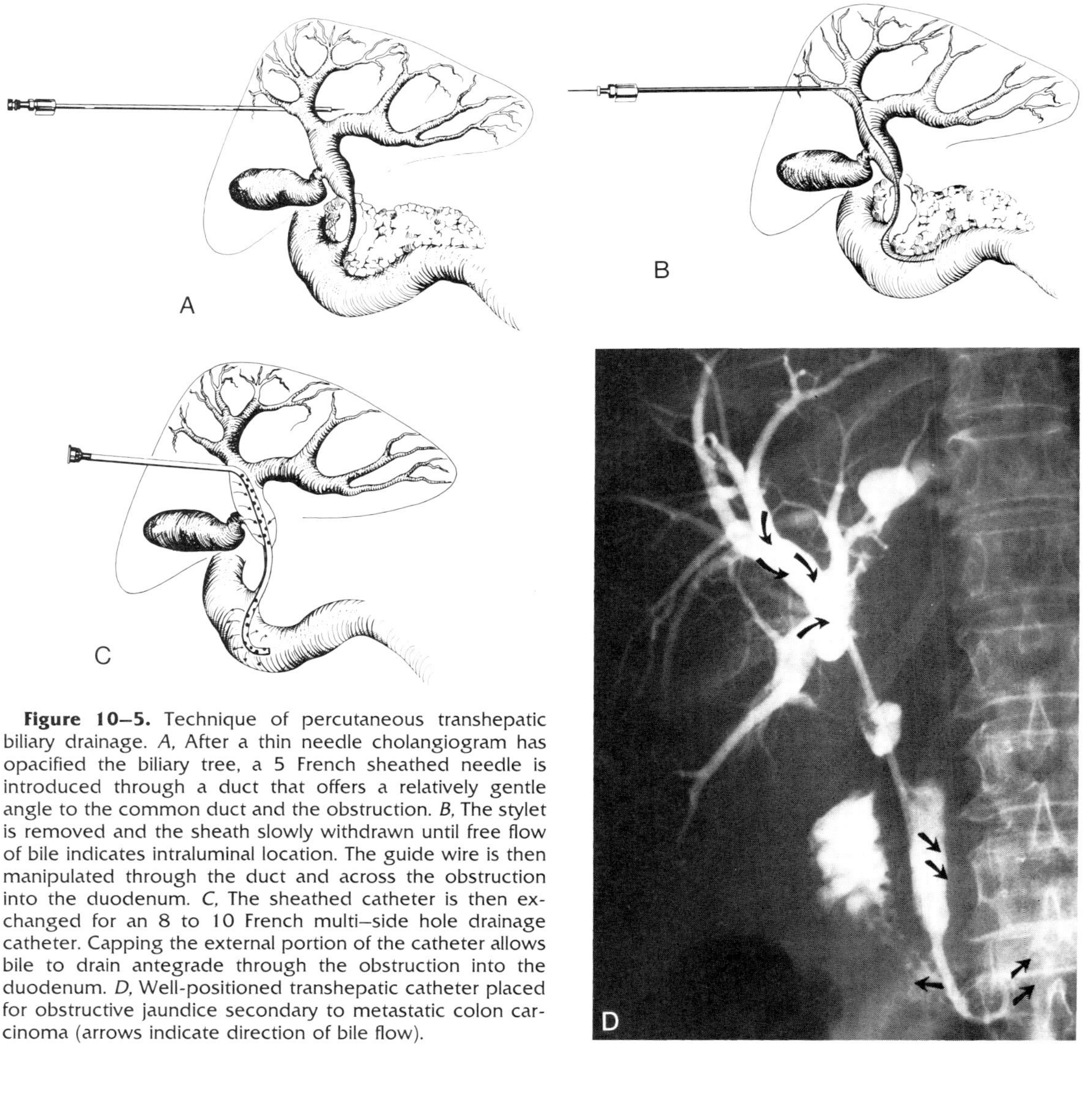

Figure 10–5. Technique of percutaneous transhepatic biliary drainage. *A,* After a thin needle cholangiogram has opacified the biliary tree, a 5 French sheathed needle is introduced through a duct that offers a relatively gentle angle to the common duct and the obstruction. *B,* The stylet is removed and the sheath slowly withdrawn until free flow of bile indicates intraluminal location. The guide wire is then manipulated through the duct and across the obstruction into the duodenum. *C,* The sheathed catheter is then exchanged for an 8 to 10 French multi–side hole drainage catheter. Capping the external portion of the catheter allows bile to drain antegrade through the obstruction into the duodenum. *D,* Well-positioned transhepatic catheter placed for obstructive jaundice secondary to metastatic colon carcinoma (arrows indicate direction of bile flow).

When the sheath has been advanced into the duodenum, a stiff guide wire is inserted, the sheath is removed, and a drainage catheter is inserted over the guide wire. The multiple side holes of the drainage catheter are positioned above and below the obstruction, which allows bile to flow into the duodenum when the tube is capped externally.

In a few patients, the obstruction cannot be crossed with the catheter. In these individuals, a catheter may be left in the biliary system proximal to the obstruction and connected externally to a drainage bag. Although this provides biliary decompression, the catheter can be easily dislodged. In addition, problems with fluid and electrolyte balance may occur with chronic external drainage.[17, 18] Fortunately, it is generally much less difficult to negotiate the catheter across the obstruction after 2 or 3 days of external drainage, and it is virtually always feasible to achieve a catheter position across the obstructing lesion.

The drainage tube is secured in place, and the patient is returned to the ward. Observation for intraperitoneal hemorrhage or sepsis is maintained for 12 hours afterwards.

Indications

Patients considered for percutaneous transhepatic biliary drainage can be divided into two groups: those requiring only temporary drainage and those requiring permanent intubation. The former group includes most patients with benign causes of biliary obstruction as well as selected patients with malignant obstruction. The latter group includes patients with advanced tumors in whom percutaneous transhepatic biliary drainage is performed exclusively for palliation.

Indications for Temporary Biliary Drainage

Malignant Obstruction. The usefulness of temporary preoperative transhepatic biliary drainage in jaundiced patients with malignant biliary obstruction is controversial. Two studies found no benefit with regard to perioperative morbidity and mortality rates in patients undergoing preoperative transhepatic biliary drainage.[19, 20] Another controlled trial of 50 patients showed that postoperative morbidity and mortality rates were decreased by preoperative decompression.[21] In the last series, serious morbidity occurred in 52 per cent of patients operated on without prior drainage compared with only 8 per cent of patients in whom PTBD was performed preoperatively.

Benign Strictures. Although benign strictures may result from external trauma and pancreatitis, most are attributable to accidental injury during biliary tract surgery. Operative repair of these strictures yields excellent results in 70 to 80 per cent of patients. Several factors (e.g., infection and elevated serum bilirubin value) have been identified as major influences on the success of surgical repair.[22, 23] With preoperative transhepatic drainage, the obstruction is relieved, biliary infection subsides, and the serum bilirubin level decreases. Moreover, placement of the catheter through the stricture into the duodenum may aid the surgeon in identifying the bile duct.

In elderly or debilitated patients or individuals for whom surgical repair of a benign stricture may be difficult or impossible, the stricture may be dilated percutaneously.[24, 25] The procedure is identical to PTBD with the exception that a balloon is positioned and inflated at the site of the stricture. This is usually followed by several months of stenting. As yet there is insufficient experience to evaluate the long-term efficacy of stricture dilatation. Preliminary reports have not been encouraging with regard to the long-term treatment of extrahepatic bile duct strictures, for the cure rate has been only 20 per cent.[25] However, dilatation of postoperative stenoses at sites of choledochal-intestinal anastomoses may be more effective than dilatation of unrepaired strictures (Fig. 10–6).

Cholangitis. Emergent surgical decompression of the bile duct in patients with acute obstructive cholangitis carries a mortality rate of 50 per cent to 75 per cent.[26–28] Using PTBD, bile can be obtained for culture, the ducts can be partially decompressed, and medical management of the sepsis can be facilitated in most cases. In addition, after sepsis is controlled, tube cholangiography can be used to demonstrate the obstruction. An elective surgical procedure may be performed subsequently to remove or bypass the obstructing lesion when the patient's condition has improved. Using this approach, a 17 per cent mortality rate was reported in one series of 18 patients with acute obstructive cholangitis.[29]

As an alternative, obstructive biliary sepsis from common duct calculi may be treated by endoscopic sphincterotomy, which, if success-

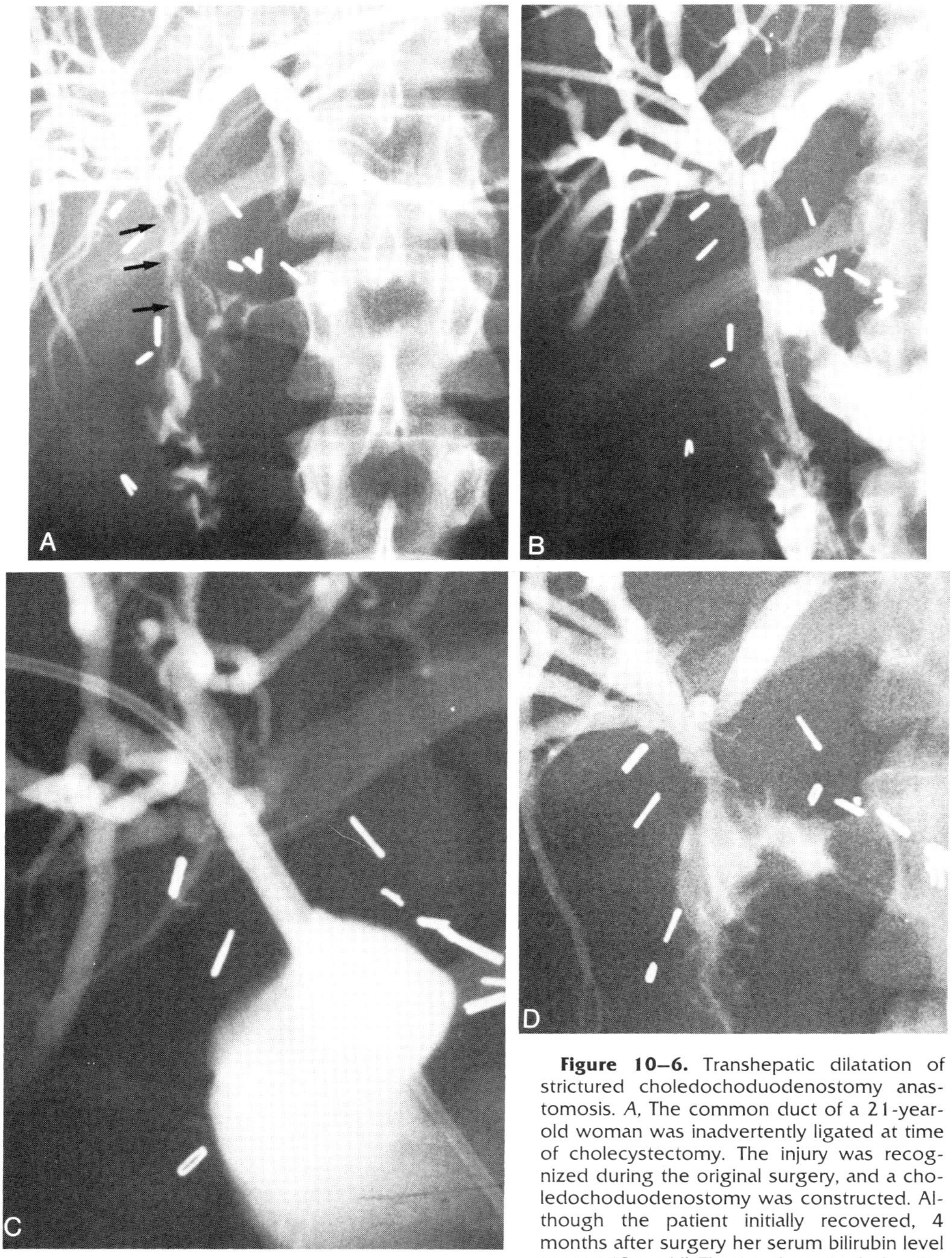

Figure 10–6. Transhepatic dilatation of strictured choledochoduodenostomy anastomosis. *A,* The common duct of a 21-year-old woman was inadvertently ligated at time of cholecystectomy. The injury was recognized during the original surgery, and a choledochoduodenostomy was constructed. Although the patient initially recovered, 4 months after surgery her serum bilirubin level rose to 12 mg/dl. The transhepatic cholangiogram demonstrates the stricture at the anastomosis (*arrows*). *B,* Antegrade drainage was established transhepatically, and the patient was discharged from the hospital. *C,* Three months later, the woman was readmitted for balloon dilatation of the stricture. The transhepatic catheter was replaced with 4 mm dilating balloon catheter, which was inflated in the narrowed area several times until it moved freely. The next day, the stricture was dilated with a 6 mm balloon and the third day with an 8 mm balloon. A catheter was left in the intrahepatic duct. A cholangiogram performed on the day after dilatation revealed wide patency through the anastomosis. The catheter was "parked" in an intrahepatic duct, and the patient was discharged from the hospital. *D,* Cholangiograms were performed at monthly intervals for the next 6 months. Since there was no evidence of recurrence of the stricture, the transhepatic catheter was removed 6 months after dilatation. The woman remains asymptomatic and anicteric 2 years later.

ful, usually provides excellent drainage of the duct.

Facilitation of Endoscopic Sphincterotomy. Endoscopic sphincterotomy has become an important technique in the management of postcholecystectomy choledocholithiasis.[30] Although technically successful in 90 per cent of patients,[31, 32] the procedure occasionally fails because of inability to pass the sphincterotome into the distal common bile duct. In this situation, temporary PTBD may be useful.

A transhepatic catheter is placed into the biliary system and advanced into the descending duodenum. The catheter is then exchanged for a retrieval basket sheath over a guide wire. The guide wire is withdrawn, and the basket is inserted into the duodenum and opened. The endoscopist guides the sphincterotome into the basket, the basket is closed, and the sphincterotome is pulled with gentle traction into the distal common bile duct and released. A sphincterotomy is performed; the transhepatic drainage catheter is temporarily left in place. When a follow-up tube cholangiogram reveals a widely patent sphincter and no residual calculi, the transhepatic drainage catheter is removed.

Sclerosing Cholangitis. Management of this disease is extremely difficult, often requiring cooperative medical, surgical, and radiologic techniques. In some patients, temporary PTBD may be useful in relieving acute episodes of cholangitis. However, because the ducts are rarely distended, standard-sized transhepatic drainage catheters may obturate the duct lumen and aggravate the cholangitis.[33] Therefore, proper patient selection and precise positioning of drainage catheters are critical when PTBD is used for this condition.

Transhepatic catheterization may be performed for balloon dilatation of strictures in patients with sclerosing cholangitis. Although the experience to date is meager, it is encouraging.[34, 35]

Catheterization for drainage and balloon dilatation may be performed through a T-tube tract. Access to the ducts may also be obtained by percutaneous puncture of a choledochojejunostomy, provided the end of the jejunal loop is affixed to the abdominal wall and is marked with metal clips. The jejunum may then be punctured under fluoroscopic guidance, and stricture dilatation, stone removal, and drainage procedures may be performed periodically as needed. When the patient's clinical condition has improved, the catheters may be removed.

Indications for Prolonged Transhepatic Biliary Drainage. Some patients with neoplastic obstructions are best treated by transhepatic drainage without operation. Examples include symptomatic patients with advanced malignancy, elderly and debilitated patients who are poor surgical candidates, and a few patients with unresectable proximal obstructions.

Pancreatic Carcinoma. Although it was hoped that the recent advances in abdominal imaging would lead to earlier diagnosis and increased cure rates for pancreatic carcinoma, most malignancies are unresectable at the time of presentation. The greatest contribution of the imaging modalities has been their ability to demonstrate features such as encasement of the superior mesenteric artery and extrapancreatic metastases that categorically rule out the possibility of cure by surgery, thereby eliminating the need for exploratory laparotomy for staging. In patients with advanced unresectable disease, surgery is associated with a high mortality rate[36, 37] and morbidity rate,[38] hardly worth the limited palliation that is possible.

In comparison, PTBD can be performed in these patients with a mortality rate of less than 2 per cent,[39] and the average length of hospitalization is little more than 1 week and may be as short as 3 days.

Cholangiocarcinoma. Because primary tumors of the extrahepatic bile ducts are often resectable, surgical exploration is usually indicated for this disease.[40] However, with lesions of the proximal extrahepatic ducts, resection is often impossible,[41] and catheter drainage may be the only means of palliation.

Cholangiocarcinoma grows slowly and metastasizes late. Therefore, if adequate drainage can be maintained, survival is occasionally prolonged.[42] In most patients it is necessary to establish percutaneous drainage of both the right and left duct (Fig. 10–7). This can be accomplished by Y- and U-tubes, which drain both lobes of the liver and are easy to replace.

Metastatic Disease. Patients with widespread malignancies are obviously poor surgical candidates. In many cases, limited support is the most that is called for, but when intense pruritus complicates obstructive jaundice, percutaneous biliary drainage may be justified. The pruritus generally disappears in the first 48 hours after adequate drainage has been achieved, even when the serum bilirubin level is still very high.

PTBD may also be indicated for patients

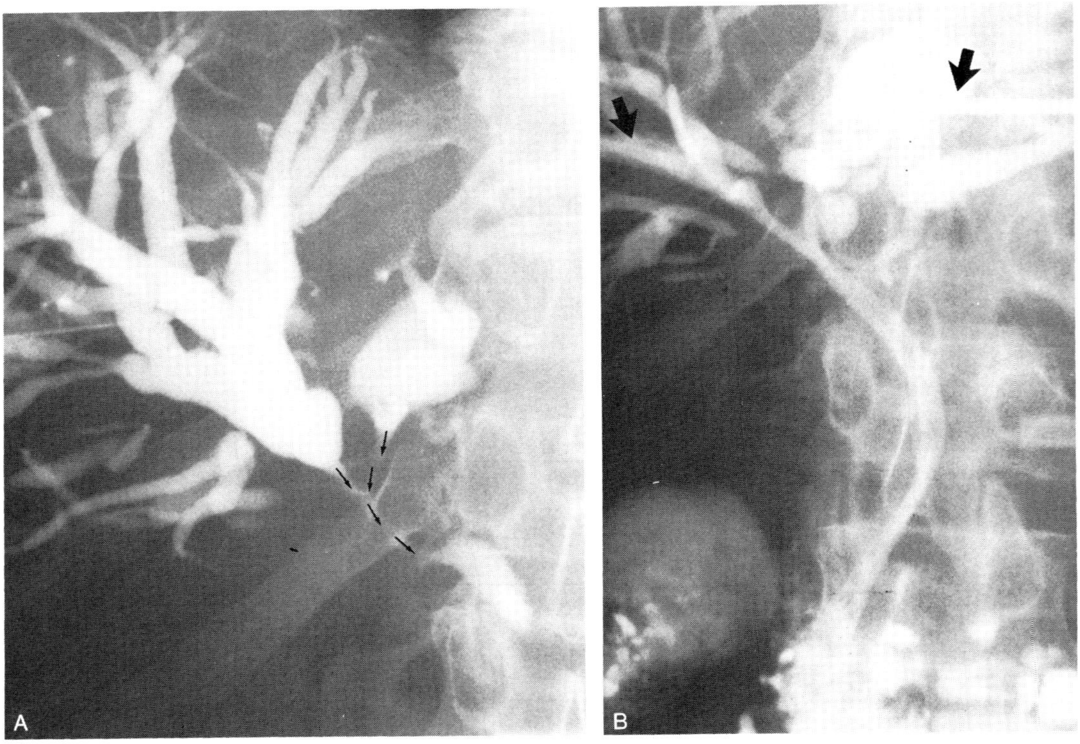

Figure 10–7. Transhepatic drainage with two catheters for nonresectable cholangiocarcinoma of the upper common hepatic duct that extends into the right and left intrahepatic ducts (Klatzkin tumor). *A*, Thin needle cholangiogram reveals separate obstructions of right and left ducts. *B*, Transhepatic catheters were introduced from each side and advanced into the duodenum so that antegrade drainage could be established for both lobes (*arrows*). Patients with this type of malignancy can live for several years if bile flow can be maintained. Decompression of only one lobe will relieve jaundice, but the undrained segment commonly becomes infected.

whose tumors are responsive to chemotherapeutic agents excreted in bile. Because these agents may be hepatotoxic when administered in the presence of biliary obstruction, percutaneous biliary drainage may be essential prior to their use.

Contraindications

Clinical Contraindications

Severe Bleeding Diathesis. Because PTBD can require several hepatic punctures, patients with bleeding diatheses deserve special consideration. Moderate or marked prolongation of the prothrombin time or partial thromboplastin time and a platelet count under 50,000/ml are relative contraindications. Vitamin K, fresh frozen plasma, or platelet transfusions are necessary to improve the coagulation status before the procedure.

Ascites. The presence of moderate or massive ascites creates several problems. First, the procedure is technically more difficult, as guide wires and catheters tend to buckle within the peritoneal cavity, making the application of coaxial force much more difficult. Second, the risk of hemorrhage related to the procedure is greater. Finally, even after satisfactory drainage is achieved, ascitic fluid tends to leak around the catheter. In some cases, relief of the biliary obstruction is followed by a decrease in the ascites, but in other cases ascites persists. Therefore, PTBD should be performed in patients with ascites only when clinical indications are compelling and other alternatives have failed.

Minimal Symptoms. The absence of severe treatable symptoms is the principal contraindication to PTBD in terminally ill patients. Although the morbidity and mortality rates are low, the procedure and the presence of the catheters are uncomfortable, and the catheters serve as constant reminders of the disease. Therefore, the presence of pruritus, severe anorexia, or infection is a prerequisite for recommending PTBD.

Anatomic Contraindications

Multiple Intrahepatic Obstructions. With catheters in the ducts, the bile always becomes colonized with bacteria, and unless complete drainage of the biliary system is achieved, recurrent cholangitis is the rule in the incompletely drained segments of duct. With multiple intrahepatic obstructions, it is impossible to establish complete biliary drainage with one or two percutaneous catheters. Theoretically, this problem can be handled by inserting still more catheters, but the quality of life becomes so severely compromised that the wisdom of this approach is questionable. It is our policy to perform percutaneous decompression only when effective drainage can be established by one or two tubes. When more than two tubes would be required, we do not consider PTBD a practical alternative.

Intraductal Tumor. Some neoplasms—rare cholangiocarcinomas, intraductal papillomas, sarcomas, and some metastatic lesions—infiltrate diffusely throughout the ductal system. When the ducts are filled with tumor, biliary drainage by any route is ineffective, and percutaneous drainage should not be attempted.

Results

The effectiveness of percutaneous biliary drainage in lowering the serum bilirubin level and relieving symptoms of obstructive jaundice has been well documented.[43–46] The success of the procedure, defined as establishment of effective bile drainage, in most series exceeds 90 per cent. Although statistics vary, the obstructing lesion can be negotiated and the catheter passed into the duodenum in over 95 per cent of cases. Pruritus nearly always resolves within 24 to 48 hours, and cholangitis improves within 18 to 24 hours.[43]

After adequate biliary decompression, serum bilirubin values decrease following first-order kinetics at an average rate of 8 per cent per day in patients without serious liver disease.[46, 47] The rate is not appreciably influenced by the type of disease, the length of time the patient has been jaundiced, or the absolute level of the serum bilirubin. On the other hand, the rate of decrease of serum alkaline phosphatase in response to relief of the obstruction is haphazard and of little diagnostic import.[47] Although the serum bilirubin level eventually returns to normal in patients without underlying hepatic disease, the level may remain high in patients with extensive hepatic metastases or hepatic parenchymal dysfunction. For example, a decline of the serum bilirubin of 10 mg/dl per cent or more was observed in 76 per cent of patients with malignant obstruction, and a decline of 5 mg/dl to 10 mg/dl in 10 per cent of patients in one series.[44]

Complications

The most frequent serious complication of transhepatic biliary drainage is sepsis, which occurs to some degree in slightly over 10 per cent of patients.[39, 48] However, septic shock is unusual (less than 2 per cent of cases).

Although a little bleeding is encountered in most patients, serious hemorrhage is rare, occurring in less than 2 per cent of cases.[48] Bleeding can be divided into two types: biliary (hemobilia) and intraperitoneal.

Hemobilia, which is not uncommon, occurs when a side hole of the biliary drainage catheter is malpositioned in the hepatic parenchyma. This can be corrected by advancing the catheter to a point at which all of the side holes are within the ducts. If this is unsuccessful, hepatic arteriography should be performed; if a hepatic arterial branch has been lacerated, it may be embolized. For further details on catheter-induced hemobilia, the reader is referred to Chapter 42.

A tear of the hepatic capsule is the usual cause of intraperitoneal bleeding. In addition, if an improper entry site has been selected immediately below the rib, the possibility of intercostal artery bleeding must be considered. In most cases, intraperitoneal bleeding requires prompt surgical management.

Death from severe bleeding is very rare but, unfortunately, has occurred. Of the 200 cases of bleeding reported by Mueller,[39] two patients died from uncontrolled hemorrhage. Death has also been reported from inadvertent transpleural puncture complicated by pneumothorax and bilious pleural effusion and from bile emboli to the lung, which occurs by a mechanism just the reverse of hemobilia.[49] Other infrequent (less than 1 per cent) complications have been observed, such as bile leakage into the peritoneal cavity, hepatic or perihepatic abscess formation, and pancreatitis.

When internal drainage cannot be established, fluid and electrolyte loss may become a problem. This is most often observed in the first 2 or 3 days following biliary drainage, during which a postdrainage choleresis may develop.

Late complications, including local skin infections and granulomata at the catheter entry site, are common but easily managed in most cases. Plugging of the catheter can be prevented by flushing the tube with 3 to 5 ml of sterile saline daily. The catheter should be changed every 2 to 3 months to prevent build-up of biliary sludge and debris within the lumen.

A few reports of carcinomatous extension along the transhepatic catheter tracts have appeared, but this complication is rare. Skin implantation as well as peritoneal seeding has been documented.[50, 51]

Insertion of Completely Indwelling Biliary Stents

History

The development of percutaneous biliary drainage in the mid-1970s stimulated interest in the feasibility of transhepatic insertion of completely indwelling biliary stents. In 1978, Pereiras developed a practical endoprosthesis that he inserted successfully in a small group of patients.[52] Subsequently, other prostheses were developed that were easier to insert, and they were evaluated in larger numbers of patients.[53–55] Currently, transhepatic insertion of biliary stents is a common procedure and is performed in most medical centers in the United States and Europe.

Technique

Before insertion of a completely indwelling biliary stent, a standard percutaneous transhepatic drainage is performed. In most cases, the transhepatic tube is left in place for 1 to 2 weeks before insertion of the endoprosthesis. The procedure, which entails little discomfort, is usually performed on an outpatient basis. As with any catheterization of the bile ducts, the patient is prepared by administration of prophylactic broad-spectrum antibiotics and a liquid diet.

The patient is positioned supine on the fluoroscopic table, and a cholangiogram is performed through the transhepatic drainage catheter. A stiff guide wire is inserted through the tube into the duodenum, and the drainage catheter is removed. Using coaxial Teflon dilators, the tract is enlarged to 12F or 16F.

An endoprosthesis of the appropriate length is selected and advanced through the tract with a pushing catheter. Once in position, the guide wire is removed and a cholangiogram is performed. In most cases, a temporary transhepatic drainage catheter is left indwelling for the first 24 hours to evacuate any blood clots that may have formed during the procedure. This catheter is then removed, and the transhepatic tract heals in 2 or 3 days.

Two types of biliary stents have been designed to ensure that migration of the endoprosthesis will not occur. The most commonly used stent is a 12F to 16F Teflon tube with eccentric flaps at its proximal end to anchor the catheter.[53] The flaps collapse as the stent is advanced through the transhepatic tract. When the flaps reach the ductal system, they spring open, anchoring the endoprosthesis in proper position (Fig. 10–8).

An alternative system involves a short piece of suture connected to the proximal end of the stent. The suture is fixed to a small plastic button buried subcutaneously at the time of stent insertion. The suture provides continuous traction, effectively preventing distal migration.

Indications

There are several advantages to utilizing completely indwelling biliary stents. The large end hole efficiently conducts bile into the duodenum. There is no associated discomfort, and the patient does not need to perform any routine tube maintenance. Most important, the quality of life is dramatically improved by not having the nuisance of a percutaneous drainage tube.

For these reasons, completely indwelling stents are indicated for all patients with malignant biliary obstruction in whom endoprosthesis placement is technically feasible. This includes patients with obstructing lesions of the extrahepatic bile duct as well as those with obstruction of the main right and left hepatic ducts. In the latter case, two stents are necessary to achieve drainage of the isolated left and right systems.

As an alternative to placement of a transhepatic biliary stent, endoscopically guided retrograde placement is available.[56–58] Previously, this technique was of limited value as the largest stent size was 6F because of endoscopic design. However, recent improvements in instrumentation have allowed placement of 10F stents by experienced endoscopists. Because this technique avoids the discomfort and morbidity of transhepatic ma-

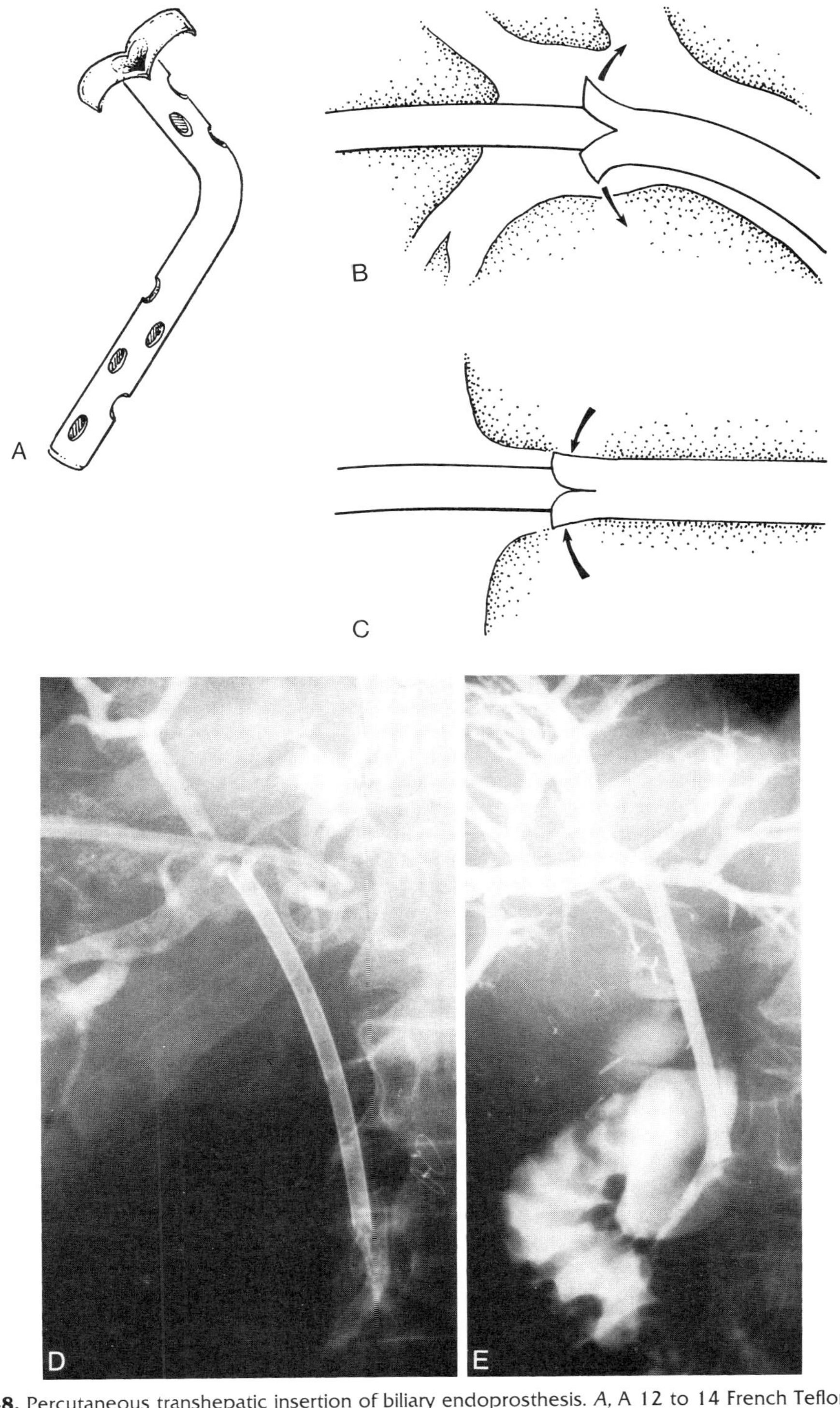

Figure 10–8. Percutaneous transhepatic insertion of biliary endoprosthesis. *A*, A 12 to 14 French Teflon tube is used for the endoprosthesis. Flaps at the proximal end serve to anchor the prosthesis above the obstruction. *B*, Flaps close like a "toggle bolt" while passing through the liver parenchyma. *C*, On entering the ductal system, the flaps open. *D*, After the endoprosthesis has been positioned, a pigtail catheter is placed to clear any clots or debris. *E*, Cholangiogram on the following day demonstrates free flow through the endoprosthesis, and the pigtail catheter is removed.

nipulation, it should be considered the procedure of choice for obstructing lesions of the mid- and distal bile duct. Transhepatic drainage and stent placement may still be used if endoscopic placement is unsuccessful.

Interestingly, a technique has been developed by which large-bore stents can be placed by the retrograde approach using fluoroscopic guidance.[59] However, because this procedure requires transhepatic puncture, it is not as attractive as endoscopically guided retrograde stent placement.

Results

Transhepatic insertion of biliary stents is successful in most individuals. In one series of 62 patients reported by Coons,[55] bilirubin levels returned to normal in 60 per cent. The remaining 40 per cent had a mean decrease in the serum bilirubin level of 8.0 mg/dl. Excellent stent patency was noted: All but one stent remained open until the time of death, which averaged 5 months in these patients with advanced malignant disease. The stents remained patent for as long as 15 months.

Complications

The complications of endoprosthesis placement include those associated with percutaneous transhepatic biliary drainage. In addition, there are two unique complications, stent migration and stent occlusion.

Stent migration was common during the early experience with endoprosthesis placement, but with improved design and catheter positioning, this complication is now unusual. In a series of 71 stent placements,[55] only two instances of migration into the duodenum occurred. If it does migrate, the prosthesis usually passes without difficulty through the alimentary canal, but another stent must then be inserted into the bile duct.

Occlusion of indwelling stents by biliary sludge and debris is also uncommon, having occurred only once in the 71 cases.[55] When it does happen, the stent must be removed, either by advancing it into the duodenum or by pulling it back out through the hepatic parenchyma. A new stent must be inserted. Finally, because endoprostheses are used to treat malignant neoplasms, progression of disease can occlude the stent, which would require it to be repositioned or replaced. However, most patients die of other manifestations of the neoplasm before obstructive jaundice recurs.

Percutaneous Cholecystostomy

History

Percutaneous puncture of the gallbladder is not a new procedure. It was first performed in the early 1920s for diagnostic purposes.[60] However, because of the risks of intraperitoneal spillage of infected bile, percutaneous catheter decompression was not attempted until recently. In 1979, a case report indicated that the procedure was feasible.[61] By 1982, it had been successfully performed in a series of 13 patients.[62]

Technique

The patient is prepared with a liquid diet and broad-spectrum antibiotics. Ultrasonic guidance is used to find the optimal position for puncture, a point anterior to where the edge of the liver separates the anterior abdominal wall and gallbladder. The needle is passed through the hepatic parenchyma into the gallbladder wall where the latter attaches to the liver. This minimizes the possibility of peritoneal spillage of bile.

After the entry site is selected, it is infiltrated with a local anesthetic. The puncture is made with an 18-gauge sheathed needle, and the stylet is removed. When the gallbladder is entered and bile returns freely, a guide wire is advanced through the sheath and coiled within the gallbladder. The sheath is removed, and a 10 or 12F drainage tube is inserted over the guide wire. The drainage tube is then secured in place.

Indications

The indications for percutaneous cholecystostomy are the same as for surgical cholecystostomy—elderly or debilitated patients with acute cholecystitis who are poor candidates for immediate cholecystectomy.

After percutaneous cholecystostomy, three management alternatives are possible. If the patient's medical condition improves substantially, an elective cholecystectomy may be performed. As an alternative, the percutaneous tract may be dilated and the gallbladder stones removed under fluoroscopic guidance (Fig. 10–9). Finally, in some patients, permanent tube drainage of the gallbladder may be warranted.

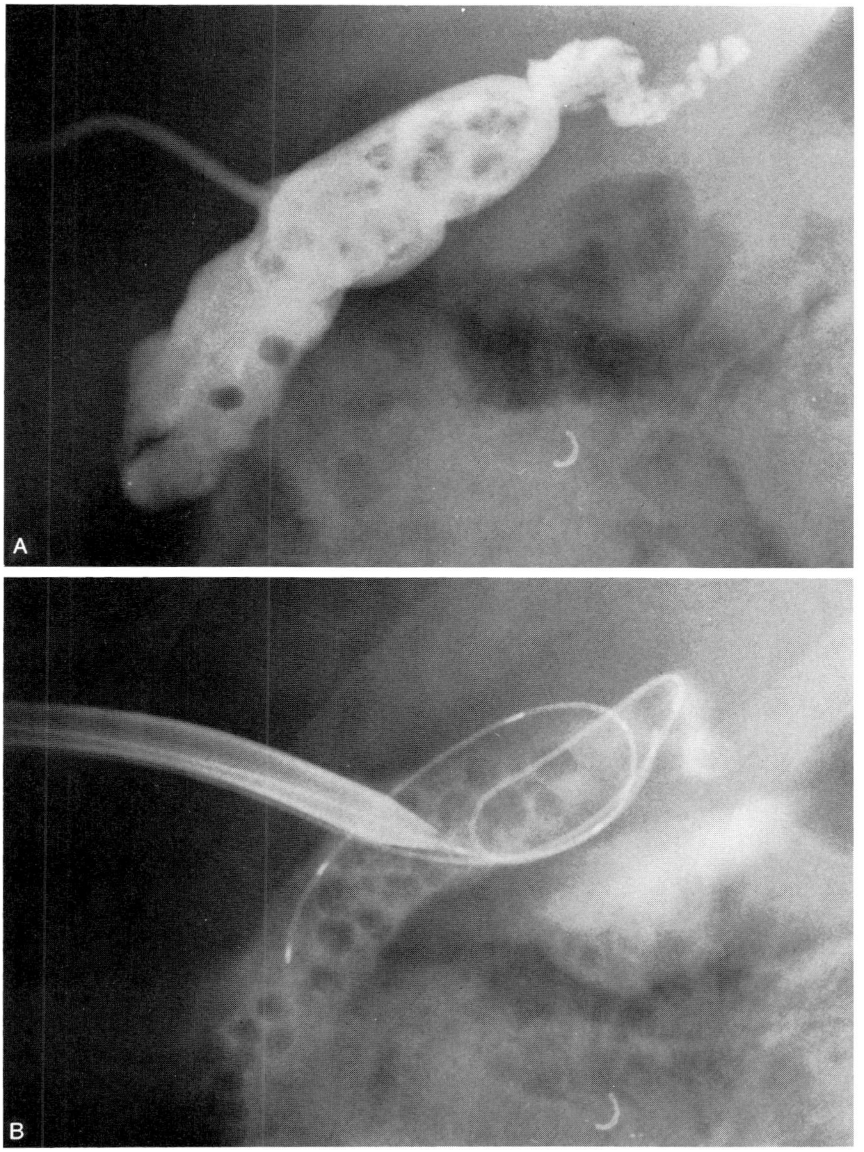

Figure 10–9. Percutaneous cholecystostomy and stone removal. *A*, A 12 French catheter has been inserted to drain the gallbladder of a 64-year-old woman with acute cholecystitis and advanced malignancy. *B*, After 1 week of drainage, the tract is dilated to a 24 French catheter.

Illustration continued on following page

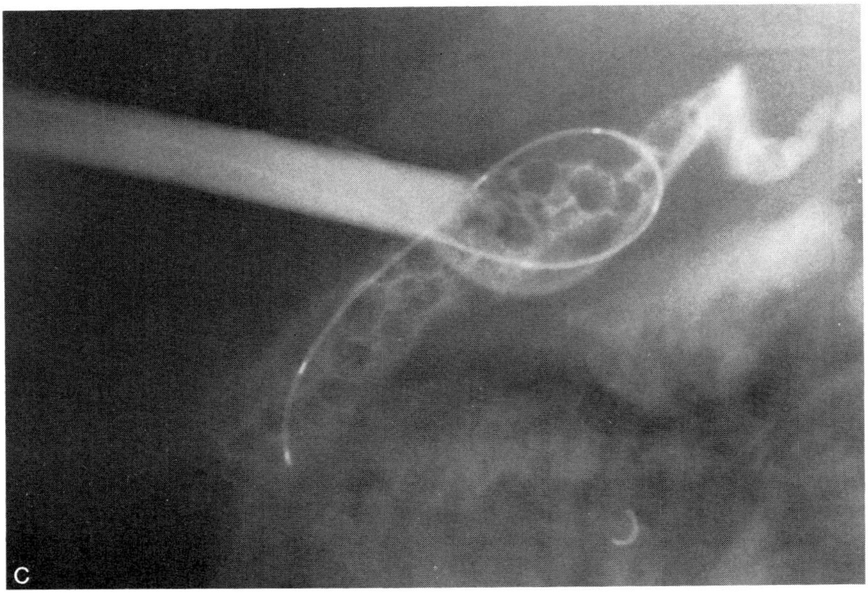

Figure 10–9 *Continued. C,* After 1 week of additional drainage and maturation of the tract, a 30 French sheath is passed through the percutaneous tract into the gallbladder. Stones can then be removed with a Dormia basket.

Results

The procedure is not technically difficult and is nearly always successful. In the largest series to date, it was accomplished without complications in 13 consecutive patients.[62] Four of five patients treated for acute cholecystitis had resolution of pain and sepsis. Temporary drainage was established in the remaining eight patients.

Complications

Bile leakage is rarely a major problem with percutaneous cholecystostomy when the catheter has been placed securely into the gallbladder. Fatal bile peritonitis has been reported in one patient, in whom the drainage catheter became dislodged outside the gallbladder. This complication can be avoided by secure fixation of the tube.

Sepsis, which is common in patients who are candidates for percutaneous cholecystostomy, may be transiently aggravated by the procedure. Therefore, contrast medium injections should be limited and used only to confirm catheter placement.

SUMMARY

A wide variety of therapeutic procedures involving the biliary tract can be performed under fluoroscopic guidance using surgical tracts or direct percutaneous punctures. The therapeutic procedures include removal of biliary calculi, establishment of external or internal biliary drainage, and dilatation of benign biliary strictures. These procedures generally entail less morbidity and mortality than do comparable surgical techniques.

We thank Gala FitzGerald for editorial assistance in manuscript preparation.

REFERENCES

1. Wendth AJ, Lieberman RC, Alpert M: Nonsurgical removal of a retained common bile duct calculus. Radiology 1972;*103*:207.
2. Mazzariello R: Review of 220 cases of residual biliary tract calculi treated without reoperation: An eight-year study. Surgery 1973;*73*:299.
3. Burhenne JH: Percutaneous extraction of retained biliary stones: 661 patients. AJR 1980;*134*:889.
4. Burhenne HL: Nonoperative roentgenologic instrumentation techniques of the post-operative biliary tract. Treatment of biliary stricture and retained stones. Am J Surg 1974;*128*:111.
5. Lear JL, et al: Percutaneous transhepatic electrohydraulic lithotripsy. Radiology 1984;*150*:260.
6. Burhenne HJ: Complications of nonoperative extraction of retained common duct stones. Am J Surg 1976;*131*:260.
7. Polack EP, Fainsinger NH, Bonnano SV: A death following complications of roentgenologic nonoperative manipulation of common bile duct calculi. Radiology 1977;*123*:585.
8. Crummy AB, Turnipseed WD: Percutaneous replacement of a biliary T-tube. AJR 1977;*128*:869.

9. Huard P, Do-Xuan-Hop: La ponction transhepatique des canaux biliaires. Bull Soc Med Chir Indoch 1937;*15*:1090.
10. Arner O, Hagberg S, Seldinger SI: Percutaneous transhepatic cholangiography: puncture of dilated and nondilated bile ducts under roentgen television control. Surgery 1962;*52*:561.
11. Drake CT, Beal JM: Percutaneous cholangiography. Arch Surg 1965;*91*:558.
12. Ferrucci JR Jr, Mueller PR, Harbin WP: Percutaneous transhepatic biliary drainage: technique, results and applications. Radiology 1980;*135*:1.
13. Thomas MJ, Pellegrini CA, Way LW: Usefulness of diagnostic tests for biliary obstruction. Am J Surg 1982;*144*:102.
14. Molnar W, Stockum AE: Relief of obstructive jaundice through percutaneous transhepatic catheter—a new therapeutic method. AJR 1974;*122*:356.
15. Hoevels J, Lunderquist A, Ihse I: Percutaneous transhepatic intubation of bile ducts for combined internal-external drainage in preoperative and palliative treatment of obstructive jaundice. Gastrointest Radiol 1978;*3*:23.
16. Ring EJ, Oleaga JA, Freiman DB, et al: Therapeutic applications of catheter cholangiography. Radiology 1978;*128*:333.
17. Kaude JV, Weidenheimer CH, Agee OF: Decompression of bile ducts with the percutaneous transhepatic technique. AJR 1969;*93*:59.
18. Tylen U, Hoevels J, Vang J: Percutaneous transhepatic cholangiography with external drainage of obstructive biliary lesions. Surg Gynecol Obstet 1977;*144*:13.
19. Norlander A, Kalin B, Sundblad R: Effect of percutaneous transhepatic drainage upon liver function and postoperative mortality. Surg Gynecol Obstet 1982;*155*:161.
20. Hatfield ARW, Terblanche J, Fataar S, et al: Preoperative external biliary drainage in obstructive jaundice. Lancet 1982;*2*:896.
21. Gundry SR, Strodel WE, Knol JA, et al: Efficacy of preoperative biliary tract decompression in patients with obstructive jaundice. Arch Surg 1984;*119*:703.
22. Braasch JW, Warren KW, Blevins PK: Progress in biliary stricture repair. Am J Surg 1975;*129*:34.
23. Warren KW, Mountain JC, Midell AL: Management of strictures of the biliary tract. Surg Clin North Am 1971;*51*:71.
24. Teplick SK, Goldstein RC, Richardson PA, et al: Percutaneous transhepatic choledochoplasty and dilatation of choledochoenterostomy strictures. JAMA 1980;*244*:1240.
25. Salomonowitz E, Castañeda-Zuniga WR, Lund G, et al: Balloon dilatation of benign biliary strictures. Radiology 1984;*151*:613.
26. Dow RW, Lindenauer SM: Acute obstructive suppurative cholangitis. Ann Surg 1969;*169*:272.
27. Ostermiller W Jr, Thompson RJ Jr, Carter R, et al: Acute obstructive cholangitis. Arch Surg 1965;*90*:392.
28. Boey JH, Way LW: Acute cholangitis. Ann Surg 1980;*191*:264.
29. Kadir S, Baassiui A, Barth KH: Percutaneous biliary drainage in the management of biliary sepsis. AJR 1982;*138*:25.
30. Safrany L, Coton PB: Endoscopic management of choledocholithiasis. Surg Clin North Am 1982; *62*:825.
31. Cotton PB, Vallon AG: British experience with duodenoscopic sphincterotomy for treatment of bile duct stones. Br J Surg 1981;*68*:373.
32. Safrany L: Endoscopic treatment of biliary tract diseases. Lancet 1978;*2*:983.
33. Oleaga JA, et al: Interventional biliary radiology. *In* Ring EJ, McLean GK (eds): Interventional Radiology: Principles and Techniques. Boston, Little Brown, 1981, p 301.
34. Martin EC, Fankuchen EL, Schultz RW, et al: Percutaneous dilatation in primary sclerosing cholangitis: two experiences. AJR 1981;*137*:603.
35. LaRusso NF, et al: Primary sclerosing cholangitis. N Engl J Med 1984;*310*:899.
36. Brooks JR, Culebras JM: Cancer of the pancreas: Palliative operations for carcinoma of the pancreas. Arch Surg 1971;*103*:330.
37. Buckwalter JA, Lawton RL, Tidrick RT: Bypass operations for neoplastic biliary tract obstruction. Am J Surg 1965;*109*:100.
38. Feduska NJ, Dent TL, Lindenauer SM: Results of palliative operations for carcinoma of the pancreas. Arch Surg 1971;*103*:330.
39. Mueller PR, van Sonnenberg E, Ferrucci JT: Percutaneous biliary drainage: technical and catheter related problems in 200 procedures. AJR 1982; *138*:17.
40. Braasch JW: Carcinoma of the bile duct. Surg Clin North Am 1973;*53*:1217.
41. Klatzkin G: Adenocarcinoma of the hepatic duct at its bifurcation within the porta hepatis: an unusual tumor with distinct clinical pathologic features. Am J Med 1965;*38*:241.
42. Terblanche J, Saunders SJ, Louw JH: Prolonged palliation in carcinoma of the main hepatic duct junction. Surgery 1972;*71*:720.
43. Pollock TW, Ring EJ, Oleaga A, et al: Percutaneous decompression of benign and malignant biliary obstruction. Arch Surg 1979;*114*:148.
44. Ferrucci JT, Mueller PR, Harbin WP: Percutaneous transhepatic biliary drainage. Radiology 1980;*135*:1.
45. Greenfield AJ: Percutaneous biliary drainage. *In* Athanasoulis CA (ed): Interventional Radiology. Philadelphia, WB Saunders, 1982, p 550.
46. Clark RA, Mitchell SE, Colley DP, et al: Percutaneous catheter biliary decompression. AJR 1981; *137*:503.
47. Pellegrini CA, Thomas MJ, Way LW: Bilirubin and alkaline phosphatase values before and after surgery for biliary obstruction. Am J Surg 1982;*143*:67.
48. Ferrucci JT, et al: Percutaneous biliary drainage. *In* Ferrucci JT, Wittenberg J (eds): Interventional Radiology of the Abdomen. Baltimore, Williams & Wilkins, 1981, p 87.
49. Dawson SL, Neff CC, Mueller PR, et al: Fatal hemothorax after inadvertent transpleural biliary drainage. AJR 1983;*141*:33.
50. Oleaga JA, Ring EJ, Freiman DB, et al: Extension of neoplasm along the tract of a transhepatic tube. AJR 1980;*135*:841.
51. Miller GA Jr, Heaston DK, Moore AV Jr, et al: Peritoneal seeding of cholangiocarcinoma in patients with percutaneous biliary drainage. AJR 1983;*141*:561.
52. Pereiras RV Jr, Rheingold OJ, Hutson D, et al: Relief of malignant obstructive jaundice by percutaneous insertion of a permanent prosthesis in the biliary tree. Ann Intern Med 1978;*89*:589.
53. Ring EJ, Schwarz W, McLean GK, et al: A simple, indwelling biliary endoprosthesis made from commonly available catheter material. AJR 1982; *139*:615.
54. Hoevels J, Lunderquist A, Owman T, et al: A large-bore Teflon endoprosthesis with side holes for non-

operative decompression of the biliary tract in malignant obstructive jaundice. Gastrointest Radiol 1980;*5*:361.

55. Coons HG, Carey PH: Large-bore, long biliary endoprostheses (biliary stents) for improved drainage. Radiology 1983;*148*:89.

56. Soehendia N, Reynders-Frederix V: Palliative bile duct drainage—a new endoscopic method of introducing a transpapillary drain. Endoscopy 1980;*12*:8.

57. Zimmon DS: Endoscopic diagnosis and management of biliary and pancreatic disease. Curr Probl Surg 1979;*16*:3.

58. Zimmon DS, Clemett AR: Endoscopic stents and drains in the management of pancreatic and bile duct obstruction. Surg Clin North Am 1982;*62*:837.

59. Kerlan RK Jr, et al: Biliary endoprosthesis: insertion using a combined peroral-transhepatic method. Radiology 1984;*150*:828.

60. Burkhardt H, Mueller W: Versuche uber die Punktion der Gallenblase und ihre Roentgen-darstellung. Deut Zschr Chiwig 1921;*161*:168.

61. Elyaderani M, Gabriele OF: Percutaneous cholecystostomy and cholangiography in patients with obstructive jaundice. Radiology 1979;*130*:601.

62. Shaver RW, Hawkins IF, Soong J: Percutaneous cholecystostomy. AJR 1982;*138*:1133.

HOWARD SHAPIRO, M.D.

11

Endoscopic Retrograde Cholangiography

Endoscopic retrograde cholangiopancreatography (ERCP) was first described in 1968 by McCune et al.,[1] but its widespread use awaited the availability of new duodenoscopes in 1970. Within 2 years there were worldwide reports on the use of this new duodenoscope to facilitate the radiographic visualization of the pancreatic duct and biliary tree.[2–8] The pioneer investigators' initial concern was with the technical feasibility of ERCP. It soon became apparent that it was adequate: As early as 1972 most major groups worldwide were reporting success rates of 70 to 90 per cent in visualizing the desired duct system.[9–13] Historically the next major concern was with the safety of ERCP. In 1975 and 1976, two excellent surveys reported an acceptably low complication rate in experienced hands.[14, 15] With improvement in equipment and radiologic techniques, ERCP today is capable of providing detailed and accurate information regarding the anatomy of the biliary tract and pancreas that is often invaluable in the planning of operations in these sites.

TECHNIQUE

Instruments

The endoscopic equipment has changed very little since the introduction of the long, side-viewing duodenoscope. The major improvement has been an increase in the arc of tip deflection. This aids in selective cannulation of the two ductal systems. The most recent models have an insulated tip that increases the safety of electrosurgery (endoscopic retrograde sphincterotomy). Standard adult forward-viewing and oblique lens panendoscopes are not suitable except following choledochoduodenostomy, when the anastomosis is encountered en face on the posterior wall of the duodenal bulb, or following Billroth II gastrojejunostomy, when the papilla is approached from below via the afferent loop.[16–18]

Instrument damage is inevitable and adds to the cost of ERCP. The tip deflector guide wires and cannula elevator are subject to breakage. Radiation damage to the fiberoptic bundles is inevitable and requires periodic replacement of these bundles.

Miniature color television cameras that permit large audiences to view the endoscopic portion of ERCP are available. This is an invaluable teaching aid for conferences as well as small tutorial groups and has enabled more rapid training of endoscopists in this rather difficult technique. Videotape recording allows permanent documentation of endoscopic findings.

The catheter system has changed little over the past decade. The basic 1.6 mm, 180 cm Teflon catheter has been improved with the addition of graduated tip markings that accurately gauge the depth of cannulation and act as an endoscopic measuring stick. A permanent guide wire within the cannula improves its durability, aids in its maneuverability, and helps prevent the injection of air into the ductal systems. Incorporation of a manometer in the injection system has been recommended as a safety feature but is not in common use.[19]

Medication

Some degree of sedation is important; we use diazepam and meperidine given intravenously to the point of cooperative somnolence.[20] In the elderly and frail the medication must be given slowly in small increments to prevent cardiorespiratory complications.[21] After the endoscope has entered the duodenum, ileus is imperative. Anticholinergic agents have been the standard in producing duodenal atony. However, in the past 5 years our preference has been to administer small intravenous increments of glucagon (0.2 mg) to attain this end and thereby avoid anticholinergic side effects.[23]

Endoscopic Technique[24]

Any skilled endoscopist can learn to use the lateral viewing duodenoscope for visualization of the distal stomach and proximal duodenum. In some cases, such as for lesions of the lesser curvature of the antrum or medial wall of the descending duodenum, the side-viewing duodenoscope is superior to the standard end-viewing endoscope. The major factor in becoming expert in ERCP is having a sufficient number of patients to learn the technique and then to maintain expertise. This requires the endoscopist to be affiliated with a major tertiary care hospital. Such a hospital will provide an adequately equipped x-ray suite and a trained gastrointestinal radiologist, both necessary supports for quality films and interpretations. These, after all, are the final determinants of successful ERCP.

After adequate sedation is achieved, the side-viewing duodenoscope is passed, with the patient lying in the left lateral decubitus position. Once the tip is in the stomach, air is inflated to distend it and enhance the view. Generally the first structure visualized is the angulus. With the tip flexed, the fundus and body of the stomach can be inspected. With the tip extended, the antrum and pylorus are usually easily brought into view. The duodenoscope is advanced with the pylorus in center view. When it is close, the tip of the duodenoscope is straightened and the scope advanced into the duodenal bulb. The junction of the bulb and descending duodenum is generally directly posterior; by rotation of the duodenoscope clockwise through 90 to 180 degrees the tip usually enters the descending duodenum with ease. At this point the patient is turned prone, and by rotation of the scope counterclockwise to the 12 o'clock position, a tubular view of the descending duodenum is obtained.

Although the papilla of Vater is generally located on the posteromedial wall of the middle third of the descending duodenum, variability in its location is to be expected, and it may be found anywhere on the medial wall of the descending duodenum. It may vary in configuration from flat to protuberant, and it often has a hoodlike covering in continuity with a circular fold (see Chapter 25, Fig. 25–3). Generally, however, it is found at the superior aspect of a vertical fold. Often, the cephalic intramural portion of the common bile duct appears as a prominent intraduodenal bulge.

One should not attempt to introduce the cannula until an "en face" view of the papilla is obtained. This can be done in two ways. One may continue to introduce a greater length of duodenoscope into the patient, thus forming a large loop along the greater curvature of the stomach. Ultimately the tip of the duodenoscope advances to an "en face" view of the ampulla. This position has the disadvantage of decreased tip mobility and sluggishness of response to the biplane tip deflection controls. In addition, it allows more of the duodenoscope to be exposed to radiation damage. A preferred maneuver is to straighten the scope by hooking the tip upward toward the papilla and slowly pulling out the scope. This reduces the intragastric loop and allows the scope to lie along the lesser curvature of the stomach. As the straightening maneuver is started the tip of the scope will frequently advance. Then by gentle withdrawal the papilla will again come into view, with about 60 cm of the instrument remaining in the patient. This latter position affords more sensitive control of the distal tip and reduces radiation exposure to the instrument.

With the papilla viewed "en face," the cannula is introduced into the papillary orifice. This introduction is facilitated by finely adjusting the biplane controls, instrument depth, and cannula elevator. The pancreatic duct is entered more readily than the common bile duct. If cholangiography is desired, an attempt should be made to place the cannula in the roof of the papilla, bowed so that it is angled upward toward the liver. Eighty per cent of the time a common channel will be encountered, but this may be as short as 1 mm. Frequently a septum divides the two ducts, and the bile duct will be more cephalad. Initially, success rates of 70 per cent were reported for selective cholangiography; today, in experienced hands, this should be near 90 per cent. However, occasionally even experts fail.

Failures are usually associated with major pathology or previous surgery. Prior Billroth II gastrectomy lowers the success rate, but ERCP is usually possible with a forward-viewing scope advanced into the afferent loop.[17, 18] Periampullary duodenal diverticula pose no barrier unless the papilla is actually within the diverticulum. Tumor involvement of the papilla or impacted common duct stones may result in radiologic failure, but the endoscopic appearance is generally diagnostic. In patients with a prior choledochoduodenostomy the anastomosis is usually easily accessible with the forward-viewing duodenoscope. Following sphincteroplasty or sphincterotomy, common duct cannulation is enhanced, but it may be difficult to obtain a pancreatogram.

Radiologic Technique[25]

The endoscopist and radiologist must work together to obtain the best possible radiographs. This requires first-rate fluoroscopic and radiographic equipment and adequate space for personnel and endoscopic equipment. Optimally the radiologist and endoscopist form a closely integrated team, sensitive to one another's needs with a minimum of words. This sets the stage for obtaining high-quality radiographs. Interpretation of technically perfect films can be difficult, and an inferior radiograph may render the entire procedure useless. Standard water-soluble contrast material is used; there is no evidence that any particular contrast material is better than another. Whatever contrast agent is used should be diluted 50 per cent if a dilated bile duct is encountered. If the contrast is too concentrated, small filling defects may be missed. The radiology table must tilt from upright to at least 15 per cent reverse Trendelenburg. This permits erect films, which are essential in layering gallstones or floating inadvertently injected air bubbles. Trendelenburg films are helpful in filling the intrahepatic biliary radicles. The volume of contrast material injected varies according to duct size and depth of cannulation. Enough dye is injected to provide excellent radiographs as judged by careful fluoroscopic monitoring of the injection process.

CONTRAINDICATIONS

Contraindications are few. The uncooperative patient is an absolute contraindication to ERCP. Such a patient can cause irreparable damage to himself, the duodenoscope, or the endoscopist. Should this situation be encountered, one should give additional sedatives or abandon the procedure. The remainder of the contraindications are relative and depend on a clinical judgment as to whether the information gained is worth the risks involved. Patients with cardiac or pulmonary disease are at risk from the medication given and must be monitored closely. Cannulation in patients with acute pancreatitis used to be thought of as hazardous. Several studies have now reported that the incidence of complication is minimal even in patients with an attack of pancreatitis.[26–28] Acute hepatitis A, B, or non-A, non-B is not a contraindication.[29, 30] Recent epidemiologic studies have failed to substantiate a single case of endoscope-transmitted hepatitis. The duodenoscope, however, should be thoroughly cleaned following suspected exposure. Allergy to iodinated dye is an indication rather than a contraindication for ERCP. In the study of ERCP complications published by Bilbao et al. in 1976, mild urticarial reaction to contrast material occurred in only 3 of 8861 patients.[15]

COMPLICATIONS

The best means of avoiding the complications of ERCP is not to do it. The best way to encourage the complications of ERCP is to do it infrequently. Once committed to performing ERCP, the best way to minimize complications is to do as many procedures as possible. It has been shown quite clearly that the complication rate falls dramatically with operator experience.[15, 31, 32] The clear implication of this finding is that ERCP should be performed only in major medical centers. The potential complications relate to medication, endoscopy, cannulation, and injection of contrast agent.[14, 15] In experienced hands, a complication rate of 1 to 3 per cent may be anticipated, with a mortality rate of 0.1 per cent. The major complications are pancreatitis and sepsis.

The serum amylase value frequently increases to significant levels following successful pancreatography.[33] When looked for, this occurs in 25 to 75 per cent of patients. It is generally asymptomatic, and the amylase level returns to normal in 1 to 4 days. Severe abdominal pain with the clinical picture of acute pancreatitis is rare, occurring in approximately 2 per cent of ERCPs.[31, 32, 34] Fortunately, this generally is mild, and in the Bilbao survey there were no deaths reported in 94 cases of pancreatitis following ERCP. This complication usually occurs in patients with recurrent pancreatitis. Clinical pancreatitis generally follows successful filling of the pancreatic duct and probably results from parenchymal overfilling. Accordingly, the pressure and volume of pancreatic duct filling must be carefully monitored. This may be done by injecting slowly, with constant fluoroscopic monitoring of duct filling. Injection should stop as soon as the secondary branch ducts are seen clearly.

Pancreatic sepsis is a lethal complication, with an incidence of 0.3 per cent. In the 25 patients reported in Bilbao's survey, 8 had partial duct obstruction and 17 had pseudocysts. The death rate was an alarming 20 per cent. If partial duct obstruction or pseudocyst is encountered, high-dose antibiotic coverage should be initiated immediately and early decompressive surgery urged. It has been our practice to screen all patients with relapsing pancreatitis and suspected pseudocyst with abdominal sonography or computerized tomographic scan prior to ERCP. These modalities are quite sensitive to the presence of a pseudocyst or even a dilated pancreatic duct.[35, 36] Then, if ERCP is deemed necessary, it can be performed just prior to definitive surgery. No attempt should be made to outline the cyst in its entirety. We have not been inclined to add antibiotics to the contrast medium, although this has been recommended by some.[37, 38]

Cholangitis is a relatively frequent complication (0.8 per cent) of ERCP but almost always occurs in the presence of a partially obstructed bile duct. The clinical onset of cholangitis may be delayed as much as 72 hours following the procedure. Although opinions to the contrary have been expressed,[39] it is our practice to administer parenteral broad-spectrum antibiotics to patients suspected of having dilated intrahepatic ducts by pre-ERCP noninvasive techniques, such as CT scan or abdominal sonography, and to those patients found to have a blocked bile duct in the process of ERCP. If a blocked duct is anticipated, pre-ERCP surgical consultation should be obtained, with definitive decompression planned for the following 24 to 48 hours. If there is choledocholithiasis, immediate endoscopic sphincterotomy and stone extraction will be curative.[21, 32] When strictures are encountered, just enough contrast medium should be injected to document the disordered anatomy and aid in the planning of definitive surgery. There is no compelling need to use antibiotics in the contrast medium. If one follows these guidelines, the incidence of cholangitis should be diminished appreciably.

Cardiopulmonary complications, instrument injuries, and drug reactions should become extremely rare as one becomes more experienced and less medication is required in the performance of ERCP.

The most significant complication of ERCP is an erroneous interpretation of the radiographs obtained.[40] This complication concerns the major worth of this diagnostic procedure and will be considered in the next section.

DIAGNOSTIC VALUE

ERCP has greatly improved the diagnostic accuracy in almost all biliary tract disorders.[21] In the differentiation of surgical from nonsurgical biliary tract disease, the demonstration of a normal cholangiogram may prevent needless operations. Perhaps the greatest value of ERCP is reducing the number of "exploratory" laparotomies. Fortunately, radiographs of the biliary tree are familiar to radiologists and clinicians, and their interpretation usually poses no problem. However, in order to recognize the abnormal, one must have standards of normality.

The Normal Cholangiogram (Fig. 11–1)

Lasser et al. evaluated the endoscopic cholangiograms of 49 patients with normal cholangiograms and liver function tests and 25 patients with known liver disease but normal extrahepatic ducts.[41] They found that the normal mean maximum duct width is 4.6 mm and that the upper limit of normal is 9 mm. There is no significant difference in the duct diameter, whether it be in the intrapancreatic portion just distal to the insertion of the cystic duct or between the cystic duct and the bifurcation. They found a slight increase in the common hepatic duct size with increased age and in patients with significant liver disease. Belsito et al., in comparing common bile duct diameters as measured by intravenous cholangiography and ERCP in

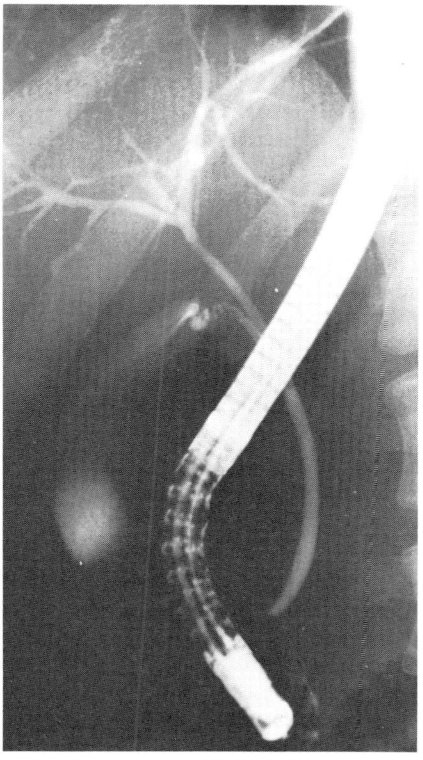

Figure 11–1. Normal cholangiogram. The common duct is of uniform caliber throughout. Good visualization of right and left hepatic ducts and their secondary branches has been obtained. The gallbladder is not completely filled.

29 patients with normal and abnormal biliary trees, found that the measurements consistently are approximately 3 mm greater on ERCP.[42]

On occasion, there is difficulty in visualizing both hepatic ducts during ERCP. This may be due to patient position, the greater specific gravity of the contrast medium with respect to bile, or inadequate filling pressure during technically difficult cannulation. If this problem is encountered, rotating the patient in a longitudinal axis or placing him in a head-down position may aid in its resolution.[25] If the cystic duct is patent, gallbladder filling should occur in an adequate cannulation (Fig. 11–2). Nonfilling suggests cystic duct obstruction but should be interpreted with caution unless one is certain that the cannulation and filling pressures are technically correct.

The common bile duct does not dilate following cholecystectomy, and in interpreting large-diameter postcholecystectomy bile ducts, comparison with an operative cholangiogram is most helpful.[43] If, indeed, on ERCP there has been postoperative dilatation, there may be partial common bile duct obstruction.[44] A helpful maneuver in this situation is to obtain delayed films, since a normal postcholecystectomy bile duct should completely drain in 30 to 45 minutes. Delay beyond this time suggests obstruction. The presence of a gallbladder invalidates any assessment of drainage time, since it provides a reservoir that may retain dye for hours.

Interpretations of abnormalities of the distal 1 to 2 cm of common bile duct are often equivocal. A prominent contraction of the sphincter of Boyden may mimic a stone. Continued fluoroscopic observation of the distal bile duct after the cannula has been removed allows one to observe periodic sphincter relaxation and thus avoid this pitfall. Benign webs in this area may mimic tumor. The common bile duct and pancreatic duct join to form a common channel in approximately 80 per cent of cases, but the length of the channel may vary from 1 to 17 mm.[45] In one patient we have observed this channel to be 2.8 cm in length.

Patients with Jaundice

ERCP facilitates the anatomic diagnosis in many patients with cholestatic jaundice.[9, 10, 12, 13, 46–49] Its precise role in relation to other

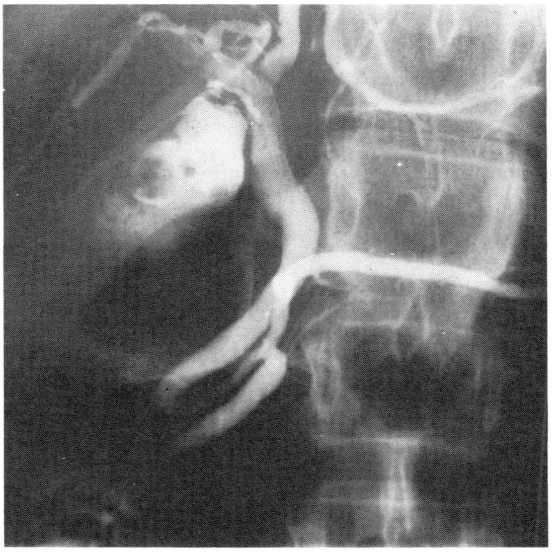

Figure 11–2. Gallstones. There are multiple radiolucencies in the gallbladder. The normal common duct is partially obscured by a normal pancreatic duct that was filled via a common channel.

diagnostic tests, such as abdominal sonography, computerized tomographic (CT) scan, isotope scans, and percutaneous transhepatic cholangiography (PTC), is discussed in Chapter 13. Intravenous cholangiography is of limited use in nonjaundiced patients (see Chapter 7); it generally lacks sufficient definition to rule out gallstones or tumor with confidence.[50] Its major virtue is simplicity. It is of no use in the clinically jaundiced patient. Abdominal sonography can generally detect dilated intrahepatic bile ducts, dilatation of the gallbladder, and stones within the gallbladder.[35, 51, 52] It may be helpful in demonstrating a pancreatic mass lesion[53] and in assessing the size of the extrahepatic biliary tree. Its interpretation is totally dependent on the expertise of the technician and radiologist. CT scans are equally sensitive in detecting intrahepatic duct or gallbladder dilatation and more sensitive in demonstrating pancreatic mass lesions.[36, 54–56] Localization of the exact level of extrahepatic duct obstruction is often difficult. Isotopic scans of the liver and pancreas are helpful to define mass lesions within the liver but are not accurate in detecting dilatation of the bile ducts unless this process is far advanced.

Because of the relative lack of precision of these noninvasive tests, we generally use them for preliminary screening of patients with cholestatic jaundice and follow with direct cholangiography. If dilated bile ducts are found, PTC will be successful in localizing the level of obstruction in approximately 80 to 90 per cent of cases and may allow placement of stents or preoperative biliary drainage.[47, 57] If the bile ducts are not dilated, PTC is less likely to be successful.[58] ERCP succeeds in visualizing the biliary tree in 75 to 90 per cent of cases, independent of dilatation of the ducts. ERCP has the additional benefit of being safe in patients with bleeding diatheses or allergy to iodinated dyes; of gathering supplemental information in the direct visualization (with biopsy potential) of the distal stomach, duodenal sweep, and papilla of Vater; and of allowing the simultaneous visualization of the pancreatic duct.[59]

The specific radiologic tests employed are dependent on the facilities of the hospital and the expertise of the personnel available to perform these procedures. This will vary from center to center, so no absolute priorities can be given, only general principles. As a rule, however, one cannot rest with the supposition that the bile duct is probably dilated or probably not dilated. One should attempt to define clearly the anatomy of the biliary tree and the level of the obstruction, if present. We have frequently had the experience of seeing partial or even complete bile duct obstruction in the presence of a nondilated biliary tree. If this scheme is followed, a precise diagnosis will be made in several days rather than several weeks and appropriate medical or surgical therapy will follow.

Diseases of the Intrahepatic Biliary Tract[59–67]

Although the primary intent of ERCP was to evaluate extrahepatic biliary obstruction, it has proved useful in the evaluation of the intrahepatic ducts as well. In order to make valid interpretations, complete filling of the biliary tree is essential, since underfilling can produce artifacts that simulate disease. If there are abnormalities, one can assume severe disease to be present; a normal intrahepatic cholangiogram does not exclude minimal or moderate disease. The abnormalities may be nonspecific and must be interpreted in light of the clinical setting. "Blind" reading of the radiographs is likely to be erroneous.

Sclerosing cholangitis may occur in its primary form or, more commonly, in association with ulcerative colitis. Although originally described as involving the extrahepatic bile ducts, primarily intrahepatic involvement has been seen in increasing numbers of patients. The lesion is similar in both areas and consists of irregular beading of the ducts due to the diffuse presence of strictures. The sclerosing process may progress to the total obliteration of major ducts. Large sacculations may be seen proximal to tight strictures. A shaggy, irregular contour to the common bile duct as well as to its branches is usual (Fig. 11–3).

Hepatic cirrhosis produces cholangiographic changes in advanced disease. These consist of intrahepatic duct tortuosity and crowding due to reduced liver volume and areas of focal duct stenosis with proximal dilatation (Fig. 11–4). They are secondary to fibrosis and nodular regeneration. In primary biliary cirrhosis, the liver may be massively enlarged. We have seen one case of selective enlargement of the caudate lobe causing total obstruction of the bile duct at its bifurcation, simulating tumor. In cirrhosis the extrahepatic biliary tree is normal unless there is associated disease, such as gallstones.

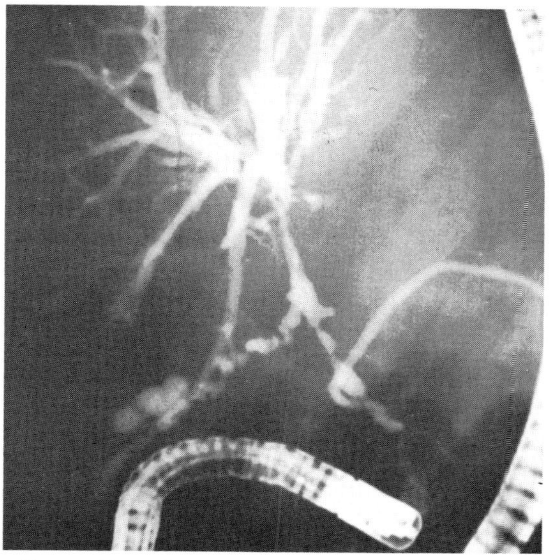

Figure 11–3. Sclerosing cholangitis. There is irregular beading and dilation throughout the biliary tree The intrahepatic ducts are moderately dilated secondary to irregular stricture formation, which is especially prominent in the proximal common bile duct. The sclerotic process also involves the cystic duct and gallbladder. The pancreatic duct filled via a common channel and is normal.

Cholangiocarcinoma of the intrahepatic ducts may involve only the right or left hepatic duct but more commonly involves both at the level of the bifurcation of the common duct. The cholangiographic appearance is that of an irregular stenosis (Fig. 11–5). If incomplete, proximal bile duct dilatation may be apparent.

Hepatoma will displace, invade, or encase the intrahepatic bile ducts. There may be dilatation proximal to a partially obstructing lesion. ERCP may be of value in the preoperative determination of extent of disease.

Metastatic lesions produce cholangiographic abnormalities only if they are of sufficient size or if they directly impinge on the intrahepatic bile ducts. The cholangiographic changes include displacement, encasement, stenosis, obstruction, and separation.

The changes associated with sarcoidosis, amyloidosis, parasitic diseases, and other infiltrative or inflammatory diseases have not yet been adequately defined.

Diseases of the Extrahepatic Biliary Tract

Gallstones

Choledocholithiasis with or without an intact gallbladder is the most common cause of extrahepatic bile duct obstruction. The bile duct may be dilated or normal even in the

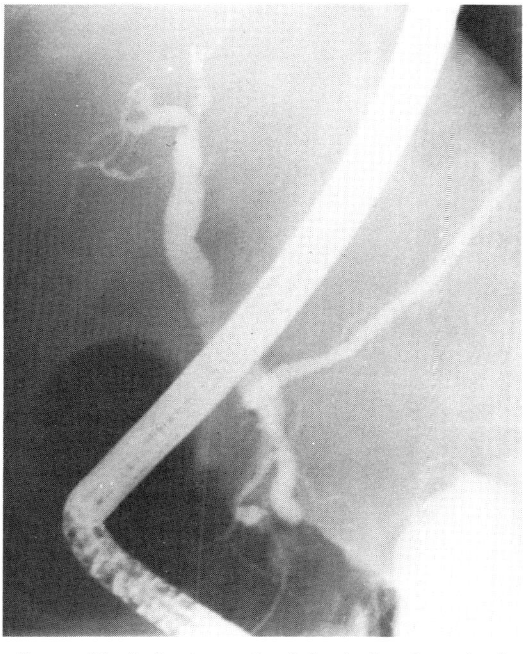

Figure 11–4. Postnecrotic cirrhosis. Intrahepatic duct crowding and tortuosity are due to reduced liver volume. The common bile duct and pancreatic duct are normal. The gallbladder is absent.

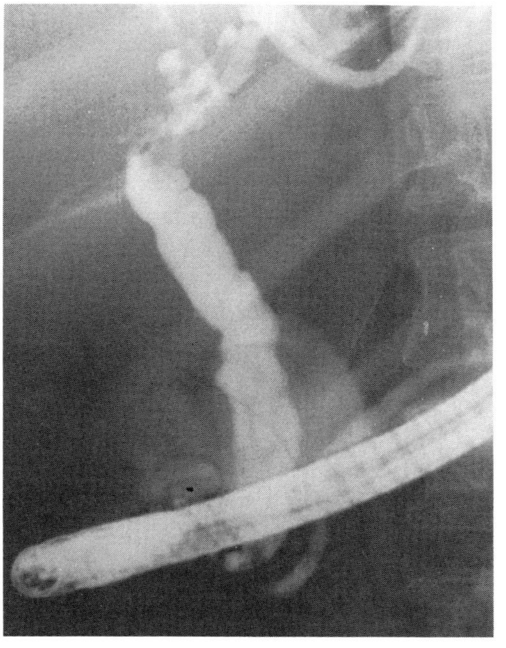

Figure 11–5. Carcinoma of the bifurcation of the common duct. There is an intraluminal mass in the proximal bile duct that partially obstructs the left hepatic duct and totally occludes the right hepatic duct. The pancreatic duct is normal. The gallbladder has been removed.

presence of marked jaundice. When it is not dilated, it is a major cause of false negative interpretations of abdominal sonography or CT scans. This lends emphasis to the point previously made that these techniques serve only to screen and must be followed by definitive cholangiography. Scarring from recurrent cholangitis is a common reason for the failure of a duct to dilate in the presence of obstruction; however, we have seen this situation in the absence of a history suggestive of cholangitis. Stones vary in number, size, and contour. They may be faceted or smooth. If smooth, they may be difficult to distinguish from air bubbles (Fig. 11–6). In general, changing the patient's position to include erect films makes the differentiation possible, since bubbles float up into the intrahepatic tree and stones generally wash down when the cannula is removed (Fig. 11–7).[25] If a filling defect with a smooth meniscus is encountered, every effort should be made to visualize the proximal bile duct to better define the defect. We have seen tumors with smooth distal menisci simulating stones. Now that endoscopic retrograde sphincterotomy and stone extraction have become the treatment of choice for patients with common duct stones, it seems reasonable to perform ERCP rather than PTC as the definitive diagnostic test.[68–71] The sphincterotomy can be performed immediately following the diagnostic cannulation. (For further details on endoscopic sphincterotomy see Chapter 25.) Concomitant stricture or tumor must be excluded. They may coexist with gallstones and may be the primary cause of obstructive jaundice.

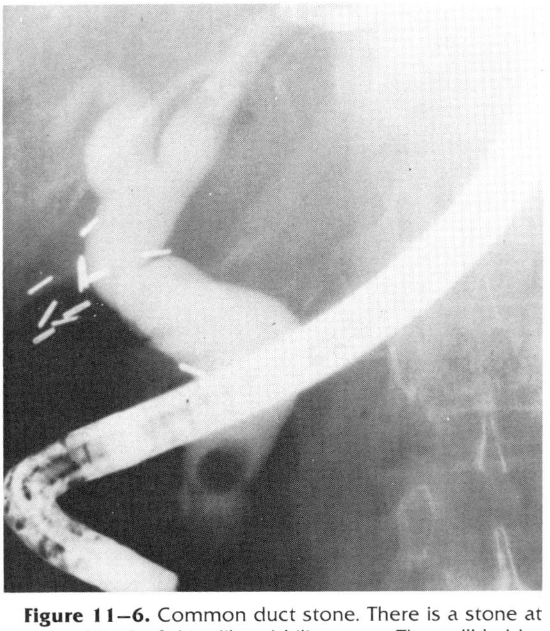

Figure 11–6. Common duct stone. There is a stone at the distal end of this dilated biliary tree. The gallbladder has been removed.

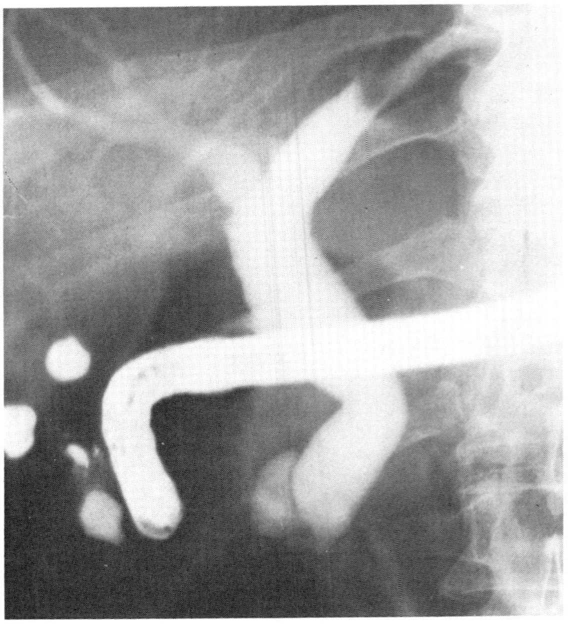

Figure 11–7. Common duct stone. This stone has been displaced into the left hepatic duct, a common consequence of forceful injection of contrast material into the distal duct.

Strictures[72, 73]

These may be benign or malignant and may cause total or incomplete obstruction of the common bile duct. The degree of duct dilatation bears no steady relationship with either the degree or the duration of the obstruction. This, as in the case of common duct stone, has led us to reserve judgment on a "negative" CT scan or abdominal sonogram, since nondilated intrahepatic ducts can be found in patients with a high degree of common duct obstruction.

Strictures of the mid-duct are almost always malignant if there has been no prior biliary tract surgery or trauma. Those due to cholangiocarcinoma generally have an abrupt cutoff or a "rat-tailed" appearance (Fig. 11–8). Those due to metastatic disease of the porta hepatis (Fig. 11–9), lymphoma, or locally invasive carcinoma of the pancreas or gallbladder are generally more smoothly ta-

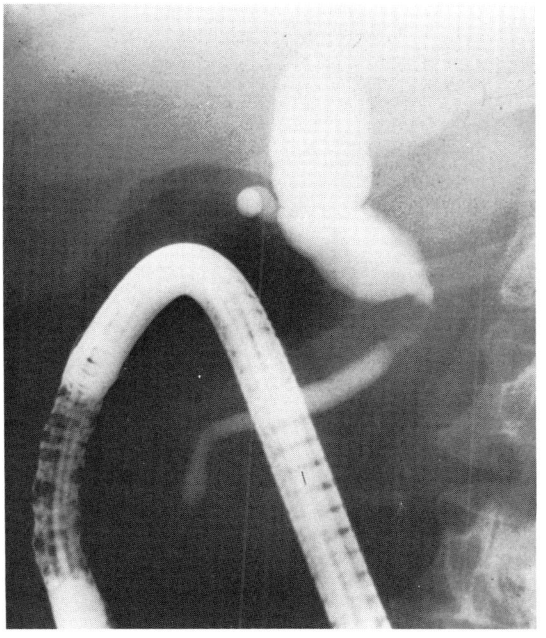

Figure 11–8. Cholangiocarcinoma. There is an irregular stricture of the mid–common duct with proximal duct dilatation. A small cystic duct remnant is present.

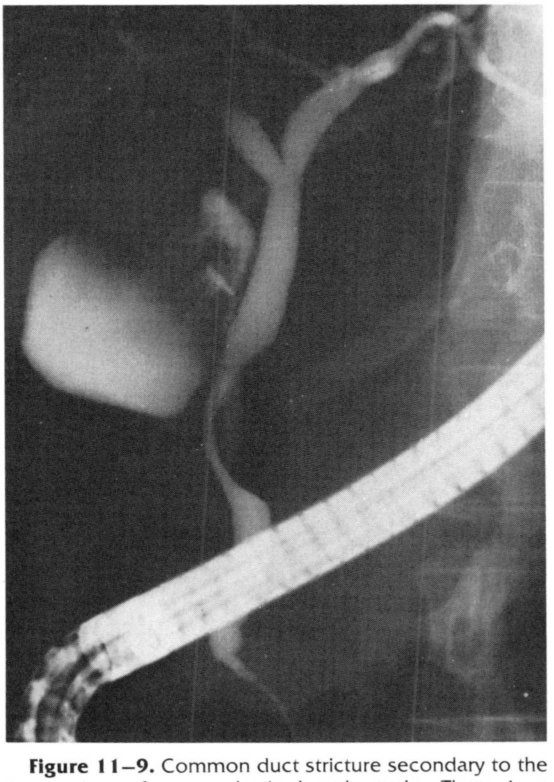

Figure 11–9. Common duct stricture secondary to the impression of a neoplastic lymph node. There is a smoothly tapered mid-duct stricture with lateral displacement of the lumen. Despite obstructive jaundice, the caliber of the intrahepatic and proximal common bile ducts is normal and the gallbladder is not enlarged.

pered. If there has been prior biliary tract surgery, the most common cause of mid-duct stricture is secondary to that surgery; its appearance may be smoothly tapered (Fig. 11–10) or abrupt with sharp margins. The distinction from malignant stricture on radiographic interpretation alone may be difficult (Fig. 11–11).

There are several criteria to differentiate benign from malignant strictures of the distal common duct. However, these are not strictly defined. One cannot rely on criteria of length, symmetry, contour, or margin irregularity. We have seen benign strictures that appeared malignant and malignant strictures that appeared benign. An attempt to obtain a simultaneous pancreatogram is mandatory, for this often assists in the establishment of a correct differential diagnosis. Changes on the pancreatogram consistent with carcinoma of the pancreas suggest encasement or direct tumor extension when there is a distal bile duct stricture (Figs. 11–12 and 11–13). Concomitant changes of chronic pancreatitis (Fig. 11–14) or the presence of a pseudocyst (Fig. 11–15) suggest a benign stricture.

In carcinoma of the papilla of Vater the diagnosis will be apparent on endoscopy and will be confirmed by target biopsy. In some patients it may be necessary to perform a

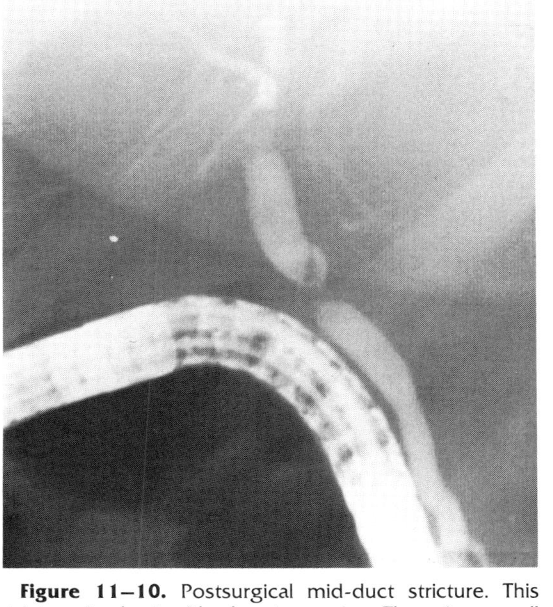

Figure 11–10. Postsurgical mid-duct stricture. This stricture is short with abrupt margins. There is a small stone proximal to the stricture. Despite intense obstructive jaundice at the time of this study the caliber of the intrahepatic and proximal bile ducts is normal.

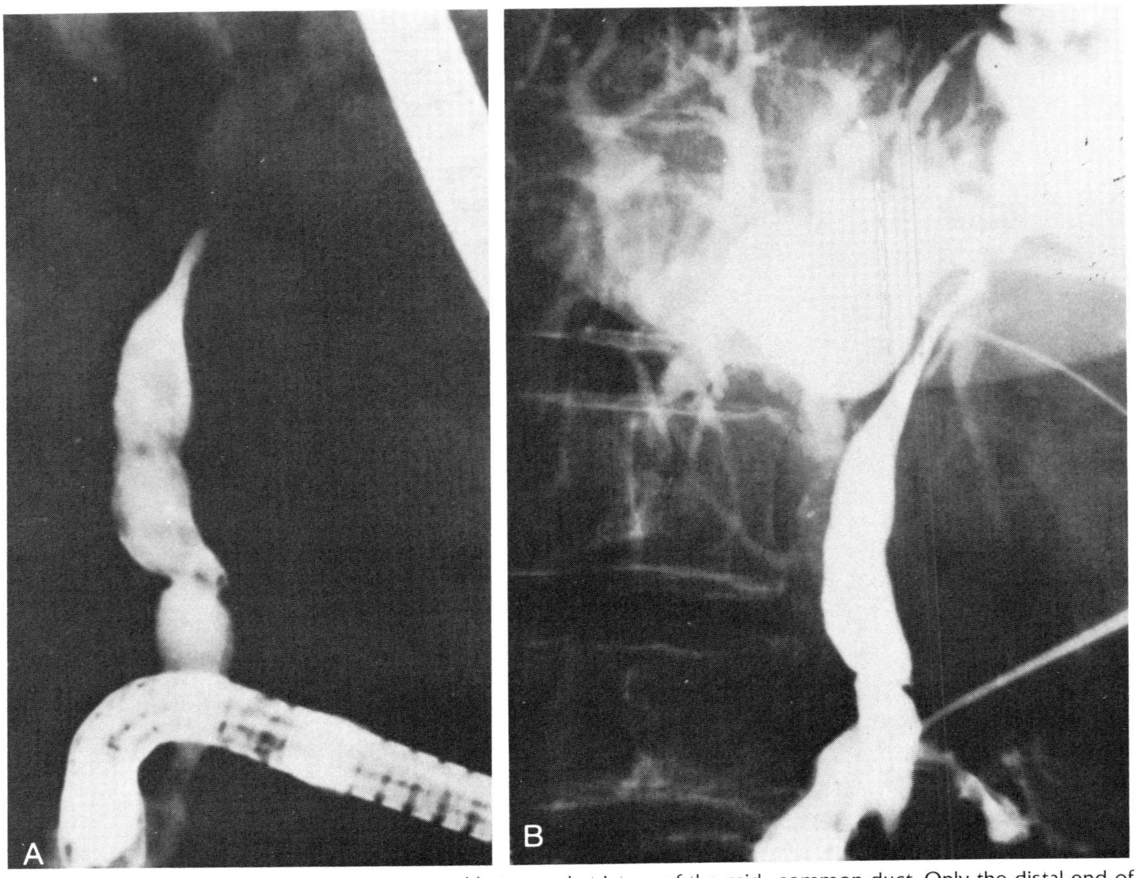

Figure 11–11. *A*, ERC demonstrating a smoothly tapered stricture of the mid–common duct. Only the distal end of the stricture is visualized. *B*, PTC demonstrating massively dilated intrahepatic ducts and the proximal end of the benign stricture. These radiographs were obtained within 10 minutes of one another and, in a complementary way, completely defined the pathologic anatomy.

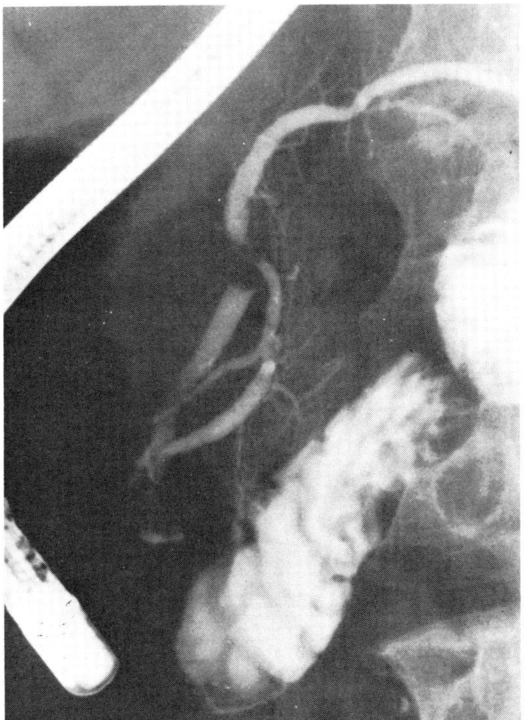

Figure 11–12. Carcinoma of the pancreas. The intrapancreatic portion of the common bile duct is completely obstructed. If the cholangiogram were seen alone, the sharp meniscus of the obstructing lesion would suggest a common duct stone. The pancreatogram, however, demonstrated a small intraluminal defect quite close to the common duct obstruction and led to the correct diagnosis of carcinoma. A large amount of contrast medium has refluxed into the intestinal lumen.

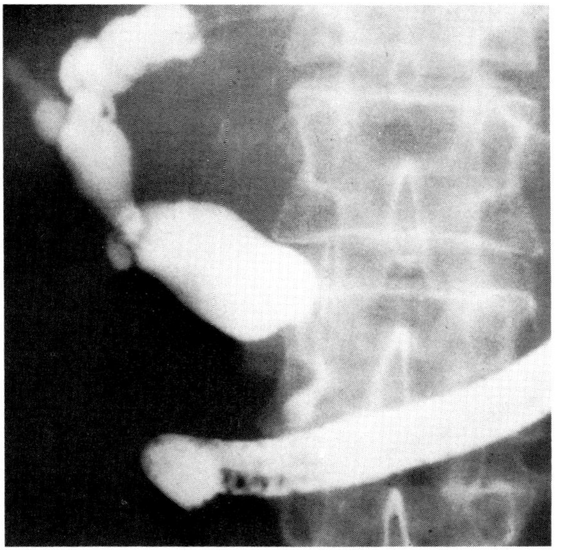

Figure 11–13. Carcinoma of the pancreas. There is an irregular stricture of the common bile duct, with marked dilatation of the intrahepatic and common bile ducts proximal to the stricture. The pancreatic duct was completely blocked. The tumor precluded obtaining a simultaneous pancreatogram.

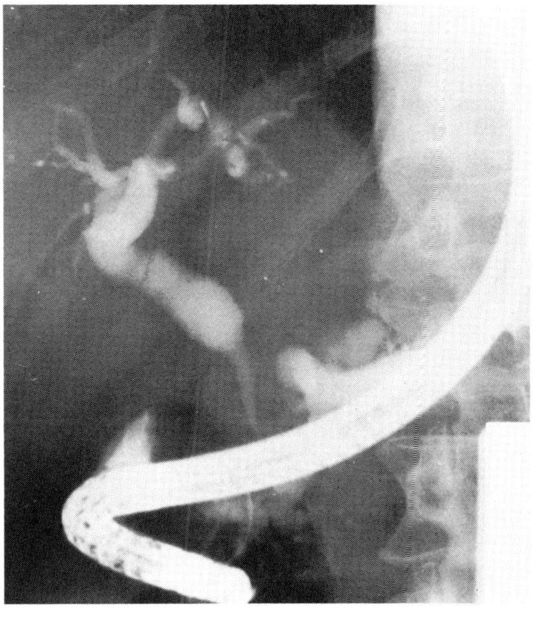

Figure 11–14. Common duct stricture secondary to chronic pancreatitis. There is a smoothly tapered concentric stricture of the distal common bile duct. A markedly dilated pancreatic duct with ectasia of its secondary branches is partially obscured by the duodenoscope.

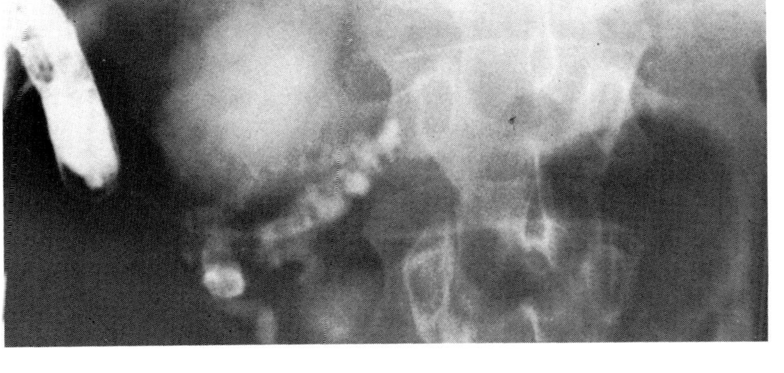

Figure 11–15. Pancreatic pseudocyst. There is a 3.5 cm communicating pseudocyst of the head of the pancreas. Irregular dilatation of the main pancreatic duct with intraluminal stones can be seen in the head of the pancreas. No attempt was made to visualize the upstream portion of the pancreatic duct for fear of overfilling the pseudocyst and its potential septic complications. This patient's presenting complaint was painless jaundice. The pseudocyst was an unexpected finding but, nonetheless, the cause of his obstructive jaundice.

small papillotomy to expose an ampullary tumor for subsequent biopsy.[85, 86] If cannulation is possible, endoscopic sphincterotomy or stent placement for palliative decompression of the biliary tree can be done.

Stenosis of the papilla of Vater often presents with a definite cholestatic episode. If the cholangiogram does not reveal stones, sludge, or a stricture, if the common duct is dilated, and if there is delayed drainage of the common duct, the diagnostic criteria for this entity have been met. A pancreatogram, when obtained, often shows symmetric dilatation of the main and secondary pancreatic ducts (Fig. 11–16). Endoscopic sphincterotomy may be curative.[71]

Following Common Duct Diversion

Anastomosis of the common bile duct with the posterior aspect of the apex of the duodenal bulb, either side-to-side or end-to-side, is frequently used in patients with benign or malignant distal bile duct strictures or advanced gallstone disease. Some patients develop cholestasis, usually with associated cholangitis, after surgery. This is most often due to stricture of the anastomosis. ERCP with the end-viewing duodenoscope facilitates establishing this diagnosis both by direct inspection of the anastomosis and by the diagnostic cholangiogram (Fig. 11–17).[84] The use of a balloon catheter may improve visualization of the biliary tract in those with an open stoma.[74] Direct dilatation of the strictured anastomosis with biopsy forceps or balloon-tipped catheters is frequently successful. In the presence of a widely patent side-to-side choledochoduodenostomy, patients may also develop cholestatic episodes and sepsis.[75] This is due to the collection of vegetable debris or stones in the distal common bile duct between the widely patent anastomosis and the papilla of Vater. This "blind loop" and the debris act as a nidus for recurrent infection, the so-called sump syndrome. This situation can be diagnosed with certainty by ERCP (Fig. 11–18) and treated effectively by endoscopic sphincterotomy.[76–78]

In several of our patients, at surgery, following choledochojejunostomy, the Roux-en-Y loop has been brought close to the skin of the anterior abdominal wall. In the event of subsequent stenosis at the anastomotic site, it has been possible to obtain ERCP via the Roux-en-Y jujunal loop and to perform retrograde dilatation of the anastomotic stricture.

Abdominal Pain

Many patients will have histories that strongly suggest cholelithiasis and yet have repeatedly negative oral cholecystograms, abdominal sonograms, and biliary drainage with examination for cholesterol crystals. ERCP may be of help under these circumstances.[79] In addition to being able to diagnose cystic duct obstruction or small gallbladder stones with certainty (see Fig. 11–2), ERCP allows the visual inspection of the distal

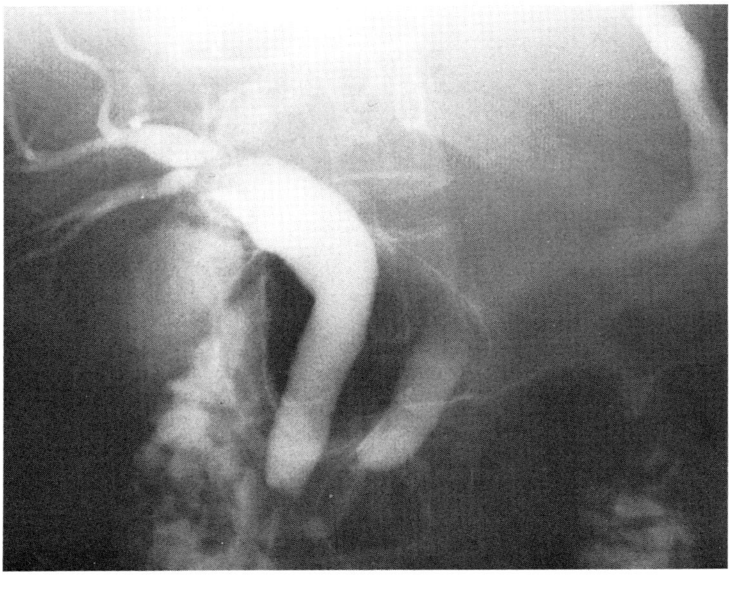

Figure 11–16. Stenosis of the papilla of Vater. There is smooth dilation of both the biliary tree and the entire pancreatic duct. Endoscopic sphincterotomy was curative.

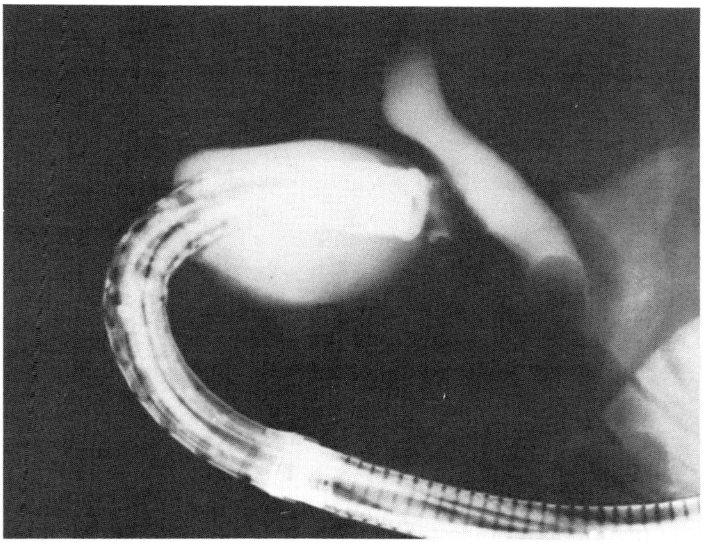

Figure 11–17. Retained common duct stone post choledochoduodenostomy. Despite a widely patent choledochoduodenostomy this patient had recurrent cholangitis. The stone has a smooth meniscus and is distal to the anastomosis. Contrast medium has refluxed into the duodenal bulb. A Roux-en-Y choledochojejunostomy was curative.

stomach and proximal duodenum for mucosal abnormalities, including peptic ulcer disease. Simultaneous pancreatography may detect occult pancreatic disease, such as early pancreatic cancer or chronic pancreatitis. If the ERCP is normal, it may prevent an exploratory laparotomy.

Following cholecystectomy, some patients complain of pain. Even in the absence of jaundice, intravenous cholangiography is often nondiagnostic and ERCP is the test of choice. It will demonstrate definitely whether residual stones, stricture, or papillary stenosis are responsible for this postcholecystectomy pain syndrome.[80] Some of these patients may have no discernible disease on ERCP, but disordered motility of the sphincter of Oddi. Endoscopic manometry provides an investigational approach to defining this disorder.[81–83]

NEW DEVELOPMENTS

With the rapid changes in clinical applications of ERCP, current interpretive criteria may become obsolete or erroneous, and standards of health and disease will require redefinition in compliance with expanding knowledge and experience. Minor variations in ERCP technique allow physiologic studies that will prove useful in defining the patho-

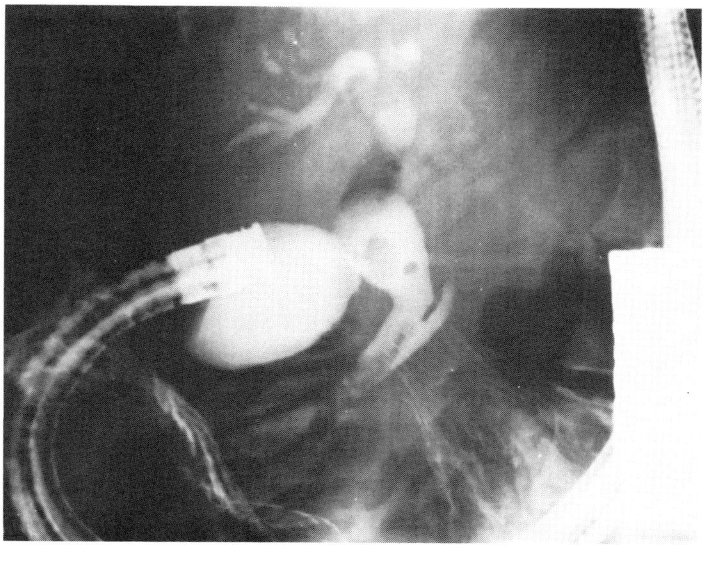

Figure 11–18. "Succotash" cholangitis post choledochoduodenostomy ("sump syndrome"). Despite a widely patent choledochoduodenostomy this patient had recurrent episodes of cholangitis. There are irregular filling defects in the distal common duct, which at surgery proved to be fragments of peas, corn, carrots, and spinach. Contrast medium has refluxed into the duodenal bulb and distal pancreatic duct.

physiology of diseases of the liver and biliary tree. Manometry of the sphincter of Oddi has already provided some insights into the altered physiology that accompanies stenosis of the sphincter of Oddi. It also permits a reliable means of quantitating the effect of sphincterotomy.[71, 81] This techniques should also enable scrutiny of the elusive syndrome of "biliary dyskinesia." Long catheters can be left within the bile duct after removal of the endoscope. The development of a balloon-tipped catheter allows the long-term quantitative collection of uncontaminated bile.[22] This technique should be useful in studies of the biliary excretion of bilirubin under different conditions, of drugs and their metabolites, and of the variations in solubility potential of bile for cholesterol. The retention catheter may also be used for the introduction of chemicals aimed at dissolution of common duct stones. It is possible that these newer developments of clinical research will prove more exciting than the diagnostic radiologic applications of endoscopic retrograde cholangiography.

REFERENCES

1. McCune WS, Shorb PE, Moscovitz H: Endoscopic cannulation of the ampulla of Vater; a preliminary report. Ann Surg 1968;*167*:752.
2. Oi I: Fiber duodenoscopy and endoscopic pancreatocholangiography. Gastrointest Endosc 1970;*17*:59.
3. Takagi K, Ikeda S, Nakagawa Y, Kumakura K, Maruyama M, Someya N, Takada T, Takekoshi T, Kin M: Retrograde pancreatography and cholangiography by fiber-duodenoscopy. Gastroenterology 1970;*59*:445.
4. Cotton PB: Cannulation of the papilla of Vater by endoscopy and retrograde cholangiopancreatography (ERCP). Gut 1972;*13*:1014.
5. Classen M, Koch H, Fruhmorgen P, Grabuer W, Demling L: Results of retrograde pancreatic cholangiography. Acta Gastroenterol Jpn 1972;*7*:131.
6. Vennes JA, Silvis SE: Endoscopic visualization of bile and pancreatic ducts. Gastrointest Endosc 1972;*18*:149.
7. Huelly F, Gaucher P, Laurent J, Vicari F, Fagi J, Bigart M-A, Jeanpierre R: La duodenoscopie et le catheterisme des voies biliares et pancreatiques. Nouv Presse Med 1972;*1*:313.
8. Ingelfinger FJ: Endoscopic pancreatocholangiography: progress and problem (Editoral). N Engl J Med 1972;*287*:879.
9. Ogoshi K, Niwa M, Hara Y, Nebel O: Endoscopic pancreatocholangiography in the evaluation of pancreaticobiliary disease. Gastroenterology 1973; *64*:210.
10. Cotton PB: Endoscopic retrograde cholangiopancreatography (ERCP). *In* Truelove JC, Trowell HC (eds): Topics in Gastroenterology. Vol 2. Oxford, Blackwell, 1975, pp 53–64.
11. Nebel OT: Its the CP in ERCP that counts. Gastrointest Endosc 1975;*21*:137.
12. Myren J: Retrograde endoscopic cholangiopancreatography (ERCP). Scand J Gastroenterol 1975; *10*:229.
13. Cotton PB: ERCP. Gut 1977;*18*:316.
14. Nebel OT, Silvis SE, Rogers G, Sugawa C, Mandelstam P: Complications associated with endoscopic retrograde cholangiopancreatography. Results of the 1974 ASGE survey. Gastrointest Endosc 1975;*22*:34.
15. Bilbao MK, Dotter CT, Lee TG, Katon RM: Complications of endoscopic retrograde cholangiopancreatography. A study of 10,000 cases. Gastroenterology 1976;*70*:314.
16. Safrany L: Endoscopy and retrograde cholangiopancreatography after Billroth II operation. Endoscopy 1972;*4*:198.
17. Katon RM, Bilbao MK, Parent JA, Smith FW: Endoscopic retrograde cholangiopancreatography in patients with gastrectomy and gastrojejunostomy (Billroth II), a case for the forward look. Gastrointest Endosc 1975;*21*:124.
18. Forbes A, Cotton PB: ERCP and sphincterotomy after Billroth II gastrectomy. Gut 1984;*25*:971.
19. Kasugai T, Kano N, Kizu M: Manometric endoscopic retrograde pancreatocholangiography: technique, significance and evaluation. Am J Dig Dis 1974;*19*:485.
20. Shapiro HA: Endoscopic diagnosis and treatment of biliary tract disease. Surg Clin North Am 1981;*61*:843.
21. Salmon PR: Re-evaluation of endoscopic retrograde cholangiopancreatography as a diagnostic method. Clin Gastroenterol 1978;*7*:651.
22. Shapiro HA, Cotton PB: Leaving a balloon tip catheter in the bile duct at duodenoscopy. Lancet 1975;*2*:13.
23. Silvis SE, Vennes JA: The role of glucagon in endoscopic cholangio-pancreatography. Gastrointest Endosc 1975;*21*:162.
24. Vennes JA: Endoscopic technique. *In* Stewart ET, Vennes JA, Geenen JE (eds): Atlas of Endoscopic Retrograde Cholangiopancreatography. St Louis, CV Mosby, 1977, pp 4–18.
25. Goldberg HI, Bilbao MK, Stewart ET, Rohrmann CA, Moss AA: Endoscopic retrograde cholangiopancreatography (ERCP): radiographic technique. Am J Dig Dis 1976;*21*:270.
26. Rosseland AR, Solhaug JH: Early or delayed endoscopic papillotomy (EPT) in gallstone pancreatitis. Ann Surg 1984;*199*:165.
27. van der Spuy S: Endoscopic sphincterotomy in the management of gallstone pancreatitis. Endoscopy 1981;*13*:25.
28. Roesch W, Demling L: Endoscopic management of pancreatitis. Surg Clin North Am 1982;*62*:845.
29. McDonald GB, Silverstein PE: Can gastrointestinal endoscopy transmit hepatitis B to patients? Gastrointest Endosc 1976;*22*:168.
30. Centers for Disease Control: Minimizing the risk of hepatitis B transmission by flexible fiberoptic endoscopy: recommendations for use, routine cleaning and disinfection. Hepatitis Surveillance Report No 41. Washington DC, September 1977.
31. Winstanley PA, Ellis WR, Hamilton J, Lintott DJ, Axon ATR: Medium term complications of endoscopic sphincterotomy. Gut 1983;*26*:730.
32. Safrany L, Cotton PB: Endoscopic management of cholelithiasis. Surg Clin North Am 1982;*62*:825.

33. Skude G, Wehlin L, Maruyama T, Ariyama J: Hyperamylasaemia after duodenoscopy and retrograde cholangiopancreatography. Gut 1976;*17*:127.
34. Ghazi A, McSherry CK: Endoscopic retrograde cholangiopancreatography and sphincterotomy. Ann Surg 1984;*199*:21.
35. Taylor KJW, Carpenter DH, McCready UR: Ultrasound and scintigraphy in the differential diagnosis of obstructive jaundice. J Clin Ultrasound 1974;*2*:105.
36. Stephen DH, Dottery RR, Sheedy PF: Computed tomography of the abdomen. Radiology 1976; *119*:331.
37. Kasugai T, Kuno N, Kobayashi S, Hattori K: Endoscopic pancreatocholangiogram. Gastroenterology 1972;*63*:227.
38. Koch H, Belohlavek D, Schaffner O, Tympner F, Rosch W, Demling L: Prospective study for the prevention of pancreatitis following endoscopic retrograde cholangio-pancreatography (ERCP). Endoscopy 1975;*7*:221.
39. Hershey SD, Choichi S, Cushing R, Ledgerwood AM, Lucas CE: The value of prophylactic antibiotic therapy during endoscopic retrograde cholangiopancreatography. Surgery 1982;*155*:801.
40. Cotton PB, Reuben A: Observer variation in pancreatogram interpretation. Gastrointest Endosc 1977;*23*:225.
41. Lasser RB, Silvis SL, Vennes JA: The normal cholangiogram. Am J Dig Dis 1978;*23*:586.
42. Belsito AA, Morta JB, Kramer GG: Measurements of the biliary tract size and drainage time. Comparison of endoscopic and intravenous cholangiography. Radiology 1977;*122*:65.
43. Wakim KG, Mahair GH: Pathophysiologic consequence of cholecystectomy. Surg Gynecol Obstet 1971;*133*:113.
44. Wise RE: Intravenous Cholangiography. Springfield, Ill, Charles C Thomas, 1962.
45. Hand BH: Anatomy and function of the extrahepatic biliary system. Clin Gastroenterol 1973;*2*:3.
46. Blumgart LH, Salmon PR, Cotton PB: Endoscopy and retrograde cholangiopancreatography in the diagnosis of the patient with jaundice. Surg Gynecol Obstet 1974;*138*:565.
47. Elias E: Progress report: Cholangiography in the jaundiced patient. Gut 1976;*17*:801.
48. Vennes JA, Jacobson JR, Silvis SE: Endoscopic cholangiography for biliary system diagnosis. Ann Intern Med 1974;*80*:61.
49. Shapiro HA: Cholestasis in ulcerative colitis. Radiographic evaluation. D. Retrograde cholangiography. Gastroenterology 1977;*73*:367.
50. Osnes M, Larsen S, Lowe P, Gronseth K, Lotwest T, Nordshus T: Comparison of endoscopic retrograde and intravenous cholangiography in diagnosis of biliary calculi. Lancet 1978;*2*:230.
51. Leopold GR, Sokoloff J: Ultrasonic scanning in the diagnosis of biliary disease. Surg Clin North Am 1973;*53*:1043.
52. Malini S, Sabel J: Ultrasonography in obstructive jaundice. Radiology 1977;*123*:429.
53. Doust BD: Ultrasonic examination of the pancreas. Radiol Clin North Am 1975;*13*:467.
54. Havrilla TR, Haaga JR, Alfidi RJ, et al: Computed tomography and obstructive biliary disease. Am J Roentgenol 1977;*128*:765.
55. Stanley RJ, Sagel SS, Levitt RG: Computed tomographic evaluation of the pancreas. 1977;*124*:715.
56. Thomas MJ, Pellegrini CA, Way LW: Usefulness of diagnostic tests for biliary obstruction. Am J Surg 1982;*144*:102.
57. Okuda K, Tanikawa K, Emwa T, Kuratomi S, Urabe K, Sumikoshi T, Kanda Y, Kukuyama Y, Muska H, Mori LT, Shimokawa Y, Yakushiju F, Matsuura Y: Non-surgical percutaneous transhepatic cholangiography: Diagnostic significance in medical problems of the liver. Am J Dig Dis 1974;*19*:21.
58. Alias E, Hamlyn AH, Jain S, Long RG, Summerfield MB, Dick MB, Sherlock S: A randomized trial of percutaneous transhepatic cholangiography with the Chiba needle versus endoscopic retrograde cholangiography for bile duct visualization in jaundice. Gastroenterology 1976;*71*:439.
59. Ayoola EA, Vennes JA, Silvis SE, Rohrmann CA, Ansel HJ: Endoscopic retrograde intrahepatic cholangiography in liver disease. Gastrointest Endosc 1976;*22*:156.
60. Rohrmann CA, Ansel HJ, Ayoola EA, Silvis SE, Vennes JA: The endoscopic retrograde intrahepatic cholangiogram; radiographic findings in intrahepatic disease. Am J Roentgenol Radium Ther Nucl Med 1977;*128*:45.
61. Summerfield JA, Elias E, Hungerford GD, Nikapota VLB, Dick R, Sherlock S: The biliary system in primary biliary cirrhosis: A study by endoscopic retrograde cholangiopancreatography. Gastroenterology 1976;*70*:240.
62. Rohrmann CA, Silverstein FE, Templeton FE: Intrahepatic condition of the biliary tree. *In* Stewart ET, Vennes JA, Geenen JE (eds): Atlas of Endoscopic Retrograde Cholangiopancreatography. St Louis, CV Mosby 1977, pp 236–240.
63. Danzi JT, Makipour H, Farmer RG: Primary sclerosing cholangitis. Am J Gastroenterol 1976;*65*:109.
64. Blackstone MO, Nemchausky BA: Cholangiographic abnormalities in ulcerative colitis associated pericholangitis which resembles sclerosing cholangitis. Am J Dig Dis 1978;*23*:579.
65. Seifert E, Safrany L, St Stender I-J, Lesch P, Luska G, Misaki F: Identification of bile duct tumors by means of endoscopic retrograde pancreato-cholangiography (ERCP). Endoscopy 1974;*6*:152.
66. Elias E, Summerfield JA, Dick R, Sherlock S: Endoscopic retrograde cholangiography in the diagnosis of jaundice associated with ulcerative colitis. Gastroenterology 1974;*67*:907.
67. Falkenstein DB, Riccoboni C, Sidhu G, Abrams RM, Seliger G, Zimmon DS: The endoscopic intrahepatic cholangiogram. Clinico pathologic correlation with post mortem cholangiograms. Invest Radiol 1975;*10*:358.
68. Mazzeo RJ, Jordan FT, Strasius SR: Endoscopic papillotomy for recurrent common bile duct stones and papillary stenosis. Arch Surg 1983;*118*:693.
69. Safrany L: Duodenoscopic papillotomy and gallstone removal. Gastroenterology 1977;*72*:338.
70. Classen M, Ossenberg FW: Nonsurgical removal of common bile duct stones. Gut 1977;*18*:760.
71. Geenen JE, Hogan WK, Shaffer RD, Stewart ET, Dodds WJ, Arndorfer RC: Endoscopic electrosurgical papillotomy and manometry in biliary tract disease. JAMA 1977;*237*:2075.
72. George P: Disorders of the extrahepatic bile ducts. Clin Gastroenterol 1973;*2*:127.
73. Scott J, Summerfield JA, Elias E, Dick R, Sherlock S: Chronic pancreatitis: a cause of cholestasis. Gut 1977;*18*:196.
74. Ikeda S, Tanaka M, Yoshimoto H, Itoh H, Nakayama F: Improved visualization of intrahepatic bile

ducts by endoscopic retrograde balloon catheter cholangiography. Ann Surg 1981;*194:*171.
75. Shapiro HA, Carlson B: "Succotash" cholangitis—diagnosis by retrograde endoscopic cholangiography. Gastroenterology 1974;*86:*824.
76. Siegel JH: Duodenoscopic sphincterotomy in the treatment of the "sump syndrome." Dig Dis Sci 1981;*26:*922.
77. Barkin JS, Silvis S, Greenwald R: Endoscopic therapy of the "sump syndrome." Dig Dis Sci 1980;*25:*597.
78. Tanaka M, Ikeda S, Yoshimoto H: Endoscopic sphincterotomy for the treatment of biliary sump syndrome. Surgery 1983;*93:*264.
79. Venu RP, Geenen JE, Toouli J, Stewart E, Hogan WJ: Endoscopic retrograde cholangiopancreatography. JAMA 1983;*249:*758.
80. Silvis SE: What is the post cholecystectomy pain syndrome? Gastrointest Endosc 1985;*31:*401.
81. Nebel OT: Manometric evaluation of papilla of Vater. Gastrointest Endosc 1975;*21:*126.
82. Matsushiro T, Nagashima H, Yamamoto K, Hariu T: Perfusion cholangiomanometry with papillary stimulation by dilute hydrochloric acid. Surgery 1984;*95:*96.
83. Toouli J, Hogan J, Geenen JE, Dodds WJ, Arndorfer RC: Action of cholecystokinin-octapeptide on sphincter of Oddi basal pressure and phasic wave activity in humans. Surgery 1982;*92:*497.
84. Reuben A, Jourdan MH, Isaacs PET, McColl I: Spontaneous closure of choledochoduodenostomy diagnosis by endoscopy and ERCP. Br J Surg 1980;*67:*283.
85. Nako NL, Siegel JH, Stenger RJ, et al: Tumors of the ampulla of Vater—early diagnosis by intraampullary biopsy during endoscopic cannulation. Gastroenterology 1982;*83:*459.
86. Siegel JH, Yatto RP: Endoscopic evaluation and therapy of periampullary adenoma. Am J Gastroenterol 1983;*78:*225.

ROBERT C. STADALNIK, M.D.
PAUL B. HOFFER, M.D.

12

Radioisotopic Evaluation of Biliary Function

The liver can be imaged best by using radionuclides that localize in the reticuloendothelial system. These agents provide a fairly good image of the liver parenchyma, but evaluation of the biliary tract is indirect, through the changes in the liver. The biliary tract can be imaged directly by using radionuclides that are excreted into the bile. These agents, while not as useful in the evaluation of the liver, make possible a direct assessment of the bile flow through the intra- and extrahepatic bile ducts and the upper gastrointestinal tract.

RETICULOENDOTHELIAL IMAGING

The most common scanning agent is ^{99m}Tc sulfur colloid. This agent consists of small radiolabeled particles, 100 mμ to about 1 μ in diameter, which are preferentially extracted from the blood by the reticuloendothelial cells of the liver, the spleen, and the bone marrow. Reticuloendothelial cells represent approximately 15 per cent of the hepatic parenchyma and are distributed uniformly throughout the liver. About 80 to 90 per cent of the ^{99m}Tc sulfur colloid injected intravenously localizes in the liver. Its extraction from the blood is very efficient, as virtually 100 per cent is cleared on a single pass through the liver.

The primary value of the ^{99m}Tc sulfur colloid liver scan is to detect hepatic masses as well as parenchymal disease. Normally, the biliary tract is not seen, since ^{99m}Tc sulfur colloid is not taken up by hepatocytes or excreted in the bile. However, when the bile ducts are dilated or the gallbladder is very distended, they may produce changes in the liver scan. For example, dilatation of the gallbladder may produce a prominent indentation in the inferior margin of the liver image.[1] This should not be confused with a prominent gallbladder fossa, seen in some normal individuals. On the other hand, dilated biliary ducts may be recognized based on one or more of the following[2]: (1) a mass or defect in the region of the junction of the right and left lobes of the liver; (2) linear defects that do not reach the periphery in the right lobe; (3) a linear defect in the left lobe oriented obliquely to the junction of the right and left hepatic lobes; (4) a stellate pattern of decreased activity in the mid–right lobe or at the interlobar junction (Fig. 12–1). These changes are not specific, as only about 45 per cent of patients with dilated ducts show the abnormal findings described. Therefore, imaging of the liver using reticuloendothelial agents should not be recommended as a primary test in the differential diagnosis of suspected biliary duct disease. Knowledge of the liver scan findings in biliary duct dilatation is important, however, as the colloid liver scan is commonly used to diagnose other hepatic diseases and the detection of dilated ducts on the scan may direct further attention to the biliary ducts.

BILIARY IMAGING

The agents used for biliary imaging are cleared from the blood by the hepatocytes and excreted into the biliary ducts. Unlike the colloids, this type of radionuclide provides a direct image of the biliary ducts and the gallbladder. These agents are used to evaluate the patency of the biliary tract. They have been found to be highly sensitive and specific for the diagnosis of acute cholecystitis and occasionally useful to differentiate biliary tract obstruction from hepatocellular disease.

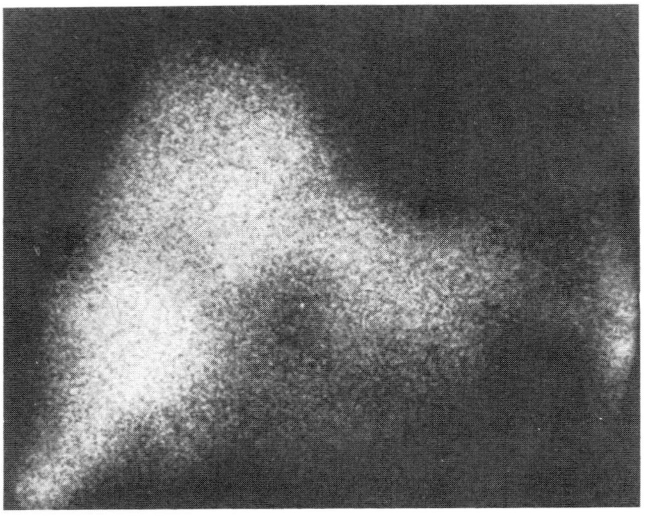

Figure 12–1. Dilated biliary ducts as seen on Tc-99m sulfur colloid imaging. There is a defect in the region of the junction between right and left lobes with an accompanying stellate pattern of decreased activity.

Rose bengal sodium I-131 was the first radiopharmaceutical used to image the hepatobiliary system.[3–5] Rose bengal was found to have several advantages over reticuloendothelial imaging agents: It is rapidly secreted into the biliary channels; it is concentrated like bile in the gallbladder; and it enters the duodenum through the common bile duct. There is no conjugation or other transformation of the dye in its passage through the liver, and there is little, if any, enterohepatic circulation. However, ^{131}I provides a low-photon flux per unit of radiation and is slowly concentrated in the biliary system. The images obtained with safe radiation exposure are, therefore, suboptimal.

In the mid-1970s a new series of ^{99m}Tc-labeled radiopharmaceuticals was developed to image the biliary tract.[6–13] While ^{99m}Tc has all the advantages of ^{131}I rose bengal, it gives a very high counting rate, it has a short (6-hour) half-life, and the radiation dose to the patient is relatively low. The introduction of two derivatives of iminodiacetic acid (methyliminodiacetic acid [MIDA] and 2, 6 dimethylphenylcarbamoylmethyl iminodiacetic acid [HIDA]) in 1977 was a major step forward in biliary imaging.[14, 16] A variety of ^{99m}Tc iminodiacetic (IDA) derivatives have since been developed (Table 12–1), and the technique of cholescintigraphy using these agents has become popular.[19–24]

These agents are all taken up by the hepatocytes and immediately excreted unconjugated into the biliary tract. The analogs differ in the amount of hepatocyte uptake, renal excretion, and rate of transport from the liver cell into the biliary tract. Although they all perform well in normal and in mildly jaundiced patients, some are more desirable in moderate to severe jaundice because of the lesser renal elimination and the greater hepatocyte uptake. Because all the agents work when the serum bilirubin level is normal (whereas only a few are useful at higher bilirubin levels), the selection of an individual agent should be based on the knowledge of serum bilirubin level. Those most commonly used are listed in Table 12–1.[17] ^{99m}Tc para-isopropyl and parabutyl analogs are more resistant to displacement by bilirubin than is dimethyl IDA. The resistance is attributed to their greater protein-binding capacity, which reduces urinary and enhances hepatic excretion.[25, 34] Although some have reported good excretion of these two agents with bilirubin levels as high as 15 mg/dl, biliary imaging should usually not be recommended if the bilirubin level is above 6 to 7 mg/dl. The initial evaluation of these patients is better done with ultrasound or computed tomography. However, if ultrasound or computed tomography is either unavailable or unsuccessful, hepatobiliary radionuclide imaging may still be worthwhile. Ongoing radiopharmaceutical research is likely to provide newer agents that may be used in severely jaundiced patients.

Table 12–1 Tc-99m ALKYL-SUBSTITUTED IMINODIACETIC ACID (IDA) DERIVATIVES

2,6-dimethyl (lidofenin, HIDA)
2,6-diethyl
p-ethoxy
p-butyl (butilfenin)
p-isopropyl (iprofenin, PIPIDA)
diisopropyl (disofenin, DISIDA)

Table 12–2 TECHNIQUE FOR Tc-99m BILIARY SCINTIGRAPHY

1. NPO or only clear liquid diet for *at least* 2 hours prior to study
2. Inject 2–5 mCi nonjaundiced patients.
   Inject 5–10 mCi jaundiced patients.
3. Use of multi-image formator serial images recorded during the first hour of the study.
4. Additional images obtained at 2–6 and 24 hours post injection if:
   a. obstruction suspected.
   b. biliary system or intestine not visualized at 1 hour.

The technique of ^{99m}Tc IDA biliary scintigraphy is outlined in Table 12–2. Using 5 mCi of any of the agents mentioned, the whole-body radiation absorbed dose is approximately 0.1 rad.[17] The scintillation camera is the instrument of choice for all biliary imaging studies. Anterior views are routinely taken. Left anterior oblique and right lateral views are used to separate biliary from renal overlap when needed. In order to prevent false positive studies due to gallbladder emptying, either nothing by mouth or only a clear liquid diet is permitted for at least 2 hours prior to the study.[11, 13]

Characteristics of a Normal Study
(Fig. 12–2)

A few minutes after injection, the radiopharmaceutical begins to concentrate within the liver. Fifteen to 20 minutes after the injection, most of the radioactivity has been removed from the blood stream and is con-

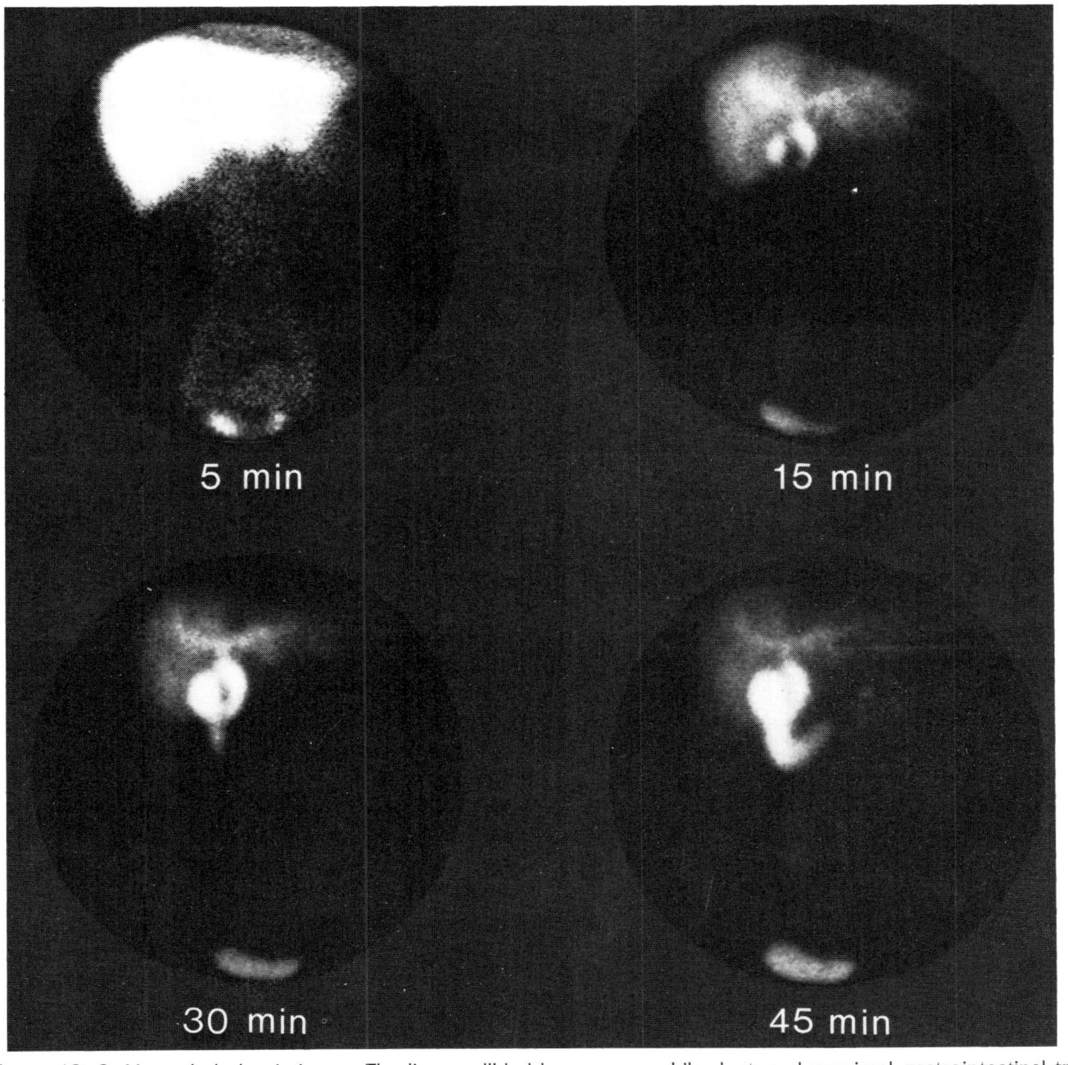

Figure 12–2. Normal cholescintigram. The liver, gallbladder, common bile duct, and proximal gastrointestinal tract are visualized 30 minutes postinjection. Bladder activity is seen in the inferior portion of the image.

TABLE 12–3 CLINICAL INDICATIONS FOR Tc-99m BILIARY TRACT IMAGING

1. Obstruction of cystic duct (cholecystitis, calculous or acalculous)
2. Evaluation of "cold" defects seen on routine Tc-99m sulfur colloid imaging
3. Study of biliary kinetics
4. Evaluation of postsurgical biliary system, bile leakage, gallbladder perforation, or cholecystocolic fistula, biliary-enteric anastomoses
5. Pediatrics
   a. Infants—Biliary atresia vs. neonatal hepatitis (pretreat with phenobarbital, 5 mg/kg/day × 5 days)
   b. Choledochal cyst
   c. Visceral heterotaxy (Ivemark's syndrome)
6. Evaluation of intrahepatic lithiasis (important in the Orient)
7. Enterogastric reflux
8. Predictive value in patients with nonvisualization of gallbladder after oral cholecystography
9. Detection of liver disease; dissociation of reticuloendothelial and hepatocyte function

centrated within the liver. This is followed by concentration of radioactivity within the biliary ducts and gallbladder. The hepatic ducts are frequently well seen in the normal patient. Thirty to 60 minutes after the injection, the gallbladder is typically well seen and radioactivity is also identified in the gastrointestinal tract. The time of optimal gallbladder filling changes from subject to subject. In 48 normal volunteers the gallbladder was clearly seen in 50 per cent of the subjects within 15 minutes, in 80 per cent within 20 minutes, and in 100 per cent within 50 minutes.[25]

Clinical Applications of Biliary Scintigraphy (Table 12–3)

Diagnosis of Acute Cholecystitis (Table 12–4)

The major use of these ^{99m}Tc-labeled biliary compounds is in the diagnosis of acute cholecystitis.[28–40] In patients with acute cholecystitis, the liver, common duct, and gastrointestinal tract are seen within 60 minutes, but the gallbladder is *not* seen (Fig. 12–3). Filling of the gallbladder implies patency of the cystic duct; therefore; the scan effectively excludes the presence of acute cholecystitis, since the precipitating cause of acute cholecystitis is obstruction of the cystic duct in about 98 per cent of patients. False negative scans (the gallbladder fills, but there is acute cholecystitis) are occasionally seen in patients with acalculous acute cholecystitis.[34–37] On the other hand, if at the end of 1 hour, there is visualization of the common bile duct and gut but not of the gallbladder, delayed views at 2 and 4 hours should be obtained. Persistent nonfilling of the gallbladder is considered positive for acute cholecystitis, whereas a delayed appearance of the gallbladder is considered a negative study. Although failure of the gallbladder to fill despite normal excretion into the small intestine has been considered pathognomonic of acute cholecystitis, experience has shown that in addition to obstruction of the cystic duct, chronic cholecystitis, carcinoma of the gallbladder, pancreatitis, prolonged fasting, total parenteral nutrition, and alcoholism may occasionally lead to nonfilling of the gallbladder. Choy et al.[41] suggested that in patients in whom the gallbladder is not seen within 40 minutes, a small intravenous dose of morphine (0.04 mg/kg) be administered. This is done with the idea of closing the sphincter of Oddi and enhancing gallbladder flow of bile.[41] When the gut is not visualized, absence of gallbladder uptake is not diagnostic, and the scan should be interpreted as indeterminate for acute cholecystitis.[26]

Several studies have now shown that the sensitivity and specificity of cholescintigraphy for acute cholecystitis are approximately 95 per cent.[20, 25–33] In patients suspected of having acute cholecystitis, cholescintigraphy provides the kind of information that used to be

TABLE 12–4 DIAGNOSIS OF ACUTE CHOLECYSTITIS WITH Tc-99m CHOLESCINTIGRAPHY

Author	Number of Patients	Sensitivity (%)	Specificity (%)	Accuracy (%)
Fonseca et al[77]	113	100	100	100
Freitas and Gulati[78]	186	97	87–95*	94–96
Matolo et al[34]†	341	92	97	95
Stadalnik and Matolo[43]	120	100	100	100
Szlabick et al[33]	117	100	97.6	99.2
Weissmann et al[36]	296	95.2	99.2	97.6

*Specificity varies with criteria for diagnosis of acute cholecystitis at surgery or by histopathologic determination. Specificity is 95 per cent if criteria of other series are used.

†Acute *and* chronic cholecystitis

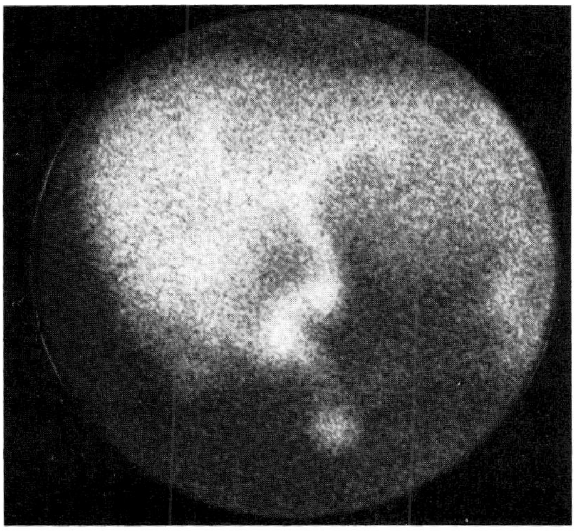

Figure 12–3. Acute cholecystitis. The liver, common bile duct, and duodenum are visualized on the 30-minute scan. The gallbladder is *not* seen.

expected from intravenous cholangiography, but at much lower risk.[19, 20] It has thus entirely replaced the use of intravenous cholangiography for this purpose. With this safe, easy-to-perform test, exclusion of the diagnosis of acute cholecystitis can be made as early as 30 minutes and the confirmation usually made within 3 hours.

Although cholescintigraphy is the diagnostic test of choice to establish patency of the cystic duct, prospective analysis of the efficacy of ^{99m}Tc IDA cholescintigraphy and cholecystosonography has shown that both are excellent techniques for assessing patients with suspected acute cholecystitis. Consequently, the choice of test should depend on other factors, including the quality of equipment and the availability of personnel. In addition, cholecystosonography is better able to assess the presence of acute cholecystitis in patients with jaundice, since biliary secretion of the radionuclide is impaired and additional information regarding the size of the ducts may be obtained.[29, 39]

It should be stressed that nonvisualization of the gallbladder implies cholecystitis, but not necessarily acute cholecystitis. About half the patients with chronic cholecystitis do not fill their gallbladders with the radiolabeled bile.[17, 38] Most studies of accuracy of cholescintigraphy in the diagnosis of acute cholecystitis focus on patients with acute right upper quadrant pain, fever, and leukocytosis who are suspected of having acute cholecystitis (Table 12–5). Nonvisualization of the gallbladder in an asymptomatic subject implies failure to fill the gallbladder during the test, not necessarily acute cholecystitis.

TABLE 12–5 CAUSES OF RIGHT UPPER QUADRANT ABDOMINAL PAIN WITHOUT BILIARY TRACT DISEASE[76]

Acute myocardial infarction	Infrahepatic abscess
Addison's disease	Leukemia
Appendicitis	Ovarian cyst
Arteriosclerotic heart disease	Pancratitis
Bowel obstruction	Peptic ulcer disease
Carcinoid tumor of appendix	Pleurisy
Cystic teratoma of ovary	Pneumonia
Diabetes	Scleroderma
Gastritis	Septic shock
Hepatic flexure colonic carcinoma	Unknown etiology
	Ureterolithiasis
Hepatitis	Urinary tract infection
Ileus	
Incarcerated umbilical hernia	

Diagnosis of Gallbladder Motor Disorders

Some patients with a normal cholecystogram have dyspeptic complaints similar to those of patients with gallstones. These symptoms have been variously termed biliary dyskinesia, acalculous chronic cholecystitis, and the cystic duct syndrome. Although there is no uniform agreement, it appears that in some patients who have no gallstones detected by conventional studies, abdominal pain similar to biliary colic is the result of abnormal gallbladder filling and emptying.[53, 54] Gallbladder contraction and emptying can be measured by quantitative cholescintigraphy. After a bolus injection, the tracer can be followed as it enters the gallbladder, and gallbladder contraction can be elicited by the intravenous injection of CCK, CCK octapeptide (sincalide), a medium-chain triglyceride (Lipomul), or a fatty meal. The response of the gallbladder can then be followed by using time-activity curves generated by a computer.[47–52] These studies have provided a new insight into the physiology of the gallbladder (see Chapter 3).

Identification of these patients, who may be cured by cholecystectomy, is made possible by quantitative cholescintigraphy.

Assessment of Cholangiointestinal Anastomoses and Gastroenterostomies

Patients who have had surgery on the biliary tract may be difficult to evaluate with ultrasonography or computed tomography, since the normal anatomic landmarks may be

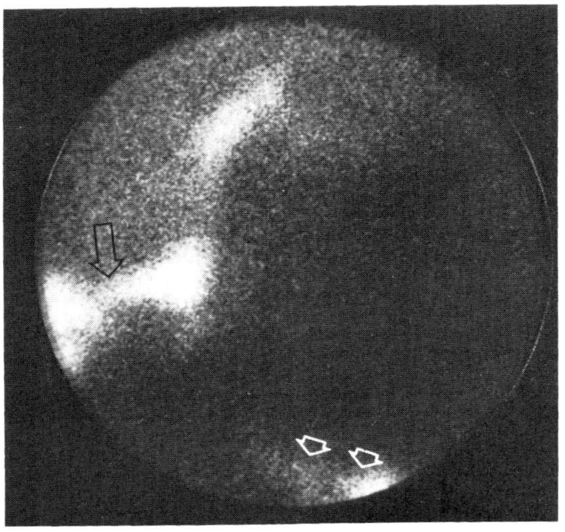

Figure 12–4. Evaluation of the biliary tract after surgery. A fistula to the skin (*single arrow*) is well demonstrated in a postcholecystectomy patient. Drainage distally into the bowel is also documented (*double arrows*).

quite distorted.[42, 43] The direction and dynamics of bile flow can be traced by serial ^{99m}Tc IDA imaging, which provides useful physiologic and anatomic information, especially regarding drainage of the biliary tract into the intestine. Leakage of bile (Fig. 12–4),[62] gallbladder perforation[59, 79] cholecystocolic fistula,[60] and gastrobiliary fistula[61] can also be evaluated.

Other Uses of Biliary Scintigraphy

Biliary scintigraphy may be useful for evaluating cold defects seen on colloid images (Fig. 12–5).[63–66] Defects in the region of the porta hepatis on colloid scan may be associated with biliary disease, masses due to tumor, or anatomic variations in gallbladder position. Using biliary scintigraphy it is possible to determine if the defect seen on the ^{99m}Tc sulfur colloid scan is due to a tumor, an obstructed and dilated gallbladder, or a normal variation in gallbladder position.

Biliary scintigraphy may be of use in the differential diagnosis of jaundice provided that hepatocyte excretion is not totally abolished. In jaundice caused by hepatocellular disease, visualization of the liver and bile ducts usually occurs at serum bilirubin levels below 5 mg/dl (Fig. 12–6). In patients with serum bilirubin levels greater than 4 to 5 mg/dl; visualization of the liver and biliary ducts with hepatobiliary agents is variable (Fig. 12–7). The initial evaluation of these patients is best accomplished with ultrasound or computed tomography. In patients with complete extrahepatic biliary obstruction, no activity will be seen in the biliary ducts or gastrointestinal tract up to 24 hours following the injection. An area of decreased activity may be seen in the region of the gallbladder. Immediate and intense secretion of radionuclide into the genitourinary system may occur.[10, 11, 18, 22–24, 44] If incomplete extrahepatic biliary obstruction is present, the appearance of activity in the gastrointestinal tract is delayed. The distended biliary ducts are seen. In addition, the gallbladder may appear dilated (Fig. 12–8).[10, 11, 18, 22, 23, 40, 43]

Biliary scintigraphy can also help distinguish neonatal jaundice due to hepatocellular disease from extrahepatic biliary duct atresia.[43] In these patients, pretreatment with

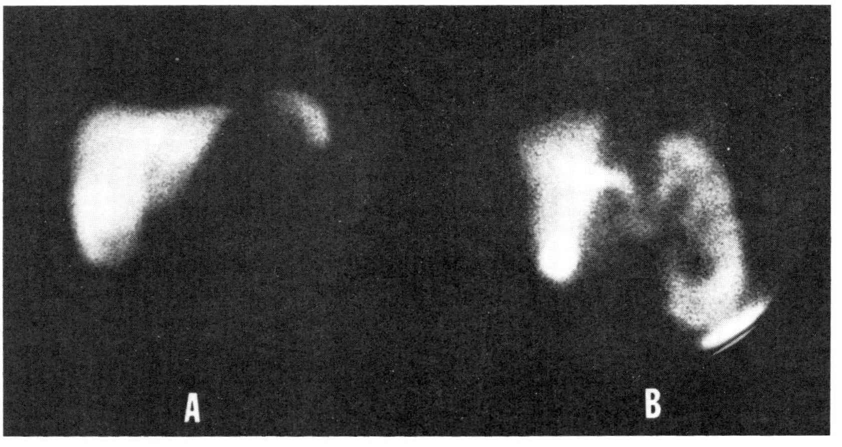

Figure 12–5. Evaluation of "cold" defect seen on Tc-99m sulfur colloid imaging. *A*, "Cold" defect seen in inferior aspect of right lobe of liver on Tc-99m sulfur colloid image. *B*, Following administration of Tc-99m biliary imaging agent, showing that the gallbladder was the cause of the defect.

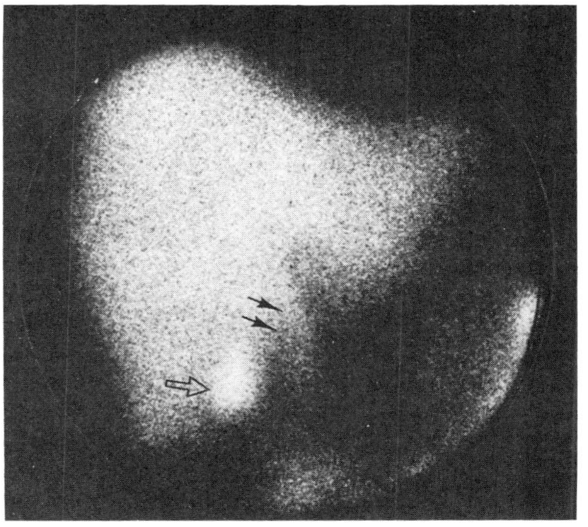

Figure 12–6. Hepatitis (serum bilirubin 4.4 mg/dl). Scintigram at 1 hour post injection shows the liver, gallbladder (*open arrow*), and common duct (*arrows*) to be adequately defined. Radioactivity is also seen in the gastrointestinal tract.

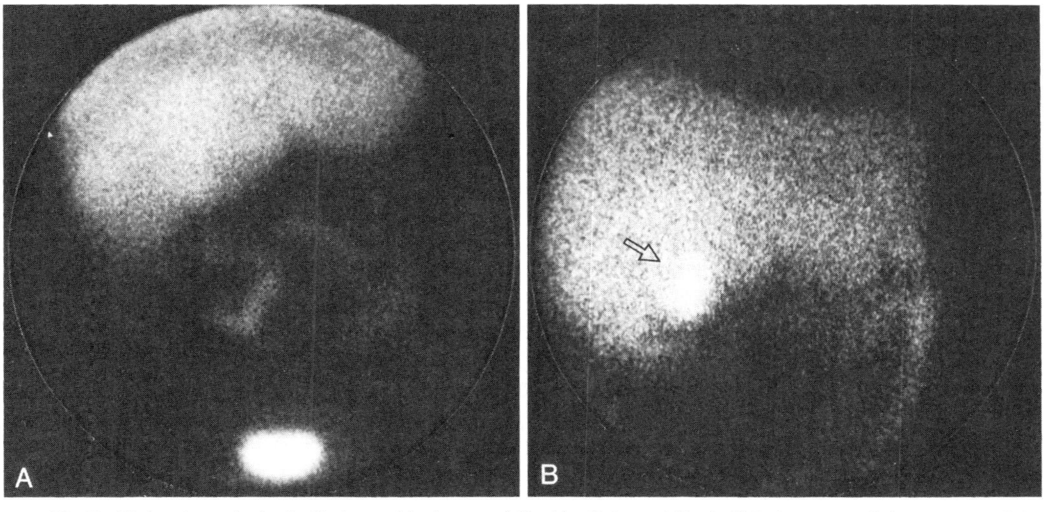

Figure 12–7. Cirrhosis and alcoholic hepatitis (serum bilirubin 8.1 mg/dl). *A*, Scintigram at 3 hours post injection shows the liver well defined as well as radioactivity in the gastrointestinal tract and bladder. *B*, Delayed scintigram shows the liver and gallbladder (*arrow*) well defined.

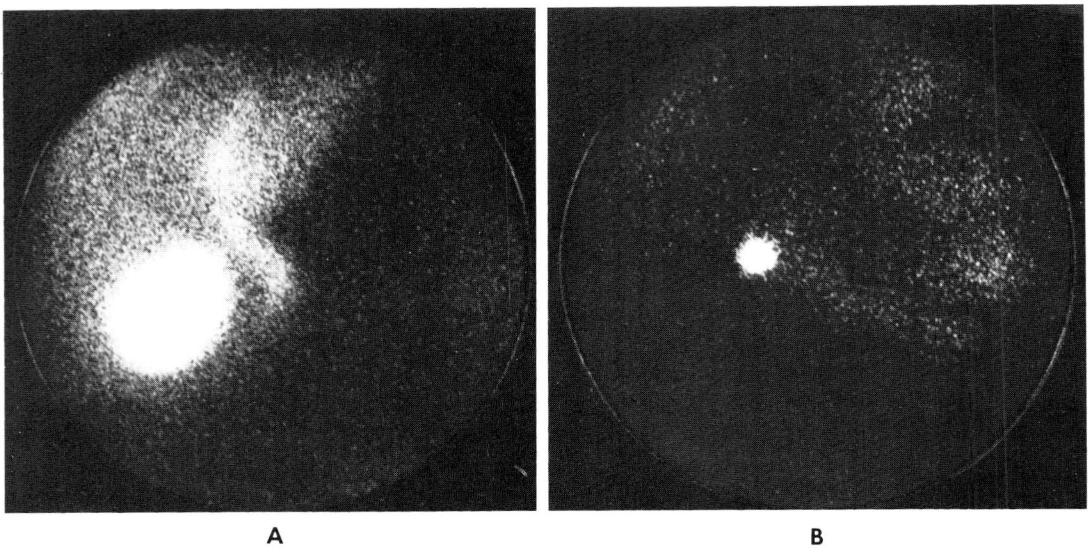

Figure 12–8. Incomplete obstruction. *A*, The prominent gallbladder and proximal common duct are visualized at 5½ hours post injection. No activity is seen in the gastrointestinal tract. *B*, Radioactivity is identified in the gastrointestinal tract 24 hours post injection. Hot spot is due to cobalt marker on umbilicus.

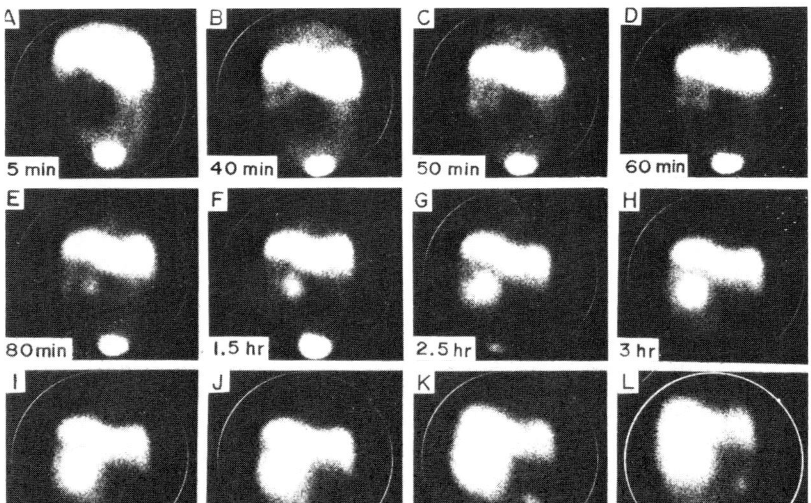

Figure 12–9. Serial supine abdominal scintiphotos. The choledochal cyst is demonstrated as a round cold area as the result of total body and liver radioactivity on early scintiphotos (*A* to *C*), with subsequent filling of the gallbladder (*B* to *D*) and cyst (*E* to *K*). Note visualization of bowel radioactivity at 8 and 24 hours (*K* to *L*). Urinary bladder is also demonstrated 5 minutes to 5 hours. (From Yeh SH, Stadalnik RC, DeNardo GL, et al: Clin Nucl Med 1978; *3*:50. Used by permission.)

phenobarbital reduces the number of false positive scans.[67, 68] The procedure is also useful to evaluate patients with Kasai portoenterostomy[43, 67] and to detect congenital abnormalities of the ducts, such as choledochal cysts (Fig. 12–9),[45, 46, 69, 70] congenital hepatic fibrosis,[71] and Ivemark's syndrome.[72]

Segmental biliary obstruction and intrahepatic gallstones can be detected using ^{99m}Tc cholescintigraphy.[5] Small "muddy" stones impacted at the bifurcation of intrahepatic ducts, which may be missed by endoscopic retrograde cholangiography and percutaneous transhepatic cholangiography,[73–75] can also be diagnosed by cholescintigraphy.

^{99m}Tc cholescintigraphy is able to separate patients with significant gallbladder disease from those without following abnormal oral cholecystography.[58] Positive ^{99m}Tc cholescintigraphy predicted significant gallbladder disease in 80 per cent of these patients, whereas a normal study ruled out significant gallbladder disease with a specificity of 78 per cent in this group.

SUMMARY

The conventional ^{99m}Tc sulfur colloid liver scan frequently demonstrates changes when biliary duct dilatation is present. However, this test is neither sensitive nor specific.

The new ^{99m}Tc biliary imaging agents are highly sensitive and specific in detecting biliary tract disease, especially cholecystitis, in patients with mild to moderate jaundice. The advantages of biliary imaging include availability, safety, simplicity, and accuracy. In addition, these tests can be performed in patients who are allergic to iodinated contrast agents.

REFERENCES

1. Oppenheim BE, Gottschalk A, Hoffer PB: Liver scanning. *In* Gottschalk A, Potchen EJ (eds): Diagnostic Nuclear Medicine. Baltimore, Williams & Wilkins, 1976, pp 399–455.
2. Heck LL, Gottschalk A: The appearance of intrahepatic biliary duct dilatation on the liver scan. Radiology 1971;*99*:135.
3. Handmaker H: Nuclear medicine in the evaluation of the patient with jaundice. JAMA 1975;*231*:1172.
4. Silverberg M, Rosenthall L, Freeman LM: Rose bengal excretion studies as an aid in the differential diagnosis of neonatal jaundice. Semin Nucl Med 1973;*111*:69.
5. Winston MA, Blahd WH: ^{131}I rose bengal imaging techniques in differential diagnosis of jaundiced patients. Semin Nucl Med 1972;*11*:167.
6. Chiotellis E, Subramanian G, McAfee JG: Preparation of Tc^{99m} labeled pyridoxal–amino acid complexes and their evaluation. Int J Nucl Med Biol 1977;*4*:29.
7. Kato M, Hazue M: Tc^{99m} (Sn) pyridoxylideneaminates: preparation and biologic evaluation. J Nucl Med 1978;*19*:397.
8. Kubota H, Eckelman WC, Poulase KP, et al: ^{99m}Tc pyridoxylideneglutamate, a new agent for gallbladder imaging: comparison with ^{131}I rose bengal. J Nucl Med 1976;*17*:36.
9. Papadimitriou J, Fotopoulas A, Koutoulidis C, et al: Evaluation of Tc^{99m} pyridoxal-phenylalanine as a hepatobiliary agent. Part 2. Clinical Tests. J Nucl Med 1977;*18*:1194.
10. Ronai PM, Baker RJ, Bellen JC, et al: ^{99m}Tc-pyridoxylidene-glutamate: A new hepatobiliary radiopharmaceutical. II. Clinical aspects. J Nucl Med 1975;*16*:728.
11. Stadalnik RC, Matolo NM, Jansholt A-L, et al: Technetium-99m-pyridoxylideneglutamate (P.G.) cholescintigraphy. Radiology 1976;*121*:657.
12. Winston BW, Subramanian G, Van Heertum RL, et al: An evaluation of 99mTc-labeled hepatobiliary agents. J Nucl Med 1977;*18*:455.
13. Baker RJ, Marion MA: Biliary scanning with Tc-99m-pyridoxylideneglutamate—the effect of food in normal subjects: concise communication. J Nucl Med 1977;*18*:793.
14. Loberg MD, Cooper M, Harvey E, et al: Development of new radiopharmaceuticals based on *N*-substitution of iminodiacetic acid. J Nucl Med 1976;*17*:633.
15. Ryan J, Cooper M, Loberg M, et al: Technetium-99m-labeled *N*-(2, 6-dimethylphenylcarbamoylmethyl) iminodiacetic acid (Tc-99m HIDA): A new radiopharmaceutical for hepatobiliary imaging studies. J Nucl Med 1977;*18*:995.
16. Eikman EA: Radionuclide hepatobiliary procedures: When can HIDA help? J Nucl Med 1979;*20*:358.
17. Rosenthall L: An update on radionuclide imaging in hepatobiliary disease. JAMA 1981;*245*:2065.
18. Rosenthall L, Shaffer EA, Lisbona R, et al: Diagnosis of hepatobiliary disease by ^{99m}Tc-HIDA cholescintigraphy. Radiology 1978;*126*:467.
19. Pare P, Shaffer EA, Rosenthall L: Nonvisualization of the gallbladder by ^{99m}Tc-HIDA cholescintigraphy as evidence of cholecystitis. CMA Journal 1978;*118*:384.
20. Stadalnik RC, Kraus JF, Matolo NM, et al: The validity of technetium-99m-pyridoxylideneglutamate (P.G.) cholescintigraphy as a diagnostic test for cholecystitis. Clin Nucl Med 1978;*3*:142.
21. Lubin E, Rachima M, Oren V, et al: Tc-99m-pyridoxylideneglutamate in jaundiced patients. J Nucl Med 1978;*19*:24.
22. Matolo NM, Stadalnik RC, Krohn KA, et al: Biliary tract scanning with ^{99m}Tc-pyridoxylideneglutamate: a new gallbladder scanning agent. Surgery 1976;*80*:317.
23. Matolo NM, Stadalnik RC, Wolfman EF Jr: Clinical evaluation of ^{99m}Tc-pyridoxylideneglutamate for hepatobiliary scanning. Am J Surg 1976;*132*:716.
24. Matolo NM, Stadalnik RC, Wolfman EF Jr: Hepatobiliary scanning using Tc-99m-pyridoxylideneglutamate. Am J Surg 1977;*133*:116.
25. Krishnamurthy GT: Acute cholecystitis: the diag-

nostic role for current imaging tests. West J Med 1982;*137*:87.
26. Mauro MA, McCartney WH, Melmed JR: Hepatobiliary scanning with ^{99m}Tc-PIPIDA in acute cholecystitis. Radiology 1982;*142*:193.
27. Matolo NM, Stadalnik RC, McGahan JP: Comparison of ultrasonography, computerized tomography, and radionuclide imaging in the diagnosis of acute and chronic cholecystitis. Am J Surg 1982;*144*:676.
28. Zeman RK, Burrell MI, Cahow CE, et al: Diagnostic utility of cholescintigraphy and ultrasonography in acute cholecystitis. Am J Surg 1981;*141*:446.
29. Ralls PW, Colletti PM, Halls JM, et al: Prospective evaluation of ^{99m}Tc-IDA cholescintigraphy and grayscale ultrasound in the diagnosis of acute cholecystitis. Radiology 1982;*144*:369.
30. Worthen NJ, Uszler JM, Funamura JL: Cholecystitis: Prospective evaluation of sonography and ^{99m}Tc-HIDA cholescintigraphy. AJR 1981;*137*:973.
31. Suarez CA, Block F, Bernstein D, et al: The role of H.I.D.A./P.I.P.I.D.A. scanning in diagnosing cystic duct obstruction. Ann Surg 1980;*191*:391.
32. Duch G, Nielsen A, Axelsson CK: The value of ^{99m}Tc-cholescintigraphy as compared with infusion cholecystography for diagnosing acute cholecystitis. Scand J Gastroenterol 1981;*16*:993.
33. Szlabick RE, Catto JA, Fink-Bennett D, et al: Hepatobiliary scanning in the diagnosis of acute cholecystitis. Arch Surg 1980;*115*:540.
34. Matolo NM, Stadalnik RC, Dixon SM: Value and limitations of scanning of the biliary tract. Surg Gynecol Obstet 1980;*150*:521.
35. Ohrt HJ, Posalaky IP, Shafer RB: Normal gallbladder scintigraphy in acute cholecystitis. Clin Nucl Med 1983;*8*:97.
36. Weissmann HS, Berkowitz D, Fox MS, et al: The role of technetium-99m iminodiacetic acid (IDA) cholescintigraphy in acute acalculous cholecystitis. Radiology 1983;*146*:177.
37. Echevarria RA, Gleason JL: False-negative gallbladder scintigram in acute cholecystitis. J Nucl Med 1980;*21*:841.
38. Shuman WP, Mack LA, Rudd TG, et al: Evaluation of acute right upper quadrant pain: sonography and ^{99m}Tc-PIPIDA cholescintigraphy. AJR 1982; *139*:61.
39. Samuels BI, Freitas JE, Bree RL, et al: A comparison of radionuclide hepatobiliary imaging and real-time ultrasound for the detection of acute cholecystitis. Radiology 1983;*147*:207.
40. Bennett MT, Shildon MI, dos Remedios LV, et al: Diagnosis of acute cholecystitis using hepatobiliary scan with technetium-99m PIPIDA. Am J Surg 1981;*142*:338.
41. Choy D, Shi EC, McLean RG, et al: Cholescintigraphy in acute cholecystitis: use of intravenous morphine. Radiology 1984;*151*:203.
42. Rosenthall L, Fonseca C, Arzoumanion A, et al: ^{99m}Tc-HIDA following upper abdominal surgery. Radiology 1979;*130*:735.
43. Stadalnik RC, Matolo NM: Radionuclide imaging of the biliary tree. Surg Clin North Am 1981;*61*:827.
44. Pors Nielsen S, Trap-Jensen J, Lindenberg J, et al: Hepatic-biliary scintigraphy and hepatography with Tc-99m diethyl-acetanilido-iminodiacetate in obstructive jaundice. J Nucl Med 1978;*19*:452.
45. Brown RG, Gilday DL, Ash JM: Tc^{99m}-pyridoxylideneglutamate quality control and clinical aspects in pediatric nuclear medicine. J Nucl Med 1976; *17*:555.
46. Yeh SH, Stadalnik RC, DeNardo GL, et al: Definitive diagnosis of choledochal cyst by ^{99m}Tc-pyridoxylideneglutamate sequential scintiphotography. Clin Nucl Med 1978;*3*:113.
47. Krishnamurthy GT, Bobba VR, Kingston E, et al: Measurement of gallbladder emptying sequentially using a single dose of ^{99m}Tc-labeled hepatobiliary agent. Gastroenterology 1982;*83*:773.
48. London JW, Guenberg A, Alavi A, et al: Automated calculation of gallbladder ejection fraction. Eur J Nucl Med 1983;*8*:307.
49. Wiener I, Inoue K, Fagan CJ, et al: Release of cholecystokinin in man. Correlation of blood levels with gallbladder contraction. Ann Surg 1981; *194*:321.
50. Maton PN, et al: Infusion of cholecystokinin octapeptide in man: relation between plasma cholecystokinin concentrations and gallbladder emptying rates. Eur J Clin Invest 1984;*14*:37.
51. Van Der Linden W, Kempi V, Edlund G: Function of liver, gallbladder and sphincter of Oddi after major surgery studied by computer-assisted cholescintigraphy and real-time ultrasonography. Br J Surg 1983;*70*:497.
52. Forgacs IC, et al: Influence of gallstones and ursodeoxycholic acid therapy on gallbladder emptying. Gastroenterology 1984;*87*:299.
53. Davis GB, Berk RN, Scheible FW, et al: Cholecystokinin cholecystography, sonography and scintigraphy: Detection of chronic acalculous cholecystitis. AJR 1982;*139*:1117.
54. Frommhold W, Wolf F: Radiological and radionuclide methods for the diagnosis of biliary disorders. Clin Gastroenterol 1983;*12*:65.
55. Freeman LM, Sugarman LA, Weissmann HS: Role of cholecystokinetic agents in 99mTc-IDA cholescintigraphy. Semin Nucl Med 1981;*11*:186.
56. Krishnamurthy GT, Bobba VR, Kingston E: Radionuclide ejection fraction: a technique for quantitative analysis of motor function of the human gallbladder. Gastroenterology 1981;*80*:482.
57. Spellman SJ, Shaffer EA, Rosenthall L: Gallbladder emptying in response to cholecystokinin. Gastroenterology 1979;*77*:115.
58. Topper TE, Tyerson TW, Nora PF: Quantitative gallbladder imaging following cholecystokinin. J Nucl Med 1980;*21*:694.
59. Brunetti JC, Van Heertum RL: Preoperative detection of gallbladder perforation. Clin Nucl Med 1980;*5*:347.
60. Edell SL, Milunsky C, Garren L: Cholescintigraphic diagnosis of cholecystocolic fistula. Clin Nucl Med 1981;*6*:303.
61. Henderson RW, Telfer N, Halls JM: Gastrobiliary fistula: pre- and postoperative assessment with 99mTc-PIPIDA. AJR 1981;*137*:163.
62. Weissman HS, Chun KJ, Frank M, et al: Demonstration of traumatic bile leakage with cholescintigraphy and ultrasonography. AJR 1979;*133*:843.
63. Brown ML, Freitas JE, Wahner HW: Useful hepatic parenchymal imaging in hepatobiliary scintigraphy. AJR 1981;*136*:893.
64. Floyd JL, Weiland FL, Hale AS, et al: Hepatic imaging: a comparison of Tc-99m-sulfur colloid and PIPIDA in the detection of defects. Clin Nucl Med 1981;*6*:53.
65. Rao BK, Pastakia B, Lieberman LM: Evaluation of focal defects on technetium-99m sulfur colloid scans with new hepatobiliary agents. Radiology 1980; *136*:497.

66. Weissman HS, Sugarman LA, Frank MS, et al: Serendipity in technetium-99m-dimethyl-iminodiacetic acid cholescintigraphy. Radiology 1980;*135*: 449.
67. Majd M, Reba RC, Altman RP: Hepatobiliary scintigraphy with ^{99m}Tc-PIPIDA in the evaluation of neonatal jaundice. Pediatrics 1981;*67*:140.
68. Majd M, Reba RC, Altman RP: Effect of phenobarbital on ^{99m}Tc-IDA scintigraphy in the evaluation of neonatal jaundice. Semin Nucl Med 1981;*11*:194.
69. Han BK, Babcock DS, Gelford MH: Choledochal cyst with bile duct dilatation: sonography and 99mTc-IDA cholescintigraphy. AJR 1981;*136*:1075.
70. Sugihara M, Yokoyama S, Namba S, et al: Radionuclide imaging in the diagnosis of choledochal cyst and intrahepatic duct dilation. Clin Nucl Med 1979;*4*:325.
71. Masuda Y, Sawa H, Kim OH, et al: A case of congenital hepatic fibrosis: usefulness of hepatobiliary scintigraphy. Clin Nucl Med 1980;*5*:359.
72. Pastakia B, Lieberman LM, Moodie D, et al: ^{99m}Technetium pyridoxylidene-glutamate imaging in visceral heterotaxy (Ivemark's syndrome). Gastroenterology 1979;*77*:1105.
73. Zeman RK, Gold JA, Cluck L, et al: Tc-99m-HIDA scintigraphy in segmental biliary obstruction. J Nucl Med 1980;*22*:456.
74. Huang M-J, Liaw Y-F, Wu C-S: Comparison of intravenous radionuclide cholescintigraphy and endoscopic retrograde cholangiography in the diagnosis of intrahepatic gallstones. Br J Radiol 1981;*54*:302.
75. Yeh SH, Liu OK, Huang MJ: Sequential scintiphotography with technetium-99m-pyridoxylideneglutamate in the detection of intrahepatic lithiasis: concise communication. J Nucl Med 1980;*21*:17.
76. Stadalnik RC, Matolo NM, Jansholt AL, et al: Clinical experience with 99mTc-disofenin as a cholescintigraphic agent. Radiology 1981;*140*:797.
77. Fonseca C, Greenburg D, Rosenthall L, et al: Assessment of the utility of gallbladder imaging with ^{99m}Tc-IDA. Clin Nucl Med 1978;*3*:437.
78. Freitas JE, Gulati RM: Rapid evaluation of acute abdominal pain by hepatobiliary scanning. JAMA 1980;*244*:1585.
79. Mesgarzadeh M, et al: Diagnosis of clinically unsuspected gallbladder perforation in an obsese patient by Tc99m-IDA cholescintigraphy. J Nucl Med 1983;*24*:1028.

BRUCE F. SCHARSCHMIDT, M.D.
*LAWRENCE W. WAY, M.D.**

13

The Jaundiced Patient: Differential Diagnosis and Clinical Approach

Jaundice is a condition in which the sclerae, mucous membranes, and skin become abnormally yellow as a result of an increased concentration of bilirubin in the blood, usually greater than 3 mg/dl. This "threshold" for clinical detection of jaundice depends upon whether the bilirubin level is rising or falling, as it requires time for the bilirubin to accumulate in tissues. In darkly pigmented patients, icterus may be most easily detected in the mucous membranes, tympanic membranes, or sclerae.

Jaundice can result from a variety of causes ranging from life-threatening hemolytic or hepatobiliary disorders to innocuous impairment of hepatic bilirubin transport. Its differential diagnosis is therefore an important and challenging clinical problem. The most important task of the clinician is the timely identification of disorders, such as biliary obstruction, for which specific therapy is required.

The purpose of this chapter is to outline an approach to the patient with jaundice, with an emphasis on clinical and laboratory findings helpful in differential diagnosis, as well as an overall approach to the patient. It includes a strategy for the use of the various techniques currently available for imaging the liver and biliary tract; however, detailed discussion of these techniques is presented in Chapters 8 through 11.

NORMAL BILIRUBIN METABOLISM
(Fig. 13–1)

In order to understand the differential diagnosis of jaundice, it is helpful to review normal bilirubin metabolism.[1–3] Daily bilirubin production in humans averages approximately 250 to 300 mg, of which about 70 per cent is produced in the reticuloendothelial system (spleen, bone marrow) from the catabolism of heme released from senescent erythrocytes. The remaining 30 per cent results largely from the breakdown of nonhemoglobin hemoproteins mainly present in the liver, of which cytochrome P-450 is quantitatively the most important.[1–3] A small fraction of daily bilirubin production results from premature destruction of newly formed erythrocytes, a process termed ineffective erythropoiesis. Heme is first converted to biliverdin by the microsomal enzyme heme oxygenase. Biliverdin is then converted very rapidly to unconjugated bilirubin by the enzyme biliverdin reductase. It is currently thought that heme oxygenase and biliverdin reductase exist as a single complex inside the cell, an arrangement that presumably allows for tightly coordinated conversion of heme to bilirubin.[3] Unconjugated bilirubin circulates in plasma tightly bound to albumin.

The hepatic uptake of unconjugated bilirubin shows characteristics of carrier-mediated transport, including saturability and competition by other organic anions.[4] Entry into liver cells is presumably facilitated by large fenestrations in the endothelial cells lining the hepatic sinusoids that permit direct contact between albumin-bound bilirubin and the surface of the liver cell. Once in hepatocytes, bilirubin binds to cytosolic proteins, such as ligandin, which probably decreases the amount of bilirubin available for reflux back into plasma and facilitates delivery of bilirubin to the endoplasmic reticulum. Water-insoluble unconjugated bilirubin is conjugated in the endoplasmic reticulum of the hepatocyte by joining glucuronic acid, and occasionally other sugars, in ester linkage to one or both propionic acid groups, thereby

*Recipient of NIH Research Career Development and Award 5 K04 AM-00323. This work was also supported in part by NIG Liver Center Grant PSO AM-18520, NIH Research Grant AM-26270, and The Walter C. Pew Fund.

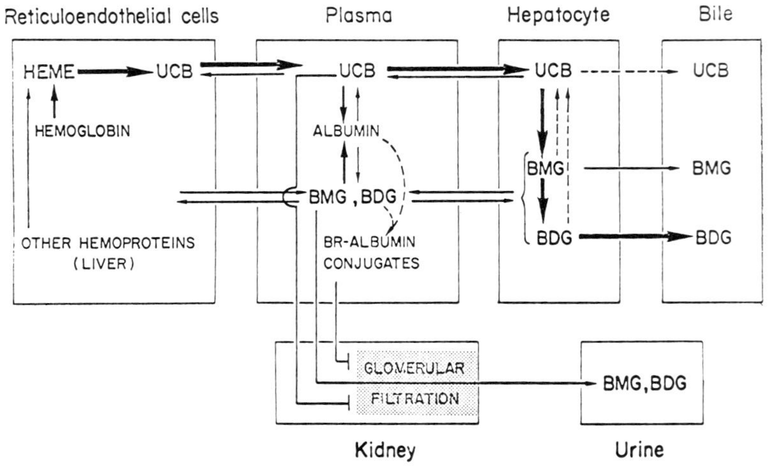

Figure 13–1. Overview of normal bilirubin metabolism and transport. Heme from hemoglobin and other hemoproteins is converted to biliverdin and then to bilirubin in extrahepatic tissues, predominantly the reticuloendothelial cells of the spleen and bone marrow. The unconjugated bilirubin (UCB) released into the plasma, which normally is tightly but reversibly bound to albumin, is taken up by hepatocytes and converted very efficiently to bilirubin monoglucuronide (BMG) and bilirubin diglucuronide (BDG). Both BMG and BDG can reflux into plasma and normally account for less than 5 per cent of total serum bilirubin. BMG in the liver is largely converted to BDG, which is then excreted in bile. Trace amounts of conjugated bilirubin are also deconjugated back to UCB. BMG and BDG in plasma also bind reversibly to albumin, but less tightly than UCB. When present in abnormally high concentrations for a long period of time, BMG and/or BDG bind irreversibly with albumin to form BR-albumin conjugates. While UCB, BMG, BDG, and BR-albumin conjugates all enter the kidney via the blood stream, only BMG and BDG appear in urine, presumably because they are most loosely bound to albumin and therefore most able to be filtered at the glomerulus.

converting bilirubin to a water-soluble molecule.[1–3] Formation of the mono- and diglucuronide is catalyzed by the microsomal enzyme UDP-glucuronyltransferase. Conjugated bilirubin is then transported across the canalicular membrane into bile. Approximately 80 per cent of the bilirubin excreted into bile is of the diglucuronide form; most of the remainder is present as the monoglucuronide. Unconjugated bilirubin is normally present in bile in trace amounts only. Bilirubin moves from the bile through the intestine to the terminal ileum and colon, where it is deconjugated and subsequently converted by bacterial enzymes to colorless compounds called urobilinogens. About 20 per cent of urobilinogen is reabsorbed, and 90 per cent of the reabsorbed fraction is re-excreted in the bile, with the remainder being excreted in the urine. For a more detailed discussion of bilirubin metabolism and transport, the reader is referred to references 1 to 3.

DIFFERENTIAL DIAGNOSIS OF JAUNDICE
(Table 13–1)

Hyperbilirubinemia results from bilirubin overproduction or decreased bilirubin clearance, or a combination of the two.[5]

Bilirubin Overproduction. Bilirubin overproduction is most commonly caused by hemolysis. The following guidelines are useful in assessing the role of hemolysis in hyperbilirubinemia.[5] First, chronic steady-state hemolysis does not, by itself, usually account for a sustained bilirubin concentration greater than 4 to 5 mg/dl. Concentrations consistently above this level usually indicate the presence of hepatic dysfunction. In contrast, acute hemolysis can result in a bilirubin production rate that transiently exceeds the excretory capacity of even a normal liver and may cause striking elevation of bilirubin values.

Transfusions are an important and often overlooked cause of increased bilirubin production. For example, 20 per cent of a unit (250 ml) of bank blood stored for 3 weeks or more hemolyzes within 24 hours of transfusion, acutely releasing as much bilirubin as is normally produced in a single day.[3] Resorption of large hematomas is another cause of

Table 13–1 CAUSE OF HYPRBILIRUBINEMIA

I. *Increased Bilirubin Production*
   Examples: Hemolysis, ineffective erythropoiesis, reabsorption of hematomas, transfusion
II. *Decreased Bilirubin Clearance*
   A. *Selective Defects in Hepatic Bilirubin Clearance*
      Examples: Gilbert's syndrome, Crigler-Najjar syndrome, Dubin-Johnson syndrome, Rotor's syndrome
   B. *Cholestasis*
      1. *Hepatocellular Disease*
         Examples: Drug-induced or viral hepatitis, pregnancy, sepsis
      2. *Biliary Tract Obstruction*
         Examples: Choledocholithiasis, tumor, sclerosing cholangitis, pancreatitis

Adapted from reference 7.

increased bilirubin production. Ineffective erythropoiesis, which may be increased in certain diseases, can also produce hyperbilirubinemia. Examples of this include megaloblastic anemia from either vitamin B_{12} or folic acid deficiency, iron deficiency anemia, sideroblastic anemia, thalassemia minor, polycythemia vera, aplasia, and lead poisoning.[1–3, 5]

Selective Congenital Defects in Hepatic Bilirubin Metabolism or Transport. (Table 13–2). Hyperbilirubinemia and, less frequently, jaundice may also result from decreased hepatic bilirubin clearance due to a hereditary defect in either the hepatic metabolism or the transport of bilirubin. Gilbert's syndrome is present in 5 to 7 per cent of white adults in the United States and Western Europe.[1–3, 5] Gilbert's syndrome results from decreased hepatic clearance of unconjugated bilirubin, but the precise mechanism remains unclear. Serum bilirubin concentrations in these patients may rise two to three fold with fasting or dehydration, or following the administration of nicotinic acid. The serum bilirubin concentration decreases following the administration of phenobaribital owing to the induction of UDP-glucuronyltransferase.

Gilbert's syndrome may present as mild scleral icterus in the second or third decade of life. More commonly, though, the bilirubin elevation is not high enough to produce clinical jaundice, and patients with Gilbert's syndrome present with unconjugated hyperbilirubinemia identified first on routine multiphasic biochemical screening or after fasting, as occurs pre- or postoperatively. Although many symptoms have been associated with the disorder, they are nonspecific and probably not attributable to Gilbert's syndrome itself. The diagnosis of Gilbert's syndrome can be established by the repeated demonstration of normal liver function tests in an asymptomatic individual with a mild elevation in the serum concentration of unconjugated bilirubin and no evidence of overt hemolysis.[5] Although liver biopsy permits structural liver disease to be ruled out and is employed in a few special centers to demonstrate reduced activity of UDP-glucuronyltransferase, it is unnecessary in routine cases. Opacification of the biliary tract is also usually unnecessary. Normal fasting and postprandial concentrations of bile acids have been shown to be helpful in excluding liver disease.[8] The major reason to establish the diagnosis of Gilbert's syndrome is to reassure the patient and to avoid unnecessary operations (e.g., cholecystectomy, splenectomy).

Crigler-Najjar syndrome (congenital nonhemolytic jaundice) is an uncommon cause of unconjugated neonatal hyperbilirubinemia caused by the absence of (Type I) or markedly reduced (Type II) glucuronyltransferase activity.[1–3, 5] Most patients with Type I Crigler-Najjar syndrome develop kernicterus and die in the neonatal period. Patients with Type II disease, and occasional survivors with the Type I syndrome, may reach adulthood. These patients have bilirubin concentrations of 5 to 40 mg/dl, all of which is unconjugated (Table 13–2). Liver function is otherwise normal, and patients with the Type II syndrome are usually asymptomatic. A diagnostic trial of phenobarbital should produce a drop in the bilirubin level in patients with Type II, but not in those with Type I, Crigler-Najjar syndrome.

Hereditary transport defects (Dubin-Johnson syndrome, Rotor's syndrome) resulting in conjugated hyperbilirubinemia are more easily confused with hepatobiliary disease.[1–3] These rare syndromes are characterized by mild jaundice and serum bilirubin levels between 1 and 5 mg/dl, mostly conjugated. Liver function tests are normal with the exception of increased retention of sulfobromophthalein. The two syndromes may be distinguished by the presence of black pigment in the liver in Dubin-Johnson syndrome, by differences in urinary coproporphyrin excretion, and by differences in plasma sulfobromophthalein disappearance (Table 13–2).

Cholestasis. In most patients, jaundice reflects the presence of cholestasis, that is, impaired bile formation or bile flow resulting from extrahepatic biliary tract obstruction or hepatic parenchymal disease. Even in cholestasis, however, increased bilirubin production may be an important contributing factor (e.g., hemolysis complicating viral hepatitis, ineffective erythropoiesis caused by folate deficiency in the alcoholic patient).

Cholestasis can be subdivided into intrahepatic and extrahepatic causes (See Table 13–1). Intrahepatic causes are conditions in which the hepatocyte is unable to excrete bile even though the major ducts are patent. These include acute and chronic viral hepatitis of any etiology, alcoholic hepatitis, drug- or toxin-induced liver injury, primary biliary cirrhosis, congestive heart failure, sepsis, pregnancy, infiltrative diseases of the liver,

Table 13–2 HEREDITARY DEFECTS IN BILIRUBIN TRANSPORT

	Gilbert's Syndrome	Crigler-Najjar Syndrome (Congenital Nonhemolytic Jaundice) *Type I*	*Type II*	Dubin-Johnson Syndrome	Rotor's Syndrome
Incidence	≤ 7% of population	Rare	Uncommon	Rare, up to 1:1300 in Iranian Jews	Rare
Identified defects in bilirubin metabolism	Decreased hepatic uptake Decreased glucuronyl transferase activity	Absent glucuronyl transferase activity	Markedly decreased or absent glucuronyl transferase activity	Impaired bilirubin excretion	Impaired bilirubin excretion
Plasma bilirubin concentration (mg/dl)	Total: ≤ 3 in absence of hemolysis or fasting Conjugated: ≤ 0.1 by new assays	Total: 17–50 (usually > 20) Conjugated: 0	Total: 6–45 (usually < 20) Conjugated: 0	Total: 1–25 (usually < 7) Conjugated: averages 60% of total	Total: 1–20 (usually < 7) Conjugated: averages 60% of total
Inheritance	? Autosomal dominant	Autosomal recessive	? Autosomal dominant with variable penetrance	Autosomal recessive	Autosomal recessive
Physical findings	Usually none; occasional scleral icterus	Jaundice, neurologic findings of kernicterus in infants	Jaundice, findings of kernicterus only rarely present	Jaundice occasional hepatomegaly	Jaundice
Plasma BSP disappearance rate	Decreased in some patients (45 min retention ≤ 15%)	Normal	Normal	Slow initial disappearance in some patients (45 min retention < 20%); frequent secondary rise at 90–120 min)	Markedly slow initial disappearance (45 min retention 30–50%); no secondary rise
Diagnosis	Clinical and laboratory findings; no elevation in serum conjugated bilirubin by newer fractionation techniques; measurement of serum bile acids if available; liver biopsy not routinely necessary	Clinical and laboratory findings; absence of bilirubin conjugates in serum by newer fractionation techniques; no reduction in plasma bilirubin concentration by phenobarbital	Clinical and laboratory findings; absence of bilirubin conjugates in serum by newer fractionation techniques; partial reduction in plasma bilirubin concentration by phenobarbital	Clinical and laboratory findings, including BSP disappearance and urinary coproporphyrins; liver biopsy shows coarse dark pigment in centrolobular cells	Clinical and laboratory findings, including BSP disappearance and urinary coproporphyrins; liver biopsy shows no dark pigment
Treatment	Phenobarbital rarely indicated	No generally effective, practical, and safe treatment available	Phenobarbital if indicated	No specific treatment available; avoid estrogens	No specific treatment available
Prognosis	Normal	Usually death in infancy; rarely, later onset of neurologic damage	Usually normal; kernicterus occurs only rarely	Probably normal	Probably normal

Modified from references 2, 6, and 7.

and liver disease in infancy. Indeed, the list of causes of intrahepatic cholestasis is very long. The second major cause of cholestasis is extrahepatic biliary obstruction, most commonly due to gallstones or a neoplasm. These conditions are discussed extensively in Chapters 18, 19, 26, and 30 to 34.

APPROACH TO THE PATIENT

The cause of jaundice in an individual patient can be diagnosed or at least suspected from the clinical history, physical examination, and routine laboratory tests.[9, 10] A practical approach to the patient with jaundice is outlined in Figure 13–2.[11] Although such an algorithm is useful as an illustration of a systematic approach, it is important to emphasize that no algorithm is applicable to all patients. Under some circumstances, it may be appropriate to skip certain steps or move in directions not indicated by the algorithm. Certain such situations will be illustrated by example in the discussion to follow.

Clinical Evaluation. The patient's *history* usually provides important diagnostic clues.

The presence of itching should alert one to the presence of cholestasis. While the identity of the "pruritogen(s)" is controversial, bile salts in the skin are the most likely candidates. A history of dark urine indicates that the jaundice stems from increased levels of conjugated bilirubin in the serum (see Fig. 13–1) and suggests the presence of cholestasis, Rotor's syndrome, or Dubin-Johnson syndrome. The presence of clay-colored (acholic) stools suggests severe cholestasis. The initial conclusion that this resulted from diminished fecal bilirubin and urobilinogen excretion is probably not correct, since patients with Type I Crigler-Najjar syndrome excrete minimal bilirubin into bile but have normal-colored feces. Stools of normal color and appearance may also be present in cases of high-grade extrahepatic bile duct obstruction, however, and light pigmentation can result from dietary changes, steatorrhea, and other factors. Consequently, changes in stool color are not very reliable as an index of biliary obstruction. The presence of abdominal pain or a history of prior biliary tract disease or surgery should alert one to a diagnosis of biliary disease.

Acute infectious hepatitis is mainly a disease of young (i.e., under age 45) persons,

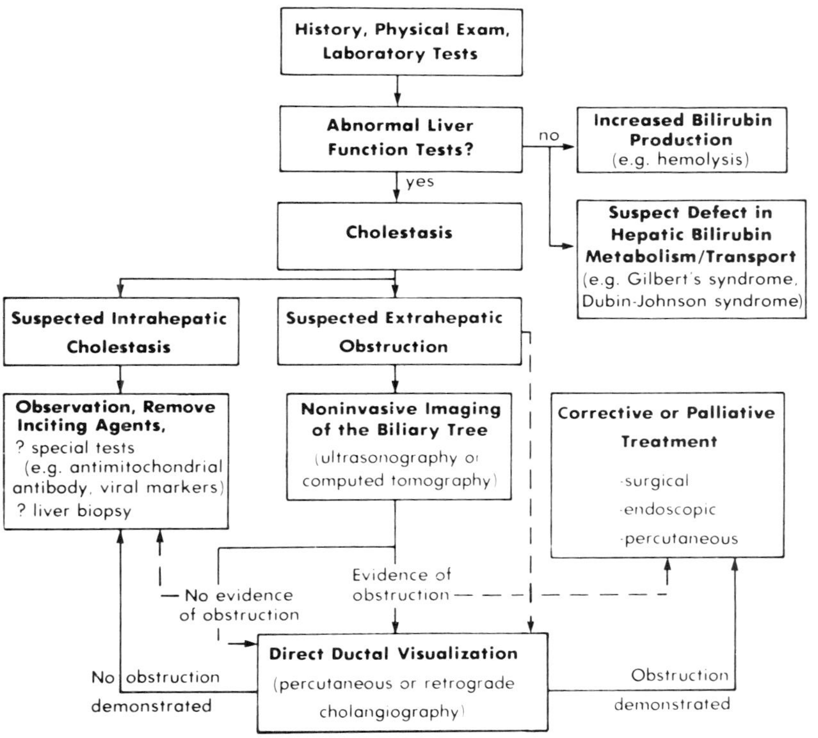

Figure 13–2. Outline of a clinical approach to the patient with jaundice. (From Lake JR, Scharschmidt BF. *In* Conn RS (ed): Current Diagnosis. Philadelphia, WB Saunders, 1985.)

and this diagnosis should be entertained with caution in others. The insidious appearance of deep jaundice over a few weeks should suggest neoplastic obstruction. Jaundice that fluctuates in intensity, especially if accompanied by fever and abdominal pain, is characteristic of gallstone disease. A history of neoplastic disease elsewhere in the body (e.g., breast, colon, stomach) indicates the possibility of hepatic metastases. Mild to moderate jaundice without other clinical findings (i.e., fever, weight loss, pain) may reflect drug-induced cholestasis, and in any case the history should always include questions about exposure to alcohol, drugs, and other potential hepatotoxins.

The *physical examination* may also be useful. For example, estimates of the degree of hyperbilirubinemia may be obtained. As mentioned previously, a level of 3 mg/dl or greater is usually required for the detection of scleral icterus. Mucous membrane or cutaneous icterus generally requires higher concentrations. The presence of occult blood in the stool may represent a clue to a periampullary neoplasm or hemobilia. Prolonged cholestasis, for example, that due to primary biliary cirrhosis, also may produce markedly elevated cholesterol levels and cutaneous xanthomas. Spider hemangiomas, ascites, and splenomegaly suggest alcoholic cirrhosis. Hepatic enlargement may reflect the presence of tumor, abscess, alcoholic injury, bile duct obstruction, cysts, and so forth. A palpable nontender gallbladder in a jaundiced patient (Courvoisier's sign) usually reflects the presence of a periampullary neoplasm or gallbladder cancer.

Laboratory Tests. Laboratory studies are often helpful in the work-up of patients with jaundice. Recommended laboratory studies include a complete blood count (CBC), reticulocyte count, and examination of the peripheral blood smear in cases of suspected hemolysis, and liver function tests, including measurement of serum bilirubin concentration and serum transaminase and alkaline phosphatase activities. If other liver function tests are normal, hemolysis, ineffective erythropoiesis, or a selective defect in hepatic bilirubin transport, such as Gilbert's syndrome, is likely to be responsible for increased bilirubin levels. Lactate dehydrogenase activities (particularly isoenzyme 1), decreased serum haptoglobin concentration, or the presence of urinary hemosiderin may also be useful in the evaluation of suspected hemolysis. If the patient is anemic and the reticulocyte count is inappropriately low, this should suggest ineffective erythropoiesis. If the CBC, reticulocyte count, and liver function tests are normal, Gilbert's syndrome should be considered. The increase in serum bilirubin concentration that accompanies Gilbert's syndrome and disorders associated with hemolysis or ineffective erythropoiesis is characteristically unconjugated, particularly if the new assays are employed (see Fig. 13–1 and following discussion.) In contrast, the hyperbilirubinemia that accompanies the Dubin-Johnson or Rotor syndrome or cholestasis is partially or predominantly conjugated (see Table 13–2).

If liver function tests are abnormal, the jaundice is very likely to be a manifestation of cholestasis. The elevation in serum bilirubin concentration that accompanies cholestasis is due largely to an increase in the conjugated fraction. Cholestasis is characteristically accompanied by increased serum activities of gamma glutamyltranspeptidase (GGT), 5′-nucleotidase, leucine aminopeptidase, and alkaline phosphatase. Unlike bilirubin or bile acids, an elevated alkaline phosphatase activity in serum does not reflect diminished biliary excretion, but rather increased synthesis and possibly increased release of this enzyme into the circulation.[12, 13] This same mechanism may be operational for the other enzymes, such as 5′-nucleotidase or leucine aminopeptidase, which are also located on the hepatocyte plasma membrane and are possibly released into plasma by the detergent effects of bile acids.[14–17] Although increased activity of these enzymes is characteristic of cholestasis, elevations may occur in other situations. Alkaline phosphatase activity may be increased in certain bone disorders and in pregnancy. GGT activity may be increased by numerous enzyme-inducing drugs, as well as alcohol, even in the absence of liver or biliary disease. It is not found in bone, and a normal GGT value therefore suggests that an elevated alkaline phosphatase activity is of bony origin. Leucine aminopeptidase is also present in virtually all tissues, but elevated serum levels are seen only in hepatobiliary disease, particularly biliary obstruction and cholestasis associated with pregnancy. Again, the principal use of this enzyme is in evaluating the significance of an elevated alkaline phosphatase activity. Other laboratory abnormalities that may accompany cholestasis include elevated concentrations of cholesterol and lipoprotein X in serum.

Other tests that are often abnormal include

the serum albumin level and the prothrombin time.

Laboratory Tests of Special Value

Serum Bilirubin. The normal concentration of bilirubin in the serum of adults is less than 1.0 mg/dl.[1–3, 5] Serum bilirubin is conventionally measured by a diazo reaction, in which bilirubin couples with a reagent such as diazotized sulfanilic acid to form a colored product that is quantified spectrophotometrically. Conjugated bilirubin tends to react "directly" in this assay, that is, without the addition of an "accelerator" such as alcohol or urea. Total bilirubin is obtained by performing the assay in the presence of an "accelerator" that facilitates the reaction of unconjugated bilirubin with the diazo reagent. The indirect fraction is calculated by subtracting the direct fraction from the total bilirubin concentration.

More sensitive and specific techniques have recently become available for measuring serum concentrations of unconjugated bilirubin, monoconjugated bilirubin, diconjugated bilirubin and, in pathologic sera, the presence of bilirubin-albumin conjugates.[19–22] Clinical evaluation of these new assays, which are not yet generally available, and comparison of the results with the conventional diazo assay, have revealed interesting and clinically relevant findings.

First, measurements of direct- and indirect-reacting bilirubin by the conventional diazo assay are very inaccurate for obtaining the concentrations of conjugated and unconjugated bilirubin, respectively, in serum. Normally, less than 5 per cent of total serum bilirubin is conjugated.[20]

Second, in most patients with hyperbilirubinemia due to cholestasis, fractionation of serum bilirubin by either the conventional or the newer techniques is of little value; that is, it does not help in distinguishing parenchymal liver disease from biliary obstruction.[20] In contrast, when dealing with a patient with mild hyperbilirubinemia, in whom Gilbert's syndrome, hemolysis, and subclinical hepatobiliary disease are diagnostic possibilities, fractionation of serum bilirubin by the newer techniques is often of value. This is also a situation in which the conventional assay is particularly unreliable.[20] As can be appreciated by examination of Figure 13–1, Gilbert's syndrome and hemolysis are accompanied either by no elevation of conjugated bilirubin levels or by an elevation that is proportional to the increase in total bilirubin; that is, conjugated bilirubin will still be 5 per cent or less of the total serum bilirubin, as in normal individuals. In contrast, a disproportionate elevation of the conjugated bilirubin level indicates cholestasis or hereditary conjugated hyperbilirubinemia (see Table 13–2).[20–22]

Third, the sera of patients with prolonged, conjugated hyperbilirubinemia typically has bilirubin-albumin conjugates, that is, conjugated bilirubin bound irreversibly to albumin (see Fig. 13–1).[22] These conjugates appear to form in serum by direct, nonenzymatic coupling of albumin and conjugated bilirubin (analogous to the formation of glycosylated hemoglobin in patients with diabetes mellitus). In contrast to conjugated bilirubin, which is excreted promptly by the normal liver and appears in urine, these complexes have a serum half-life comparable to that of albumin (2 to 3 weeks) and do not appear in urine.[22, 23] These complexes may account for up to 80 per cent of total serum bilirubin in patients with prolonged obstruction, and their presence helps to explain two important clinical observations: (1) the prolonged persistence of direct-reacting hyperbilirubinemia in patients with resolving obstruction due to the long half-life of the complexes; and (2) the lower renal threshold for conjugated bilirubin in patients with the recent onset of hepatobiliary disease in whom conjugates are just beginning to form, as compared with patients with resolving liver disease, in whom conjugates may account for most of the serum bilirubin.[22]

Thus, while total bilirubin measured by the conventional diazo assay remains adequate for most patients, the shortcomings of the assay are important to appreciate. The newer assays, which provide information of value in selected patients, should be more readily available in the near future.

Serum Bile Acids. With either parenchymal liver disease or biliary obstruction, the normally efficient hepatic clearance of bile acids from portal venous blood is impaired.[18] Indeed, elevation of serum bile acids is a more sensitive index of cholestasis than is hyperbilirubinemia. Although a normal bile acid level is helpful in excluding a cholestatic disorder and may aid in making a diagnosis of Gilbert's syndrome, elevated values are nonspecific and are not useful in the differential diagnosis of cholestasis. Measurement of serum bile acid levels is currently not available in most laboratories.

Table 13–3 CLINICAL CLUES TO EXTRAHEPATIC OBSTRUCTION

History
Abdominal pain suggestive of biliary disease or pancreatitis
Previous biliary surgery
Prolonged or intermittent cholestasis
Absence of exposure to hepatitis or potential hepatotoxins (e.g., drugs) and absence of hepatitis-like symptoms
Physical Examination
Palpable gallbladder or abdominal mass
High fever suggestive of cholangitis
Occult blood in stool
Absence of stigmata of chronic liver disease
Abdominal tenderness
Laboratory Studies
Disproportionate elevation of bilirubin, alkaline phosphatase
Elevated amylase
Complete normalization of a prolonged prothrombin time following parenteral administration of vitamin K
Negative serologic markers for viral hepatitis, chronic active hepatitis, primary biliary cirrhosis

Adapted from references 6 and 7.

DISTINGUISHING INTRAHEPATIC FROM EXTRAHEPATIC CHOLESTASIS

Clinical Clues. The differential diagnosis of cholestasis is the most common and perhaps most important distinction faced by the clinician in evaluating a jaundiced patient. It is particularly important that patients with biliary obstruction be correctly identified so that appropriate treatment can be instituted. Clinical clues to the presence of extrahepatic obstruction are outlined in Table 13–3. The value of the patient history, physical examination, and routine laboratory tests in the differential diagnosis of jaundice has been reaffirmed by a recent prospective study in which over 90 per cent of cases of proven obstructive jaundice were correctly suspected on the basis of clinical evaluation alone.[10] Laboratory tests of particular value in the differential diagnosis of cholestasis include serologic tests for hepatitis B virus infection, antimitochondrial antibodies (positive in 85 per cent or more of patients with primary biliary cirrhosis at some time during the course of the disease), and serum amylase activity (often elevated with pancreatic or biliary tract disease).

Although the distinction between intra- and extrahepatic causes of cholestasis can usually be made on the basis of a thorough clinical evaluation, it is important to be aware of hepatic parenchymal disorders that may present with prominent cholestasis suggestive of extrahepatic obstruction (Table 13–4). The most important causes of intrahepatic cholestasis to identify are those that are potentially treatable or reversible on withdrawal of the offending agent. In some instances (e.g., alcoholic hepatitis, amyloidosis), liver biopsy may permit a specific diagnosis. However, in most instances (e.g., cholestatic viral hepatitis, drug- or estrogen-induced cholestasis, benign recurrent cholestasis, cholestasis related to sepsis) liver biopsy demonstrates only cholestasis with variable hepatocellular necrosis, findings that by themselves do not permit a specific diagnosis.

It is worth emphasizing that biliary and hepatocellular disease often coexist. For example, the incidence of gallstones is known to be increased in cirrhotics, and about 40 per cent of patients with primary biliary cirrhosis have gallbladder stones.[24] Thus, known hepatocellular disease should not dissuade one from pursuing possible biliary disease suspected on clinical grounds.

Episodic mild jaundice associated with abdominal pain and fever is typical of cholangitis due to choledocholithiasis. If an ultrasound scan demonstrates gallbladder stones and the bilirubin value is in the range of 3 to 10 mg/dl, the diagnosis of choledocholithiasis is highly probable. Attacks of cholangitis in a patient who has had previous biliary surgery may also suggest biliary stricture as a possible cause. Stricture would be unlikely, however, if the course after the original operation had been entirely uncomplicated

Table 13–4 CAUSES OF LIVER DYSFUNCTION THAT CAN MIMIC EXTRAHEPATIC OBSTRUCTION

Viral hepatitis	Primary biliary cirrhosis
Alcoholic hepatitis	Postoperative cholestasis
Benign recurrent cholestasis	Parenteral nutrition
Pregnancy	Hodgkin's disease
Sepsis	Drugs (e.g., estrogens, phenothiazines, rifampin)
Infiltrative liver disease (e.g., amyloidosis, sarcoidosis)	Inherited disorders (e.g., arteriohepatic dysplasia)
Hepatic neoplasia	Sickle cell disease
Hepatic abscess	Hereditary hyperbilirubinemia (e.g., Dubin-Johnson syndrome)

Adapted from references 6 and 7.

(e.g., by jaundice excessive bile drainage, or cholangitis). It is also rare for the initial symptoms of a stricture to appear more than a few years after the original biliary operation.

Neoplastic obstruction of the bile duct usually results in intense jaundice and pruritus and, in most cases, weight loss. The bilirubin value in patients with neoplastic obstruction averages about 18 mg/dl[75] and nearly always exceeds 5 mg/dl. These patients seldom present with manifestations of biliary infection, and the jaundice and hyperbilirubinemia rarely fluctuate appreciably. The abdominal pain in neoplastic obstruction is deep-seated and aching, unlike the more acute pain typical of common duct stones.

It is important in making a differential diagnosis to recognize the significance of the absolute level of the serum bilirubin. Levels above 10 mg/dl are so uncommon as a result of gallstone obstruction that, even if gallbladder stones are demonstrated on ultrasound scans, hyperbilirubinemia of this degree will more often be caused by an obstructing tumor than by stones in the duct.[75] Consequently, with a bilirubin concentration of 10 mg/dl or greater direct cholangiography would almost always be indicated, whereas with lower values choledocholithiasis may be assumed to be the cause of ductal obstruction if stones have been demonstrated in the gallbladder by ultrasound scans or cholecystograms.

Techniques for Imaging the Biliary Tree. If extrahepatic obstruction is suspected from the clinical findings, further evaluation to determine the site and nature of the obstruction is warranted (see Fig. 13–2).[11] An appropriate next step in many patients is the use of a noninvasive study such as ultrasonography or computed tomography to determine whether or not the intra- and extrahepatic biliary systems are dilated, implying mechanical obstruction. Ultrasonography and computed tomography (CT) will demonstrate ductal dilatation in 85 per cent or more of patients with jaundice due to biliary obstruction.[11, 25–36] Both techniques may yield additional information, such as the presence of stones in the gallbladder or the presence of a pancreatic mass. If the presumptive diagnosis from the clinical findings is choledocholithiasis, ultrasonography is preferred to computed tomography. If neoplastic obstruction is suspected, computed tomography is preferable to ultrasonography[37] because it is at least as sensitive as ultrasonography in detecting ductal dilatation and is superior in identifying the site of obstruction (i.e., whether or not the extrahepatic bile duct is also dilated), the presence of metastases to the liver or nearby lymph nodes, and direct extension of a tumor into adjacent structures (e.g., the splanchnic vessels, portal vein, inferior vena cava).[38, 39]

False negative examinations occur with both modalities, and errors in interpretation, especially, are frequent with ultrasonography.[11] False negative results may also occur in the presence of sclerosing cholangitis or cirrhosis, presumably because of poor distensibility of the bile ducts and hepatic parenchyma. Common duct stones, which typically produce only partial or intermittent biliary obstruction, often fail to cause ductal dilatation.[32, 36, 40–45] CT and ultrasound are usually unable to detect stones in the common duct.[32, 43–46]

If dilated bile ducts are detected, it is generally appropriate to further define the obstruction with direct cholangiography, either endoscopic retrograde cholangiography or percutaneous transhepatic cholangiography. Because the ducts may fail to dilate in some cases of obstruction, direct cholangiography is indicated if the clinical suspicion of biliary obstruction is high even when scans are negative. Indeed, in certain situations, such as recurrent symptoms in patients who have had cholecystectomy, cholangiography may be appropriate as the first procedure, bypassing scans.[44, 47] For a detailed description of retrograde and percutaneous cholangiography, along with their specific indications and risks, the reader is referred to Chapters 10 and 11.

Preoperative cholangiography usually is not required in patients whose clinical presentation is typical of common duct stones (i.e., mild to moderate jaundice in the presence of gallbladder stones). Here, cholangiography will not provide information that will affect the decision to operate, and the remaining details are readily obtained once the abdomen is opened.

Other Tests. Many other tests (discussed also in Chapters 9 through 12), are sometimes employed in the work-up of the jaundiced patient. Because they lack sensitivity and specificity, as compared with the techniques described earlier, they are not routinely indicated, although they may be helpful under certain circumstances. *Technetium-*

99m sulfur colloid scans are useful primarily in the detection of intrahepatic mass lesions, which occasionally may produce striking cholestasis when strategically located. Overall, the diagnostic yield of a liver scan in the work-up of jaundice is low compared with computed tomography and ultrasonography, and the test is falling into disuse.

Several reports have suggested that *hepatobiliary scintigraphy* with Technetium-99m dimethylacetanilide iminodiacetic acid (HIDA) or related biliary radionuclides may be useful in the evaluation of jaundice. HIDA is taken up by hepatocytes and excreted into bile in detectable amounts even in patients with moderately severe cholestasis and hyperbilirubinemia. The detection of HIDA in the bile ducts but not in the gallbladder is a generally reliable indicator of cystic duct obstruction in a previously healthy individual. False negative examinations occur frequently, however, in alcoholic patients, those receiving parenteral nutrition, and those with severe systemic illness.[48, 49] Prospective studies have indicated that the utility of scanning with HIDA or related compounds in the differential diagnosis of cholestasis is limited,[10, 36, 50] and the use of opioid drugs may cause an excretory pattern that mimics obstruction.[51] Moreover, radionuclide scans are unable to provide the kind of resolution available with direct cholangiography, and complete failure of the extrahepatic ducts to be imaged is of little help in distinguishing intra- from extrahepatic cholestasis.

Intravenous cholangiography, although generally classified as noninvasive, is associated with a 5 per cent incidence of adverse reactions, including a 1 per cent incidence of serious hypersensitivity reactions. Moreover, even in patients with a serum bilirubin concentration < 3 mg/dl, duct opacification is not adequate to permit a definitive reading in up to 45 per cent of cases, and no ductal opacification is generally achieved when the bilirubin concentration exceeds 3 mg/dl. Thus, intravenous cholangiography has no role in the routine evaluation of jaundice.[52, 53] Oral cholecystography is also of no value in the work-up of the jaundiced patient. It will usually not opacify the gallbladder when the serum bilirubin concentration exceeds 3 mg/dl.

Despite anecdotal reports suggesting that liver biopsy in patients with biliary obstruction might be associated with an inordinate risk of complications such as peritonitis, large series suggest that the risk of liver biopsy is not greatly increased so long as the prothrombin time (< 3 sec prolonged) and platelet count (> 80,000/mm^3) are acceptable.[54] Nonetheless, liver biopsy is not indicated in the routine work-up of jaundice because (1) histologic findings diagnostic of obstruction are often absent in patients with proven obstruction, and (2) even if histologic changes suggestive of biliary obstruction are present, the biopsy generally provides no information regarding the location or nature of the obstruction.[54, 55] The principal role of a liver biopsy in the jaundiced patient is in the differential diagnosis of difficult or confusing cases of intrahepatic cholestasis.

MANAGEMENT OF THE PATIENT WITH ESTABLISHED BILIARY OBSTRUCTION

In most instances the treatment for patients with biliary obstruction is surgical. However, a variety of therapeutic alternatives, including percutaneous or endoscopic passage of a stent and endoscopic sphincterotomy, are available. These obviate the need for surgery, either emergently or altogether, in selected patients. The surgical and nonsurgical approaches to treatment of patients with biliary obstruction are described in detail elsewhere and will not be reviewed here. However, selected points are discussed in the following section.

Establishing a Plan. Consideration of therapeutic options should generally begin even before a precise diagnosis is established. That is, if, on the basis of clinical evaluation—often coupled with a noninvasive imaging technique such as ultrasonography—biliary obstruction appears highly likely, it is reasonable to make projections regarding the most probable diagnosis and the most appropriate form of therapy. Although such projections are occasionally incorrect and may need to be modified as further information becomes available, they help avoid the use of tests that are unnecessary, dangerous, or redundant and thus minimize risk and expense to the patient as well as the time required to establish a diagnosis and begin appropriate treatment.

This approach can be illustrated by the following examples.

1. Given an otherwise healthy patient who underwent cholecystectomy for gallstones 3 months ago and now presents with episodic

right upper quadrant pain, fever, and biochemical evidence of cholestasis, a retained stone is a very likely possibility. In this instance, endoscopic sphincterotomy represents the preferred therapy;[56] endoscopic retrograde cholangiography, which could then be accompanied by sphincterotomy and stone extraction, is the key diagnostic test (see Chapter 25). Noninvasive imaging of the biliary tract is unnecessary in many such patients.

2. Given a similar patient without prior history of cholecystectomy in whom an ultrasound examination reveals gallbladder stones, a dilated common bile duct with or without stones, and no other abnormalities (e.g., no pancreatic mass), laparotomy for an anticipated cholecystectomy with common bile duct exploration is a reasonable next step without further evaluation. If the preoperative diagnosis of gallstones with choledocholithiasis was incorrect, the correct diagnosis may be made at the time of surgery and appropriate measures taken. Apart from such situations, in which the diagnosis of distal common duct obstruction due to choledocholithiasis seems very likely, it is usually not appropriate to perform a laparotomy on the basis of ultrasonographic findings alone.[37, 57]

3. Given a middle-aged or elderly patient with severe, prolonged cholestasis, in whom noninvasive imaging reveals dilated intrahepatic ducts without dilatation of the common duct or gallbladder, proximal obstruction due to tumor is likely. Percutaneous cholangiography would be a reasonable next test to confirm the diagnosis and obtain a specimen of bile for cytologic study (which is positive in about 30 per cent of patients with Klatskin tumors). Useful information is also obtained on the intrahepatic extent of the lesion and the prospects for obtaining decompression by stents in the event that the patient is not a candidate for resection.

A variety of other general examples could be outlined, and individual patients very often present special problems and considerations. Often, the efficient work-up can be determined using a team approach involving the primary physician, gastroenterologist, surgeon, and interventional radiologist.

Assessing the Benefits and Risks of Biliary Decompression. High-grade biliary obstruction is obviously an undesirable situation. Deficiency of bile acids in the intestinal lumen results in malabsorption of fat and fat-soluble vitamins. Products normally secreted in bile, such as bile acids, bilirubin, and cholesterol, accumulate in the blood stream and may result in severe, often disabling pruritus. Moreover, the elevated biliary pressure results in regurgitation of bile into the blood stream, probably through intracellular junctions between hepatocytes (see Chapter 6). This is particularly dangerous when the bile is infected, as it may result in cholangitis-biliary sepsis. Finally, prolonged obstruction, even when so mild as to be unaccompanied by overt jaundice, may result in liver damage and ultimately cirrhosis.[58] Complete relief of obstruction can potentially reverse all these abnormalities. However, it should be noted that complete return to normal of the serum bilirubin concentration may not occur or may be delayed in patients with coexisting liver disease.[59–62] Even when no significant liver disease exists, bilirubin concentration in serum may require weeks to return to normal owing to the presence of bilirubin-albumin conjugates (see earlier).

Bile duct obstruction also affects renal, cardiovascular, and immune function and, possibly, wound healing. Jaundice is associated with decreased peripheral vascular resistance, impaired left ventricular performance, and a diuretic effect, the sum of which may be a chronically depleted blood volume. Paradoxically, the renal vascular bed constricts. These changes set the stage for renal dysfunction following hypotension caused by a blood loss during surgery that would be well tolerated by the nonjaundiced patient.

The foregoing considerations make the merits of biliary decompression—particularly complete and permanent decompression—self-evident. By comparison, the merits of temporary decompression are often more ambiguous and must be carefully weighed against the associated risks. Several[59–61] but not all[62] retrospective analyses have suggested that temporary percutaneous biliary drainage reduces subsequent operative morbidity and mortality in patients with malignant biliary obstruction. Prospective studies have failed to confirm these findings.[63, 64] It is noteworthy that the control groups in reports claiming a beneficial effect of preoperative biliary decompression are characterized by relatively high (e.g., 20 per cent) operative mortality rates. The advent of percutaneous stents for treating patients with obstruction due to advanced malignancy, however, has removed the highest-risk patients from the surgical pool, and operative mortality rates in jaundiced patients should now be closer to 5 per cent (Bongard and Way, unpublished results). In this setting, preoperative decompression has little chance of being helpful. By contrast, the advantages of nonoperative biliary drainage in the patient with toxic cholangitis are less controversial. In conjunction with appropriate antibiotic therapy, nonoperative drainage allows surgery to be delayed until the patient can be resuscitated and stabilized.

The benefits of biliary drainage in the patient with inoperable malignancy of the biliary tract must also be carefully considered. In such instances, the objective is palliation, and the symptoms directly attributable to the cholestasis are thus of paramount importance. In the minimally symptomatic patient with mild or absent pruritus, there is little reason for performing invasive (i.e., risky) procedures to establish drainage; indeed, the risks of percutaneous drainage may well outweigh the benefits.[66, 67] Intervention can be postponed until warranted by the patient's symptoms. In this regard, the physician must consider not only the obvious risks and benefits of nonoperative drainage (see Chapter 10), but also the psychologic impact on the patient and his family, attributable either to the therapy itself (e.g., an exterior drainage catheter requires care and serves as a reminder of the patient's terminal illness) or to the failure of the physician to undertake any therapy at all.

Medical Treatment. While removing or bypassing the biliary obstruction is the most desirable objective, this unfortunately is not possible in all instances. It is particularly in such patients that medical measures may be necessary to deal with the consequences of of cholestasis.

Pruritus can be particularly disturbing and disabling. Although the pathogenesis is not altogether clear, use of the binding resin cholestyramine rests on the assumption that bile acids, or other substances that undergo enterohepatic circulation, are responsible.[68, 69] Therapy is typically begun with 12 to 16 gm daily, given orally in divided doses with meals. Because the resultant depletion of the bile acid pool may further impair absorption of dietary fats, attention must be paid to diet and vitamin supplementation. While frequently helpful in patients with partial biliary obstruction, cholestyramine would not be expected to benefit patients with complete obstruction and therefore absence of intestinal bile acids.

Other methods of treating pruritus are generally less successful. Phenobarbital (120 to 250 mg per day)[70] is reportedly helpful in some patients, but controlled observations have not demonstrated relief of pruritus.[71] Neither conventional antihistamines (H_1-receptor blockade) nor H_2-receptor blockers have been found beneficial in controlled trials.[72] A variety of other modalities have been tried, including the use of 17α-alkyl substituted androgens, phototherapy, and plasma exchange or plasma perfusion through adsorbents such as charcoals.[6] Although these techniques are reportedly effective in some patients, controlled observations are lacking.

Malabsorption of fat and fat-soluble vitamins is a frequent manifestation of severe cholestasis. Such malabsorption may manifest itself as flatulence, diarrhea, night blindness (vitamin A deficiency), osteomalacia (vitamin D deficiency), hypoprothrombinemia (vitamin K deficiency), and possibly, in children, neurologic dysfunction (vitamin E deficiency).[73] Symptomatic steatorrhea responds to restriction of dietary fat to less than 40 gm daily and, if necessary, supplementation with medium-chain triglycerides, but this is rarely necessary in patients with only obstruction of the bile duct.

Bone disease is particularly common in patients with cholestatic liver disease, such as primary cirrhosis; in many such patients, osteoporosis rather than osteomalacia is the sole or predominant disorder.[74] Although no treatment has yet been shown to reverse this poorly understood form of osteoporosis, dietary calcium supplementation would seem to be a prudent recommendation. Bone biopsy may be necessary to define precisely the nature of the bone disorder and formulate a rational approach to therapy.

REFERENCES

1. Wolkoff A: Bilirubin metabolism and hyperbilirubinemia. Semin Liver Dis 1983;*3*:1.
2. Scharschmidt BF, Gollan JL: Bilirubin metabolism and hereditary hyperbilirubinemia. *In* Popper H, Schaffner F (eds) Progress in Liver Diseases. New York, Grune & Stratton, 1979, pp 187–212.
3. Gollan JL, Schmid R: Bilirubin metabolism and hyperbilirubinemic disorders. *In* Wright R (ed): Liver and Biliary Disease. Philadelphia, WB Saunders 1982, pp 255–295.
4. Scharschmidt BF, Waggoner JG, Berk PD: Hepatic

organic anion uptake in the rat. J Clin Invest 1975;*56:*1280.

5. Berk PD, Martin JF, Blaschke TF, et al: Unconjugated hyperbilirubinemia. Ann Intern Med 1975; *82:*552.
6. Scharschmidt BF: Jaundice. *In* Sleisenger MH, Fordtran JS (eds): Gastrointestinal Disease: Pathophysiology, Diagnosis, Management. Philadelphia, WB Saunders, 1983, pp 355–368.
7. Lake JR, Scharschmidt BF: Jaundice. *In* Conn RS (ed): Current Diagnosis. Philadelphia, WB Saunders, 1985, pp 54–61.
8. Vierling JM, Berk PD, Hofmann AF, et al: Normal fasting-state levels of serum cholyl–conjugated bile acids in Gilbert's syndrome. An aid to the diagnosis. Hepatology 1982;*2:*340.
9. Schenker S, Balint J, Schiff L: Differential diagnosis of jaundice: Report of a prospective study of 61 proved cases. Am J Dig Dis 1962;*7:*449.
10. O'Connor KW, Snodgrass PJ, Swonder JF, et al: A blinded prospective study comparing four current non-invasive approaches in the differential diagnosis of medical versus surgical jaundice. Gastroenterology 1983;*84:*1498.
11. Scharschmidt BF, Goldberg HI, Schmid R: Approach to the patient with cholestatic jaundice. N Engl J Med 1983;*308:*1515.
12. Simon FR, Sutherland E: Hepatic alkaline phosphatase isoenzymes: characterization, and differential alteration. Enzyme 1977;*22:*80.
13. Righetti ABB, Kaplan MM: Effects of actinomycin D on rat liver alkaline phosphatase. Proc Soc Exp Biol Med 1971;*136:*491.
14. Hatoff DE, Hardison WGM: Bile acids modify alkaline phosphatase induction and bile secretion pressure after bile duct obstruction in the rat. Gastroenterology 1981;*80:*66.
15. Scharschmidt BF, Keeffe EB, Blankenship NM, et al: In vitro effects of bile salts on ATPase activity and lipid fluidity of liver plasma membranes. Hepatology 1981;*1:*137.
16. DeBroc ME, Borgers M, Wieme RJ: The separation and characterization of liver plasma membrane fragments circulating in the blood of patients with cholestasis. Clin Chim Acta 1975;*59:*369.
17. Hatoff DE, Hardison WGM: Induced synthesis of alkaline phosphatase by bile acids in rat liver cell culture. Gastroenterology 1979;*77:*1062.
18. Scharschmidt BF: Bile formation and cholestasis, metabolism and enterohepatic circulation of bile acids, and gallstone formation. *In* Zakim D, Boyer T (eds): Hepatology. Philadelphia, WB Saunders, 1982, pp 297–351.
19. Lauff JJ, Kaspar ME, Ambrose RT: The separation of bilirubin species in serum and bile by high performance reversed phase liquid chromatography. J Chromatogr 1981;*226:*391.
20. Scharschmidt BF, Blanckaert N, Farina F, et al: Measurement of unconjugated and diconjugated bilirubin in the serum of patients with hepatobiliary disease. Gut 1982;*2:*643.
21. Muraco M, Blanckaert N: Liquid chromatographic assay and identification of mono and diester conjugates of bilirubin in normal serum. Clin Chem 1983;*29:*1767.
22. Weiss JS, Gautam A, Lauff JJ, et al: The clinical importance of a protein-bound fraction of serum bilirubin in patients with hyperbilirubinemia. N Engl J Med 1983;*309:*147.
23. Gautam A, Seligson HS, Gordon DR, et al: Irreversible binding of conjugated bilirubin to albumin in cholestatic rats. J Clin Invest 1984;*73:*873.
24. Summerfield JA, Elias E, Hungerford GD, et al: The biliary system in primary biliary cirrhosis. Gastroenterology 1976;*70:*240.
25. Vallon AG, Lees WR, Cotton PB: Grey-scale ultrasonography in cholestatic jaundice. Gut 1979;*20:*51.
26. Lapis JL, Orlando RC, Mittelstaedt CA, Staab EV: Ultrasonography in the diagnosis of obstructive jaundice. Ann Intern Med 1978;*89:*61.
27. Morris AI, Fawcett RA, Wood R, et al: Computed tomography, ultrasound, and cholestatic jaundice. Gut 1978;*19:*685.
28. McKay AJ, Duncan JG, Lam P, et al: The role of grey-scale ultrasonography in the investigation of jaundice. Br J Surg 1979;*66:*162.
29. Goldberg HI, Filly RA, Korobkin M, et al: Capability of CT body scanning and ultrasonography to demonstrate the status of the biliary ductal system in patients with jaundice. Radiology 1978;*129:*731.
30. Malini S, Sabel J: Ultrasonography in obstructive jaundice. Radiology 1977;*123:*429.
31. Vicary FR, Cusick G, Shirley IM, et al: Ultrasound and jaundice. Gut 1977;*18:*161.
32. Berk RN, Cooperberg PL, Gold RP, et al: Radiography of the bile ducts. Radiology 1982;*145:*1.
33. Taylor KJW, Rosenfield AT, Spiro HM: Diagnostic accuracy of gray scale ultrasonography for the jaundiced patient: A report of 275 cases. Arch Intern Med 1979;*139:*60.
34. Bolondi L, Gandolfi L, Rossi A, et al: Ultrasound in the diagnosis of cholestatic jaundice. Am J Gastroenterol 1979;*71:*168.
35. Baron RL, Stanley RJ, Lee JK, et al: A prospective comparison of the evaluation of biliary obstruction using computed tomography and ultrasonography. Radiology 1982;*145:*91.
36. Matzen P, Malchow-Moller A, Brun B, et al: Ultrasonography, computed tomography, and cholescintigraphy in suspected obstructive jaundice—a prospective comparative study. Gastroenterology 1983; *84:*1492.
37. Way LW: Diagnosis of pancreatic and other periampullary cancers. *In* Reber HA (ed): Surgical Diseases of the Pancreas. Philadelphia, Lea & Febiger, in press.
38. Nix GAJJ, Schmitz PIM, Wilson JHP, et al: Carcinoma of the head of the pancreas. Therapeutic implications of endoscopic retrograde cholangiopancreatography findings. Gastroenterology 1984; *87:*37.
39. Jafri SZH, Aisen AM, Glazer GM, et al: Comparison of CT and angiography in assessing resectability of pancreatic carcinoma. AJR 1984;*142:*525.
40. Zeman RK, Dorfman GS, Burrell MI, et al: Disparate dilatation of the intrahepatic and extrahepatic bile ducts in surgical jaundice. Radiology 1981; *138:*129.
41. Fried AM, Bell RM, Bivens BA: Biliary obstruction in a canine model: Sequential study of the sonographic threshold. Invest Radiol 1981;*16:*317.
42. Shimizu H, Ida M, Takayama S, et al: The diagnostic accuracy of computed tomography in obstructive biliary disease: A comparative evaluation with direct cholangiography. Radiology 1981;*138:*411.
43. Cronan JJ, Mueller PR, Simeone JF, et al: Prospective diagnosis of choledocholithiasis. Radiology 1983;*146:*467.
44. Gross BH, Harter LP, Gore RM, et al: Ultrasonic evaluation of common bile duct stones: Prospective

comparison with endoscopic retrograde cholangiopancreatography. Radiology 1983;*146*:471.
45. Laing FC, Jeffrey RB Jr: Choledocholithiasis and cystic duct obstruction: Difficult ultrasonographic diagnosis. Radiology 1983;*146*:475.
46. Laing FC, Jeffrey RB, Wing VW: Improved visualization of choledocholithiasis by sonography. AJR 1984;*143*:949.
47. Vennes JA, Bond JH: Approach to the jaundiced patient. Gastroenterology 1983;*84*:1615.
48. Shuman WP, Gibbs P, Rudd TG, et al: PIPIDA scintigraphy for cholecystitis: False positive in alcoholism and total parenteral nutrition. AJR 1982; *138*:1.
49. Kalff V, Froelick JW, Lloyd R, et al: Predictive value of an abnormal hepatobiliary scan in patients with severe intercurrent illness. Radiology 1983;*146*:191.
50. Scott BB, Evans JA, Unsworth J: The initial investigation of jaundice in a district general hospital: A study of ultrasonography and hepatobiliary scintigraphy. Br J Radiol 1980;*53*:557.
51. Jochl RJ, Koch KL, Nahrwald DL: Opioid drugs cause bile duct obstruction during hepatobiliary scans. Am J Surg 1984;*147*:134.
52. Osnes M, Larsen S, Lowe P, et al: Comparison of endoscopic retrograde and intravenous cholangiography in the diagnosis of biliary calculi. Lancet 1978;*2*:230.
53. Goodman MW, Ansel JH, Vennes JA, et al: Is intravenous cholangiography still useful? Gastroenterology 1980;*79*:642.
54. Morris JS, Gallo GA, Schener PJ, et al: Liver biopsy in "difficult" jaundice. Gastroenterology 1975; *68*:750.
55. Lance P, Bevan PG, Hoult JG, et al: Rapid and accurate diagnosis of acute cholecystitis with ^{99m}Tc-HIDA cholescintigraphy. Br Med J 1977;*2*:236.
56. Allen B, Shapiro H, Way LW: Management of recurrent and residual common duct stones. Am J Surg 1981;*142*:41.
57. Eyre-Brook RA, Ross B, Johnson AG: Should surgeons operate on the evidence of ultrasound alone in jaundiced patients? Br J Surg 1983;*70*:587.
58. Afroudakis A, Kaplowitz N: Liver histopathology in chronic common bile duct stenosis due to chronic alcoholic pancreatitis. Hepatology 1981;*1*:65.
59. Nakagama T, Ikeda A, Okuda K: Percutaneous transhepatic drainage of the biliary tract. Gastroenterology 1978;*74*:554.
60. Denning DA, Ellison EC, Carey LC: Preoperative percutaneous transhepatic biliary decompression lowers operative morbidity in patients with obstructive jaundice. Am J Surg 1981;*141*:61.
61. Gobien RP, Stanley JH, Souceh CD, et al: Routine preoperative drainage: Effect on management of obstructive jaundice. Radiology 1984;*152*:353.
62. Norlandes A, Kalin B, Sunblad R: Effects of percutaneous transhepatic drainage upon liver function and postoperative morbidity. Surg Gynecol Obstet 1982;*155*:161.
63. Hatfield ARW, Terblanche J, Fataar S, et al: Preoperative external biliary drainage in obstructive jaundice: A prospective controlled clinical trial. Lancet 1982;*2*:846.
64. McPherson GAD, Benjamin IS, Hodgson HJF, et al: Preoperative percutaneous transhepatic biliary drainage: The results of a controlled trial. Br J Surg 1984;*71*:371.
65. Gundry SR, Strodel WE, Knol JA, et al: Efficacy of preoperative biliary tract decompression in patients with obstructive jaundice. Arch Surg 1984;*119*:703.
66. McPherson GAD, Benjamin IS, Habib NA, et al: Percutaneous transhepatic drainage in obstructive jaundice: Advantages and problems. Br J Surg 1982;*69*:261.
67. Stambuch EC, Pitt HA, Pais SO, et al: Percutaneous transhepatic drainage. Arch Surg 1983;*118*:1388.
68. Carey JB, Williams G: Relief of the pruritus of jaundice with a bile-acid sequestering resin. JAMA 1961;*176*:432.
69. Schaffer F, Klion FM, Latuff AJ: The long term use of cholestyramine in the treatment of primary biliary cirrhosis. Gastroenterology 1965;*48*:293.
70. Bloomer JR, Boyer JL: Phenobarbital effects in cholestatic liver disease. Ann Intern Med 1975; *82*:310.
71. Metreau JM, Lecompte Y, Arondel J, et al: Phenobarbital therapy in intrahepatic and extrahepatic cholestatis in adults. Digestion 1976;*14*:471.
72. Harrison AR, Littenberg G, Goldstein L, et al: Pruritus, cimetidine and polycythemia (letter). N Engl J Med 1979;*300*:433.
73. Rosenbaum JL, Keating JP, Prensky AL, et al: A progressive neurologic syndrome in children with chronic liver disease. N Engl J Med 1981;*304*:503.
74. Matloff DS, Kaplan MM, Neer RM, et al: Effects of 25-hydroxyvitamin D_3 treatment. Gastroenterology 1982;*82*:97.
75. Pellegrini CA, Thomas MJ, Way LW: Bilirubin and alkaline phosphatase values before and after surgery for biliary obstruction. Am J Surg 1982;*143*:67.

SECTION III

GALLSTONE DISEASE

LAWRENCE W. WAY, M.D.

14

Cholelithiasis and Chronic Cholecystitis

Gallstones do not inevitably cause disease. Some remain asymptomatic, some give rise to minor symptoms, and others cause serious complications. This chapter will cover the epidemiology and natural history of gallstone disease and will describe the clinical conditions associated with nonacute gallstone disease of the gallbladder.

EPIDEMIOLOGY OF GALLSTONE DISEASE

Approximately 20 million people in the United States have gallstones, and about 300,000 operations are performed yearly for this disease and its complications. Each year about one third as many individuals are surgically treated for gallstones as newly acquire the disease.

The incidence of gallstone disease is influenced by age, sex, and a variety of cultural, ethnic, and medical factors.[1–9] Cholesterol gallstone disease is two to three times as common in women as in men. The difference begins at puberty, increases until menopause, and then declines. Gender has no influence, however, on the frequency of pigment gallstone disease.

Estimates of the prevalence of gallbladder disease vary depending on the methods and criteria used to make the diagnosis. Most epidemiologic studies have relied on questionnaires or interviews, basing the diagnosis on a history of cholecystectomy or imaging tests positive for gallstone disease. Studies of this kind have given prevalence rates such as those in Table 14–1.[4]

The figures in Table 14–1 show that racial background has a major influence on the prevalence of gallstones. Blacks are relatively less susceptible, Caucasians have intermediate susceptibility, and American Indians are markedly susceptible. Mexican-Americans, a racially mixed group, have a prevalence between that of American Indians and Caucasians. The relative susceptibility of blacks, Caucasians, and American Indians in the United States is about 1, 1.5, and 3, respectively.

As might be expected, autopsy studies and cholecystographic or ultrasonographic surveys produce prevalence estimates that are two to three times higher than those derived from patient histories. Representative data from such studies, by Godrey et al.,[5] Bateson,[10] Sampliner et al.,[11] and a group from Rome,[8] are given in Table 14–2.

In most epidemiologic studies, obesity has been found to increase the risk of gallstone disease.[12–15] Bernstein et al.[12] stratified a group of 62,739 American women into five cohorts of different body weights and found a strong progressive correlation between the risk of gallstone disease and increasing levels of obesity. The relative risk of gallstone disease in the most overweight women in the 20- to 29-year-age group was 6.75 compared with women of the same age of normal

Table 14–1 PREVALENCE OF GALLBLADDER DISEASE BY AGE[4]

Age Group	Framingham, Mass. (%)	Pima Indians (%)	Mexican-Americans (%)	Caucasians (%)	Blacks (%)
15–19			0	0	0
20–29			4	3	0
30–39	2	36	18	8	3
40–49	6	40	25	25	12
50–59	10	34	33	16	13

Table 14–2 PREVALENCE OF GALLBLADDER DISEASE BY AGE

	Pima Indians[11]		Italian[8]		England[5]		Scotland[10]		Sweden[7]	
Age	*Men*	*Women (%)*	*Women (%)*	Age	*Men*	*Women (%)*	*Men*	*Women (%)*	*Men*	*Women (%)*
15–24	0	13	2.5	20–29					6	14
25–34	4	73	6	30–39	3	0			4	33
35–44	11	71	11	40–49	0	13	4	0	13	15
45–54	32	76	18	50–59	4	21	10	28	18	40
55–64	66	62	25	60–69	9	20	16	32	27	53
≥65	68	90		70–79	17	21	23	34	36	63
				80–89	19	27	26	43	45	63

weight. The relative risk associated with obesity remained elevated in all age levels examined (i.e., up to age 60) but was greatest in the 20- to 29-year-old cohort.

Layde et al.,[6] using data from a family planning clinic in Oxford, England, found obesity to be the major factor governing variations in the prevalence of gallstone disease in women aged 25 to 39 years. The relative risk (6.6) for the most overweight group in this study was similar to that in the report by Bernstein et al.[12]

Williams and Johnston[9] reported that the principal risk factor for gallstones in persons living in a rural Canadian community was obesity. In one study from Australia,[15] the effect of obesity was confined to women under age 50.

Gallstone disease is an ancillary finding in a large percentage of persons who present for surgical therapy of morbid obesity.[16, 17] Thiet et al.[17] calculated the incidence of symptomatic cholelithiasis to be about 70 per cent in a series of 477 morbidly obese patients who had gastric or intestinal bypass operations for obesity. The excess prevalence of gallstone disease in these patients was confined to the women. Because of the technical insensitivity of preoperative ultrasound and cholecystography in the morbidly obese, Thiet et al.[17] and Herbst et al.[18] have found that operative ultrasonography is the most practical and reliable means of diagnosing gallstones in these patients.

The effect of parity has not been conclusively settled. Bernstein et al.,[12] Layde et al.,[6] and a group from Rome[8] found a relationship between increasing parity and gallstone disease, but others have not.[4, 11] When a positive effect has been found, the contribution of parity appears to be moderate compared with the more striking influence of obesity.

Oral contraceptives do not appear to increase the overall incidence of gallstone disease, but they accelerate the onset so that the disease occurs at a younger age.[19, 20] The influence of some other factors, such as obesity and parity, may also be at least partly explained in this way.

Dietary studies[21, 22] have given conflicting data on the relationship of total energy intake to the risk of gallstone formation; the influence of fat intake could not be separated from total caloric intake. Smith and Gee[22] thought that there might be a relationship between cholelithiasis and a diet low in protein, fat, and crude fiber. Scragg et al.[15] found that sugar intake had an influence, and Capron et al.[23] implicated prolonged fasting as a possible risk factor in some persons.

Along with gallstones and obesity, diabetes mellitus is a common finding in American Indian women. Diabetes has variously been reported to have either a positive effect[4, 23, 24] or no effect[11] on gallstone formation. Bennion and Grundy[25] reported that the cholesterol saturation of bile increased in response to insulin therapy in patients with diabetes. The very high prevalence of gallstones in American Indians cannot be explained as a result of the effects of obesity or diabetes. After all other risk factors are taken into account, an inherited predisposition remains as the major determinant.

Other factors identified as increasing the incidence of gallstone disease in individual studies include smoking,[6] low socioeconomic status and education level,[26] low calcium intake,[9] and sedentary lifestyle.[9] Moderate drinking (i.e., 20 gm alcohol daily) was found in one report[27] to have a protective effect.

Cirrhosis of the liver has been noted to be associated with a markedly increased risk of pigment gallstone formation.[28, 29] Diseases known to produce increased rates of hemoglobin turnover (e.g., congenital spherocytosis, sickle cell anemia) have a high incidence of associated pigment gallstone disease; the explanation for the association with cirrhosis may be related to hypersplenism. The incidence of pigment gallstone disease in cirrhotics with known portal hypertension (40 per cent), for example, was even higher than in cirrhotics without portal hypertension (30 per cent).[29]

NATURAL HISTORY OF GALLSTONE DISEASE

Although estimates vary, of the 70 to 90 per cent of people with gallstones who never come to surgical treatment, about two thirds have mild symptoms or no symptoms at all. Since gallstone disease is so common, the diagnosis is occasionally made in such persons during the course of an evaluation for some other medical problem, and then the question arises as to whether treatment should be recommended. If prophylactic treatment of these cases could be shown to have major health benefits, it would be possible by ultrasound screening to detect the large numbers of subclinical cases of gallstone disease so that treatment could be instituted before more severe manifestations develop.

To decide how these mild cases would best be treated the following information is required: (1) the rate at which symptoms (e.g., colic, dyspepsia) develop in asymptomatic persons; (2) the rate at which complications (e.g., acute cholecystitis, cholangitis, pancreatitis, carcinoma) develop; (3) the likelihood that a complication rather than uncomplicated symptoms will be the initial clinical manifestation; (4) whether the answers to the previous two questions differ in patients with no symptoms compared with those who have symptoms; (5) the mortality rate of elective cholecystectomy; (6) the mortality rate of complications; and (7) the cost of treatment.

The reports from the 1960s on the natural history of gallstone disease, which were once considered authoritative, have now been superseded by better data. These older articles by Lund[30] and Wenckert and Robertson[31] traced the natural history of a total of 1307 unoperated patients and reported that 30 per cent of patients experienced attacks of colic, 20 per cent experienced complications, and 50 per cent remained asymptomatic. Concluding that the average patient with gallstone disease had a 50 per cent chance of experiencing significant clinical problems in the next few years, these authors recommended cholecystectomy for all patients regardless of the severity of their symptoms except when ancillary conditions that increased the risks of operation were present.

The patients who formed the basis of these reports, however, are not as representative of asymptomatic and mildly symptomatic disease as was once assumed. They had all been hospitalized for symptomatic gallstone disease before their course was followed, and many of them (50 to 90 per cent) had nonopacifying gallbladders on oral cholecystography. The latter is a reflection of more advanced disease, seen in less than 30 per cent of asymptomatic persons with gallstones diagnosed by screening examinations.

The natural history of asymptomatic or mildly symptomatic patients is more accurately described in the recent reports from Gracie and Ransohoff,[32] McSherry et al.,[33] and Thistle et al.[34]

Gracie and Ransohoff[32] followed 123 asymptomatic patients with gallstones diagnosed by screening oral cholecystograms. The group comprised 110 men and 13 women, whose average age was 54 years (range 29 to 87 years). The gallbladder opacified on cholecystography in 108 patients (88 per cent) and did not opacify in 15 (12 per cent). Follow-up, which was complete for all patients, ranged from 11 to 24 years. During this time biliary pain developed in 13 per cent (16) of the patients, and complications developed in 2 per cent (3). All three instances of complications followed episodes of uncomplicated biliary colic. Biliary pain developed in 10 ± 3 per cent of patients within 5 years, 15 ± 4 per cent at 10 years, and 18 ± 4 per cent at both 15 and 20 years. Therefore, among asymptomatic patients, pain developed initially in about 2 per cent per year; at 10 years the rate decreased; and after about 15 years, patients who were still asymptomatic were likely to remain so.

McSherry et al.[33] reported the outcome of expectant management in 691 patients with gallstone disease (65 per cent women, 35 per cent men) who were followed for an average of 78 ± 62 months. Upon entry into the study, 556 (80 per cent) of the patients had experienced biliary symptoms, and 135 (20 per cent) had been asymptomatic. Symptoms developed in 10 per cent of the asymptomatic patients over an average of 5 years of follow-up. Only two deaths related to gallstone disease occurred in the entire group of 691 patients, both in patients with chronic symptoms. Therefore, as in the study by Gracie and Ransohoff,[32] asymptomatic patients had about a 2 per cent chance of experiencing colic per year of follow-up. Complications such as acute cholecystitis and pancreatitis were very uncommon, and in 90 per cent of instances they followed rather than preceded the appearance of colic.

Additional information was provided by the National Cooperative Gallstone Study, a randomized trial that compared chenodeoxycholate with placebo in the treatment of gallbladder gallstone disease. Data describing the natural history of the disease among the 305 patients in the placebo group were reported by Thistle et al.[34] In order to qualify for entry into the study, the patients initially were required to have opacification of the gallbladder on oral cholecystograms, no calcium in the gallstones seen on plain films, and no symptoms for the 3 months preceding therapy. During the 24 months of follow-up, biliary colic occurred in 13 per cent of the 305 patients given placebo, and an episode of pain lasting for more than 5 hours occurred in only 2 per cent. Those who had had an attack of biliary colic in the 12-month period before the study began were more likely than the asymptomatic patients to have an attack during the 24-month follow-up period. Twelve patients (4 per cent), three of whom had gangrenous acute cholecystitis, required cholecystectomy because of biliary symptoms. No deaths occurred as a result of the gallstone disease or its surgical treatment.

Insights into the natural history of gallstone disease can also be gleaned from autopsy studies.[3, 5, 7, 10] They demonstrate, for example, that only 10 to 20 per cent of autopsied persons with gallstone disease had surgical treatment (i.e., cholecystectomy) before they died, and of those who had not, the gallstones contributed to death in only a few (2 to 5 per cent). The deaths attributable to untreated gallstone disease were almost entirely confined to elderly people and were reasonably well balanced by the few unexpected deaths that followed elective cholecystectomies.

The obvious conclusions from these natural history data are that most persons with gallstones either have no symptoms or have symptoms so mild that treatment is not sought. The morbidity of asymptomatic gallbladder disease is low, and when clinical manifestations appear, they usually consist of colic rather than life-threatening complications. Furthermore, the overall mortality rate of unheralded complications exclusive of carcinoma (i.e., acute cholecystitis, jaundice, or pancreatitis) is below 10 per cent, so even when complications arise, the outcome of treatment is likely to be good.

Nevertheless, the risks of surgical therapy are also low, so careful calculations are required to assess the merits of treatment versus no treatment in asymptomatic or mildly symptomatic patients.

Ransohoff et al.[35] subjected the issue of prophylactic cholecystectomy in asymptomatic persons to decision analysis. The morbidity statistics used in calculating the risks of expectant management were obtained from their earlier article[32] (subsequently supported by the data from McSherry et al.),[33] which had demonstrated about a 2 per cent per year rate of conversion from an asymptomatic to a symptomatic state. The risks of elective and emergency surgery were obtained from 11 representative reports in the literature.

The decision analysis showed that prophylactic cholecystectomy for a 50-year-old man would result in an average loss of 18 days of life expectancy. Choosing cholecystectomy over expectant management for a 30-year-old woman, a 30-year-old man, and a 50-year-old woman would decrease life expectancy by 1, 4, and 12 days, respectively. If operative mortality rates could be reduced to zero, recalculation showed that the outcome would now favor surgery, but life expectancy would be increased in this theoretical situation by only 6 to 7 days in 30-year-old patients. Taking inflation into account, the costs would be more than sixfold greater with prophylactic surgery than with expectant management.

What all this means is that little is accomplished by aggressive therapy of asymptomatic or mildly symptomatic gallstone disease. Considering the number of affected persons, it is obvious that the health care system would be totally overwhelmed by any plan to screen and treat a major proportion of persons who have gallstones, and the costs would amount to billions of dollars. Fortunately, the natural history of the disease proves to be benign in all but a small fraction of cases, so expectant management is not only safe but also preferable to surgical treatment in the average case.

On the other hand, although gallstones pose little threat to the average person, severe, even lethal, disease is occasionally en-

Table 14–3 RELATIONSHIP OF RACE AND GALLBLADDER CANCER

Race and Sex	Mean Age at Dx Gallbladder Cancer	Gallbladder Cancer Incidence (100,000/yr)	Relative Risk	Cancer Risk per 20 Years (%)	No. Cholecystectomies to Prevent One Cancer
Blacks/Women	72.5	3.0	4.5	0.15	667
Caucasians/Women	73.9	11.5	4.3	0.50	200
American Indian/Women	64.4	46.4	12.2	1.50	67

countered. The next question, therefore, is whether high-risk groups who do not follow the typical course can be identified.

Studies on the epidemiology of gallbladder cancer[36, 37] demonstrate a close association of this tumor with gallstone disease, and it is clear that gallstones constitute a precancerous state. However, the strength of this relationship varies considerably among various ethnic groups (Table 14–3).[38, 39]

The figures in Table 14–3 show that gallbladder cancer, just like gallstone disease, is much more common in American Indians than in other United States ethnic groups. They further demonstrate that cancer occurs at an earlier age in American Indians than in other ethnic groups and that it affects a higher proportion of those who have gallstone disease. One other report noted that the frequency of invasive carcinoma or carcinoma in situ found incidentally in gallbladders removed for symptomatic gallstone disease was 0.5 to 1.5 per cent in Caucasians but was as high as 3 to 5 per cent in Mexicans.

Diehl and Beral[41] reported epidemiologic data from various countries suggesting that the incidence of gallbladder cancer was inversely proportional to the cholecystectomy rate of the preceding year. Nevertheless, in most patients the threat of gallbladder cancer is too small and remote to have an important influence on the natural history of gallstone disease and to be considered a cogent argument for early therapy of the gallstones. Considering the data in Table 14–3, however, the situation may be different for American Indians, Mexican-Americans, and other racially mixed groups that share a similar genetic background. Weiss et al.[38] noted, for example, that the chances of gallbladder cancer developing in American Indian women with gallstone disease is greater than the risk of lung cancer in cigarette smokers. Such data suggest that a more aggressive policy of cholecystectomy may be justified in persons of American Indian ancestry who have gallstone disease, in order to prevent this fatal illness.

Amaral and Thompson[16] and Thiet et al.[17] reported that in morbidly obese patients the natural history of gallstone disease seemed to be more aggressive than in others, and for these patients prophylactic cholecystectomy was recommended at the time of gastric bypass if gallstones were present. Calcification in the wall of the gallbladder (Fig. 14–1), an uncommon condition, is associated with gallbladder carcinoma and probably should be handled as if it were a premalignant state.[42, 43] There is also evidence that large gallstones (>2.5 cm) are more likely to precipitate an attack of acute cholecystitis[44] or give rise to gallbladder cancer[45] than are smaller stones. However, there are no good epidemiologic

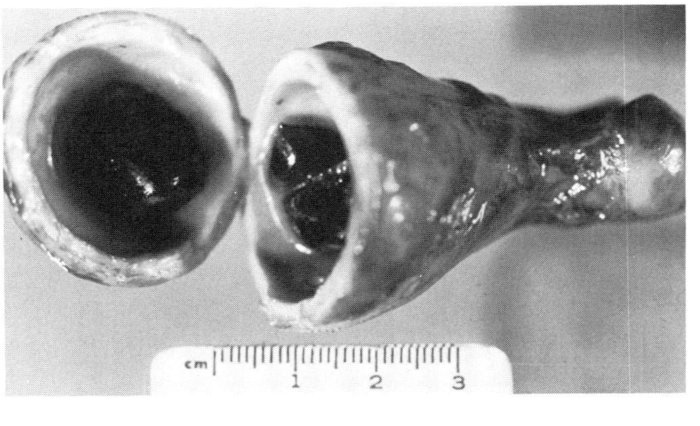

Figure 14–1. Calcified gallbladder in a patient with right upper quadrant pain. There was no sign of cancer in this gallbladder.

data on the natural history of large stones that would indicate whether these increased risks are great enough to be of clinical importance.

It is commonly assumed that small stones, which can more easily enter the cystic and common ducts, pose a greater potential problem than do larger stones. For example, Houssin et al.[46] recommended cholecystectomy for patients whose gallstones are 3 mm or smaller in diameter because of the risk of pancreatitis. This retrospective study, however, suffers from the same shortcomings as do previous surgical assessments of natural history; if the thesis were valid, support for it might have been expected from the aforementioned observations of Gracie and Ransohoff,[32] McSherry et al.,[33] and Thistle et al.[34]

Asymptomatic patients with stones in the common duct do not appear to have as benign a course as do those with stones confined to the gallbladder. Little has been written on the natural history of choledocholithiasis, and no prospective studies, similar to the ones for gallbladder stones, exist. Post-mortem surveys indicate, however, that in patients who are found at autopsy to have choledocholithiasis, the ductal stones have contributed to the patient's death in about half the cases.[3, 10] Thus, the threat of untreated choledocholithiasis appears to be considerably greater than that of untreated gallbladder stones, and expectant management could not ordinarily be justified for this condition.

Cholelithiasis may occur in children,[47–52] in whom cholecystectomy is probably indicated regardless of the severity of symptoms. In most children with gallstones a specific etiologic factor can be identified, the most common ones being prolonged total parenteral nutrition, congenital hemolytic disease, and disease of the ileum. Patients without special risk factors resemble their adult counterparts in many ways, since they tend to be female, obese, and older than the others.

Pigment gallstone disease, a result of hemolysis, is seen in about 50 per cent of patients above the age of 10 years with sickle cell disease.[53, 54] The abdominal crises of sickle cell disease consist of pain, jaundice, right upper quadrant tenderness, fever, and leukocytosis—a syndrome that may be impossible to distinguish from acute cholecystitis. Because of the similarities between sickle cell crises and acute cholecystitis, coupled with the knowledge that elective—but not emergency—operations are well tolerated in sickle cell disease, prophylactic cholecystectomy is usually recommended for gallstones even in the absence of symptoms.[55–57]

One commonly accepted notion introduced into the surgical literature 20 to 30 years ago is that associated diabetes mellitus raises the risks of gallstone disease. It is widely believed that complications, such as acute cholecystitis, are more common with this combination and that when complications occur, they are more likely to be fatal than in the absence of diabetes. More representative statistics fail to support this contention, however.[58–60] Morbidity is moderately increased in patients with diabetes, but this can be explained by an increased prevalence of cardiorespiratory and renal disease in these patients. In fact, diabetes seems to be well tolerated in association with a wide variety of surgical conditions, and contrary to previous teaching, it does not by itself seem to increase the morbidity of biliary disease or its surgical treatment.[58]

Consequently, if an individual patient is accidentally discovered to have gallstones, the indolent natural history of the disease should be explained. A few patients may wish to proceed with cholecystectomy or therapy with chenodiol (chenodeoxycholic acid). This is acceptable if only to decrease anxiety, since the risks of either form of treatment are low. In a few patients, special considerations, such as choledocholithiasis, may warrant stronger recommendations for therapy. However, there is no justification for urging treatment in the average patient with gallbladder stones in the hope of preventing complications in the future. In general, the urgency for treatment in gallbladder disease parallels the severity of symptoms.

BILIARY COLIC AND CHRONIC CHOLECYSTITIS

Biliary colic is the principal complaint in the majority of symptomatic patients with gallstones. Although patients with gallstone disease are usually said to have "chronic cholecystitis," this is not an entirely accurate designation because gallstone formation, not inflammation, is the earliest step in gallbladder disease. Gallstones, as noted previously, are not inevitably symptomatic; except for patients with advanced disease there is little correlation between the severity and frequency of colic, on the one hand, and the pathologic changes in the gallbladder, on the other.[61, 62] In patients who have never had acute cholecystitis, the histologic changes in the gallbladder wall consist of fibrosis and round cell infiltration with minimal thickening. The mucosa is usually intact. Bacteria can be cultured from gallbladder bile or gallstones in about 10 per cent of patients, but bacterial infection is not thought to contribute to the symptoms or pathologic findings in nonacute gallbladder disease.

Biliary colic, a visceral pain, is the result of transient obstruction of the cystic duct by a stone[63] and, except in patients with acute cholecystitis, is not accompanied by acute inflammation. Therefore, it is possible to have colic with a grossly normal or mildly abnormal gallbladder or to have no symptoms despite advanced gallbladder scarring.

Clinical Manifestations

About 75 per cent of patients with gallstone disease seek medical attention because of episodic pain (biliary colic). Although the symptoms are not pathognomonic for biliary disease, it is usually possible, when all aspects of the illness are considered, to make a fairly accurate diagnosis from the history. Confirmation of the original impression must then be obtained by demonstrating the presence of gallstones.

In a typical case, the patient experiences episodes of upper abdominal pain, usually in the epigastrium or right upper quadrant but sometimes in other upper abdominal locations.[64, 65] The pain may be precipitated by eating a meal, but more commonly there is no inciting event, and the pain can even begin at night, although this is uncommon.

Biliary colic is a steady rather than an intermittent pain, as suggested by the word "colic."[64] A typical attack consists of gradually increasing pain over 15 minutes to an hour, which remains at a plateau for an hour or more, and then diminishes slowly. In a third of patients the pain has a sudden onset, and, less often, relief is also sudden. Pain lasting more than 5 to 6 hours should suggest acute cholecystitis.

In order of decreasing frequency, the pain is felt maximally in the epigastrium, right upper quadrant, left upper quadrant, and various parts of the precordium or lower abdomen.[64, 65] It is incorrect to think that pain located elsewhere than in the right upper quadrant is "atypical" of gallstone disease. In over one half of patients, the pain radiates to other parts of the abdomen or the back, often to the scapula, the middle of the back, or the tip of the right shoulder. The attack is associated with vomiting and sweating in most individuals, and vomiting occasionally affords some relief. The vomiting is rarely as protracted as in intestinal obstruction, however. As with other kinds of visceral pain, the patient with biliary colic is usually restless and active during an attack.

The interval between attacks may be weeks, months, or years, and the unpredictability of their timing is a hallmark of the disease. As shown in the studies of Thistle et al.,[34] the activity of the disease tends to remain about the same over long periods. If the patient has been experiencing frequent attacks, they usually continue with the same frequency.

Dyspepsia is a general term used to refer to a group of ill-defined symptoms associated with gallstone disease and many other abdominal conditions.[66–70] Dyspepsia includes fatty or other kinds of food intolerances; excessive belching or flatus; postprandial abdominal bloating, fullness, and discomfort; inability to finish a normal-sized meal; epigastric burning; regurgitation of bitter fluid (water brash); and nausea and vomiting. One or more of these symptoms are present in about 80 per cent of patients with gallstones who seek medical care. About 25 per cent of patients experience some relief from antacids. About one third of patients have heartburn, some of whom have positive acid infusion (Bernstein) tests.

Prospective studies of middle-aged women have shown that the frequency and severity of dyspeptic complaints are unrelated to the presence of gallstones.[68] This suggests, on the one hand, that dyspepsia is randomly distributed in relation to gallstone disease and is not a direct consequence of the stones. On the other hand, most patients with gallstones and dyspepsia obtain some relief following cholecystectomy,[67, 69] which suggests that the two are, at least to some extent, related. Several investigators[65, 66, 68, 69] have noted an inverse correlation between the extent of chronic inflammatory changes in the gallbladder and the magnitude of preoperative dyspepsia. If gallstones are associated with poor function on the oral cholecystogram, dyspepsia is less likely to be cured by cholecystectomy than if the gallbladder functions well.

The physical examination is usually normal, but a few patients have tenderness in the region of the gallbladder during an attack of biliary colic.

Chronic distention of the gallbladder due to hydrops may occur with chronic cystic duct obstruction.[71, 72] The gallbladder in this condition contains an uninfected clear mucoid fluid. Patients with hydrops may or may not have symptoms. Hydrops must not be confused with empyema of the gallbladder, which presents as an acute toxic illness.

Diagnosis

About 15 per cent of gallstones contain enough calcium to be seen on plain films of the abdomen, but without additional studies it is not possible to be sure that the stones are actually within the gallbladder.

Ultrasonography and Oral Cholecystography[73–82]

The principal methods of imaging gallstones are ultrasonography and oral cholecystography. The specificity (about 98 per cent) and sensitivity (about 95 per cent) of both tests are very high.

Ultrasound scans may show gallstones (echogenic objects that produce an acoustic shadow) or sludge (echogenic material that layers and does not produce an acoustic shadow).[75] Very small stones may fail to produce shadows and therefore either may be missed or may be confused with sludge. Rarely, advanced scarring and contraction of the gallbladder around gallstones make it impossible to locate the gallbladder or the stones, a finding that should also raise the possibility of gallbladder cancer. Combining oral cholecystography with ultrasonic scanning may occasionally be useful, for the presence of the dense contrast medium in the gallbladder may cause small stones to float, facilitating their detection by ultrasound.[83]

Sludge, which consists of precipitated calcium bilirubinate, may be seen in association with gallstones or in any condition causing bile stasis.[84, 85] Sludge is common in persons receiving total parenteral nutrition. By itself, sludge is not an indication for cholecystectomy, although it often occurs in conjunction with a surgical lesion such as bile duct obstruction.

Oral cholecystography is an excellent method of diagnosing gallstones, but ultrasonography is just as accurate and requires no preparation of the patient, involves no ionizing radiation, and is simpler to perform. Oral cholecystography, however, shows whether the gallbladder functions and whether the stones are calcified—information of value if treatment with chenodiol is being contemplated. Because the gallbladder fails to opacify in about 40 per cent of patients in response to the initial dose of contrast agent, ultrasound is much more likely to provide a correct diagnosis during the first examination.

Although ultrasound is the first test ordered in most cases, oral cholecystography must not be considered an outmoded test. If the ultrasound results are negative and gallstone disease still seems to be a possibility, an oral cholecystogram should be obtained. If oral cholecystography is done first, ultrasound may be used if the cholecystogram fails to opacify or if the cholecystogram unexpectedly appears normal.[86–88] It must be remembered that both tests give false negative results in about 5 per cent of cases; since gallstone disease is so common, difficulties in diagnosis can be expected occasionally by all physicians who see patients with this disease.

About 60 per cent of oral cholecystograms opacify on the initial study.[89] When a single-dose study fails to opacify and there is no reason to suspect problems with intestinal absorption or hepatic excretion of the contrast agent, the patient may be given a second dose and x-rays repeated on the following day. This brings about opacification of the gallbladder in about two thirds of the remaining patients. Persistent nonopacification at this point is more than 95 per cent reliable as an indication of gallbladder disease.[89] It is usually easier, however, to study patients with nonopacification by ultrasound rather than to proceed with a double-dose oral cholecystogram.[90]

Prolonged opacification of the gallbladder on oral cholecystography is no longer considered to be significant as was once claimed.[91]

If both ultrasonography and oral cholecystography are normal and symptoms are highly suggestive, the next test should be either an endoscopic retrograde cholangiogram (with filling of the gallbladder) or an examination of duodenal bile for cholesterol crystals or bilirubinate granules.

Endoscopic Retrograde Cholangiography (ERCP)

Venu et al.[92] reported the results of ERCP in 195 patients who were thought clinically to have biliary pain but who had no stones on oral cholecystograms or ultrasound studies of the gallbladder. Thirty-two of these patients had had mild, transient abnormalities of liver function tests that coincided with the attacks of pain. No liver function abnormalities had been detected in the other 163 patients. ERCP demonstrated gallstones in 25 (78 per cent) of the 32 with abnormal test results but in only 4 (25 per cent) of the remainder. The most common ERCP finding in the first group was a layer of very small (3 to 7 mm) stones at the interface between the bile and the contrast medium. The ability of ERCP to partially displace gallbladder bile with contrast medium, which creates an interface where small stones can float, was credited with the success of this study.

Duodenal Drainage

Duodenal drainage studies are cumbersome compared with ultrasonography, but they may be useful in diagnosing gallstones when other tests have failed. The test involves duodenal intubation and sampling of gallbladder bile, which is then examined for the presence of cholesterol crystals or calcium bilirubinate granules. This method of diagnosis was first described about 30 years ago, but only recently have the methods been refined, the theory supported with sound evidence, and the reliability validated.[93–95]

The following technique was developed by Strasberg and his colleagues at the University of Toronto.[96] A tube is placed under radiographic control into the duodenum, and another tube is placed in the stomach. During the test, gastric secretions are aspirated from the gastric tube and discarded. The duodenal tube is allowed to drain by siphonage, placing the end of the fluid-filled tube below the patient, where it can empty into a collecting receptacle. The patient is given an IV injection of cholecystokinin (CCK) (1.5 U/kg over 3 minutes) or CCK-octapeptide (0.02 μg/kg over 1 minute). After the hormone is given, bile issuing from the duodenal tube will be noted to be light yellow (A bile), then dark (B bile), and then light again (C bile). The sequence consists of common duct bile, gallbladder bile, and hepatic bile.

The B bile, which comes from the gallbladder, is used for the examination. A sample is centrifuged at 2000 rpm for 10 minutes, and the pellet is examined by light and polarizing microscopy. Cholesterol crystals have typical platelike parallelogram shapes, which are birefringent under polarized light (Fig. 14–2). Calcium bilirubinate appears as small red-brown granules in clusters (Fig. 14–3). If gastric acid has not been excluded from the duodenum, a precipitate that resembles calcium bilirubinate granules may appear, so it is important to make sure that the pH of the specimen is above 5.0.

A positive duodenal drainage test consists of ten or more cholesterol or calcium bilirubinate crystals per slide. A finding of between one and ten crystals is considered suggestive but not diagnostic.

Scientific support for using the presence of cholesterol crystals in diagnosing gallstone disease comes from the observations of Sedaghat and Grundy.[95] These workers noted the presence of cholesterol crystals in bile specimens from 25 of 28 patients with cholesterol gallstones but in none of the specimens from 72 patients without cholesterol gallstones, even though the latter group included some patients whose bile was supersaturated with cholesterol. Subsequently, Burnstein[93] and Delchier[94] and their coworkers showed prospectively in a total of 114 patients that the presence of cholesterol crystals or bilirubinate granules in gallbladder bile obtained by duodenal intubation was sensitive and specific for the diagnosis of gallstones in patients with normal cholecystograms and ultrasound studies. Thus, the duodenal drainage test seems to be both useful and reliable and probably deserves wider use.

*Cholecystokinin Cholecystography**

There is some evidence that gallbladder disease can be detected if abdominal pain or abnormalities in gallbladder motor function occur in response to an intravenous injection of cholecystokinin.

Nathan et al.[97] and Davis et al.[98] showed that pain occurs in only 1 per cent of normal subjects when CCK is given during oral cholecystography, so that pain during this test

---

*See also Chapters 3 and 7 for discussions on this subject.

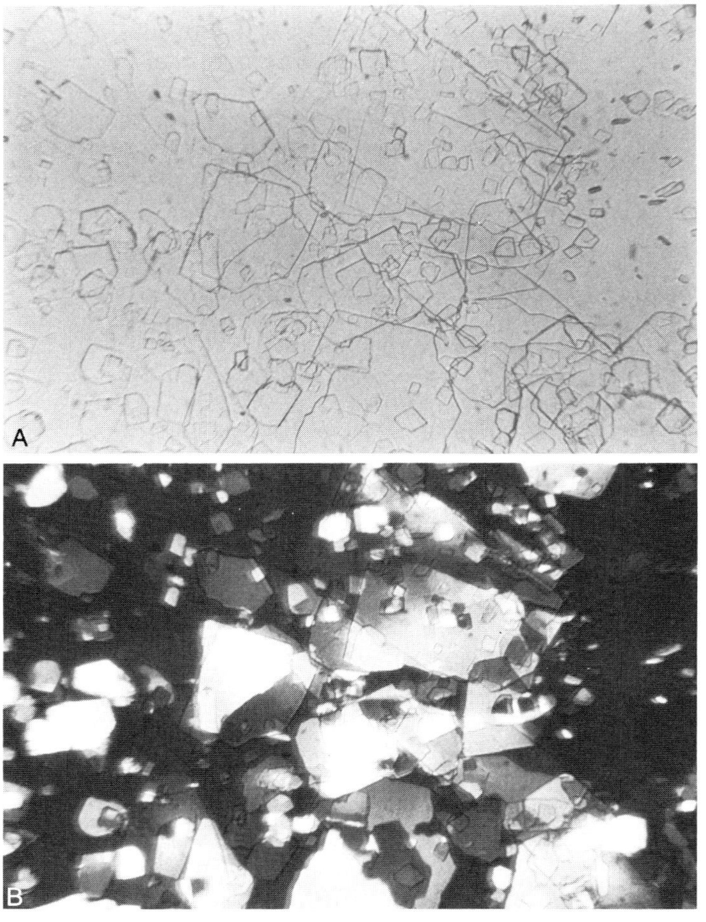

Figure 14–2. *A*, Cholesterol crystals as seen under ordinary light microscopy. *B*, Cholesterol crystals as seen under polarized light microscopy.

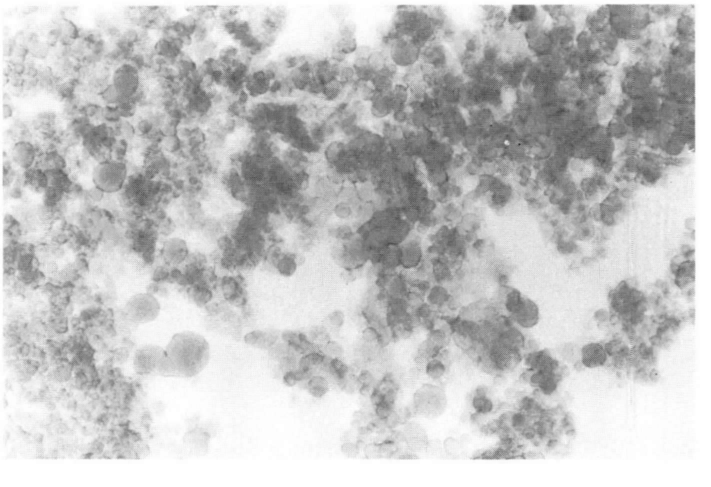

Figure 14–3. Calcium bilirubinate granules as seen under light microscopy.

could be of significance in the diagnosis of gallbladder disease. This is the theory of the cholecystokinin cholecystogram, which involves using fluoroscopy to observe the response of the opacified gallbladder to an injection of CCK (or CCK-octapeptide) and correlating abnormalities in gallbladder emptying with the patient's symptoms. Burnstein et al.[93] combined performance of CCK cholecystography with the duodenal drainage test. It can also be performed using Tc-iminodiacetic acid derivatives instead of radiopaque contrast media to image the gallbladder.

According to Burnstein et al.,[93] the CCK cholecystogram should be considered abnormal if less than 20 per cent (hypocontraction) or more than 80 per cent (hypercontraction) of gallbladder bile is emptied in response to CCK. In their experience, hypercontraction correlated with the presence of abnormal bile (88 per cent specific) on duodenal drainage. Hypocontraction was a less sensitive and specific finding. A "fighting gallbladder," defined as a gallbladder that develops a rounded shape in response to CCK but fails to empty, has also been said to be an important sign.

The diagnostic usefulness of CCK cholecystography is unsettled. Dunn et al.[99] studied the test prospectively in 74 patients with normal cholecystograms who had symptoms of gallbladder disease. Seventeen (85 per cent) of 20 patients who had reproduction of their pain in response to CCK were relieved or improved by cholecystectomy, but a similar response to cholecystectomy occurred in six (67 per cent) of nine patients with no pain after CCK. There was also a high incidence (14 to 36 per cent) of false positive results in a group of control subjects. These authors concluded that the CCK cholecystogram was of uncertain value, a sentiment shared by Davis et al.[98] Others, however, claim that since a positive test is usually associated with a good clinical result after cholecystectomy, CCK cholecystography can be used clinically as long as it is realized that false negative tests may occur.[93, 100–104]

Differential Diagnosis

Because the symptoms of chronic cholecystitis are not highly specific, the patient's history, the findings on physical examination, and the laboratory data must all be carefully evaluated. An upper gastrointestinal series,[105] barium enema, or intravenous pyelogram may be indicated preoperatively in some patients, but ordering an upper gastrointestinal series in the absence of clinical suspicions of gastroduodenal disease, which was routine in the past, has been shown to be unrewarding.[106] The most common diseases to be considered in the differential diagnosis are gastritis, peptic ulcer, reflux esophagitis, pancreatitis, renal disease, lesions of the colon (diverticulitis and carcinoma), radiculitis, and angina pectoris.

An upper gastrointestinal series may show reflux esophagitis with or without a hiatus hernia or peptic ulcer disease. Endoscopy of the upper gastrointestinal tract may be indicated in some patients with symptoms of reflux. When available, pH measurements of the lower esophagus may be helpful.

The pain of angina pectoris is of shorter duration than the average episode of biliary colic, but the location of the pain is not as specific for each of these conditions as is sometimes thought. An electrocardiogram should be performed, in some cases during exercise.

The question of whether gallbladder disease may have a direct influence on cardiac disease has been debated for some time. The basis for thinking so has been that arrhythmias or episodes of angina pectoris occasionally subside following cholecystectomy.[107, 108] Experimentally, distention of the bile ducts sometimes induces cardiac arrhythmias, premature ventricular contractions, or angina. However, prospective clinical studies suggest that gallbladder disease only rarely affects the heart, so cholecystectomy should not be performed specifically in the hope of improving cardiac disease.

Patients with chronic pancreatitis, many of whom are alcoholics, may have vague upper abdominal complaints similar to those of patients with gallstone disease. Even though gallstones may cause acute pancreatitis, gallstone pancreatitis (in contrast with alcoholic pancreatitis) rarely leads to chronic scarring with endocrine and exocrine dysfunction. Special studies (such as a glucose tolerance test, endoscopic retrograde pancreatography, or tests of exocrine function) may be required if the history or plain films suggest the possibility of pancreatitis. Nevertheless, if a symptomatic patient is discovered to have both chronic pancreatitis and gallstones, cholecystectomy should usually be performed as a first attempt to provide pain relief.

The irritable colon syndrome, which may produce postprandial abdominal pain, should be considered in the differential diagnosis, especially if there is a distinct relationship of symptoms to bowel movements. When both diseases are present, cholecystectomy will probably be indicated because it is usually impossible to exonerate the gallbladder as a cause of the symptoms.

Because colonic function increases after eating (gastrocolic reflex), colonic lesions such as adenocarcinoma or diverticular disease may be associated with postprandial discomfort. When the discomfort is on the right side of the abdomen, as it may be with right-sided neoplasms, the syndrome may closely mimic gallstone disease. Awareness of this problem should lead to more thorough study of the colon in appropriate cases.

Renal stones or infection may produce right-sided abdominal pain, but if a urinalysis is obtained routinely and abnormal results are further investigated by intravenous pyelography, renal disease should rarely be overlooked.

Radiculitis from osteoarthritis or peripheral nerve tumors may produce symptoms that resemble those produced by gallstones. Thoracic spine films and, occasionally, myelograms should be obtained in selected patients in whom radicular pain cannot be explained on the basis of the clinical examination.

Treatment

Cholecystectomy is the only definitive treatment and is indicated for most symptomatic patients (Figs. 14–4 and 14–5). The other forms of treatment to be discussed are currently experimental, impractical, or both. Therapeutic diets (e.g., a low-fat diet), anticholinergic drugs, and antacids are of no value in preventing attacks of colic, although they may provide some relief from dyspeptic symptoms. In fact, gallbladder contraction is just as complete after ingestion of a low-fat meal as after a high-fat meal.[109]

Cholecystectomy (See also Chapter 21)

Cholecystectomy usually relieves preoperative pain if other abdominal disease has been ruled out and if stones are not left behind in the bile duct.[110, 111] It is less possible to be sure that dyspepsia will be eliminated by cholecystectomy, although, as indicated earlier, some relief can be expected in most cases. When dyspepsia is the major complaint and pain is not present, the results are unpredictable, so that dyspepsia by itself is not an accepted indication for surgery.

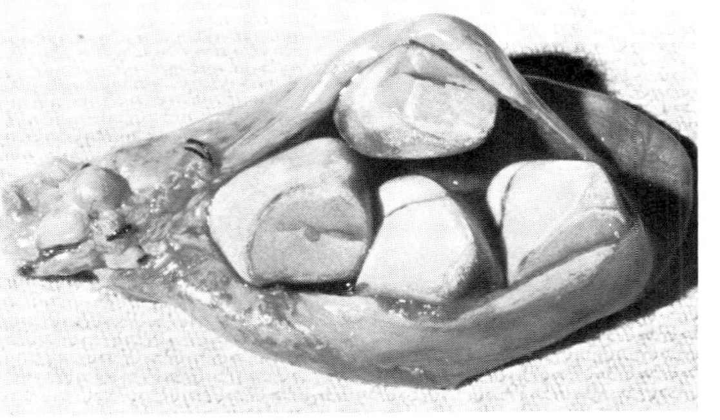

Figure 14–4. Typical faceted cholesterol gallstones in a gallbladder removed for symptomatic chronic cholecystitis.

In a collected series the overall mortality rate of elective cholecystectomy without common duct exploration or other ancillary procedures was 0.20 per cent (6 deaths in 2756 cholecystectomies).[112–115] These reports[112–114] were chosen because they give detailed mortality statistics and the cause of death in each patient. Mortality rates in this range can be expected only when the surgery is performed by fully trained surgeons. In the large experience from The New York Hospital–Cornell Medical Center,[116] the gross mortality rate of cholecystectomy in patients under age 50 years was 0.1 per cent and in patients over age 50, 0.8 per cent. Cardiovascular complications were the principal cause of death in the latter group.

Many reports on the mortality rates of operations for gallstone disease fail to distin-

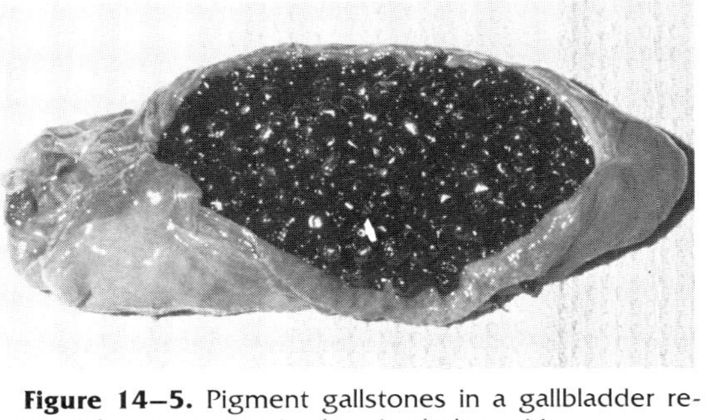

Figure 14–5. Pigment gallstones in a gallbladder removed for symptomatic chronic cholecystitis.

guish between routine operations and cholecystectomy done as an ancillary procedure during laparotomy for some other serious disease, such as carcinoma of the pancreas.[115–117] In other instances the mortality rate of operations performed for acute cholecystitis is not separated from that of cholecystectomies done electively,[118] or the results of simple cholecystectomy are included among those for cholecystectomy plus common duct exploration. These practices inflate the mortality rates attributed to "cholecystectomy" and have sometimes been used inappropriately to estimate the risks of an elective operation in otherwise healthy persons with minimal disease.

Age by itself is not a contraindication to elective cholecystectomy.[119–121] The risks in the elderly are the result of the ancillary diseases that are so often present in this age group. The increased risks in patients with diabetes mellitus are a result of the increased prevalence of renal and cardiovascular disease in individuals with this disease.[58–60] Elective cholecystectomy is considerably more hazardous in patients with cirrhosis of the liver than in others, and surgery should be undertaken only if the symptoms are severe or the cirrhosis mild.[122–124]

Cholecystectomy produces no alterations in digestion and absorption, and, perhaps surprisingly, the concentration of bile acids in intestinal chyme remains in the physiologic range after removal of the gallbladder.[125] There is no need for special diets (e.g., a low-fat diet) or vitamin supplements postoperatively.

In summary, deaths and major complications after cholecystectomy are encountered primarily in the elderly or others who have serious disease in other organ systems.

*Dissolution Therapy**

Chenodeoxycholic acid (CDCA, chenodiol) (12 to 15 mg/kg body weight/day) will lower the cholesterol saturation of bile enough to bring about gradual dissolution of cholesterol stones in some patients.[126–130] Chenodeoxycholic acid treatment is unsuccessful or otherwise contraindicated in the presence of any of the following: (1) pigment stones, (2) calcified stones, (3) large (>1.5 cm) stones, (4) nonopacifying gallbladder, (5) women who might become pregnant, (6) concomitant liver disease, (7) symptoms too severe to tolerate 2 years of therapy, (8) obesity (it is difficult to desaturate the bile in obese persons), and (9) absence of signs of dissolution on oral cholecystogram following 9 months of treatment. About 85 to 90 per cent of patients now being treated by cholecystectomy would be excluded from consideration for chenodeoxycholic acid therapy for one or more of these reasons.[131]

In the controlled trial of this treatment in the United States, the stones dissolved in 15 per cent of selected patients during 2 years of continuous therapy.[128] Other studies indicate that more stringent selection criteria and higher doses of the drug would increase the chance of success to 30 to 50 per cent of treated patients.[129]

Ursodeoxycholic acid (UDCA) (10 mg/kg body weight/day) is preferable to CDCA because it is equally effective but does not produce diarrhea or liver dysfunction.[132–136] A combination of CDCA and UDCA may be more effective than either alone.[137] Ursodeoxycholic acid is not yet available in the United States, however.

A major weakness of dissolution therapy is the tendency for gallstones to recur in most successfully treated patients after the drug is discontinued.[138, 139] This may be prevented by giving a chronic nighttime maintenance dose of the drug,[139] but the safety of this approach has not been proved.

At present the indications for dissolution therapy are unclear. More information is needed on its efficacy and on whether the selection of patients can be improved to increase the success rate. Based upon the data available, CDCA or UDCA might be preferable to surgery in appropriately selected patients with serious ancillary disease that increases the risks of surgery. Most such patients would be over 65 years of age. In others, cholecystectomy would be superior.

Lithotripsy

Gallstones, like kidney stones, can be fragmented by exposure to extracorporeal shock waves.[140, 141] The stones are broken into pieces that range in size from small granules to about 8 mm, which increases the efficacy of dissolution by cheno- or ursodeoxycholic acid.

In the report by Sauerbruch et al.,[140] gallbladder stones were eliminated within 1 to

*Dissolution therapy is discussed in greater detail in Chapter 4, The Formation and Dissolution of Gallstones.

25 weeks in six of nine patients treated by 600 to 1500 shock waves followed by a combination of UDCA plus CDCA, each given in a daily dose of 7 to 8 mg/kg. Painful episodes in two patients, one of whom developed mild pancreatitis, were thought to coincide with passage of stone fragments through the common duct. The following were considered contraindications to this therapy: stones greater than 25 mm in diameter, more than three stones, calcified stones, nonopacifying gallbladder on oral cholecystogram, concurrent common bile duct stone, and poor general condition of the patient.

There is a possibility, therefore, that the ability to fragment gallstones may augment the effectiveness of dissolution therapy. However, this is extremely complex and expensive technology, which seems to have the potential of complications to adjacent organs, and, as with CDCA given alone, recurrent stone formation can be expected in most patients. Furthermore, with the present list of exclusions, less than 10 per cent of patients with gallstones are candidates for shock wave treatment.

This treatment is currently in its infancy, and experience is too scant to know what its efficacy and safety will be. Although the technology is basically the same, it is not possible to use the machines that were designed for kidney stones to treat gallbladder stones; the positioning and monitoring systems are different. This is a major drawback, since the machines for kidney stones cost 2 million dollars plus the expense of installing them.

Percutaneous Dissolution

Allen et al.[142] reported dissolving cholesterol gallbladder stones in four patients using methyl tert-butyl ether (MTBE) instilled through a catheter inserted percutaneously into the gallbladder. With CT scans used for guidance, the catheter was passed through the liver and hepatic surface of the gallbladder into the gallbladder lumen. MTBE was chosen as a solvent because it dissolves cholesterol rapidly, and, unlike diethyl ether, it remains liquid at body temperature. No serious side effects were described in these four patients, in three of whom the stones were successfully dissolved. A common bile duct stone was also dissolved in one of the patients.

More information will have to be developed concerning the safety and efficacy of this approach before its place in the therapy of gallstone disease can be determined.

Incidental Cholelithiasis and Incidental Cholecystectomy

Sometimes patients scheduled for an operation on some other organ are discovered preoperatively or intraoperatively to have gallstones, and a decision must be made concerning whether it is important and safe to remove the gallbladder as an incidental procedure. As mentioned earlier, cholecystectomy should probably be performed in conjunction with gastric bypass operations in morbidly obese patients who have gallstones, and this has become fairly standard practice.[16, 17] In other patients, the natural history of untreated gallstones would not be expected to pose risks greater than the minimal ones documented by Gracie and Ransohoff[32] and McSherry et al.,[33] a subject discussed in detail previously.

Cholecystectomy, however, would add few additional risks to most abdominal operations, and there is good evidence that an incidental cholecystectomy is acceptable as long as the incision is adequate and the patient stable and reasonably healthy.[143–145] Specific discussions have supported incidental cholecystectomy in the elderly[146] and during colectomy,[147] gynecologic operations,[148] and insertion of arterial grafts.[149, 150]

McSherry and Glenn[144] pointed out that it is also safe to treat other abdominal diseases incidentally discovered during planned biliary tract surgery.

CHOLESTEROLOSIS

Cholesterolosis of the gallbladder consists of deposits of cholesterol esters in submucosal macrophages and epithelial cells.[151–154] As viewed from the mucosal surface, the submucosal cholesterol produces a fine yellow reticular pattern on a red background, an appearance similar to a ripe strawberry (Fig. 14–6). The saturation of bile with cholesterol in patients with cholesterolosis is in the range of what is seen in normal subjects, and the pathogenesis of this condition probably differs from that of cholesterol gallstones.[152, 155] Gallstones and cholesterolosis are more often found independent of one another than together.[7] Methyl sterols (cholesterol precursors) are increased in hepatic and gallbladder bile of patients with cholesterolosis, presumably as a result of increased hepatic production.[155] It has been postulated that cholesterolosis results from absorption

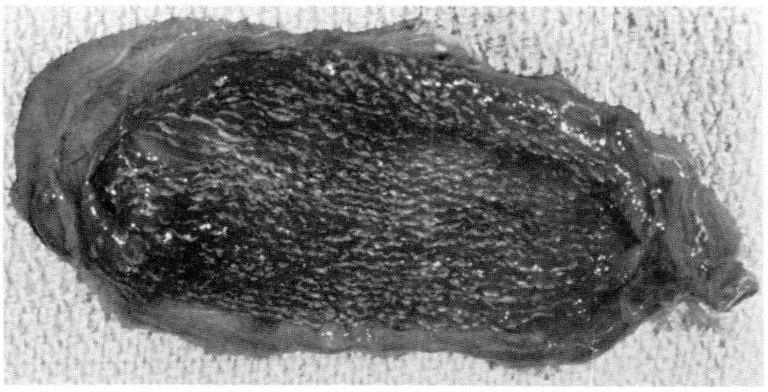

Figure 14–6. Cholesterolosis and chronic cholecystitis in a patient with episodic abdominal pain who had had several negative oral cholecystograms and ultrasound studies. The patient had been referred to a psychiatrist on the assumption that her symptoms had no organic source. The gallbladder contained several tiny (1 mm) stones (not shown). She has had no symptoms in the 7 years since cholecystectomy was performed.

of these free sterols from gallbladder bile by the gallbladder mucosa, followed by accumulation in submucosal macrophages.

In 80 per cent of cases the cholesterol deposits are confined to the mucosa (planar cholesterolosis).[152] In 20 per cent of cases, however, the lesions grow to assume a polypoid configuration, and then the cholesterol polyps may separate from their mucosal attachments and behave like ordinary gallstones. The planar form is usually asymptomatic, but polypoid cholesterolosis may be responsible for biliary colic or biliary pancreatitis. Planar and polypoid cholesterolosis are not distinct conditions but just different degrees of the same process. Because the stones that form from cholesterolosis are usually very small, they may be difficult to detect on oral cholecystograms or ultrasound scans. In some cases the oral cholecystogram may reveal decreased concentration of the contrast medium or one or more small mucosal excrescences (cholesterol polyps) that remain fixed as the patient changes position. Duodenal drainage studies may also be helpful in diagnosis. Symptomatic cases should be treated by cholecystectomy (Fig. 14–6).

GALLSTONE DISEASE, CHOLECYSTECTOMY, AND CANCER

The prevalence of gallstone disease in various cultures has been shown by Lowenfels et al. to correlate with the prevalence of cancer of the uterus, large intestine, and stomach.[156] These findings have been interpreted to suggest that common environmental factors, thought most likely to involve dietary habits, influence the rates of all these diseases. In an autopsy study, Lowenfels[157] measured the relationship between the prevalence of gallstone disease and death from colorectal cancer. There was a 13-fold increase in the prevalence of gallstones in women under age 50 with colorectal cancer, but no correlations were found in other groups.

In another case-controlled study,[158] gallstone disease was found to be more prevalent among subjects who died from cancer compared with subjects who died from other causes. When the analysis was restricted to 89 women under age 50 who died from cancer of the breast, reproductive system, or colon, the odds ratio reached its highest value (3.3).

Linos et al.[159] found a relative risk for colon cancer of 1.52 among patients with cholelithiasis. They attributed this result to case-finding bias, however, since the positive correlation was confined to patients whose gallstones were asymptomatic.

Therefore, there is evidence that gallstone disease is more common in societies with a high prevalence of various cancers, but it is not clear that correlations exist for these diseases among the individuals in these societies.

There are also theoretical reasons to think that changes in the enterohepatic circulation of bile acids following cholecystectomy may increase the incidence of colon cancer.[160] Cholecystectomy increases cycling of the enterohepatic circulation, which results in greater exposure of bile acids to intestinal bacteria and increased conversion of primary to secondary bile acids. Deoxycholate, the principal secondary bile acid, has been implicated as a possible cofactor in the pathogenesis of several carcinomas. Furthermore, in experimental animals, either cholecystectomy or the feeding of bile acids increases the frequency of colonic neoplasms in response to exogenous carcinogens.

In recent years, several reports have linked cholecystectomy in man to an increased risk of colon cancer 10 to 15 years later. Vernick and Kuller[161] performed a case-controlled study of 150 patients with adenocarcinoma of the cecum or ascending colon. Two control groups were used: carcinoma of the left colon and neighborhood controls. Compared with the control groups, the relative risk for right-sided colon cancer was 1.86 in patients who had had cholecystectomies.

Linos et al.[162] traced the health of 1681 residents of Rochester, Minnesota, who had

had cholecystectomies an average of 13 years previously. The relative risk for right-sided colon cancer in the women was found to be 2.1. There was no association in the men.

Turunen and Kivilaakso[163] calculated that the relative risk of developing colon cancer after cholecystectomy was 1.59 compared with controls and was 3.00 for cancer of the right colon. They found no correlation in autopsied subjects between unoperated gallstones and colon cancer.

Dissenting views concerning a cancer-promoting effect of cholecystectomy are as numerous, however. In well-controlled studies, Weiss,[164] Adami,[165] Abrams,[166] and Spitz[167] and their coworkers found no relationship between previous cholecystectomy and cancer of the colon in general, or of the right colon in particular.

Therefore, it is possible that cholecystectomy increases the risk of carcinoma of the right colon, but the data are by no means conclusive, and the effect, if it truly exists, is slight.

REFERENCES

1. Bainton D, Davies GT, Evans KT, et al: Gallbladder disease. Prevalence in a South Wales industrial town. N Engl J Med 1976;*294*:1148.
2. Barker DJP, Gardner MJ, Power C, et al: Prevalence of gall stones at necropsy in nine British towns: a collaborative study. Br Med J 1979; *2*:1389.
3. Bateson MC, Bouchier IAD: Prevalence of gall stones in Dundee: a necropsy study. Br Med J 1975;*4*:4271.
4. Diehl AK, Stern MP, Ostrower VS, et al: Prevalence of clinical gallbladder disease in Mexican-American, Anglo, and Black women. South Med J 1980;*73*:438.
5. Godrey PJ, Bates T, Harrison M, et al: Gall stones and mortality: a study of all gall stone related deaths in a single health district. Gut 1984;*25*:1029.
6. Layde PM, Vessey MP, Yeates D: Risk factors for gall-bladder disease: a cohort study of young women attending family planning clinics. J Epidemiol Community Health 1982;*36*:274.
7. Lindstrom CG: Frequency of gallstone disease in a well-defined Swedish population. A prospective necropsy study in Malmo. Scand J Gastroenterol 1977;*12*:341.
8. Rome Group for the Epidemiology and Prevention of Cholelithiasis (GREPO): Prevalence of gallstone disease in an Italian adult female population. Am J Epidemiol 1984;*119*:796.
9. Williams CN, Johnston JL: Prevalence of gallstones and risk factors in Caucasian women in a rural Canadian community. Can Med Assoc J 1980; *120*:664.
10. Bateson MC: Gallbladder disease and cholecystectomy rate are independently variable. Lancet 1984;*2*:621.
11. Sampliner RE, Bennett PH, Comess LJ, et al: Gallbladder disease in Pima Indians. Demonstration of high prevalence and early onset by cholecystography. N Engl J Med 1979;*283*:1358.
12. Bernstein RA, Giefer EE, Vieira JJ, et al: Gallbladder disease. II. Utilization of the life table method in obtaining clinically useful information. A study of 62,739 weight-conscious women. J Chron Dis 1977;*30*:529.
13. Honore LH: Cholesterol cholelithiasis in adolescent females. Its connection with obesity, parity, and oral contraceptive use—a retrospective study of 31 cases. Arch Surg 1980;*115*:62.
14. Layde PM, Vessey MP, Yeates D: Risk factors for gall-bladder disease: a cohort study of young women attending family planning clinics. J Epidemiol Community Health 1982;*36*:274.
15. Scragg RKR, McMichael AJ, Baghurst PA: Diet, alcohol, and relative weight in gall stone disease: a case-control study. Br Med J 1984;*288*:1113.
16. Amaral JF, Thompson WR: Gallbladder disease in the morbidly obese. Am J Surg 1985;*149*:551.
17. Thiet MD, Mittlestaedt CA, Herbst CA Jr, et al: Cholelithiasis in morbid obesity. South Med J 1984;*77*:416.
18. Herbst CA, Mittelstaedt CA, Staab EV, et al: Intraoperative ultrasonography evaluation of the gallbladder in morbidly obese patients. Ann Surg 1984;*200*:691.
19. Boston Collaborative Drug Surveillance Programme: Oral contraceptives and venous thromboembolic disease, surgically confirmed gallbladder disease, and breast tumours. Lancet 1973;*1*:1399.
20. Royal College of General Practitioners' Oral Contraception Study: Oral contraceptives and gallbladder disease. Lancet 1982;*2*:957.
21. Sarles H, Hauton J, Planche NE, et al: Diet, cholesterol gallstones, and composition of the bile. Dig Dis 1970;*15*:251.
22. Smith DA, Gee MI: A dietary survey to determine the relationship between diet and cholelithiasis. Am J Clin Nutr 1979;*32*:1519.
23. Capron JP, Delamarre J, Herve MA: Meal frequency and duration of overnight fast: a role in gall-stone formation? Br Med J 1981;*283*:1435.
24. Hanis CL, Ferrell RE, Tulloch BR, et al: Gallbladder disease epidemiology in Mexican Americans in Starr County, Texas. Am J Epidemiol 1985; *122*:820.
25. Bennion LJ, Grundy SM: Effects of diabetes mellitus on cholesterol metabolism in man. N Engl J Med 1977;*296*:1365.
26. Diehl AK, Rosenthal M, Hazuda HP, et al: Socioeconomic status and the prevalence of clinical gallbladder disease. J Chron Dis 1985;*38*:1019.
27. Thornton J, Symes C, Heaton K: Moderate alcohol intake reduces bile cholesterol saturation and raises HDL cholesterol. Lancet 1983;*2*:819.
28. Bouchier IAD: Postmortem study of the frequency of gallstones in patients with cirrhosis of the liver. Gut 1969;*10*:705.
29. Nicholas P, Rinaudo PA, Conn HO: Increased incidence of cholelithiasis in Laennec's cirrhosis. A postmortem evaluation of pathogenesis. Gastroenterology 1972;*63*:112.
30. Lund J: Surgical indications in cholelithiasis: prophylactic cholecystectomy elucidated on the basis of long-term follow up on 526 nonoperated cases. Ann Surg 1960;*151*:153.

31. Wenckert A, Robertson B: The natural course of gallstone disease. Eleven-year review of 781 nonoperated cases. Gastroenterology 1966;*50*:376.
32. Gracie WA, Ransohoff DF: The natural history of silent gallstones. The innocent gallstone is not a myth. N Engl J Med 1982;*307*:798.
33. McSherry CK, Ferstenberg H, Calhoun WF, et al: The natural history of diagnosed gallstone disease in symptomatic and asymptomatic patients. Ann Surg 1985;*202*:59.
34. Thistle JL, Cleary PA, Lachin JM, et al: The natural history of cholelithiasis: the National Cooperative Gallstone Study. Ann Intern Med 1984;*101*:171.
35. Ransohoff DF, Gracie WA, Wolfenson LB, et al: Prophylactic cholecystectomy or expectant management for silent gallstones. Ann Intern Med 1983;*99*:199.
36. Diehl AK: Epidemiology of gallbladder cancer: a synthesis of recent data. J Natl Cancer Inst 1980;*65*:1209.
37. Lowenfels AB, Lindstrom CG, Conway MJ, et al: Gallstones and risk of gallbladder cancer. J Natl Cancer Inst 1985;*75*:77.
38. Weiss KM, Ferrell RE, Hanis CL, et al: Genetics and epidemiology of gallbladder disease in new world native peoples. Am J Hum Genet 1984;*36*:1259.
39. Strom BL, Hibberd PL, Soper KA, et al: International variations in epidemiology of cancers of the extrahepatic biliary tract. Can Res 1985;*45*:5165.
41. Diehl AK, Beral V: Cholecystectomy and changing mortality from gallbladder cancer. Lancet 1981;2:187.
42. Polk HC Jr: Carcinoma and the calcified gallbladder. Gastroenterology 1966;*50*:582.
43. Ashur H, Siegal B, Oland Y, et al: Calcified gallbladder (porcelain gallbladder). Arch Surg 1978;*113*:594.
44. Schein CJ, Hurwitt ES, Rosenblatt MA: The significance of calculus size in determining the indication for elective cholecystectomy. Gastroenterology 1955;*29*:377.
45. Diehl AK: Gallstone size and the risk of gallbladder cancer. JAMA 1983;*250*:2323.
46. Houssin D, Castaing D, Lemoine J, et al: Microlithiasis of the gallbladder. Surg Gynecol Obstet 1983;*157*:20.
47. Adye B, Ryand JA Jr: Cholecystitis in teenage girls. West J Surg 1983;*139*:471.
48. Henschke CI, Teele RL: Cholelithiasis in children: recent observations. J Ultrasound Med 1983;*2*:481.
49. Lau GE, Andrassy RJ, Mahour GH: A 30-year review of the management of gallbladder disease at a children's hospital. Am Surg 1983;*49*:411.
50. Pokorny WJ, Saleem M, O'Gorman RB, et al: Cholelithiasis and cholecystitis in childhood. Am J Surg 1984;*148*:742.
51. Shafer AD, Ashley JV, Goodwin CD, et al: A new look at the multifactorial etiology of gallbladder disease in children. Am Surg 1983;*49*:314.
52. Takiff H, Fonkalsrud EW: Gallbladder disease in childhood. Am J Dis Child 1984;*138*:565.
53. Lachman BS, Lazerson J, Starshak RJ, et al: The prevalence of cholelithiasis in sickle cell disease as diagnosed by ultrasound and cholecystography. Pediatrics 1979;*64*:601.
54. Sarnaik S, Slovis TL, Corbett DP, et al: Incidence of cholelithiasis in sickle cell anemia using the ultrasonic gray-scale technique. J Pediatr 1980;*96*:1005.
55. Cameron JL, Maddrey WC, Zuidema GD: Biliary tract disease in sickle cell anemia: surgical considerations. Ann Surg 1971;*174*:702.
56. Flye MW, Silver D: Biliary tract disorders and sickle cell disease. Surgery 1972;*72*:361.
57. Stephens CG, Scott RB: Cholelithiasis in sickle cell anemia. Surgical or medical management. Arch Intern Med 1980;*140*:648.
58. Walsh DB, Eckhauser FE, Ramsburgh SR, et al: Risk associated with diabetes mellitus in patients undergoing gallbladder surgery. Surgery 1982; *91*:254.
59. Hjoryrup A, Sorensen C, Dyremose E, et al: Influence of diabetes mellitus on operative risk. Br J Surg 1985;*72*:783.
60. Sandler RS, Maule WF, Baltus ME: Factors associated with postoperative complications in diabetes following biliary tract surgery. Gastroenterology 1986;*91*:157.
61. Edlund Y, Zettergren L: Histopathology of the gallbladder in gallstone disease related to clinical data. Acta Chir Scand 1959;*116*:450.
62. Nahrwold DL, Rose RC, Ward SP: Abnormalities in gallbladder morphology and function in patients with cholelithiasis. Ann Surg 1976;*184*:415.
63. Sullivan FJ, Eaton SB Jr, Ferrucci JT Jr, et al: Cholangiographic manifestations of acute biliary colic. N Engl J Med 1973;*288*:33.
64. French EB, Robb WAT: Biliary and renal colic. Br Med J 1963;*3*:135.
65. Gunn A, Keddie N: Some clinical observations on patients with gallstones. Lancet 1972;*2*:7771.
66. Johnson AG: Cholecystectomy and gallstone dyspepsia. Clinical and physiological study of a symptom complex. Ann R Coll Engl 1975;*56*:69.
67. Kingston RD, Windsor WO: Flatulent dyspepsia in patients with gallstones undergoing cholecystectomy. Br J Surg 1975;*62*:231.
68. Price WH: Gall-bladder dyspepsia. Br Med J 1963;2:138.
69. Rhind JA, Watson L: Gall stone dyspepsia. Br Med J 1968;*1*:32.
70. Earlam RJ, Thomas M: The clinical significance of gallstones and their radiological investigation. Br J Surg 1978;*65*:164.
71. Gambill EE, Hodgson JR, Priestley JT: Painless obstructive cholecystopathy. Arch Intern Med 1962;*110*:442.
72. Gambill EE, Hodgson JR, Priestley JT: Obstructive cholecystography or primary roentgenographic shadow of the gallbladder. Report on 262 patients. Am J Dig Dis 1965;*10*:939.
73. Bartum RJ, Crow HC, Foote SR: Ultrasonic and radiographic cholecystography. N Engl J Med 1977;*296*:538.
74. Boutkan H, Butzelaar RMJM, Davies G: The diagnosis of gallstones—a prospective comparison of oral cholecystography and real-time ultrasound. Neth J Surg 1984;*36*:124.
75. Cooperberg P, Golding RH: Advances in ultrasonography of the gallbladder and biliary tract. Radiol Clin North Am 1982;*20*:611.
76. Cooperberg P, Burhenne HJ: Real-time ultrasonography. Diagnostic technique of choice in calculous gallbladder disease. N Engl J Med 1980; *302*:1277.
77. Detwiler RP, Kim DS, Longerbeam JK: Ultrason-

ography and oral cholecystography. A comparison of their use in the diagnosis of gallbladder disease. Arch Surg 1980;*115*:1096.
78. Escallon A Jr, Rosales W, Aldrete JS: Reliability of pre- and intraoperative tests for biliary lithiasis. Ann Surg 1985;*201*:640.
79. Ferrucci JT Jr, Fordtran JS, Cooperberg PL, et al: The radiological diagnosis of gallbladder disease. Radiology 1981;*141*:49.
80. Krook PM, Allen FH, Bush WH Jr, et al: Comparison of real-time cholecystosonograpy and oral cholecystography. Radiology 1980;*135*:145.
81. Lee JKT, Melson GL, Koehler RE, et al: Cholecystosonography: accuracy, pitfalls and unusual findings. Am J Surg 1980;*139*:223.
82. Mogensen NB, Madsen M, Stage P, et al: Ultrasonography versus roentgenography in suspected instances of cholecystolithiasis. Surg Gynecol Obstet 1984;*159*:353.
83. Lebensart PD, Bloom RA, Meretyk S, et al: Oral cholecystosonography: a method for facilitating the diagnosis of cholesterol gallstones. Radiology 1984;*153*:255.
84. Allen B, Bernhoft R, Blanckaert N, et al: Sludge is calcium bilirubinate associated with bile stasis. Am J Surg 1981;*141*:51.
85. Filly RA, Allen B, Minton MJ, et al: In vitro investigation of the origin of echoes within biliary sludge. J Clin Ultrasound 1980;*8*:193.
86. Fiegenschuh WH, Loughry CW: The false-normal oral cholecystogram. Surgery 1977;*81*:239.
87. McCluskey PL, Prinz RA, Guico R, et al: Use of ultrasound to demonstrate gallstones in symptomatic patients with normal oral cholecystograms. Am J Surg 1979;*138*:655.
88. Somerville KW, Rose DH, Bell GD, et al: Gallstone dissolution and recurrence: are we being misled? Br Med J 1982;*284*:1295.
89. Mujahed Z, Evans JA, Whalen JP: The nonopacified gallbladder on oral cholecystography. Radiology 1974;*112*:1.
90. Bartrum RJ Jr, Crow HC, Foote SR: Ultrasound examination of the gallbladder. An alternative to "double-dose" oral cholecystography. JAMA 1976;*236*:1147.
91. Jacob CO, Modan M, Itzchak Y, et al: Prolonged opacification of the gallbladder after oral cholecystography: a reevaluation of its clinical significance. Gastroenterology 1981;*81*:938.
92. Venu RP, Geenen JE, Toouli J, et al: Endoscopic retrograde cholangiopancreatography. Diagnosis of cholelithiasis in patients with gallbladder x-ray and ultrasound studies. JAMA 1983;*249*:758.
93. Burnstein MJ, Vassal KP, Strasberg SM: Results of combined biliary drainage and cholecystokinin cholecystography in 81 patients with normal oral cholecystograms. Ann Surg 1982;*196*:627.
94. Delchier JC, Benfredj P, Preaux AM, et al: The usefulness of microscopic bile examination in patients with suspected microlithiasis: a prospective evaluation. Hepatology 1986;*6*:118.
95. Sedaghat A, Grundy SM: Cholesterol crystals and the formation of cholesterol gallstones. N Engl J Med 1980;*302*:1274.
96. Strasberg SM: Personal communication, 1986.
97. Nathan MH, Newman A, Murray DJ: Normal findings in oral and cholecystokinin cholecystography. JAMA 1978;*240*:2271.
98. Davis GB, Berk FN, Scheible FW, et al: Cholecystokinin cholecystography, sonography, and scintigraphy: detection of chronic acalculous cholecystitis. AJR 1982;*139*:1117.
99. Dunn FH, Christensen EC, Reynold J, et al: Cholecystokinin cholecystography. Controlled evaluation in the diagnosis and management of patients with possible acalculous gallbladder disease. JAMA 1974;*228*:997.
100. Nora PF, Davis RP, Fernandez MJ: Chronic acalculous gallbladder disease: a clinical enigma. World J Surg 1984;*8*:106.
101. Griffen WO, Bivins BA, Rogers EL, et al: Cholecystokinin cholecystography in the diagnosis of gallbladder disease. Ann Surg 1980;*191*:636.
102. Proudfoot R, Mattingly SS, Snodgrass S, et al: Cholecystokinin cholecystography: Is it a useful test? South Med J 1985;*78*:1443.
103. Pickleman J, Peiss RL, Henkin R, et al: The role of sincalide cholescintigraphy in the evaluation of patients with acalculous gallbladder disease. Arch Surg 1985;*120*:693.
104. Rajagopalan AE, Pickleman J: Biliary colic and functional gallbladder disease. Arch Surg 1982;*117*:1005.
105. Choctaw WT, Pollack EW, Wolfman EF Jr: Evaluation of associated upper gastrointestinal pathology prior to elective cholecystectomy. Am J Surg 1978;*135*:620.
106. Max MH, Polk HC Jr: Routine preoperative upper gastrointestinal series (UGIS) in patients with biliary tract disease: a plea for more selectivity. Surgery 1977;*82*:334.
107. Friedman GD: The relationship between coronary heart disease and gallbladder disease. A critical review. Ann Intern Med 1968;*68*:222.
108. Palmer ED: Gallbladder disease and the cardiac status. JAMA 1975;*234*:97.
109. Mogadam M, Albarelli J, Ahmed SW, et al: Gallbladder dynamics in response to various meals: is dietary fat restriction necessary in the management of gallstones? Am J Gastroenterol 1984;*79*:745.
110. Bremner DN, McCormick JSC, Thomson JWW, et al: A study of cholecystectomy. Surg Gynecol Obstet 1974;*138*:752.
111. Gunn AA, Foubiser G: Biliary surgery. A 5-year follow-up. R Coll Surg Edinb 1978;*23*:292.
112. MacLean LD, Goldstein M, MacDonald JE, et al: Results of cholecystectomy in 1000 consecutive patients. Can J Surg 1975;*18*:459.
113. Martin JK Jr, van Heerden JA: Surgery of the liver biliary tract, and pancreas. Mayo Clin Proc 1980;*55*:333.
114. Seltzer MH, Steiger E, Rosato FE: Mortality following cholecystectomy. Surg Gynecol Obstet 1970;*130*:64.
115. Glenn F, McSherry CK: Etiological factors in fatal complications following operations upon the biliary tract. Ann Surg 1963;*157*:695.
116. McSherry CK, Glenn F: The incidence and causes of death following surgery for nonmalignant biliary tract disease. Ann Surg 1980;*191*:271.
117. Weckesser EC: Surgery for gallbladder disease in Ohio. A survey of 3,085 operations. Am J Surg 1961;*102*:695.
118. National Halothane Committee: Summary of the National Halothane Study. Possible association between halothane anesthesia and postoperative hepatic necrosis. JAMA 1966;*197*:775.
119. Houghton PWJ, Jenkinson LR, Donaldson LA: Cholecystectomy in the elderly: a prospective study. Br J Surg 1985;*72*:220.

120. Huber DF, Martin EW Jr, Cooperman M: Cholecystectomy in elderly patients. Am J Surg 1983;*146*:719.
121. Sullivan DM, Hood TR, Griffen WO Jr: Biliary tract surgery in the elderly. Am J Surg 1982; *143*:216.
122. Aranha GV, Sontag SJ, Greenlee HB: Cholecystectomy in cirrhotic patients: a formidable operation. Am J Surg 1982;*143*:55.
123. Bloch RS, Allaben RD, Walt AJ: Cholecystectomy in patients with cirrhosis. A surgical challenge. Arch Surg 1985;*120*:669.
124. Castaing D, Houssin D, Lemoine J, et al: Surgical management of gallstone in cirrhotic patients. Am J Surg 1983;*146*:310.
125. Simmons F, Bouchier IAD: Intraluminal bile salt concentrations and fat digestion after cholecystectomy. S Afr Med J 1972;*46*:2089.
126. Tangedahl T: The present status of agents for dissolving gallstones. Am J Gastroenterol 1985;*80*:64.
127. Kogut K, Aragoni T, Ackerman NB: Cholecystectomy in patients with mild cirrhosis. Arch Surg 1985;*120*:1310.
128. Schoenfield LJ, Lachin JM, Baum RA, et al: Chenodiol (chenodeoxycholic acid) for dissolution of gallstones: the National Cooperative Gallstone Study. Ann Intern Med 1981;*95*:257.
129. Maton PN, Iser JH, Reuben A, et al: Outcome of chenodeoxycholic acid (CDCA) treatment in 125 patients with radiolucent gallstones. Factors influencing efficacy, withdrawal, symptoms and side effects and post-dissolution recurrence. Medicine 1982;*61*:86.
130. Fisher MM, Roberts EA, Rosen IE, et al: The Sunnybrook gallstone study: a double-blind controlled trial of chenodeoxycholic acid for gallstone dissolution. Hepatology 1985;*5*:102.
131. Johansson G: A prospective study of the clinical significance of the treatment of gallstones with chenodeoxycholic acid. Surg Gynecol Obstet 1984;*154*:127.
132. Erlinger S, Go AL, Husson JM, et al: Franco-Belgian Cooperative Study of ursodeoxycholic acid in the medical dissolution of gallstones. A double-blind, randomized, dose-response study, and comparison with chenodeoxycholic acid. Hepatology 1984;*4*:308.
133. Roda E, Bazzoli F, Morselli AM, et al: Ursodeoxycholic acid vs. chenodeoxycholic acid as cholesterol gallstone–dissolving agents: a comparative randomized study. Hepatology 1982;*2*:804.
134. Fromm H, Roat JW, Gonzalez V, et al: Comparative efficacy and side effects of ursodeoxycholic and chenodeoxycholic acids in dissolving gallstones. A double-blind controlled study. Gastroenterology 1983;*85*:1257.
135. Meredith TJ, Williams GV, Maton PN, et al: Retrospective comparison of "cheno" and "urso" in the medical treatment of gallstones. Gut 1982;*23*:382.
136. Stiehl A, Raedsch R, Rudolph G, et al: Effect of ursodeoxycholic acid in biliary bile acid and bile lipid composition in gallstone patients. Hepatology 1984;*4*:107.
137. Podda M, Zuin M, Dioguardi ML, et al: A combination of chenodeoxycholic acid and ursodeoxycholic acid is more effective than either alone in reducing biliary cholesterol saturation. Hepatology 1982;*2*:334.
138. Ruppin DC, Dowling RH: Is recurrence inevitable after gallstone dissolution by bile-acid treatment? Lancet 1982;*1*:181.
139. Gleeson D, Ruppin DC, British Gallstone Study Group: Discrepancies between cholecystography and ultrasonography in the detection of recurrent gallstones. J Hepatol 1985;*1*:597.
140. Sauerbruch T, Delius M, Paumgartner G, et al: Fragmentation of gallstones by extracorporeal shock waves. N Engl J Med 1986;*314*:818.
141. Mulley AG Jr: Shock-wave lithotripsy. Assessing a slam-bang technology. N Engl J Med 1986; *314*:845.
142. Allen MJ, Borody TJ, Bugliosi TF, et al: Rapid dissolution of gallstones by methyl tert-butyl ether. N Engl J Med 1985;*312*:217.
143. Kovalcik PJ, Burrell MJ, Old WL Jr: Cholecystectomy concomitant with other intra-abdominal operations. Assessment of risk. Arch Surg 1983; *118*:1059.
144. McSherry CK, Glenn F: Biliary tract surgery concomitant with other intra-abdominal operations. Ann Surg 1981;*193*:169.
145. Thompson JS, Philben VJ, Hodgson PE: Operative management of incidental cholelithiasis. Am J Surg 1984;*148*:821.
146. Schreiber H, Macon WL IV, Pories WJ: Incidental cholecystectomy during major abdominal surgery in the elderly. Am J Surg 1978;*135*:196.
147. Shennib H, Fried GM, Hampson LG: Does simultaneous cholecystectomy increase the risk of colonic surgery? Am J Surg 1986;*151*:266.
148. Stevens ML, Hubert BC, Wenzel FJ: Combined gynecologic surgical procedures and cholecystectomy. Am J Obstet Gynecol 1984;*149*:350.
149. Ouriel K, Ricotta JJ, Adams JT, et al: Management of cholelithiasis in patients with abdominal aortic aneurysm. Ann Surg 1983;*196*:717.
150. Tompkins WC, Chavez CM, Conn JH, et al: Combining intra-abdominal arterial grafting with gastrointestinal or biliary tract procedures. Am J Surg 1973;*126*:598.
151. Salmenkivi K: Cholesterosis of the gall-bladder. A clinical study based on 269 cholecystectomies. Acta Chir Scand (Suppl) 1964;*324*:1.
152. Holzbach RT, Marsh M, Tang P: Cholesterolosis: physical-chemical characteristics of human and diet-induced canine lesions. Exp Mol Pathol 1977;*27*:324.
153. Koga A, Todo S, Nishimura M: Electron microscopic observations on the cholesterol distributed in the epithelial cells of the gallbladder. Histochemistry 1975;*44*:303.
154. Koga A: Fine structure of the human gallbladder with cholesterosis with special reference to the mechanism of lipid accumulation. Br J Exp Pathol 1985;*66*:605.
155. Tilvis RS, Aro J, Strandberg TE, et al: Lipid composition of bile and gallbladder mucosa in patients with acalculous cholesterolosis. Gastroenterology 1982;*82*:607.
156. Lowenfels AB, Schwaetz R, Pitchumoni C: Cholelithiasis and cancer. Gastroenterology 1981;*80*:1218.
157. Lowenfels AB: Gallstones and the risk of cancer. Gut 1980;*21*:1090.
158. Lowenfels AB, Domellof L, Lindstrom L, et al: Cholelithiasis, cholecystectomy, and cancer: a case-control study in Sweden. Gastroenterology 1982;*83*:672.

159. Linos DA, O'Fallon WM, Thistle JL, et al: Cholelithiasis and carcinoma of the colon. Cancer 1982;*50*:1015.
160. Schottenfeld D, Winawer SJ: Cholecystectomy and colorectal cancer. Gastroenterology 1983;*85*:966.
161. Vernick LJ, Kuller LH: Cholecystectomy and right-sided colon cancer: an epidemiological study. Lancet 1981;*2*:381.
162. Linos DA, Beard CM, O'Fallon WM, et al: Cholecystectomy and carcinoma of the colon. Lancet 1981;*2*:379.
163. Turunen MJ, Kivilaakso EO: Increased risk of colorectal cancer after cholecystectomy. Ann Surg 1981;*194*:639.
164. Weiss NS, Daling JR, Chow WH: Cholecystectomy and the incidence of cancer of the large bowel. Cancer 1982;*49*:1713.
165. Adami HO, Meirik O, Gustavsson S, et al: Colorectal cancer after cholecystectomy: absence of risk increase within 11–14 years. Gastroenterology 1983;*85*:859.
166. Abrams JS, Anton JR, Dreyfuss DC: The absence of a relationship between cholecystectomy and the subsequent occurrence of cancer of the proximal colon. Dis Colon Rectum 1983;*26*:141.
167. Spitz MR, Russell NC, Guinee VF, et al: Questionable relationship between cholecystectomy and colon cancer. J Surg Oncol 1985;*30*:6.

CARLOS A. PELLEGRINI, M.D.
LAWRENCE W. WAY, M.D.

15

Acute Cholecystitis

Acute cholecystitis is one of the more common abdominal emergencies, especially among middle-aged women. It is most often a complication of cholelithiasis, it occurs in 10 to 20 per cent of patients with symptomatic gallstones, and it is associated with considerable morbidity and mortality.[1–5] The incidence of acute cholecystitis increases with each decade of life.

PATHOGENESIS

The mechanisms responsible for the development of acute cholecystitis are not totally understood, but it appears that several factors are involved.

Cystic Duct Obstruction

In 95 per cent of patients, acute cholecystitis is associated with cystic duct obstruction from cholelithiasis. Some of these patients have a small stone inside the cystic duct obturating the lumen, and some a gallstone firmly impacted in Hartmann's pouch, producing external compression of the cystic duct.[6–8]

Obstruction of the cystic duct changes the absorptive capacity of the gallbladder mucosa. For example, 12 hours after ligation of the cystic duct, the gallbladder ceases to absorb fluid (rabbit) or produces a net secretion (dog) into the lumen.[9, 10] Three days after cystic duct ligation, calcium bilirubinate particles (sludge) and, in some cases, pigment stones form in the gallbladder of the dog.[11]

Obstruction of the cystic duct in dogs, however, most often produces hydrops or chronic inflammation instead of acute cholecystitis.[12, 13] The inability to reproduce acute cholecystitis consistently by obstruction of the cystic duct in animals is not surprising because hydrops, chronic inflammation, and acute cholecystitis are also among the spectrum of results that follows cystic duct obstruction in man.

In about 5 per cent of patients, acute cholecystitis develops in the absence of cholelithiasis (acute acalculous cholecystitis). Cystic duct obstruction may not be the initiating event in these cases. Instead, gallbladder bile stasis is implicated most often, frequently as a result of prolonged fasting.[14–25] Increased cholesterol saturation of bile, which occurs during fasting, may be a contributing factor. The stasis leads to inspissation of bile[26, 27] and the formation of sludge and pigment stones.[11] Whether these events produce cystic duct obstruction secondarily is not known.

Therefore, while most cases of acute cholecystitis are associated with sudden obstruction of the cystic duct by a stone, acute cholecystitis occasionally develops in the absence of obstruction. On the other hand, obstruction of the cystic duct does not always cause acute cholecystitis; several other factors play a role in the development of the acute inflammatory process.

Mediators of the Inflammatory Response

Bile acids have been identified as possible initiators of the inflammatory response. For example, studying the gallbladder of the rabbit in vitro, Heuman found that permeability to passage of dextran through the gallbladder wall was markedly increased by exposure to taurodeoxycholate and, to a lesser degree, taurocholate, effects that could be inhibited by the addition of lecithin.[28] In the dog gallbladder, taurodeoxycholate can completely abolish transepithelial water movement, an effect also eliminated by the addition of lecithin.[29] At low concentrations, bile acids alter transport mechanisms in the cell membrane, and at higher concentrations they produce lysis of the membrane and release of intracellular enzymes, which may further damage adjacent cells. Lecithin may protect against the deleterious effects of bile salts by tying up the bile salts in mixed micelles. Since bile from patients with gallstones contains more deoxycholate and less lecithin than that from controls, these findings could be relevant to the pathogenesis of acute cholecystitis.[30]

Another factor thought to predispose to acute cholecystitis is the presence of *lithogenic bile*. Gallbladders exposed to lithogenic bile become inflamed, and acute cholecystitis has been reported to result from ligation of the cystic duct in prairie dogs fed a cholesterol-supplemented diet even before gallstones develop.[31] These findings may be relevant to the pathogenesis of acalculous cholecystitis in man. In fact, lithogenic bile is present in most patients after prolonged fasting (e.g., hyperalimentation). Cholesterol crystals, which have been shown to produce inflammation in other tissues, could be the injurious agent.

Acute cholecystitis has been produced following the introduction of *pancreatic juice* into the gallbladder lumen. The resulting acute inflammation was believed to be due to the action of trypsin. However, it is hardly possible that pancreatic juice could gain access to the gallbladder in vivo.

Lysolecithin induces structural changes in biologic membranes, and after ligation of the cystic duct, injection of lysolecithin into the lumen of the gallbladder causes acute cholecystitis.[32] Lysolecithin originates from hydrolysis of lecithin and is present in small amounts in normal bile. In patients with acute cholecystitis the ratio of lysolecithin to lecithin in bile is increased, and it has been postulated that lysolecithin is a key factor in the pathogenesis of acalculous cholecystitis.[28, 33] After damaging the epithelium of the gallbladder, lysolecithin is thought to be partially absorbed by the damaged mucosa. High concentrations of lecithin protect against the effects of lysolecithin.

The conversion of lecithin to lysolecithin is catalyzed by *phospholipase A,* an enzyme present in lysosomes in the mucosal cells of human gallbladder but normally absent from gallbladder bile. Sjodahl et al.[33] proposed that phospholipase A may be released from the damaged epithelium when a stone becomes impacted in the neck of the gallbladder. Incubation of bile in the presence of extracts from gallbladder epithelium increases the lysolecithin:lecithin ratio, suggesting that bile stasis may also release phospholipase A. Lysolecithin activity in bile is also increased by exposure of the mucosa to β-glucuronidase,[34] and increased β-glucuronidase activity in the bile from *E. coli* or other sources could augment lysolecithin release.

Prostaglandins are another candidate for a role in the pathogenesis of cholecystitis: (1) Prostaglandins mediate inflammation in a number of human tissues; (2) a high concentration of prostaglandins is present in the wall of the inflamed gallbladder;[35] and (3) prostaglandin E_1 can convert absorption in the gallbladder to secretion,[36, 37] which could explain the gallbladder distention seen in acute cholecystitis. Indomethacin, a prostaglandin synthetase inhibitor, reverses mucosal secretion in experimental acute cholecystitis[10] and relieves the pain of acute cholecystitis in humans, presumably by ameliorating gallbladder distention.[38] The role of gastric and pancreatic secretion, drugs,[39] and other factors in the pathogenesis of cholecystitis remains unclear.

Bacteria can be cultured from the gallbladder in about 20 per cent of patients with cholelithiasis (and no acute inflammation) and in about 50 per cent of patients with acute cholecystitis.[40, 41] It seems likely that the source of bacteria is the intestine, since enteric organisms are most frequently found.[41] Whether these organisms reach the biliary tract via the splanchnic lymphatics, via the common duct, or from the portal blood remains a matter of speculation. Injection of *E. coli*, clostridia, and other bacterial species into the gallbladder lumen, however, fails to produce acute cholecystitis when the cystic duct is patent, although when the duct is ligated, suppurative cholecystitis results. A few cases of acalculous cholecystitis are caused by primary biliary infection with *E. coli*, clostridia, or *Salmonella typhi*.

The weight of evidence favors a secondary role for bacteria in human cholecystitis. Nevertheless, the suppurative complications, such as empyema, perforation, emphysematous cholecystitis, and septicemia, cause much of the morbidity of this disease.

Evolution of Acute Cholecystitis

Edema of the gallbladder wall is the earliest manifestation of acute cholecystitis. Edema is thought to stem from obstruction of the venous and lymphatic outflow due to inflammation of the cystic duct pedicle caused by the impacted stone. If the stone dislodges and patency of the gallbladder outflow is restored, the symptoms and the local inflammatory reaction subside promptly. In fact, it is often difficult to decide whether attacks of relatively short duration should be considered mild acute cholecystitis or biliary colic without inflammation.

If the stone remains obstructing the gallbladder, the evolution of the illness is dictated by whether or not ischemia of the wall develops and by the presence of secondary infection. When obstruction of the cystic duct does not result in gallbladder inflammation, ischemia, or infection, hydrops of the gallbladder develops. In hydrops, bile pigments are absorbed and the gallbladder contents become a clear mucoid fluid. On the other hand, when ischemia develops, the inflammation worsens, and the fundus may become necrotic. This complication is most frequent in the second week of the illness, rarely before the third day. The slower pace of the evolution of acute cholecystitis contrasts with that of acute appendicitis, which if untreated ends in perforation within hours rather than days.

The severity of the symptoms may not correlate well with the severity of the inflammatory process in the gallbladder. This is especially true in the elderly and in individuals with diabetes mellitus. Gangrene of the gallbladder may develop rapidly, and perforation of the distended gallbladder can occur with minimal symptoms in these patients. While the clinical manifestations may subside within several days, the acute inflammatory process tends to persist for weeks.

The Pathogenesis of Ischemia. Because advanced acute cholecystitis demonstrates ischemic necrosis, it has been suggested that the inflammation surrounding Hartmann's pouch may occlude the cystic artery. However, arteriography during acute cholecystitis in humans shows the cystic artery to be patent and the gallbladder to be hypervascular.[42] Furthermore, attempts at producing necrotizing cholecystitis by ligation of the cystic artery in experimental animals have not been successful, probably because there are so many arterial anastomoses between the terminal branches of the cystic artery and the liver capsule.[8] It does not appear, therefore, that occlusion of the cystic artery or vein contributes to the early events in acute cholecystitis in man.

Ischemia of the gallbladder wall and, eventually, necrosis are probably caused by a different mechanism. With increasing gallbladder distention due to secretion of fluid into the lumen, pressure in the gallbladder rises to as high as 25 to 55 cm H_2O,[43] and blood flow drops progressively (e.g., at 60 mm Hg, flow is only 25 per cent of baseline levels).[44] The decrease in flow is disproportionately great in the mucosa. The predilection for perforation to occur in the fundus may be due to its large diameter and the greater tension that would result in this area, according to Laplace's law. In fact, injection of arterial vessels of acutely inflamed human gallbladders has shown small vessel thrombosis adjacent to areas of necrosis in the fundus. Since cholelithiasis and chronic cholecystitis produce tortuosity and occlusion of small vessels and loss of the normal anastomotic net, it is possible that they may render the gallbladder more susceptible to acute ischemia. Diseases with pre-existing lesions of the small blood vessels (e.g., diabetes mellitus) are known to predispose to perforation.

In summary, the pathophysiology of acute cholecystitis in humans has not been entirely deciphered, and the etiology is probably multifactorial. The empirical evidence suggests that sudden occlusion of the cystic duct in the presence of saturated bile in the gallbladder can alter absorptive function of the mucosa, activate inflammatory mediators, and damage the mucosa. The acutely inflamed gallbladder then becomes susceptible to secondary infection. Finally, the blood supply may be compromised by high luminal pressures, and necrosis or perforation may ensue.

PATHOLOGY

On gross examination the gallbladders of patients with acute cholecystitis are distended and filled with colorless bile (Fig. 15–1). The gallbladder wall is thickened, owing to submucosal and subserosal edema, and is hyperemic (Fig. 15–2). In a later stage, the fundus may become necrotic and may perforate (Fig. 15–3).

The pathologic change most characteristic of acute cholecystitis is edema, which may be of help to the surgeon when developing a cleavage plane between the gallbladder and the liver. Because edema tends to disappear with fixation, the gross specimen is usually more strikingly abnormal than are histologic sections (Figs. 15–1 to 15–3).

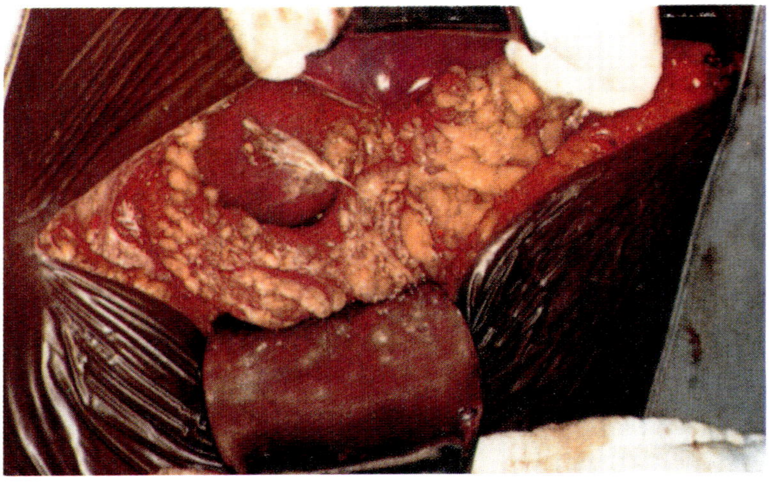

Figure 15–1. Acute cholecystitis. The gallbladder is distended and surrounded by an inflamed omentum.

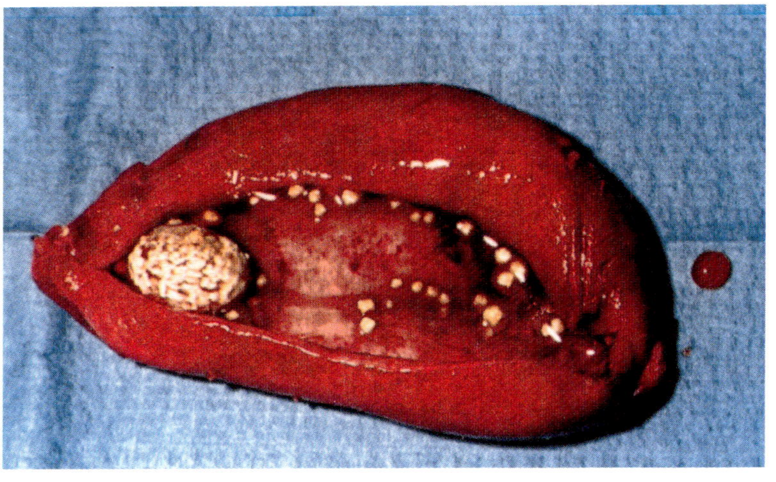

Figure 15–2. Acute cholecystitis. The gallbladder is opened, and there is marked edema of the wall. There are multiple cholesterol stones of various sizes.

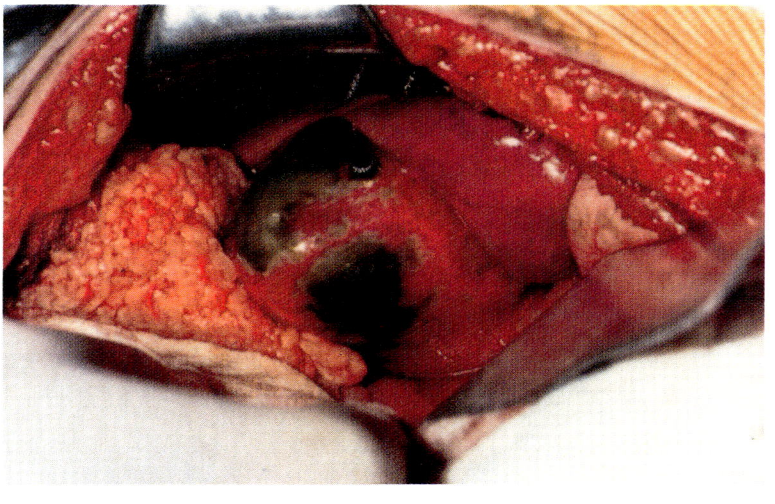

Figure 15–3. Acute cholecystitis. The gallbladder is surrounded by the omentum. The fundus is necrotic.

Mucosal ulcerations are frequent at the site of impaction of the stone, but the epithelial lining otherwise may look remarkably intact. The submucosa is infiltrated with polymorphonuclear leukocytes, and the venules and lymphatics are dilated. Occasionally, small vessels are thrombosed and fibrin deposits are found on the serosal surface. In addition to acute inflammation, the gallbladder wall in 95 per cent of patients with acute cholecystitis has evidence of chronic inflammation: flattening of the columnar epithelium, metaplasia of the mucosal lining, increased numbers of goblet cells, and lymphocytic infiltration of the submucosal layer. In cases that resolve spontaneously, acute inflammation has largely cleared by 4 weeks, but some residual evidence of inflammation may last for several months.

DIAGNOSIS

Clinical Findings

In most cases, the diagnosis of acute cholecystitis is suggested by the clinical findings. The disease is more common in women and the middle-aged or elderly. About 75 per cent of patients have had bloating and attacks of biliary colic in the past. In the remainder, acute cholecystitis is the first clinical manifestation of gallstone disease. The patient may give a history of dietary indiscretion shortly before the attack of upper abdominal pain. It is important to distinguish acute cholecystitis from biliary colic, as most patients with biliary colic may be safely treated as outpatients.

The pain in acute cholecystitis is located in the right subcostal area, over the gallbladder, but it may begin as a less well localized discomfort in the right upper quadrant or the epigastrium. Epigastric distress in the early stages of cholecystitis is a visceral pain resulting from distention of the gallbladder; it is similar in its cause and character to the attacks of biliary colic of chronic gallbladder disease. As inflammation develops and the peritoneal surfaces become involved, the pain is more precisely related to the gallbladder in the right upper quadrant. Once the pain reaches its peak, it tends to remain steady, unlike the pain of ureteral colic or intestinal obstruction.

On physical examination there is localized tenderness in the right upper quadrant. The tenderness is exacerbated during subcostal palpation by deep inspiration, which produces inspiratory arrest (Murphy's sign). Although direct and rebound tenderness may be present, it is often impossible to detect a distended gallbladder in the very obese patient or when abdominal guarding is present. The gallbladder can be felt as a tender palpable mass in the right upper quadrant in 20 to 25 per cent of patients; when associated with typical symptoms, this is almost pathognomonic of acute cholecystitis. Percussion over the anterior right costal margin and the posterior lower portion of the right rib cage may aggravate the pain in the gallbladder area.

The physical findings, however, vary from patient to patient. Sometimes a distended gallbladder is palpable in a patient with very few abdominal complaints. Other patients have severe epigastric pain consistent with acute cholecystitis, but tenderness in the gallbladder region may not be striking. Tenderness and the ability to discern a mass depend on the proximity of the gallbladder to the overlying peritoneum. For example, an organ scarred from chronic disease may be buried within or beneath the liver substance, protected from contact with the parietal peritoneum.

Laboratory Findings

The most important laboratory aids are the leukocyte count and liver function tests. Leukocytosis is common in acute cholecystitis and exceeds 10,000/dl in 75 per cent of cases.

Liver chemistry tests are helpful but nonspecific. Serum glutamic or pyruvic transaminase values are often mildly elevated but rarely to levels suggestive of hepatitis. In approximately 40 per cent of patients, one or both enzymes will be abnormal.[45–47] The akaline phosphatase concentration is elevated in 15 per cent of cases even in the absence of a common duct stone.

Jaundice is present in about 10 per cent of cases, but the serum bilirubin level is abnormal in 25 per cent. Jaundice does not necessarily imply the presence of a common duct stone, although the incidence of choledocholithiasis is higher in acute cholecystitis than in chronic cholecystitis.[45, 46, 48] Rarely, the stone impacted in Hartmann's pouch may produce secondary obstruction of the common duct by direct compression or edema (Mirizzi's syndrome).[49–51] In addition to common duct stones, inflammation of the liver adjacent to the gallbladder, spasm of the choledochal sphincter, or pancreatitis may cause hyperbilirubinemia.

Serum amylase levels are often elevated. While some patients have associated pancreatitis, most do not. The normal amylase-creatinine clearance ratio is below 4; if it exceeds 8, pancreatitis should be suspected. Cholecystectomy should not be delayed simply because the serum amylase level is elevated.

Blood sugar should be measured before beginning the administration of intravenous fluids. On occasion, undiagnosed diabetes mellitus will be first detected during an attack of acute cholecystitis.

Blood urea nitrogen and creatinine levels should be obtained at the time of admission. Sepsis associated with biliary tract infection will occasionally result in acute tubular necrosis and may be prevented with adequate hydration. Azotemia at the time of admission is an ominous sign and should be corrected, if at all possible, before operation.

Radiographic Findings

In approximately 20 per cent of patients with gallstones, the stones contain enough calcium to be seen on plain films. If stones are seen, it is important to distinguish them from renal calculi, and an intravenous pyelogram may be helpful. If stones are not seen, plain films may only show signs of ileus.

Oral cholecystography is not useful: It would take several hours to do, and most patients have been unable to eat or to retain food for several hours before admission to the hospital, which prevents opacification even in the case of a normal gallbladder.[52, 53]

Ultrasonography is the test of choice.[54–57] In addition to cholelithiasis, it will show a distended gallbladder, thickening and edema of the gallbladder wall, and, occasionally, pericholecystic fluid.[58–60] The ultrasonographer can tell that the tenderness is over the gallbladder. Sonography is especially useful in pregnant women with right upper quadrant pain, since it avoids exposure to ionizing radiation (for further details on sonography in the diagnosis of acute cholecystitis see Chapter 8).

Radionuclide cholescintigraphy to image the bile ducts and gallbladder is very useful. A Tc-99m derivative of iminodiacetic acid (e.g., HIDA, PIPIDA, DISIDA) is injected intravenously and is excreted by the liver into bile. The gamma-emitting radionuclide images the liver, bile ducts, and gallbladder even with bilirubin levels as high as 5 to 6 mg/dl. Each study gives about 20 to 50 per cent of the radiation exposure from a single abdominal roentgenogram.

A positive study (diagnostic of acute cholecystitis) consists of *no* imaging of the gallbladder in the presence of radioactivity in the duodenum.[62–68] This pattern reflects obstruction of the cystic duct. Obstruction of the cystic duct can be shown in about 95 per cent of cases of acute cholecystitis. Rarely (1 per cent of cases), a normal gallbladder will fail to be imaged.[69, 70] In some cases, this may be due to the presence of residual Telepaque (the contrast material used for oral cholecystography) in the gallbladder. It may also be the result of gallbladder emptying induced by a meal given within 2 hours of the study. Therefore, it is important to keep these patients *without* food or liquids 4 to 6 hours before the biliary scan and to perform the test before doing oral cholecystography. False positive results may also occur in patients with biliary pancreatitis and in those who have chronic cholecystitis with chronic obstruction of the cystic duct. False negative findings may occur in acute acalculous cholecystitis. (Cholescintigraphy in acute cholecystitis is discussed in Chapter 12.) CT scanning is of little value.[57] Endoscopic retrograde cholangiopancreatography is not indicated in suspected acute cholecystitis but should be reserved for other biliary tract conditions in which acute infection is less likely.

Intravenous cholangiography may be of benefit. If the gallbladder fills, there is reasonable assurance that the patient does not have acute cholecystitis.[61] However, this study has been largely replaced by HIDA scans, which provide much more accurate information (IV cholangiography in acute cholecystitis is discussed in Chapter 7).

Differential Diagnosis

The differential diagnosis includes other causes of acute abdominal pain. *Acute pancreatitis* must always be considered. As mentioned earlier, some patients with acute cholecystitis have elevated amylase levels. On the other hand, some patients with biliary pancreatitis have distended gallbladders, so that the differentiation between cholecystitis and pancreatitis may be difficult. Although the two diseases may coexist, this is uncommon. Pancreatitis causes pain and tenderness close to the midline and, on ultrasound, none of the manifestations of acute cholecystitis. The amylase levels are higher than in acute cholecystitis. If pancreatitis is seriously considered, a CT scan should be obtained, which would be expected to demonstrate pancreatic swelling. (For diagnosis of pancreatitis, refer to Chapter 20.)

A *perforated peptic ulcer,* especially in association with a slow leak down the right gutter, may make the differential diagnosis most difficult. A history of ulcer adds to the difficulty. Upright and left lateral decubitus x-ray films generally show the presence of free air if a perforated ulcer is present.

Appendicitis is the condition most often mistaken for acute cholecystitis. A large inflamed gallbladder may extend far enough into the right lower quadrant to mimic acute appendicitis, or a high appendix may be thought to represent cholecystitis. The distinction can usually be made by ultrasound and HIDA scans.

A *kidney stone* on the right side can also produce severe pain in the right upper quadrant. Usually the pain radiates downward into the genitalia, and the pain and tenderness are most severe in the region of the right costovertebral angle.

Acute hepatic congestion or alcoholic hepatitis may be very difficult to differentiate from acute cholecystitis. Hepatic cysts, abscesses, and primary and metastatic hepatic tumors near the gallbladder may simulate cholecystitis. Hepatic adenomas near the gallbladder may mimic acute cholecystitis. Hemorrhage into the adenoma produces symptoms and physical findings that are highly suggestive of acute cholecystitis.

The Fitz-Hugh–Curtis syndrome is an infrequent mimic of acute cholecystitis. It is caused by gonococcal perihepatitis and occurs in a sexually active female, typically 2 to 3 weeks following an episode of gonococcal salpingitis.

At times it is difficult to differentiate between acute cholecystitis and *coronary occlusion.* Nocturnal attacks, particularly in obese patients who complain of severe epigastric or substernal distress associated with shortness of breath, may produce a diagnostic challenge. Electrocardiograms are essential, and enzyme studies should be obtained.

COMPLICATIONS

The major complications of acute cholecystitis are empyema and perforation.

Empyema. The gallbladder contains stones and pus, and for this reason the disease has been called suppurative cholecystitis. The patient usually has high fever, chills, and leukocytosis greater than 15,000/dl. This complication is probably more common among diabetics. Hypotension, shock, and septicemia may lead to rapid deterioration and death. After aggressive resuscitation with intravenous fluids, the patient should undergo emergent surgery, either cholecystectomy or cholecystostomy.[5]

Perforation. Perforation of the gallbladder is the result of progressive ischemia and necrosis of the wall. Infection of the gallbladder contents may enhance the process. Depending on other variables, the perforation may occur (1) free into the peritoneal cavity (early perforation before adjacent viscera have walled off the area); (2) into an adjacent viscus (late perforations that involved the wall of another viscus previously adherent to the gallbladder); or (3) perforation within a relatively well walled off area, giving rise to pericholecystic abscess. Fortunately, free perforation is uncommon. The omentum and adjacent viscera adhere to the gallbladder, and when the gallbladder wall is finally breached, the contents are confined to the immediate region. (See also Chapter 16.)

Pericholecystic abscess, the most common form of perforation,[4, 71] presents with findings similar to those of empyema (i.e., sepsis), often with a palpable right upper quadrant mass. Differentiation from empyema may be impossible, although ultrasound may show a pericholecystic collection of fluid. Treatment consists of cholecystostomy or cholecystectomy.

TREATMENT

Initial Management

The clinical diagnosis of acute cholecystitis is enough to justify immediate hospitalization. The course of the disease is unpredictable, and the diagnosis is rarely certain until corroborative tests have been performed.

If fever or leukocytosis is present, a blood culture should be among the initial diagnostic tests. Nasogastric intubation should be performed early. The right upper quadrant inflammatory process often diminishes duodenal peristalsis, with resulting functional gastric outlet obstruction. Other supportive measures should be appropriate to the severity of the illness. Prerenal azotemia and elevated hematocrit levels should be treated by fluid replacement. Antibiotics are usually given, although controlled trials have shown they have no influence on the course of the disease. The rationale for antibiotics is (1) as a prophylactic measure to prevent wound infection in patients treated surgically, and (2) as therapy of suppurative complications. For most patients, a cephalosporin (cefazolin 2 to 4 gm daily) suffices. However, for patients with severe disease or diabetes mellitus, a regimen consisting of penicillin, clindamycin, and an aminoglycoside is indicated.[41, 72] Antibiotics are given preoperatively and for 48 hours postoperatively if an operation is performed during the acute attack.

After initial resuscitation a decision has to be made whether to perform early surgery or to treat the patient nonoperatively.

Timing of Surgery

There are two schools of thought concerning treatment of acute cholecystitis: (1) expectant management of the acute attack followed by elective cholecystectomy 6 to 8 weeks later, and (2) early surgery during the acute attack (i.e., within the first 24 to 48 hours of admission).

The expectant management regimen consists of nasogastric suction and antibiotics, with surgery reserved for those whose disease progresses. Examples of the manifestations that might justify a shift from nonoperative to operative therapy are increasing pain, tenderness, fever, leukocytosis, or development of a subcostal mass where one was not present when the patient was admitted. The early surgery approach involves cholecystectomy for all uncomplicated cases unless there are specific contraindications to operation, such as serious concomitant disease.

Table 15–1 CONTROLLED TRIALS COMPARING EARLY AND DELAYED (INTERVAL) CHOLECYSTECTOMY FOR ACUTE CHOLECYSTITIS

Author	Timing of Cholecystectomy (No. of Patients) Early	Delayed
van der Linden and Sunzel[73]	70	58
McArthur et al. (1975)[74]	15	15
Lahtinen et al. (1978)[75]	49	44
Jarvinen and Hastbacka (1980)[76]	80	75
Total	214	192

The rationale for conservative management is that most cases of cholecystitis will resolve on expectant management; early surgery may spread localized infection into the general peritoneal cavity; operation may be more difficult and complications more frequent because the anatomy is obscured; and exploration of the common duct, if needed, may be more hazardous.

However, four controlled trials carried out within the last 15 years[73–76] (Table 15–1) have all concluded that early surgery is preferable: The incidence of operative complications was the same, the total duration of illness was reduced by about 30 days and the length of hospitalization by about 1 week, and the death rate was slightly lower (Table 15–2). The last point suggests that, in some patients, early surgery aborted the illness and avoided serious complications. In addition, with early surgery the overall cost of treating the disease is lowered substantially.[77–80]

In patients who are fit for abdominal surgery and in whom the diagnosis is clear, we advocate early operation. About two thirds of patients with acute cholecystitis satisfy the criteria for early definitive operation. Because elderly patients and those with diabetes do not respond to medical therapy as other patients do and tend to develop serious complications more often,[81–84] we advocate early surgery even more strenuously for them. Of

Table 15–2 CONSOLIDATED RESULTS OF THE FOUR CONTROLLED TRIALS LISTED IN TABLE 15–1

Timing of Cholecystectomy	Patients	Deaths	Duct Injuries	Total Mean Hospital Stay (Days)	Failure of Regimen (%)*
Early	214	0	0	10.9	9
Delayed	192	5	0	20.1	19

*Means that cholecystectomy was not performed as planned.

course, early operation should be performed in patients who have evidence of complications.

Therefore, if a patient is thought to have acute cholecystitis, the diagnosis should be confirmed by ultrasound or Tc-99-HIDA scanning and preparation made for early operation. The operation is not handled as if it were an emergency. It is performed on the next operative schedule after the patient has been adequately prepared. On the other hand, if the patient's general condition is poor, surgery is postponed. Elective cholecystectomy is then performed 6 to 8 weeks after the acute attack if the patient's condition can be improved.

Nonoperative Management

If the patient is not fit for operation, or if the decision is made to treat the patient conservatively, nasogastric suction and intravenous fluids are continued until the abdominal symptoms subside. Antibiotics should be given for 5 to 7 days. The key to this approach is to monitor the response to treatment carefully, so that if complications arise, they are detected as early as possible.

Frequent examination of the patient is essential. The abdominal findings should be carefully recorded by the initial examiner. If a mass is present over the gallbladder region, it may be useful to outline its limits with a skin pencil. The white blood cell count, pulse, and temperature are charted, and narcotic requirements are reviewed periodically. Increasing pain, fever, and white blood cell count or the appearance of signs of sepsis would be reasons for changing plans and intervening early. An enlarging, tender mass indicates impending or actual perforation. Changes on ultrasound scan may reveal progression of the disease.

Approximately two thirds of the patients respond favorably to nonoperative treatment. They should remain in the hospital until they are well enough to eat and drink. The disease progresses in about one third of patients. These individuals require narcotics with increasing frequency because of the severe inflammatory process in the right upper quadrant and the increasing size of the mass in the gallbladder region. Such patients require emergency surgical intervention.

Thus, patients with acute cholecystitis treated conservatively may be clinically classified into one of three groups. One group, who do well almost from the start and steadily improve, constitute approximately 60 per cent of all patients. A second group of about 30 per cent show little improvement or may worsen. The third group show advanced disease (e.g., suppurative cholecystitis) when first admitted and require emergency operation.

Operative Management

Cholecystectomy

This is the operation of choice, and it is possible in 90 per cent of patients with acute cholecystitis. Cholecystectomy should be carried out following the general principles described in Chapter 21. Certain aspects of the operation that apply to patients with acute cholecystitis will be discussed here.

The first step of the operation is aspiration of the contents of the gallbladder using a large trocar. This facilitates cholecystectomy and provides a sample of bile for culture and sensitivity studies. The omentum, which frequently surrounds the gallbladder (see Figs. 15–1 and 15–3), can usually be separated from its wall by blunt finger dissection. We prefer to start the cholecystectomy from the fundus and proceed downward, because with an inflamed, distended gallbladder, early exposure of the region of the cystic duct may be difficult and hazardous.

In most cases, cholecystectomy can be performed quite easily following an edematous cleavage plane between the serosa and the muscularis. Finger dissection may be useful in some areas to avoid injury to adjacent structures. Even an impacted stone can be dislodged, and the ampulla of the gallbladder can be dissected free from the region of the common duct by finger dissection. The cystic duct may be friable, and thus it is often unwise to dissect it down as far as is usually done in cases of chronic cholecystitis.

Operative cholangiography should be performed unless the exposure is hazardous, gross contamination from an abscess has occurred, or the patient is a poor surgical risk. It was formerly believed that a solitary calculus blocking the cystic duct or the lower end of the gallbladder precluded the presence of a common duct stone, but this is an unreliable assumption. The overall incidence of common duct stones in association with acute cholecystitis is about 15 to 20 per cent.[45–47]

At the completion of the operation one or two closed suction drains should be left adjacent to the foramen of Winslow. The drains, and the T-tube if the common duct was explored, are brought out through stab wounds below the right costal margin. The omentum is tucked into the area of dissection to seal off the general abdominal cavity, and the wound is closed in a routine manner.

Cholecystostomy

Cholecystostomy is not required very often, but it may be lifesaving.[85–88] It may be the best procedure for elderly patients who are poor surgical risks and who present a well-defined mass in the right upper quadrant.[85] It may be a planned procedure, performed with local infiltration anesthesia. Less frequently, it may be decided upon when cholecystectomy was planned but seemed hazardous owing to technical difficulties in obtaining a satisfactory exposure, particularly in the region of the neck of the gallbladder. The technique of cholecystostomy is discussed in Chapter 21. In some very high-risk patients, percutaneous transhepatic cholecystostomy[86–88] may be used (see Chapter 10).

Postoperatively, the output from the cholecystostomy tube should be inspected regularly and the amount measured. A cholangiogram should be obtained 5 to 8 days postoperatively to check for residual calculi. The decision to remove the gallbladder some weeks later will depend upon the evaluation of the surgical risk, the age of the patient, and the technical difficulties anticipated. If the gallbladder is left in place, gallstones and symptoms will recur in about 50 per cent of patients. However, it may be years before this occurs. Thus, while it may be desirable in young patients to plan cholecystectomy within a month or 6 weeks, operation is unnecessary in poor-risk or elderly patients.

Partial Cholecystectomy

Rarely, it may be advisable to split the inferior surface of the acutely inflamed gallbladder, remove the offending calculus, and leave intact a portion of the gallbladder adjacent to the liver. This choice might be appropriate if cholecystectomy appears hazardous because of the extent of inflammation or because an abscess is encountered. This procedure is sometimes useful if the gallbladder is deeply buried within the liver substance and if the structures in the region of the cystic duct cannot be easily identified or separated from the common duct.

An incision is made in the midportion of the gallbladder, and all the stones, including the impacted calculus, are removed. No effort is made to dissect the region of the ampulla of the gallbladder from the adjacent common duct. The redundant gallbladder wall outside the liver bed is carefully excised. The mucosa of the gallbladder should be curetted with electrocautery. If possible, a catheter should be inserted into the cystic duct. One or two drains are placed in the area of the remaining gallbladder and, along with the cystic duct catheter, are brought out through a separate stab wound.

POSTOPERATIVE CARE

The care of the patient after operation for acute cholecystitis depends, of course, upon the patient as a surgical risk in terms of associated illnesses, age, and obesity, the degree of inflammation of the gallbladder, and the technical difficulties encountered. Antibiotic therapy should be adjusted as soon as the results of the culture and sensitivity determinations are returned. Nasogastric suction is advisable to treat paralytic ileus and gastric retention. In patients who fail to show satisfactory progress, a CT scan to evaluate for an intra-abdominal or liver abscess should be done.

PROGNOSIS

The overall death rate from acute cholecystitis is 5 per cent. Nearly all the deaths are in patients over 60 years of age[80–85] and those with diabetes mellitus. Secondary cardiovascular and pulmonary complications contribute to the morbidity in these patients. Sepsis, peritonitis, intrahepatic abscess formation, cholangitis, and pancreatitis are serious complications. Patients who develop empyema or perforation are less likely to recover.

ACUTE ACALCULOUS CHOLECYSTITIS

Acute cholecystitis in the absence of gallstones accounts for 5 to 10 per cent of cases in adults. Although the pathogenesis is not clear, bile stasis and increased bile lithogenicity appear to play an important role.[89–91] Patients recovering from trauma,[12, 14–16, 19, 22] severe systemic illnesses, or recent major surgery[17–21, 92–94] are more susceptible to acalculous cholecystitis. Gallstones are not present in about 50 per cent of children with acute cholecystitis.[95]

Although the signs and symptoms are usually similar to those of acute cholecystitis associated with calculous disease, the diagnosis may be difficult, as associated illnesses often cloud the picture, particularly since gallstones cannot be demonstrated. Most of the errors in the diagnostic tests used for acute cholecystitis are seen in patients with the acalculous form of the disease.[96–98]

Acute cholecystitis occurring in the postoperative period is a particularly dangerous form of the illness.[17, 19, 69, 89] The diagnosis is often obscured by the previous operative procedure. In most instances, the first clue is the development of unexplained fever. Only one patient in four complains of epigastric or right upper quadrant pain. Some authors have suggested that the onset tends to coincide with resumption of oral intake, but others have not found such a relationship. In general, the diagnosis is obscure until right upper quadrant tenderness or a palpable mass becomes evident.

Perforation, gangrene, empyema, and cholangitis are much more frequent than in the usual case of acute cholecystitis. These severe complications are present in more than 50 per cent of cases of postoperative acute cholecystitis.

Cholecystectomy is the treatment of choice, and because of the rapid progression of the disease, must be done as early as the diagnosis is made. The mortality varies between 30 and 50 per cent.[19]

EMPHYSEMATOUS CHOLECYSTITIS

Emphysematous cholecystitis is a rare condition in which bubbles of gas from anaerobic infection appear in the lumen of the gallbladder, its wall, the pericholecystitic space, and, on occasion, the bile ducts. *Clostridium* species are the most commonly implicated organisms, but other gas-forming anaerobes such as *E. coli* or anaerobic streptococci may be found. Three times as many men as women are affected, and 20 per cent of all patients have diabetes mellitus. In contrast to the usual form of acute cholecystitis, the disease probably is a bacterial infection from the start. In many cases, the gallbladder contains no stones. The characteristics suggest the possibility that cystic artery occlusion and ischemia may initiate emphysematous cholecystitis.

The disease begins with sudden and rapidly progressive right upper quadrant pain. Fever and leukocytosis reach high levels quickly, and the patient is considerably more toxic than is usually the case in acute cholecystitis. On examination, a mass can usually be found in the right upper quadrant.

Plain films of the abdomen show tissue emphysema outlining the gallbladder and, in some cases, an air-fluid level in the lumen. The clinical and x-ray pictures are characteristic enough so that the diagnosis is usually obvious. If the changes on plain films are equivocal, a CT scan may bring them out.

The patient should be treated with high doses of antibiotics effective against clostridia and the other species mentioned. Emergency surgical treatment should follow the initial resuscitative measure. Cholecystectomy can be safely performed in most cases, but those who are most critically ill might fare better with cholecystostomy. The types of complications are the same as in other forms of acute cholecystitis, but the illness is more severe and death rates higher.

TORSION OF THE GALLBLADDER

Torsion of the gallbladder is a very rare condition,[99] with fewer than 200 cases recorded in the world literature since the first case was reported by Wendel in 1898. Two conditions have been associated with torsion. The first and most common arises when the gallbladder is entirely free except for the cystic duct and artery. The second occurs when the gallbladder has a mesentery long enough to allow the organ to become twisted. Although the first condition appears always to be congenital, the second may be acquired. Partial torsion may produce a puzzling recurrent clinical picture, whereas complete torsion produces an acute illness with early gangrene. The preoperative diagnosis usually is acute cholecystitis. The condition is most common past the age of 60 years and is treated by cholecystectomy.

GALLBLADDER INFARCTION

Infarction of the gallbladder is a rare cause of acute cholecystitis. It has been reported in association with hepatic artery ligation, hypertension, bacterial endocarditis, cystic vein thrombosis, hepatic artery emboli, and periarteritis nodosa.

Although periarteritis nodosa may produce complete gallbladder infarction, more often it results in patchy necrosis of the mucosa with ulceration. Complaints may be of recurrent right upper abdominal pain or of an acute unremitting illness. In some instances, periarteritis is first diagnosed by the microscopic findings in the excised gallbladder.

With increased use of hepatic artery ligation in the treatment of liver trauma with bleeding and hepatic arterial cannulation for the administration of cancer chemotherapeutic agents, there is an increased incidence of hepatic artery thrombosis.[100–102] Gallbladder infarction is a possibility in both instances, and cholecystectomy should probably be done in those cases in which the hepatic artery is ligated or cannulated at laparotomy. Other causes of gallbladder infarction are principally anecdotal. The patients either have developed acute abdominal pain and evidence of right upper quadrant peritonitis or have been found to have unsuspected gallbladder infarction at autopsy.

REFERENCES

1. Wenckert A, Robertson B: The natural course of gallstone disease. Eleven-year review of 781 nonoperated cases. Gastroenterology 1966;*56*:376.
2. Glenn F: Trends in surgical treatment of calculous disease of the biliary tract. Surg Gynecol Obstet 1975;*140*:877.
3. Mitchell A, Morris PJ: Hospital admissions for acute cholecystitis: changes in the age and sex distribution in Oxford in the post-war period. Br J Surg 1982;*69*:26.
4. Roslyn J, Busuttil RW: Perforation of the gallbladder: a frequently mismanaged condition. Am J Surg 1979;*137*:307.
5. Fry DE, Cox RA, Harbrecht PJ: Empyema of the gallbladder: a complication in the natural history of acute cholecystitis. Am J Surg 1981;*141*:366.
6. Byrne JJ, Berger RL: The pathogenesis of acute cholecystitis. Arch Surg 1960;*81*:812.
7. Edlund YA, Olsson OJ: Acute cholecystitis. II. Timing of cholecystectomy. Acta Chir Scand 1958;*115*:284.
8. Thomas CG Jr, Womack NA: Acute cholecystitis, its pathogenesis and repair. Arch Surg 1952; *64*:590.
9. Kent SJS, Segal MB: The effect of biliary obstruction on the concentrating activity of the rabbit gallbladder. J Physiol 1975;*251*:33.
10. Svanvik J, Pellegrini CA, Allen B, Bernhoft RA, Way LW: Transport of fluid and biliary lipids in the canine gallbladder in experimental cholecystitis. J Surg Res. In press.
11. Bernhoft RA, Pellegrini CA, Broderick WC, Way LW: Biliary sludge and stone formation in the acutely ligated dog gallbladder. Gastroenterology 1983;*85*:1166.
12. Morris CR, Hoft RP, Ivy AC: An experimental study of the role of stasis in the etiology of cholecystitis. Surgery 1952;*32*:673.
13. Womack NA, Bricker EM: Pathogenesis of cholecystitis. Arch Surg 1942;*44*:658.
14. McDermott MW, Scudamore CH, Boileau LO, Snelling CFT, Kramer TA: Acalculous cholecystitis: Its role as a complication of major burn injury. Can J Surg 1985;*28*:529.
15. Herlin P, Ericsson M, Holmin T, Jonsson P-E: Acute acalculous cholecystitis following trauma. Br J Surg 1982;*69*:475.
16. Flancbaum L, Majerus TC, Cox EF: Acute posttraumatic acalculous cholecystitis. Am J Surg 1985;*150*:252.
17. Devine RM, Farnell MB, Mucha P: Acute cholecystitis as a complication in surgical patients: Arch Surg 1984;*119*:1389.
18. Gately JF, Thomas EJ: Acute cholecystitis occurring as a complication of other diseases. Arch Surg 1983;*118*:1137.
19. Ullman M, Hasselgren P-O, Tveit E: Posttraumatic and postoperative acute acalculous cholecystitis. Acta Chir Scand 1984;*150*:507.
20. Long TN, Heimbach DM, Carrico CJ: Acalculous cholecystitis in critically ill patients. Am J Surg 1974;*136*:31.
21. Glenn F, Becker CG: Acute acalculous cholecystitis: an increasing entity. Ann Surg 1982;*195*:131.
22. Alawneh I: Acute non-calculous cholecystitis in burns. Br J Surg 1978;*65*:243.
23. Howard RJ: Acute acalculous cholecystitis. Am J Surg 1981;*141*:194.
24. Orlando R III, Gleason E, Drezner AD: Acute acalculous cholecystitis in the critically ill patient. Am J Surg 1983;*145*:472.
25. Massie JD, Moinuddin M, Phillips JC: Acute calculous cholecystitis with patent cystic duct. AJR 1983;*141*:39.
26. Glenn F: Acute acalculous cholecystitis. Ann Surg 1979; *189*:458.
27. Petersen SR, Sheldon GF: Acute acalculous cholecystitis: A complication of hyperalimentation. Am J Surg 1979;*138*:814.
28. Heuman R, Norrby S, Sjodahl R, Tiselius HG, Tagesson C: Altered gallbladder bile composition in gallstone disease. Relation to gallbladder wall permeability. Scand J Gastroenterol 1980;*15*:581.
29. Ammon HV: Effect of taurine conjugated bile salts with and without lecithin in water and electrolyte transport in the canine gallbladder *in vivo*. Gastroenterology 1979;*76*:778.
30. Ho KJ, Ho LC, Hsu SC: Bile acid pool size in relation to functional status of gallbladder and biliary lipid composition in Chinese. Am J Clin Nutr 1980;*33*:1026.
31. Roslyn JJ, DenBesten L, Thompson JE Jr, Silverman BF: Roles of lithogenic bile and cystic duct occlusion in the pathogenesis of acute cholecystitis. Am J Surg 1980;*140*:126.

32. Sjodahl R, Wetterfors J: Lysolecithin and lecithin in the gallbladder wall and bile; their possible roles in the pathogenesis of acute cholecystitis. Scand J Gastroenterol 1974;*9*:525.
33. Sjodahl R Tagesson C, Wetterfors J: On the pathogenesis of acute cholecystitis. Surg Gynecol Obstet 1978;*146*:199.
34. Ho KJ, Ho LHC, Kruger R: Characterization and determination of the activity of biliary B(Beta)-glucuronidase in rats. J Lab Clin Med 1979;*93*:916.
35. Wood JR, Stamford JF: Prostaglandin in chronic cholecystitis. Prostaglandin 1977;*13*:97.
36. Svanvik J, Allen B, Way L: An experimental method to study the inflammatory secretion in the gallbladder. Gastroenterology 1979;*76*:1257.
37. Jansson R: Effects of gastrointestinal hormones on concentrating function and motility in the gallbladder. An experimental study in the cat. Acta Physiol Scand (Suppl) 1978;*456*:1.
38. Thornell E, Jansson R, Kral JG, Svanvik J: Inhibition of prostaglandin synthesis as a treatment for biliary pain. Lancet 1979;*1*:584.
39. Rosenberg L, Shapiro S, Slone D, Kaufman DW, Miettinen OS, Stolley PD: Thiazides and acute cholecystitis. N Engl J Med 1980;*303*:546.
40. Bourgault AM, England DM, Rosenblatt JE, Forgacs P, Bieger C: Clinical characteristics of anaerobic bactibilia. Arch Intern Med 1979;*139*:1346.
41. Claesson B, Holmlund D, Matzch T: Biliary microflora in acute cholecystitis and the clinical implications. Acta Chir Scand 1984;*150*:229.
42. Rosch J, Grollman JH Jr, Steckel RJ: Arteriography in the diagnosis of gallbladder disease. Radiology 1969;*92*:1485.
43. Csendes A, Sepulveda A: Intraluminal gallbladder pressure measurements in patients with chronic or acute cholecystitis. Am J Surg 1980;*139*:383.
44. Ruf W, Suehiro GT, Suehiro A, Pressler V, McNamara JJ: Intestinal blood flow at various intraluminal pressures in the piglet with closed abdomen. Ann Surg 1980;*191*:157.
45. Pitluk HC, Beal JM: Choledocholithiasis associated with acute cholecystitis. Arch Surg 1979;*114*:887.
46. Jarvinen H: Abnormal liver function tests in acute cholecystitis; the predicting of common duct stones. Ann Clin Res 1978;*10*:323.
47. Stryker SJ, Beal JM: Acute cholecystitis and common-duct calculi. Arch Surg 1983;*118*:1063.
48. Reiss R, Pikelnies S, Engleberg M: The value of early surgery and routine operative cholangiography in the management of acute cholecystitis. World J Surg 1979;*3*:107.
49. Montefusco P, Spier N, Geiss AC: Another facet of Mirizzi's syndrome. Arch Surg 1983;*118*:1221.
50. McSherry CK, Ferstenberg H, Virshup M: The Mirizzi syndrome: suggested classification and surgical therapy. Surg Gastroenterol 1982;*3*:219.
51. Witte CL: Choledochal obstruction by cystic duct stone. Am Surg 1984;*50*:241.
52. Rosenbaum HD: An evaluation of oral cholecystography. JAMA 1974;*229*:76.
53. Zboralske FF, Amberg JR: Cholecystocholestasis: A cause of cholecystographic error. Am J Dig Dis 1962;*7*:339.
54. Dillon E, Parkin GJS: The role of upper abdominal ultrasonography in suspected acute cholecystitis. Clin Radiol 1980;*31*:175.
55. Worthen NJ, Uszler JM, Funamura JL: Cholecystitis: prospective evaluation of sonography and ^{99m}Tc-HIDA cholescintigraphy. AJR 1981;*137*:973.
56. Zeman RK, Burrell MI, Cahow CE, Caride V: Diagnostic utility of cholescintigraphy and ultrasonography in acute cholecystitis. Am J Surg 1981;*141*:446.
57. Krishnamurthy GT: Acute cholecystitis: the diagnostic role for current imaging tests. West J Med 1982;*137*:87.
58. Berger M, Smith E, Holm HH, Mascatello V: Utility of ultrasound in the differential diagnosis of acute cholecystitis. Arch Surg 1977;*112*:273.
59. Bloom RA, Fisher A, Pode D, Asaf Y: Shifting intramural gas — A new ultrasound sign of emphysematous cholecystitis. J Clin Ultrasound 1984;*12*:40.
60. Jeffrey R, Laing B, Wong W, Callen A: Gangrenous cholecystitis: diagnosis by ultrasound. Radiology 1983;*148*:219.
61. Dykes EH, Stewart I, Gray SH, Simpson C, Davidson S, McArdle CS: Infusion cholecystography in the early diagnosis of acute gallbladder disease. Br J Surg 1984;*71*:854.
62. Down RHL: More on radionuclide scanning in the diagnosis of acute cholecystitis. Gastroenterology 1981;*80*:417.
63. Duch G, Nielsen A, Axelsson CK: The value of ^{99m}Tc-cholescintigraphy as compared with infusion cholecystography for diagnosing acute cholecystitis. Scan J Gastroenterol 1981;*16*:993.
64. Choy D, Shi EC, McLean RG, Hoschi R, Murray IPC, Ham JM: Cholescintigraphy in acute cholecystitis: use of intravenous morphine. Radiology 1984; *151*:203.
65. Fink-Bennett D, Freitas JE, Ripley SD, Bree RL: The sensitivity of hepatobiliary imaging and real-time ultrasonography in the detection of acute cholecystitis. Arch Surg 1985; *120*:904.
66. Mauro MA, McCartney WH, Melmed JR: Hepatobiliary scanning with ^{99m}TC-PIPIDA in acute cholecystitis. Radiology 1982;*142*:193.
67. Cabellon S, Brown JM, Cavanaugh DG: Accuracy of the hepatobiliary scan in acute cholecystitis. Am J Surg 1984;*148*:607.
68. Gill T, Dillon E, Leahy L, Reeder A, Peel ALG: Ultrasonography, HIDA scintigraphy or both in the diagnosis of acute cholecystitis? Br J Surg 1985;*72*:267.
69. Pare P, Shaffer EA, Rosenthall L: Nonvisualization of the gallbladder by ^{99m}Tc-HIDA cholescintigraphy as evidence of cholecystitis. Can Med Assoc J 1978;*118*:384.
70. Ohrt HJ, Posalaky IP, Shafer RB: Normal gallbladder scintigraphy in acute cholecystitis. Clin Nucl Med 1983;*8*:97.
71. Felice PR, Trowbridge PE, Ferrara JJ: Evolving changes in the pathogenesis and treatment of the perforated gallbladder: a combined hospital study. Am J Surg 1985;*149*:466.
72. Jarvinen H, Renkonen OV, Palmu A: Antibiotics in acute cholecystitis: Ann Clin Res 1978;*10*:247.
73. van der Linden W, Sunzel H: Early versus delayed operation for acute cholecystitis: a controlled clinical trial. Am J Surg 1970;*120*:7.
74. McArthur P, Cuschieri A, Sells RA, Shields R: Controlled clinical trial comparing early with interval cholecystectomy for acute cholecystitis. Br J Surg 1975;*62*:850.
75. Lahtinen I, Alhava EM, Auke S: Acute cholecystitis treated by early and delayed surgery. A controlled clinical trial. Scand J Gastroenterol 1978;*13*:673.
76. Jarvinen HJ, Hastbacka J: Early cholecystectomy

for acute cholecystitis: a prospective randomized study. Ann Surg 1980;*191*:501.

77. van der Linden W, Edlund G: Early versus delayed cholecystectomy: the effect of a change in management. Br J Surg 1982;*68*:753.
78. Salleh HBM, Balasegaram M: Treatment of acute cholecystitis by routine urgent operation. Br J Surg 1974;*61*:705.
79. Alinder G, Herlin P, Lindgren B, Holmin T: The cost-effectiveness of early or delayed surgery in acute cholecystitis. World J Surg 1985;*9*:329.
80. Fowkes FGR, Gunn AA: The management of acute cholecystitis and its hospital cost. Br J Surg 1980;*67*:613.
81. Glenn F: Surgical management of acute cholecystitis in patients 65 years of age and older. Ann Surg 1981;*183*:56.
82. Morrow DJ, Thompson J, Wilson SE: Acute cholecystitis in the elderly. A surgical emergency. Arch Surg 1978;*113*:1149.
83. Houghton PWJ, Jenkinson LR, Donaldson LA: Cholecystectomy in the elderly: a prospective study. Br J Surg 1985;*72*:220.
84. van Rensburg LCJ: The management of acute cholecystitis in the elderly. Br J Surg 1984;*71*:692.
85. Glenn F: Cholecystostomy in the high risk patient with biliary tract disease. Ann Surg 1977;*185*:185.
86. Elyaderani MK, McDowell DE, Gabriele OF: A preliminary report of percutaneous cholecystostomy under ultrasonography and fluoroscopy guidance. J Clin Gastroenterol 1983;*5*:277.
87. Pearse DM, Hawkins IF, Shaver R, Vogel S: Percutaneous cholecystostomy in acute cholecystitis and common duct obstruction. Radiology 1984;*152*:365.
88. Eggermont AM, Lameris JS, Jeekel J: Ultrasound-guided percutaneous transhepatic cholecystostomy for acute acalculous cholecystitis. Arch Surg 1985;*120*:1354.
89. Fox MS, Wilk PJ, Weissmann HS, Freeman LM, Gliedman ML: Acute acalculous cholecystitis. Surg Gynecol Obstet 1984;*159*:13.
90. Flati G, Flati D, Jonsson PE, Porowska B Tuscano D, Amicucci G, Negro P, Carboni M: Role of cholesterol and calcium bilirubinate crystals in acute postoperative acalculous cholecystitis. Ital J Surg Sci 1984;*14*:333.
91. Deitch EA, Engel JM: Acute acalculous cholecystitis. Am J Surg 1981;*142*:290.
92. Ottinger LW: Acute cholecystitis as a postoperative complication. Ann Surg 1976;*184*:162.
93. Deshmukh N, Nagpal NC: Postoperative cholecystitis. Am J Gastroenterol 1985;*80*:284.
94. Orlando R, Gleason E, Drezner AD: Acute acalculous cholecystitis in the critically ill patient. Am J Surg 1983;*145*:472.
95. Pieretti R, Auldist AW, Stephens CA: Acute cholecystitis in children. Surg Gynecol Obstet 1975;*140*:16.
96. Shuman WP, Rogers JV, Rudd TG, Mack LA, Plumley T, Larson EB: Low sensitivity of sonography and cholescintigraphy in acalculous cholecystitis. AJR 1984;*142*:531.
97. Weissman HS, Berkowitz D, Fox MS, Gliedman ML, Rosenblatt R, Surgarman LA, Freeman LM: The role of technetium-99m iminodiacetic acid (IDA) cholescintigraphy in acute acalculous cholecystitis. Radiology 1983;*146*:177.
98. Ramanna L, Brachman MB, Tanasescu DE, Berman DS, Waxman AD: Cholescintigraphy in acute acalculous cholecystitis. Am J Gastroenterol 1984;*79*:650.
99. Wetstein L, Attkiss M, Aufses AH Jr: Acute torsion of the gallbladder: Review of the literature and report of a case. Am Surg 1976;*42*:138.
100. Carrasco H, Freeny PC, Chuang VP, Wallace S: Chemical cholecystitis associated with hepatic artery infusion chemotherapy. AJR 1983;*141*:703.
101. Marymont JV, Dakhil SR, Travers H, Housholder DF: Chemical cholecystitis associated with hepatic arterial chemotherapy delivered by a permanently implanted pump. Hum Pathol 1985;*16*:986.
102. Kuroda C, Iwasaki M, Tanaka T, Tokunaga K, Hori S, Yoshioka H, Nakamura H, Sakurai M, Okamura J: Gallbladder infarction following hepatic transcatheter arterial embolization. Radiology 1983;*149*:85.

JOHN H.C. RANSON, B.M., B.Ch., FACS

16

Perforation of the Gallbladder

INTRODUCTION

Spontaneous perforation of the gallbladder with extravasation of its contents is a relatively uncommon complication of biliary disease. Since it is encountered infrequently in the individual experience of many physicians, it has sometimes been considered to be a curiosity requiring little serious attention.[1, 2] Reviews of large groups of patients with biliary disease have shown, however, that perforation is one of the most commonly lethal inflammatory complications affecting the gallbladder.[3, 4] Failure to consider the possibility of perforation is a major factor contributing to the high mortality of this condition.

History

In the seventeenth century, Riolanus[5] described rupture of the gallbladder, which he attributed to "violent motion in vomiting." At that time, perforation was recognized clinically when bile and gallstones drained from an abdominal abscess or fistula.[6] The first detailed description of free rupture of the gallbladder into the peritoneal cavity was given in 1844 by James Duncan[7] of Edinburgh, who reported bile peritonitis secondary to gangrenous cholecystitis in a patient who died following repair of a femoral hernia. During the closing years of the nineteenth century, gallbladder perforation was reported with increasing frequency, and in 1912, McWilliams[8] of New York collected and analyzed descriptions of 108 patients who had been treated surgically for spontaneous bile peritonitis. In 94 per cent of cases, peritonitis was due to perforation of the gallbladder or cystic duct, and in 74 per cent, the perforation was related to biliary calculi. Most of the conclusions of McWilliams' study have been confirmed by observations over the past 70 years, and many of the principles of surgical management that he described remain valid today.

Classification

In 1934, Niemeier[9] grouped perforations of the gallbladder into the following three categories: Type I, acute perforations that result in general peritonitis (Fig. 16–1); Type II, subacute perforations, in which adhesions from prior inflammation protect the general peritoneal cavity and lead to a localized abscess (Fig. 16–2); and Type III, chronic perforations, in which long-standing inflammation leads to fistula formation between the gallbladder and another viscus (Fig. 16–3). Some patients, such as those with rupture of a pericholecystic abscess into a viscus or into the general peritoneal cavity, do not fit read-

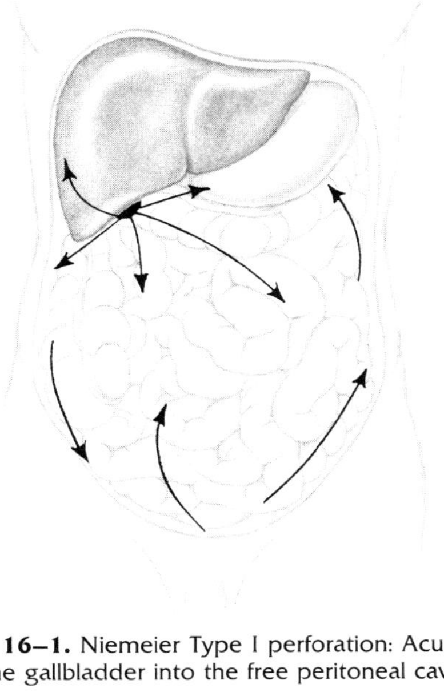

Figure 16–1. Niemeier Type I perforation: Acute rupture of the gallbladder into the free peritoneal cavity.

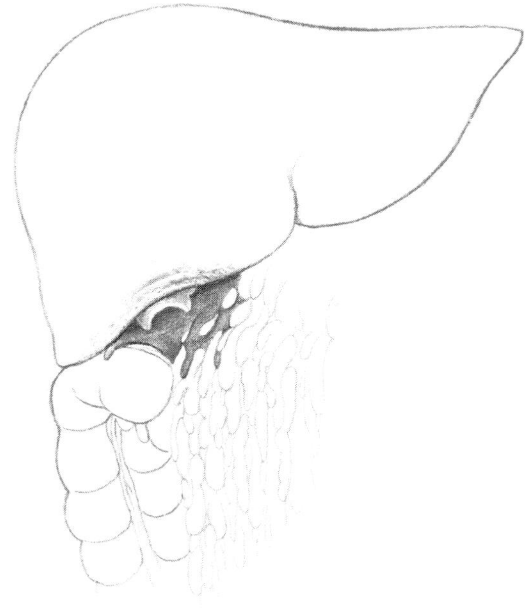

Figure 16–2. Niemeier Type II perforation: Subacute rupture of the gallbladder, localized by adjacent liver, colon, and omentum to form a pericholecystic abscess.

ily into one of these groups. Nonetheless, the Niemeier classification is widely accepted and has proved valuable in analyses of the incidence, natural history, clinical presentation, and treatment of gallbladder perforations. Biliary fistulae (Type III perforations) and their consequences are discussed in Chapters 17 and 38.

INCIDENCE

Most perforations of the gallbladder either occur spontaneously as a complication of cholecystitis or are related to abdominal trauma.

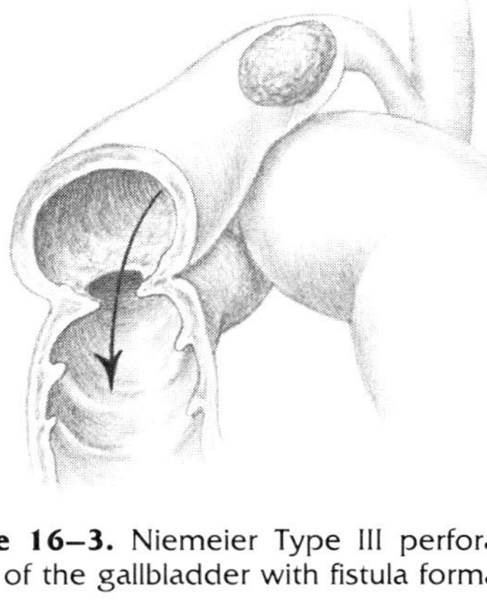

Figure 16–3. Niemeier Type III perforation: Chronic rupture of the gallbladder with fistula formation.

Spontaneous Perforation

Perforation of the gallbladder is found in 1 to 3 per cent of patients treated surgically for inflammatory gallbladder disease.[10, 11] The reported incidence of perforation in patients with acute cholecystitis ranges from 5 per cent to 25 per cent.[3, 10, 12–17, 41] This variation reflects differences in criteria used to define acute cholecystitis as well as differences in patient population. The average frequency of perforation in patients with acute cholecystitis is 10 per cent (Fig. 16–4).[14]

Extravasation of gallbladder contents is limited, and a localized pericholecystic abscess forms in approximately 50 per cent of patients (Niemeier Type II). In many of these patients, the abscess is in the hepatic bed of the gallbladder. In the remainder, it is walled off from the peritoneal cavity by adhesions between the gallbladder, omentum, and adjacent viscera. In 30 per cent of perforations, the gallbladder contents drain into the free peritoneal cavity, resulting in generalized peritonitis (Niemeier Type I). Approximately 20 per cent of perforations occur slowly and lead to a fistula between the gallbladder and other organs, most commonly the duodenum, colon, and stomach (Niemeier Type III).[10, 11, 14, 15, 40]

The frequency of gallbladder perforation is related to the patient's age and sex.[3, 15, 16, 18, 40] Perforation may occur at any age, but 65 per cent of cases are in patients over age 60 years. The sex incidence of perforation is approximately equal, but because cholelithiasis is far more common in women than in men, perforation is *relatively* more common in men.

In addition, there is an apparent association between perforation and the presence of diabetes mellitus.[18] Perforation occurs in 20 per cent of patients in whom acute cholecystitis is recognized during a postoperative or post-traumatic period,[19] and it appears to be more common in acalculous acute cholecystitis than in calculous acute cholecystitis. In patients with acute cholecystitis caused by typhoid infection, the incidence of perforation may be as high as 50 per cent.[20]

Traumatic Perforation (See Chapter 41)

Traumatic perforation is uncommon, occurring in only 2 to 5 per cent of major abdominal injuries. Ninety per cent of such perforations are due to penetrating trauma,

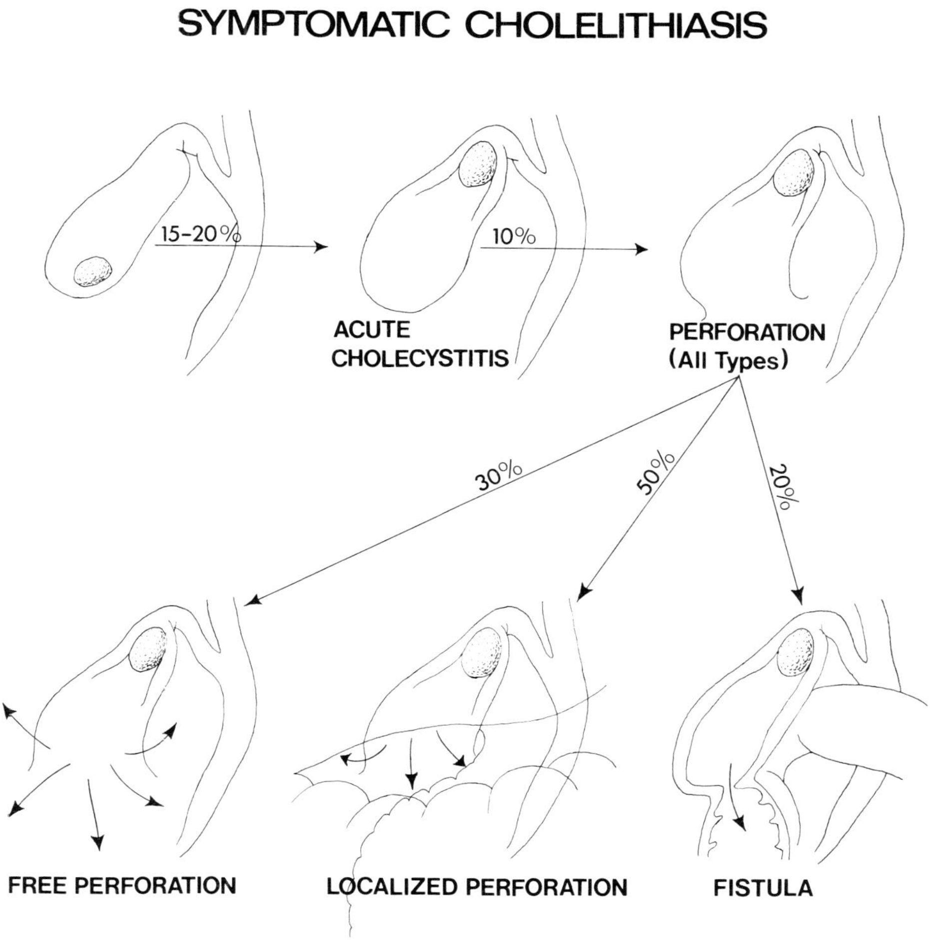

Figure 16–4. The incidence of acute cholecystitis and perforation of the gallbladder in patients with symptomatic cholelithiasis.

and 80 per cent are associated with other significant intra-abdominal injuries.[46, 47]

PATHOLOGY

Biliary Pathology

The conditions associated with perforation of the gallbladder are listed in Table 16–1.

Trauma

In most traumatic perforations, immediate disruption of the gallbladder and spillage of bile occur. Rarely, blunt abdominal injury may cause avulsion of the gallbladder from its hepatic bed with interruption of blood supply and delayed ischemic rupture.[21]

Cholecystitis

In most patients, perforation is a complication of cholecystitis, usually associated with cholelithiasis.

Gross Findings. In patients with a cholecystenteric fistula (Type III perforation), the acute inflammation has frequently resolved by the time of diagnosis. In patients with a free perforation or localized abscess (Types I and II), the gallbladder is usually inflamed and edematous with focal areas of gangrene. Calculous cystic duct obstruction is frequent. The perforation is usually located in the gallbladder fundus.[17, 22]

Microscopic Findings. Histologic examination of perforated gallbladders usually shows chronic inflammation with fibrosis and chronic inflammatory cell infiltration. Rokitansky-Aschoff sinuses are present in 60 per

TABLE 16–1 ETIOLOGIC FACTORS IN PERFORATION OF THE GALLBLADDER

Traumatic	Penetrating Blunt	
Inflammatory	*Acute cholecystitis*	Cholelithiasis Acalculous Post-traumatic Idiopathic Infectious (typhoid)
Neoplastic	Gallbladder carcinoma Colon or stomach carcinoma	
Miscellaneous	Intramural hemorrhage Penetrating peptic ulcer "Spontaneous"	

cent of patients. In peritonitis, acute inflammation is also present with edema and polymorphonuclear cell infiltrates. The gallbladder mucosa is completely destroyed in 20 per cent of cases. Intramural hemorrhage or abscesses may be seen, and vascular obstruction with infarction is common.[14, 15, 17, 22, 23]

Pathogenesis. Since perforation is often associated with cystic duct obstruction, it has been postulated that inflammation of the gallbladder wall and continued mucus secretion lead to increasing intraluminal pressure within the obstructed gallbladder. As intraluminal pressure increases, it is thought that lymphatic, venous, and, eventually, arterial insufficiency occurs, leading to infarction and rupture.[14, 15, 23] Measurements of intraluminal pressure in patients with biliary disease have shown, however, that there is little correlation between pressure levels and the occurrence of gangrene of the gallbladder wall. The most marked increases in intraluminal pressure have been recorded in patients with uninflamed hydropic gallbladders.[3]

Examination of the blood supply of human gallbladders following injection of the cystic artery has demonstrated that in chronic cholecystitis, there is gross distortion of the arterial pattern with focal areas of greatly reduced vascularity. By contrast, in hydropic gallbladders the arterial supply is essentially normal.[24] In experimental studies, obstruction of the cystic duct or the cystic artery alone leads to little or no inflammatory change in the gallbladder wall.[39] Gangrenous cholecystitis requires combined vascular and cystic duct obstruction.[25] It is probable, therefore, that in most patients, the pathogenesis of gallbladder perforation involves a combination of acute inflammation related to cystic duct obstruction and vascular insufficiency due to chronic cholecystitis.

No single mechanism explains all the clinical observations, and other factors of importance are infection and direct pressure by gallstones upon the gallbladder wall. Infection is present in most gallbladders at the time of perforation and is the primary cause of perforation in typhoid cholecystitis. Finally, the presence of concentrated bile salts or pancreatic enzymes within the gallbladder lumen may influence the severity of cholecystitis and may contribute to perforation in some patients.[8, 14, 22, 25, 26] In perforations complicating acute acalculous cholecystitis, infarction of the gallbladder wall has been attributed to primary vascular, suppurative, or chemical causes.[19, 20]

In rare instances, perforation of the gallbladder with bile peritonitis is encountered in the absence of acute cholecystitis or biliary obstruction.[54] The perforations in these cases have been attributed to rupture of a microabscess within the gallbladder wall, possibly occurring in Rokitansky-Aschoff sinuses. In addition, localized ischemic infarcts of the gallbladder wall secondary to spontaneous intramural hemorrhage have been described.[23, 27–29]

Neoplasm

Carcinoma of the gallbladder is occasionally found in association with perforation.[10, 17, 30, 60] In some cases, the perforation may be related to tumor necrosis, but more commonly it is a consequence of cholelithiasis.[17] Chronic perforation and fistula formation are rarely caused by invasion of the gallbladder by tumors of the transverse colon or stomach.

Miscellaneous

A variety of inflammatory diseases affecting organs adjacent to the gallbladder may occasionally result in a fistulous communication with the gallbladder. The most common are penetrating peptic ulcer and granulomatous disease of the bowel.

Sequelae of Acute Perforation

The consequences of gallbladder perforation are related to the site of perforation, the rate at which rupture occurs, the presence of infection within the gallbladder, and the presence of cystic duct obstruction. Twenty to 50 per cent of the gallbladder wall is covered by liver, and perforation of this area usually leads to a relatively small contained abscess. Occasionally, perforation of the hepatic surface of the gallbladder may track deep into the liver substance and result in an intrahepatic abscess (Fig. 16–5). Perforation of the peritoneal surface of the gallbladder usually results in a localized abscess walled off by adjacent structures (Niemeier Type II), but it may result in general peritonitis (Niemeier Type I). In patients with persistent cystic duct obstruction, rupture of the gallbladder into the peritoneal cavity leads to a purulent peritonitis. If the cystic duct is patent, however, perforation results in bile peritonitis.

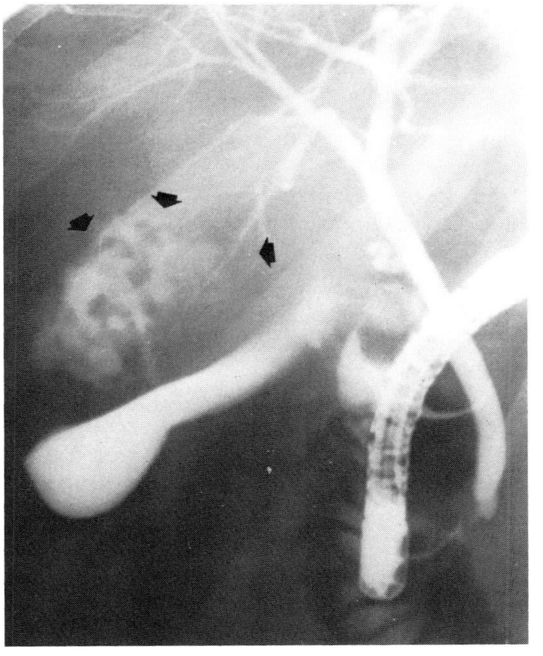

Figure 16–5. Endoscopic retrograde cholangiogram demonstrating a small perforation of the hepatic surface of the gallbladder. The perforation is associated with a large intrahepatic abscess (*arrow*).

Bile Peritonitis

Factors responsible for the highly lethal consequences of bile peritonitis include the toxic effects of bile, either locally within the peritoneal cavity or systemically, following absorption into the blood stream; the presence of concomitant infection; and the reflux of pancreatic enzymes into the peritoneal cavity, which causes rapid accumulation of intraperitoneal fluid and a fall in plasma volume and hemoconcentration with resulting hypovolemia. These changes are due to local effects of bile on the permeability of the peritoneum and underlying vasculature. Bile salts may have direct toxic effects, and the severity of the local changes is directly related to their concentration. Intravenous infusion of bile produces hemolysis but no rapid fluid shifts. Since intravascular hemolysis is not a prominent feature of experimental bile peritonitis, binding of bile salts by proteins in peritoneal exudate may protect against this complication.[31]

If the intravascular volume is maintained, sterile bile peritonitis is relatively well tolerated in experimental animals.[32, 33] A bland form of sterile bile peritonitis is occasionally observed in humans when a traumatic gallbladder perforation is not immediately diagnosed.[21]

The addition of bacterial infection in experimental bile peritonitis is associated with a sharply increased mortality[8, 23]; in perforation complicating acute cholecystitis, the gallbladder contents are almost invariably infected. The bacteria most frequently identified in clinical bile peritonitis are *Escherichia coli, Streptococcus,* and *Enterococcus.*[10, 17, 18] One factor contributing to the seriousness of infected bile peritonitis may be an inhibitory effect of bile on phagocytosis and the complement system.[8]

Finally, reflux of pancreatic secretions into the gallbladder has been documented in some patients, and the presence of active intraperitoneal trypsin increases the virulence of experimental bile peritonitis. The frequency with which active pancreatic enzymes are present in the peritoneal exudate in clinical bile peritonitis is unknown, but it is probably not a major factor in most patients.[34]

DIAGNOSIS OF ACUTE PERFORATION

Clinical Features

The diagnosis of perforation of the gallbladder in patients with acute cholecystitis is notoriously difficult to make and is frequently reached only at operation or autopsy. A correct preoperative diagnosis is achieved in only 10 per cent of patients.[3, 10, 14]

The most common clinical findings are abdominal pain, nausea and vomiting, and right upper quadrant abdominal tenderness. The same findings are present in uncomplicated acute cholecystitis but are usually more marked in the presence of perforation.

Free Perforation. In patients with free perforation, generalized abdominal tenderness and guarding may suggest widespread peritonitis, but this is present in only 30 per cent of cases. The temperature is normal or subnormal in about 50 per cent of patients, and a right upper quadrant abdominal mass is usually not palpable. Leukocytosis may be absent or mild, but jaundice is detectable in 20 to 50 per cent of patients.[11, 15, 18, 35, 36] Since the diagnosis is often obscure, paracentesis may demonstrate intraperitoneal bile and indicate the need for operation. Of course, a negative paracentesis does not exclude the possibility of a localized perforation.

Localized Perforation. A right upper quadrant abdominal mass is palpable in 60 per cent of patients with a localized perforation. The white blood cell count is above 10,000/cu mm in 75 per cent of patients and above 20,000/cu mm in 30 per cent. Fever is greater than 101° F.[10, 11, 15, 17]

Radiology

Free Perforation. In patients with free perforation, plain abdominal radiographs frequently show signs of peritoneal irritation, with loss of soft tissue markings and an intestinal gas pattern indicating paralytic ileus.[11, 35] In patients who have no associated cystic duct obstruction, the free perforation may be detected by ^{99m}Tc cholescintigraphy.[50–53, 55]

Localized Perforation. In patients with a localized perforation, plain radiographs of the abdomen may show radiopaque gallstones in the right upper quadrant and displacement of the colonic gas pattern by a soft tissue mass. Plain films will rarely distinguish between perforation and uncomplicated acute cholecystitis. Abdominal ultrasonography will usually identify gallstones, a distended gallbladder, and a thickened gallbladder wall.[43, 44] A fluid-filled pericholecystic mass may be seen if the abscess is large enough.[42, 45, 49, 56–59] In patients with hypoalbuminemia or ascites, these studies must be interpreted with caution, because gallbladder distention, thickening of the gallbladder wall, and pericholecystic fluid may be observed in the absence of intrinsic biliary disease.[37] Opacification of the biliary tree by intravenous, percutaneous transhepatic, or endoscopic retrograde cholangiography usually demonstrates only cystic duct obstruction; the perforation itself is rarely shown.

Since the clinical and radiologic findings are nonspecific, the possibility of perforation must be considered in every patient being evaluated for acute cholecystitis. If nonoperative management for acute cholecystitis is undertaken, a lack of prompt improvement, the development of general abdominal tenderness, a persistent or expanding abdominal mass, high fever, or marked leukocytosis strongly suggests gallbladder perforation.

PREVENTION OF GALLBLADDER PERFORATION

Seventy-five to 90 per cent of patients with perforation of the gallbladder give a history of previous biliary symptoms.[10, 12, 16, 40, 41] With the increasing safety of elective biliary surgery, it may be possible to decrease the frequency of perforation by performing cholecystectomy early in patients with symptomatic gallbladder disease.

Since most perforations are complications of acute cholecystitis, early cholecystectomy for acute cholecystitis has been proposed as a means to reduce the frequency of this complication.[3, 14, 16, 41] Unfortunately, perforation has already occurred in many patients at the time medical advice is sought, and the preventive value of early surgery during acute cholecystitis is uncertain. Nonetheless, difficulty in diagnosing perforation and delay in instituting appropriate treatment contribute significantly to the morbidity of this condition.[8, 12, 17] Early operative treatment of acute cholecystitis allows an accurate diagnosis and reduces the possibility of complications resulting from a delay in treatment.

TREATMENT OF ACUTE PERFORATION

Free perforation of the gallbladder requires emergency resuscitation and operative treatment. Vigorous correction of hypovolemia with close monitoring of intravascular volume is essential, and broad-spectrum antibiotics should be administered. Operative treatment is undertaken as soon as the patient's condition allows and forms part of the resuscitative management.

In patients with a localized pericholecystic abscess, a short period of intravenous fluid therapy, nasogastric suction, and antibiotic administration may result in substantial clinical improvement. The wait for improvement to occur should not, however, be prolonged, since that would further delay operative treatment. During elective biliary surgery, rare instances are encountered in which gallstones are found in the pericholecystic area, indicating healing of a localized perforation either spontaneously or following nonoperative treatment. More commonly, however, delay in surgical intervention is followed by clinical deterioration and an increased mortality.[8, 12, 22, 41]

Surgical Treatment

Operative treatment should aim to remove as much peritoneal contamination as possible and to correct the underlying biliary disease.

Cholecystostomy. Since many patients with perforation are elderly and critically ill, cholecystostomy has been widely employed in the past. Cholecystostomy is appropriate for some perforations that follow penetrating trauma, and it may be the only feasible treatment for perforation in patients with an unresectable gallbladder carcinoma. Cholecystostomy may also be appropriate when other conditions, such as portal hypertension or acute pancreatitis, make definitive surgery hazardous, or when the inflammation is so severe that the surgeon feels that cholecystectomy would be too risky. Unfortunately, however, cholecystostomy may leave a partially devitalized organ within the peritoneal cavity, and it frequently does not adequately drain the common bile duct in patients with choledocholithiasis. With current anesthetic management and supportive care, additional surgical intervention and anesthesia are, in general, less dangerous to the patient than the risk of continued infection.

Cholecystectomy. The preferred operation for perforation associated with acute cholecystitis is cholecystectomy. Choledocholithiasis is present in 15 to 20 per cent of patients, and cholangiography or common bile duct exploration should be performed as indicated. If the duodenum is involved in severe inflammation or infection, duodenotomy should not be performed at this time.[11] Occasionally, bile peritonitis is encountered in the absence of a grossly evident gallbladder perforation. In this situation, cholangiography is essential, since peritonitis may originate from an easily overlooked rupture of the intrahepatic biliary tree.

In patients with a free perforation, the peritoneal cavity should be irrigated copiously with saline, and particular attention should be paid to aspirating fluid collections in the subphrenic areas and pelvis. The subhepatic space should be drained through a separate incision in all patients.

Postoperative management includes parenteral antibiotic administration, as indicated by the cultures obtained during surgery, and maintenance of nasogastric decompression until gastrointestinal function returns.

RESULTS OF TREATMENT

The mortality of free and localized perforations of the gallbladder is summarized in Table 16–2. Among 100 patients with free perforation collected from the recent literature, the overall mortality was 31 per cent. The diagnosis was made at autopsy in 11 per cent of these patients. Of the 89 patients who were treated surgically, the mortality was 22 per cent. Among 39 patients with a localized

TABLE 16–2 MORTALITY ASSOCIATED WITH ACUTE PERFORATIONS OF THE GALLBLADDER

Treatment	Free Perforations (Type I)[3, 11, 15, 18, 35, 38]		Localized Perforations (Type II)[3, 11, 15, 38]	
	Number	*Mortality (%)*	*Number*	*Mortality (%)*
Surgical	89	22	34	6
Medical	11	100	5	100
Total	100	31	39	18

TABLE 16–3 RELATIONSHIP BETWEEN TYPE OF SURGICAL TREATMENT AND MORTALITY IN ACUTE PERFORATION OF THE GALLBLADDER*

Surgical Treatment	Number	Mortality (%)
Incision and drainage alone	6	67
Cholecystostomy	62	26
Cholecystectomy	123	15
Cholecystectomy + common bile duct exploration	39	15

*Niemeier Types I and II[11, 12, 15, 16, 18, 35, 38]

perforation, the mortality was 18 per cent. The diagnosis was first made at autopsy in 13 per cent, and among 34 patients treated operatively, the mortality rate was 6 per cent.

The influence of the type of surgical treatment on survival is summarized in Table 16–3. In six patients with localized pericholecystic abscesses, drainage of the subhepatic area without attempts to correct the underlying biliary disease was associated with a mortality of 67 per cent. In 62 patients treated by cholecystostomy and drainage, the mortality was 26 per cent. The best results followed definitive correction of the underlying biliary disease by cholecystectomy. Of 162 patients treated in this way, the mortality was 15 per cent. Twenty-four per cent of this group had a common bile duct exploration in addition to cholecystectomy, without increased mortality.

The increased mortality rate following cholecystostomy is heavily influenced by the patient population for whom this procedure was selected. Nevertheless, experience supports the contention that early definitive correction of the underlying biliary disease is superior to cholecystostomy in patients with perforation of the gallbladder.

CONCLUSIONS

Perforation of the gallbladder may complicate a variety of traumatic, inflammatory, and neoplastic conditions. It is seen most commonly in acute calculous cholecystitis. Perforation occurs in about 10 per cent of cases of acute cholecystitis. About 50 per cent of perforations are contained by adherent liver, colon, and omentum as a localized pericholecystic abscess. Thirty per cent of perforations produce free peritonitis, and 20 per cent produce a cholecystenteric fistula.

The clinical diagnosis of gallbladder perforation is difficult to make, and delay in treatment is a major factor responsible for the high mortality rate. The morbidity of perforation may be reduced by greater awareness of this condition and early surgical correction of the underlying biliary disease.

REFERENCES

1. Oglivie H: Men of two worlds. Arch Surg 1950;*61*:7.
2. Lee AE: The management of acute cholecystitis. Br J Surg 1957;*45*:523.
3. Reisenfeld G: Perforation of the gallbladder. Int Surg 1969;*52*:218.
4. Gagic N, Frey CF, Gaines R: Acute cholecystitis. Surg Gynecol Obstet 1975;*140*:868.
5. Riolanus J: A Sure Guide; or the Best and Nearest Way to Physick and Chyurgery. London, John Streeter, 1671, p 60.
6. Fitchett CW: Spontaneous external biliary fistula. Va Med Mon 1970;*97*:538.
7. Duncan J: Femoral hernia; gangrene of the gallbladder; extravasation of bile; peritonitis; death. North J Med 1844–45;*2*:151.
8. McWilliams CA: Acute, spontaneous perforation of the biliary system into the free peritoneal cavity. Ann Surg 1912;*55*:235.
9. Niemeier OW: Acute free perforation of the gallbladder. Ann Surg 1934;*99*:922.
10. Cowley LL, Harkins HN: Perforation of the gallbladder. Surg Gynecol Obstet 1943;*77*:661.
11. Butler RM, Harkins HN: Perforation of the gallbladder with special reference to cholecystenteric fistulas. Am J Surg 1961;*101*:717.
12. Friley M: Perforation of the gallbladder. Rev Surg 1972;*29*:377.
13. Morse L, Krynski B, Wright AR: Acute perforation of the gallbladder. Am J Surg 1957;*94*:772.
14. Strohl EL, Diffenbaugh WG, Baker JH, et al: Gangrene and perforation of the gallbladder. Int Abstr Surg 1962;*114*:1.
15. Isch JH, Finneran JC, Nahrwold DL: Perforation of the gallbladder. Am J Gastroenterol 1971;*55*:451.
16. McEachern CG, Sullivan RE: Perforation of the gallbladder. Arch Surg 1963;*87*:489.
17. Pines B, Rabinovitch J: Perforation of the gallbladder in acute cholecystitis. Ann Surg 1954;*140*:170.
18. Abu-Dalu J, Urca I: Acute cholecystitis with perforation into the peritoneal cavity. Arch Surg 1971;*102*:108.
19. Ottinger LW: Acute cholecystitis as a postoperative complication. Ann Surg 1976;*184*:162.
20. Uthman SM: Acalculous acute typhoid cholecystitis. Leb Med J 1972;*25*:503.
21. Penn I: Injuries of the gall-bladder. Br J Surg 1962;*49*:636.
22. Bussmann JF, Loewe KR, Kohler-Heurich H: Die freier Gallenblassenperforation und die perforations lose gallige Peritonitis. Langenbecks Arch Chir 1973;*333*:133.
23. Glenn F, Moore SW: Gangrene and perforation of the wall of the gallbladder. Arch Surg 1942;*446*:677.
24. Gordon KCD: Cystic arterial patterns in diseased human gall bladders. Gut 1967;*8*:565.

25. Thomas CG, Womack NA: Acute cholecystitis, its pathogenesis and repair. Arch Surg 1952;*64*:590.
26. Ellis H, Adair HM: Bile peritonitis—a report of fifteen patients. Postgrad Med J 1974;*50*:713.
27. Mouzas GL, Briggs JH: Perforation of gall-bladder during prednisone treatment. Br Med J 1957;*2*:450.
28. Schour L, Malin J: Spontaneous perforation of the normal gallbladder. Arch Surg 1973;*107*:465.
29. Ellis H: Bile peritonitis. Br J Surg 1960;*48*:166.
30. Kotorac V: Biliary peritonitis resulting from a perforated carcinomatous gallbladder. Gastroenterology 1972;*63*:328.
31. Thoren L: Bile peritonitis—an experimental study in rabbits. Acta Chir Scand 1958;(Suppl)*230*:1.
32. Thoren L: Bile peritonitis II—experimental studies of plasma volume loss, haptoglobin concentration in serum and kidney lesions in bile peritonitis. Acta Chir Scand 1963;*126*:114.
33. Cain JL, Labat JA, Cohn I: Bile peritonitis in germ-free dogs. Gastroenterology 1967;*53*:600.
34. Elmslie RG, White TT: Experimental inquiry into the significance of trypsin in bile peritonitis, with particular reference to the human secretions. Br J Surg 1966;*53*:1063.
35. Dale G, Solheim K: Bile peritonitis in acute cholecystitis. Acta Chir Scand 1975;*141*:764.
36. Roslyn J, Busuttil RW: Perforation of the gallbladder: a frequently mismanaged condition. Am J Surg 1979;*137*:307.
37. Raghavendra BN, Feiner HD, Subramanyam BR, et al: Acute cholecystitis: sonographic-pathologic analysis. AJR 1981;*137*:327.
38. Essenhigh DM: Perforation of the gall-bladder. Br J Surg 1968;*55*:175.
39. Bernhoft RA, et al: Pigment sludge and stone formation in the acutely ligated dog gallbladder. Gastroenterology 1983;*85*:1166.
40. Lennon F, Green WER: Perforation of the gallbladder. J R Coll Surg Edinb 1983;*28*:169.
41. Paul GJ: Perforation of the gallbladder: analysis of 22 cases. J Med Soc NJ 1980;*77*(2):97.
42. Madrazo BL, Francis I, Hricak H, et al: Sonographic findings in perforation of the gallbladder. AJR 1982;*139*:491.
43. Kane RA: Ultrasonographic diagnosis of gangrenous cholecystitis and empyema of the gallbladder. Radiology 1980;*134*:191.
44. Sanders RC: The significance of sonographic gallbladder wall thickening and its relation to cholecystitis. J Clin Ultrasound 1980;*8*:143.
45. Sty JR, Starshak RJ, Gorenstein L: Gallbladder perforation in a case of Kawasaki disease: image correlation. J Clin Ultrasound 1983;*11*:381.
46. Wiener I, Watson LC, Wolma FJ: Perforation of the gallbladder due to blunt abdominal trauma. Arch Surg 1982;*117*:805.
47. Soderstrom CA, Mackawa K, DuPriest RW Jr, et al: Gallbladder injuries resulting from blunt abdominal trauma. An experience and review. Ann Surg 1981;*193*:60.
48. Spigos DG, Tan WS, Larson G, et al: Diagnosis of traumatic rupture of the gallbladder. Am J Surg 1981;*141*:731.
49. Gottesman L, Marks RA, Khoury PT, et al: Diagnosis of isolated perforation of the gallbladder following blunt trauma using sonography and CT scan. J Trauma 1984;*24*:280.
50. Mesgarzadeh M, Haines JE, Bobba VR: Diagnosis of clinically unsuspected gallbladder perforation in an obese patient, by Tc-99m IDA cholescintigraphy. J Nucl Med 1983;*24*:1028.
51. Caride VJ, Gibson DW: Noninvasive evaluation of bile leakage. Surg Gynecol Obstet 1982;*154*:517.
52. Weissman HS, Byun KJ, Freeman LM: The role of Tc99m IDA scintigraphy in the evaluation of hepatobiliary trauma. Semin Nucl Med 1983;*13*:199.
53. Zeman RK, Lee CH, Stahl R, et al: Strategy for the use of biliary scintigraphy in non-iatrogenic biliary trauma. Radiology 1984;*151*:771.
54. Thornton JG: Spontaneous perforation of the gallbladder without gallstones. Br J Surg 1984;*71*:314.
55. Powers TA, Melton RE: Diagnosis of gallbladder perforation by Tc-99m disofenin cholescintigraphy. Clin Nucl Med 1982;*7*:201.
56. Fleischer AC, Muhletaler CA, Jones TB: Sonographic detection of gallbladder perforation. South Med J 1982;*75*:606.
57. Hutton L, Lamki N, Rankin R: Halo around the gallbladder—a prognostic sign? J Can Assoc Radiol 1982;*33*:80.
58. van den Broek HA: Sonographic findings in a case of acute cholecystitis with gallbladder perforation. A case report. Diagn Imaging 1983;*52*:219.
59. Wilson DG, Lieberman LM: Perforation of the gallbladder diagnosed preoperatively. Eur J Nucl Med 1983;*8*:145
60. Klamer TW, Max MH: Carcinoma of the gallbladder. Surg Gynecol Obstet 1983;*156*:641.

LAWRENCE W. WAY, M.D.

17

Gallstone Ileus

Gallstone ileus consists of obstruction of the intestine by a gallstone. The stone usually enters the gut through a cholecystoduodenal fistula and then passes distally until it reaches a point where it is too large to pass any farther. Gallstones responsible for causing gallstone ileus are usually 2.5 cm or more in diameter, which corresponds to the diameter of the narrowest part of the intestine, the ileum.

The disease is uncommon and may be decreasing in frequency, although there is disagreement on the latter point. Even though gallstone ileus is not encountered very often, it is important to consider this syndrome in any elderly patient with intestinal obstruction. Awareness of gallstone ileus is a prerequisite to diagnosis, and early diagnosis is critical in minimizing the death rate.

Because no one surgeon or institution has a large experience with this disease, most articles on gallstone ileus report only a few cases. Therefore, in the preparation of this chapter, the English-language literature between 1950 and 1985 was reviewed (including 23 cases treated in our medical center) in order to generate data that thoroughly describe the disease. In this process, all articles that covered an institution's entire experience over a period of several years were included. This amounted to 67 articles describing a total of 1061 patients.[1–67]

EPIDEMIOLOGY

About 85 per cent of people who develop gallstone ileus are women, and the female to male ratio is considerably higher than that for gallstone disease in general. The preponderance of women is higher in patients under age 65 years than in those over age 65. The disease characteristically occurs in the elderly. The age range in the collected series of 1061 patients was 13 to 93 years, with a median of about 70 years.

Gallstone ileus has been estimated to be responsible for 1 to 2 per cent of all cases of obstruction of the small intestine. In patients older than 65 years who have intestinal obstruction, the chance of gallstone ileus being the cause is about 25 per cent, and the diagnosis is even more likely if the patient does not have an incarcerated abdominal wall hernia and gives no history of a previous abdominal operation.

The frequency of the disease is subject to two influences that would be expected to have opposite effects. First is the increasing tendency, compared with 30 to 40 years ago, for patients with symptomatic gallstone disease to be treated by cholecystectomy early in their illness. This would have the effect of decreasing the numbers of patients whose gallstones grow to such a large size. Second, however, is the increasing longevity of the population, which places greater numbers of elderly persons at risk. No figures are available on the incidence of gallstone ileus, and although one group noted no decline in recent years,[68] our impression is that the disease is less common now than it was 20 years ago.

PATHOLOGY

The gallstone usually enters the intestine through a cholecystenteric fistula. In about 90 per cent of cases the fistula is between the gallbladder and the second portion of the duodenum. The next most common type of fistula is cholecystocolonic, with the gallstone giving rise to large bowel obstruction. Occasional cases have been seen in which the fistula was between the gallblader and the jejunum or stomach. Gallstone ileus has also been seen rarely in patients who have previously had a cholecystectomy, in whom the gallstone entered the duodenum through the ampulla of Vater or a choledochoduodenal fistula.[69] The latter is probably the explanation in most such cases.

It is important to note that a cholecystenteric fistula does not by itself usually give rise to symptoms. Anastomoses between the gallbladder and intestine are often made deliberately to route bile around a distal common duct obstruction, and in the absence of obstruction these patients do not develop cholangitis. This is true for fistulas into the colon as well as for those into the small intestine.

Although chronic cholecystitis is present in all patients with gallstone ileus, it is surprising that most of them have not had especially severe symptoms of gallbladder disease before they presented with intestinal obstruction.[3,16,50] Overall, about 50 per cent of patients give a history of ordinary biliary colic, but only 25 per cent have had an attack within the year preceding the development of gallstone ileus. Furthermore, acute cholecystitis rarely accompanies or immediately precedes the intestinal obstruction. This suggests that the fistula represents the end point of an indolent erosion by the heavy gallstone through the gallbladder wall, rather than the culmination of an attack of acute inflammation.

Usually just one large stone enters the intestine, but there may be more than one; during surgery it is important to check for additional stones proximal to the one causing the obstruction in order to avoid the possibility of an immediate postoperative recurrence. A second large stone can be found in the intestine in about 10 per cent of cases; three and even four large stones have been recovered in rare cases. The presence of a facet on one surface of the obstructing stone is an important clue to the existence of a second stone.

Once it enters the duodenum, the stone moves slowly in an aboral direction. Most gallstones that find their way into the intestine are small and are passed rectally without causing symptoms. Only the larger ones have a chance of producing symptoms, and with few exceptions those causing gallstone ileus are more than 2.5 cm in diameter. This is the approximate threshold size for stones to obstruct the human small intestine. About two thirds of obstructing stones are found lodged in the ileum, the narrowest part of the gut and the part with the least vigorous peristalsis. To obstruct the colon, either the gallstone must be very large or, more often, unrelated disease (usually diverticulitis) has produced a fixed narrowing of the colonic lumen at the point where the stone hangs up. The largest recorded stone responsible for gallstone ileus measured 17.5 cm in its longest diameter and obstructed the transverse colon.[70]

Among the 1061 cases surveyed in the literature review,[1–67] information on the site of gallstone obstruction was available for 913. The locations of these 913 gallstones were as follows: ileum, 608 (64 per cent); jejunum, 218 (23 per cent); colon, 37 (4 per cent); stomach, 10 (1 per cent); and other or unknown, 40 (4.2 per cent). Among the last group were stones that had been passed rectally after transiently causing small bowel obstruction, and one stone that was vomited after producing symptoms by obstructing the pylorus.

Gastrointestinal bleeding develops as a complication of gallstone ileus in a few patients. The site of the bleeding is usually at the cholecystoduodenal fistula or at the point of impaction of the stone in the intestine. The rare case of massive bleeding, manifested by hematemesis or melena, usually requires cholecystectomy if the origin of bleeding is the cholecystenteric fistula, or small bowel resection if the origin is at the point of impaction.

CLINICAL MANIFESTATIONS

The clinical presentation is mainly that of small bowel obstruction, without distinguishing features that separate gallstone ileus from other forms of small bowel obstruction. Abdominal pain is present in most cases, and abdominal distention develops in patients with distal obstruction as the obstruction becomes more complete. The clinical findings are often confusing, however, and a delay of 3 to 4 days between hospitalization and laparotomy is typical.

One reason for delay in diagnosis is that in the early stages the obstruction is often incomplete and the symptoms intermittent as the stone moves down the length of the small bowel. This has been referred to as a tumbling obstruction, a pattern manifested by bloating, vomiting, and constipation that waxes and wanes. Both the physician and the patient may be lured into thinking that the problem, unrecognized as gallstone ileus, is likely to resolve. Eventually, the obstruction becomes unremitting, but by then the patient's overall strength has diminished. The result is that in addition to delay by the patient in seeking care, another 2 to 7 days' delay (average 4 days) is typical before the diagnosis is made and the need for surgery becomes clear.

The combined effects of inability to eat, vomiting, and delay in therapy as well as a high frequency of associated diseases result in dehydration, electrolyte imbalance, renal dysfunction, and, often, aggravation of the associated disease. Elderly patients cannot tolerate this much stress, which is the principal reason for the high death rate of gallstone ileus. Nevertheless, management of patients with this disease seems to have improved in recent years, for the death rate has been dropping.

Many patients give a history of previous abdominal pain from gallstones, but it may be difficult to make a connection between these symptoms and the current illness. As mentioned earlier, only a few patients experience right upper quadrant pain or symptoms of cholangitis in conjunction with the gallstone ileus. Jaundice is also uncommon.

In most cases, abdominal distention, hyperactive bowel sounds, and diffuse abdominal tenderness are the principal abnormalities on physical examination. Right upper quadrant tenderness may be present but usually is not. In an occasional patient the gallstone can be felt as a mobile mass on abdominal or rectal examination, but it rarely is identified correctly.

X-RAY FINDINGS

Plain films of the abdomen may be diagnostic, but unless they are inspected carefully with the possibility of gallstone ileus in mind, important abnormalities may be overlooked. The changes, first described by Rigler et al.,[71] are (1) signs of small bowel obstruction, (2) the presence of a large gallstone remote from the gallbladder area, (3) changing position of the gallstone on sequential films, and (4) air in the biliary tree. In practice, identifying air in the biliary tree (Fig. 17–1) or an ectopic gallstone in addition to small bowel obstruction is the key to diagnosis on plain films. The biliary air shadows may be subtle, masked to some extent by the large amounts

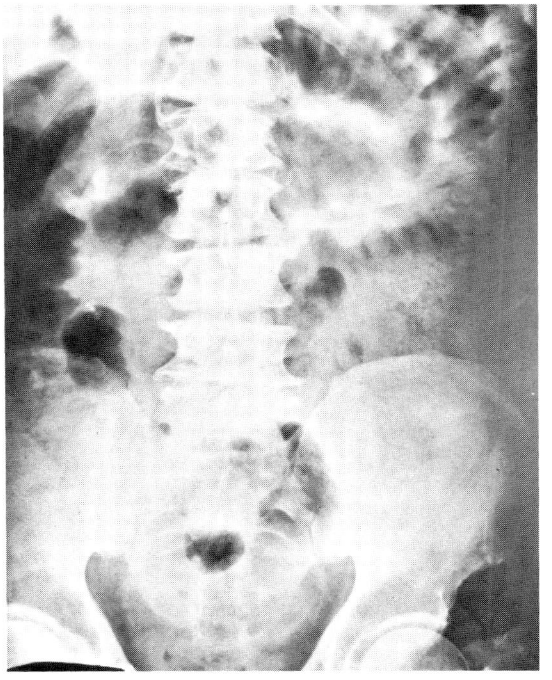

Figure 17–1. Supine film of the abdomen in a patient with gallstone ileus. The air-filled gallbladder can be seen in the right upper quadrant.

of small bowel gas. Air is noted in the gallbladder or bile ducts in about 50 per cent of patients before surgery,[4, 16, 50] but retrospectively, after the diagnosis is known, it can be found in even more of them.[39] In 80 per cent of cases the gallstone contains too little calcium to be seen on plain films, but if it is seen, the diagnosis should be readily apparent.

Barium upper gastrointestinal x-rays may be of great help.[50, 64] Barium outlines the cholecystoduodenal fistula, the gallbladder, and, often, the bile ducts (Fig. 17–2). If the ducts are not opacified, the image of the gallbladder must be differentiated from a giant duodenal ulcer or a duodenal diverticulum. The barium also may pass down the small intestine and demonstrate the gallstone as a circular negative shadow in the intestinal lumen (Fig. 17–3).

LABORATORY FINDINGS

Laboratory tests contribute little to the diagnosis in the average case. The only tests likely to suggest the presence of biliary disease are measurements of serum bilirubin

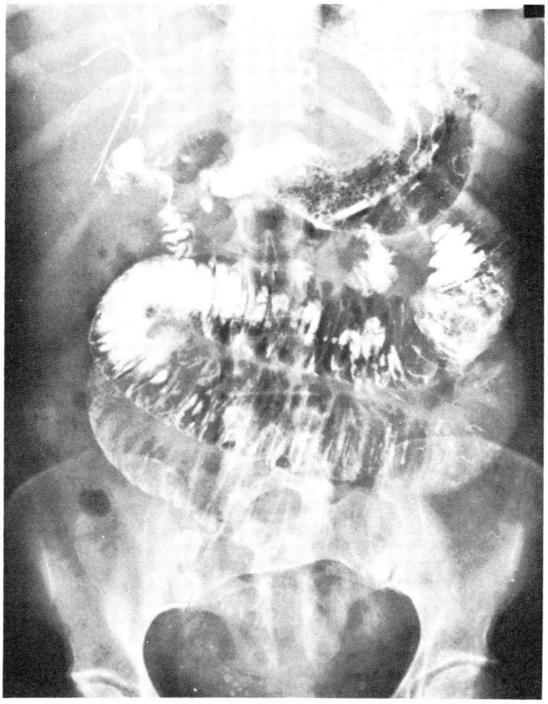

Figure 17–2. Upper gastrointestinal series in a patient with gallstone ileus. The gallbladder and bile ducts have been opacified by barium.

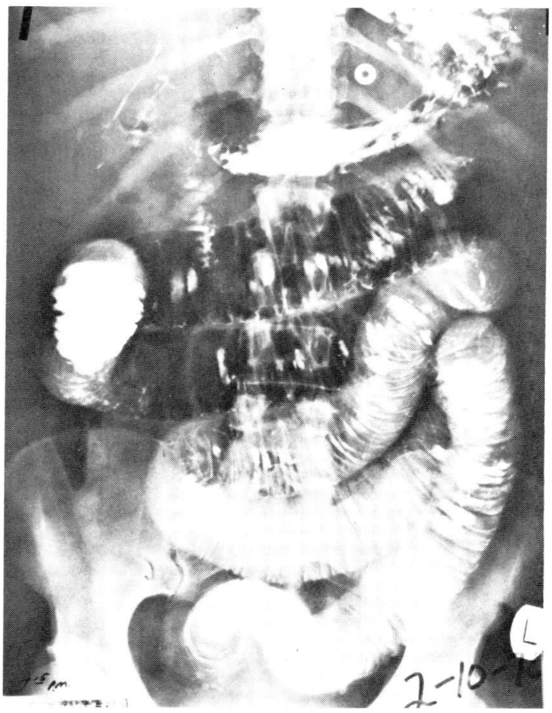

Figure 17–3. A later phase of the upper gastrointestinal series shown in Figure 17–2. The gallstone has been outlined by barium

and alkaline phosphatase, which are abnormal in 15 to 20 per cent of patients. The changes are rarely marked, however, and are also compatible with nonspecific alterations in liver function as a result of stressful illness.

The white blood cell count is usually slightly elevated. Electrolyte abnormalities from vomiting consist of hyponatremia, hypochloremia, and hypokalemia. The creatinine and BUN levels may be elevated.

TREATMENT

The diagnosis of gallstone ileus is being made preoperatively nowadays in about half the cases, and the other half are diagnosed preoperatively as intestinal obstruction. Operation is performed in a few patients with a preoperative diagnosis of appendicitis or other miscellaneous conditions.

Once the diagnosis of gallstone ileus is made, surgery should be performed as soon as the patient has been rehydrated and electrolyte abnormalities have been corrected. There is no reason to delay in the belief that the stone may pass spontaneously. As mentioned before, much of the morbidity of gallstone ileus can be attributed to surgery being performed relatively late in the illness.

At laparotomy the gallstone should be milked into healthy bowel a short distance proximal to where it has lodged, and then removed through an enterotomy. It is unusual for an intestinal resection to be required; when resection is necessary, the rate of complications and death is higher.[50] Nevertheless, intestinal perforation or gangrene with impending perforation usually requires a resection.

The entire intestine must be carefully examined for a second stone, which is present in about 10 per cent of cases. A few patients even have a third stone big enough to cause obstruction. These additional gallstones must also be removed.

Other ways proposed to manage the obstructing stone are less advisable. For example, it has been reported that milking the stone distally into the cecum may then put it in a position where it can pass spontaneously, and an enterotomy can be avoided. This is a potentially dangerous maneuver, however, because the distal small bowel may be traumatized during the milking efforts, with the result that a resection now becomes necessary. There are also examples in which the stone, having been milked into the cecum, was subsequently unable to pass through the sigmoid colon.[3]

It has also been suggested that the stone may be crushed by manual pressure applied from outside the bowel. The fragments, too small to cause obstruction, could then pass. This technique is also much too likely to damage the bowel wall, and it cannot be recommended.

There has been considerable debate about whether or not to remove the gallbladder at the same time as the intestinal obstruction is treated. The arguments in favor of this approach[5, 15, 63] are that it eliminates (1) the need for a second laparotomy to remove the gallbladder; (2) the possibility of cholangitis due to reflux of intestinal contents into the bile ducts; (3) the possibility of recurrent gallstone ileus due to residual stones in the gallbladder; and (4) the risk of gallbladder carcinoma.

The merits of limiting the operation to removal of no more than the obstructing gallstone are that the patient is spared the potential morbidity of an additional procedure, which on occasion can be technically difficult and time-consuming. After the gallstone has passed into the intestine, the gallbladder itself usually presents no immediate problem; the reasons for removing it are as prophylaxis against relatively uncommon late problems that are rarely life-threatening.

The principal argument for simultaneous cholecystectomy has been to prevent recurrent gallstone ileus, but the available data show that this is an uncommon event. Of 782 patients with gallstone ileus[1–68] who were treated by lithotomy alone and then followed, only 25 experienced recurrent gallstone ileus, a crude incidence of recurrence of 3.3 per cent. If those patients who died in the postoperative period are eliminated from the calculation, the risk of recurrence becomes 4 per cent. Of these 25 recurrent cases, only 2 patients (8 per cent) died. It appeared that when the patient presented with a history of a previous episode of gallstone ileus, the diagnosis was made with less difficulty the second time, institution of treatment was more expeditious, and the death rate was lower.

Thus, if cholecystectomy were advocated as a standard accompaniment of lithotomy, the main purpose would be to improve upon a 1 in 25 risk of recurrence and a 1 in 333 risk of death from recurrence. Looked at in this way, it seems likely that a liberal policy of prophylactic cholecystectomy would almost certainly result in more complications and deaths than if cholecystectomy were done infrequently.[34] For example, among the 23 patients with gallstone ileus treated at our hospital, 4 died; one of these deaths followed complications resulting from breakdown of the duodenal closure after a technically difficult, simultaneous cholecystectomy.[64] The gallbladder posed no immediate threat, and after it had been removed it was found to contain no additional gallstones.

For these reasons the majority of authors who have written about the treatment of gallstone ileus have recommended that the gallbladder be left undisturbed at the initial operation.[3, 16, 27, 34, 50, 64] Of 909 patients in the collected series in which adequate detail was provided, only 59 (6.5 per cent) had cholecystectomy in conjunction with the enterolithotomy. Even if the opposite approach were favored, one must admit that the risks of leaving the gallbladder alone are very low, and it would be difficult to justify prolonging the operation to remove the gallbladder in an old fragile patient or to tackle a challenging edematous right upper quadrant mass. Cholecystectomy would be reasonable only in a stable patient whose gallbladder exhibited more chronic than acute inflammation.

On the other hand, if the gallbladder were discovered by palpation to contain another stone, this would be a more compelling indication for simultaneous cholecystectomy. Operative ultrasonography might also be helpful in checking for residual gallbladder stones, although there have been no reports on its use in patients with gallstone ileus. Malt[72] recommended cholecystolithotomy as a technically simpler alternative to cholecystectomy. In practice, palpable gallbladder stones seem to be encountered only rarely, for this situation has not often been mentioned in articles on gallstone ileus.

The next question is whether an interval cholecystectomy should be performed after the patient recovers from lithotomy without cholecystectomy. Our policy is to recommend expectant management in elderly people if they have few or mild symptoms. Younger people (eg, those under age 65) are encouraged to undergo cholecystectomy regardless of their symptomatic status.

DUODENAL OBSTRUCTION

The clinical picture can be very puzzling when the gallstone fails to pass down the intestine but instead obstructs the duodenum (Bouveret's syndrome).[73–76] In this situation vomiting is prominent, but abdominal distention depends on the extent to which the stomach becomes dilated, since the syndrome is essentially a form of gastric outlet obstruction. The stone is typically located in the duodenal bulb or, less often, in the descending duodenum or at the duodenojejunal flexure.

Physical examination occasionally reveals a right upper quadrant mass. The diagnosis can be made by endoscopy or upper gastrointestinal barium studies. On endoscopy, the gallstone is visible in the duodenal bulb, just past the pylorus.[77, 78] Its character can often be ascertained by probing with the end of the scope. Upper gastrointestinal series demonstrates the gallstone as a filling defect in the duodenal bulb, and it also outlines the fistula and the biliary tree. At this point the diagnosis becomes clear. In a few cases, CT scans have demonstrated the gallstone in the duodenum. Treatment usually consists of cholecystectomy, extraction of the gallstone, and repair of the fistula. Some cases have been managed by milking the stone into the stomach, where it can be removed through a gastrotomy.

GASTRIC OBSTRUCTION

A large gallstone that has entered the stomach through a pyloric fistula has another kind of presentation.[79] In this case, gastric outlet obstruction occurs when the stone obstructs the pylorus, but the symptoms may be intermittent as the stone moves around inside the stomach. The patient may experience relief by lying on the left side or manipulating the upper abdomen, which dislodges the stone from its position of obstruction. Some patients have been cured when they spontaneously vomited the stone. Most often, it must be removed through a gastrotomy.

COLONIC OBSTRUCTION

Gallstone obstruction of the colon usually occurs when a stone becomes impacted in the sigmoid colon at a site narrowed by diverticular disease.[80, 81] In most cases the stone reaches the colon by passing through the small intestine, but direct entry via a cholecystocolonic fistula occurs in about one third of patients.

The clinical presentation consists of large bowel obstruction, which is often thought initially to be caused by a neoplasm or diverticulitis. Barium enema may outline the gallstone, which may be mistaken for a fecal mass. In some cases it can be seen on colonoscopy. Occasionally, the stone eventually negotiates the sigmoid narrowing and then is evacuated or can be manually removed from the rectum. Most often, laparotomy is required, at which time the sigmoid should be resected, and a proximal colostomy and closure of the distal colon performed.

RECURRENT GALLSTONE ILEUS

The overall risk of recurrent gallstone ileus is about 4 per cent.[1–67] Recurrences may appear early or late. Of 23 cases in which the interval between the first and second attacks of gallstone ileus was known, seven (30 per cent) occurred within 2 weeks, nine (40 per cent) occurred between 2 weeks and 8 weeks, and seven (30 per cent) occurred between 2 months and 12 months.[1–67]

Early recurrences most often result from a second stone that has already entered the lumen of the small bowel at the time of the initial operation. Careful inspection of the bowel proximal to the obstructing stone will disclose the second stone, which can be removed, thus preventing recurrence.

Late cases undoubtedly result from additional stones that initially remain within the gallbladder. Although late recurrences could be prevented by cholecystectomy either at the time of the initial operation or shortly thereafter, the overall risks in most patients weigh in favor of expectant management in the absence of symptoms of biliary disease.

PROGNOSIS

The overall death rate is 20 per cent (215 deaths out of 1061 cases), but better general management of elderly patients and a trend toward earlier diagnosis have led to improvements in recent years. About 15 per cent of the deaths represent patients who are moribund upon admission to the hospital and who die without surgery. The other 85 per cent of deaths occur postoperatively, usually as the result of abdominal sepsis or cardiopulmonary or renal complications. Nonlethal postoperative complications, such as wound infection and pneumonia, are common. Gallbladder carcinoma is subsequently found in a few patients. A second gallstone ileus occurs in 4 per cent of patients, almost always within 12 months of the first attack.

REFERENCES

1. Agner O, Hansen LK, Iversen OH: Gallstone ileus. Dan Med Bull 1961;*8*:84.
2. Aldridge RT: Gallstone ileus. NZ Med J 1962; *61*:595.
3. Anderson RE, Woodward N, Diffenbaugh WG, et al: Gallstone obstruction of the intestine. Surg Gynecol Obstet 1967;*125*:540.
4. Andersson A, Zederfeldt B: Gallstone ileus. Acta Chir Scand 1969;*135*:713.
5. Beck AR: Gallstone ileus. Mt Sinai Hosp J 1966; *33*:165.
6. Berliner SD, Burson LC: One-stage repair for cholecyst-duodenal fistula and gallstone ileus. Arch Surg 1965;*90*:313.
7. Bridenbaugh RB, Bridenbaugh JH, Berg HM: Gallstone ileus. Report of four cases. AJR 1957;*77*:684.
8. Brockis JG, Gilbert MC: Intestinal obstruction by gall-stones. A review of 179 cases. Br J Surg 1957;*44*:461.
9. Brown DB, Kerr IF, Livingstone DJ: Gall-stone obstruction. Br J Surg 1966;*53*:672.
10. Buetow GW, Crampton RS: Gallstone ileus. A report of 23 cases. Arch Surg 1963;*86*:174.
11. Camacho E, Whitcomb JG, Evans DM: Gallstone ileus. Henry Ford Hosp Med Bull 1958;*6*:345.
12. Carter DC, Macleod DAD: Obturation obstruction of the small intestine. R Coll Surg Edinb 1970;*15*:13.
13. Coffey RJ, Willox GD: Gallstone obstruction of the intestinal tract. Am Surg 1952;18:286.
14. Collins GM, Claxton RC: Gall-stone intestinal obstruction: a review of the literature and presentation of new cases. Med J Aust 1966;*1*:578.
15. Cooperman AM, Dickson ER, ReMine WH: Changing concepts in the surgical treatment of gallstone ileus: a review of 15 cases with emphasis on diagnosis and treatment. Ann Surg 1968;167:377.
16. Day EA, Marks C: Gallstone ileus. Review of the literature and presentation of thirty-four new cases. Am J Surg 1975;*129*:552.
17. Deckoff SL: Gallstone ileus. A report of 12 cases. Ann Surg 1955;*152*:52.
18. Dorr TW: The roentgen diagnosis of gallstone ileus. Radiology 1954;*62*:363.
19. Esposito JJ: Roentgen diagnosis of gallstone ileus. Conn Med 1964;*28*:745.
20. Fjermeros H: Gall-stone ileus. Case reports and review of 178 cases from Scandinavia and Finland. Acta Chir Scand 1964;*128*:186.
21. Foley TJ, Selzer J: Gallstone ileus. Seven cases with two recurrences. Wisc Med J 1958;*57*:253.
22. Fox PF: Planning the operation for cholecystoenteric fistula with gallstone ileus. Surg Clin North Am 1970:*50*:93.
23. Fraser WJ: Intestinal obstruction by gall-stone. Br J Surg 1954;*42*:210.
24. Gibson JM Jr, Westerly RI: Gallstone ileus. Arch Surg 1963;*86*:161.
25. Greenlee RM, Berry WH: Intestinal obstruction due to gallstones. NY State J Med 1953;*53*:1342.
26. Haffner JFW, Semb LS, Aakhus T: Gallstone ileus. A report of 22 cases. Acta Chir Scand 1969;*135*:707.
27. Hesselfeldt P, Jess P: Gallstone ileus. A review of 39 cases with emphasis on surgical treatment. Acta Chir Scand 1982;*148*:431.
28. Hudspeth AS, McGurit WF: Gallstone ileus. A continuing surgical problem. Arch Surg 1970;*100*:668.
29. Jekler J: Intestinal obstruction caused by impacted gallstones. Surgery 1959;*46*:858.
30. Jenkins HP, Evans R, Kollert W: Gallstone ileus. Surg Clin North Am 1961;*41*:71.
31. Jenssen C Fr: Gallstone ileus. Acta Chir Scand 1955;*109*:116.
32. Karaharju EO, Rannikko S: Intestinal obstruction caused by gallstones. Ann Chir Gynaecol Fenn 1972;*61*:181.
33. Karlin S, Miller WC: Gallstone obstruction of the small bowel. Louisiana State Med J 1954;*106*:391.
34. Kasahara Y, Umemura H, Shiraha S, et al: Gallstone ileus. Review of 112 patients in the Japanese literature. Am J Surg 1980;*140*:437.
35. Kelly TR, Getty PA: Gallstone ileus at a community hospital. Ohio State Med J 1969;*65*:143.
36. Kirkland KC, Croce EJ: Gallstone intestinal obstruction. A review of the literature and presentation of 12 cases, including 3 recurrences. JAMA 1961; *176*:116.
37. Kolstad P: The clinical and roentgenological diagnosis of gallstone ileus. Report of five cases. Acta Chir Scand 1954;*107*:269.
38. Koskinen EVS: The importance of the liver changes in intestinal obstruction caused by gallstones. Report of eleven cases. Ann Chir Gynaecol Fenn 1958;*47*:439.
39. Kurtz RJ, Heimann TM, Kurtz AB: Gallstone ileus: a diagnostic problem. Am J Surg 1983;*146*:314.
40. Kvist E: Gallstone ileus. A retrospective study. Acta Chir Scand 1979;*145*:101.
41. Levine RM, Ripstein CB: The diagnosis and surgical management of gall stone ileus. Can Med Assoc J 1952;*66*:113.
42. McCune WS, Salzberg AM: Gallstone ileus. Am Surg 1955;*21*:334.
43. McLaughlin CW JR, Raines M: Obstruction of the alimentary tract from gallstones. Am J Surg 1951;*81*:424.
44. Miller HR, Araj JS: Gallstone ileus. A report of five cases. Ohio State Med J 1963;*59*:163.
45. Moore TC, Baker WH: Operative and radiologic relief of gallstone intestinal obstruction. Surg Gynecol Obstet 1963;*116*:189.
46. Morlock CG, Shocket E, ReMine WH: Intestinal obstruction due to gallstones. Gastroenterology 1956;*30*:462.
47. Nemir P Jr: Gallstone ileus. Report of eight cases. Surg Gynecol Obstet 1952;*94*:469.
48. Piedad OH, Wels PB: Spontaneous internal biliary fistula, obstructive and nonobstructive types: twenty-year review of 55 cases. Ann Surg 1972;*175*:75.
49. Pierson JC, Mekanik EA: Gallstone ileus. Observations based on three recent cases. Del State Med J 1951;*23*:304.

50. Raf L, Spangen L: Gallstone ileus. Acta Chir Scand 1971;*137*:665.
51. Raiford TS: Intestinal obstruction caused by gallstones. Am J Surg 1962;*104*:383.
52. Ramanujam P, Shabeeb N, Silver JM: Unusual manifestations of gallstone migration into the gastrointestinal tract. South Med J 1983; *76*:30.
53. Rogers FA, Carter R: Gallstone intestinal obstruction. Calif Med 1958;*88*:140.
54. Ruby RH, Nine-Curt J: Intestinal obstruction due to gallstones. Mo Med Assoc J 1952;*49*:341.
55. Safaie-Shirazi S, Printen KJ: Gallstone ileus: review of forty cases. J Am Geriatr Soc 1972;*20*:335.
56. Sanders RL, Pool RM: Gallstone obstruction of the intestine. South Med J 1952;*45*:328.
57. Shore S, Jacob HH, Cannon JA: Intestinal obstruction resulting from biliary calculi (gallstone ileus). Arch Surg 1952;*64*:301.
58. Smith C Jr, Gratiot JH: Intestinal obstruction due to gallstones. Calif Med 1957;*86*:44.
59. Stanistreet RH: Gall-stone ileus. Aust NZ J Surg 1953;*23*:73.
60. Stitt RB, Heslin DJ, Currie DJ: Gall-stone ileus. Br J Surg 1967;*54*:673.
61. Svartholm E, Andren-Sandberg A, Evander A, et al: Diagnosis and treatment of gallstone ileus. Report of 83 cases. Acta Chir Scand 1982;*148*:435.
62. Thomas HS, Cherry JK, Averbook BD: Gallstone ileus. JAMA 1962;*179*:131.
63. Warshaw AL, Bartlett MK: Choice of operation for gallstone intestinal obstruction. Ann Surg 1966;*164*:1051.
64. Way LW, Dunphy JE: Gallstone ileus. Bull Soc Int Chir 1975;*34*:647.
65. Whitesell FB Jr: Gallstone ileus. Am Surg 1970;*36*:317.
66. Wiley JW, Henderson AJ: Acute intestinal obstruction due to gallstones. Seven cases reported—one recurrent. West J Surg Gynecol Obstet 1956; *64*:213.
67. Wright PJM, Trafford PA: Gall-stone ileus. Br J Surg 1953;*41*:6.
68. Kurtz RJ, Heimann TM, Beck AR, et al: Patterns of treatment of gallstone ileus over a 45-year period. Am J Gastroenterol 1985;*80*:95.
69. Masters RG, Wellington JL: Gallstone ileus in the absence of the gallbladder: case report and review of the literature. Can J Surg 1985;*28*:65.
70. Turner GG: A giant gall-stone impacted in the colon and causing acute obstruction. Br J Surg 1932;*20*:26.
71. Rigler LG, Borman CN, Noble JF: Gallstone obstruction: pathogenesis and roentgen manifestations. JAMA 1941;*117*:1753.
72. Malt RA: Experience with recurrent gallstone ileus applied to management of the first attack. Am J Surg 1964;*108*:92.
73. Halasz NA: Gallstone obstruction of the duodenal bulb (Bouveret's syndrome). Am J Dig Dis 1964;*9*:856.
74. Milstoc M, Berger AR, Finkel J: Gallstone obstruction of the second portion of the duodenum. Am J Dig Dis 1969;*14*:143.
75. Printen JK, Safaie-Shirazi S: Duodenal obstruction caused by gallstones: report of six cases. Am Surg 1973;*39*:688.
76. Thomas TL, Jaques PF, Weaver PC: Gallstone obstruction and perforation of the duodenal bulb. Br J Surg 1976;*63*:131.
77. Oakland DJ, Denn PG: Endoscopic diagnosis of gallstone ileus of the duodenum. Dig Dis Sci 1986;*31*:98.
78. Torgerson SA, Greening GK, Juniper K Jr, et al: Gallstone obstruction of duodenal cap (Bouveret's syndrome) diagnosed by endoscopy. Am J Gastroenterol 1979;*72*:165.
79. Redding ME, Anagnostopoulos CE, Wright HK: Cholecystopyloric fistula with gastric outlet obstruction: a rare form of gallstone ileus and its management. Ann Surg 1972;*176*:210.
80. Milsom JW, MacKeigan JM: Gallstone obstruction of the colon. Report of two cases and review of management. Dis Col Rectum 1985;*28*:367.
81. Pryor JH: Gall-stone obstruction of the sigmoid colon with particular reference to aetiology. Br J Surg 1959;*47*:259.

LAWRENCE DENBESTEN, M.D.

18 Choledocholithiasis

Common duct stones are present in 10 to 15 per cent of the 500,000 patients undergoing cholecystectomy in the United States each year. About 1 per cent of these patients require a second procedure to remove a stone overlooked at the first operation, and 2 per cent require two or more additional procedures related to common duct stones. Common duct stones should be removed because they may lead to cholangitis, liver abscesses, pancreatitis, or biliary cirrhosis.

Recent technologic advances have improved the management of choledocholithiasis. Accurate preoperative diagnosis is usually possible. Ultrasound and percutaneous or endoscopic retrograde cholangiography, monitored by x-ray units capable of image amplification, television monitoring, videotape recording and spot x-ray films, provide accurate preoperative information. Use of the choledochoscope during common bile duct exploration allows detailed examination of the biliary tree to rule out the presence of tumors or residual stones. Stones remaining or newly formed in the bile ducts can usually be removed through the T-tube tract or by endoscopic transduodenal section of the ampulla of Vater.

ETIOLOGY

Common duct stones are the end result of a breakdown in the normal mechanism by which bile solutes are maintained in solution.[1-3] The primary bile solutes are cholesterol, phospholipid, bile acids, and bilirubin. Gallbladder stones and common duct stones are formed principally from cholesterol or bilirubin. Stones in the common duct, with rare exceptions, are chemically similar to coexisting stones in the gallbladder.[4] In other words, patients with cholesterol common duct stones have cholesterol gallbladder stones and patients with pigment common duct stones will be found to have pigment gallbladder stones. The pathogenesis of gallbladder stones is discussed in detail in Chapter 4.

Common duct stones may originate in the gallbladder or the bile ducts. Cholesterol stones formed in the gallbladder vary in size from a few millimeters to several centimeters. The larger stones are faceted, carrying the imprint of adjacent stones. Their color varies from white to yellow to dark brown. Pigment stones that originate in the gallbladder are commonly 2 to 3 mm in diameter, black, and irregular, but the appearance of pigment stones varies greatly, and large heterogeneous pigment stones are occasionally seen in the gallbladder. Large pigment stones formed principally of calcium bilirubinate are frequently found in the common duct. Small cholesterol and pigment stones may pass from the gallbladder through the cystic duct into the common bile duct. Occasionally, even larger stones can pass through a dilated cystic duct. Less commonly, large stones may pass through a fistula between the gallbladder and bile duct that is caused by pressure necrosis of the adjacent walls.

Common duct stones that have originated in the gallbladder are often small, and those composed of cholesterol are usually faceted (as a result of contact with adjacent stones). Stones that originate in the duct are referred to as primary stones. They are often soft, smooth, yellowish tan, and round like the duct. The frequency with which stones found in the common duct arise primarily in the duct (primary stones) or result from the passage of gallbladder stones through the cystic duct (secondary stones) is still being debated.[4-6] Most surgeons believe that all but 10 to 15 per cent of common duct stones form originally in the gallbladder and secondarily come to reside in the duct. Madden,[5, 6] however, believes that the frequency of primary duct stones is much higher. Using morphologic criteria originally proposed by Aschoff,[7] he concluded that 56 (52 per cent) of 107 consecutive patients operated on for common duct stones had primary stones (Table 18–1).[6] Of those patients classified as having primary stones, 68 per cent had a single common duct stone, whereas single stones were present in only 25 per cent of those classified as having secondary stones. In addition, 47 per cent of the 60 patients with primary stones had had one or more previous common bile duct explorations, and 50 per cent were judged to have a stricture (distal common bile duct calibrated with a No. 3 Bakes dilator) of the ampulla. These conclusions have been criticized because they assume that morphologic features are valid indices of stone origin and that ampullary stricture is satisfactorily defined by this calibration technique.

Other observations showing that stones can form primarily in the duct are as follows: Ten per cent of patients with common duct stones have none in the gallbladder.[4, 8] Twenty per cent of humans without a gallbladder (agenesis of the gallbladder) have common duct stones.[9] In a 10-year study of the natural history of 91 patients who had had common duct stones removed, Thurston found that the frequency of appearance of other stones decreased during the first year after operation and then rose again sharply during the third postoperative year.[10] Twenty-six per cent of patients presented with their second stones 10 years or more after the first operation.

Bernhoft et al.[4] analyzed the chemical composition of common duct stones and compared the results with the gross characteristics of the stones and the clinical features of the patient's illness. The gallbladder and common duct stones in individual patients were compared. These investigators found that cholesterol stones from the duct were almost always indistinguishable (chemically and visibly) from cholesterol stones found in the gallbladder. Pigment stones in the duct, however, often varied substantially from their counterparts in the gallbladder. Pigment common duct stones contained proportionally more calcium bilirubinate and less bilirubin polymers than did pigment gallbladder stones. Bernhoft et al.[4] concluded that the evidence supported a gallbladder origin for virtually all cholesterol common duct stones. Pigment stones were thought in most cases to have originated in the gallbladder and to have entered the duct secondarily. It was clear, however, that pigment stones could also form de novo in the duct in the presence of stasis. It was thought that some pigment common duct stones might develop as the result of fine pigment precipitates from the gallbladder passing through the cystic duct and becoming compacted into stones only after arriving in the common duct. After inspecting a wide variety of common duct and associated gallbladder stones, it was apparent that no morphologic variant was pathognomonic of primary common duct stones. Earthy stones, which some surgeons have considered to be almost certainly of duct origin, were found in situations in which they were most likely to have been of gallbladder origin. It was also noted by these authors that pigment common duct stones were more often accompanied by serious complications, such as cholangitis, than were cholesterol common duct stones. Pigment stones were more likely to be found in men and in an older age group.

Although the exact incidence of primary and secondary stones remains controversial, it may be higher than the 10 to 15 per cent figure that is generally accepted. It is important to identify patients with primary stones, because their rate of recurrent stones after choledocholithotomy alone is high. Contributing factors may include obstruction of the distal duct, errors in the metabolism of hemoglobin or cholesterol, or bacteria proliferating in a partially obstructed duct. Prevention of recurrent primary stones is best guaranteed by providing a widely patent communication between the common bile duct and the intestinal tract, as will be discussed later in the section on treatment.

The possible involvement of functional abnormalities in the pathogenesis of common duct stones was studied by Toouli et al,[11] who compared the motor behavior of the common duct in patients with common duct stones

Table 18–1 CLASSIFICATION OF COMMON DUCT STONES

Type	Number	Per Cent
Primary	60*	56.1
Secondary	40	37.4
Combined	7	6.5
Total	107	100.0

*No stones in gallbladder: 12 (20.0 per cent)

and in normal subjects. Pressures in the choledochal sphincter were found to be the same in both groups, but a higher percentage of contractions in the patients with stones propagated in a retrograde direction. Toouli et al.[11] postulated that this abnormality might predispose to stasis within the duct and foster the development or retention of common duct stones. These findings could not be reproduced by De Masi and his colleagues,[12] however. Guelrud et al.[13] presented evidence that the subgroup of patients who had pancreatitis due to common duct stones had abnormally high resting pressures within the choledochal sphincter and elevated pressure gradients between the sphincter and the duodenum.

Intrahepatic Stones

The location, number, consistency, and behavior of primary common duct stones are different than for secondary stones (i.e., stones that originate in the gallbladder). Intrahepatic stones in Western countries are most often associated with long-standing ductal obstruction or congenital dilatation of the intrahepatic ducts. Neglected common duct stones, traumatic strictures, slow-growing tumors, and sclerosing cholangitis are common causes of obstruction in such patients. When recurrent cholangitis is superimposed on obstruction, deposition of cellular debris, deconjugated bilirubin, and bile salts contribute to stone formation. Cystic dilatation of the right and left hepatic ducts and their main branches (Caroli's disease), an uncommon familial disease often associated with cystic disease of the kidneys, may lead to stone formation by producing stasis with secondary cholangitis in the cystic areas.

Intrahepatic stones are frequently encountered in persons native to Western China or Hong Kong. The disease that causes this, recurrent pyogenic cholangitis (Oriental cholangiohepatitis), is discussed in detail in Chapter 35.

Intrahepatic stones are manifested by bouts of abdominal pain and cholangitis. The diagnosis often remains obscure until the segmentally dilated ducts containing stones are identified by cholangiography. Intrahepatic stones frequently contain enough calcium to be identified by CT scans but rarely enough to be seen on plain films of the abdomen.

The treatment of intrahepatic stones includes antibiotics for cholangitis, removal of stones via the common duct, and, rarely, resection of portions of the liver if the process is segmental. For poorly understood reasons, recurrent pyogenic cholangitis more often involves the ducts to the left lobe of the liver than those to the right lobe. Intrahepatic stones resulting from common or hepatic duct strictures are best treated by early removal of the stones and procedures to decompress the ducts proximal to the stricture. If the cholangitis is allowed to continue to the point at which numerous segmental strictures have occurred, continued morbidity must be anticipated, and death from uncontrollable sepsis may result.

PATHOPHYSIOLOGY OF COMMON DUCT STONES

Dynamics of Bile Flow

When pressure in the bile duct resulting from obstruction to the passage of bile exceeds 40 cm of water, bile refluxes from canaliculi into the blood stream.[14] Bile pressure, normally about 15 cm H_2O, is generated by the bile secretory mechanism and can reach this high level with complete ductal obstruction. During the interdigestive period, bile enters the gallbladder, where water and electrolytes are absorbed. Gallbladder bile remains isotonic with hepatic bile but becomes concentrated 20 to 30 times. In the resting common bile duct, rhythmic fluctuations of pressure occur at a rate of two to six per minute and generate pressures of up to 30 cm of water. The origin of these contraction waves was traditionally credited to the gallbladder, since the common bile duct contains almost no muscle fibers. However, cholecystectomy does not affect pressure dynamics in the duct, and it is now known that intermittent relaxation and contraction of the ampullary sphincter is the cause.[15] When gastric chyme enters the duodenum, these rhythmic contractions are replaced by tonic contractions of the same magnitude that last 5 to 30 minutes. The tonic contractions are normally accompanied by relaxation of the ampulla of Vater, which drops resting pressure in the duct from 15 cm to 10 cm H_2O. Sphincter pressure does not approach zero even with maximal stimulation by cholecystokinin (CCK). The gallbladder empties 50 to 75 per cent of its contents within 30 minutes of the onset of stimulation.

The normal gallbladder and sphincter of Oddi respond to a large number of substances that release CCK from the duodenum and that increase the concentration of cyclic AMP in the wall of the gallbladder.[16] Parenterally administered CCK causes the gallbladder to contract within 1 to 2 minutes. Exposure of the upper intestine to acid gastric chyme containing dietary fats and essential amino acids results in gallbladder contraction within 10 to 30 minutes. Magnesium hydroxide is also a potent stimulant of gallbladder contraction. Parasympathetic stimulation increases, and sympathetic stimulation decreases gallbladder contraction. Although secretin increases bile flow into the duodenum by relaxing the sphincter of Oddi, other gastrointestinal hormones, such as glucagon and insulin, have no effect except in pharmacologic doses. The question of whether these neurohumoral stimulators of bile flow, sphincter tone, and gallbladder contraction act directly on biliary muscle or through CCK release, and the place of cyclic AMP as a mediator of their action, remain the subject of investigation.

These physiologic questions are discussed further in Chapter 3.

Differing Patterns of Common Bile Duct Obstruction

The orderly flow of bile from the common duct into the duodenum is altered when the duct is obstructed. Obstruction may result from stones occluding the distal common duct, scarring or stricture of the ampulla of Vater, or extrinsic compression of the duct from inflammatory processes or neoplasms. Other causes include duodenal ulcer and metastatic neoplasms. See Chapter 43 for a discussion of other rare causes.

When obstruction is sudden and complete, bile flow stops, as intraductal pressure exceeds the maximal secretory pressure of the liver (i.e., about 40 cm H_2O). If the obstruction is located above the level of the cystic duct or if the gallbladder has been removed, regurgitation of bile into the venous system will be manifested as jaundice within 4 to 6 hours. If the obstruction is below the cystic duct, the gallbladder accepts and concentrates bile, and jaundice does not appear for 36 to 48 hours. In the meantime, the patient experiences biliary colic, often referred to the back and the tip of the scapula, followed by a deep, dull, and often nauseating sensation. If bacteria are present in bile, chills, fever, and leukocytosis follow quickly. If obstruction is relieved because of passage or dislodgment of a stone, or because smooth muscle spasm induced by the stone in the gallbladder or ampulla of Vater subsides, the pain, chills, and fever disappear within an hour or two. If complete obstruction persists and the bile is infected, life-threatening septic cholangitis may follow quickly (see Chapter 19).

Gradual, progressive obstruction is often accompanied by only mild symptoms, such as anorexia, and jaundice may not be apparent until the degree of obstruction passes a threshold 4 to 6 months later. The first symptom in such cases may be pruritus without jaundice, and the alkaline phosphatase level may be very high while the bilirubin level is normal. Occasionally, such a patient may first come to medical attention with manifestations of biliary cirrhosis, such as pruritus, variceal bleeding, or liver failure.

The kidney eliminates bilirubin regurgitated into the blood stream when the bile duct becomes obstructed. As the serum bilirubin concentration rises, the kidney clears a fixed fraction of pigment circulating through it. Consequently, the bilirubin concentration rises rapidly during the early phases of sudden complete obstruction, but thereafter the rate of rise slows and finally reaches a plateau. Complete obstruction results in a plateau bilirubin level between 15 and 30 mg/dl. Higher levels usually indicate concomitant sepsis, renal failure, hemolysis, or operative stress. When obstruction is relieved, 10 to 15 days are required before the bilirubin concentration approaches normal.[17]

Duct obstruction may be associated with cholangitis of varying severity. Cholangitis may be manifested as chills and fever, right upper quadrant pain, and jaundice (Charcot's triad), which resolve spontaneously or after antibiotic treatment.

Obstruction in a patient with transient attacks is often incomplete or only transiently complete as the stone becomes dislodged or spasm of the sphincter subsides. For further details on the pathophysiology of biliary obstruction see Chapter 6.

CLINICAL MANAGEMENT OF COMMON DUCT STONES

Natural History

The natural history of choledocholithiasis is diverse.[18] Some stones may be present for years without causing problems. Rarely, the stones first become apparent only after secondary biliary cirrhosis is well established, and the patient experiences liver failure or variceal bleeding. Other stones may become impacted in the ampulla and cause pain, chills, and fever, requiring hospitalization and an emergency operation.

Many small stones that enter the common duct from the gallbladder pass into the duodenum and are evacuated in the stool, often without producing symptoms. Stones can be recovered from the stools of about 10 per cent of patients with asymptomatic cholelithiasis.[19, 20] Stones less than 3 mm in diameter are probably unable to produce clinical manifestations unless many accumulate simultaneously, or the stone encounters an abnormally narrow distal duct or ampulla. Kelly[20] recovered stones ranging in size from 1 to 12 mm from the feces of 38 of 45 patients (84 per cent) with recurrent gallstone pancreatitis. All the patients had relief of pain and jaundice before the stones were recovered from the stools. Stones that exceed the diameter of the ampulla may remain for years, causing minimal difficulty, or they may, without warning, cause severe cholangitis. Unfortunately, there is no way to determine which stones will cause difficulty. Because knowledge of the natural history of common duct stones is incomplete and it is impossible to predict which patients will develop serious problems,[18] removal of all common duct stones is accepted therapy.[6]

Clinical Presentation

Most often, common duct stones are first diagnosed from operative findings at the time of cholecystectomy;[21] the surgeon feels stones in the duct or the operative cholangiogram shows filling defects. A second common presentation consists of chills and fever, jaundice, and biliary colic (Charcot's triad). Nausea and vomiting are frequently associated with biliary colic, and the pain may radiate to the back and the tip of the scapula. A third common presentation consists of a serum bilirubin elevation two or three times normal and a minimal elevation of the alkaline phosphatase level. If the interval between these minimal findings and a definitive diagnosis of choledocholithiasis exceeds 4 to 5 years, biliary cirrhosis may develop. Other patients present with cholangitis accompanied by positive blood cultures, which usually resolves spontaneously or after antibiotic treatment. A few patients present with obstructive suppurative cholangitis, which has a mortality rate of 30 to 50 per cent. These patients are in septic shock, manifested by mental confusion, hypotension, acidosis, and, often, death.[23] When the duct in these patients is opened, infected bile escapes under pressure. Unrelieved biliary obstruction complicated by infection is a common cause of liver abscess formation. The abscesses are usually scattered throughout the liver parenchyma and frequently herald a fatal outcome.

Physical Signs

The physical signs of choledocholithiasis vary depending on whether the obstruction occurs suddenly or gradually, whether it is partial or complete, and whether the bile is minimally or heavily colonized with bacteria. As previously noted, the appearance of jaundice may follow the onset of symptoms by as much as 48 hours when a functioning gallbladder is present, or 4 hours or less when the gallbladder is absent. Jaundice is most easily detected by examining the sclerae and the mucous membranes of the mouth, especially the palate. In natural light, icterus can be detected when the bilirubin level reaches about 2 mg/dl. Artificial (yellow) light may obscure jaundice even with serum bilirubin levels of 4 to 5 mg/dl.

Most often, the gallbladder cannot be felt on abdominal examination in patients with jaundice caused by common duct stones. However, if the onset of common duct obstruction coincides with an attack of cholecystitis, a mass may be detected in the right subcostal region. In this situation the mass mostly represents inflamed omentum or loops of small bowel, and it is often tender. Liver tenderness secondary to obstructed outflow from the distal common bile duct or accompanying cholangitis may be mistaken for a tender palpable gallbladder. If choledocholithiasis is accompanied by pancreatitis, epigastric tenderness is usually present, and a mass or fullness may be felt over the pancreas.

Laboratory Diagnosis

Laboratory examinations may be normal in patients with nonobstructing common bile duct stones.[21] In patients with symptoms, laboratory tests reflect the degree of bile duct obstruction and the severity of secondary infection.[23] Thus, the white blood count may be normal, elevated to 15,000 or 18,000/mm^2 in cholangitis, or depressed to 2000 to 3000/mm^2 in overwhelming sepsis. Choledocholithiasis commonly produces an elevation of the serum alkaline phosphatase concentration.[17] The rise may be transient if the obstruction is transient, but the height of the alkaline phosphatase does not correlate with the degree of obstruction or the level of the serum bilirubin. A normal serum alkaline phosphatase concentration is evidence against a common duct stone as the cause of a patient's symptoms. The serum transaminase levels (SGOT and SGPT) are often transiently elevated to 200 to 500 units. The serum transaminases have a half-life of only a few hours. Transient, very high levels of these enzymes may follow acute injury, shock, congestive heart failure, or hypoxia. Transient elevations lasting 24 to 48 hours associated with a rise in the alkaline phosphatase value are very suggestive of common duct obstruction. Marked and more prolonged elevation of serum transaminases is more characteristic of viral hepatitis; prolonged, milder elevations are typical of chronic hepatitis, cirrhosis, or alcoholic liver disease. LDH levels may also rise to as high as ten times normal, higher than is usually recorded during viral hepatitis. A mild elevation of the serum bilirubin level (less than 3 mg/dl) occurs in roughly 30 per cent of patients with acute cholecystitis.[24] Higher levels usually indicate the presence of a common duct stone (Figure 18–1).[17,21,23,25] Serum bilirubin levels rarely exceed 10 mg/ml in patients with choledocholithiasis. Serum bilirubin levels above 15 mg/ml are almost always indicative of a stricture (benign or malignant) or parenchymal disease of the liver.[17] Although liver enzyme determinations may suggest choledocholithiasis as the cause for jaundice, liver biopsy is usually necessary to rule out causes other than common duct stone when the diagnosis is uncertain.

Special Diagnostic Tests

Ultrasonography has largely replaced intravenous cholangiography (IVC) as the primary screening examination for patients with

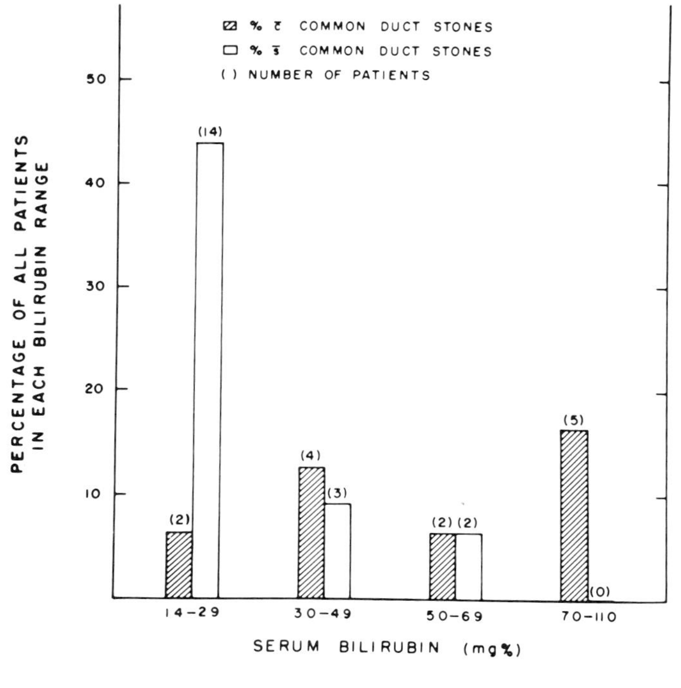

Figure 18–1. Distribution of 32 patients with and without common duct stones according to degree of elevation of serum bilirubin levels.

suspected common duct stones.[21, 23] Although the diagnostic accuracy of IVC may approach 70 per cent when the bilirubin value is less than 2.5 mg/dl, the test has a low reliability and occasionally is followed by a serious allergic reaction.[26] Ultrasonography is inexpensive, widely available, and detects gallbladder stones and dilated ducts with an accuracy approaching 90 per cent.[27] It is very accurate in detecting gallbladder stones but rarely locates stones in the duct (other than indirectly by demonstrating dilatation). Even when the examination is inconclusive, the sonogram often provides the information needed to select the best confirmatory examination (i.e., percutaneous or endoscopic retrograde cholangiography).

Computerized axial tomography gives information similar to that of ultrasound scans, but CT is less accurate in detecting gallbladder stones, is considerably more expensive, and because of the radiation exposure, cannot be used repeatedly to follow changes in a lesion.

An upper gastrointestinal barium x-ray study may show encroachment of an obstructing tumor on the duodenum, a diverticulum at the ampulla of Vater, or unrelated but surgically significant upper gastrointestinal abnormalities.

Percutaneous transhepatic cholangiography successfully opacifies the biliary tract in 65 per cent of normal subjects and in over 90 per cent of patients with bile duct obstruction.[28] Although endoscopic retrograde cholangiography (ERCP) requires special skills and is relatively expensive, it has the advantage of opacifying both the pancreatic and the bile duct in most cases.[23, 29, 30] The size of the duct cannot be accurately determined by this technique, since the injection of contrast medium may dilate the duct beyond its resting size.

Treatment

The presence of a stone in the common bile duct is sufficient indication for its removal. A controversy, if one exists today, concerns the timing and method by which the removal should be performed. In general, the greater the patient risk, the greater is the urgency of definitive management. Patients with diabetes mellitus, debilitation, or advanced age tolerate cholangitis or an emergency operation poorly.

Preoperative Preparation

An accurate preoperative diagnosis and careful preoperative preparation are important for the safe management of patients with biliary tract obstruction. The risks of an unnecessary or wrong operation and the increased morbidity and mortality from inadequate preoperative preparation are substantial. The current emphases on shortening hospitalization time, decreasing the number of diagnostic tests, and avoiding unnecessary antibiotic therapy are appropriate for many patients coming to operation. However, failure to obtain accurate information on the morphology of the obstructed bile duct, to correct metabolic abnormalities, and to rule out alternative causes of the patient's problem may increase mortality and morbidity. Although intraoperative cholangiography usually gives adequate information on the size of the ducts, the site and cause of obstruction, and the number and location of stones, obtaining this information with the patient under general anesthesia prolongs the operation, requires critical decisions to be made at the operating table, and may subject a small number of patients to an unnecessary operation. Thus, preoperative cholangiography is often indicated except in the most routine cases.

Correction of fluid and electrolyte abnormalities can almost always be accomplished within 4 to 6 hours and will be time well spent, even in patients with septic cholangitis. A urine flow of at least 20 ml/hour should be established preoperatively. Patients with unstable hemodynamics often require monitoring of central venous and right heart pressures. Use of a Swan-Ganz catheter also permits simultaneous monitoring of cardiac output using thermodilution techniques. In general, changes in pressure and cardiac output in an individual patient are more important than specific deviations from normal values, which have been largely derived from postcardiotomy patients. Septic patients with low serum albumin concentrations may present with central venous pressures of 2 or 3 mm Hg, mean right heart pressures of 3 or 4 mm Hg, and cardiac outputs of 13 or 14 liters. If one administers intravenous crystalloid and colloid solutions in an effort to obtain more "normal" readings, pulmonary edema or heart failure may develop. A doubling of venous and right heart pressures often represents adequate volume replacement.

Parenteral vitamin K will correct clotting abnormalities in most patients unless liver function is seriously deranged. Oral vitamin K is poorly absorbed from the gastrointestinal tract of jaundiced patients because it is fat-soluble and requires bile salts for absorption. If the prothrombin time fails to return toward normal after three daily doses of 5 mg, the presence of hepatic parenchymal dysfunction should be assumed.

Perioperative antibiotics should be routinely administered to patients undergoing operations for choledocholithiasis. Approximately 80 per cent of patients with obstruction secondary to stones have infected bile, and the incidence is 100 per cent in patients with cholangitis. Bacterial colonization of bile is less frequent in patients with obstruction secondary to neoplasms. The cephalosporins are secreted in bile and are effective against most strains of *E. coli,* the most common organism.[31] Parenteral cefazolin provides an equivalent concentration of antibiotic in bile within 1 hour at half the dosage of cephalothin, and its half-life in bile is twice as long. None of the antibiotics reaches therapeutic levels in bile when the duct is osbtructed, so therapeutic effects depend on tissue levels. A dose should be given 4 to 6 hours preoperatively, during operation, and 6 hours postoperatively. Suppurative cholangitis should be treated with antibiotics effective against aerobic and anaerobic organisms, and these drugs should be continued postoperatively and modified in response to the results of bile cultures.[32] It may also be helpful to perform a Gram stain of bile during operation.

Choledochotomy

Choledochotomy and choledocholithotomy are the principal therapy for choledocholithiasis. If the operation is performed primarily for cholecystolithiasis and common duct stones are suspected, an intraoperative cholangiogram should be performed via the cystic duct. The study may give useful information even when stones are known to be present in the duct. Operative cholangiography gives information on the location and number of stones, but there is a tendency to underestimate the number.[21] It has been shown that operative cholangiography has the power to decrease the incidence of negative common duct explorations (from 65 to 35 per cent) and missed common duct stones (from 15 to 8 per cent).[21, 33]

The role of manometry and flow studies in addition to intraoperative cholangiography through the cystic duct remains to be defined. The unobstructed ampulla of Vater has an opening pressure of less than 15 cm H_2O and a flow rate greater than 10 ml/minute at a duct pressure of 30 cm H_2O.[33] If one or both of these limits are exceeded, common duct exploration has been recommended. White reports that flow and pressure studies are as accurate as intraoperative cholangiography.[33] Furthermore, they have the advantage of identifying patients for whom sphincteroplasty or choledochoenteric bypass are necessary because of ampullary stenosis or stricture of the lower end of the duct. Data from a study comparing intraoperative cholangiography with pressure and flow determinations are summarized in Table 18–2.[29] We consider these data to be preliminary and in need of confirmation before they can be recommended as having a bona fide place in biliary surgery.

The absolute indications for exploring the common bile duct are the following: (1) a positive intraoperative cholangiogram; (2) preoperative diagnosis of common duct stones; (3) stone palpable in the common bile duct; and (4) active cholangitis (Figure 18–2).[21] A history of previous jaundice or pancreatitis, small stones, or a dilated duct, the so-called relative indications for common duct exploration, usually require a positive operative cholangiogram before exploration

Table 18–2 INTRAOPERATIVE COMMON DUCT ASSESSMENT

	Uninterpretable	False Negative	False Positive	Accuracy
Cholangiography	0	3/183	9/183	12/183 (93%)
Resting pressure only	0	11/79	7/179	18/179 (90%)
Flow only	0	5/91	3/91	8/91 (91%)
Flow and pressure	3	5/89	2/89	7/89 (92%)
Flow, pressure and cholangiography	0	0/158	3/158	3/158 (98%)

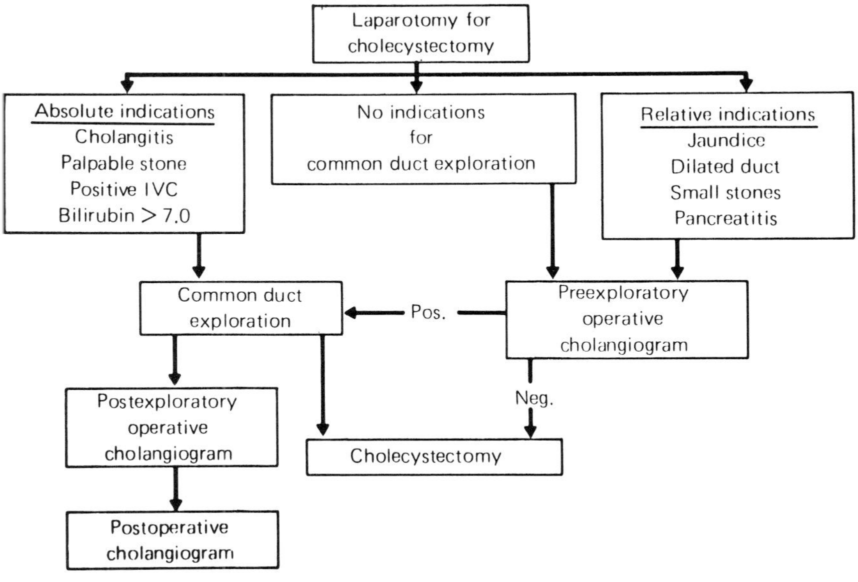

Figure 18–2. Choledocholithiasis: Indications for common duct exploration.

is undertaken. If the cholangiogram is positive, technically faulty, or does not clearly rule out stones, duct exploration should be performed.

Common duct exploration should follow a carefully established routine. The technique is described in Chapter 22. The 8 to 10 per cent incidence of overlooked stones following duct exploration can be decreased to 2 to 4 per cent by the use of choledochoscopy.[34] The choledochoscope allows a thorough inspection of the distal common duct and the primary, secondary, and tertiary ducts proximally. A T-tube should be left in the duct to allow intraoperative cholangiography before terminating the operation, postoperative decompression of the biliary tract, and a tract for removal of any overlooked stones. After 7 days of gravity drainage, a postoperative cholangiogram will verify absence of stones, free flow of contrast material in the duodenum, and the absence of a leak from the choledochotomy. The T-tube is then left to gravity drainage for 24 hours, when either it is pulled or the patient is discharged to have the tube removed 7 to 14 days later. Drains placed at the time of choledochotomy and brought through a stab wound in the flank may be removed in 36 to 48 hours if there is no bile drainage.

The treatment of retained stones detected on postoperative T-tube cholangiograms is discussed in Chapter 10.

Endoscopic Sphincterotomy

Endoscopic transduodenal sphincterotomy to remove common duct stones is the procedure of choice for most patients with choledocholithiasis who have had a previous cholecystectomy.[35–37] The technique involves passing a wire via an endoscope into the distal common duct and using cautery to create a 1 cm sphincterotomy. Retained stones usually pass spontaneously into the duodenum. Endoscopy and endoscopic cholangiography are repeated in 7 to 14 days to verify that the stones have passed. If the stones fail to pass through the enlarged ampulla, they may be removed using specially designed instruments. Endoscopic sphincterotomy for residual or recurrent stones was successful in 86 per cent of patients in the hands of Shapiro.[35] A detailed discussion of endoscopic therapy is contained in Chapter 25.

Drainage Procedures

Drainage procedures are indicated at the time of choledochotomy in specified situations. Allen et al.[35] recommend performing a drainage procedure when: (1) many stones are present in the duct, (2) there has been a previous choledocholithotomy, (3) the duct is greater than 2 cm in diameter, (4) not all stones can be removed from the duct, and (5) the duct is strictured distal to the choledochotomy. Each of these clinical situations is associated with a high rate of recurrent stones after choledocholithotomy alone. For instance, the recurrence rate after choledocholithotomy without a drainage procedure in patients with primary duct stones, abnormal ducts, or previous choledocholithotomy was about 30%.[35, 38]

Duct decompression may be by transendoscopic sphincterotomy, by transduodenal sphincteroplasty, or by duct-enteric anastomosis. Sphincteroplasty is favored when the duct is small or its distal segment stenotic. Otherwise, I prefer an end-to-side anastomosis of the duct to a Roux-en-Y limb of jejunum for drainage. In my opinion, side-to-side choledochoduodenostomy, although technically simple and satisfactory in patients with a short life expectancy, is too often associated with stenosis, bouts of ascending cholangitis, and inspissation of food in the distal duct (sump syndrome).

Conclusions

The overall results of surgical treatment of choledocholithiasis are excellent. To achieve the best results, however, it is important to perform a drainage procedure when the aforementioned indications are present. Endoscopic sphincterotomy has proved to be a simpler and equally successful technique for treating choledocholithiasis in patients who have had a previous cholecystectomy, and it is often of immediate value to bring acute cholangitis under control in patients who still possess their gallbladders.

REFERENCES

1. Admirand WH, Small DM: Physiochemical basis of cholesterol gallstone formation in man. J Clin Invest 1968;*47*:1043.
2. Carey MC, Small DM: The physical chemistry of cholesterol solubility in bile. J Clin Invest 1978;*61*:998.
3. Holan KR, Holzbach RT, Hermann RE, et al: Nucleation time: A key factor in the pathogenesis of cholesterol gallstone disease. Gastroenterology 1979;*77*:611.
4. Bernhoft RA, Pellegrini CA, Motson RW, et al: Composition and morphologic and clinical features of common duct stones. Am J Surg 1984;*148*:77.
5. Madden J: The nature and significance of common duct stones. Surg Gynecol Obstet 1968;*126*:3.
6. Madden J: Common duct stones, their origin and surgical management. Surg Clin North Am 1973;*53*:1095.
7. Aschoff L: Lectures in Pathology. New York, Paul B. Hoever, 1924.
8. Colcock BP, Perey B: Exploration of the common bile duct. Surg Gynecol Obstet 1964;*118*:20.
9. Gerwig WH, Countryman LK, Gomez AC: Congenital absence of the gallbladder and cystic duct. Ann Surg 1961;*153*:113.
10. Thurston OG, McDougall RM: The effect of hepatic bile on retained common duct stones. Surg Gynecol Obstet 1976;*143*:625.
11. Toouli J, Geenen JE, Hogan WJ, et al: Sphincter of Oddi motor activity: a comparison between patients with common bile duct stones and controls. Gastroenterology 1982;*82*:111.
12. De Masi E, Corazziari E, Habib FI, et al: Manometric study of the sphincter of Oddi in patients with and without common bile duct stones. Gut 1984;*25*:275.
13. Guelrud M, Mendoza S, Vicent S, et al: Pressures in the sphincter of Oddi in patients with gallstones, common duct stones, and recurrent pancreatitis. J Clin Gastroenterol 1983;*5*:37.
14. Huang T, Bass JA, Williams RD: The significance of biliary pressure in cholangitis. Arch Surg 1969;*98*:629.
15. Ashkin JR, Soloway RD: Factors affecting delivery of bile to the duodenum in man. Gastroenterology 1978;*74*:560.
16. Lin TN: Actions of gastrointestinal hormones and related peptides on the motor function of the biliary tract. Gastroenterology 1975;*69*:1006.
17. Pellegrini CA, Thomas MJ, Way LW: Bilirubin and alkaline phosphatase values before and after surgery for biliary obstruction. Am J Surg 1982;*143*:67.
18. Way LW: Retained common duct stones. Surg Clin North Am 1973;*53*:1139.
19. Acosta JN, Ledesma CL: Gallstone migration as a cause of acute pancreatitis. N Engl J Med 1974;*290*:484.
20. Kelly T: Gallstone pancreatitis: Pathophysiology. Surgery 1976;*80*:488.
21. Way LW, Admirand WH, Dunphy JE: Management of choledocholithiasis. Ann Surg 1972;*176*:347.
22. Thomas MJ, Pellegrini CA, Way LW: Usefulness of diagnostic tests for biliary obstruction. Am J Surg 1982;*144*:102.
23. Welch JP, Donaldson G: The urgency of diagnosis and surgical treatment of acute suppurative cholangitis. Am J Surg 1976;*131*:527.
24. Dumont AE: Significance of hyperbilirubinemia in acute cholecystitis. Surg Gynecol Obstet 1976; *142*:855
25. Rosoff L: Biochemical tests for hepatobiliary disease. Surg Clin North Am 1977;*57*:257.
26. Goodman MW, Ansel HJ, Vennes JA, et al: Is intravenous cholangiography still useful? Gastroenterology 1980;*79*:642.
27. Goldstein LI, Sample WF, et al: Gray-scale ultrasonography and thin-needle cholangiography. JAMA 1977;*238*:1041.
28. Elias E, Hamlyn AN, Jain S, et al: A randomized trial of percutaneous transhepatic cholangiography with the Chiba needle versus endoscopic retrograde cholangiography for bile duct visualization in jaundice. Gastroenterology 1976;*71*:439.
29. Shapiro HA: Endoscopic diagnosis and treatment of biliary disease. Surg Clin North Am 1981;*61*:843.

30. Ghazi A, McSherry CK: Endoscopic retrograde cholangiopancreatography and sphincterotomy. Ann Surg 1984;*199*:21.
31. Williams MMK, Regamey C: Pharmacokinetics of cefazolin compared with four other cephalosporins. J Infect Dis 1973;*128*:5341.
32. Keighley MRE, McLeish AR, Alexander-Williams J, et al: Identification of the presence and type of biliary microflora by immediate Gram stains. Surgery 1977;*81*:469.
33. White TW, Bordley J: One percent incidence of recurrent stones six to eight years after manometric cholangiography. Ann Surg 1978;*188*:562.
34. Tompkins RK, Johnson J, Longmire WP: Operative endoscopy in the management of biliary tract neoplasms. Am J Surg 1976;*132*:174.
35. Allen B, Shapiro H, Way LW: Management of recurrent and residual common duct stones. Am J Surg 1981;*142*:41.
36. Mazzeo RJ, Jordan FT, Strasius ST: Endoscopic papillotomy for recurrent common bile duct stones and papillary stenosis. A community hospital experience. Arch Surg 1983;*118*:693.
37. Cotton PB: Endoscopic management of bile duct stones; (apples and oranges). Gut 1984;*25*:587.

HENRY A. PITT, M.D.
JOHN L. CAMERON, M.D.

19

Acute Cholangitis

In 1877 Charcot[1] provided the first detailed description of cholangitis when he wrote that "intermittent hepatic fever" developed secondary to ". . . stagnant bile." He also stated very astutely that stones, benign strictures, and malignancies were responsible for this clinical syndrome. This statement, of course, remains true more than 100 years later. Only in very recent years, however, has the phenomenon of cholangitis following nonoperative biliary manipulations been added to Charcot's list of stones, strictures, and tumors as a common cause of cholangitis.

Since Charcot's initial description, the triad of intermittent fever and chills, jaundice, and abdominal pain that bears his name has become widely recognized as the hallmark of cholangitis. Not until 1959 did Reynolds and Dargan[2] add central nervous system depression and shock to Charcot's triad. These authors suggested that this pentad was characteristic of a virulent form of cholangitis that became known as acute "suppurative" cholangitis. They also felt that this severe form of cholangitis was due to complete, as opposed to partial, biliary obstruction and was associated with pus in the bile ducts.

In recent years, however, it has become clear that not all patients with Reynolds' pentad have pus in their bile ducts and, vice versa, that suppuration within the biliary tree is not always associated with mental depression and shock. Thus, the term "suppurative cholangitis" technically should be reserved for those patients found to have biliary pus and should not be used to characterize clinical symptoms. Perhaps a better term for those patients with the most severe clinical forms of biliary sepsis might be "acute toxic cholangitis."

PATHOPHYSIOLOGY

The two factors necessary for the initiation of clinical cholangitis are (1) the presence of significant numbers of bacteria within the biliary tree and (2) elevation of intraductal pressure sufficient to cause a reflux of bacteria or endotoxin into the blood stream (Fig. 19–1). Obstruction plays a key role in the pathogenesis of acute cholangitis because it has the dual effect of increasing the concentration of bacteria due to stasis and of causing an increase in intraductal pressure. The presence of a foreign body, such as a gallstone or parasite, within the biliary tree is almost always associated with bacterial growth and can readily cause obstruction.

Bacterial Factors

Cultures of normal gallbladder and common duct bile are almost always sterile. When gallstones are present, however, gallbladder bile and gallbladder wall cultures are positive at least 50 per cent of the time.[3, 4] In addition, when a stone is present in the common duct, cultures are positive in 75 to 90 per cent of patients, despite the fact that many of these patients may be asymptomatic.[5–8] With partial common duct obstruction due to choledocholithiasis, benign biliary strictures, or a previous biliary-intestinal anastomosis, common duct bile cultures yield organisms in 90 to 100 per cent of patients.[3, 5, 6, 8] However, with complete ductal obstruction, commonly seen with malignancy, only 25 to 40 per cent of bile cultures are positive for bacteria.[8–10] Thus, infected bile appears to correlate with the presence of a foreign body (stones or

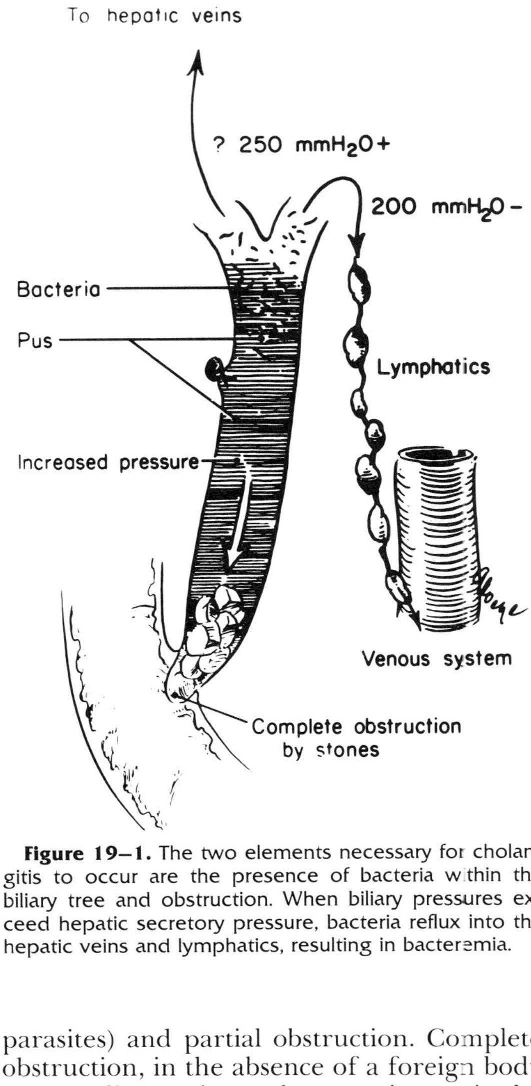

Figure 19–1. The two elements necessary for cholangitis to occur are the presence of bacteria within the biliary tree and obstruction. When biliary pressures exceed hepatic secretory pressure, bacteria reflux into the hepatic veins and lymphatics, resulting in bacteremia.

parasites) and partial obstruction. Complete obstruction, in the absence of a foreign body or any diagnostic or therapeutic manipulation, is less apt to be associated with infected bile or acute cholangitis.

The incidence of positive bile cultures has also been shown to have a direct correlation with advancing age.[6, 8, 11, 12] The organisms most commonly cultured in the bile are *E. coli, Klebsiella pneumoniae,* and *Streptococcus faecalis* (enterococcus). These organisms are similar to those seen in the upper intestinal tract.[13] Prior to 1975, there was a striking absence of anaerobic bacteria cultured from the bile in most published series. The absence of anaerobes within the biliary tree may have been a reflection of (1) inhibition of their growth by bile salts[14, 15] or (2) inadequate culturing techniques. However, since 1975, numerous reports[8, 16–21] have documented the presence of anaerobes, including *Bacteroides fragilis* in bile cultures. Careful analysis of these reports, however, suggests that those patients most likely to harbor anaerobes include (1) the elderly, (2) those with complex biliary problems, and (3) those who present with cholangitis.

The fact that patients presenting with cholangitis are most likely to have anaerobes in their bile is supported by an analysis by Pitt and his colleagues[7] of patients with choledocholithiasis (Table 19–1). Twenty-seven per cent of patients with common duct stones who presented with cholangitis had anaerobes recovered from operative bile cultures. In comparison, only 5 per cent of patients with no preoperative fever had anaerobes in their bile. This difference was statistically significant ($p < 0.01$). A more complete discussion of specific bacteria recovered in patients with cholangitis can be found in the section on laboratory data.

The pathway by which bacteria reach the biliary tree is still not entirely clear. Possibilities include (1) the ascending route, through the common duct from the duodenum; (2) through gastrointestinal and biliary tract lymphatics; (3) via the hepatic artery; (4) via the portal vein; and (5) from a chronically infected gallbladder. The ascending route through the bile duct was proposed by Edlund et al.[5] in 1959 by a process of elimination and because their work, that of Taylor,[22] and that of Orloff and associates[23] showed very little support for the portal vein bacteremia route. Moreover, the fact that acute cholangitis is uncommon in the face of complete common duct obstruction is supportive circumstantial evidence for the ascending route. Although the ascending route at first seems quite logical, there are no experimental or clinical data to confirm reflux with a normal sphincter mechanism.

Table 19–1 BILE CULTURE DATA IN 73 PATIENTS WITH CHOLEDOCHOLITHIASIS

Bile Culture	Preoperative Cholangitis: *Yes (%) (n=33)*	Preoperative Cholangitis: *No (%) (n=40)*
Positive	88*	65
Gram-negative aerobes	76†	38
Gram positive aerobes	45	45
Anaerobes	27†	5

*$p < 0.025$
†$p < 0.01$
Adapted from Pitt HA, Postier RG, Cameron JL: Surgery 1983;*94*:447.

Investigators have shown that Evans blue dye injected into the duodenum will extend along the common bile duct lymphatics to the gallbladder,[5] but no experimental evidence suggests that bacteria can pass from ductal lymphatics back into bile. In addition, experimental work in guinea pigs by Dineen[24] demonstrated that the number of bacteria reaching the bile was insignificant if the bacteria were introduced via duodenal lymphatics. His studies showed that the flow of lymph around the common duct was toward periduodenal and celiac lymph nodes and away from the liver.

Multiple small abscesses can develop within the liver in cases of severe sepsis. Presumably, these bacteria reach the liver via the hepatic artery. However, no clinical or experimental data suggest that this route is a frequent source of biliary bacteria. Edlund and associates[5] initially thought that the portal vein was an unlikely source of bacteria in the bile. However, Dineen[24] subsequently showed that this pathway was by far the most significant and efficient mechanism for deliverying bacteria to bile in his experimental model. Dineen's studies also demonstrated that obstruction of bile flow increased the number of bacteria recovered from the bile after introduction of bacteria into the portal vein.

Initial clinical studies showed a very low incidence of positive portal vein cultures in normal individuals. However, subsequent reports have documented portal vein bacteremias in a variety of circumstances. In 1955 Schatten and associates[25] found a 32 per cent incidence of positive portal vein cultures in patients undergoing upper abdominal operations. In 1958 Brooke and Slaney[26] showed a high incidence of portal vein bacteremia in patients with ulcerative colitis. Ong[27] in 1962 reported a 40 per cent incidence of positive portal vein cultures from 33 patients with recurrent pyogenic cholangitis who were in an acute phase of the disease. Peripheral vein blood samples taken at the same time revealed only a 15 per cent incidence of positive cultures. In contrast, portal vein cultures taken from 64 patients operated upon during a quiescent phase of recurrent pyogenic cholangitis were positive in only 6 per cent.

The portal vein theory assumes that small numbers of enteric bacteria frequently enter the portal circulation. Some of these organisms are removed by the reticuloendothelial system within the liver, and some are excreted into the bile. With a normal biliary tree these organisms pass innocently back into the intestinal tract. However, in the presence of a foreign body such as a stone, and particularly with obstruction to the flow of bile, bacteria that have survived this route are able to multiply.

One potential objection to the portal vein theory is that the low incidence of anaerobes recovered from the bile does not reflect the flora seen in the lower intestinal tract. However, the fact that bile salts inhibit anaerobic growth may be a partial explanation. Moreover, the recent observation that anaerobes are found in approximately one fourth of patients with cholangitis refutes this potential objection. The fact that anaerobes are able to flourish when obstruction is present may be due to diminished secretion and concentration of bile salts in the bile of these patients.

Thus, most investigators agree that the portal vein is the most likely route of bacterial invasion of the biliary tree. However, Scott and Khan[28] in 1967 suggested that organisms in an infected common bile duct may be derived from a chronically infected gallbladder. These authors argued that gallbladder wall infection is initiated by the hematogenous route, although others subsequently suggested that organisms may reach the gallbladder via the portal vein route. Within the gallbladder, stasis may promote bacterial growth in both the bile and the gallbladder wall. This combined theory is supported by the fact that the same organisms are almost always cultured from the gallbladder wall and the common duct bile in an individual patient. This theory also explains the low incidence of common bile duct infection seen with complete obstruction due to a tumor. The portal vein–infected gallbladder theory would be further supported if it could be shown that the 25 to 40 per cent of patients with complete obstruction due to a tumor who do have positive bile cultures also had gallstones or a chronically infected gallbladder.

Obstructive Factors

Flemma and his colleagues[3] demonstrated quite convincingly in 1967 that the presence of bacteria in the bile, even in concentrations greater than 10^5 organisms/ml, is not sufficient to produce cholangitis without concomitant obstruction. They showed that cholangitis could be precipitated by cholangiography and felt that the syndrome of clinical cholangitis with fever and chills was the result of disruption of the biliary tract mucosa with a direct entry of bacteria from the biliary system into the blood stream producing a septicemia.

As early as 1947, Mixer and his associates[29] demonstrated that particles the size of bacteria or viruses could be transferred to the blood stream in association with cholangiography. They also observed that biliary pressures in the range of 20 cm of water were necessary to initiate reflux from the biliary system into the blood stream. In 1953 Edlund and Hanzon[30] demonstrated by fluorescent microscopic studies a direct communication between terminal bile duct canaliculi and liver sinusoids. The existence of this communication was also confirmed by electron microscopic studies done by Rouiller in 1956[31] and by Hampton in 1958.[32]

Further support for the direct anatomic communication between biliary canaliculi and liver sinusoids came in 1962, when Hultborn and his associates[33] demonstrated reflux of radioactive-labeled saline, dye, albumin, and gold when these substances were injected into an obstructed common bile duct. Reflux occurred so rapidly that these authors concluded that the communication must have been a direct one with the venous, as opposed to the lymphatic, system. In this study, particles of up to 200 or 300 Å, slightly larger than the size of a virus, could be regurgitated into the blood stream at relatively low biliary pressures.

Studies by Jacobsson et al.,[34] also published in 1952, demonstrated that radioactive-labeled bacteria refluxed into the blood stream at pressures that were only slightly higher than the secretory pressure of the liver (15 cm of water). In this experiment the majority of bacteria were filtered off in the liver, but approximately 10 per cent of injected organisms entered the blood stream. In 1969 Huang et al.[35] demonstrated in dogs that hepatic vein blood and thoracic duct lymph remained sterile if the pressure within an infected common bile duct remained less than 20 cm of water. When pressures were raised above 25 cm of water, organisms appeared rapidly in both the blood and the lymph. Moreover, the concentrations of bacteria in both these systems were directly proportional to the bile duct pressure. These authors stressed that increased biliary pressure associated with obstruction was the key factor in the pathogenesis of the bacteremia in cholangitis.

In 1952 Mallet-Guy[36] determined that normal biliary pressures ranged from 7 to 14 cm of water. This finding was confirmed in canine studies by Williams et al.[37] in 1967. With partial common duct obstruction, however, the average intraductal pressure increased to 18 cm of water, and this pressure increased even further to 29 cm of water with complete obstruction. Hopton and White[38] confirmed the presence of increased resting biliary tract pressures in patients with a diseased common bile duct.

With complete obstruction resting pressures are higher than with partial obstruction. Cholangitis, however, is more commonly associated with partial than with complete obstruction. This apparent discrepancy is explained by the fact that bile is more frequently infected in patients with partial obstruction, which is usually associated with biliary calculi. Total obstruction, on the other hand, is more often associated with a malignancy. Moreover, acute cholangitis is more likely to occur when a sudden increase in intraductal pressure occurs with choledocholithiasis or during cholangiography. The gradual obstruction that accompanies a tumor is less likely to result in bacterial reflux.

Thus, the clinical symptoms of fever and chills associated with cholangitis are due to a systemic bacteremia caused by a cholangiovenous or a cholangiolymphatic reflux of organisms that results from a rise in intrabiliary pressure. The presence of infected bile without obstruction or of obstruction without infection is not sufficient to produce clinical cholangitis. Thus, both infection and obstruction are necessary, and the presence of a foreign body within the biliary tree enhances both of these factors.

Until very recently, in the vast majority of series, common duct stones were the most common cause of biliary obstruction resulting in acute cholangitis. In fact, in a collected series of 303 patients with cholangitis described by Pitt and Longmire[39] in 1980 nearly 80 per cent of the cases were due to choledocholithiasis (Table 19–2). Benign strictures, obstructed biliary anastomoses, and malignant strictures accounted for most of the other cases. However, a recent analysis by Thompson et al.[40] from UCLA suggests that malignant obstruction and congenital problems are now frequent causes of cholan-

Table 19–2 CHANGING ETIOLOGY OF CHOLANGITIS AT TERTIARY REFERRAL CENTERS

	Literature[39] 1960–1980 (%)	UCLA[40] 1970–1980 (%)	UCLA[41] 1984–1985 (%)
Choledocholithiasis	79	25	22
Benign strictures*	10	53	4
Malignant strictures	9	19	39
Nonoperative manipulations	—	—	35

*Includes iatrogenic and anastomotic strictures, congenital anomalies, and sclerosing cholangitis.

gitis at selected tertiary referral centers. Moreover, a more recent study[41] from the same institution suggests that nonoperative biliary manipulations, often in patients with end-stage malignancies, have become a leading cause of cholangitis.

With the increased utilization of transhepatic, T-tube, and endoscopic retrograde cholangiography as well as percutaneous transhepatic drainage and endoprosthesis placement, cholangitis following biliary manipulation has become a frequent occurrence. In a series of 100 consecutive T-tube cholangiograms performed at the Johns Hopkins Hospital, nine patients developed documented instances of bacteremia.[16] In a series of 75 patients undergoing transhepatic cholangiography,[3] five developed cholangitis. Bacteremia has also been reported following endoscopic retrograde cholangiography[42] and nonoperative extraction of biliary calculi through T-tube tracts.[43]

CLINICAL PRESENTATION

As with many disorders, all degrees of severity of bacterial cholangitis can occur. In some instances the entity may be so mild and of such short duration that the episode resolves without the patient seeking medical aid. At the opposite end of the spectrum is the patient who presents moribund with a picture of septic shock and who, at the time of surgery or autopsy, is found to have gross pus under pressure in the bile ducts as well as multiple liver abscesses (Fig. 19–2). These latter patients should be categorized as having acute toxic cholangitis. This entity, however, represents one end of a particularly broad spectrum of pathology that is termed cholangitis.

The clinical presentation of a patient with cholangitis can be quite variable. Not all patients with cholangitis present with Charcot's triad of fever and chills, jaundice, and abdominal pain, and not all patients with this triad have cholangitis. Pancreatitis, acute cholecystitis, pyelonephritis, or sepsis from a variety of sources may at times present with fever and chills, jaundice, and some degree of abdominal pain. In addition, many patients with cholangitis do not have one or more of the triad that is classically seen with cholangitis. Thus, as Rogers[44] pointed out in 1903, "this condition . . . is of considerable importance on account of the very great difficulty of diagnosis. . . ."

This difficulty in diagnosis is apparent from a series of 180 hospitalized patients with the clinical diagnosis of cholangitis seen at the Johns Hopkins Hospital between 1952 and 1974.[45] On close inspection, only 78 of the 180 patients had enough clinical, laboratory, radiographic, operative, or post-mortem data to support the diagnosis with any surety. Moreover, in a series of 36 patients with cholangitis seen at the University of

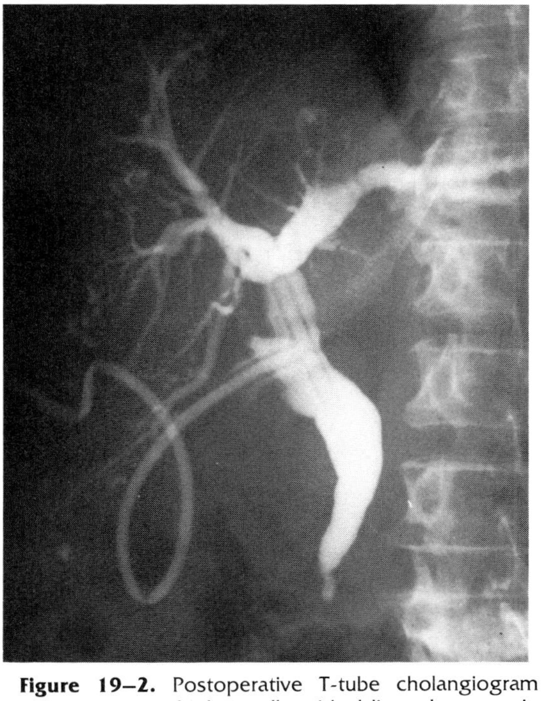

Figure 19–2. Postoperative T-tube cholangiogram demonstrating multiple small residual liver abscesses in a patient who had presented with "suppurative" cholangitis.

California at San Diego (UCSD), the diagnosis was made prospectively in only 18 patients, the remaining being diagnosed at surgery or at autopsy.[40]

In recent years most authors have focused on the most severe form of cholangitis, and little attention has been paid to the less severe varieties of the disease. Often, in taking a history from a patient with gallstones, an episode of fever, chills, and jaundice is described. The patient may state that the episode lasted for 24 hours and abated without medical aid being sought. In addition, patients with benign strictures frequently will have recurrent episodes of cholangitis that are easily managed at home with oral antibiotics. With more severe forms of cholangitis, however, most patients are ill enough to seek medical aid, and most require hospitalization. At the far end of the spectrum is the patient with toxic cholangitis who may be admitted in septic shock and who may die before surgery can be undertaken.

Patients who present with cholangitis tend to be in an older age group than is ordinarily seen with biliary tract disease. The average age of the 78 patients in a series from Johns Hopkins was 61 years, with a range of 30 to 87 years.[45] In another series of 73 consecutive patients with choledocholithiasis seen at the Johns Hopkins Hospital, the mean age of the 33 patients presenting with cholangitis was 61 years.[7] In comparison, the mean age of the 40 patients in this series with common duct stones and no preoperative cholangitis was only 48 years ($p < 0.001$). Among 36 patients with cholangitis reported from UCSD, 16 were older than 70 years, and 11 were older than 80 years.[46] Despite the fact that biliary calculi are more frequent in females than in males, the sex ratio of patients with cholangitis is approximately equal. Forty of the 78 patients in the earlier series from Johns Hopkins[45] were males, and in the series from UCSD, two thirds of the patients were males.

The classic presentation of fever and chills, abdominal pain, and jaundice is by no means always present (Table 19–3). Although all 78 patients presenting to Johns Hopkins had a history of recent fever, only 51 (65 per cent) actually had a temperature of more than 100°F on admission.[45] In 29 of the patients in this series the admission temperature was greater than 102°F, and in 8 it was greater than 104°F. Chills had been present by history in 58 (74 per cent) of the patients. Both abdominal pain and jaundice were present in 79 per cent of the patients in this analysis. However, in many instances the abdominal pain was mild, and 16 patients had no complaint of any abdominal discomfort. This observation is not unusual for cholangitis, and an initial complaint of severe abdominal pain should alert the clinician to consider other diagnoses. Thus, Charcot's triad was complete in less than 60 per cent of the 78 Hopkins patients who had well-documented cholangitis.

Table 19–3 CLINICAL PRESENTATION IN ACUTE CHOLANGITIS

Sign or Symptom	Patients (%)
Fever*	65
Chills	79
Abdominal pain*	79
Jaundice*	79
Abdominal tenderness	81
Nausea/vomiting	51
Septic shock	5
Loss of bowel sounds	3

*Charcot's triad complete in <60 per cent of patients.
Adapted from Saharia PC, Cameron JL: Surg Gynecol Obstet 1975;*142*:369.

Physical examination of the abdomen can also be quite variable. Sixty-three of the 78 patients (81 per cent) in the Johns Hopkins series had mild to moderate abdominal tenderness in the right upper quadrant.[45] However, 15 patients had no evidence of abdominal tenderness on examination. In addition, only 35 of the patients had evidence of peritoneal irritation. Nineteen patients had right upper quadrant guarding, and 16 patients had rebound tenderness in the right upper quadrant. In 76 of the 78 patients, bowel sounds were recorded as normal. Thus, not only is severe abdominal pain unusual in cholangitis, but also marked generalized abdominal findings on physical examination are unusual. If generalized or severe abdominal findings are present, the physician should seriously consider other diagnoses in addition to acute cholangitis. Many of the errors in diagnosis of cholangitis hinge on the mistaken concept that patients invariably have severe abdominal pain and significant abdominal findings. In fact, the opposite is true.

A comprehensive review of acute cholangitis was published by Pitt and Longmire in 1980.[39] These authors analyzed 303 patients with acute cholangitis reported in the literature. They compared 112 patients who presented with shock with 191 reported patients who were not hypotensive. Fifty-two per cent of the 303 patients were older than 70 years, and the subgroup who presented with shock were only slightly older than those who were not in shock. More than 70 per cent of each subgroup had a history of biliary tract disease. Likewise, these two groups differed very little in their clinical presentation. For the entire series, 88 per cent had chills and fever, 93 per cent were jaundiced, and 83 per cent had right upper quadrant pain. However, patients presenting with shock were more likely to have a white blood cell count greater than 20,000/mm^3.

An interesting study was carried out by Andrew and Johnson[47] in an attempt to identify preoperatively those patients presenting with acute "suppurative" cholangitis. These authors compared 39 patients admitted to their hospital with Charcot's classic triad resulting from choledocholithiasis with 17 patients from their institution who were found at operation to have acute "suppurative" cholangitis. Mean age was similar in both groups. Prior common bile duct surgery, including biliary-intestinal anastomoses and sphincteroplasties, was more common in the group of patients with acute "suppurative" cholangitis. Chills and fever on admission were actually seen more frequently in the patients with nonsuppurative cholangitis. The incidence of jaundice and right upper quadrant pain was similar in both groups. Septic shock, a temperature of 104°F or greater, and rebound tenderness were seen in a much higher proportion of patients with "suppurative" cholangitis. The mean white count in patients with acute "suppurative" cholangitis was 22,000/mm^3, and in "nonsuppurative" cholangitis it was 14,000/mm^3. The average serum bilirubin was 9 mg/dl in the patients with "suppurative" cholangitis and 6 mg/dl in the patients with "nonsuppurative" cholangitis. Blood cultures were positive in 43% of the patients with "suppurative" cholangitis and in only 8 per cent of those with "nonsuppurative" cholangitis.

A similar analysis by Boey and Way[48] suggested that patients with "suppurative" cholangitis were more likely to present with shock, a fever greater than 102°F, and a bilirubin value greater than 4 mg/dl. Andrew and Johnson[47] also collected reports from the literature of 86 patients with acute "suppurative" cholangitis. Fifty-eight per cent were found to have leukocytosis greater than 20,000/mm^3, and the average serum bilirubin was 10.2 mg/dl. Both these figures are significantly greater than one usually encounters in patients with "nonsuppurative" acute cholangitis. Interestingly, Andrew and Johnson found that in the 86 cases collected from the literature, 69 per cent of patients developed liver abscesses.

Thus, with acute "suppurative" cholangitis, prior common duct surgery, a temperature above 104°F with a picture of septic shock, rebound tenderness, a marked leukocytosis, significant hyperbilirubinemia, and positive blood cultures are more frequent. All these findings obviously will alert the clinician to the fact that he is dealing with a markedly ill patient who has a high chance of having pus in the common duct. As pointed out by Boey and Way, however, severe systemic symptoms are not always associated with suppuration, and pus in the biliary tree does not always result in severe systemic sepsis.[48] The presence of septic shock that does not respond rapidly is a clinical situation that we have termed acute toxic cholangitis, and we believe that it requires urgent biliary decompression.

DIAGNOSIS

As with most acute intra-abdominal problems, the diagnosis of acute cholangitis frequently cannot be made on the basis of clinical and laboratory findings alone. However, certain laboratory changes occur often enough to aid confirmatory evidence to support the clinical diagnosis. Some authorities would argue that bacteremia occurs in essentially all patients with cholangitis. However, bacteremia is proved by positive blood cultures in less than half of well-documented cases. Nevertheless, in those patients with blood cultures positive for typical biliary bacteria, especially when the same organism is recovered from the bile, a diagnosis of cholangitis can be made with reasonable assurance. Confirmatory radiologic evidence for underlying biliary pathology adds to the confidence of diagnosis. Although usually not necessary, histologic evidence of extrahepatic or intrahepatic bile ducts containing numerous polymorphonuclear leukocytes and bacteria, with inflammatory infiltration in the surrounding portal triads, proves the diagnosis of cholangitis.

Laboratory Findings

In a series of 78 patients presenting to the Johns Hopkins Hospital[45] with acute cholangitis, 50 (63 per cent) had leukocyte elevations greater than 10,000/mm^3 (Table 19–4). Five of these patients (6 per cent) had leukocyte counts greater than 20,000/mm^3, and two were leukopenic. Those patients presenting with normal leukocyte counts in most instances had significant shifts to the left. These observations have also been made at the University of California at San Francisco (UCSF) by Boey and Way,[48] who noted that one quarter of their patients had normal white blood cell count and a left shift. In a series of 36 patients presenting to UCSD, 35 (97 per cent) were found to have leukocyte counts in excess of 10,000/mm^3.[46]

Even though most patients with acute cholangitis have hyperbilirubinemia, the degree of bilirubin elevation is quite variable. Among the 78 patients presenting to Johns Hopkins[46] with acute cholangitis, 5 (6 per cent) had normal serum bilirubin levels (Table 19–4). An additional 10 patients (13 per cent) had minimal bilirubin elevations, between 1 and 2 mg/dl. Thus, almost 20 per cent of the patients in this series had serum bilirubin levels of 2 mg/dl or less. Boey and Way[48] reported that 16 of their 74 patients had a serum bilirubin of less than 2 mg/dl. Saik and colleagues[46] stated that 3 of 36 patients (8 per cent) with acute cholangitis had normal serum bilirubin levels; whereas in the remaining 92 per cent an elevated serum level was detected.

Alkaline phosphatase levels are usually elevated in patients with cholangitis (Table 19–4). In the Johns Hopkins series, 92 per cent of patients with acute cholangitis had an elevated serum alkaline phosphatase value. In the series from UCSD reported by Saik and colleagues,[46] 89 per cent had alkaline phosphatase elevations. Serum glutamic-oxaloacetic transaminase (SGOT) levels are also raised in the great majority of patients presenting with acute cholangitis. In the Johns Hopkins series, SGOT and SGPT values were elevated in 93 per cent and 98 per cent, respectively (Table 19–4).

Thus, the trio of blood tests consisting of bilirubin, alkaline phosphatase, and transaminase levels may provide a degree of confirmatory evidence for the clinical diagnosis of acute cholangitis. Acute cholangitis is invariably associated with some degree of obstruction of the biliary tract. Thus, elevations of these three serum tests would be expected. Although they by no means make the diagnosis of acute cholangitis, to see acute cholangitis in the absence of such serum abnormalities would be distinctly unusual.

Serum amylase determinations were performed in 54 of the 78 patients in the Johns Hopkins series.[45] In 19 of the patients (35 per cent) the serum levels were elevated (Table 19–4). Moreover, in six patients (11 per cent) the amylase was greater than 1000 Caraway units/dl. Thus, a serum amylase elevation may provide clinical evidence of calculous disease in the common duct and, thereby, further support the clinical diagnosis of acute cholangitis.

Table 19–4 LABORATORY FINDINGS IN ACUTE CHOLANGITIS

Laboratory Finding	Patients (%)
White blood count (per mm^3)	
>10,000	63
>20,000	6
Bilirubin (mg/dl)	
>1.5	94
>2.0	81
>5.0	53
SGOT (IU/L)	
>20	93
>100	29
SGPT (IU/L)	
>20	97
>100	31
Alkaline phosphatase	
Abnormal	92
Amylase (Caraway units)	
>200	35
>1000	11

Adapted from Saharia PC, Cameron JL: Surg Gynecol Obstet 1976;*142*:369.

Bacteriologic Findings

Blood cultures were obtained shortly following admission in 50 of the 78 patients presenting to Johns Hopkins[45] with acute cholangitis. In 20 patients (40 per cent) the blood cultures were positive. In 9 of the 20 patients (45 per cent), *E. coli* was the organism grown; in 8 patients (40 per cent), *Klebsiella pneumoniae* was cultured. Thus, in 85 per cent of the patients with positive blood cultures, the organisms were *E. coli* or *Klebsiella pneumoniae*. In one patient each, *Streptococcus faecalis* (enterococcus), a paracolon, and *Bacteroides fragilis* were cultured. Blood cultures were positive in 36 of 84 patients (44 per cent) reported from UCSF.[48] In the series of 36 patients with acute cholangitis from UCSD, 17 (47 per cent) had positive blood cultures.[46] In each of these three series, *E. coli* and *Klebsiella* species were the most frequent organisms obtained on blood culture.

At the time of surgery, bile cultures were obtained in 35 patients with acute cholangitis in the series of patients from Johns Hopkins.[45] All cultures were positive. In 21 of the patients (60 per cent), multiple organisms were found. However, as would be expected from the preoperative blood culture data, *E. coli* and *Klebsiella pneumoniae* were the most frequently cultured organisms. In 26 of the 35 patients (74 per cent), *E. coli* was present in the infected bile; in 14 (40 per cent), *Klebsiella pneumoniae* was present. Enterococcus was cultured in the bile from 11 of the patients (31 per cent).

Bile cultures were positive in 79 of 86 patients (92 per cent) studied by Boey and Way.[48] In 38 of their patients (48 per cent), multiple organisms were isolated from the bile. In the series of 36 patients with cholangitis presented by Saik and associates,[46] 28 underwent surgery and had common duct cultures performed. In 26 patients (93 per cent), the cultures were positive. In 16 of the 26 patients (61 per cent), multiple organisms were grown. In 17 of the 26 positive cultures (65 per cent), *E. coli* was isolated. *Klebsiella pneumoniae* was present in 13 of the positive cultures (50 per cent). Enterococcus was the next most commonly cultured organism, being found in seven bile samples (27 per cent). Thus, the bile culture data from these three series are almost identical. In each of these series a large number of other organisms were infrequently cultured. However, *E. coli* and *Klebsiella pneumoniae* were the most commonly found organisms, with entercoccus being cultured in a significant number.

Of note is the fact that in each of these large series of patients with acute cholangitis, anaerobic organisms were only infrequently cultured in the blood or bile. One possible explanation for the paucity of anaerobes reported in these series is that anaerobic culturing techniques may not have been routinely employed during the period of these studies. In comparison, anaerobes were isolated from the bile of 9 of 33 patients (27 per cent) with choledocholithiasis and preoperative cholangitis seen at Johns Hopkins between 1976 and 1979.[7] During this same period, anaerobes were isolated from the bile of only 2 of 40 patients (5 per cent) with common duct stones and no preoperative cholangitis ($p < 0.025$). The anaerobic organism most frequently recovered in this group of patients was *Bacteroides fragilis*.

Radiographic Findings

Plain abdominal x-rays are generally not helpful in evaluating the patient who presents with acute cholangitis. In the series from Johns Hopkins,[45] 52 of the 78 patients had plain abdominal x-rays, and only eight abnormalities were seen. In five of these eight patients the nonspecific finding of ileus or a sentinel loop was present. In two patients radiopaque gallstones were seen, and in one patient air was noted in the biliary tree. In the remaining 44 patients the abdominal x-rays were normal or demonstrated only nonspecific changes.

Because of hyperbilirubinemia at the time of presentation, oral cholecystography is of no help in most patients with cholangitis. Intravenous cholangiography is rarely indicated because of low yield, occasional severe allergic reactions, and availability of other, newer tests. In those patients who present with a clinical picture of cholangitis, ultrasound (US) and computerized tomography (CT) may be quite helpful in demonstrating the presence of stones, dilated bile ducts, or small liver abscesses (Fig. 19–3). These techniques have the advantage of being noninvasive and may aid in confirming the diagnosis in ill patients.

Ultrasound, of course, is more accurate than CT in the detection of gallstones, but neither is particularly helpful in diagnosing choledocholithiasis, a more likely cause of cholangitis. Both US and CT can diagnose biliary dilatation, but CT may be slightly more accurate in this regard.[49] Moreover, in comparison with CT, US has the disadvantage of poor visualization of the distal bile duct and pancreas. CT has the further advantage of better resolution within the liver for detection of small abscesses but has the disadvantages of ionizing radiation and higher cost.

In summary, either US or CT may be a useful test in confirming the suspicion of a biliary source of sepsis by demonstrating biliary dilatation or liver abscesses. However, neither is particularly accurate in determining the site or cause of obstruction.[49] The use of radionuclide scanning of the biliary tree with ^{99m}Tc HIDA and other iminodi-

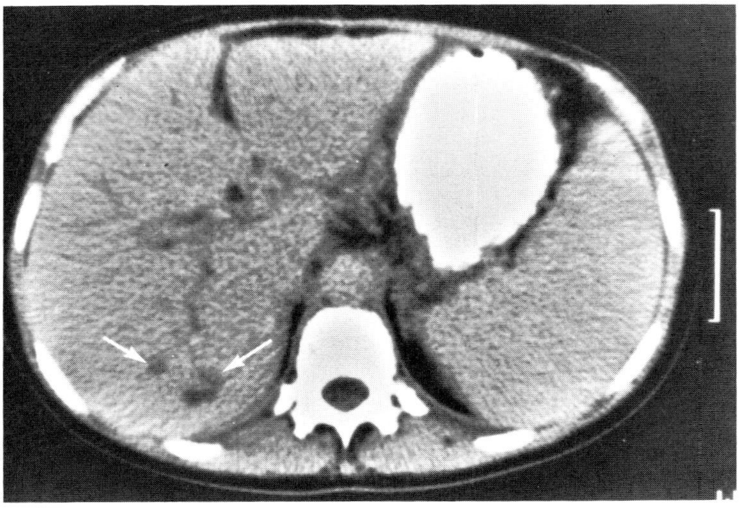

Figure 19–3. Computerized tomogram demonstrating dilated intrahepatic ducts and two small liver abscesses (*arrows*) posteriorly in the right lobe of the liver in a patient with recurrent pancreatic cancer.

acetic acid derivatives has the same advantage as US and CT of being noninvasive. However, although cholescintigraphy is quite useful in the diagnosis of acute cholecystitis, this technique lacks the resolution necessary to accurately define biliary anatomy.[50]

As will be discussed in more detail later, most patients with acute cholangitis will eventually require surgery. Before surgery, most patients will need transhepatic or endoscopic retrograde cholangiography to adequately define biliary anatomy (Fig. 19–4). Although both these techniques can very accurately depict the biliary anatomy, they are associated with a small incidence of complications. In performing either procedure in a patient with a recent episode of cholangitis, timing of the cholangiogram and of antibiotic coverage is critical.

Before a patient with a recent episode of cholangitis undergoes either of these procedures, he should have received an adequate course of systemic antibiotics and have been afebrile for several days. Transhepatic cholangiography (THC) is associated with an approximate 5 per cent incidence of cholangitis and 0.25 per cent mortality. In a series of 75 patients undergoing THC with no antibiotic coverage, Flemma and his colleagues[3] reported a 7 per cent incidence of cholangitis. In a more recent series by Okuda and associates,[51] a 4 per cent incidence of cholangitis was observed among 315 patients undergoing THC with antibiotic coverage.

The overall incidence of complications after endoscopic retrograde cholangiography (ERC) is approximately 3 per cent, with a mortality of approximately 0.2 per cent. The incidence of cholangitis following ERC reported in 1975 from the Johns Hopkins Hospital was 5 per cent among 75 consecutive patients.[52] However, in a collected series of over 10,000 patients undergoing ERC, Bilboa et al.[52] reported an incidence of cholangitis of only 0.8 per cent.

In a large series of ERC by Zimmon et al.,[53] cholangitis was not seen in those patients with a normal biliary tree but occurred in 5

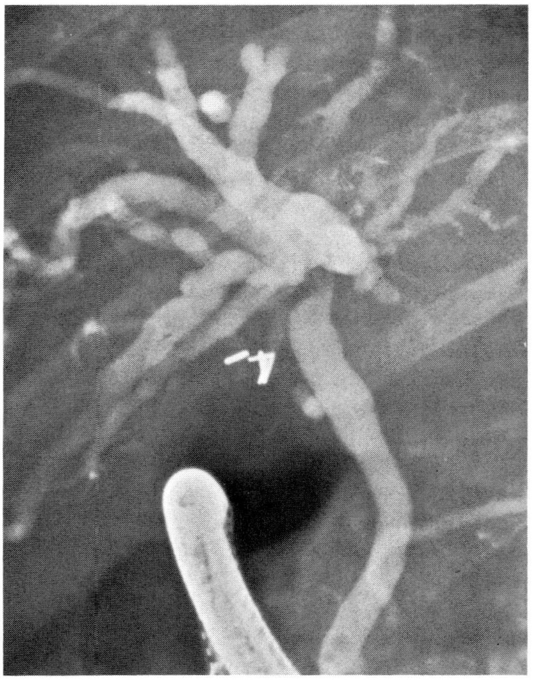

Figure 19–4. Endoscopic retrograde cholangiogram demonstrating a hilar stricture due to a cholangiocarcinoma. Preoperative knowledge of this lesion will aid the surgeon at operation.

per cent of the patients with biliary obstruction. Kasagai and associates[54] performed ERC on 405 patients who were covered with systemic antibiotics, with a 0.7 per cent incidence of cholangitis. When these authors added thiamphenicol aminoacetate HCl (Neomycon G) to the contrast medium, they reported no cholangitis among 252 patients who were also covered with systemic antibiotics. Therefore, either THC or ERC can be performed reasonably safely in patients with a recent episode of cholangitis if (1) adequate antibiotic therapy has been carried out prior to the performance of the cholangiogram, and (2) systemic antibiotic coverage is provided during the study. The addition of antibiotics to the contrast medium in these high-risk patients needs further investigation with respect to toxicity of specific antibiotics to biliary mucosa.

Differential Diagnosis

A variety of disorders can present with fever and chills, abdominal pain, and jaundice. The clinical entity that is most frequently confused with acute cholangitis, however, is acute cholecystitis (Table 19–5). As with cholangitis, patients who develop acute cholecystitis tend to be elderly, and both are seen as frequently in men as in women.[55] While fever is present in almost all patients with acute cholecystitis, chills are less common and more suggestive of cholangitis. Almost all patients with acute cholecystitis have right upper quadrant pain and tenderness, symptoms and physical findings that are present somewhat less often in patients with cholangitis.

Table 19–5 DIFFERENTIATION OF ACUTE CHOLANGITIS AND ACUTE CHOLECYSTITIS

	Cholangitis	Cholecystitis
Presentation		
Age	60s	50s
Female:Male	1:1	3:2
Fever	90%	90%
Chills	75%	50%
Jaundice	95%	30%
RUQ pain	80%	95%
RUQ tenderness	80%	95%
Laboratory Findings		
WBC> 10,000	70%	70%
WBC> 20,000	10%	5%
Bilirubin> 1.5	95%	30%
Bilirubin> 5.0	55%	5%
Alkaline phosphatase ↑	90%	40%
SGOT/SGPT ↑	95%	50%
Amylase ↑	35%	15%

Jaundice may be seen in both cholecystitis and cholangitis but is more common in acute cholangitis. Although hyperbilirubinemia may be present in as many as 25 to 30 percent of patients with acute cholecystitis, the level of bilirubin is usually less than 5 mg/dl.[55] In contrast, over 90 percent of patients who present with cholangitis have hyperbilirubinemia, and in 55 percent of these patients the bilirubin will be greater than 5 mg/dl.[45] Nausea and vomiting may be seen with both illnesses and is not helpful in the differential diagnosis.

Abdominal tenderness is present in the vast majority of patients with acute cholecystitis, and peritoneal signs are frequent. On occasion a palpable, tender gallbladder or a positive Murphy's sign will also be present in acute cholecystitis. While the majority of patients with acute cholangitis have some abdominal tenderness, it is usually mild, and peritoneal signs are seen in fewer than half the patients. The presence or absence of bowel sounds on physical examination does not differentiate between these two entities.

The white blood cell count is frequently, but not invariably, elevated in both illnesses. A marked leukocytosis (>20,000/mm^3) or a leukopenia suggests a septicemia and is more apt to be associated with acute cholangitis. The alkaline phosphatase is elevated in most patients with cholangitis, but as many as 40 percent with acute cholecystitis will also have an elevated serum level.[55] Mild elevations in the SGOT or SGPT are seen in almost all patients with cholangitis. However, these enzymes are also elevated in approximately 50 percent of patients with acute cholecystitis.[55] The serum amylase may also be elevated in both conditions.

Plain abdominal x-rays are normal in most patients with acute cholangitis or acute cholecystitis, and the presence of gallstones on plain abdominal films does not differentiate between the two. Air either within the biliary tree or within the gallbladder may be helpful, but these x-ray findings are rare. Ultrasonography can demonstrate gallstones and biliary duct dilatation. However, because of problems with overlying gas and the failure to detect stones in the distal common duct, US will not always differentiate cholecystitis from cholangitis. Similarly, cholescintigraphy can document cystic duct obstruction and acute cholecystitis but usually does not give enough information regarding the extrahepatic ducts to accurately diagnose cholangitis.

Thus, the differentiation between acute cholecystitis and cholangitis may be difficult and in some cases impossible. The physical examination of the right upper quadrant and the level of bilirubin yield the two most important differentiating characteristics. The patient with true peritoneal signs in the right upper quadrant and a normal or only minimally elevated bilirubin is more likely to have acute cholecystitis. A patient presenting with less in the way of abdominal findings, but with a bilirubin of 5 mg/dl or greater and a septic picture, is more likely to have cholangitis.

Other diseases in and around the liver that might be confused with cholangitis are hepatitis, liver abscesses, and pancreatitis. Patients with viral or alcoholic hepatitis may present with fever, right upper quadrant pain, and jaundice. In comparison with patients with acute cholangitis, those with hepatitis usually have a more chronic presentation, absence of chills, and higher elevations of serum transaminase. The presence of multiple microscopic liver abscesses may be an extension of acute "suppurative" cholangitis. However, liver abscesses of other than biliary tract origin may also present in a fashion identical to cholangitis. Moreover, the physical examination and laboratory findings may be very similar. These patients can be differentiated preoperatively with the use of ultrasound, radionuclide scanning, or computerized tomography.

The clinical presentation of pancreatitis may also be very similar to that of acute cholangitis. Bilirubin elevations are common with both entities. Elevations in serum amylase are present in most patients with pancreatitis but also can be seen in as many as one third of patients presenting with acute cholangitis.[45] The abdominal findings in acute pancreatitis, however, are almost always more severe than in acute cholangitis. Penetrating or perforated ulcers may also present with fever, right upper quadrant pain, hyperamylasemia, and a mild elevation in bilirubin secondary to sepsis.

Among other illnesses that might be confused with cholangitis are right-sided diverticulitis or pyelonephritis, appendicitis, a right lower lobe pneumonia or pulmonary infarct, and bacterial endocarditis. Jaundice is generally not associated with diverticulitis or appendicitis. However, if sepsis occurs, mild bilirubin elevations can result. If untreated, these diseases can also result in pylephlebitis and multiple liver abscesses. Patients with acute pyelonephritis or right lower lobe pneumonia are usually not jaundiced. However, if severe sepsis accompanies these problems, an elevated bilirubin may be seen secondary to hemolysis. Patients with bacterial endocarditis can develop multiple abscesses in many organs, including the liver and spleen. Mild jaundice is also common in these patients.

TREATMENT

Once the clinical diagnosis of acute cholangitis is suspected, the initial treatment in most instances will be systemic antibiotics. Depending upon the severity of the episode and the nature of the clinical presentation, other general supportive measures may be required. Biliary decompression is, perhaps, the most important aspect of treatment for patients with cholangitis. Until recent years, surgical decompression was the only option. However, percutaneous transhepatic drainage and endoscopic sphincterotomy are alternative methods that are now available for decompression of selected patients. Considerable debate continues, however, about the most appropriate method for drainage, the timing of biliary decompression, and the choice of antibiotics. These aspects of treatment will be considered in more detail following a discussion of general supportive measures.

General Supportive Measures

For the patient who presents with chills and a low-grade fever and no other systemic signs or symptoms, antibiotic therapy alone may be sufficient. For the patient who presents with fever and chills, vomiting, a tender abdomen, and absent bowel sounds, intravenous fluids and nasogastric decompression may also be indicated. For the infrequent patient who presents in septic shock, more intensive monitoring and therapy will be necessary. All such patients will require a central venous catheter, and some of them will need a Swan-Ganz catheter to monitor the central venous and pulmonary wedge pressures.

Initial treatment of the hypotension, which

generally is secondary to peripheral vasodilatation, should be carefully monitored volumes of crystalloids. Most patients will not be anemic, but if the hemoglobin is very low, blood should also be administered. If the patient does not respond by an elevation of arterial pressure prior to an increase in central venous or pulmonary wedge pressure, an ionotropic drug, such as dopamine, should be started. Large doses of steroids should also be considered for patients in septic shock. Hypoglycemia has been documented in patients with acute toxic cholangitis and may be, in part, responsible for the central nervous system depression seen with this entity. Therefore, blood glucose levels should be monitored and intravenous glucose administered.

For patients with severe cholangitis, a Foley catheter is also required for hourly monitoring of urinary output. A minimum of 30 ml of urine per hour is desired to ensure that the cardiac output and renal blood flow are adequate. Since some patients with cholangitis may have biliary cirrhosis secondary to long-standing biliary tract problems, coagulation studies should be obtained and vitamin K administered if the prothrombin time is prolonged.

Antibiotic Therapy

For the majority of patients presenting with acute cholangitis, antibiotic therapy will be the mainstay of treatment. No general agreement exists in the literature, however, as to the most appropriate antibiotic regimen to use in acute cholangitis. In choosing an antibiotic or antibiotics for treatment of biliary infections, several factors must be considered. Important antibiotic properties include (1) antibacterial spectrum, (2) biliary excretion, (3) serum and tissue levels, (4) toxicity, and (5) cost.

When considering the antibacterial spectrum, let us assume that approximately 70 percent of patients with cholangitis will have gram-negative aerobes in their bile, approximately 30 percent will grow enterococcus, and approximately 10 percent will harbor *Bacteroides fragilis*.[7, 8] For many years, the combination of a penicillin and an aminoglycoside was recommended by many experts for treatment of biliary infections.[7, 40, 48] This regimen was chosen because of the broad spectrum provided against common biliary pathogens. Theoretically, the synergistic action of these antibiotics against enterococcus and the gram-negative aerobic coverage of the aminoglycoside would provide adequate antibacterial coverage for 85 to 90 percent of patients with cholangitis.[7, 8] The addition of an antibiotic with coverage for *Bacteroides fragilis*, such as clindamycin or metronidazole, would provide nearly complete antibacterial coverage for these patients.

Many of the third-generation cephalosporins provide excellent coverage for the gram-negative aerobes, and some also inhibit the growth of anaerobes. However, this group of antibiotics is, in general, not effective against enterococcus. The one cephalosporin with the best enterococcal coverage, cefoperazone, also achieves extremely high levels in bile. However, in a recent comparative trial[41] this agent, when used alone, was not as effective as the combination of ampicillin and tobramycin in treating patients with cholangitis. Whether the addition of ampicillin, for enterococcal coverage, to a third-generation cephalosporin would be of any benefit is at present an unanswered question.

The recent introduction of broad-spectrum penicillins, such as piperacillin and imipenem, adds an option that would be expected to provide coverage for most biliary pathogens. These agents are effective against gram-negative aerobes, enterococci, and anaerobes. However, the question of whether these agents used alone will be as effective as the combination of a penicillin and an aminoglycoside has yet to be adequately studied. Thus, numerous antibiotic options that theoretically would inhibit nearly all biliary pathogens are currently available. In choosing an antibiotic, therefore, other factors should also be considered.

Although several antibiotics are preferentially excreted into bile, numerous studies have shown that biliary antibiotic levels are markedly diminished in the face of bile duct obstruction. For cholangitis to develop, both bile duct obstruction and bactibilia are required. Thus, the very situations in which high biliary levels of an antibiotic may be important are also those in which high levels are unlikely to be achieved because of biliary obstruction. This paradox probably explains why Keighley and his associates[56] found that an aminoglycoside with broad antibacterial spectrum and poor biliary excretion was more efficacious in preventing infections following biliary surgery than rifamycin, which has excellent biliary excretion but a limited antibacterial spectrum.

Nevertheless, knowledge of the biliary excretion of commonly employed antibiotics may be important (1) when biliary obstruction is partial and (2) when obstruction has been relieved. If both the peak bile levels and the ratio of peak bile to peak serum levels are considered, antibiotic excretion into bile can be classified as low, moderate, high, and very high (Table 19–6). The biliary excretion of the aminoglycosides as a group is low. In comparison, most of the older penicillins have moderate biliary excretion, with the exception of nafcillin, which achieves very high biliary levels, and ampicillin, which has higher levels in bile than in serum. This property is also true for the first-generation cephalosporins, cefoxitin, the macrolides, clindamycin and erythromycin, and the tetracyclines. A relatively small group of antibiotics are actively excreted into and achieve very high levels in bile. Of note is the fact that several of the newer broad-spectrum penicillins, which have excellent antibacterial spectra against biliary organisms, are also actively secreted into bile (Table 19–6).

While high biliary excretion may be a theoretical advantage in certain situations, other pharmacokinetic properties, such as liver, tissue, and serum levels and half-life, are also important considerations when choosing an antibiotic for treatment of cholangitis. For example, in patients with cholangitis who are totally obstructed, serum and liver levels sufficient to protect against sepsis and hepatic abscess are extremely important. Examples of agents with poor biliary excretion, but adequate serum and liver levels to protect against septicemia and abscess formation, include chloramphenicol and the aminoglycosides.

Since several antibiotic combinations with broad antibacterial coverage against biliary organisms are now available, the relative toxicity of these agents has assumed greater importance. One of the major concerns in this regard, of course, is the potential nephrotoxicity of the aminoglycosides. Patients with cholangitis or multiple liver abscesses resulting from biliary obstruction are at increased risk for developing renal failure because of sepsis, obstructive jaundice, and age-related, pre-existing renal disease. In a recent study of 33 patients presenting with cholangitis secondary to choledocholithiasis, Pitt and his colleagues[7] found that one third developed a postoperative increase in serum creatinine. These patients had received an average of 10 days of aminoglycoside therapy, and renal problems had developed despite careful monitoring of serum aminoglycoside levels. The postoperative hospital stay of patients who developed renal problems was significantly longer than in similar patients who had no postoperative renal difficulties.

Although nephrotoxicity has been a major concern with the aminoglycosides, the alternatives—the newer penicillins and cephalosporins—are not entirely innocuous. Both groups of drugs, of course, must be used with caution or avoided entirely in patients with a history of penicillin hypersensitivity. Some of the third-generation cephalosporins have also been associated with an increased incidence of bleeding complications. Disorders of hemostasis may result from hypo-

Table 19–6 BILIARY EXCRETION OF ANTIBIOTICS

	Low	Moderate	High	Very High
Peak Bile/Serum Ratio:	< 1	1–2	2–20	> 20
Peak Bile Level (μg/ml):	< 5	5–20	20–100	> 100
	Amikacin	Amoxicillin	Ampicillin	Azlocillin
	Bacitracin	Carbenicillin	Cefazolin	Cefamandole
	Chloramphenicol	Methicillin	Cefotaxime	Cefoperazone
	Colistimethate	Metronidazole	Cefoxitin	Mezlocillin
	Gentamicin	Oxacillin	Cephradine	Nafcillin
	Kanamycin	Penicillin	Clindamycin	Piperacillin
	Netilmicin	Sulfamethoxazole	Erythromycin	Rifamycins
	Streptomycin	Sulfathiazole	Imipenem	
	Tobramycin	Ticarcillin	Moxalactam	
	Vancomycin	Trimethoprim	Tetracyclines	

prothrombinemia, platelet dysfunction, and, rarely, immune-mediated thrombocytopenia. Since patients with biliary obstruction may already have hypoprothrombinemia or portal hypertension or both, these newer cephalosporins must be used cautiously in these individuals.

Another form of toxicity that has been observed with the newer broad-spectrum cephalosporins has been bacterial and, in particular, enterococcal superinfection. In comparison, problems with bleeding and superinfection have occurred less frequently with the newer broad-spectrum penicillins. These agents, therefore, provide good coverage for biliary organisms, excellent biliary excretion, and a potential advantage in terms of toxicity. Many clinicians, however, have been concerned about the efficacy of these agents when used alone and are still awaiting comparative data from ongoing randomized trials.

The proliferation of antibiotics suitable for patients undergoing biliary surgery has been paralleled by escalating costs for these drugs. Now that agents with relatively equal antibacterial spectra, biliary excretion, and potential toxicity are available, cost must also be considered. The least expensive agents that have been recommended by some experts for patients undergoing biliary surgery include penicillin G, ampicillin, and gentamicin. Among the aminoglycosides other than gentamicin, tobramycin is the least expensive, while netilmicin costs slightly more. Amikacin, on the other hand, is twice as expensive as netilmicin. Although the newer penicillins, piperacillin and mezlocillin, are all more expensive than penicillin G and ampicillin, even the most expensive, piperacillin, is less costly than any of the currently available third-generation cephalosporins. Clindamycin is approximately equal in cost to piperacillin; therefore, antibiotic combinations that include clindamycin are more expensive than piperacillin alone.

Taking all these factors into account, combinations that include a penicillin, an aminoglycoside, and an agent effective against *Bacteroides fragilis* remain the standard of care for patients with the most severe forms of cholangitis. However, whenever an aminoglycoside is administered to a patient with cholangitis, very careful monitoring of serum antibiotic levels is mandatory. If blood or bile cultures indicate that less nephrotoxic agents will suffice, aminoglycoside therapy should be discontinued. In addition, prolonged postoperative administration of aminoglycosides to patients whose biliary obstruction has been alleviated and whose fever has abated is not warranted.

Combinations including an aminoglycoside are probably not necessary, however, for patients with cholangitis who present with only a transient fever and no other signs of sepsis. For patients who are less severely ill, newer, less toxic antibiotics, such as piperacillin, should provide adequate antibacterial coverage. Whether piperacillin or imipenem alone is adequate therapy for severe cholangitis remains an unanswered question. Until randomized trials provide these data, we recommend that initial antibiotic therapy for patients with biliary sepsis be individualized on the basis of the severity of the presenting symptoms.

Biliary Decompression

The majority of patients presenting with acute cholangitis will respond to antibiotic therapy. Within 24 to 48 hours temperature and liver function tests will return toward normal. However, if the patient does not respond initially, surgical, radiographic, or endoscopic decompression should be carried out within hours of admission.

At the time of surgery in patients with toxic cholangitis, a distended common duct will be encountered. Upon performing a choledochotomy, pus under pressure will be found. With gross purulence in the common duct, minimal biliary tract manipulation should be carried out. Any stones evident in the immediate vicinity of the choledochotomy should be removed. In this setting the surgeon should be extremely careful not to elevate pressures within the biliary tree by irrigation, as this may facilitate further egress of bacteria from the bile ducts into the blood stream. A T-tube should then be inserted and the operation terminated.

In operating on patients in septic shock, no attempt should be made to completely rid the biliary tree of calculi or to perform operative cholangiography. If the patient's condition allows, a cholecystectomy should be performed. Under no circumstances, however, should a cholecystostomy be used as a means of duct decompression. Cholecystostomy alone has proved to be totally inadequate as a means of decompressing a common duct in the face of toxic cholangitis and carries an extremely high mortality.[46, 57] When operating on these severely ill patients, the surgeon should carefully palpate the liver to ascertain whether liver abscesses are present. In the face of a benign or malignant biliary stricture, one has to be certain that the T-tube or stent is placed above the point of obstruction. In most instances, however, no further treatment should be carried out for the stricture at the time of exploration for toxic cholangitis. Following emergency duct decompression, secondary biliary tract procedures can be carried out weeks or months later under elective conditions.

For the majority of patients with less severe forms of cholangitis, initial nonoperative therapy will be satisfactory. Since all patients will have some degree of obstruction secondary to biliary tract pathology, most will require work-up of the biliary tract and subsequent surgery. For occasional patients, particularly those who have had multiple benign stricture repairs and in whom further biliary tract surgery would be risky and perhaps unsuccessful, one may choose nonoperative management. This approach may be especially appropriate when attacks of cholangitis are infrequent and mild. In such an instance, chronic administration of an oral antibiotic secreted in high concentration in bile may be necessary. In this setting the combination of trimethoprim and sulfamethoxazole has been used in recent years because of adequate gram-negative aerobic coverage and moderate biliary excretion. Ampicillin, tetracycline, and the cephalosporins have also been used as oral agents with moderate success despite their less than ideal coverage.

The majority of patients presenting with less severe forms of cholangitis, however, have biliary tract pathology that requires surgical, radiologic, or endoscopic intervention. Once the patient has responded adequately to the initial antibiotic therapy, biliary tract pathology should be accurately defined prior to operative or nonoperative manipulation. In recent years, with the widespread availability of endoscopic retrograde and transhepatic cholangiography, there is no longer any need to surgically explore a patient following an episode of acute cholangitis without knowing the anatomic pathology with a great deal of accuracy.

The importance of accurately defining the obstructive pathology following an attack of acute cholangitis, but prior to operative intervention, was demonstrated in a series of 78 patients presenting with acute cholangitis to the Johns Hopkins Hospital.[45] Eleven patients in this series died. Six of the 11 deaths resulted from continuing or recurrent cholangitis and sepsis following surgery, often after an initial period of improvement. An autopsy was performed in these six patients, and in each case retained stones or persistent strictures inadequately stented were found. In each instance the unsuccessful biliary tract procedure was secondary to incomplete information concerning the biliary tract pathology. If a patient with acute cholangitis does not respond rapidly to initial antibiotic therapy, emergency surgical decompression of the biliary tree should be carried out. However, for the vast majority of patients who do respond, one has adequate time to define the patient's biliary tract pathology.

Sixty-four of the 78 patients in the series from Johns Hopkins underwent surgical intervention.[45] In only 13 patients was the surgery carried out within the first 48 hours of admission. In 33 patients the surgery was carried out between 2 and 10 days after admission, and in 18 patients a lapse of more than 10 days occurred before the corrective biliary tract surgery was performed. In none of the patients in whom surgery was delayed for two or more days following admission to the hospital did a recurrent attack of cholangitis develop prior to operations. Similar observations have been made by Thompson et al.[40]

In patients who respond to antibiotic therapy, one can proceed with the biliary tract work-up without the threat of recurrent sepsis. This work-up should proceed after the patient has been afebrile for at least 48 hours. Cholangiography should be performed under the continuing coverage of antibiotics having a broad spectrum of activity against the common biliary organisms. Moreover, one has to be careful that the biliary tree pressure is not elevated excessively during transhepatic or endoscopic retrograde cholangiography. If obstructive pathology is demonstrated and adequate drainage of contrast medium cannot be attained after cholangiography, surgery should be performed on an urgent basis to avoid sepsis.

Response to therapy for most patients with acute cholangitis is prompt and gratifying. The overall mortality in the group of 78 patients from the Johns Hopkins Hospital was 14 percent.[45] Two of these 11 deaths were in patients who were admitted to the hospital in a state of severe septic shock and who died within 8 hours of admission without being stabilized to the point at which an operation seemed reasonable. Six patients, previously mentioned, died of recurrent cholangitis following surgery because of inadequate surgical decompression. The development of a hepatic abscess considerably worsens the prognosis. Four of the 11 deaths in this series were in patients who developed this complication. The overall mortality in the group of 36 patients from UCSD was 22 percent.[40] Sixteen of the 99 patients (16 percent) with acute cholangitis reported by Boey and Way[48] died. If one extracts from these series, however, patients who present in septic shock with toxic cholangitis, the mortality of acute nontoxic cholangitis is much less.

Acute toxic cholangitis carries a very high mortality. In the review compiled by Pitt and Longmire,[39] 29 deaths occurred among 191 patients (15 percent) who presented with cholangitis but without shock. Of these patients, 178 underwent surgical decompression, with a mortality rate of 9 percent. In comparison, 60 of 112 patients (55 percent) presenting in shock with acute toxic cholangitis failed to survive. Thirty-four of these patients never came to surgery, and all 34 died.

In the collective review of 86 patients by Andrew and Johnson,[47] all patients who did not have surgery died, and the mortality in those patients undergoing ductal decompression was in the range of 50 percent. These authors felt, on the basis of their review, that the most important factor leading to demise in acute toxic cholangitis was failure to establish the correct diagnosis and to perform surgical decompression of the biliary tree as an emergency. Thus, if one is to manage the rare patient with acute toxic cholangitis successfully, a high index of suspicion is necessary. If a patient with a clinical picture of cholangitis presents and fails to respond to initial therapy, immediate biliary decompression should be undertaken.

In recent years several authors have suggested that percutaneous transhepatic drainage (PTD) may be a reasonable option for decompression of patients with cholangitis (Fig. 19–5). In 1978 Nakayama and colleagues[58] reported 11 patients with acute suppurative cholangitis in whom percutaneous transhepatic drainage was achieved. Two of these patients had multiple liver abscesses of biliary origin. Only 1 of these 11 patients died. In 1982 Kadir et al.[59] reported that PTD had been performed on 18 patients with biliary sepsis at the Johns Hopkins Hospital. Fifteen of these patients had a favorable response; however, three elderly patients with carcinoma of the pancreas died.

Of 95 patients undergoing PTD at UCLA, 37 had a temperature greater than 100.4°F and 9 had a bacteremia before the procedure.[60] Complications following PTD were no higher when patients with pre-PTD fever or bacteremia were compared with those who were afebrile or nonbacteremic beforehand. However, when these same 95 patients were considered as "preoperative" or "palliative" patients, those with end-stage malignancies had a significantly higher 30-day mortality.

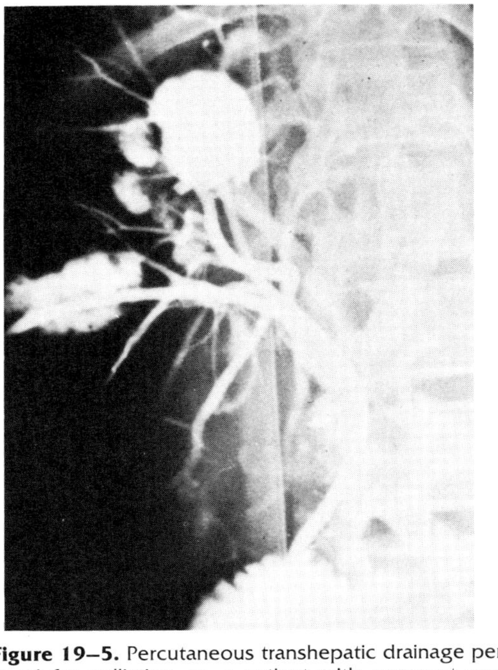

Figure 19–5. Percutaneous transhepatic drainage performed for palliation on a patient with recurrent pancreatic cancer (see Fig. 19–3) who developed a strictured choledochojejunostomy and liver abscesses.

Table 19–7 COMPARISON OF ENDOSCOPIC SPHINCTEROTOMY AND SURGERY PERFORMED EMERGENTLY FOR GALLSTONE PANCREATITIS

Procedure	Number of Patients	Number of Deaths	Mortality (%)
Endoscopic sphincterotomy[62–65]	72	5	6.9
Surgery[66, 67]	143	7	4.9

This analysis suggests that in predicting outcome following PTD the patient's underlying disease process is more important than is preprocedure cholangitis. These authors suggest that PTD may be an appropriate approach for patients with severe cholangitis who do not respond to antibiotics. In the absence of expert radiologists familiar with PTD, however, surgery remains the decompressive method of choice.

Despite large series demonstrating that endoscopic sphincterotomy can be performed safely and effectively, few data are available to document the results of this nonoperative approach in patients with acute cholangitis. Numerous reports have documented that endoscopic sphincterotomy is associated with a 1.0 to 1.5 percent mortality, an 8 to 10 percent morbidity, and a 90 to 95 percent success rate. However, very few data document the results of endoscopic sphincterotomy in those patients at highest risk for surgery—those with severe cholangitis or unresolving gallstone pancreatitis.

One recent series,[61] however, reports that when endoscopic sphincterotomy was performed for acute cholangitis in 19 patients, one died, a mortality rate of 5 per cent, not 1 per cent. Similarly, when endoscopic sphincterotomy has been performed emergently for gallstone pancreatitis, a mortality rate of 7 per cent can be calculated from available reports (Table 19–7). Interestingly, when surgical sphincterotomy or sphincteroplasty has been done emergently for gallstone pancreatitis, reported hospital mortality is only 5 per cent. These data suggest that when endoscopic sphincterotomy is performed for cholangitis, morbidity and mortality are significantly higher than usually quoted and are not necessarily any better than results obtained with surgery. In this regard, prospective, randomized studies will be necessary to determine the best method of decompression for patients with severe cholangitis secondary to choledocholithiasis.

REFERENCES

1. Charcot JM: Leçons sur les maladies du foie des voies biliaires et des veins. Paris, Faculté de Médecine de Paris. Recueillies et publiées par Bourneville et Sevestre, 1877.
2. Reynolds BM, Dargan EL: Acute obstructive cholangitis. A distinct clinical syndrome. Ann Surg 1959;*150*:299.
3. Flemma RJ, Flint LM, Osterhout S, et al: Bacteriologic studies of biliary tract infection. Ann Surg 1967;*166*:563.
4. Fukunaga FH: Gallbladder bacteriology, histology, and gallstones. Arch Surg 1973;*106*:169.
5. Edlund YA, Mollstedt BO, Ouchterlong O: Bacteriological investigation of the biliary system and liver in biliary tract disease correlated to clinical data and microstructure of the gallbladder and liver. Acta Chir Scand 1959;*116*:461.
6. Keighley MRB, Flinn R, Alexander-Williams J: Multivariate analysis of clinical and operative findings associated with biliary sepsis. Br J Surg 1976;*63*:528.
7. Pitt HA, Postier RG, Cameron JL: Consequences of preoperative cholangitis and its treatment on the outcome of surgery for choledocholithiasis. Surgery 1983;*94*:447.
8. Pitt HA, Postier RG, Cameron JL: Biliary bacteria: Significance and alterations after antibiotic therapy. Arch Surg 1982;*117*:445.
9. O'Connor MJ, Schwartz ML, McQuarrie DG, et al: Cholangitis due to malignant obstruction to biliary outflow. Ann Surg 1981;*193*:341.
10. Keighley MRB, Lister DM, Jacobs SI, et al: Hazards of surgical treatment due to micro-organisms in the bile. Surgery 1974;*75*:578.
11. Mason GR: Bacteriology and antibiotic selection in biliary tract surgery. Arch Surg 1968;*97*:533.
12. Chetlin SH, Elliott DW: Biliary bacteremia. Arch Surg 1971;*102*:303.
13. Gorbach SL, Plant AG, Nahas L, et al: Studies of intestinal microflora. II. Micro-organisms of the small intestine and their relations to oral and fecal flora. Gastroenterology 1967;*53*:856.
14. Binder HJ, Filburn B, Flock M: Bile acid inhibition of intestinal anaerobic organisms. Am J Clin Nutr 1975;*28*:119.
15. Williams RC, Showalter R, Kern F Jr: *In vivo* effect of bile salts and cholestyramine on intestinal anaerobic bacteria. Gastroenterology 1975;*69*:483.
16. Pitt HA, Postier RG, Cameron JL: Bacteremia after tube cholangiography. Ann Surg 1980;*191*:30.
17. Nielsen NL, Justensen T: Anaerobic and aerobic bacteriological studies in biliary tract disease. Scand J Gastroenterol 1976;*11*:437.
18. England DM, Rosenblatt JE: Anaerobes in human biliary tracts. J Clin Microbiol 1977;*6*:494.
19. Shimada K, Inamatsu T, Yamashiro M: Anaerobic bacteria in biliary disease in elderly patients. J Infect Dis 1977;*135*:850.
20. Bergan T, Dobloug I, Liavag I: Bacterial isolates in cholecystitis and cholelithiasis. Scand J Gastroenterol 1979;*14*:625.
21. Jackaman FR, Hilson GRF, Marlow LS: Bile bacteria in patients with benign bile duct stricture. Br J Surg 1980;*67*:329.
22. Taylor FW: Blood-culture studies of the portal vein. Arch Surg 1956;*72*:889.
23. Orloff MJ, Peskins GW, Ellis HL: A bacteriological

study of human portal blood. Ann Surg 1956; *148*:738.
24. Dineen P: The importance of the route of infection in experimental biliary tract obstruction. Surg Gynecol Obstet 1964;*119*:1001.
25. Schatten WE, Desprez JD, Holden WD: A bacteriologic study of portal vein blood in man. Arch Surg 1955;*71*:404.
26. Brooke BN, Slaney G: Portal bacteraemia in ulcerative colitis. Lancet 1958;*1*:1206.
27. Ong GB: A study of recurrent pyogenic cholangitis. Arch Surg 1962;*84*:63.
28. Scott AJ, Khan GA: Origin of bacteria in bile duct bile. Lancet 1967;*2*:790.
29. Mixer HW, Rigler LG, Gonzales-Oddone MV: Experimental studies on biliary regurgitation during cholangiography. Gastroenterology 1947;*9*:64.
30. Edlund Y, Hanzon V: Demonstration of the close relationship between bile capillaries and sinusoid walls. Acta Anat 1953;*17*:105.
31. Rouiller C: Les canalicules biliaires: étude au microscope électronique. Acta Anat 1956;*26*:94.
32. Hampton JC: An electron microscope study of the hepatic uptake and excretion of microscopic particles injected into the blood stream and into the bile duct. Acta Anat 1958;*32*:262.
33. Hultborn A, Jacobsson B, Rosengren B: Cholangiovenous reflux during cholangiography. Acta Chir Scand 1962;*123*:111.
34. Jacobsson B, Kjellander J, Rosengren B: Cholangiovenous reflux. Acta Chir Scand 1962;*123*:316.
35. Huang T, Bass JA, Williams RD: The significance of biliary pressures in cholangitis. Arch Surg 1969;*98*:629.
36. Mallet-Guy P: Value of preoperative manometric and roentgenographic examination in the diagnosis of pathologic changes and functional disturbances of the biliary tract. Surg Gynecol Obstet 1952; *94*:385.
37. Williams RD, Fish JC, Williams DD: The significance of biliary pressure. Arch Surg 1967;*95*:374.
38. Hopton D, White TT: An evaluation of manometric operative cholangiography in 100 patients with biliary disease. Surg Gynecol Obstet 1971;*133*:949.
39. Pitt HA, Longmire WP Jr: Suppurative cholangitis. *In* Hardy JM (ed): Critical Surgical Illness, 2nd ed. Philadelphia, WB Saunders, 1980, pp 380–408.
40. Thompson JE, Tompkins RK, Longmire WP Jr: Factors in management of acute cholangitis. Ann Surg 1982;*195*:137.
41. Muller EL, Pitt HA, Thompson JE, et al: Antibiotics in biliary infections: A randomized trial of ampicillin/tobramycin, cefoperazone, and piperacillin. In preparation.
42. Davis JL, Milligan FD, Cameron JL: Septic complications following endoscopic retrograde cholangiopancreatography. Surg Gynecol Obstet 1975;*140*: 365.
43. Burhenne HJ: Complications of nonoperative extraction of retained common duct stone. Am J Surg 1976;*131*:260.
44. Rogers L: Biliary abscesses of the liver with operation. Br Med J 1903;*2*:706.
45. Saharia PC, Cameron JL: Clinical management of cholangitis. Surg Gynecol Obstet 1976;*142*:369.
46. Saik RP, Greenburg AG, Farris JM, et al: Spectrum of cholangitis. Am J Surg 1975;*130*:143.
47. Andrew DJ, Johnson SE: Acute suppurative cholangitis. A medical and surgical emergency. Am J Gastroenterol 1970;*54*:141.
48. Boey JH, Way LW: Acute cholangitis. Ann Surg 1980;*191*:264.
49. Tompkins RK, Pitt HA: Surgical management of benign lesions of the bile ducts. Curr Probl Surg 1982;*19*:322.
50. Rosenthal L, Shaffer ER, Lisboner R, et al: Diagnosis of hepatobiliary disease by ^{99m}Tc HIDA cholescintigraphy. Radiology 1978;*126*:467.
51. Okuda K, Tanikawa K, Emara T, et al: Nonsurgical percutaneous transhepatic cholangiography. Diagnostic significance in medical problems of the liver. Am J Dig Dis 1974;*19*:21.
52. Bilboa MK, Dotter CT, Lee TG, et al: Complications of endoscopic retrograde cholangiopancreatography (ERCP): A study of 10,000 cases. Gastroenterology 1976;*70*:314.
53. Zimmon DS, Fulkenstein DG, Riccobono C, et al: Complications of endoscopic retrograde cholangiopancreatography: Analysis of 300 consecutive cases. Gastroenterology 1975;*69*:303.
54. Kasagai T, Kuno N, Kizu M: Manometric endoscopic retrograde pancreatocholangiography. Am J Dig Dis 1974;*19*:485.
55. Raine PAM, Gunn AA: Acute cholecystitis. Br J Surg 1975;*62*:697.
56. Keighley MRB, Drysdale RB, Quoraishi AH, et al: Antibiotics in biliary disease: The relative importance of antibiotic concentrations in the bile and serum. Gut 1976;*17*:495.
57. Glenn F, Moody FC: Acute obstructive suppurative cholangitis. Surg Gynecol Obstet 1961;*113*:265.
58. Nakayama T, Ikeda A, Okuda K: Percutaneous transhepatic drainage of the biliary tract: Technique and results in 104 cases. Gastroenterology 1978; *74*:554.
59. Kadir S, Baassiri A, Barth KH, et al: Percutaneous biliary drainage in the management of biliary sepsis. Am J Roentgenol 1982;*138*:25.
60. Lois JF, Grace PA, Gomes AS, et al: The risk of transhepatic drainage in patients with cholangitis. Submitted for publication.
61. Neoptolemos JP, Harvey MH, Slate ND, Carr-Locke DL: Abdominal wall bile staining and 'biliscrotum' after retroperitoneal perforation following endoscopic sphincterotomy. Br J Surg 1984;*7*:684.
62. Siegel JH: Endoscopic papillotomy in the treatment of biliary tract disease: 258 procedures and results. Dig Dis Sci 1981;*26*:1057.
63. van der Spuy S: Endoscopic sphincterotomy in the management of gallstone pancreatis. Endoscopy 1981;*13*:25.
64. Safrany L, Cotton PB: A preliminary report: Urgent duodenoscopic sphincterotomy for acute gallstone pancreatitis. Surgery 1981;*89*:424.
65. Delmotte JS, Pommelet P, et al: Initial duodenoscopy sphincterotomy in patients with acute cholangitis or pancreatitis complicating biliary stones. Gastroenterology 1982;*82*:1042.
66. Acosta JM, Pellegrini CA, Skinner DB: Etiology and pathogenesis of acute biliary pancreatitis. Surgery 1980;*88*:118.
67. Stone HH, Fabian TC, Dunlop WE: Gallstone pancreatitis: Biliary tract pathology in relation to time of operation. Ann Surg 1981;*194*:305.

CARLOS A. PELLEGRINI, M.D.

20

Biliary Pancreatitis

Approximately 5 per cent of patients with cholelithiasis develop acute pancreatitis.[1, 2] By contrast, about 50 per cent of patients with acute pancreatitis have gallstones.[1, 3–5] Although biliary pancreatitis can occur at any age, the peak incidence is between 50 and 70 years. Women are affected twice as often as men.[3] The proportion of patients with alcoholic pancreatitis to those with gallstone pancreatitis varies from one institution to another and from one country to another, depending on the relative prevalence of gallstones and alcoholism. Gallstone pancreatitis is more frequent than alcoholic pancreatitis in England,[3, 4, 6] Germany,[7] and Israel,[8, 9] whereas alcoholic pancreatitis predominates in France[1, 10] and in county and Veterans Administration hospitals in the United States.[1]

PATHOGENESIS

The association of pancreatitis and biliary tract disease was first made in 1856 by Claude Bernard. He showed that the injection of bile in the pancreatic duct of dogs induced pancreatitis.[11] A few years later, Lancereaux proposed that acute pancreatitis in humans was the result of reflux of bile into the pancreatic duct.[12] The implication of gallstones in the development of acute pancreatitis was introduced at the turn of the century by Opie, a pathologist at Johns Hopkins, who found an impacted stone in the ampulla of Vater of a patient who had died of acute pancreatitis.[13] Based on this observation and in experiments that he carried out in dogs, he proposed the "common channel theory." This theory postulated that in patients in whom the common bile duct and the pancreatic duct joined before entering the duodenum, the impaction of a stone at the ampulla of Vater produced reflux of bile into the pancreatic duct, which activated the pancreatic enzymes and gave rise to pancreatitis.[14]

The common channel theory did not hold for long, however, as it was shown that in humans, bile rarely refluxes into the pancreatic duct (the pressure in the pancreatic duct rises to higher levels than that in the bile duct if both are occluded); gallstones are rarely found impacted at the ampulla in patients who die of necrotizing pancreatitis; and not all patients with acute pancreatitis and cholelithiasis have common duct stones at the time of operation.[2]

In 1974 Acosta and Ledesma, in a landmark paper, reported the results of a study in which the stools of patients with biliary pancreatitis were screened for the presence of gallstones. They found gallstones in the stools of 34 of the 36 patients with acute pancreatitis within 10 days of the attack, and in 3 out of 36 patients with cholelithiasis but no pancreatitis. Most patients with pancreatitis had elevation of serum bilirubin levels associated with the attack, and the finding of the gallstone in the stool was preceded by relief of symptoms and a sudden decrease in the serum amylase and bilirubin levels. In most cases, there was only one stone in the stool, but two or more stones (up to 80) were found in ten patients. Most gallstones retrieved from the stool were small. These findings gave rise to the concept that biliary pancreatitis was frequently caused by *transient blockage* of the ampulla of Vater by a migrating stone.[19] In the same year, an independent study by Kelly[20] reported similar results and established beyond doubt a close temporal relationship between transampullary passage of gallstones and attack of acute pancreatitis.

Once it became established that gallstone migration was of cardinal importance in the genesis of acute pancreatitis, several questions emerged. For example, why did only 3 to 8 per cent of patients with cholelithiasis ever develop pancreatitis? Why, once they experienced the first attack, was recurrence so high (up to 50 per cent in the first 6 months)?[21, 22] Why did migration of a stone cause pancreatitis in some patients and not in others? (About 10 per cent of patients with cholelithiasis pass gallstones through the ampulla, and only very few develop acute pancreatitis.)[19, 20, 23] How did the migrating stone cause acute pancreatitis?

Several local factors determine whether gallstones are likely to induce an attack of acute pancreatitis. The size, density, and shape of stones influence their ability to travel down the cystic duct and impact at the ampulla. The functional status of the gallbladder and the caliber of the cystic duct are important in facilitating transfer of gallstones from the gallbladder into the common bile duct, and both the caliber of the ampulla and the presence of a common channel may influence the frequency and severity of resulting pancreatitis.

Physical Characteristics of the Gallstones

In most cases, the stones that migrate through the ampulla and cause pancreatitis are small (Fig. 20–1).[19, 20, 24, 25] For example, comparing 18 patients who had cholelithiasis and a history of acute pancreatitis with 28 patients who had cholelithiasis alone, McMahon and Shepta found that 78 per cent of patients with a history of pancreatitis had small, irregular or mulberry-shaped stones. This was seen in only 43 per cent of the patients in the control group. Patients with pancreatitis had more gallstones in their gallbladders, and the mean weight of their stones was half that seen in those without pancreatitis.[24] The importance of small stones as a cause of pancreatitis was underscored by Houssin et al. in a study of microlithiasis of the gallbladder. These authors found that microlithiasis (stone diameter of 3 mm or less) was present in approximately 25 per cent of their patients with cholelithiasis. The majority of these patients (76 per cent) had symptoms of biliary tract disease, and pancreatitis was much more common among these patients than among those with larger stones. For example, 15 of their 68 patients with microlithiasis had had pancreatitis before their cholecystectomy.[25]

Cystic Duct Diameter

The diameter of the cystic duct and the resistance to flow (a reflection of the degree of convolution and the number of valves of Heister) play a role in the migration of gallbladder stones. In one study, flow rates through the cystic duct in gallbladders perfused *ex-vivo* at a constant pressure were twice as large in patients with pancreatitis than in those with cholelithiasis but no pancreatitis, suggesting a larger diameter and less resistance in the cystic duct of patients with pancreatitis.[24] It has also been shown that in over two thirds of patients with previous pancreatitis, the gallstones are smaller than the cystic duct and thus may easily migrate into the common bile duct.[2]

The Common Bile Duct and the Ampulla of Vater

The frequency with which stones are found in the common bile duct of patients who have suffered an attack of pancreatitis depends on the time of observation. For example, Armstrong et al. found gallstones in the common bile duct in all patients operated on within 48 hours of the onset of pancreatitis, in 66 per cent of those operated on within 3 to 7 days, in 23 per cent of those operated on between 8 and 21 days, and in 11 per cent of those operated on beyond the twenty-second day.[2] In a prospective randomized trial of early operation in patients with acute pancreatitis, Stone et al. found choledocholithiasis in 75 per cent of patients operated on within 72 hours but in only 28 per cent of those operated on a few weeks later.[26] These findings suggest that in the majority of patients with acute pancreatitis, the stones coming from the gallbladder remain only transiently in the common bile duct, and give further support to the theory of gallstone migration. However, in some patients the primary source of stones is the common bile duct. Indeed, Kelly has shown that, following cholecystectomy, residual or recurrent stones can give rise to pancreatitis.[27] In this study, over 90 per cent of patients with previous pancreatitis who had residual or recurrent choledocholithiasis experienced another attack of pancreatitis.

The finding of an impacted stone at the ampulla is also related to the time of observation. We found a stone at the ampulla of

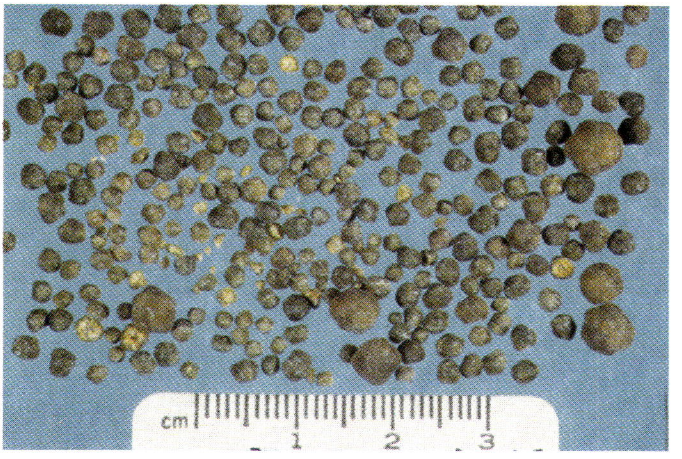

Figure 20–1. Multiple cholesterol stones from the gallbladder of a patient with several previous attacks of biliary pancreatitis. Note the predominance of small stones, 2 to 3 mm in diameter. There are several stones less than 1 mm in diameter.

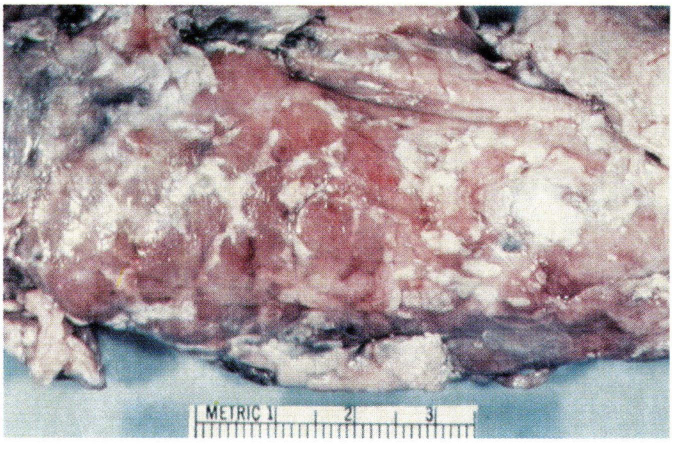

Figure 20–2. Pancreas from a patient who died of acute necrohemorrhagic pancreatitis. Dark areas of ischemic necrosis and hematoma alternate with white areas of fat necrosis on a background of diffuse hemorrhage, giving the characteristic mottled appearance.

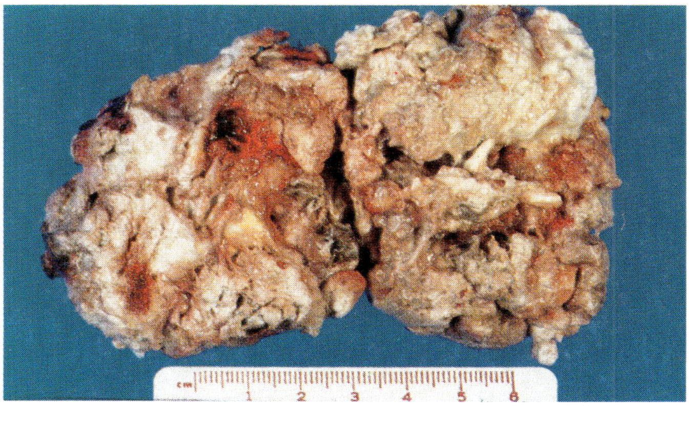

Figure 20–6. Large amounts of devitalized tissue removed from the retroperitoneum of a patient who had postoperative pancreatitis. She returned to the operating room for further debridement 3 weeks later and eventually recovered.

Vater in 75 per cent of a group of 55 patients operated on within 48 hours of the attack of pancreatitis. The majority of these patients were operated on during the initial 24 hours.[15] Contrary to this observation, Coppa et al. were unable to find ampullary obstruction in a group of 14 patients who underwent transhepatic cholangiography during the acute phase of biliary pancreatitis.[28] However, there is now plenty of evidence to support the concept of temporary ampullary impaction of a stone in patients with biliary pancreatitis. For example, Kelly reported finding stones impacted in 62 per cent of patients operated on within 48 hours of the onset of pancreatitis;[29] in Armstrong's large prospective study, ampullary obstruction was found in 67 per cent of patients operated on within 48 hours, 33 per cent of those operated on between 3 and 7 days, and 5 per cent of those operated on after the eighth day.[2] Although Stone found ampullary obstruction by a stone in only 6 per cent of patients operated on within 72 hours of the attack, he found the offending stone in the duodenum in 31 per cent of them, and an edematous ampulla with intense inflammation of the distal common bile duct in the majority of patients.[26] As experience with endoscopic papillotomy in the acute phase of pancreatitis is mounting, impacted stones or evidence of recent dislodgment are seen in almost every patient who undergoes this procedure within a few hours of the initiation of pancreatitis.[30–34]

Patients with previous pancreatitis tend to have larger common bile ducts than those without such a history.[35] The duct is sometimes dilated even in the absence of choledochal calculi, implying either previous temporary obstruction of the biliary tree or a dilated duct of other cause.[2] In a study of patients with choledocholithiasis, we found that 17 per cent of those with pigment stones had a history of previous pancreatitis, whereas none of those with cholesterol common duct stones did.[36] This underscores the fact that in some patients with pancreatitis there is a primary common bile duct disorder.

Indeed, there is evidence that the function of the sphincter of Oddi in patients with previous pancreatitis differs from that of patients with cholelithiasis but no pancreatitis. For example, Guelrud et al. have shown that the basal sphincter of Oddi pressure, the pressure gradient between common duct and duodenum, and the amplitude of the pressure waves at the ampulla are higher in patients with previous pancreatitis than in those with choledocholithiasis alone.[37] In addition, Cuschieri et al. have shown that the sphincter of Oddi of patients with pancreatitis fails to relax in response to ceruletide.[38] Whether or not this apparent sphincter dysfunction increases the chance of a stone getting caught at the ampulla is not yet clear.

Pancreatic Duct Reflux

Several authors have shown that pancreatic duct reflux on operative cholangiography at the time of elective cholecystectomy is more frequently observed in patients with previous biliary pancreatitis than in those without.[2, 15, 39–41] In order for reflux to occur between the bile duct and the pancreas, a common channel must be present. However, this is the case in over 90 per cent of patients with or without pancreatitis. It has been postulated that those who develop biliary pancreatitis have a larger channel and that, in these patients, pancreatic juice enters the bile duct and mixes with bile. Then the pancreatic-biliary mixture (with a high concentration of unconjugated bile salts) enters the pancreatic duct and produces pancreatitis. Whatever the reason, reflux into the pancreatic duct appears to be a factor that predisposes to pancreatitis.

A particularly severe form of pancreatitis associated with biliary tract disease, but with a different pathogenesis, is that observed immediately following an operation for cholelithiasis. Indeed, the most common cause of postoperative pancreatitis is an operation on the biliary tract.[42] Operative trauma to the ampulla of Vater—not the gallstones—is usually responsible for the development of pancreatitis in these patients.

The normal ampulla is 2 to 4 mm in diameter. Dilatation of the ampulla of Vater with Bakes dilators greater than 4 to 5 mm may lead to injury that creates edema and inflammation of the periampullary tissues, causing obstruction of the pancreatic and common ducts. False passage of a Bakes dilator or other instruments at the time of common duct exploration may lead to inflammation of the periampullary structures. Use of the long-limb T-tube, with the lower limb passing through the ampulla into the duodenum, may compress and obstruct the pancreatic duct and is a recognized cause of acute pancreatitis.[43] Likewise, acute pancreatitis has been reported in about 5 per cent of patients who have percutaneous stents placed through the ampulla to treat malignant biliary obstruction.[44]

In summary, a growing body of clinical and experimental work suggests that the character of gallstones and the anatomy and motor function of the biliary tract play a role in determining who is likely to develop biliary pancreatitis. Patients at risk are those with functioning gallbladders that harbor numerous small stones. In these patients the cystic ducts are larger, and small stones migrate through the common duct to the ampulla. There they become impacted temporarily and eventually find their way into the duodenum. Anatomic and functional differences at the ampullary region may explain why these stones are caught, whereas they pass without incidence in others. It is clear that once an episode of pancreatitis has occurred, the stage is set for subsequent episodes of gallstone migration through the cystic duct; new episodes will occur unless cholelithiasis is treated.[21, 22]

PATHOLOGY

The Pancreas

The changes in the pancreas with biliary pancreatitis consist of edema, necrosis, and hemorrhage. These processes may coexist, and the severity of pancreatitis depends to a great extent on the relative extent of each one.

Interstitial edema, with infiltration of polymorphonuclear leukocytes, is the most common finding. In this form of pancreatitis the exocrine, endocrine, and ductular cells are not damaged; recovery from the inflammation is complete, with no functional or morphologic sequelae to the gland. Indeed, 6 to 8 weeks after an attack of pancreatitis the pancreas looks completely normal in most patients.

Necrotizing pancreatitis implies coagulation necrosis of glandular elements and the surrounding fatty tissue. Necrosis usually does not affect the gland uniformly: dark, friable areas of frank necrosis with bleeding, grayish zones of ischemic necrosis, and white areas indicating fat necrosis with deposition of calcium soaps alternate with regions of preserved architecture to give the pancreas a mottled appearance (Fig. 20–2). Most cases of necrotizing pancreatitis are associated with subcapsular hematomas of varying size. Hemorrhage and necrosis are thought to be related to the same underlying lesion: disruption and thrombotic occlusion of blood vessels. An enlarged, inflamed pancreas containing patchy areas of necrosis has been called a pancreatic phlegmon.[46]

The Peripancreatic Tissues

The extension of the inflammatory process into adjacent tissues, very common in the severe forms of biliary pancreatitis, is important, for it determines the outcome in many patients who recover from the acute attack of pancreatitis. The absence of a well-developed pancreatic capsule allows the inflammatory process to spread freely and affect adjacent organs, such as the duodenum, the colon and mesocolon, the proximal small bowel and its mesentery,[47, 48] the splenic vessels, the terminal common bile duct, the celiac and superior mesenteric ganglia, the lesser omental sac, the pararenal spaces, and even the posterior mediastinum (Fig. 20–3). Tissue debris, inflammatory exudate, pancreatic juice from ruptured canaliculi, blood, and

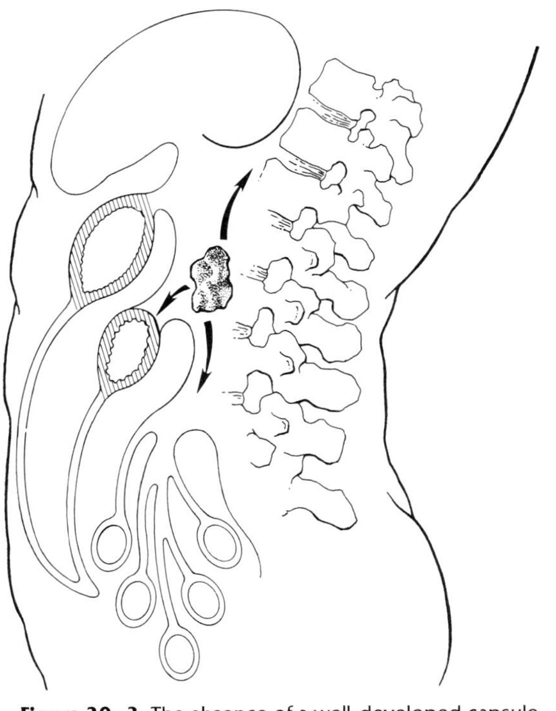

Figure 20–3. The absence of a well-developed capsule around the pancreas allows the inflammatory process to extend to the transverse mesocolon, the mesentery, and the retroperitoneum.

necrosed tissues collect around the pancreas and may eventually give rise to pseudocysts, abscesses, fistulae, and bowel obstruction. Extravasated blood dissects along tissue planes in the retroperitoneum and at the base of the transverse mesocolon. In some patients with large hematomas, it may lead to discoloration and diffuse induration of the costovertebral angle (Turner's sign) or the periumbilical area (Cullen's sign).

Fluid collections that arise within or, more commonly, adjacent to the pancreas (Fig. 20–4) extend throughout the retroperitoneum, the transverse mesocolon, and occasionally the small bowel mesentery for varying distances. Peripancreatic fluid may find its way into the peritoneal cavity. Ascites associated with acute pancreatitis is usually blood-stained and slightly dark and has a high amylase content. The fluid may reach the chest through the diaphragmatic lymphatics and cause a pleural effusion. Most peripancreatic effusions disappear as pancreatic inflammation subsides. Persistence of sterile collections of fluid and debris leads to the formation of pancreatic pseudocysts.

Areas of fat necrosis are common in the retroperitoneal area. The result of the precipitation of calcium salts of free fatty acids liberated by pancreatic lipase, they appear opaque and yellow. The natural history of the *necrosed areas* of the gland and adjacent tissues is determined by their size and the development of infection.[49] If they remain uninfected, they may heal by reabsorption, fibrosis, calcification, or sequestration, a process whereby the necrotic segment is isolated and excluded through the development of a capsule from granulation tissue. Larger segments may become incorporated in pseudocysts, as the surrounding fluid is eventually contained by a capsule, and it is not rare to find relatively large sloughs of necrotic tissue floating freely inside a pseudocyst. Infection of necrotic tissue brings about the development of a pancreatic abscess.

PATHOPHYSIOLOGY

Triggering Mechanism

Biliary pancreatitis is most often the result of sudden, complete obstruction of the pancreatic duct. Pancreatic duct obstruction may result from direct compression by an impacted stone or from traumatic periampullar inflammation caused by the migrating stone. For example, operative cholangiograms done within hours of the onset of pancreatitis rarely demonstrate reflux of contrast medium into the pancreatic duct despite free flow into the duodenum, suggesting persistent, complete obstruction of the pancreatic duct.[26] Papillotomy, in these patients, produces a sudden "gush" of pancreatic juice as soon as the sphincter is dilated or cut, suggesting considerable pancreatic duct hypertension.[15, 26, 40]

As most attacks of gallstone pancreatitis occur shortly after meals, it is thought that pancreatic ductal hypertension may be exacerbated by the postprandial stimulation of pancreatic secretion.[15] Indeed, in experimental studies, continuous stimulation of the pancreas by cerulein alone is sufficient to produce pancreatitis and damage to canalicular cells; in the isolated perfused canine pan-

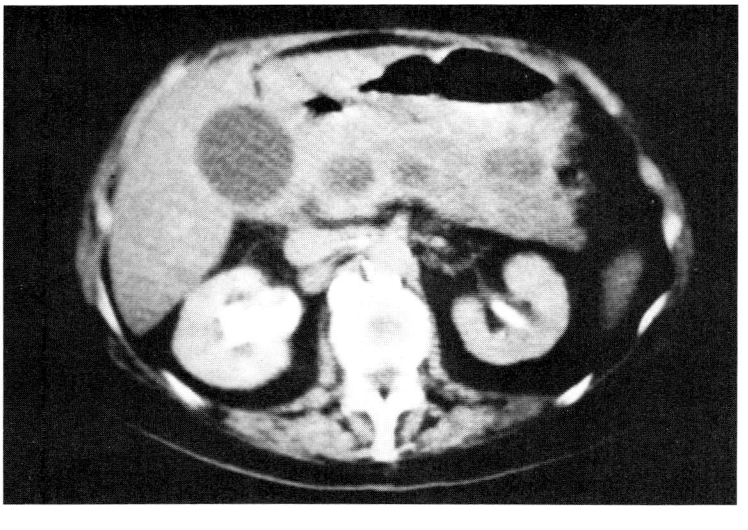

Figure 20–4. CT scan of the pancreas 2 weeks after an attack of acute pancreatitis. The gland is enlarged, the fat planes are erased, and there are several loculated fluid collections in and around the gland. The gallbladder is dilated.

creas, acute pancreatitis can be produced by obstruction of the pancreatic duct and secretin stimulation.[50]

Exactly how the migrating stone triggers premature activation of zymogens that initiate autodigestion of the pancreas is not known. Pancreatic juice contains several inactive zymogens that normally undergo activation only after entering the duodenum. There, trypsinogen is transformed into trypsin by enterokinase, an enzyme attached to the brush border membrane of duodenal mucosa. Trypsin then activates the other pancreatic zymogens, including chymotrypsinogens, proelastases, procarboxypeptidases, and prophospholipases. During episodes of pancreatitis, however, activated proteolytic enzymes, such as elastase and trypsin, can be found in pancreatic juice and within the gland itself. The enzymes are thought to play an important role in the development of pancreatitis.

Although it is not clear what leads to the premature activation of enzymes, speculation has centered around two theories: (1) Duodenal contents, including enterokinase, reflux into the pancreatic duct and activate trypsinogen, and (2) pancreatic ductal hypertension, resulting from continued secretion into the obstructed duct, leads to rupture of peripheral canaliculi, extravasation of pancreatic juice, and intraparenchymal activation of digestive enzymes.[45] The first possibility is supported by the development of pancreatitis in dogs with a closed duodenal loop or by injection of duodenal juice into the pancreatic duct. In patients with biliary pancreatitis, the evidence suggests that pancreatic ductal hypertension is more likely to explain the process of enzyme activation.

However, recent findings cast doubt on the concept that enzyme activation occurs in the pancreatic duct or intercellular space. Instead, these findings suggest that activation of enzymes may occur within the pancreatic acinar cell itself, subsequent to exposure of digestive zymogens to lysosomal hydrolases.[52, 57] Both proteins are normally synthesized by ribosomes in the endoplasmic reticulum, but when synthesis is completed, digestive zymogens are stored into membrane-enclosed intracellular spaces that contain potent trypsin inhibitors, the zymogen granules. Activation of zymogens by hydrolases is further prevented by storing hydrolases within lysosomes. Early stages of pancreatitis may involve merging of lysosomes and zymogen granules and intracellular activation of trypsinogen. How pancreatic ductal hypertension causes this phenomenon remains unknown. However, once it has started, the process leads to a sequence of enzymatic reactions that produce the local and systemic manifestations of acute pancreatitis.

Local Events

Obstruction of the pancreatic duct outflow causes, first, congestion of the gland, which leads to pancreatic edema.[45] Canalicular hypertension or rupture of acinar cells, or both, lead to extravasation of pancreatic juice into the interstitium. This edema fluid with its enzymatic components has been termed juice edema.[7] Stretching of the peritoneal capsule caused by the enlargement of the gland is responsible for the development of pancreatic pain, at least initially. Absorption of edema fluid, primarily through the rich net of pancreatic lymphatics, leads to an increase in the serum amylase level. If the obstruction to flow of pancreatic juice is relieved at this stage, the interstitial edema is cleared by the lymphatics and the gland returns to its original size. Because the symptoms disappear rather quickly and the anatomic changes in the pancreas are minimal, some authors have questioned whether this type of inflammatory process should be considered pancreatitis and refer to it as "biliary colic with increased serum amylase." Nevertheless, these patients do have pancreatic inflammation (the biliary tract does not produce amylase), and the mechanisms that set the process in motion are similar to those responsible for more severe pancreatitis. From a clinical standpoint, thinking of these patients as having pancreatitis leads to institution of appropriate therapy of the associated cholelithiasis.

If the process does not resolve within a short period, the autodigestive mechanism starts. Necrosis is brought about by the proteolytic enzymes (trysin, chymotrypsin, and so forth) and by the action of lipase on the neutral fat stored in fat cells.[7] Collagenase, which destroys the connective tissue that separates the lobules of the gland, facilitates tryptic necrosis and extension into the adjacent tissues. Elastase has a destructive effect on the walls of the blood vessels and is probably responsible for the hemorrhagic component.

Some authors believe that edematous pancreatitis and necrohemorrhagic pancreatitis are two different entities from the start. For instance, Wells et al. were not able to show a progression from acute interstitial pancreatitis to a necrohemorrhagic form in a dog model of biliary pancreatitis. Indeed, all their animals developed some form of necrosis, and they postulated that all cases of biliary pancreatitis—even those that macroscopically appear to be just edematous—have a component of mild necrosis.[51] In addition, overt necrosis of the gland is occasionally found in patients operated on relatively early (i.e., in the first 48 to 72 hours), raising the possibility that these individuals developed necrosis from the very beginning. However, there is good evidence that, in humans, acute edematous pancreatitis caused by gallstones may progress to a necrohemorrhagic form.[7, 52]

Whether *all* cases of necrohemorrhagic pancreatitis are preceded by an edematous form of pancreatitis—as well as the critical events that determine this progression—is less clear. We have presented evidence that suggests that the length of time the stone remains impacted at the ampulla correlates with the degree of pancreatic damage. For example, in 55 patients who had a gallstone impacted at the ampulla at the time of anatomic observation (surgery or autopsy) the degree of pancreatitis directly correlated with the duration of ampullary obstruction: Whereas all patients who had ampullary obstruction for 6 to 12 hours had edematous pancreatitis, 5 of 6 patients with a stone impacted for 72 to 96 hours had marked pancreatic necrosis. In addition, we did not observe any evidence of necrosis with obstruction periods of less than 24 hours.[15] Others, who have had an opportunity to examine the gland during this very early stage in a large group of consecutive patients with biliary pancreatitis, have reported similar findings.[26, 53] These findings suggest that in the first 24 hours of the initiation of the attack of pancreatitis, the changes in the gland are reversible in almost all patients. They also explain the relative absence of late complications (such as pancreatic pseudocysts and pancreatic abscesses) in patients in whom the patency of the pancreatic duct is restored within the first 48 hours.[15, 26, 31–34, 40, 54, 55]

Systemic Events

The systemic manifestations of acute pancreatitis, such as respiratory insufficiency, are thought to result from proteolytic enzymes (e.g., trypsin, elastase) that enter the circulation via portal vein blood and lymphatics and by absorption from the peritoneum.[56] Alpha-2-macroglobulin, the chief defense against these molecules, complexes with proteases that gain access to the blood, and the complexes are then cleared by the reticuloendothelial system. In severe pancreatitis, alpha-2-macroglobulin levels drop so low that the circulation contains free proteases, capable of activating the complement (C3) and kinin (kininogen) systems. The resulting products, activated C3 and bradykinin, initiate other harmful events, such as aggregation of granulocytes, which produce a respiratory lesion identical to that seen in the acute respiratory distress syndrome (ARDS) from other causes (e.g., trauma or sepsis). The kinins produce vasodilatation and increased vascular permeability, which contribute to the development of edema, loss of intravascular volume, and shock. In some patients the pancreatic proteases lead to the development of microthrombi, which consume clotting factors and cause disseminated intravascular coagulation. Patients with severe pancreatitis also have high concentrations of endotoxin in the serum, the origin of which is not clear. The increase in vascular permeability and the development of microthrombi are particularly evident in the parenchyma of the lung and the kidney.

In the *lung* the most prominent feature is edema. Pulmonary edema is caused by a disruption of the alveolar-capillary membrane that is usually reversible. The fluid is a transudate, and its genesis is linked to the increased permeability caused by the circulating kinins. In addition, hypoalbuminemia, phospholipase A, and high concentrations of free fatty acids alter pulmonary surfactant and further contribute to the development of pulmonary edema. The large amounts of fluid necessary to resuscitate patients with severe pancreatitis aggravate this situation.

Pulmonary edema leads to arterial hypoxemia. In the first 3 to 4 days of the attack, PA_{O_2} levels of 50 to 60 mm Hg without associated changes on chest radiographs are seen in 30 to 40 per cent of patients with biliary pancreatitis. Hypoxemia is aggravated in patients with severe pancreatitis by marked right-to-left shunting. This is caused by pulmonary intravascular microthrombi formed as a result of subclinical disseminated intravascular coagulation and by granulocyte aggregation in the pulmonary capillaries.[57–59]

Aggregated neutrophils in the lung capillaries may release oxygen-free radicals, which in combination with other inflammatory mediators (PGE_2, PGE, and so forth), contribute to the leakage of the lung capillaries. Some patients progress to a more serious pulmonary insufficiency and typical adult respiratory distress syndrome. They develop diffuse pulmonary infiltrates, seen on chest radiographs, and severe hypoxemia. The incidence of this type of ARDS rises with the increasing clinical severity of the attack, with coexisting hyperlipidemia and the development of sepsis.[57, 60]

In the *kidney,* some degree of renal dysfunction is the most common occurrence. Hypovolemia is a major factor, but mild renal failure is also seen in the absence of hypovolemia. Selective increase in renal vascular resistance, leading to a reduction in renal blood flow and oxygen uptake,[61] and decreased tubular protein reabsorption[61] have been documented in patients with pancreatitis. Histologic studies have shown thrombi in glomerular capillaries and deposits of fibrinogen and IgG in the glomerular basement membrane.[61]

Most patients with severe gallstone pancreatitis have some degree of transient *hyperglycemia.* This is thought to be caused by an excess of glucagon rather than a deficit of plasma insulin. Indeed, basal plasma glucagon concentrations have been found to be ten times above normal in patients with a first attack of pancreatitis.[63]

Transient *hypocalcemia* develops in about one third of patients with pancreatitis.[64, 65] The degree of hypocalcemia parallels the clinical severity of the disease.[65, 66] Hypocalcemia in these patients is accompanied by a decrease of ionized serum calcium.[64, 65] The exact cause of hypocalcemia is not known, but it has been linked to the hypoalbuminemia that invariably results from severe pancreatitis. Calcium sequestration in areas of fat necrosis may explain to a certain extent the fall in serum calcium, but if the homeostatic mechanisms supposed to restore calcium to normal were functioning properly, calcium should promptly return to normal after the initial fall. Some investigators have proposed that inadequate PTH secretion is partly responsible for the low calcium,[65] although appropriate rises in PTH have been found by other workers.[64, 67] It is also possible that the hypocalcemia may be related to the relative hyperglucagonemia observed in these patients.[63] Glucagon normally induces release of thyrocalcitonin, which lowers the serum level of calcium.

DIAGNOSIS

There are four aspects to the diagnosis of biliary pancreatitis: the diagnosis itself, the identification of associated biliary tract disease, the diagnosis of severity of pancreatitis, and the diagnosis of complications.

Diagnosis of Pancreatitis

Clinical Findings. The clinical findings range from mild, self-limited symptoms to a fulminant, rapidly lethal disease. Unfortunately, the clinical features of acute pancreatitis sometimes mimic those of other intra-abdominal processes, such as perforated or penetrating peptic ulcer, acute cholecystitis, acute cholangitis, intestinal obstruction, acute appendicitis, and so forth.

The most common symptom is *pain,* mostly epigastric, with frequent radiation to the back and occasionally to the flanks. The pain often begins after a heavy meal; the onset is rapid (although probably not as rapid as that seen in perforated viscus) and becomes constant shortly after it starts. Pain is sometimes relieved by sitting forward and sometimes by the knee-chest position. Most patients also have *nausea and vomiting,* and some have mild abdominal distention, although the latter is not usually seen until after 24 to 48 hours of the onset of pancreatitis.

The physical findings vary with the severity of pancreatitis. Most patients have *tachycardia* and some degree of *tachypnea,* which may worsen rapidly. Temperature and blood pressure are usually normal on admission. The abdomen has slight distention, few or absent bowel sounds, and epigastric tenderness, which may lead to the feeling of fullness.

Laboratory Findings. *Serum amylase* remains the most widely used laboratory measurement in the evaluation of patients suspected of having pancreatitis. Over 90 per cent of patients with biliary pancreatitis have elevated serum amylase levels,[68] and these values are, overall, higher than those observed in patients with alcoholic pancreatitis. One must be aware that patients with other acute abdominal conditions may have elevated serum amylase levels. However, this is not as common as was previously thought, the values are not usually as high, and elevation of serum amylase in other acute abdominal processess is not observed as early as in pancreatitis. For example, evaluating all emergency admissions to our surgical unit over a 1-year period, we found that whereas 97 per cent of patients who were eventually proven to have acute pancreatitis had elevated serum amylase levels, only 20 per cent of those with other abdominal conditions did.[69] *Serum lipase* is also elevated in these patients.

Urinary amylase output rises in parallel with serum amylase. A few years ago there was enthusiasm about the diagnostic value of the ratio of *clearance of amylase/clearance of creatinine* (normal 1 to 4 per cent). Most patients with pancreatitis have values above 6 per cent.[70] However, the use of this ratio has not lived up to expectations and is of little clinical value. Instead, efforts to increase the diagnostic accuracy of serum amylase have shifted to the study of the different *amylase isoenzymes* in the serum.[71] However, with present techniques it is not always possible to differentiate salivary from pancreatic amylases, and although potentially useful, this determination remains experimental.

As discussed earlier (see Pathophysiology), *serum glucose* is elevated in about 10 per cent of patients with biliary pancreatitis. In the absence of diabetes, hyperglycemia indicates severe pancreatitis. *Hypocalcemia,* also discussed, is an ominous finding.

Radiology. Abdominal *flat plate* and *upright films* should always be obtained in the evaluation of patients with abdominal pain. In nearly half of patients with pancreatitis there is evidence of ileus, usually localized; in one quarter of patients there is dilatation of the proximal colon with an abrupt "cutoff" at the distal transverse colon. Although these findings are nonspecific, the films are valuable in the differentiation of pancreatitis from other acute abdominal processes.

Ultrasonography is useful in the diagnosis of gallbladder disease and in the evaluation of the extrahepatic biliary tract in patients with pancreatitis.[72–74] It is not as useful in the evaluation of the pancreas and retroperitoneum, as these can be defined in only about two thirds of patients with pancreatitis because of the associated ileus. The diagnostic accuracy of ultrasonography with regard to the pancreas is greatly surpassed by CT scan.

Computed tomography provides excellent images of the pancreas and peripancreatic areas and is the diagnostic test of choice when one is trying to determine whether acute pancreatitis is present. Early in the course of pancreatitis there is diffuse pancreatic enlargement and obliteration of the peripancreatic fat planes. Occasionally, peripancreatic fluid can be detected in early stages (see Fig. 20–4). Later in the course of acute pancreatitis, CT is particularly useful when one is dealing with complications, as it is very accurate in the diagnosis of pseudocysts, abscesses, and other retroperitoneal fluid collections.[75–78]

In summary, in most patients the diagnosis of pancreatitis can be suspected by the history, clinical findings, and elevated serum amylase levels and aided by the findings of the abdominal plain film. This remains to a certain extent a diagnosis of exclusion, but it may be sufficient to treat patients with mild or moderate disease. When the patient is sicker or when it is important to make a positive diagnosis, computed tomography is the diagnostic test of choice. Although ultrasonography is of limited value in determining the presence or absence of pancreatitis, it is very useful in the diagnosis of associated cholelithiasis and evaluation of the extrahepatic biliary tree. With the use of these techniques, very few patients will need either diagnostic peritoneal lavage or celiotomy solely for the purpose of diagnosis.

Diagnosis of Associated Biliary Tract Disease

The second step in the diagnostic work-up of a patient with biliary pancreatitis is diagnosis of the associated cholelithiasis. The history and clinical findings provide some clues. Approximately 20 per cent of patients with biliary pancreatitis have been previously studied for other manifestations of cholelithiasis and know that they have gallstones.[79] When compared with those who have alcoholic pancreatitis, patients with gallstones tend to be older and are more likely to be female.[80] Patients with biliary pancreatitis more frequently have a history of jaundice and an onset of the attack with pain localized to the right upper quadrant. Direct and rebound tenderness in the right upper quadrant—rather than generalized—are also more common in patients with gallstones.[81]

Several studies have reported that patients with biliary pancreatitis have higher serum levels of glutamic-pyruvic and glutamic-oxalocetic transaminases and of alkaline phosphatase than do those with alcoholic pancreatitis.[80–85] Levels of serum bilirubin[80, 83, 84] and amylase[80, 84] are also higher in patients with biliary pancreatitis. We found that the average serum amylase value for patients admitted to our unit with biliary pancreatitis was 1600, whereas the average of those admitted with alcoholic pancreatitis was 400.[69] Although these findings may assist in the diagnosis of gallstones early in the attack of pancreatitis, confirmation of biliary tract disease requires further testing.

Early detection of cholelithiasis is best accomplished by ultrasonography.[72–74, 86] Since it is easily available, relatively cheap, and noninvasive, we recommend it for all patients with a first attack of pancreatitis. For further details on the diagnostic use of ultrasonography refer to Chapter 8. Oral cholecystography is not possible during the early stages of pancreatitis, and the gallbladder may be nonopacified, even in the absence of gallstones, for 4 to 6 weeks after the episode of pancreatitis, presumably owing to the adjacent inflammatory process. On the other hand, ultrasonography and oral cholecystography may be falsely normal, as most of these patients have very small gallstones and functioning gallbladders. Milgalter and Freund reported that in up to 36 per cent of their patients with biliary pancreatitis, oral cholecystograms and intravenous cholangiograms failed to reveal the presence of gallstones.[87] Direct cholangiography may show the gallstones when ultrasonography and oral cholecystography have failed,[88–92] and occasionally, cholecystectomy may be the only way to find the gallstones in a patient with recurrent attacks of pancreatitis. Small gallstones are frequently found in these patients, and recurrence of pancreatitis is rare after cholecystectomy.[87]

Even when a positive diagnosis of cholelithiasis has been made, this is only indirect evidence in support of the biliary origin of pancreatitis in the individual patient. It may be important in selected patients to determine beyond doubt whether an attack of pancreatitis was caused by the associated cholelithiasis or whether there are two coincident diseases. The issue is particularly relevant in the alcoholic who has cholelithiasis. *Screening of the stools* following an attack of pancreatitis, as recommended by Acosta et al., may be of help, as the chances are over 85 per cent that a gallstone will be found if it is involved in the development of the attack of pancreatitis.[93] This approach, however, requires several days. Instead, some have advocated the use of *radionuclide biliary scanning* with ^{99m}Tc-labeled HIDA during the acute attack of pancreatitis.[94] In most patients with biliary pancreatitis the gallbladder does not fill, whereas it does in most patients with other forms of pancreatitis.[94, 95] Interpretation of the results of this test must be done with care, since acute cholecystitis, which may mimic acute pancreatitis, is also expected to yield no gallbladder visualization.[96] For further details refer to Chapter 12. *Direct cholangiography* has also been proposed to determine whether a stone is involved in the attack of pancreatitis. It can be performed by the percutaneous route[28] (see also Chapter 10) or by retrograde cannulation of the ampulla (see also Chapters 11 and 25). The advantage of the latter is that it is not only diagnostic but also therapeutic, as the offending stone may be extracted after a papillotomy is performed.[30, 97]

Diagnosis of Severity of Gallstone Pancreatitis

In general, there is a correlation between the clinical severity of pancreatitis and the damage to the gland. Most patients with mild pancreatitis have edematous pancreatitis, whereas most patients who die have the necrohemorrhagic form of pancreatitis. Unfortunately, it is frequently impossible to examine the pancreas directly.

In 1974 Ranson identified 11 early objective prognostic signs, five known shortly after admission and six that developed during the first 48 hours (Table 20–1). Patients with fewer than two of these prognostic signs have minimal mortality, whereas mortality is near 15 per cent in those with three or four signs, near 40 per cent in those with five or six signs, and approaches 100 per cent for those

Table 20–1 RANSON'S CRITERIA OF SEVERITY OF ACUTE PANCREATITIS

Criteria Present Initially
Age over 55 years
White blood cell count > 16,000/ml
Blood glucose > 200 mg/dl
Serum LDH > 350 IU/L
SGOT (AST) > 250 IU/dl
Criteria Developing During First 48 Hours
Hematocrit fall of greater than 10 percentage points
BUN rise of more than 5 mg/dl
Serum CA^{2+} < 8 mm Hg
Arterial Po_2 < 60 mm Hg
Base deficit > 4 mEq/l
Estimated fluid sequestration > 6000 ml

with seven or eight signs.[66] These signs are useful not only to determine the prognosis but also to identify patients who are likely to develop complications and who should be closely monitored.

McMahon et al.[98] reported that the severity of pancreatitis may be estimated by the volume and color of peritoneal fluid obtained by early paracentesis. Other studies have found that serum methemalbumin and cAMP levels may have prognostic value.[99]

Diagnosis of Complications

The diagnosis of complications is based on careful daily evaluation and a series of biochemical and radiologic studies to monitor the progression of those patients with severe disease. Computed tomography of the abdomen, at intervals of a week or so, provides invaluable information regarding the evolution of the process in the pancreas and peripancreatic tissues. It is the best diagnostic aid when one is trying to find the cause of persistent fever or septicemia 2 to 3 weeks into the course of pancreatitis (Fig. 20–5).

NATURAL HISTORY AND CLINICAL COURSE

The majority of patients with biliary pancreatitis have a relatively benign course. Pancreatitis is edematous only, and rapid resolution of the abdominal pain and the ileus is the rule. However, about 15 per cent of patients with gallstone pancreatitis develop hemorrhagic necrosis of the pancreas and become seriously ill. Mortality in this group reaches 50 per cent.

The clinical course of severe pancreatitis can be divided into two phases: the inflammatory phase and the septic phase.

Inflammatory Phase

This phase lasts 7 to 10 days. During this time the predominant clinical problem is fluid loss. Inflammation of the pancreas and the retroperitoneum mimics a severe burn sequestering a large amount of fluid. In addition, the ileus that invariably accompanies this form of pancreatitis contributes to the fluid loss. Acute renal failure from hypovolemia used to be the most common cause of death during this phase of pancreatitis.[100] Since vigorous hydration became an established part of treatment, acute renal failure is not seen as frequently, and most patients who die during this phase do so from respiratory failure. Unfortunately, the large volumes of fluid needed to resuscitate these patients aggravate their severe pulmonary edema.

Septic Phase

Patients who survive the inflammatory phase of pancreatitis may, by the second or third week, develop sepsis. Sepsis is usually secondary to infection of necrotic tissues. Septic complications are more common among patients with biliary pancreatitis than among those with alcoholic pancreatitis. Although patients with biliary pancreatitis are

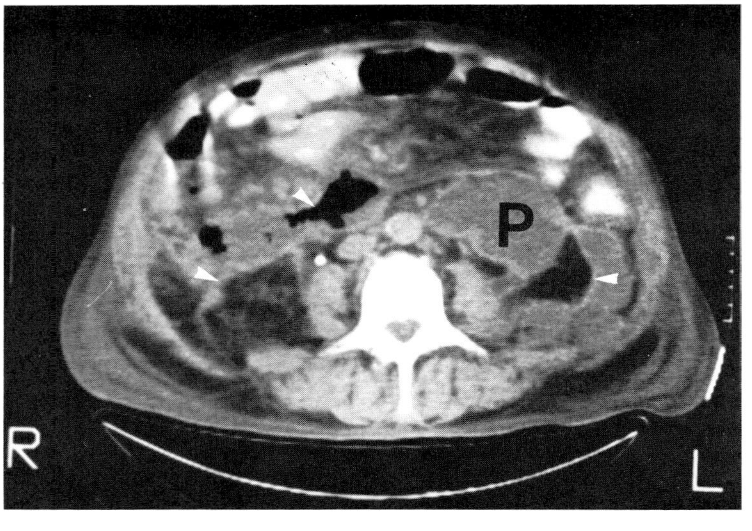

Figure 20–5. CT scan of the abdomen of a patient who developed a pancreatic abscess after an attack of pancreatitis. The body of the gland (P) is large and displaces the stomach anteriorly. There are several areas of air and fluid collection in the retroperitoneum and around the duodenal sweep (arrowheads).

usually older (by 15 to 20 years) than those with alcoholic pancreatitis, they survive the inflammatory phase of hemorrhagic pancreatitis more often than their alcoholic counterparts do, and thus there are proportionally more patients with gallstone pancreatitis who develop pancreatic abscesses.[49] Patients with biliary pancreatitis may also develop pancreatic pseudocysts. In general, however, pseudocysts arising from biliary pancreatitis are uncommon, as most are secondary to pancreatitis caused by alcohol abuse.

Death occurs in 2 to 8 per cent of patients with biliary pancreatitis. In a study of 116 patients who died of pancreatitis, Storck et al. found that all but two died during the first attack. About 50 per cent of all fatalities occurred within the first week, the majority during the first few days. Early death was more common among the alcoholic patients. Patients with biliary pancreatitis who died had a protracted clinical course and eventually succumbed to infection.[100]

Clinical Course After an Attack of Biliary Pancreatitis

After resolution of acute pancreatitis the course of the patient is dictated by whether or not cholelithiasis is treated. Recurrent bouts of pancreatitis will occur in one third to two thirds of patients within 3 to 6 months after the initial attack unless the biliary tract pathology is eliminated.[1, 20–22, 39] After adequate treatment of the biliary tract disease, however, only 2 to 5 per cent of patients will ever experience another attack of acute pancreatitis. Most of these individuals have residual or recurrent common bile duct stones, and further recurrences are common in this group.[27]

It is important to recognize that whereas alcoholic pancreatitis frequently leads to chronic pancreatitis, progressive fibrosis of the gland is not seen in patients with gallstone pancreatitis. In fact, residual sequelae either to the parenchyma of the pancreas or to exocrine or endocrine function is rarely observed after gallstone pancreatitis, even in patients who survived a very severe attack.

MANAGEMENT OF PATIENTS WITH GALLSTONE PANCREATITIS

The comments made in this section apply primarily to patients with severe pancreatitis, as those with mild disease tend to recover rapidly regardless of treatment. However, it is not always possible to differentiate one group from the other at the time of admission, especially when it is the first admission for pancreatitis. It is therefore wise to consider all these patients as potentially being very sick and to carefully monitor their fluid and electrolyte requirements as well as the respiratory status until it is obvious that they are recovering well from the attack.

The goal in managing patients with gallstone pancreatitis is to provide initial resuscitation and supportive care, early detection of complications, and definitive treatment of the associated cholelithiasis. The first two goals are accomplished by nonoperative management; the third requires operative intervention. Local complications, such as pancreatic abscesses and pseudocysts, almost always require intervention. The treatment of these complications is similar to that of patients with other forms of pancreatitis and is beyond the scope of this chapter.

Nonoperative Management

Since no single agent has proved effective in ameliorating the course of pancreatitis or preventing the development of complications, nonoperative management should focus on fluid and electrolyte resuscitation, treatment of pain and associated ileus, respiratory and nutritional support, and treatment of associated biliary tract infection.

Fluid and Electrolytes. During the initial phase of severe pancreatitis the loss of intravascular fluid into the retropancreatic tissues and the intestine is considerable. Intravascular volume must be carefully restored and maintained, and this usually requires large amounts (i.e., 5000 to 6000 ml/24 h) of crystalloid solutions. Thus, it is advisable to measure central venous pressure and to catheterize the urinary bladder. When there is associated respiratory insufficiency, it may be wise to measure pulmonary artery wedge pressure to determine the filling pressures of the left atrium. Albumin and fresh frozen plasma may be used but are not generally required. Transfusions of blood may be required to compensate for the hemorrhage around the pancreas. In general, the hematocrit tends to be low in these patients because of the high volume of crystalloids used. Hypokalemia and hypocalcemia should be monitored and treated if necessary.

Treatment of Pain. Pain is the most common symptom in patients with pancreatitis. Because there is no relationship between the degree of pain and the prognosis, patients with mild pancreatitis may complain of severe and unremitting epigastric pain. We prefer to use meperidine (100 to 150 mg q 3 to 4 h IM) rather than morphine, as there is evidence that morphine may lead to ampullary spasm and increased pancreatic duct pressure. Splanchnic block has been recommended, but the risk of the procedure in these patients may outweigh its potential benefits. Interestingly, decompression of the stomach by a nasogastric tube alleviates the epigastric pain of pancreatitis considerably in some patients.

Treatment of Associated Ileus. All patients with pancreatitis should be left fasting until the abdominal pain has subsided. There is experimental evidence that feeding during acute pancreatitis worsens pancreatic inflammation.[68] Two previous studies on the effect of nasogastric suction on patients with pancreatitis showed that the outcome was the same whether a nasogastric tube was used or not. However, all patients included in these studies had mild pancreatitis and would have been expected to recover regardless of treatment. We institute nasogastric suction upon admission and tend to leave the tube until the pain and distention have resolved. Aspiration of gastric contents may also decrease pancreatic exocrine secretion and alleviate pancreatic inflammation.

In later stages of pancreatitis the function of the gastrointestinal tract may be affected by mechanical obstruction. The most common sites are the second portion of the duodenum, the upper jejunum close to the ligament of Treitz, and the transverse colon. Obstruction is caused by expansion of the inflammatory process (pancreatic abscess or pancreatic phlegmon) or, in later stages, by scarring of the peripancreatic tissues. The first requires prompt drainage of the abscess; the latter usually requires bypass of the obstructed segment.

Monitoring and Treatment of Respiratory Failure. As discussed earlier, nearly half of patients with pancreatitis develop arterial hypoxemia during the initial phase. In most cases this resolves rapidly, but since hypoxemia may be lethal if untreated, it is important to check arterial blood gases on admission and at intervals of 6 to 12 hours until the patient shows clear signs of improvement. In patients who deteriorate, early endotracheal intubation and ventilatory support should be instituted. Not infrequently those who require ventilatory support go on to develop ARDS, necessitating positive end-expiratory pressure. When acute respiratory insufficiency develops 2 to 3 weeks after the initial attack, one should suspect the presence of sepsis and look for retroperitoneal or intra-abdominal abscesses.

Nutritional Support. Patients who are unlikely to recover from pancreatitis within 1 week should be started on total parenteral nutrition (TPN). As the initial resuscitation is best accomplished with crystalloid solutions, and as one cannot be sure of the course for the first 2 to 3 days, we usually do not initiate TPN until 4 to 5 days after admission. The use of IV lipids has been controversial because of the association of pancreatitis with hyperlipidemia, but we have used standard doses of Intralipid 10 per cent IV Fat Emulsion in patients with biliary pancreatitis and have not noted exacerbation of pain.

Treatment of Associated Biliary Tract Infection. Previous studies have shown that ampicillin does not affect the course of mild alcoholic pancreatitis, and, by extension, many authors do not recommend antibiotics for any form of pancreatitis. We found evidence of biliary tract infection in 33 per cent of a series of patients operated on during the first 48 hours of the onset of pancreatitis[15] and thus recommend an initial short course of cephalosporins in patients with biliary pancreatitis.

Other Supportive Measures. Individuals with severe pancreatitis admitted to the intensive care unit should receive all other general supportive measures indicated for the critically ill. For example, antacids must be given regularly, as they can reduce markedly the incidence of upper gastrointestinal bleeding, a serious complication in these patients.

Treatment of Associated Biliary Tract Disease

In the early part of this century the high morbidity and mortality of operations on the biliary tract precluded the routine recommendation of cholecystectomy following an attack of biliary pancreatitis. However, it became clear that recurrence of pancreatitis was high when cholelithiasis remained untreated.[21, 22] As fluid and anesthetic management improved, several authors recommended that these patients be operated on 6 to 8 weeks after the attack of pancreatitis to prevent a recurrent attack. The problem with this approach was twofold: A second hospital admission was required, and several authors reported that in the relatively brief period between the attack and the elective operation 25 to 56 per cent of the patients experienced a second attack[29, 101–104] and even death[103] from recurrent biliary pancreatitis.

In 1964 Glenn and Frey suggested that correction of the associated biliary tract disease could be accomplished during the initial admission for pancreatitis, with a relatively low mortality.[105] Although their strategy was challenged temporarily,[4] the concept of operative correction of the associated biliary tract disease during the initial hospitalization as soon as the acute signs of pancreatitis have resolved is almost universally supported.[5, 16, 18, 20, 29, 101, 103, 106, 107]

In 1978 we proposed that patients with pancreatitis associated with gallstones might benefit from operative treatment of cholelithiasis within 48 hours after the onset of symptoms.[43] It was our belief that removal of an impacted gallstone blocking the orifice of the pancreatic duct would prevent the development of pancreatic necrosis and subsequent infection. We hypothesized that, in some patients, persistent calculous obstruction of the ampulla of Vater was responsible for progression of pancreatic inflammation. In a group of 46 patients operated on within 48 hours of the onset of pancreatitis over a 3-year period we had only one death (2.9 per cent), which compared favorably with the 16 per cent mortality we had observed in the previous 8 years. Of particular interest was the fact that none of these patients developed pancreatic abscesses or other local complications associated with pancreatic necrosis.

Several subsequent studies disagreed with this strategy.[17, 29, 102, 108] For example, Ranson reported a mortality rate of 23 per cent among a group of 22 patients operated on during the first week of pancreatitis and no mortality among 58 patients treated nonoperatively until pancreatitis subsided.[102] In a follow-up study that included 133 patients, the same author reported that there was a 65 per cent mortality rate among those operated on early as opposed to an 18 per cent mortality among those treated conservatively.[17] Based on these results, Ranson recommended a conservative approach for patients with severe pancreatitis. Similarly, Kelly reported a 12 per cent mortality in patients operated on within 72 hours of the initiation of pancreatitis, which contrasted with a 5 per cent mortality among those operated on after 5 to 7 days.[29] In these studies the decision to operate or not to operate was not the result of randomization or of a systematic approach but rather was based on a number of factors, including clinical deterioration and lack of response to the conservative approach. Thus, the differences in mortality can hardly be accepted as a cogent argument against early operation.

The only prospective randomized study to date compared 36 patients with biliary pancreatitis subjected to operation within 72 hours of hospital admission with 34 similar patients who received conventional nonoperative therapy and were operated on 3 months later.[26] All patients in the early and the delayed groups underwent cholecystectomy, transduodenal sphincteroplasty, and pancreatic duct septotomy. In general, patients who underwent early operation improved rapidly. The hospital stay was 13.5 days, and the mortality was 2.9 per cent (one patient). Patients treated by delayed operation had an average hospital stay of 23 days (including both hospital admissions) and a mortality of 6.8 per cent (two patients). Curiously, both deaths in the delayed surgery group occurred at the time of elective admission for biliary tract operation. Three years later, Mercer reported on 34 consecutive patients with biliary pancreatitis operated on within 48 hours of admission, with no mortality.[53] It is of interest that none of the patients in Stone's trial[26] or in Mercer's report[53] developed pancreatic abscesses. Although Ranson's criteria for prognosis were not used in these studies, there is little doubt that most patients included in the trials of early operation[26, 40, 53] were less ill than those included in Ranson's[17, 102] or Kelly's[29] series. Whether this represents a different population or a different stage of the disease is unclear. Most patients operated on within 48 hours have been found to have very mild pancreatitis, and many of them would be considered by Ranson to have "acute biliary tract disease and hyperamylasemia" but no pancreatitis. At any rate, definitive biliary tract surgery appears to be not only possible but safe in the great majority of patients admitted with the diagnosis of biliary pancreatitis.

Early Endoscopic Sphincterotomy

The idea that early restoration of ampullary patency may ameliorate pancreatitis has now been carried one step further with the use of endoscopic sphincterotomy. As with early operation, there was initially some reluctance to perform endoscopic cannulation and contrast injection of the bile duct in patients with pancreatitis. In 1980, Safrany reported the results of early endoscopic papillotomy (following diagnostic ERCP) for biliary pancreatitis in 15 patients. He found an impacted ampullary stone in eight patients and several stones within the common bile duct in the other seven patients. The fear that instillation of hyperosmolar contrast medium into the duct of Wirsung in patients with pancreatitis might exacerbate the disease appear to be unfounded. Instead, all patients became pain-free immediately after the procedure. Rapid and marked improvement was observed over the next 2 days in all 15 patients as amylase and bilirubin values became normal.[34] Enthusiasm for this approach grew, and soon several authors reported similar findings and similar results.[30–33, 54] In a recent prospective randomized study of early diagnostic ERCP (and papillotomy if biliary disease was confirmed) versus conservative management of patients with suspected biliary pancreatitis, the authors reported a dramatic improvement in all patients following sphincterotomy. There were no deaths or major complications in 66 patients who underwent ERCP during the early phase of acute pancreatitis.[97]

Therefore, although further experience is needed, it appears that urgent papillotomy is a safe way to restore ampullary patency without the need for an urgent operation, and it may be all that is needed in the older, high-risk patient. Whether this maneuver may abort the course of pancreatitis and prevent the development of septic complications must await the results of future studies.

Elective ERCP and Endoscopic Sphincterotomy. Several studies have now shown that, in patients with recurrent pancreatitis of the kind that would have been termed idiopathic in the past, diagnostic ERCP plays a major role, as it identifies correctable lesions in up to 50 per cent of them.[88–92] The most common cause of recurrent pancreatitis in patients without a history of alcoholism is the presence of minute gallbladder stones, which not infrequently do not show up on ultrasonography or oral cholecystography. Direct opacification of the gallbladder by ERCP is diagnostic in many of these patients. Endoscopic papillotomy with transampullar stone extraction is the treatment of choice in patients with previous cholecystectomy and recurrent choledocholithiasis (see Chapters 25 and 26).

Other Treatment Options

Peritoneal Lavage

The rationale for peritoneal lavage is threefold: It may help to establish a diagnosis of pancreatitis if hemorrhagic peritoneal fluid with a high amylase content is aspirated,[68] it may help determine the severity of the attack,[98] and it may remove toxic substances released from the pancreas that are thought to be responsible for systemic complications. It was introduced in 1965 by Wall,[120] who noted marked improvement in three patients with acute pancreatitis and associated renal failure following a short course of peritoneal lavage. Peritoneal lavage can be done with percutaneously placed catheters,[17] but some authors think that positioning the catheters next to the pancreas at laparotomy offers some advantage.[109] Theoretically, this method is more efficient, since it would lavage the lesser sac more thoroughly and would allow more accurate assessment of the severity of the disease by direct examination of the pancreas. The obvious disadvantage is the need for operation.

Technique. We prefer to place the catheters under direct vision through a small infraumbilical incision. Direct percutaneous insertion carries the risk of bowel injury, since these patients have marked ileus. The catheter must be tightly secured to the fascia and the peritoneum, or else fluid may leak through the wound. Lavage is commenced immediately after insertion of the catheters. We use an isotonic electrolyte solution containing 15 gm/L of glucose, 4 mEq/L of potassium, and 500 USP/L of heparin. About 2 liters of warmed fluid are infused into the abdomen over a 20-minute period. Abdominal distention, high diaphragms, and incipient respiratory failure may mandate the use of smaller lavage volumes and may precipitate the need for endotracheal intubation and assisted ventilation. After 20 to 30 minutes the fluid is drained and the cycle is repeated. Lavage is discontinued at 48 to 72 hours to decrease the chance of infection. Respiratory function and serum glucose levels must be closely monitored during peritoneal lavage.

Results. Enthusiasm for the use of peritoneal lavage has been fueled in the United States by the results of a prospective randomized study[110] and by reports from Ranson.[17, 68] These studies suggested that a prompt improvement of cardiovascular and respiratory status could be expected in some patients, although mortality and development of complications were not markedly affected. In a relatively large, well-controlled multicenter clinical trial in England, Mayer et al. compared the course of patients treated with and without peritoneal lavage and failed to show any difference in the outcome.[111] This study, however, included several patients with idiopathic pancreatitis. Although this trial seriously challenges the routine use of peritoneal lavage, one should not overlook the fact that in some patients—especially those with marked ascites—the institution of peritoneal lavage is often followed by a striking, immediate, clinical improvement most noticeable in their respiratory status.[17, 112] Perhaps removal of the toxin-rich fluid (which often amounts to several liters) from the peritoneal cavity, and not lavage itself, is the most important step in such patients.

The indications for peritoneal lavage in patients with biliary pancreatitis are still not well defined. For example, Ranson recommends it for patients who have three or more positive signs; others limit its use to those who have evidence of major plasma volume loss, hypotension, and tachycardia and whose condition does not stabilize but continues to deteriorate after 24 hours of aggressive fluid therapy. We feel that in patients with biliary pancreatitis the critical step is the restoration of ampullary patency. We therefore concentrate our efforts in that direction but continue to use peritoneal lavage in individual patients with severe pancreatitis.

Pancreatic Resection

Total or near-total pancreatectomy early in the course of severe pancreatitis was introduced by Watts a little over 20 years ago[113] and has been used extensively in France. The idea was that in severely ill patients with necrotic pancreatitis, extirpation of the disease by removal of the pancreas would improve the chances of recovery. However, the operation carries a mortality rate of 30 to 50 per cent under these circumstances,[109, 114–117] and surprisingly, it does not prevent septic complications. The sequelae of this operation were highlighted by Nordback, who, in a follow-up study of 40 patients who underwent partial or total pancreatectomy, found that the diabetes, the state of nutrition, and the upper gastrointestinal symptoms associated with pancreatectomy made this option hardly worth considering.[117] Formal resections of the pancreas for biliary pancreatitis are therefore not recommended.

In patients who develop extensive necrosis and sepsis, and in whom the devitalized tissues must be excised, it is preferable to limit the resection to necrotic tissue (pancreatic debridement) without attempting to excise viable pancreas.[101] The debridement consists of combined blunt and sharp dissection through planes that are largely bloodless because the local vessels have thrombosed. Sometimes large amounts of partly liquefied, partly solid material can be scooped out, with apparent benefit to the patient (Fig. 20–6). Several large Silastic sumps should be left in the debrided areas. Not infrequently, pancreatic juice will leak through the sumps for some time. Additional dead tissue and sloughs of peripancreatic fat can later be evacuated by lavage through the tracts. Since the large bulk of necrotic tissue involves the retroperitoneum rather than the pancreas, late endocrine and exocrine insufficiencies are rare, even after extensive debridement. Therefore, in the rare patient with extensive pancreatic necrosis secondary to pancreatitis we prefer to use debridement rather than carry out formal pancreatic resections.

REFERENCES

1. Frey CF: Gallstone pancreatitis. Surg Clin North Am 1981;*61*:923.
2. Armstrong CP, Taylor TV, Jeacock J, Lucas S: The biliary tract in patients with acute gallstone pancreatitis. Br J Surg 1985;*72*:551.
3. Trapnell JE, Ducan EHL: Patterns of incidence in acute pancreatitis. Br Med J 1975;*2*:179.
4. Imrie CW, Whyte AS: A prospective study of acute pancreatitis. Br J Surg 1975;*62*:490.
5. Martin JK, van Heerden JA, Bess MA: Surgical management of acute pancreatitis. Mayo Clin Proc 1984;*59*:259.
6. Trapnell JE, Anderson MC: Role of early laparotomy in acute pancreatitis. Ann Surg 1967;*165*:49.
7. Becker V: Pathological anatomy and pathogenesis of acute pancreatitis. World J Surg 1981;*5*:303.
8. Freund H, Pfeffermann R, Durst AL, et al: Gallstone pancreatitis. Arch Surg 1976;*111*:1106.

9. Sharon P, Melmed S, Neuman G: Acute pancreatitis in a community with a low alcohol intake. Int Surg 1979;*64:*63.
10. Mercadier M: Surgical treatment of acute pancreatitis: Tactics, techniques, and results. World J Surg 1981;*5:*393.
11. Bernard C: Le cors de physiologie experimental. Paris, JB Baillière, 1856.
12. Lancereaux E: Traite des maladies du foie et du pancreas. Paris, O Poin, 1899.
13. Opie EL: The relationship of cholelithiasis to disease of the pancreas and fat necrosis. Johns Hopkins Hosp Bull XII, 1900;*118:*19.
14. Opie EL: The etiology of acute hemorrhagic pancreatitis. Johns Hopkins Bull 1901;*121:*182.
15. Acosta JM, Pellegrini CA, Skinner DB: Etiology and pathogenesis of acute biliary pancreatitis. Surgery 1980;*88:*118.
16. Welch JP, White CE: Acute pancreatitis of biliary origin: is urgent operation necessary? Am J Surg 1982;*143:*120.
17. Ranson JHC: Conservative surgical treatment of acute pancreatitis. World J Surg 1981;*5:*351.
18. Kim U, Sheth M: Optimal timing of surgical intervention in patients with acute pancreatitis associated with cholelithiasis. Surg Gynecol Obstet 1980;*150:*499.
19. Acosta JM, Ledesma CL: Gallstone migration as a cause of acute pancreatitis. N Engl J Med 1974;*290:*484.
20. Kelly TR: Gallstone pancreatitis. Arch Surg 1974;*109:*294.
21. Paloyan D, Simonowitz D, Skinner DB: The timing of biliary tract operations in patients with pancreatitis associated with gallstones. Surg Gynecol Obstet 1975;*141:*737.
22. Satiani R, Stone HH: Predictability of present outcome and future recurrence in acute pancreatitis. Arch Surg 1979;*114:*711.
23. Acosta JM, White TT: Gallstone migration in acute pancreatitis. Contemp Surg 1980;*17:*14.
24. McMahon MJ, Shefta JR: Physical characteristics of gallstones and the calibre of the cystic duct in patients with acute pancreatitis. Br J Surg 1980;*67:*6.
25. Houssin D, Castaing D, Lemoine J, Bismuth H: Microlithiasis of the gallbladder. Surg Gynecol Obstet 1983;*157:*20.
26. Stone HH, Fabian TC, Dunlop WE: Gallstone pancreatitis. Biliary tract pathology in relation to time of operation. Ann Surg 1981;*194:*305.
27. Kelly TR, Swaney PE: Gallstone pancreatitis: the second time around. Surgery 1982;*92:*577.
28. Coppa GF, LeFleur R, Ranson JHC: The role of Chiba-needle cholangiography in the diagnosis of possible acute pancreatitis with cholelithiasis. Ann Surg 1981;*193:*393.
29. Kelly TR: Gallstone pancreatitis. The timing of surgery. Surgery 1980;*88:*345.
30. Safrany L, Cotton PB. A preliminary report: urgent duodenoscopic sphincterotomy for acute gallstone pancreatitis. Surgery 1981;*89:*424.
31. van der Spuy S: Endoscopic sphincterotomy in the management of gallstone pancreatitis. Endoscopy 1981;*13:*25.
32. Roesch W, Demling L: Endoscopic management of pancreatitis. Surg Clin North Am 1982;*62:*845.
33. Esquivel DA, Grassano PN: Urgent endoscopic papillotomy in patients with biliary pancreatitis. Rev Argent Cirug 1982;*43:*160.
34. Safrany L, Neuhaus B, Krause S, Portocarrero G, Schott B: Endoskopische papillotomie bei akuter, biliar bedingter pankreatitis: Dtsch Med Wochenschr 1980;*105:*115.
35. Osborne DH, Harris NWS, Gilmour H, Carter DC: Operative cholangiography in gallstone associated acute pancreatitis. J Coll Surg Edinb 1983;*28:*96.
36. Bernhoft RA, Pellegrini CA, Motson RW, Way LW: Composition and morphologic and clinical features of common duct stones. Am J Surg 1984;*148:*77.
37. Guelrud M, Mendoza S, Vicent S, Gomez M, Villalta B: Pressures in the sphincter of Oddi in patients with gallstones, common duct stones, and recurrent pancreatitis. J Clin Gastroenterol 1983;*5:*37.
38. Cuschieri A, Cumming JGR, Wood RAB, Baker PR: Evidence for sphincter dysfunction in patients with gallstone associated pancreatitis: effect of ceruletide in patients undergoing cholecystectomy for gallbladder disease and gallstone associated pancreatitis. Br J Surg 1984;*71:*885.
39. Kelly TR: Gallstone pancreatitis: Pathophysiology. Surgery 1976;*80:*488.
40. Acosta JM, Rossi R, Galli MR, Pellegrini CA, Skinner DB: Early surgery for acute gallstone pancreatitis: Evaluation of a systematic approach. Surgery 1978;*83:*367.
41. Taylor TV, Rimmer S: Pancreatic-duct reflux in patients with gallstone pancreatitis. Lancet 1980;*2:*848.
42. Frey CF, Beal JH: Pancreatitis as a complication of operation. Arch Surg 1963;*87:*1053.
43. Pellegrini CA, Paloyan D, Acosta JM, Skinner DB: Acute pancreatitis of rare causation. Surg Gynecol Obstet 1977;*144:*899.
44. Luska G, Poser H: Acute pancreatitis in obstructive jaundice following combined internal and external percutaneous transhepatic bile duct drainage (PTBD). Eur J Radiol 1983;*3:*112.
45. Ofstad E: Formation and destruction of plasma kinins during experimental acute hemorrhagic pancreatitis in dogs. Scand J Gastroenterol 1970;5(Suppl):1.
46. Warshaw A: Pancreatic abscesses. N Engl J Med 1972;*287:*1234.
47. Russell JC, Welch JP, Clark DG: Colonic complications of acute pancreatitis and pancreatic abscess. Am J Surg 1983;*146:*558.
48. Abearian H, Eftaiha M, Kraft AR, Nyhus LM: Colonic complications of acute pancreatitis. Arch Surg 1979;*114:*995.
49. Frey CF, Lindenauer SW, Miller TA: Pancreatic abscess. Surg Gynecol Obstet 1979;*149:*722.
50. Broe PJ, Cameron JL: Experimental gallstone pancreatitis: Pathogenesis and response to different treatment modalities. Ann Surg 1982;*195:*556.
51. Wells AD, Imahori SC, Schenk WG Jr: Does edematous pancreatitis exist in biliary-related pancreatitis? Arch Surg 1983;*118:*1277.
52. Steer ML: Search for the trigger mechanism of pancreatitis. Gastroenterology 1984;*86:*764.
53. Mercer LC, Saltzstein EC, Peacock JB, Dougherty SH: Early surgery for biliary pancreatitis. Am J Surg 1984;*148:*749.
54. Rosseland AR, Solhaug JH: Early or delayed endoscopic palillotomy (EPT) in gallstone pancreatitis. Ann Surg 1984;*199:*165.
55. Riemann JF, Demling L: Ten years of endoscopic papillotomy. Endoscopy 1983;*15:*239.

56. Lasson A, Ohlsson K: Acute pancreatitis. The correlation between clinical course, protease inhibitors, and complement and kinin activation. Scand J Gastroenterol 1984;*19*:707.
57. Steer ML, Meldolesi J, Figarella C: Pancreatitis. The role of lysosomes. Dig Dis Sci 1984;*29*:934.
58. Kimura T, Toung JK, Simeon M, Bell WR, Cameron JL: Respiratory failure in acute pancreatitis: The role of free fatty acids. Surgery 1980;*87*:509.
59. Troyer A, Naeije R, et al: Impairment of pulmonary function in acute pancreatitis. Chest 1978;*73*:360.
60. Miller A, Lees RS, McClusky MA, et al: The natural history and surgical significance of hyperlipemic abdominal crisis. Ann Surg 1979;*190*:401.
61. Werner MH, Hayes DF, Lucas CE, Rosenberg IK: Renal vasoconstriction in association with acute pancreatitis. Am J Surg 1974;*127*:185.
62. Johnson SG, Ellis DJ, Levitt MD: Mechanism of increased renal clearance of amylase/creatinine in acute pancreatitis. N Engl J Med 1976;*295*:1214.
63. Donowitz M, Hendler R, Spiro HM, Binder HJ, Felig P: Glucagon secretion in acute and chronic pancreatitis. Ann Intern Med 1975;*83*:778.
64. Weir GC, Lesser PB, Drop LJ, Fischer JE, Warshaw AL: The hypocalcemia of acute pancreatitis. Ann Intern Med 1975;*83*:185.
65. Robertson GM Jr, Moore EW, Switz DM, Sizemore GW, Estep EL: Inadequate parathyroid response in acute pancreatitis. N Engl J Med 1976;*294*:512.
66. Ranson JHC, Rifkin KM, Roses DF, et al: Prognostic signs and the role of operative management in acute pancreatitis. Surg Gynecol Obstet 1974;*139*:69.
67. Allam BF, Imrie CW: Serum ionized calcium in acute pancreatitis. Br J Surg 1977;*64*:665.
68. Ranson JHC: Acute pancreatitis. Curr Probl Surg 1979;*16*:1.
69. Patti MG, Pellegrini CA, Way LW: Serum amylase is useful in the differential diagnosis of acute abdominal pain. Gastroenterology 1986;*90*:1580.
70. Levitt MD: Clinical use of amylase clearance and isoamylase measurements. Mayo Clin Proc 1979;*54*:428.
71. McMahon LF: Pancreatitis: Is total serum amylase misleading? J Clin Gastroenterol 1985;*7*:17.
72. Neoptolemos JP, Hall AW, Finlay DF, Berry JM, Carr-Locke DL, Fossard DP: The urgent diagnosis of gallstones in acute pancreatitis: a prospective study of three methods. Br J Surg 1984;*71*:230.
73. McKay AJ, Imrie CW, Neill J, Duncan JR: Is an early ultrasound scan of value in acute pancreatitis? Br J Surg 1982;*69*:369.
74. Previti FW, Holt RW: Cholecystosonography in the evaluation of the gallbladder in pancreatitis. Surg Gynecol Obstet 1980;*150*:81.
75. Ruben D, Quiros S, Linares CA, Chiesa D, et al: Valor de la tomografia computada en la pancreatitis aguda. Rev Argent Cirug 1985;*49*:75.
76. Siegelman SS, Copeland BE, Saba GP, Cameron JL, et al: CT of fluid collections associated with pancreatitis. AJR 1980;*134*:1121.
77. Hill MC, Barkin J, Isikoff MB, Silverstein W, Kaiser M: Acute pancreatitis: Clinical vs. CT findings. AJR 1982;*139*:263.
78. Mammoni OH: Pancreatitis aguda, enfoque diagnostico y alternativas terapeuticas. Rev Argent Cirug 1980;*39*:15.
79. Houdard PC, et al: Les complication pancreatiques de la lithiase biliaire. Ann Chir 1977;*31*:729.
80. Blamey SL, Osborne DH, Gilmour WH, O'Neill J, Carter DC, Imrie CW: The early identification of patients with gallstone associated pancreatitis using clinical and biochemical factors only. Ann Surg 1983;*198*:574.
81. Graham DF, Wyllie FJ: Prediction of gall-stone pancreatitis by computer. Br Med J 1979;*1*:515.
82. Nordback I, Auvinen O, Autio V: Clinicobiochemical factors in predicting gallstones in necrotizing pancreatitis. Surg Gynecol Obstet 1985;*161*:139.
83. McMahon MJ, Pickford IR: Biochemical prediction of gallstones early in an attack of acute pancreatitis. Lancet 1979;*2*:541.
84. Van Gossumn A, Seferian V, Rodzynek JJ, Wettendorff P, Cremer M, Delcourt A: Early detection of biliary pancreatitis. Dig Dis Sci 1984;*29*:97.
85. Linos DA, Adson MA: Gallstone pancreatitis. Int Surg 1983;*68*:153.
86. Goodman AJ, Neoptolemos JP, Carr-Locke DL, Finlay DBL, Fossard DP: Detection of gallstones after acute pancreatitis. Gut 1985;*26*:125.
87. Milgalter E, Freund HR: Exploration of the biliary system in recurrent acute pancreatitis of undetermined etiology despite normal cholecystography. J Clin Gastroenterol 1985;*7*:45.
88. Smith R, Williams R, Cotton PB: Gallstone pancreatitis with normal biliary radiology. Br J Surg 1976;*63*:861.
89. Katon RM, Bilbao MK, Eidemiller LR, Benson JA Jr: Endoscopic retrograde cholangiopancreatography in the diagnosis and management of nonalcoholic pancreatitis. Surg Gynecol Obstet 1978;*147*:333.
90. Cooperman M, Ferrara JJ, Carey LC, Thomas FB, Martin ED Jr, Fromkes JJ: Idiopathic acute pancreatitis: the value of endoscopic retrograde cholangiopancreatography. Surgery 1981;*90*:666.
91. Hamilton I, Bradley P, Lintott DJ, McMahon MJ, Axon ATR: Endoscopic retrograde cholangiopancreatography in the investigation and management of patients after acute pancreatitis. Br J Surg 1982;*69*:504.
92. Dickerson RM, Loeb P, Fry WJ: Acute and subacute pancreatitis: Role of surgery and endoscopic retrograde cholangiopancreatography. Arch Surg 1980;*115*:552.
93. Acosta MJ, Rossi R, Ledesma CL: The usefulness of stool screening for diagnosing cholelithiasis in acute pancreatitis. A description of the technique. Am J Dig Dis 1977;*22*:168.
94. Mackie CR, Wood AB, Preece PE, Cuschieri A: Surgical pathology at early elective operation for suspected acute gallstone pancreatitis: preliminary report of a prospective clinical trial. Br J Surg 1985;*72*:179.
95. Glazer G, Murphy F, Clayden GS, Lawrence RG, Craig O: Radionuclide biliary scanning in acute pancreatitis. Br J Surg 1981;*68*:766.
96. Al-Sheikh W, Serafini A, Barkin J, Spoliansky G, Hourani M: The role of hepatobiliary scintigraphy in differentiating acute cholecystitis from acute nonbiliary pancreatitis. Am J Gastroenterol 1983;*78*:502.
97. Neoptolemos JP, London N, Slater N, Carr-Locke DL, Fossard DP, Moossa AR: A prospective study of ERCP and endoscopic sphincterotomy in the diagnosis and treatment of gallstone acute pancreatitis. Arch Surg, in press.
98. McMahon MJ, Playforth MJ, Pickford LR: A comparative study of methods for the prediction of

severity of attack of acute pancreatitis. Br J Surg 1980;*67*:22.

99. Ranson JHC: Etiological and prognostic factors in human acute pancreatitis. Am J Gastroenterol 1982;*77*:33.
100. Storck G, Pettersson G, Edlund Y: A study of autopsies upon 116 patients with acute pancreatitis. Surg Gynecol Obstet 1976;*143*:241.
101. Elfström J: The timing of cholecystectomy in patients with gallstone pancreatitis. Acta Chir Scand 1978;*144*:487.
102. Ranson JHC: The timing of biliary surgery in acute pancreatitis. Ann Surg 1979;*189*:654.
103. Mayer AD, McMahon MJ, Benson EA, Axon ATR: Operations upon the biliary tract in patients with acute pancreatitis: aims, indications and timing. Ann R Coll Surg Engl 1984;*66*:179.
104. Semel L, Schrieber D, Fromm D: Gallstone pancreatitis: Support for a flexible approach. Arch Surg 1983;*118*:901.
105. Glenn GG, Frey CF: Re-evaluation of the treatment of pancreatitis associated with biliary tract disease. Ann Surg 1964;*160*:723.
106. Osborne DH, Imrie CW, Carter DC: Biliary surgery in the same admission for gallstone-associated acute pancreatitis. Br J Surg 1981;*68*:758.
107. Heij HA, Veen HF, Eggink WF, Obertop H: Timing of surgery for acute biliary pancreatitis. Am J Surg 1985;*149*:371.
108. Tondelli P, Stutz K, Harder F, Schuppisser JP, Allgower M: Acute gallstone pancreatitis: best timing for biliary surgery. Br J Surg 1982;*69*:709.
109. Kauste A, Hockerstedt K, Ahonen J, Tervaskari H: Peritoneal lavage as a primary treatment in acute fulminant pancreatitis. Surg Gynecol Obstet 1983;*156*:458.
110. Stone HH, Fabian TC: Peritoneal dialysis in the treatment of acute alcoholic pancreatitis. Surg Gynecol Obstet 1980;*150*:878.
111. Mayer D, McMahon M, Corefield A, Cooper MJ, et al: Controlled clinical trial of peritoneal lavage for the treatment of severe acute pancreatitis. N Engl J Med 1985;*312*:399.
112. Pellegrini CA: The treatment of acute pancreatitis: A continuing challenge. N Engl J Med 1985; *312*:436.
113. Watts GT: Total pancreatectomy for fulminant pancreatitis. Lancet 1963;*2*:384.
114. Kummerle F, Neher M: Management of complications after operations for acute pancreatitis. World J Surg 1981;*5*:387.
115. Hollender LF, Meyer C, Marrie A, da Costa SE, Castellanos JG: Role of surgery in the management of acute pancreatitis. World J Surg 1981;*5*:361.
116. Aldridge MC, Ornstein M, Glazer G, Dudley HAF: Pancreatic resection for severe acute pancreatitis. Br J Surg 1985;*72*:796.
117. Nordback IH, Auiven OA: Long-term results after pancreas resection for acute necrotizing pancreatitis. Br J Surg 1985;*72*:687.
118. Alexandre JH, Guerrieri MT: Role of total pancreatectomy in the treatment of necrotizing pancreatitis: World J Surg 1985;*5*:369.
119. Knol JA, Eckhauser FE, Strodel WE: Surgical treatment of necrotizing pancreatitis by marsupialization. Am Surg 1984;*50*:324.
120. Wall AJ: Peritoneal dialysis in the treatment of severe acute pancreatitis. Med J Aust 1965;2:281.

CHARLES K. McSHERRY, M.D.

21

Cholecystostomy and Cholecystectomy

When one considers the frequency with which biliary tract operations are performed today, it is difficult to appreciate that the first cholecystectomy was performed a little over 100 years ago.[35] Although attempts at surgical intervention for calculous biliary tract disease occurred in the seventeenth and eighteenth centuries, it remained for John S. Bobbs of Indiana to perform the first cholecystolithotomy on June 15, 1867.[7] His patient was a 30-year old woman with an abdominal mass presumed to be an ovarian tumor. The operation was done under chloroform anesthesia on the third floor above a drugstore. It was not until after the surgeon had incised a huge hydropic gallbladder that he realized the true nature of the lesion present. After evacuating the contents of the gallbladder, Bobbs sutured it closed. The patient's postoperative course was uneventful, and she lived to old age without recurrence of her symptoms.[5]

Total removal of the gallbladder was not successfully accomplished until 1882. Credit for the first elective cholecystectomy belongs to Karl Langenbuch of Germany.[1, 2, 35] The first cholecystectomy in the United States was performed by Justus Ohage of Minnesota in 1886.[5] In 1890, Courvoisier performed the first successful choledocholithotomy.[60] Accurate preoperative diagnosis of cholelithiasis became possible with the introduction of cholecystography by Graham and Cole.[25] The first successful cholecystogram in a human was obtained in 1924.[25] A normal gallbladder was observed in a patient who had right upper quadrant pain and was later found to have a ureteral obstruction.[5] A major step forward in the treatment of cholelithiasis occurred in 1932, when Mirizzi of Argentina introduced intraoperative cholangiography.[40] Endoscopic retrograde cholangiopancreatography (ERCP) was introduced by Kasugai et al[33] in 1972, and operative fluoroscopy and cholangiography using the image amplifier by Berci et al[6] in 1978.

Improvements in preoperative diagnosis and greater acceptance of planned elective surgery by patients are among the major factors responsible for the successful management of biliary tract disease. Indeed, operations upon the gallbladder and biliary passages are, with the exception of herniorrhaphy, the most common procedures performed by general surgeons. Approximately 500,000 patients undergo cholecystectomy annually in the United States.

PREOPERATIVE EVALUATION AND PROCEDURE OF CHOICE

Cholelithiasis and its sequelae are the most frequent indications for operation upon the biliary tract. Less common diseases that require cholecystectomy are acalculous cholecystitis, the hyperplastic cholecystoses, neoplasms, and trauma. In approximately 80 per cent of patients, biliary tract operations are elective and should therefore be done under optimal conditions. Currently available radiographic techniques and sonography should permit an accurate preoperative assessment of the nature and extent of disease and allow for preoperative planning.

The assessment of operative risk in patients with *chronic cholecystitis* must be based upon a complete history and physical examination and include sufficient laboratory studies to screen for disorders of the cardiovascular, pulmonary, and renal systems.

Age over 70 years[29, 55] or associated cirrhosis[3, 49] increases the risk of cholecystectomy. Several studies have identified cardiovascular complications as the most frequent cause of death, and pulmonary complications as the leading cause of postoperative morbidity.[22, 23, 43, 53] Correction of preoperative deficits should result in an operative mortality rate for elective cholecystectomy of 0.5 per cent or less.

In patients with *acute cholecystitis*, preoperative evaluation and the correction of metabolic deficits must often be accomplished in an abbreviated time span, frequently during the time required for radiographic confirmation of the diagnosis. The degree of urgency parallels the clinical evidence of sepsis and its response to antimicrobial therapy. A palpable gallbladder together with clinical evidence of sepsis exemplifies the type of patient who must be prepared for operation without undue delay, usually within 12 to 24 hours from the time of admission.

The operative risk is a major factor in choosing between cholecystectomy and cholecystostomy. The former almost always requires general anesthesia, whereas the latter can be safely performed with local infiltration anesthesia. Patients with severe incorrectable deficits in cardiac, pulmonary, and renal function may be able to tolerate the operative burden of local anesthesia but not that imposed by general or inhalation techniques. In patients with chronic cholecystitis and cholelithiasis, cholecystectomy has, with few exceptions, been the procedure of choice. For example, between 1932 and 1975, there were 8392 patients operated upon for nonacute biliary tract disease at The New York Hospital–Cornell Medical Center. Of this group, only 82 patients (0.97 per cent) underwent cholecystostomy. These latter patients all had severe coexisting medical illnesses, most commonly cardiac disease. They were operated upon because frequent episodes of biliary colic impaired their ability to function, and, in some instances, unduly complicated the already difficult management of their medical illnesses.

In patients with acute cholecystitis, the indications for cholecystostomy in preference to cholecystectomy are quite different. Often they are technical in nature and relate to the hazards of dissection in the face of inflammatory obliteration of the landmarks in the hepatoduodenal ligament. The decision to perform cholecystostomy in these patients is often made at the time of surgery, following assessment of the safety with which the gallbladder can be removed. The fear of common duct injury and its disastrous consequences is the usual motivation for "backing away" from cholecystectomy. Cholecystostomy is performed more frequently in patients with acute cholecystitis than in those with chronic cholecystitis.[51] From 1932 to 1975, 1489 patients underwent cholecystectomy and 291 underwent cholecystostomy (16 per cent) for acute cholecystitis at The New York Hospital–Cornell Medical Center. Cholecystostomy, in effect, reflected the severity of the acute cholecystitis and had an operative mortality of 9.2 per cent, whereas cholecystectomy was accomplished with a mortality of 1.3 per cent.

ACUTE CHOLECYSTITIS: EARLY VS DELAYED OPERATION

The timing of operation in patients with acute cholecystitis has been a matter of controversy in biliary tract surgery. Some surgeons prefer early operation and others, delayed surgical intervention. Although it is true that many patients can, and do, recover from acute cholecystitis without operation, others are not cured despite antimicrobial therapy. In patients who fail to respond to expectant management, cholecystitis may evolve to gangrene and then to perforation.[17, 44] In a group of 26,334 patients collected from selected reports[11, 16, 37, 45, 47, 54] and unpublished data from The New York Hospital, the incidence of perforation was 10 per cent, and the mortality from perforation was 21.3 per cent. Perforations of the gallbladder have been classified by Niemeier[42] into three types. Type I is perforation into the free peritoneal cavity and is the least common variety encountered. Type II perforation is characterized by pericholecystic abscess and Type III by perforation into adjacent viscera. Both Type II and Type III perforations occur with equal frequency in most reported series. (For further details on gallbladder perforation see Chapter 16.)

Unfortunately, it is usually impossible to predict which patients with acute cholecystitis will progress to perforation, and it also may be impossible to diagnose perforation preoperatively. This concern prompts most surgeons to advocate early operation in patients with acute cholecystitis.[15, 21, 41] Furthermore, several controlled clinical trials have shown that early operation results in shorter hospitalization and decreased morbidity.[30, 34, 57]

Advocates of delayed operation are of the opinion that the acute inflammatory component of the disease is best treated with antibiotics and that cholecystectomy is less hazardous after subsidence of the acute inflammatory phase. Data in support of this hypothesis are not convincing, and personal experience suggests that the technical problems associated with delayed cholecystectomy are often more difficult to solve than those encountered during the acute phase.

CHOLECYSTOSTOMY: TECHNIQUE

Operations upon the biliary tract can usually be accomplished with equal ease through subcostal or paramedian incisions. My preference in most patients is the right subcostal approach, because it provides excellent exposure and the wound heals well. In the presence of a palpable gallbladder, as often occurs with acute cholecystitis, the length of the incision can be restricted to the area directly over the fundus. This may be of some importance when the procedure is done under local anesthesia.

With the gallbladder exposed, a pursestring suture is placed in the fundus of the gallbladder (Fig. 21–1). The serosa within the area encompassed by the pursestring suture is incised (Fig. 21–2) to facilitate insertion of a trocar (Fig. 21–3*A*). The trocar is used to evacuate the fluid contents of the gallbladder, a sample of which should be sent for bacteriologic identification. After withdrawal of the obturator (Fig. 21–3*B*), bile is aspirated from the gallbladder by suction applied to the sidearm of the trocar. Manual compression of the gallbladder facilitates this process. Stone forceps (Fig. 21–4) are then used to extract the calculi from the gallbladder. With large stones, it may be necessary to lengthen the cholecystotomy incision at the fundus. Instruments such as the malleable pituitary spoons or Mayo common duct spoons may be used in preference to stone forceps if the calculi are small and multiple. It is advisable to irrigate the gallbladder with isotonic saline in an effort to flush out additional small calculi and debris that were not removed with the forceps or pituitary spoons. Exploration of the gallbladder lumen by digital palpation may minimize the occurrence of overlooked stones. This maneuver, performed simultaneously with palpation of the serosal surface of the gallbladder, is occasionally useful to locate and dislodge stones impacted in the cystic duct.

After the contents of the gallbladder have been evacuated, decompression and drainage of the biliary tree are maintained by suturing a Malecot catheter into the gallbladder (Fig. 21–5). The previously placed pursestring suture plus an additional one are used to secure the catheter at the fundus of the gallbladder. A closed drainage system (e.g., a Jackson-Pratt drain) or two Penrose drains are then

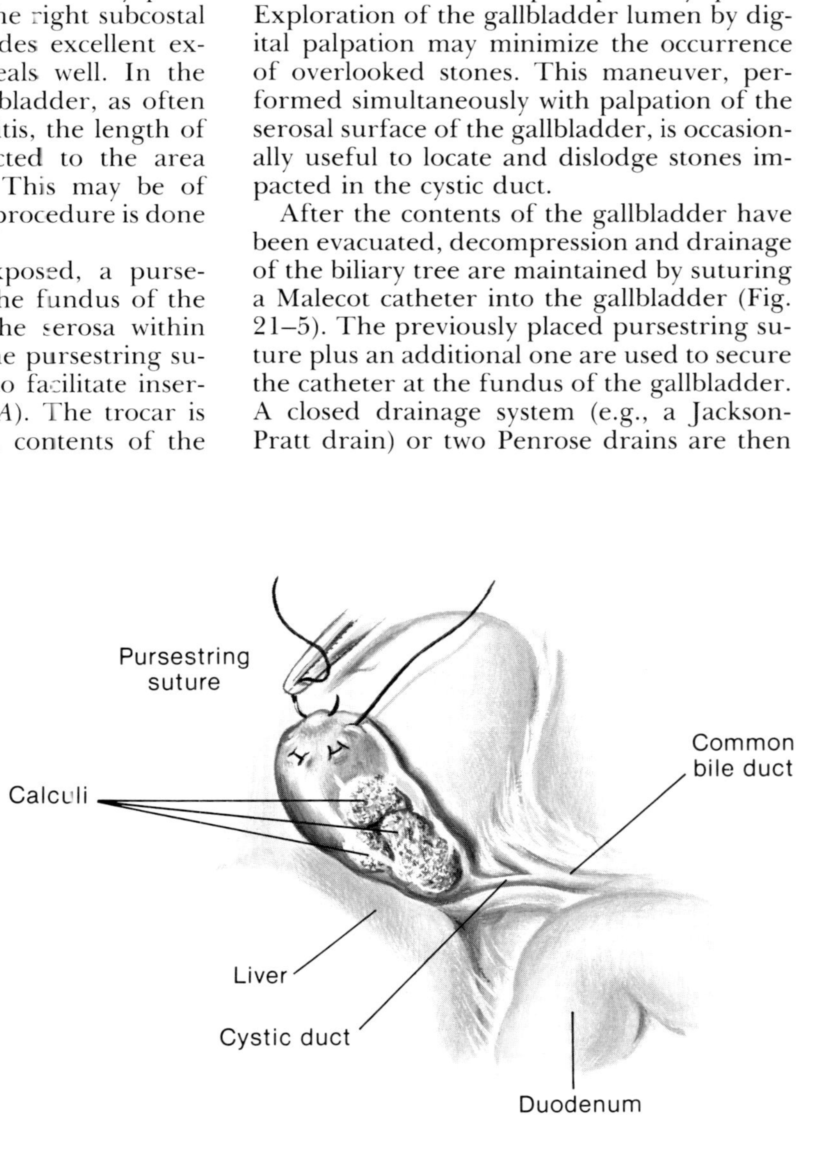

Figure 21–1. Cholecystostomy. After the fundus of the gallbladder is exposed, a pursestring suture is secured in place.

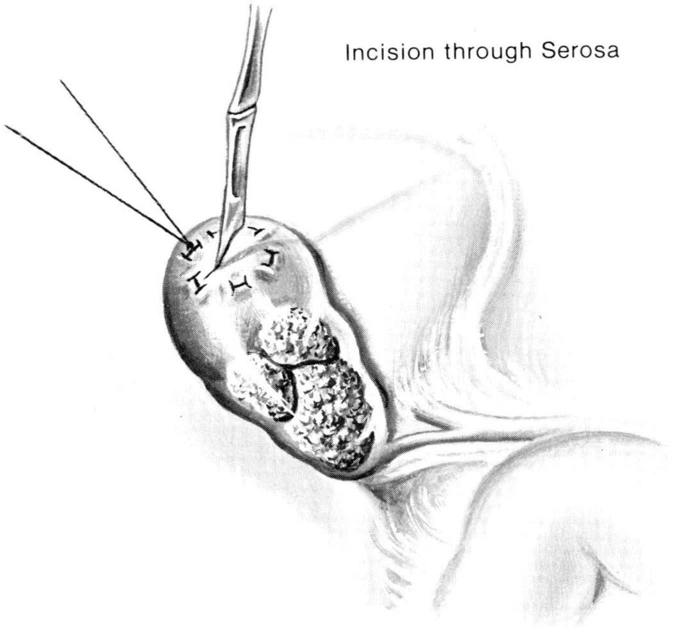

Figure 21–2. In order to facilitate the introduction of a trocar into the gallbladder, the serosa is incised within the area of the pursestring suture.

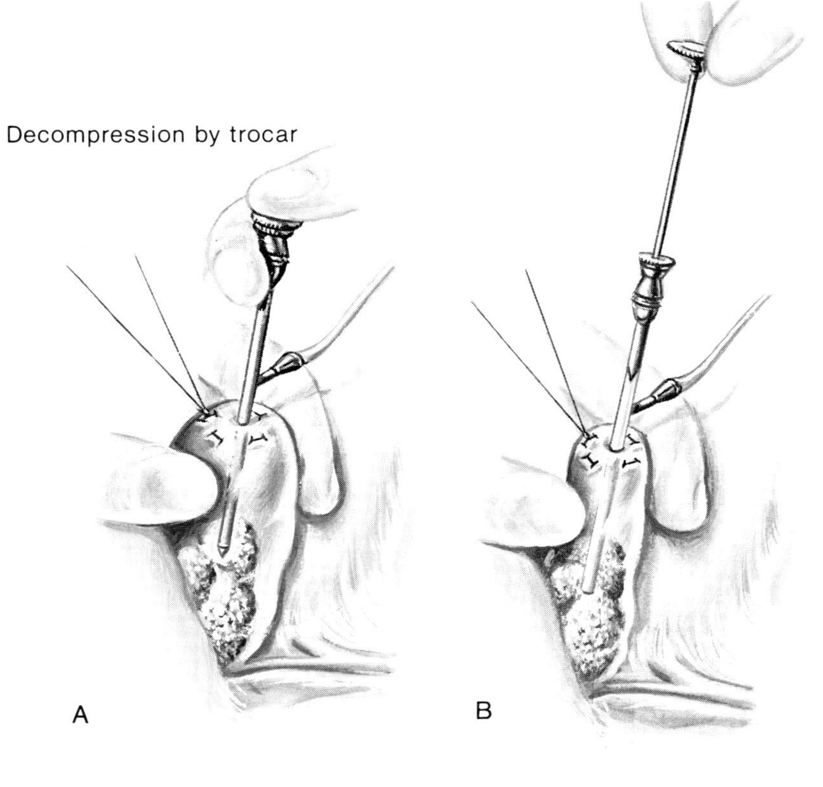

Figure 21–3. The trocar is inserted into the lumen (*A*), and then the obturator is withdrawn to permit aspiration of the gallbladder contents by suction applied to the side arm of the trocar (*B*).

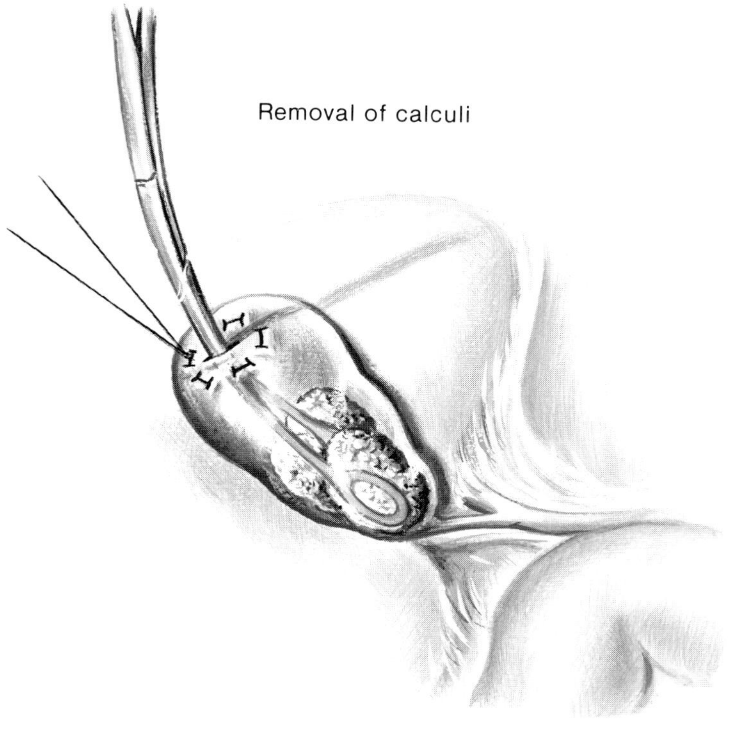

Figure 21–4. Stone forceps are used to extract the calculi from the gallbladder.

placed alongside the gallbladder. The catheter and drains are brought out through separate stab wounds and are sutured to the skin. The fundus of the gallbladder is then sutured to the adjacent overlying peritoneum and posterior rectus fascia with interrupted sutures (Fig. 21–6); this is to prevent, or at least minimize, bile leakage into the peritoneal cavity.

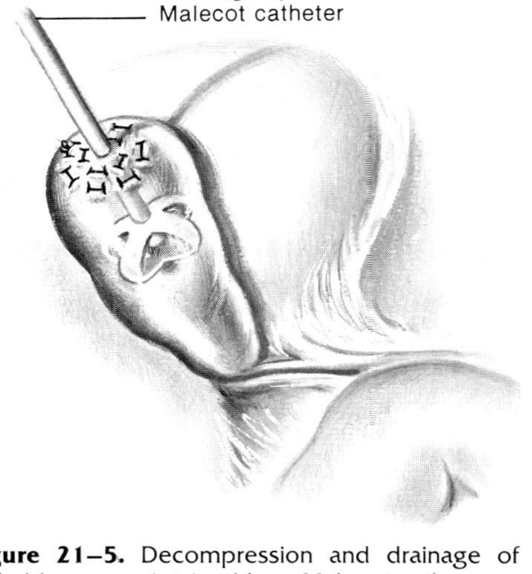

Figure 21–5. Decompression and drainage of the gallbladder are maintained by a Malecot catheter.

In some patients with acute cholecystitis, the fundus of the gallbladder may be necrotic and therefore unable to hold sutures. In this situation, the necrotic area is resected, the gallbladder calculi removed, and a Malecot catheter sutured into the lumen of the gallbladder proximal to the fundus. This precludes any efforts to secure the gallbladder remnant to the anterior abdominal wall and mandates the use of a sump drain in addition to the Penrose drains to maintain adequate bile drainage and egress of other fluids from the abdominal cavity.

Comments. Cholecystostomy in the treatment of acute cholecystitis is effective because it decompresses and drains the gallbladder. In patients who have acute cholecystitis and cholangitis (due to common duct obstruction), one should not assume that this procedure will provide drainage of the common bile duct as well as the gallbladder, a necessary goal in these patients. The cystic duct may be occluded by residual small stones or inflammatory debris or may be functionally closed by intraluminal swelling. Patency of the cystic-choledochal junction may be evi-

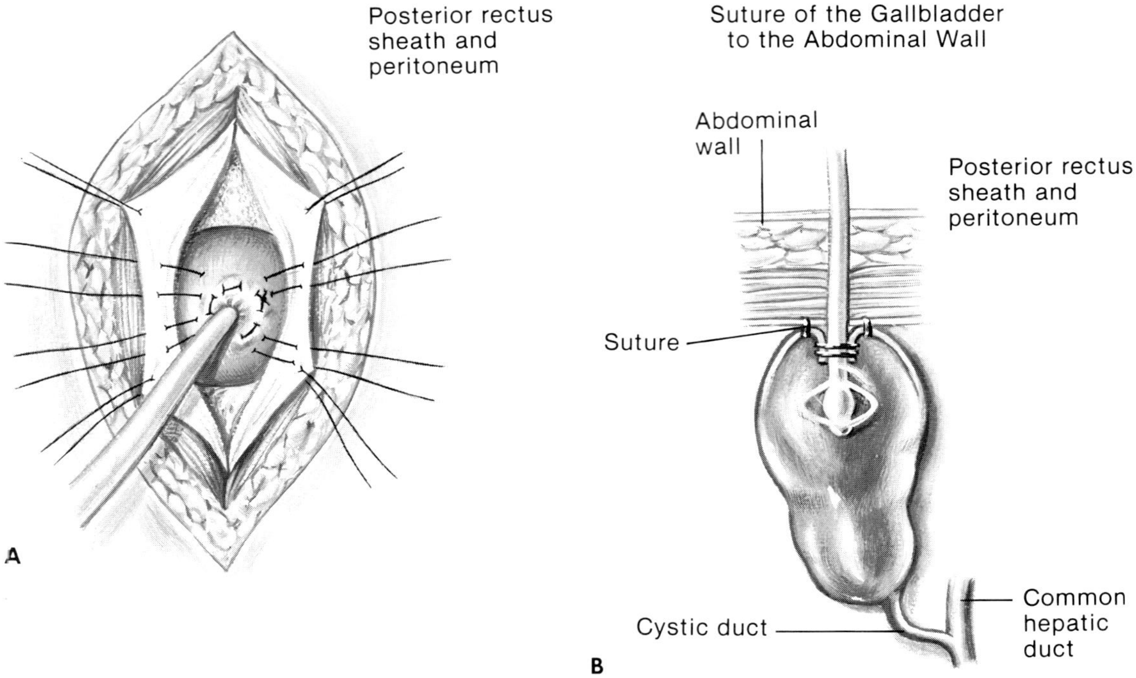

Figure 21–6. The fundus of the gallbladder is sutured to the overlying abdominal wall with interrupted sutures placed through the peritoneum and posterior rectus sheath (*A*). As illustrated in the cross-sectional view (*B*), this should prevent or minimize bile leakage into the peritoneal cavity.

dent at operation by the efflux of bile through the cystic duct, or it may be demonstrated radiographically by tube cholangiogram. Unless patency of the cystic duct is evident, T-tube drainage of the common bile duct must be established in addition to cholecystostomy in patients with clinically significant cholangitis.

It is difficult at times to distinguish the relative contributions of acute cholecystitis and cholangitis to the clinical picture of sepsis in the individual patient. There is considerable variation in the severity of cholangitis. Most patients with cholangitis respond to antimicrobial therapy with clinical improvement and defervescence of fever. Patients with distal obstruction of the common bile duct (e.g., from common duct stones or strictures) may respond poorly or not at all. Often these patients exhibit progressive jaundice. In its most severe form, the disease leads to gram-negative sepsis, which is manifested by peripheral vascular collapse, cyanosis, and mental confusion. Failure to recognize this disease is a major factor in its high mortality.

As reported by Gagic and Frey,[18] the high mortality rate associated with cholecystostomy may, in part, be due to the failure to recognize the limitations of this procedure in dealing with patients with cholangitis. Some advocate the use of percutaneous cholecystostomy in very ill patients.[13, 43, 50] The technique of percutaneous cholecystostomy is described in Chapter 10.

Although percutaneous cholecystostomy is possible and relatively safe, the technique has certain disadvantages. Cholecystolithotomy and cleansing of the gallbladder lumen are not possible, at least during the initial procedure, and a pericholecystic abscess may be overlooked. Furthermore, debris, sludge, and small stones tend to occlude the catheters fairly early on. This technique should therefore be reserved for selected patients.

The postoperative management of patients with a cholecystostomy depends in large measure on the indications for this procedure. A tube cholangiogram should be performed before removal of the Malecot catheter. If residual stones are present in the gallbladder or common bile duct, it may be advisable to leave the catheter in place until such time as the patient can be prepared for cholecystectomy (with or without choledochotomy, as dictated by the cholangiographic findings). If one elects to remove the Malecot catheter in the presence of residual stones, a persistent biliary-cutaneous fistula may result, especially if these calculi completely obstruct the cystic or common bile duct. Nonobstructing residual stones in the gallbladder may be the cause of persistent or recurrent infection at the cholecystostomy site after removal of the Malecot catheter. In any event, the presence of residual stones imparts more urgency to an interval cholecystectomy.

In the majority of patients with chronic cholecystitis subjected to cholecystostomy because of severe coexistent medical illnesses, cholecystostomy should be regarded as a definitive procedure.[51] We would recommend cholecystectomy to patients in this category only if they had a life expectancy in excess of 2 years. This recommendation is based upon the report of Hays and Glenn,[27] who noted that 49 of 78 patients (63 per cent) who did not return for elective cholecystectomy within 2 years after cholecystostomy for acute cholecystitis developed symptoms of recurrent biliary tract disease.

Patients with acute cholecystitis who are good operative risks are advised to undergo cholecystectomy 6 to 8 weeks after cholecystostomy. This interval is sufficient for subsidence of the inflammatory reaction and for safe cholecystectomy.

CHOLECYSTECTOMY: TECHNICAL CONSIDERATIONS

Two methods are accepted in the performance of cholecystectomy. One commences with identification of the structures in the hepatoduodenal ligament, namely the cystic and common hepatic ducts and the cystic artery. The cystic artery is temporarily ligated, and then the gallbladder is removed by dissecting it from the liver, starting at the fundus and proceeding to the ampulla. The cystic duct and cystic artery are not divided until after the gallbladder has been completely mobilized and the identity of these structures confirmed. The second method involves dissection and division of the cystic artery and duct, followed by removal of the gallbladder beginning at the ampullary region and proceeding toward the fundus. This technique is often referred to as the retrograde method. My preference is for the former, or antegrade, technique because of the inherent safety afforded by the more accurate identification of the biliary ducts and cystic artery.

The grave prognosis associated with injury to the common bile duct in the course of cholecystectomy is well known to all surgeons.[59] The prevention of this catastrophe requires a knowledge of all the potential hazards of the procedure as well as a degree of operative skill to accomplish it with technical precision. The ability to recognize anomalies of the ductal system and its blood supply and to deal with unexpected hemorrhage is the cornerstone of the skills required of the individual who accepts responsibility for the performance of cholecystectomy.

A right subcostal incision provides excellent exposure to the area of the gallbladder and hepatoduodenal ligament and is the incision of choice. In patients with narrow costal arches, a paramedian or midline incision may be used. More important than the type of incision is its extent; abdominal incisions should be long enough to afford adequate exposure with minimal retraction.

After the peritoneal cavity is entered, the falciform ligament is divided to enhance exposure of the upper abdomen and to permit a complete exploration of the intra-abdominal organs. The viscera that occupy the right hypochondrium adjacent to the liver are retracted to expose the gallbladder and inferior surface of the liver. The hepatic flexure of the colon is reduced into the lower abdomen and held there by moist laparotomy pads. Adhesions between the inferior surface of the gallbladder and adjacent structures are common and must be divided. The assistant then applies traction to the distal stomach and duodenum to effect tension upon and stretching of the hepatoduodenal ligament. Enhanced exposure of the superior portion of this ligament can be achieved by the careful placement of retractors—one at the level of the fundus of the gallbladder to elevate the rib margin, and the other medial to the gallbladder to elevate the inferior surface of the liver and expose the hilar structures (Fig. 21–7). With this exposure, the contents of the gallbladder can be palpated and the course of the common bile duct noted. With a finger in the foramen of Winslow, the distal common duct can be palpated for stones. The head of the pancreas should be palpated to determine its consistency. Examination of the duodenum must include palpation in the region of the ampulla of Vater, checking for the presence of a calculus or tumor.

Upon completion of these maneuvers, the peritoneum overlying the triangle of Calot is incised. This anatomic triangle is bordered

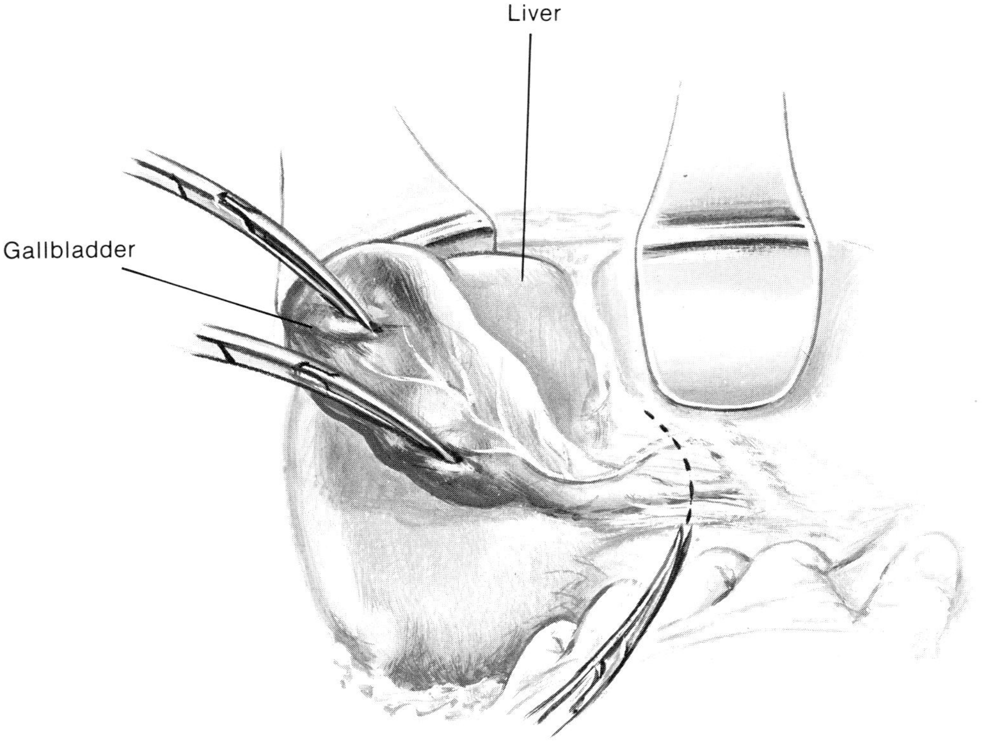

Figure 21–7. Cholecystectomy. With traction on the hepatoduodenal ligament, the peritoneum in the area of the triangle of Calot is incised.

by the cystic artery and the cystic and common hepatic ducts. The most inferior structure in the triangle, the cystic duct, is usually the first to be exposed by blunt dissection, and it should be tagged by a silk ligature (Fig. 21–8). The cystic artery is similarly exposed, and a silk ligature should be passed around it as it enters the gallbladder. This ligature is secured with a single knot to minimize blood loss during the dissection of the

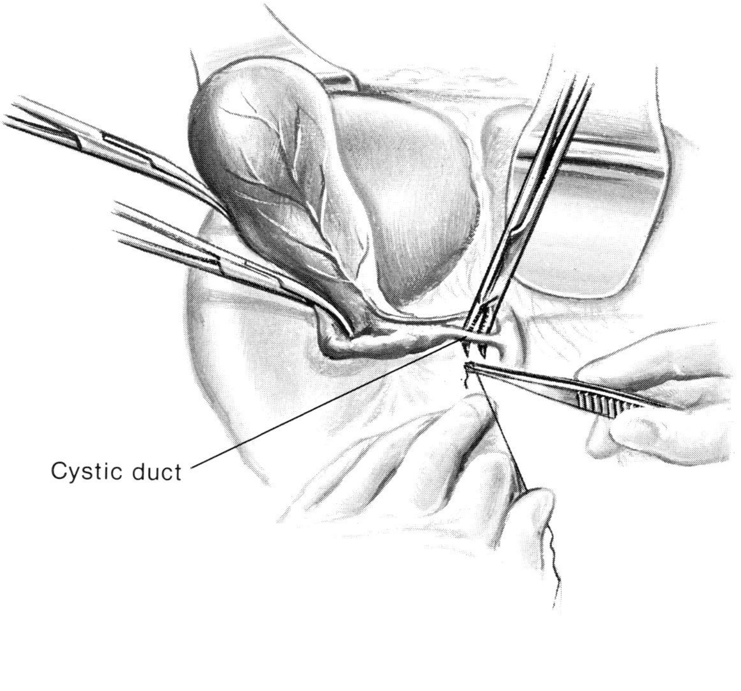

Figure 21–8. A ligature is placed around the cystic duct for purposes of identification and traction.

gallbladder from its capsule. Often there is a lymph node in the anatomic triangle that may partially obscure the cystic artery or, less commonly, the cystic duct. Excision of this node is not necessary or advisable. The peritoneum surrounding the gallbladder is incised at a distance of 1 to 1.5 cm from the liver (Fig. 21–9). The gallbladder is then dissected from its peritoneal attachment to the liver by a combination of blunt and sharp dissection beginning at the fundus (Fig. 21–10). As the dissection proceeds to the ampulla of the gallbladder, the small blood vessels and bile ducts encountered are ligated and divided. In the course of this dissection, the junction of the cystic artery and the anterior surface of the gallbladder in the ampullary segment becomes evident. This cystic artery is ligated in continuity or, more commonly, secured between two clamps and then divided (Fig. 21–11). The stump of the cystic artery is ligated with nonabsorbable suture.

Division of the cystic artery usually facilitates exposure of the cystic duct, and this structure is dissected to its junction with the common hepatic duct. The length and diameter of the cystic duct are variable, and anomalies are frequent in this area. Cholangiography should be performed at this stage of the procedure if an anomaly is suspected, or if it is deemed essential or advisable to search for additional stones in the common bile duct. An appropriate-sized straight rubber catheter or commercially prepared Cholangiocath is inserted via a small incision into the proximal cystic duct and secured with a ligature (Fig. 21–12). Dilute contrast material, for example, Hypaque 50 per cent diluted with an equal volume of saline, is allowed to flow under gravity or with minimal pressure into the ductal system. In most patients, 8 to 15 ml of contrast agent is sufficient. Care must be taken to avoid the introduction of air bubbles into the system. Following review of the radiograph, and assuming that there are no indications for choledochotomy, the Cholangiocath is removed and the cystic duct divided between clamps placed 5 to 8 mm from the junction of the cystic and common hepatic ducts (Fig. 21–

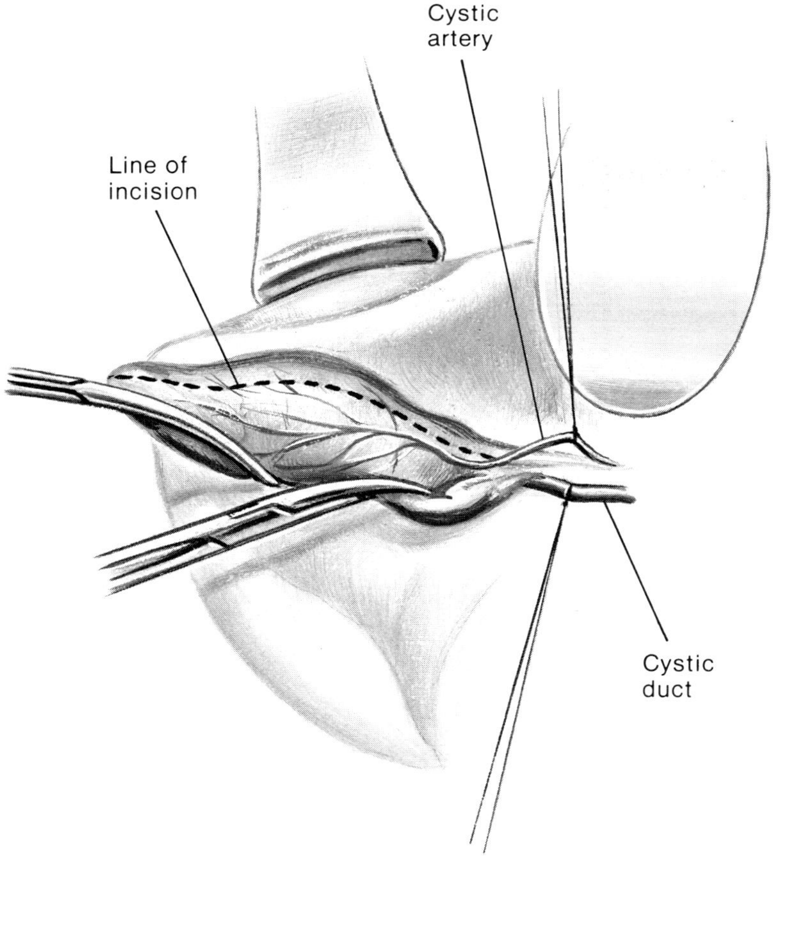

Figure 21–9. The peritoneum overlying the gallbladder is incised 1 to 1.5 cm from the liver after the cystic duct and artery have been identified.

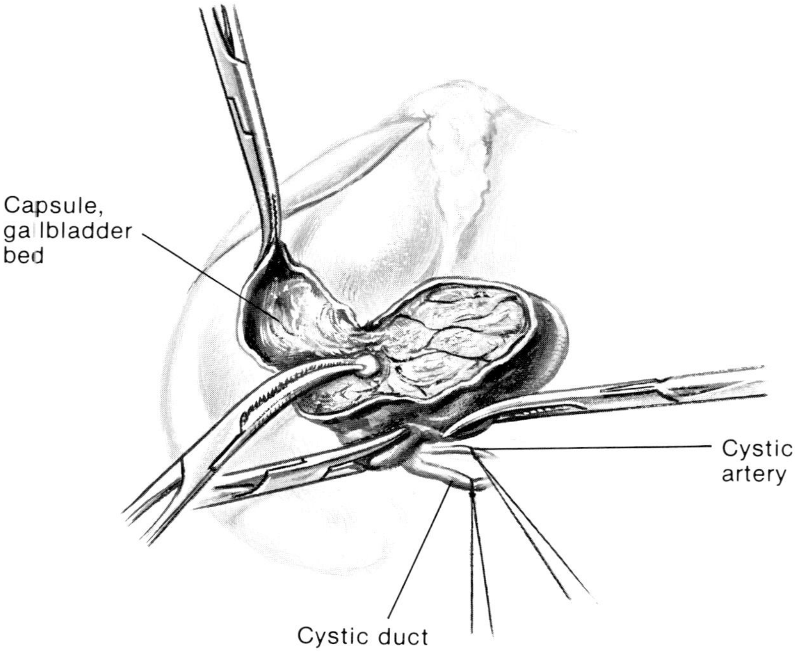

Figure 21–10. The gallbladder is dissected from its peritoneal attachments to the liver by both blunt and sharp dissection.

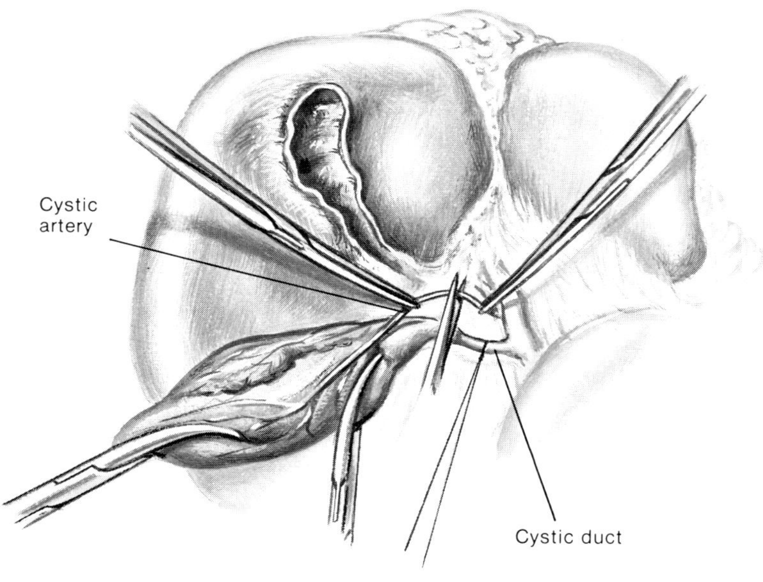

Figure 21–11. After the gallbladder has been mobilized, the cystic artery is divided between clamps as close to the gallbladder wall as possible.

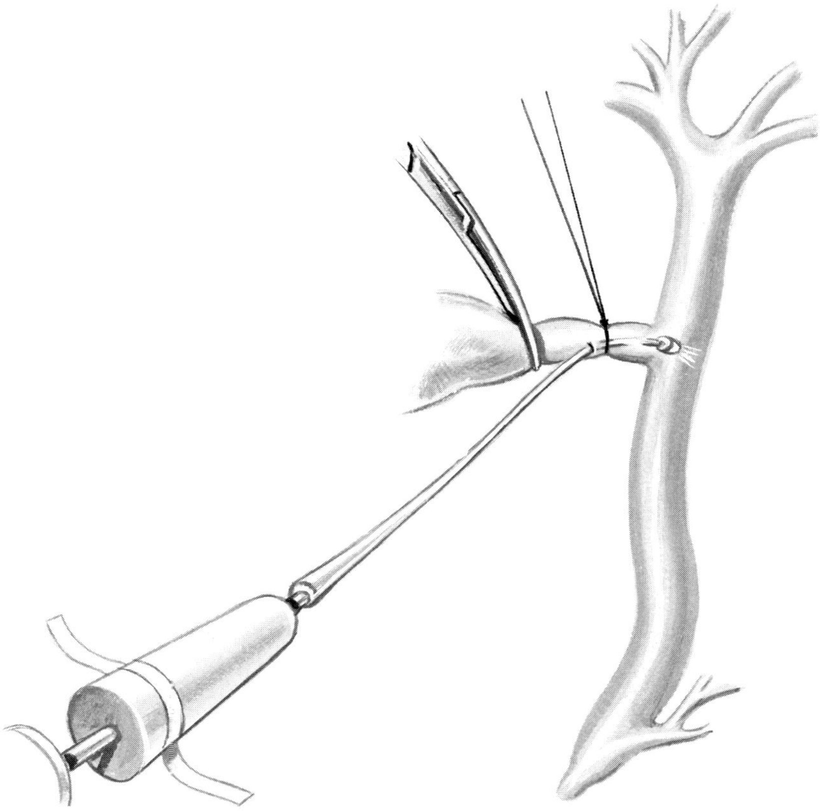

Figure 21–12. A cystic duct cholangiogram is obtained using dilute contrast material.

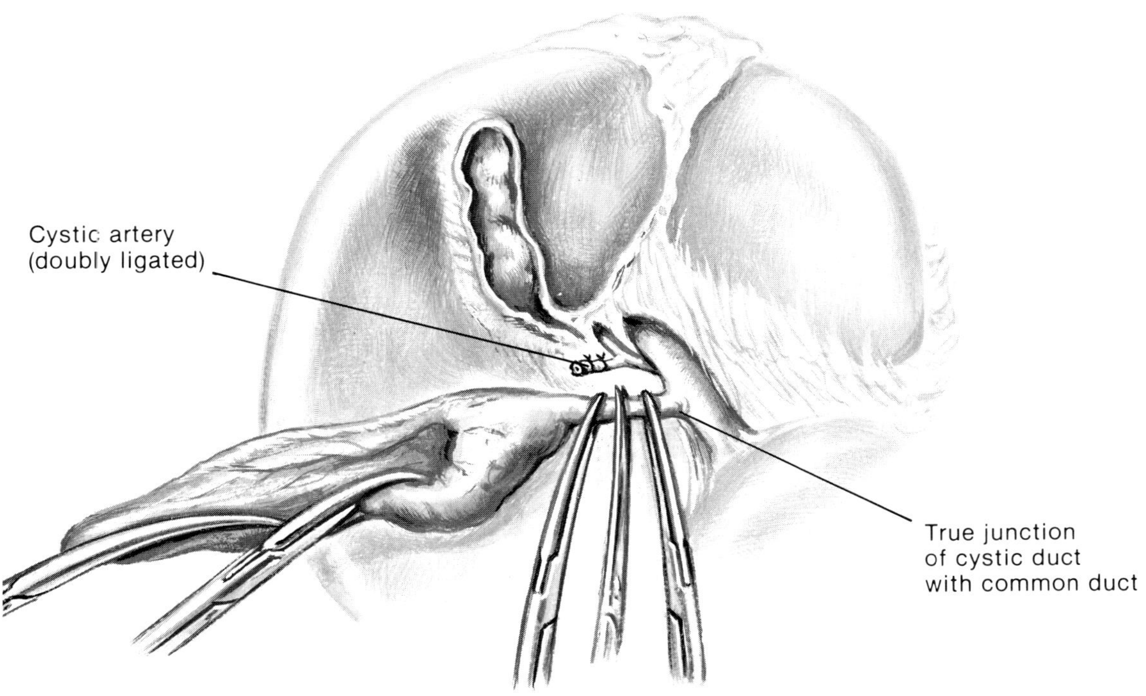

Figure 21–13. The cystic duct is divided 5 to 8 mm from its junction with the common hepatic duct.

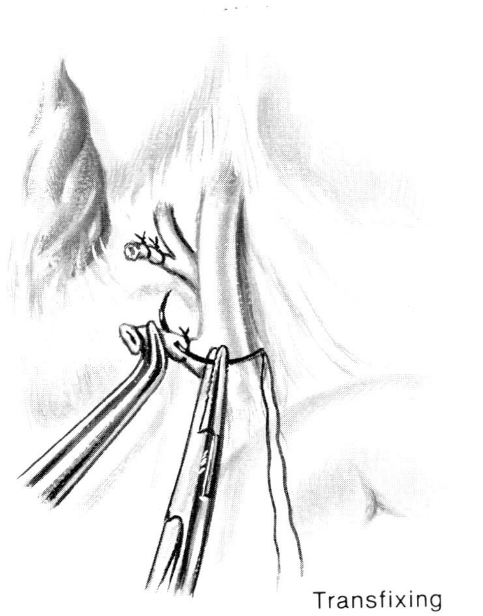

Figure 21–14. The stump of the cystic duct is secured with both a ligature and a transfixion suture of nonabsorbable material.

13). The stump of the cystic duct is secured with a ligature and a transfixion suture of nonabsorbable material (Fig. 21–14). If drainage of the gallbladder fossa is necessary, a Penrose drain or a closed system drain (e.g., Jackson-Pratt) may be placed in the region of the foramen of Winslow and allowed to emerge along the course of the gallbladder bed (Fig. 21–15). Some surgeons attempt to reperitonealize the gallbladder bed by approximating the cut edges of the so-called capsule of the gallbladder. This maneuver is reputed to minimize postoperative adhesions. This is doubtful, and we rarely attempt reperitonealization. The abdominal wound is closed in layers (Fig. 21–16) and a suitable dressing applied.

Comments: The principal hazard of cholecystectomy is injury to the common bile duct. The causes of such injuries are obviously many and varied; Figure 21–17 depicts a few of the more common ones encountered. Hemorrhage, particularly from the cystic artery and less commonly from the portal vein, is perhaps the most frequent cause of injury (Fig. 21–17*A*). With blood obscuring the operative field, blind clamping of structures in the hemorrhage area may result in inadvertent occlusion of a portion of, or all of, the common duct. Additional damage of the duct may occur with ligatures and transfixion sutures used to secure the vessel. Prevention of injury to the biliary ductal system in the face of hemorrhage requires mature judgment that resists the impulse to seek immediate control of blood loss at the expense of accurate and precise surgical technique.

A less frequent cause of ductal injury is the erosion of a stone impacted in the am-

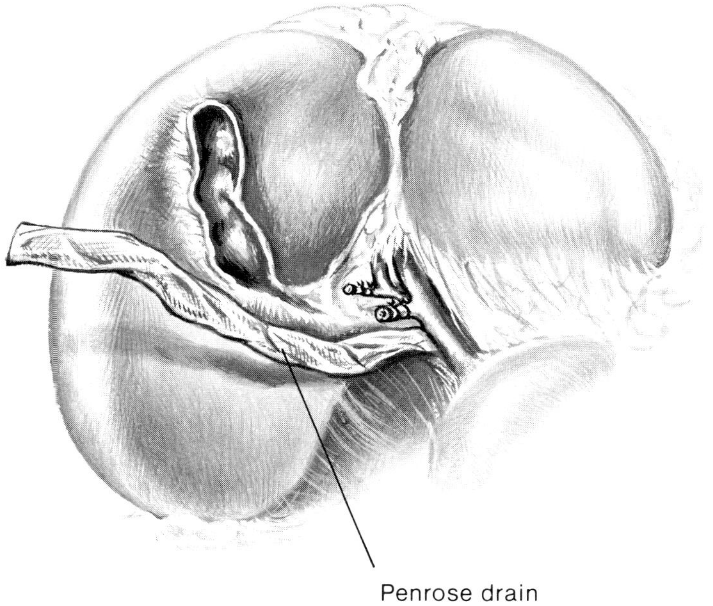

Figure 21–15. A Penrose drain is placed at the foramen of Winslow and brought out of the abdominal cavity along the gallbladder bed.

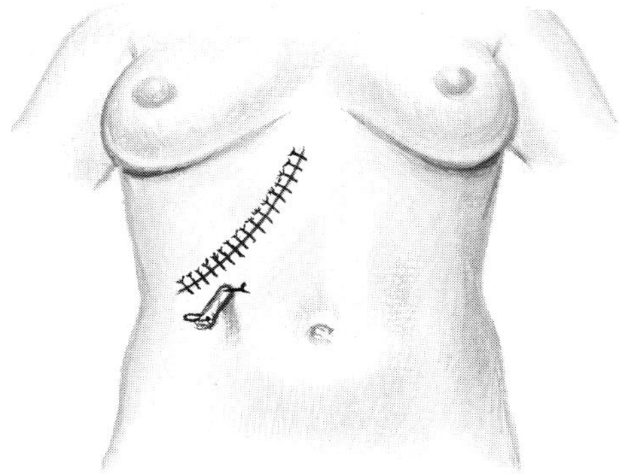

Figure 21–16. The abdominal wall is closed in layers and the drain brought out through a separate stab wound.

pulla of the gallbladder into the common duct (Fig. 21–17*B*) in patients with acute cholecystitis. Unless he recognizes it, the surgeon will mistake the common bile duct distal to the stone for the cystic duct. In patients with short cystic ducts (Fig. 21–17*C*), traction on the ampulla of the gallbladder may also convey the mistaken impression that the distal common bile duct is the cystic duct.

Although cholecystectomy is frequently performed, there is considerable variation in the pathology encountered and the technical problems that require solution. Common duct injuries are preventable but only by constant attention to detail and a respect for the potential hazards of this operation.

Many surgeons drain the subhepatic space in patients who undergo elective cholecystectomy, to prevent the accumulation of bile and blood, which, if infected, could result in a subhepatic abscess.[58] Gallbladder bile in patients without stones is usually sterile. With chronic cholecystitis, gallbladder bile cultures are positive in 30 per cent of patients. However, the presence of bactibilia does not seem to be associated with an increased incidence of infectious complications in elective cholecystectomy for chronic cholecystitis.[14] Complications attributable to the use of drains are infrequent and consist almost exclusively of superficial staphylococcal infections at the drain site. The routine use of drains following cholecystectomy for chronic cholecystitis has been challenged. Kambouris et al.[32] in 1973 reported on 500 patients who underwent biliary tract operations; drains were omitted in 62.5 per cent of these patients. Patients without drains had a shorter hospital stay and a lower incidence of postoperative complications. Similarly, Goldberg et al.[24] in 1975 reported fewer wound infections and a lower incidence of postoperative fever in 37 patients in whom drains were omitted. Three subsequent randomized prospective studies have shown that there is no benefit from routine drainage of the gallbladder bed following elective cholecystectomy.[8, 39, 56] Following cholecystectomy for acute cholecystitis, we used a closed drainage system in all patients.

Routine operative cholangiography has been advocated by increasing numbers of surgeons over the past several years. Saltzstein et al.[48] have reported their experience with cystic duct cholangiography in 423 of 506 consecutive patients undergoing cholecystectomy. Of this group, there were 79 patients with clinical indications for common duct exploration. Thirty-nine (50 per cent) had normal operative cholangiograms and, therefore, were not subjected to choledochotomy. Of 427 patients without clinical

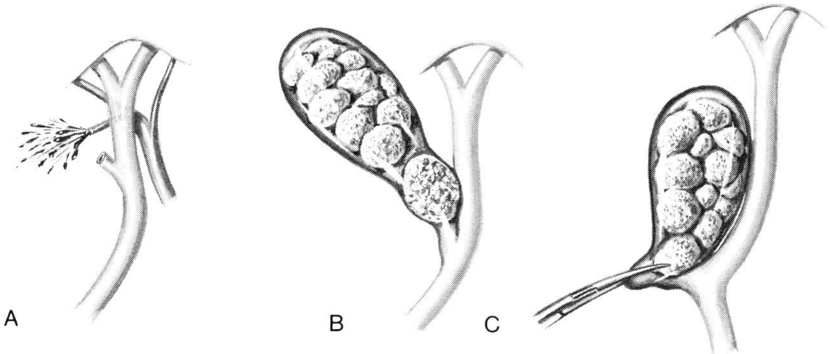

Figure 21–17. The potential causes of common duct injury include (*A*) hemorrhage from the cystic artery, (*B*) erosion of a stone through the wall of the gallbladder into the common hepatic duct, and (*C*) excessive traction on the ampulla of the gallbladder in the presence of a short cystic duct.

indications for duct exploration, unsuspected common duct stones were detected in 8 (1.8 per cent). Kakos et al.[31] in 1972 reported on the use of operative cholangiography at Ohio State University for the years 1951 through 1970. The use of this technique increased progressively from 2.9 per cent in 1951 to 93 per cent in 1970. As a result, the number of patients undergoing choledochotomy decreased from 41 per cent to 25 per cent, and the number of positive duct exploration increased from 28 per cent to 62 per cent. This experience is similar to that of the author. The indications for operative cholangiography have been progressively expanded, resulting in fewer negative common duct explorations.[9, 12, 28, 52] In my opinion, operative cholangiography does not have to be performed in all patients; Hall et al.[26] have reported on the pitfalls associated with undue reliance on operative cholangiography in the prevention of residual common duct stones. Patients with a large solitary cholesterol stone and those with very small-caliber cystic ducts are examples of patients in whom the procedure is rarely productive.[10, 20, 36] The effectiveness of operative cholangiography is also proportional to the ability and skill of the individual interpreting the radiographs.[38, 46] In this respect, surgeons should seek the expertise of a radiologist to assist them in increasing the accuracy of these studies. Further details on the use and interpretation of operative cholangiography are described in Chapter 22.

REFERENCES

1. Ammon HV, Hofmann AF: The Langenbuch paper. I. An historical perspective and comments of the translators. Gastroenterology 1983;*85*:1426.
2. Ammon HV, Hofmann AF: The Langenbuch paper. II. A translation. Gastroenterology 1983; *85*:1430.
3. Aranha GV, Sontag SJ, Greenlee HB: Cholecystectomy in cirrhotic patients: a formidable operation. Am J Surg 1982;*143*:55.
4. Arnold DJ: 28621 cholecystectomies in Ohio. Results of a survey in Ohio hospitals by the Gallbladder Survey Committee. Ohio Chapter, American College of Surgeons. Am J Surg 1970;*119*:714.
5. Beal JM: Historical perspective of gallstone disease. Surg Gynecol Obstet 1984;*158*:181.
6. Berci G, Shore JM, Hamlin JA, Morgenstern L: Operative fluoroscopy and cholangiography. The use of modern radiologic techniques during surgery. Am J Surg 1978;*135*:32.
7. Bobbs JS: Case of lithotomy of the gallbladder. Tr Indiana State Med Soc, Indianapolis, 1868, p 68.
8. Budd DC, Cochran RC, Fouty WJ Jr: Cholecystectomy with and without drainage. A randomized, prospective study of 300 patients. Am J Surg 1982;*143*:307.
9. Coelho JCU, Buffara M, Pozzobon CE, Altenburg FL, Artigas GV: Incidence of common bile duct stones in patients with acute and chronic cholecystitis. Surg Gynecol Obstet 1984;*158*:76.
10. Deitch EA, Voci VE: Operative cholangiography. The case for selective instead of routine operative cholangiography. Am Surg 1982;*48*:297.
11. Diffenbaugh WG, Sarver FE, Strohl EL: Gangrenous perforation of the gallbladder. Arch Surg 1949;*59*:74.
12. Doyle PJ, Ward-McQuaid JN, McEwen Smith A: The value of routine peroperative cholangiography—a report of 4000 cholecystectomies. Br J Surg 1982:*69*:617.
13. Elyaderani MK, McDowell DE, Gabriele OF: A preliminary report of percutaneous cholecystostomy under ultrasonography and fluoroscopy guidance. J Clin Gastroenterol 1983;*5*:277.
14. Farnell MB, van Heerden JA, Beart RW Jr: Elective cholecystectomy. The role of biliary bacteriology and administration of antibiotics. Arch Surg 1981;*116*:537.
15. Fowkes FGR, Gunn AA: The management of acute cholecystitis and its hospital cost. Br J Surg 1980;*67*:613.
16. Friley M: Perforation of the gallbladder. Rev Surg 1972:*29*:377.
17. Fry DE, Cox RA, Harbrecht PJ: Empyema of the gallbladder: a complication in the natural history of acute cholecystitis. Am J Surg 1981;*141*:366.
18. Gagic N, Frey CF: The results of cholecystostomy for the treatment of acute cholecystitis. Surg Gynecol Obstet 1975:*140*:255.
19. Gagic N, Frey CF, Gaines R: Acute cholecystitis. Surg Gynecol Obstet 1975;*140*:868.
20. Gerber A, Apt MK: The case against routine operative cholangiography. Am J Surg 1982;*143*:734.
21. Glenn F, Dillon LD: Developing trends in acute cholecystitis and choledocholithiasis. Surg Gynecol Obstet 1980;*151*:528.
22. Glenn F, McSherry CK: Etiologic factors in fatal complications following biliary tract surgery. Ann Surg 1963;*157*:695.
23. Glenn F, McSherry CK, Dineen P: Morbidity of surgical treatment for nonmalignant biliary tract disease. Surg Gynecol Obstet 1968;*126*:15.
24. Goldberg IM, Goldberg JP, Liechty RD, et al: Cholecystectomy with and without surgical drainage. Am J Surg 1975;*130*:29.
25. Graham EA, Cole WH: Roentgenologic examination of the gallbladder: preliminary report of a new method utilizing the intravenous injection of tetrabromphenolphthalein. JAMA 1924;*82*:613.
26. Hall RC, Sakiyalak P, Kim SK, Rogers LS, Webb WR: Failure of operative cholangiography to prevent retained common duct stones. Am J Surg 1973;*125*:51.
27. Hays DM, Glenn F: The fate of the cholecystostomy patient. J Am Geriatr Soc 1955;*3*:21.
28. Holliday HJ, Farringer JL Jr, Terry RB, Pickens DR Jr: Operative cholangiography. Review of 7,529 operations on the biliary tree in a community hospital. Am J Surg 1980;*139*:379.
29. Huber DF, Martin EW, Cooperman M: Cholecystectomy in elderly patients. Am J Surg 1983; *146*:719.

30. Jarvinen HJ, Hastbacka J: Early cholecystectomy for acute cholecystitis. A prospective randomized study. Ann Surg 1980;*191*:501.
31. Kakos GS, Tompkins RK, Turnipseed W, Zollinger RM: Operative cholangiography during routine cholecystectomy. Arch Surg 1972;*104*:484.
32. Kambouris AA, Carpenter WS, Allahen RD: Cholecystectomy without drainage. Surg Gynecol Obstet 1973;*137*:613.
33. Kasugai T, Kuno N, Kizu M, et al: Endoscopic pancreatocholangiography. II. The pathological endoscopic pancreatocholangiogram. Gastroenterology 1972;*63*:217.
34. Lahtinen J, Alhava EM, Aukee S: Acute cholecystitis treated by early and delayed surgery. A controlled clinical trial. Scand J Gastroenterol 1978;*13*:673.
35. Langenbuch C: Ein fall von exstirpation der gallenblase wegen chronischer cholelithiasis. Berl Klin Wochenschr 1882;*48*:725.
36. Levine SB, Lerner HJ, Leifer ED, Lindheim SR: Intraoperative cholangiography. A review of indications and analysis of age-sex groups. Ann Surg 1983;*198*:692.
37. MacDonald JA: Early cholecystectomy for acute cholecystitis. Can Med Assoc J 1974;*111*:796.
38. Machi J, Sigel B, Spigos DG, Beitler JC, Justin JR: Critical factors in the image clarity of operative cholangiography. J Surg Res 1983;*35*:480.
39. Maull KI, Daugherty ME, Shearer GR, Sachatello CR, Ernst CB, Meeker WR, Griffen WO Jr: Cholecystectomy: to drain or not to drain. A randomized prospective study of 200 patients. J Surg Res 1978:*24*:259.
40. Mirizzi PL, Losada CQ: Die untersuchung der gallenwege wahrend der operation. Dtsch Ztschr Chir 1932 *236*:755.
41. Mitchell A, Morris PJ: Trends in management of acute cholecystitis. Br Med J 1982;*284*:27.
42. Niemeier OW: Acute perforations of the gallbladder. Ann Surg 1934;*99*:922.
43. Radder RW: Ultrasonically guided percutaneous catheter drainage for gallbladder empyema. Diagn Imaging 1980;*49*:330.
44. Roslyn J, Busuttil RW: Perforation of the gallbladder: a frequently mismanaged condition. Am J Surg 1979;*137*:307.
45. Rosoff L, Robbins FG: Operative treatment of acute cholecystitis. Surg Clin North Am 1973;*53*:1079.
46. Sachatello CR, Lieber A: A simple method to determine the resolution of operative cholangiograms. Am J Surg 1982;*143*:769.
47. Salleh HBM, Balasegaram M: Treatment of acute cholecystitis by routine urgent operation. Br J Surg 1974;*61*:705.
48. Saltzstein EC, Evani SV, Mann RW: Routine operative cholangiography. Arch Surg 1973;*107*:289.
49. Schwartz SJ: Biliary tract surgery and cirrhosis: a critical combination. Surgery 1981;*90*:577.
50. Shaver RW, Hawkins IF Jr, Soong J: Percutaneous cholecystostomy. AJR 1982;*138*:1133.
51. Skillings JC, Kumai C, Hinshaw JR: Cholecystostomy: a place in modern biliary surgery? Am J Surg 1980;*139*:865.
52. Stark ME, Loughry CW: Routine operative cholangiography with cholecystectomy. Surg Gynecol Obstet 1980;*151*:657.
53. Stelzer MH, Steiger E, Rosato FE: Mortality following cholecystectomy. Surg Gynecol Obstet 1970; *130*:64.
54. Strohl EL, Diffenbaugh WG, Baker JH, Cheema MH: Collective reviews. Gangrene and perforation of the gallbladder. Int Abstr Surg 1962;*114*:1.
55. Sullivan DM, Hood TR, Griffen WO Jr: Biliary tract surgery in the elderly. Am J Surg 1982;*143*:218.
56. Trowbridge PE: A randomized study of cholecystectomy with and without drainage. Surg Gynecol Obstet 1982;*155*:171.
57. Van Der Linden W, Edlund G: Early versus delayed cholecystectomy: the effect of a change in management. Br J Surg 1981;*68*:753.
58. Van Der Linden W, Kempi V, Gedda S: A radionuclide study on the effectiveness of drainage after elective cholecystectomy. Ann Surg 1981;*193*:155.
59. Way LW, Bernhoft RA, Thomas MJ: Biliary stricture. Surg Clin North Am 1981;*61*:963.
60. Wood M: Eponyms in biliary tract surgery. Am J Surg 1979;*138*:746.

LEON MORGENSTERN, M. D.

22

Exploration of the Common Bile Duct for Stones

INTRODUCTION AND HISTORY

L. G. Courvoisier[1] is generally credited with having performed the first successful choledochotomy in 1890. Within a short time the procedure was adopted by many surgeons on the continent and in the United States. In 1898, W. S. Halsted[2] reported three successful choledocholithotomies and recommended primary closure of the explored duct. Later, however, he recommended postoperative drainage through the cystic duct. Ironically, Halsted himself succumbed in 1922 to the complications of a second choledocholithotomy for a retained common duct stone. The T-tube, still sometimes called the Kehr tube in Europe, was introduced by Hans Kehr[3] (1862–1916) of Germany.

The two major refinements in common duct exploration during the twentieth century have been the introduction of operative cholangiography for imaging the ductal system and choledochoscopy for direct visual inspection of the opened duct and its tributaries. Operative cholangiography was first performed by Mirizzi[4] of Argentina in 1931 and has since become increasingly recognized as an important diagnostic adjunct.

Choledochoscopy was first described by Bakes in 1923, who used very simple equipment, consisting of a speculum, mirror, and small light bulb in the distal duct. McIver[5] in 1941 and Wildegans[6] in 1953 independently introduced rigid instruments, incorporating telescopic, light, and irrigation systems. In 1965 Shore and Lippman[7] described a flexible, fiberoptic choledochoscope that had been used successfully to retrieve intrahepatic stones. The modern rod-lens rigid choledochoscope, employing a new optical principle, was introduced by Berci,[8] Morgenstern,[9] and Shore[10] in 1971 and has since become the principal instrument used at this time for endoscopic inspection of the biliary tract. Yamakawa et al.[11] described a flexible, fiberoptic choledochoscope with a steerable tip and instrument channel in 1976, which has given good results in subsequent clinical reports.[12]

Operative ultrasonography is the latest candidate for a role in assessing the common duct for the presence of stones.[13, 14] The instrumentation is evolving rapidly, and it is still too early to know just how much of a contribution ultrasonography will make.

Contributors to the techniques and instrumentation for common duct exploration have been legion. Nevertheless, the three major advances in the area of biliary tract surgery remain choledocholithotomy, operative cholangiography, and operative endoscopy.

SURGICAL ANATOMY AND PHYSIOLOGY OF THE BILE DUCTS OF IMPORTANCE IN EXPLORATION

Extrahepatic Ducts

The common bile duct is formed by the confluence of the right and left main hepatic ducts. The portion cephalad to the cystic duct is often called the common hepatic duct and the portion caudad to the cystic duct insertion, the common bile duct. Variations in the site of insertion of the cystic duct make this arbitrary division cumbersome. For purposes of surgical anatomy, the entire common extrahepatic duct can be considered the common bile duct.

The confluence of right and left main hepatic ducts usually takes place within 1.0 to 1.5 cm of the porta hepatis. The extrahepatic segment of the left main duct is longer than that of the right, rendering it more susceptible to extrahepatic injury during exploration. Rarely is it necessary during routine operative exploration of the duct to expose the hepatic ducts. Trauma, stricture, or neoplasm is the usual reason for operative exposure of the bifurcation.

Lying slightly to the right of the midline, the supraduodenal portion of the common bile duct descends obliquely leftward toward the duodenum. It then disappears retroduodenally, where it may be exposed by the Kocher maneuver for a distance of 1.5 to 2.0 cm before it begins its transpancreatic and transduodenal passage to terminate at the papilla of Vater.

The total length of the extrahepatic bile duct varies from 11 to 12 cm. Its average normal width at its widest portion is 0.8 to 1.0 cm; the average diameter of the duct increases slightly with advancing age. Ducts measuring over 1.2 cm in diameter are considered dilated. With no abnormal resistance to emptying, there is no appreciable increase in the diameter of the duct following cholecystectomy.

The normal common duct is blue-gray, reflecting the yellow-green bile as seen through the thin-walled duct. It is easily compressible and elastic to palpation. In contrast, the chronically obstructed and inflamed duct is grayish white, its wall obviously thickened; grossly dilated lymphatics and veins may form a plexus pattern on its surface. Neither the normal nor the obstructed duct possesses any independent motility or contractibility.

Hepatic Ducts

The anatomy of the hepatic ducts is described in Chapter 1. The direction of the major ducts and their branches must be known by the surgeon as he explores the interior of the hepatic ducts. The left hepatic duct courses obliquely upward and to the left, with no major tributaries. It dilates more easily, especially in its extrahepatic portion, and is more frequently the repository of intrahepatic calculi. The right hepatic duct arises at the junction of the ventrocranial branch and the dorsocaudal branch. The ventrocranial branch on the right is easily seen endoscopically, in contrast to the dorsocaudal branch, whose angle of entry precludes good inspection. Its orifice may be mistaken for a stone or, conversely, a stone at this point may be taken as a normal finding.

Anomalies are common,[15, 16] and the exploring surgeon must be wary. Accessory ducts are more common on the right, joining the gallbladder or the cystic duct, or both. A common anomaly and potential hazard is entry of the cystic duct into the right hepatic duct, which presents a threat of injury to the latter during dissection or ligation of the supposed cystic duct.

Considerations of bile duct physiology have little influence on the technique of exploration. Contraction of Boyden's sphincter at the terminus of the duct in response to manipulation, overzealous injection of cold contrast material, and other stimuli, may produce a "pseudocalculus" sign on cholangiography. Distention of a poorly emptying duct to 2 or 2.5 times the normal resting diameter should not necessarily be attributed to calculous obstruction.

INDICATIONS FOR COMMON DUCT EXPLORATION[17–21]

An absolute indication for common duct exploration is the proven presence of calculi or other abnormal intraductal elements, including foreign bodies and neoplasms, opacified or felt during operative and radiographic examination of the duct.

Another absolute indication is suppurative choledochitis,[22–24] which is described in Chapter 19. Patients with this syndrome are usually so ill that extended exploration of the ductal system is not indicated. Only if the cause of the obstruction can be easily identified and corrected is any manipulation indicated. Operative cholangiography and choledochoscopy are contraindicated because they may spread or aggravate the existent cholangitis. With few exceptions, any steps more definitive than T-tube decompression and rapid removal of accessible calculi are deferred until the cholangitis and sepsis have subsided.

A third absolute indication for common duct exploration is persistent jaundice and the presence of a dilated, thickened duct. We have retrieved calculi from such ducts even when operative cholangiography failed to show them. In the markedly dilated duct, cholangiography alone is not absolutely reliable to rule out the presence of stones, sludge, or calculous debris.

Absolute indications given in the past for

common duct exploration no longer apply, with the use of improved operative cholangiography and the ability in the majority of cases to rule out common duct stones when they are absent. Among indications cited in the past have been a prior history of jaundice, a gallbladder containing small stones, a wide cystic duct, a history of pancreatitis, and acalculous cholecystitis. Too often, ductal exploration for these indications yields negative results.[17–21] We have placed increasing reliance on cholangiography to obviate unnecessary ductal exploration with its attendant increased morbidity and mortality. We believe that the normal-sized common duct should be opened only when definitive evidence of intraductal calculi exists.

SURGICAL ACCESS TO THE COMMON BILE DUCT

Access to the common bile duct may be through an upper abdominal, vertical, or right subcostal incision, depending on the habitus of the patient and the preference of the surgeon. There are surgeons who prefer an upper midline incision for its ease of performance and versatility, but our impression is that it may limit access to the gallbladder, especially in obese patients. The upper right paramedian incision is useful for patients with a very acute subcostal angle. Our preference has been for a right subcostal incision extending from the midline to the anterior axillary line. This provides optimal exposure for the gallbladder and common duct with a minimum of vigorous retraction. The medial angle of the incision should extend just beyond the border of the right rectus muscle. The ligamentum teres hepatis and falciform ligament should be serially divided and ligated.

For patients in whom exposure of the extrahepatic biliary tract poses difficulties, we prefer the Kehr incision, which consists of the standard right subcostal incision extended upward at the midline to the xyphoid. It affords excellent exposure to the porta hepatis and is especially useful in very obese patients.

After the abdomen has been explored, the gallbladder and common duct areas are prepared for dissection. We employ three laparotomy pads folded in thirds for retraction of adjacent structures. One is packed over the hepatic flexure of the colon, one is placed over the distal stomach and duodenum, and the third is used superiorly to retract the right lobe of the liver cephalad. It is often necessary to divide adhesions to the diseased gallbladder or an inflamed porta hepatis before the pads are placed. Care should be taken not to tear the liver capsule with retractors while obtaining exposure, because the troublesome bleeding that ensues interferes with visibility. Hepatic bleeding produced in this way usually responds to pressure for several minutes. Occasionally, a topical hemostatic agent can save time and facilitate dissection.

Traction in two directions is the key to optimal exposure of the common duct. The gallbladder is grasped with Mayo clamps on the fundus and Hartmann's pouch (when the latter is safely exposed); the first assistant then exerts traction on the duodenum and hepatoduodenal ligament, rendering the latter taut.

The peritoneum overlying the triangle of Calot is then lifted and sharply incised in the direction of the common duct. The fat and areolar tissue that generally lie beneath the peritoneum are easily wiped with a peanut sponge in cephalic and caudal directions, thereby exposing the wall of the common duct. Occasionally, a small venous bleeder in the periductal fat requires application of a small hemoclip or control by electrocoagulation. Electrocoagulation directly on the common duct should be avoided.

In the average case, we prefer to dissect out the cystic duct before mobilizing the gallbladder, which allows operative cholangiography to be performed early in the dissection. The cystic artery is identified, and the anterior and posterior branches are ligated separately, if necessary. Although hemoclips are preferred by some surgeons for the cystic artery, we use a double ligature of 2-0 silk. With the cystic artery ligated and divided, straightening of the slightly convoluted cystic duct is more easily accomplished in readiness for operative cholangiography. In patients in whom exposure of the triangle of Calot is difficult because of severe inflammatory changes, dissection of the gallbladder from above downward is the safer approach. As soon as it can be identified with certainty near its junction with the gallbladder, the cystic duct should be occluded to prevent stones or sludge from being forced into the common duct during the dissection. For this purpose we use a medium-sized rubber vessel-loop, passed twice around the cystic duct and held taut until the cystic duct is subsequently ligated. It is important that the common duct be identified above and below the cystic duct junction. Occasionally, this is not possible because of an anomalous insertion of the cystic duct (for example, in the retroduodenal portion of the duct, or when it spirals posteriorly to insert on the left side of the common duct). In these instances it is sufficient to identify the zone of adventitial fusion rather than to embark on a potentially dangerous dissection.

With the cystic duct identified, occluded, straightened, and exposed, the stage is now prepared for operative cholangiography.

OPERATIVE CHOLANGIOGRAPHY

Equipment

Since its introduction by Mirizzi, significant improvements have been made in operative cholangiography.[25–27] Long an area neglected by radiologists and scorned by surgeons, it now plays a prominent role in biliary tract surgery. Because it delineates the ductal anatomy, a cholangiogram may demonstrate occult, nonpalpable stones or reveal otherwise hidden and potentially dangerous biliary tract anomalies. Fifteen to 20 per cent of patients manifest significant variations from normal ductal anatomy.

The principal problem with operative cholangiography today is that it is so often done by an obsolete, ineffective, and sometimes misleading technique. The conventional, static, three-film method ignores the progress of recent years. Only by bringing advanced techniques to the operating suite[28] can maximum speed and the diagnostic accuracy advantages of operative cholangiography be realized. Assessment of ductal filling and direct observation of sphincter function are provided by the use of image amplification and the ability to perform *serial, aimed* films for proper evaluation.

Our technique of operative cholangiography, which includes operative fluoroscopy, requires the following equipment (Fig. 22–1):

1. Operating table with radiolucent table top with lateral extension, allowing biaxial movement in lateral and cephalocaudal axes (floating coordinate top) as well as lateral tilt.
2. Ceiling suspended, overhead x-ray tube and collimator on an articulated arm and a three-phase generator (800–1000 mA).
3. Image amplifier with built-in rotating prism, television camera, and side-loading x-ray camera, allowing image display on television monitors. One of the latter is ceiling-mounted, the other floor-mounted. The side-loading x-ray camera records the images on 100 mm × 100 mm x-ray film.
4. Double foot switch, allowing alternation between fluoroscopy and serially aimed films, at will or at predetermined intervals (e.g., 1 to 2 films per second).
5. Small darkroom with compact 90-second film processor located in the operating suite. Dry films are available and mounted minutes after exposure (Fig. 22–2).

It is recognized that this equipment may be too expensive for most hospitals. Nevertheless, it is required for state-of-the-art cholangiography in the operating room.

Technique

Before the operation is begun, the patient is positioned on the operating table with a

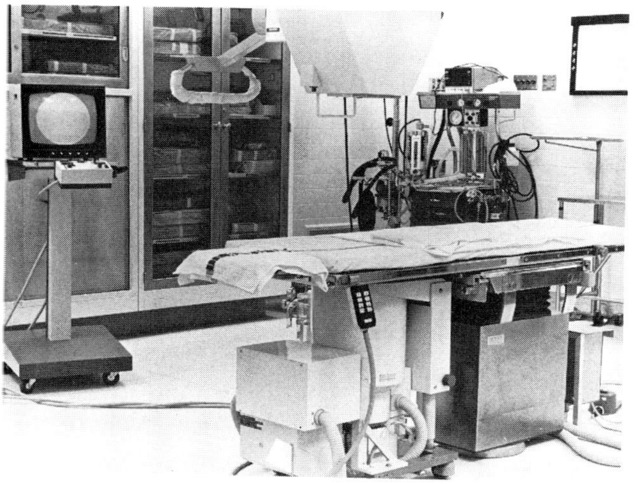

Figure 22–1. Properly equipped operative cholangiographic facility, showing overhead x-ray tube, radiolucent operating table with movable top, image amplifier (below table), and television monitor for fluoroscopic observation.

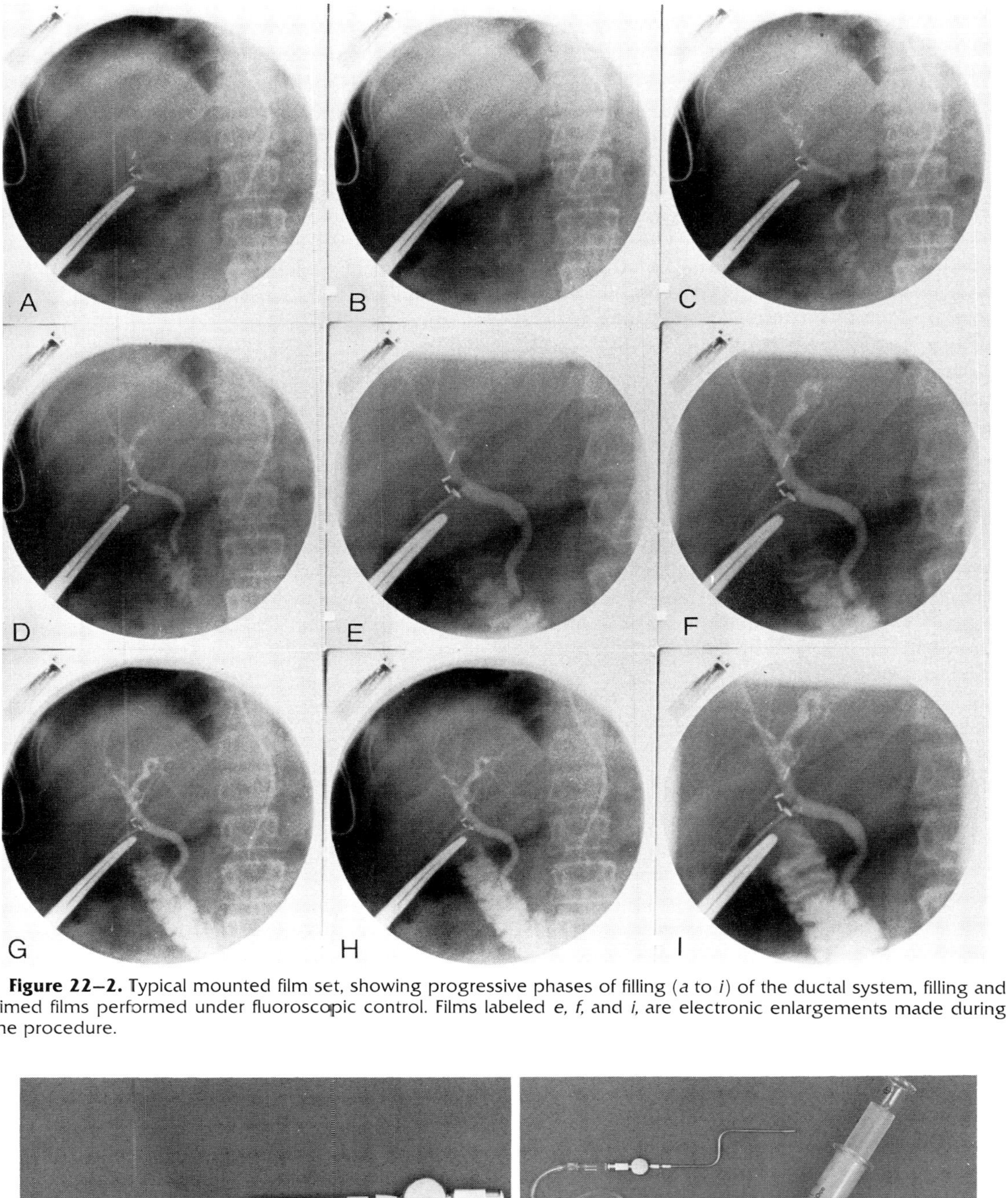

Figure 22–2. Typical mounted film set, showing progressive phases of filling (*a* to *i*) of the ductal system, filling and aimed films performed under fluoroscopic control. Films labeled *e*, *f*, and *i*, are electronic enlargements made during the procedure.

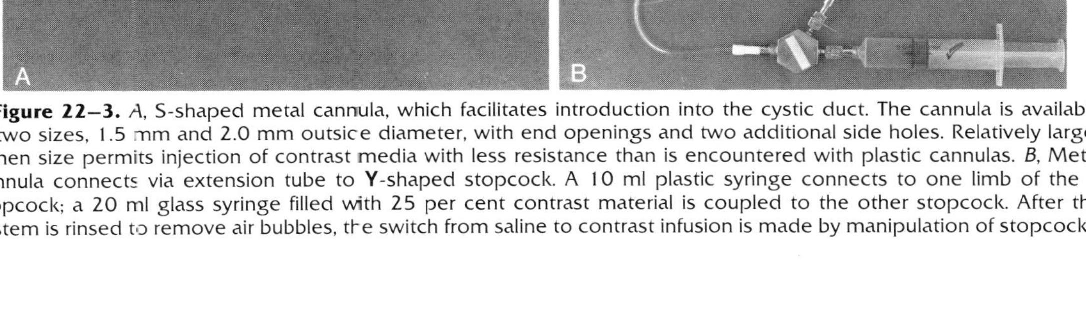

Figure 22–3. *A*, S-shaped metal cannula, which facilitates introduction into the cystic duct. The cannula is available in two sizes, 1.5 mm and 2.0 mm outside diameter, with end openings and two additional side holes. Relatively larger lumen size permits injection of contrast media with less resistance than is encountered with plastic cannulas. *B*, Metal cannula connects via extension tube to **Y**-shaped stopcock. A 10 ml plastic syringe connects to one limb of the **Y** stopcock; a 20 ml glass syringe filled with 25 per cent contrast material is coupled to the other stopcock. After the system is rinsed to remove air bubbles, the switch from saline to contrast infusion is made by manipulation of stopcocks.

radiolucent inflatable cushion beneath the left loin. The cushion is inflated during cholangiography if the duct is superimposed over the thoracic spine. Proper positioning is assured by fluoroscopy, and a scout film is taken of the right upper quadrant. The shadow of the liver edge should cross approximately at the midpoint of the film.

The cholangiographic set, consisting of a metal cannula (Fig. 22–3*A*), a venous extension tube, and a Y-shaped adapter with stopcocks and Luer-Lok receivers (Fig. 22–3*B*), is then prepared. To one of the Luer-Lok receptors, a saline-filled plastic syringe is attached; to the other, a glass syringe filled with 25 per cent Hypaque is attached. Air bubbles must be excluded from the system.

With traction on the cystic duct, a small incision is made in its anterior wall 1.0 to 1.5 cm from the junction with the common duct, using a fine Potts scissors. A small quantity of bile escapes from the cut cystic duct, which should be cultured for aerobic and anaerobic bacteria.

While a continuous flow of saline is maintained through it, a cannula is inserted carefully into the cystic duct for a few millimeters only. Its position is secured with a modified Borge clamp[29] (Fig. 22–4). By injecting saline slowly, the patency and watertight seal around the cannula is checked.

Numerous other catheters and devices are available for cannulation and infusion of dye into the cystic duct.[30–32] These are chiefly made of plastic and held in place either by a ligature or by a hemoclip. Many are too compressible or flexible to insert into the duct in many cases. Moreover, in proportion to its outer diameter, the metal cannula has a much larger inner diameter, which facilitates the injection of contrast media. For these reasons, we prefer the metal cannula shown in Figure 22–3*A*.

All extraneous clamps, laparotomy sponges, and other radiopaque items are removed from the field. The laparotomy wound is covered with a sterile towel, and the overhead x-ray tube on the articulated arm is moved into position directly over the field.

With the venous extension attached, the surgeon can inject contrast material at a safe distance from the collimated x-ray beam. The initial film is taken to demonstrate the position of the cannula before the injection is begun. Contrast medium is then slowly injected under fluoroscopic control. As soon as the first trace of contrast is visible, another film is exposed. Subsequently, serial aimed films are made with the addition of small increments of contrast under direct visual control. It is important to record the *early*

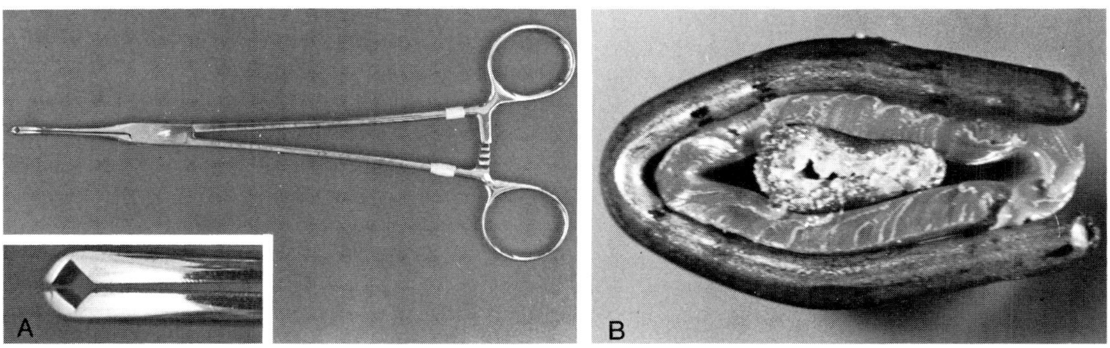

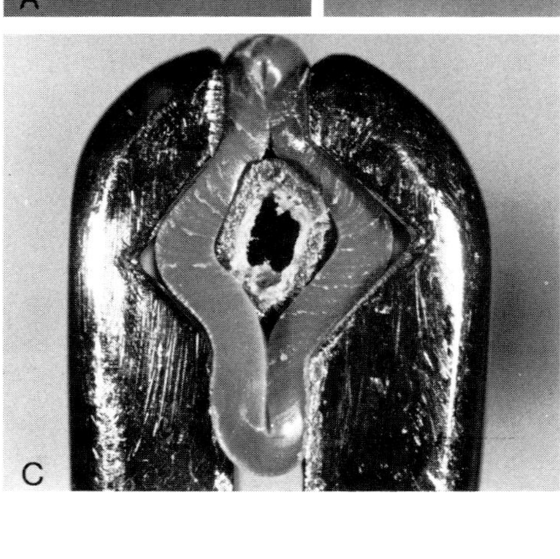

Figure 22–4. *A*, Modified Borge clamp. The jaws of the clamp (inset) are rhomboid. The flexible distal portion of the clamp permits its use in a variety of duct sizes. Fixation of the cannula is more secure with the use of this instrument than with hemoclips or sutures. Comparative fixation of the catheter in the cystic duct by hemoclip (*B*) and special Borge clamp (*C*). Note the difference in lumen size, with the unobstructed lumen of the simulated cystic duct seen in *C*.

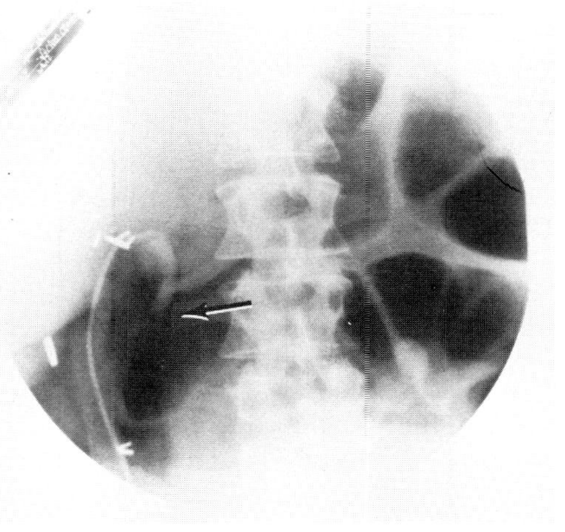

Figure 22–5. Early filling stage. A stone (*arrow*) is visible in the distal common duct. On subsequent films this stone was obscured by contrast material. Serial films with small increments of contrast material injected under visual control, with emphasis on the early filling stage, are of paramount importance.

filling stage of the duct system to demonstrate small stones that may otherwise be obscured as the density of the duct increases with the addition of more contrast medium (Fig. 22–5). In the presence of a patulous sphincter with rapid emptying into the duodenum, the injection pressure is slightly increased to purposely create sphincter spasm, and the remainder of the ductal system is filled with the necessary amount of contrast agent. During this process a number of films are exposed. Should there be less than optimal filling of the hepatic radicles, the patient is tilted into the Trendelenburg position until all ducts and intrahepatic tributaries are seen.

In the event that contrast medium does not drain into the duodenum (e.g., a holdup occurs at Boyden's sphincter), several maneuvers are possible. Intermittent fluoroscopic observation will often show transient opening and passage of the contrast material through the spastic sphincter (Fig. 22–6). Other possible steps are to (1) administer intravenous glucagon (1 mg), (2) increase injection pressure gradually, and (3) wait 2 to 3 minutes before injecting further.

Round radiolucent shadows (air bubbles) may be differentiated from stones by slowly perfusing the duct with saline, which generally removes bubbles (Fig. 22–7). Contrast material should be reinjected, and shadows from bubbles will now be gone. Anomalous (Fig. 22–8) ducts and other anatomic variations may be demonstrated, which enhances the safety and accuracy of the dissection.

Using this system and equipment, the entire process should take no longer than 5 minutes and should provide 6 to 12 well-exposed, well-centered, and informative x-ray films.

TECHNIQUE OF COMMON DUCT EXPLORATION

Incision

After being exposed, the common duct is first palpated, preferably with the operating surgeon on the left side of the patient. Impacted stones should not be dislodged before the duct is opened, lest the stone be lost in

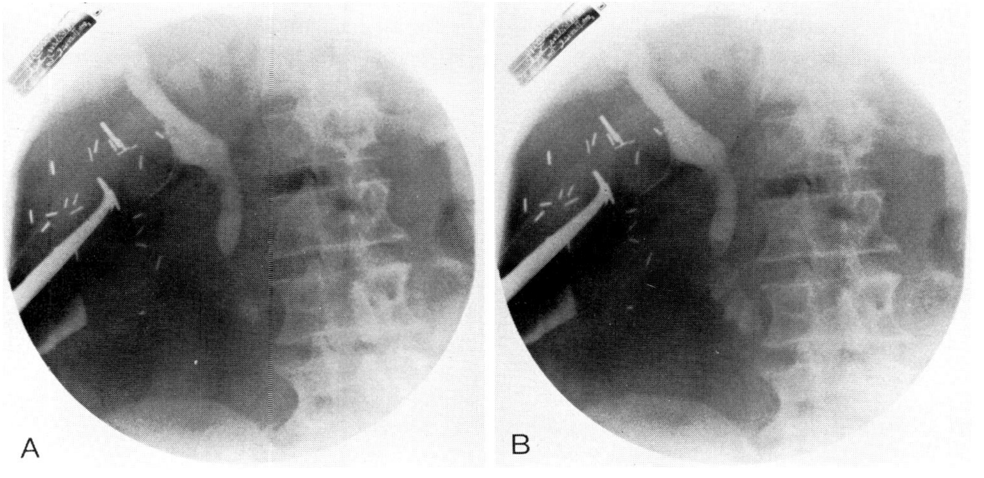

Figure 22–6. *A*, Distal duct observed during systolic phase of sphincter contraction with minimal drainage into duodenum. *B*, Same case, with serial film showing radiolucent stone during diastolic phase of sphincteric function.

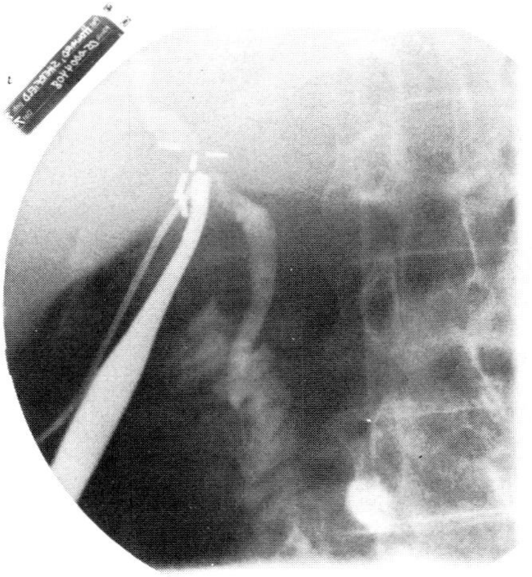

Figure 22–7. Air bubble mimicking stone. After the duct was rinsed with saline and the cholangiogram was repeated, this artifact disappeared.

dilated intrahepatic ducts. The ductal incision should be placed about 1 cm superior to the duodenum. In a thick-walled, chronically obstructed duct, it is advisable to insert two guy sutures (swedged-on 4-0 silk) in approximately the midportion of the transverse axis of the duct. The duct is then precisely incised with a No. 11 or a No. 15 scalpel blade between the guy sutures, entering the duct lumen. The incision is then enlarged cephalad for a total distance of 2 cm, which allows ample room for the exploration. Bile from the common bile duct should also be cultured. Spillage of bile is avoided by constant suction, placement of a laparotomy pad behind the duct, or use of a "stone cup." The assistant should be poised with stone forceps, ready to grasp any stones that appear at the orifice of the choledochotomy.

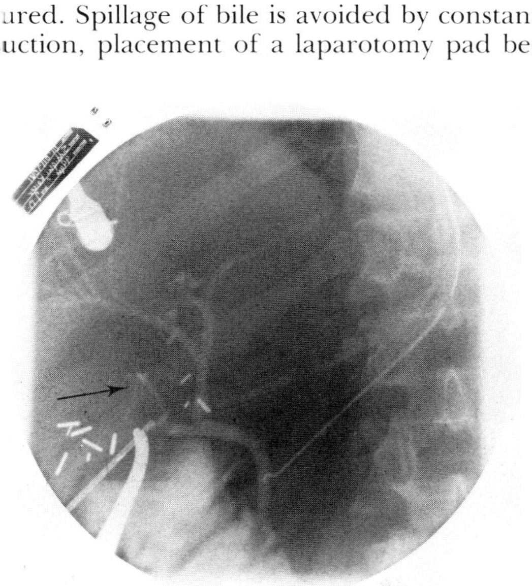

Figure 22–8. Anomalous right hepatic duct (*arrow*) entering the cystic duct nearly 2 cm from its junction with the common duct.

When the duct is thin-walled, as it might be with obstruction of recent onset or obstruction due to neoplasm, the placement of guy sutures as a preliminary procedure is not advised. Bile does not clot, and even minute openings in thin-walled ducts have a great tendency to leak. After incision with a No. 11 blade, guy sutures are placed on the cut edges of the duct wall. Traction on these sutures should be gentle to avoid tearing the duct. More than one set of guy sutures may be placed if necessary to maintain adequate intraductal exposure.

Caution should be taken not to place the incision too far to the right on the ductal circumference, since an incision here might enter an area of cystic duct fusion or a dilated cystic duct.

Instrumentation

Conventional instruments for common duct exploration include gallstone scoops, Randall stone forceps (quarter curved, half curved, three quarters curved, and full curved), Bakes dilators, and 10 F or 12 F rubber catheters with a bulb syringe for saline irrigation (Fig. 22–9). Newer exploratory devices include the Fogarty biliary balloon-tipped catheter and the choledochoscope* for biliary endoscopy.

The first gentle probing for unseen stones should be with the Randall stone forceps. The curved forceps that best fits the anatomic situation should be used. The forceps not only can grasp but also can serve as a probe with which an impacted stone can be felt. Mobilization of the duodenum and the head of the pancreas (Kocher maneuver) may facilitate instrumentation of the bile duct and the choledocholithotomy. Unfortunately, the degree to which the forceps can be opened is limited by the width of the duct. A forceps has yet to be devised that will open only the distal jaws. The limitation of the Randall forceps for larger stones is that the jaws cannot be opened wide enough to grasp or disimpact a stone. It is our practice to probe the distal duct first and then the left and right hepatic ducts, in that order.

---

*Berci-Shore choledochoscope. K. Storz Endoscopy Company, Los Angeles, CA 90048.

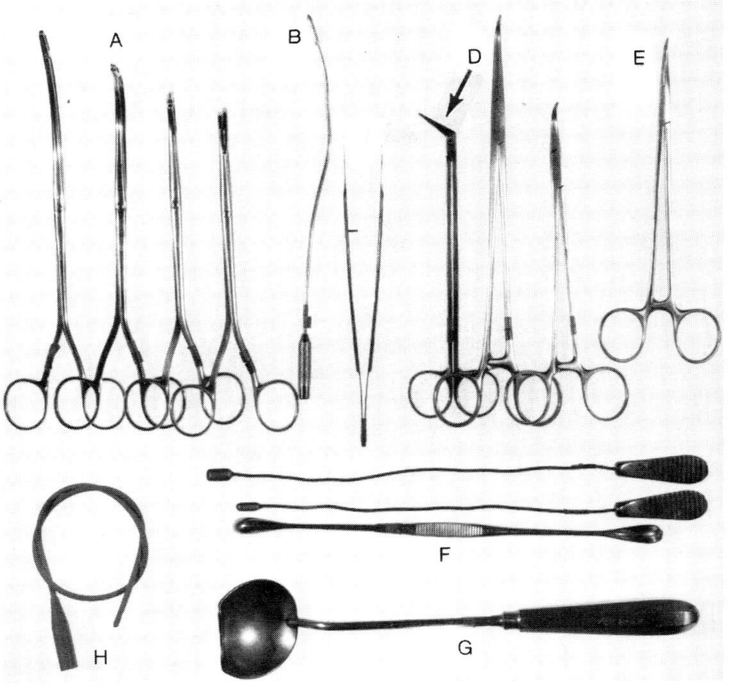

Figure 22–9. Conventional instruments for common duct exploration. *A*, Randall stone forceps. *B*, Bakes dilator (3 mm). *C*, Fine Cushing forceps. *D*, 7 inch, 45 degree Potts scissors. *E*, Fine right-angle clamps for dissection. *F*, Malleable and rigid scoops. *G*, Stone cup. *H*, 10 F catheter for irrigation.

The use of scoops should be limited. Scoops can injure the delicate choledochal mucosa and are seldom effective in extracting stones. They should never be used vigorously enough to curette the mucosa. Scoops are properly used only as a trap to withdraw stones from the duct; insertion and withdrawal should be smooth and gentle. Occasionally, they may be helpful in disimpacting a stone or in removing thick sludge.

Bakes dilators should be used only as probes and never to dilate the sphincter of Oddi.[33] Nothing larger than a 3 mm dilator should be passed through the sphincter. The shining metal tip of the dilator can be seen against the duodenal wall after having passed through the sphincter. Large dilators induce sphincter spasm, injure the sphincter, and may cause pancreatitis. Passage of the dilator through the sphincter does not prove that a stone is not located in the distal duct, lodged in a periampullary recess.

Irrigation is the next step. A 10 F or 12 F catheter, depending on the duct size, is introduced distally, and the duct is copiously irrigated with warm saline. Stones and debris float out. Next, the right and left hepatic ducts are irrigated. Observed endoscopically, unimpacted stones in the upper ducts often whirl around rather than descend during irrigation, and they must be removed under endoscopically guided control. Considerable irrigation also takes place during biliary tract endoscopy.

The Fogarty biliary catheter comes in two sizes, 5 F and 6 F. A useful tool for retrieving common duct stones, it is, however, not without dangers. Perforation, disruption of intrahepatic ducts, and bleeding have occurred from its use. We prefer to use the Fogarty catheter in conjunction with the choledochoscope, with guidance and placement under direct vision.

Choledochoscopy

The rigid choledochoscope in clinical use today owes its effectiveness to the superior optical qualities of the Hopkins rod-lens system. Irrigation, lighting, and image transmission systems are incorporated within a diameter of 5 × 3 mm, allowing the instrument to be introduced into all but the smallest ducts (Fig. 22–10A). The vertical limb measures 300 mm. The horizontal limb is available in two sizes, 40 mm and 60 mm. Attached to a fiberoptic illumination system, the instrument provides a wide angle of view, great depth of field, and a clear picture of the interior of the duct. The distal duct can be easily inspected all the way to the ampulla and the proximal main ducts to their secondary and tertiary radicles. The dorsocaudal

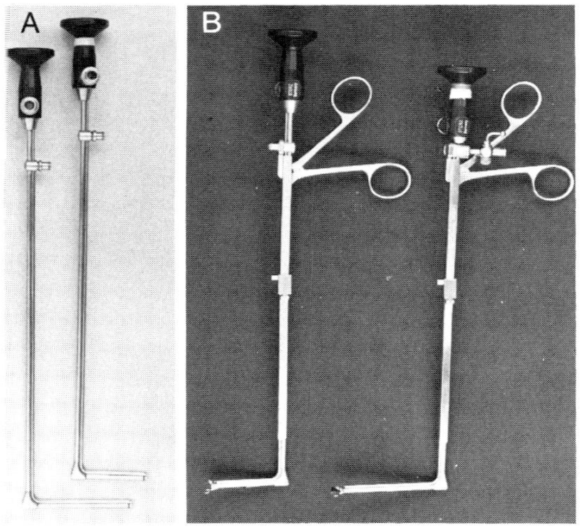

Figure 22–10. *A*, Rigid choledochoscope with two sizes of horizontal limbs, 40 and 60 mm. *B*, Instrument guide channel attached to choledochoscope for passage of stone forceps, biliary balloon catheter, and Dormia basket.

branch of the right duct, except for its orifice, is inaccessible.

Choledochoscopy is carried out in a fluid-filled system. As the duct is dilated with irrigating fluid, the view of the lumen of the duct is improved. Because the irrigation channel is narrow, the irrigating fluid, normal saline, must be delivered under pressure to provide adequate flow. The Fenwal pressure infusion system is employed, and the saline bag is held with the pressure cuff. Standard IV tubing connects the irrigating saline to the choledochoscope with the aid of sterile extension tubes. The pressure is maintained at 300 mm Hg, and 1 liter is usually required for a complete examination.

The scope should be inserted gently in a direction parallel to the duct, with the endoscopist on the left side of the patient. Although a small (10 mm) choledochotomy incision aids choledochoscopy by retaining more fluid, a 20 mm incision is preferred for the standard maneuvers. To narrow the choledochotomy aperture for purposes of choledochoscopy, the two inferior guy sutures may be crossed so more fluid is retained and the duct distends more widely. Switching off the main overhead operating room lights aids in accommodation and visualization. The eye is held a short distance from the eyepiece.

The scope is advanced toward the ampulla. In most cases it is *not* necessary to mobilize the duodenum by the Kocher maneuver to examine the distal duct completely. If the duct angles sharply retroduodenally, it may be necessary to mobilize the duodenum or to use the instrument with a 60 mm horizontal limb.

After examination of the distal duct, the scope is removed and reintroduced in the cephalic direction. The sharp bifurcation identifies the confluence of the two major ducts. Each duct is inspected, and secondary and tertiary radicles are readily visible in markedly dilated ducts.

The mucosa of the distal duct is normally a pale grayish pink with scattered shallow pits throughout its circumference. Distally the duct narrows, and the mucosa near the ampullary orifice has a finely papillary appearance. It is imperative to inspect the ampullary orifice. Its shape is variable, and its size ranges from a pinpoint opening to a fairly patulous one. The tip of the scope should *not* be passed through the sphincter.

In the opposite direction, the bifurcation between the two main ducts provides the first easily accessible landmark proximally. The angle of division of the main ducts varies in acuteness. When the angle is wide, it may be difficult to see the lumen of the left duct. The left duct extends directly upward and to the left without major tributaries. The major tributary of the right duct, the dorsocaudal branch, is not accessible endoscopically.

Inflammation produces a boggy, angry red, edematous mucosa that yields reluctantly to the pressure of the irrigation fluid. Fronds of lacy, tenacious mucus cling to the walls. The pits are obliterated. Mucoid exudate often forms a network of entrapped debris, which may be difficult to remove. Calculi are readily visible.

Stones can usually be retrieved with forceps or by other conventional methods. If the usual methods are unsuccessful, a stone forceps, Fogarty biliary catheter, or Dormia stone basket (Fig. 22–10*B*) may be passed through the guide channel of the choledochoscope. The stone forceps are suitable only for grasping small stones or stone fragments. The Fogarty biliary catheter is passed beyond the stone, the balloon is inflated, and the stone is delivered by traction toward the choledochotomy. Several passes may be necessary. Passage of the Fogarty catheter under direct visual control obviates the dangers of blind instrumentation with this device.

The Dormia basket is passed in the same way. The tip is advanced beyond the stone, the basket opened, the stone trapped, and scope and instrument-bearing channel removed with the stone.

Rigid forceps can also be used to obtain a biopsy of intraductal tumors. The use of the

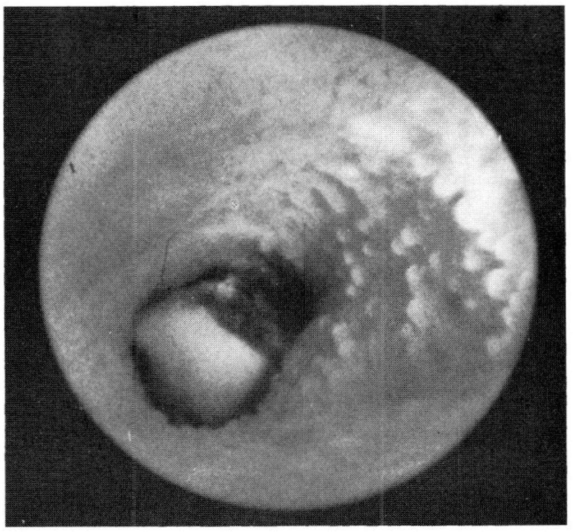

Figure 22–11. Stone outlined in an inflamed duct (film taken from motion picture frame).

choledochoscope in the identification of multiple bile duct tumors has been described by Tompkins et al.[34]

As with any instrument, use of the choledochoscope requires acquisition of a specific skill, acquaintance with intraductal anatomy, and mastering effective techniques of intraductal stone manipulation. Once the technique is learned, the dividends of choledochoscopy are great and the disadvantages negligible. We have found no increase in wound infection, nor have we had any ductal injuries.[35–37] Since the view is excellent and passage is always under direct vision, complications are rare. Choledochoscopy aids in the detection and management of overlooked stones (Fig. 22–11), shortens the time required for choledochal exploration, and frequently obviates the necessity for duodenotomy.

Closure of the Common Duct

Before the common duct is closed, a decision must be made as to the type of drainage required. Is the duct to be drained by a T-tube, or is a drainage procedure, such as choledochoduodenostomy or sphincteroplasty, necessary? Very few surgeons recommend primary closure (as Halsted did early in his surgical career), but sporadic reports by advocates of primary closure continue to appear.[38] This approach is definitely a minority view and is not recommended by this author.

The decision for an auxiliary drainage procedure, such as choledochoduodenostomy or sphincteroplasty,[39–41] may be based on several factors. The nature of the stones in the common duct or hepatic ducts may be a determinant. For example, if the stones are thought to be primary common duct stones, a drainage procedure may be indicated, particularly in large, chronically obstructed ducts.[42, 43] Stenosis of the sphincter of Oddi, as determined by probing with the Bakes dilators, may be important; passage of the 3 mm dilator indicates a nonstenotic sphincter. Failure to demonstrate adequate emptying of the duct after proper radiographic studies constitutes another indication. Recurrence of stones following one or more previous choledochotomies often reflects primary stone formation in the duct—another indication. Finally, inability to extract multiple stones from the intrahepatic ducts or to remove an impacted periampullary stone is an indication for a drainage procedure. Drainage procedures are discussed more fully in Chapters 23 and 24. For the most part, we reserve choledochoduodenostomy for elderly patients with multiple common duct stones, particularly intrahepatic stones or obvious primary duct stones.

For routine choledochotomies, in which no anastomosis to the duodenum is performed, a T-tube is inserted into the common duct through the original choledochotomy. T-tubes are ordinarily supplied with 12 inch stems and 5 inch horizontal limbs. The diameter of the tube employed depends upon the size of the duct and the presence of residual stones. T-tube sizes vary from 8 F to 22 F. Sizes 8 to 12 are used in the smallest ducts, sizes 16 to 22 in larger ducts. Rarely is it necessary to use a T-tube larger than 18 F. If the possibility of residual stones exists or postoperative instrumental stone extraction is anticipated, no tube smaller than 16 F or 18 F should be used. Whelan T-tubes are manufactured with a vertical limb 4 F size greater in diameter than the horizontal limb, which provides the radiologist or endoscopist with a larger tract postoperatively if the duct has to be instrumented. This is the T-tube of choice.

The T-tube is usually tailored before insertion. The long (5 inch) horizontal limbs are each shortened to about 2.5 cm, and the tube is guttered so that only half the circumference (nearest the T-juncture) remains (Fig. 22–12). This is not only adequate for retention within the duct but also allows for better drainage of bile than occurs through the narrow internal diameter of the original tube. Unguttered T-tubes may become coated with deposits of bile pigment, cholesterol, or mu-

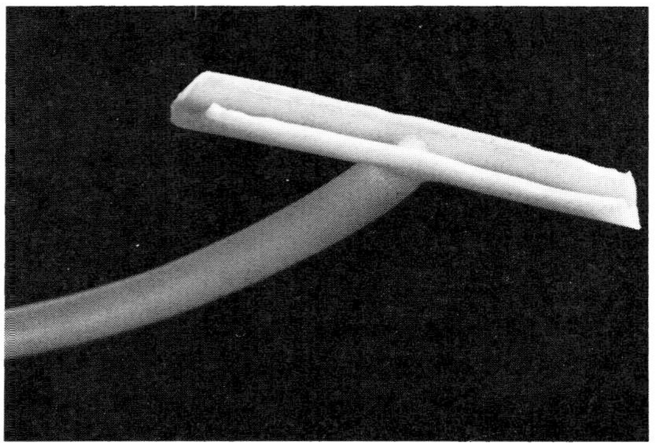

Figure 22–12. Guttered T-tube. Half the circumference of the tube has been trimmed away. Vertical limbs have been shortened to 2.5 cm each.

cus and debris and may plug. The guttered T-tube is also more easily removed, with less traction exerted on the common duct wall. Whether the T-tube exits from the lower or upper end of the choledochotomy incision is not important. The position often depends on the best fit.

The choledochotomy is closed with interrupted chromic catgut (atraumatic swedged-on gastrointestinal needles) placed at 1.0 mm or 1.5 mm intervals. For small, thin-walled ducts, 4-0 chromic catgut is recommended. For thicker-walled ducts, 3-0 chromic catgut is preferred. Other absorbable suture materials are acceptable. Nonabsorbable sutures, such as silk or synthetic monofilament or polyfilament sutures, should not be used. There is ample evidence that nonabsorbable sutures eventually are extruded *into* the lumen of the duct and may form the nidus for an intraductal calculus.[44, 45]

With the T-tube anchored firmly in the duct and the duct sutured closed, completion cholangiography is performed to rule out residual stones. Bile is allowed to flow back to fill the T-tube, and care is taken not to introduce air bubbles into the system. After the closure is tested for leakage by injection of saline, the same injection technique, solutions, fluoroscopy, aimed films, and development systems are used as described in the section on cholangiography. If accessible calculi are recognized and the patient's condition permits, the choledochotomy should be reopened and the stones retrieved. Alternatively and less preferably, the stone or stones may be left for later nonoperative extraction (see Chapters 10 and 25).

The direction and exit site of the long limb of the T-tube are of extreme importance should later stone extraction be necessary. The tube should exit laterally through a stab wound beneath the lateral angle of the subcostal wound or subcostally in the midclavicular line when other incisions are used. There should be enough intra-abdominal slack in the tube to prevent it from being pulled out of the duct postoperatively when the abdominal wall drops forward, but the tube should not execute a full circle because the resulting tract may be impossible to negotiate instrumentation, if this is required. It is axiomatic that every T-tube accidentally pulled out early in the postoperative procedure is the fault of the operating surgeon and his staff, not the fault of the patient.[46] The tube is fixed to the skin with *two* nonabsorbable (2-0 nylon, 2-0 prolene) sutures, which are tied to the skin near the stab wound and then tied securely around the tube. Additionally, the tube is fixed to the dressing with adhesive, which, in turn, is pinned to the main dressing. A plastic connecting tube attaches the T-tube to a length of sterile IV tubing, which is led to a sterile plastic collecting bag. The connecting tube should also be fixed with adhesive to the patient's skin. We have found the thigh drainage bags unwieldy and also unsatisfactory for dependent drainage when the patient is recumbent. We therefore recommend suspending the plastic collecting bag from the bed when the patient is recumbent, or pinning it to the patient's gown when the patient is ambulatory. Every precaution must be taken to prevent premature dislodgement of the tube. Irrational patients should be adequately restrained.

A T-tube is not a substitute for a drain. A Jackson-Pratt drain is placed in Morison's pouch and allowed to exit through a separate stab wound at least 3.0 cm from the T-tube exit site.

A brisk daily choleresis of 750 to 1000 ml of bile may follow decompression of a chronically obstructed duct. Conversely, a very scanty output may occur in the first 24 hours. The output averages 250 to 300 ml/24 hours, denoting partial passage of bile through the tube and the remainder through the patent sphincter. A continued scant outflow from the tube may mean that the tube is plugged, kinked, or otherwise mechanically defective. Continued profuse output of 500 to 1000 ml suggests obstruction at the distal end of the duct.

Should the T-tube be accidentally pulled or become dislodged within the first few days, operative replacement is necessary, since bile peritonitis is almost certain to supervene.

After the fourth day a suitable tract may have formed. If a tract has formed, and the accident is discovered early enough, it may be possible for the radiologist to insert a sterile 12 F or 14 F catheter through the tract into the duct and re-establish controlled drainage. A soft spiral angiographic guide wire passed under fluoroscopic control may be necessary to aid in insertion of the catheter (see Chapter 10). The catheter should be fixed in the same manner as recommended for the original T-tube.

A brief rise in bilirubin (2 to 3 mg/dl) and alkaline phosphatase levels in the immediate postoperative period is no cause for concern. It should, however, be transient, and followed by a normal decay curve. The causes of postoperative jaundice have been described by Morgenstern.[47]

T-tube management varies from surgeon to surgeon and hospital to hospital. Most surgeons order a T-tube cholangiogram by the seventh postoperative day and remove the tube (in the absence of residual stones or obstruction) by the tenth day. T-tube cholangiography should be performed slowly and without undue pressure, since postcholangiogram cholangitis can be induced if the examination is performed incorrectly.

If bile output is in the normal range (250 to 300 ml), we begin plugging the T-tube for short periods (e.g., 30 to 60 minutes) on the fifth postoperative day, in the morning, afternoon, and evening. The tube is reopened at the slightest indication of discomfort by the patient. Plugging is gradually continued with small daily increments (e.g., 2 hours, three times a day). After the T-tube cholangiogram is performed and judged to be normal, the plugging intervals are lengthened, and the tube is removed on the tenth day. The skin fixation sutures are cut, and slow gentle traction is exerted until the tube is felt to slip out of the duct. It is then pulled out the tract. The T-tube stab wound usually drains a small amount of bile for a few hours, and drainage then ceases. Rarely, even after one to several weeks, an adequate tract has not formed, and removal of the T-tube is followed by severe pain, tenderness, and fever. This calls for prompt surgical replacement of the T-tube or radiologic placement of sump drains; otherwise, generalized bile peritonitis will result.

In uncomplicated cases, the Jackson-Pratt drain is removed by the fifth or sixth day. Should there be drainage of bile from the Penrose drain, it should be left in place until the cause is explained and treated. Drainage of bile via the Penrose drain suggests that an accessory duct (to gallbladder bed, cystic duct, or hepatic duct) is open and draining, that the choledochotomy has partially disrupted, or that the T-tube has been dislodged from the duct. Small severed accessory ducts will usually seal in time, although it may take several weeks. Small choledochotomy disruptions, manifested as confined extravasations seen on T-tube cholangiography, will also seal with adequate drainage. Dislodged T-tubes may have to be reinserted operatively, or, if only partially dislodged, an adequate tract may form and allow the tube to be removed without reoperation. If T-tube cholangiography does not reveal the source of bile extravasation, injection of contrast medium into the Jackson-Pratt drain occasionally will do so. The drain should not be removed while bile still drains through it. Drainage should be collected in a sterile drainage system (e.g., Hollister) and bile output measured. Copious biliary drainage from both T-tube and drain may lead to the insidious development of a metabolic acidosis, especially in elderly patients.

Bile extravasation may produce a subhepatic collection of bile or an abscess. Collections such as this may require drainage, but frequently they will drain spontaneously through one of the drain sites. Bacterial colonization of the drain tract is not necessarily a reason for giving systemic antibiotics.

In chronically obstructed ducts the bile is usually infected with enteric organisms (*E. coli, Klebsiella, Pseudomonas, Enterobacter, Proteus, Bacteroides, Clostridium*). We employ a broad-spectrum antibiotic, such as cefazolin (every 6 to 12 hours), begun preoperatively and continued for 48 hours postoperatively. When cultures of bile taken at operation return with sensitivity studies, specific antibiotics are used only if signs of sepsis are present. Otherwise, antibiotics are discontinued.

CHOLANGIOMANOMETRY (RADIOMANOMETRY)

Manometry has been used as a diagnostic tool in a number of medical centers since its introduction and development by Caroli[48] and Mallet-Guy[49] in France and Hess[50] in Switzerland. Its use has been more popular in Europe than in the United States, although here White,[51, 52] Schein,[53] and Salomon[54] have been advocates.

Equipment varies in complexity from the original Caroli manometer, which consists of a saline reservoir mounted on a calibrated manometric column, to the complex Brucke cholangiomanometer, which allows delivery of a precise amount of saline into the duct per unit of time. There are other variations in instrumentation, which are beyond the scope of this chapter and the experience of the author.

It is claimed that intraoperative pressure studies, especially when combined with cholangiography, reflect sphincter of Oddi function and help identify occult calculi in the distal common duct. I find claims for biliary tract manometry difficult to evaluate. Its proponents present many arguments, but they have not convinced most surgeons. White[55] claimed a 1 per cent incidence of recurrent common duct stones after manometric cholangiography. We have achieved the same incidence with operative cholangiography and choledochoscopy alone.

For a description of the technique of cholangiomanometry, the reader is referred to the publications cited in the foregoing references.

REOPERATIVE SURGERY ON THE COMMON BILE DUCT

Secondary choledochotomy for recurrent or residual stones poses additional problems. Unless absolutely mandatory, re-exploration before 3 to 4 weeks is inadvisable because of postoperative inflammation. Adhesions are vascular, planes are indistinct, diffuse oozing is inevitable, and the operation is invariably difficult.

Gaining exposure of the common bile duct at a secondary operation must take into account the distorted anatomic relationships and the danger of injury to vital structures. Omentum, colon, and duodenum usually have become adherent to the gallbladder bed, the undersurface of the liver, and the porta hepatis. The foramen of Winslow is often obliterated. Because of the small but real risk of an unplanned colotomy, the colon should be mechanically prepared preoperatively.

The incision must be ample. In thin elderly patients, especially if the primary operation had been performed many years ago, there may be few adhesions, and the dilated common duct may be immediately apparent. The incision required is usually an extension of the original one. A Kehr incision is usually excellent.

After the peritoneal cavity is entered, care must be taken to avoid injury to the colon, duodenum, and right lobe of the liver. It is usually best to first mobilize the hepatic flexure and upper ascending colon medially, gradually freeing the transverse colon from the right hepatic lobe and approaching the second portion of the duodenum retrocolically. Then, it is possible to dissect the first portion of the duodenum from its adhesions to the liver and the porta hepatis. Completion of this dissection will usually succeed in exposing the dilated common bile duct.

Dense fibrosis in the porta hepatis may require the common duct to be identified by needle aspiration (a 22 gauge needle on a 5 ml syringe). Two vascular structures are at risk during re-exposure. The main hepatic artery is juxtaposed to the duct on the left, and the adventitial coats are fused. The artery may be identified by palpation and avoided. The portal vein lies immediately below the common duct. When needle aspiration yields venous blood easily, the needle is usually in the portal vein and the common duct is more superficial. Dissection behind the duct should be avoided to preclude portal vein injury.

The operation necessarily involves mobilization of the second portion of the duodenum by the Kocher maneuver, which provides adequate exposure and facilitates exploration of the duct.

When the duct is well exposed, cholangiography is performed before choledochotomy. It is not advisable to dissect out the cystic duct, even if it were identifiable, for this purpose. Cholangiography is performed by inserting a needle directly into the common duct (a ¾ inch, 21 gauge butterfly [scalp vein] needle, which comes with a short infusion set). A venous extension tube is attached to this, which, in turn, is connected to the standard cholangiographic infusion set described previously. The needle is held in place by fixing it to the duct wall with a 4-0 silk suture.

Operative cholangiography is then performed as described earlier.

LIVER BIOPSY

Liver biopsy may be indicated in patients undergoing choledochotomy. Michel et al.[56]

have described the technique and findings in a report on liver biopsies during upper abdominal procedures. Triaditis, bile duct proliferation, early stages of fibrosis, and foci of hepatocellular necrosis are but a few of the conditions encountered. They may be of importance in explaining pre- or postoperative jaundice and enzyme abnormalities. In reexplorations, the degree of hepatic structural alteration can also be assessed. We believe liver biopsy is of particular importance in patients with pre-existing jaundice whose ductal exploration has yielded negative results.

REFERENCES

1. Courvoisier LG: Kasuistisch-statistische Beiträge zur Pathologie und Chirurgie der Gallenwege. Leipzig, FCW Vogel, 1890, pp 57–58.
2. Halsted WS: Miniature hammers and the suture of the bile ducts. Bull Johns Hopkins Hosp 1898;*9*:67.
3. Kehr H: Die Praxis der Gallenwege Chirurgie, Vols 1 and 2. Munchen, Lehman, 1913.
4. Mirizzi PL: Operative cholangiography. Surg Gynecol Obstet 1937;*65*:702.
5. McIver MA: An instrument for visualizing the interior of the common duct at operation (preliminary note). Surgery 1941;*9*:112.
6. Wildegans H: Die Operative Gallengangsendoskopie. Munchen Urban and Schwarzenberg, 1960.
7. Shore JM, Lippman HN: A flexible choledochoscope. Lancet 1965;*1*:1200.
8. Berci G, Shore JM: Advances in cholangioscopy. Endoscopy 1972;*4*:29.
9. Morgenstern L, Shore JM, Berci G: Potentials of a new miniature optical system (endoscope) as a diagnostic aid. Am Surg 1972;*38*:312.
10. Shore JM, Morgenstern L, Berci G: An improved rigid choledochoscope. Am J Surg 1971;*122*:567.
11. Yamakawa T, Mieno K, Noguchi T, et al: An improved choledochofiberscope and non-surgical removal of retained biliary calculi under direct visual control. GI Endosc 1976;*22*:160.
12. Bauer JJ, Salky BA, Gelernt IM, et al: Experience with the flexible fiberoptic choledochoscope. Ann Surg 1981;*194*:161.
13. Sigel B, Coelho JCU, Nyhus LM, et al: Comparison of cholangiography and ultrasonography in the operative screening of the common bile duct. World J Surg 1982;*6*:440.
14. Sigel B, Machi J, Beitler JC, et al: Comparative accuracy of operative ultrasonography and cholangiography in detecting common duct calculi. Surgery 1983;*94*:715.
15. Benson EA, Page RE: A practical reappraisal of the anatomy of the extrahepatic bile ducts and arteries. Br J Surg 1976;*63*:853.
16. Goor DA, Ebert PA: Anomalies of the biliary tree. Report of a repair of an accessory bile duct and review of the literature. Arch Surg 1972;*104*:302.
17. Bartlett MK, Waddell WR: Indications for common duct exploration: Evaluation in 1000 cases. N Engl J Med 1958;*258*:164.
18. Way LW, Admirand WH, Dunphy JE: Management of choledocholithiasis. Ann Surg 1972;*176*:347.
19. Rolfsmeyer ES, Bubrick MP, Kollitz PR, et al: The value of operative cholangiography. Surg Gynecol Obstet 1982;*154*:369.
20. Doyle PJ, Ward-McQuaid JN, McEwen Smith A: The value of routine peroperative cholangiography—a report of 4000 cholecystectomies. Br J Surg 1982;*69*:617.
21. Levine SB, Lerner HJ, Leifer ED, et al: Intraoperative cholangiography. A review of indications and analysis of age-sex groups. Ann Surg 1983;*198*:692.
22. Reynolds BM, Dargan EL: Acute obstructive cholangitis: A distinct clinical syndrome. Ann Surg 1959;*150*:299.
23. Dow RW, Lindenauer SM: Acute obstructive suppurative cholangitis. Ann Surg 1969;*169*:272.
24. Hinchey EJ, Couper CE: Acute obstructive suppurative cholangitis. Am J Surg 1969;*117*:62.
25. Hermann RE, Hoerr SO: The value of the routine use of operative cholangiography. Surg Gynecol Obstet 1965;*121*:1015.
26. Walker JH: Operative cholangiography: The obligation of the the radiologist to the surgeon and his patient. AJR 1975;*125*:490.
27. Berci G, Steckel R: Modern radiology in the operating room. Arch Surg 1973;*107*:577.
28. Berci G, Shore JM, Hamlin JA, et al: Operative fluoroscopy and cholangiography: The use of modern radiologic technics during surgery. Am J Surg 1978;*135*:32.
29. Borge J: Operative cholangiography: New cholangiogram catheter clamp and improved technique. Arch Surg 1977;*112*:340.
30. Henzel JH, DeWeese MS: Common duct exploration with and without balloon-tipped biliary catheters. Arch Surg 1971;*103*:199.
31. Shore JM, Berci G: A simple rapid technic for cystic duct cholangiography. Am J Surg 1972;*123*:741.
32. Farha GJ, Pearson RN: Transcystic duct operative cholangiography: Personal experience with 500 consecutive cases. Am J Surg 1976;*131*:228.
33. Heimbach DM, White TT: Immediate and long term effects of instrumental dilation of the sphincter of Oddi. Surg Gynecol Obstet 1979;*148*:79.
34. Tompkins RK, Johnson J, Storm FK, et al: Operative endoscopy in the management of biliary tract neoplasms. Am J Surg 1976;*132*:174.
35. Kappes SK, Adams MB, Wilson SD: Intraoperative biliary endoscopy. Mandatory for all common duct operations? Arch Surg 1982;*117*:603.
36. Rattner DW, Warshaw AL: Impact of choledochoscopy on the management of choledocholithiasis. Experience with 499 common duct explorations at the Massachusetts General Hospital. Ann Surg 1981;*194*:76.
37. Escat J, Glucksman DL, Maigne C, et al: Choledochoscopy in surgery for choledocholithiasis. Six year experience in 380 consecutive patients. Am J Surg 1984;*147*:670.
38. Chande S, Devitt JE: T-tubes, the surgical amulet after choledochotomy. Surg Gynecol Obstet 1973; *136*:100.
39. Stuart M, Hoerr SO: Late results of side to side choledochoduodenostomy and of transduodenal sphincterotomy for benign disorders. A twenty year comparative study. Am J Surg 1972;*123*:67.
40. Jones SA, Smith LL: A reappraisal of sphincteroplasty (not sphincterotomy). Surgery 1972;*71*:565.
41. Allen B, Shapiro H, Way LW: Management of recurrent and residual common duct stones. Am J Surg 1981;*142*:41.
42. Madden JL, Chun JY, Kandalaft S, et al: Choledo-

choduodenostomy: An unjustly maligned surgical procedure? Am J Surg 1970;*119*:45.
43. Bernhoft RA, Pellegrini CA, Motson RW, et al: Composition and morphologic and clinical features of common duct stones. Am J Surg 1984;*148*:77.
44. Mackie DB, Haynes S, May RE: Unabsorbable suture material: A rare cause of recurrent stones in the common bile duct. Br J Surg 1973;*60*:23.
45. Rees BI, Jacob G: Silk sutures in the common bile duct. Br Med J 1977;*2*:1265.
46. Ger R, Duboys E, Addei KA: The mechanism of T tube dislocation and its prevention. Surgery 1982;*91*:531.
47. Morgenstern L: Postoperative jaundice: An approach to a diagnostic dilemma. Am J Surg 1974;*128*:255.
48. Caroli J: Contribution to the study of the functioning of Oddi's sphincter. *In* Delmont J (ed): The Sphincter of Oddi. Basel, S Karger, 1977.
49. Mallet-Guy P: Value of preoperative manometric and roentgenographic examination in the diagnosis of pathologic changes and functional disturbances of the biliary tract. Surg Gynecol Obstet 1952; *94*:385.
50. Hess W, Lamm H: Surgery of the Biliary Passages and the Pancreas. New York, Van Nostrand, 1965.
51. White TT, Waisman H, Hopton D, et al: Radiomanometry, flow rates, and cholangiography in the evaluation of common bile duct disease. Am J Surg 1972;*123*:73.
52. Hopton D, White TT: An evaluation of manometric operative cholangiography in 100 patients with biliary disease. Surg Gynecol Obstet 1971;*133*:949.
53. Schein CJ, Beneventano TC: Biliary manometry: Its role in clinical surgery. Surgery 1970;*67*:255.
54. Salomon J, Roseman DL: Intraoperative measurement of common duct resistance. Arch Surg 1978;*113*:650.
55. White TT, Bordley J: One percent incidence of recurrent gallstones six to eight years after manometric cholangiography. Ann Surg 1978;*188*:562.
56. Michel SL, Lipsky R, Morgenstern L: "Routine" liver biopsy in upper abdominal surgery. Arch Surg 1977;*112*:959.

STANLEY O. HOERR, M.D.
ROBERT E. HERMANN, M.D.

23

Choledochoduodenostomy

When a biliary bypass is indicated, there are several procedures from which to choose. If the gallbladder is present and suitable, many surgeons use a cholecystoenterostomy for this purpose; under these circumstances we prefer a simple end-to-side cholecystojejunostomy. However, if the gallbladder is absent or if it is scarred and shrunken, the common bile duct must be used instead. A direct anastomosis between the common bile duct and the duodenum may on occasion be the easiest and best method for the surgeon to provide internal diversion of bile. The anastomosis may be an end-to-side or a side-to-side choledochoduodenostomy.

Surgeons in the United States have been reluctant to abandon the complicated and more difficult end-to-side choledochoduodenostomy or the even more complicated and time-consuming Roux-en-Y choledochojejunostomy in favor of the simpler side-to-side choledochoduodenostomy. The principal fear has been that following the side-to-side procedure, the common bile duct distal to the anastomosis will act as a blind pouch, favoring retention of products of digestion with resultant stasis, infection, and disabling cholangitis. This problem has been called the sump syndrome. While this concern is understandable, our experience has shown that cholangitis is rare following a side-to-side choledochoduodenostomy, even in the occasional patient in whom calculi or food debris accumulate in the duct distal to the anastomosis. When cholangitis does occur, it is almost always due to development of a stricture of the anastomosis.

We have participated in a number of studies of side-to-side choledochoduodenostomy, all of which support the belief that cholangitis is a comparatively rare late complication. In a series of 48 patients who had side-to-side choledochoduodenostomies performed between 1950 and 1970 for malignant obstruction, there were no instances of late cholangitis among the 43 patients who survived the operation.[1] All patients were followed until they died of their disease; in 11 patients this period exceeded 1 year. Similar findings were reported by Kaminski, et al. in 33 patients who had choledochoduodenostomies for malignant obstruction of the biliary tree.[2]

In another study, side-to-side choledochoduodenostomy was compared with transduodenal sphincterotomy in the treatment of various benign conditions, such as chronic choledocholithiasis.[3] Results were satisfactory in 33 (80 per cent) of 41 patients having side-to-side choledochoduodenostomies who were followed for 6 months to 20 years (median, 7 years); the unsatisfactory outcomes were not a result of cholangitis or sepsis. In another study of patients with strictures of the common bile duct, the best results were obtained in 49 cases of reconstruction by choledochoduodenostomy; 94 per cent of patients were classified as having excellent or good results.[4] Our most recent study compared choledochoduodenostomy, cholecystojejunostomy, and sphincteroplasty for biliary and pancreatic disease.[5] This confirmed the good, long-term results of choledochoduodenostomy performed for a variety of benign and malignant conditions. Seventy-six of 84 patients who survived operation were regarded as having good results. Two patients had poor results and required reoperation for strictures of the anastomosis.

A number of other studies from this country and abroad support the view that side-to-side choledochoduodenostomy has a low incidence of recurrent cholangitis if performed correctly and for sound indications. Nearly all authors stress that the procedure should be reserved for distal obstruction of the common bile duct, that the duct should be enlarged to a diameter of at least 2 cm, and that the anastomotic stoma should be at least

2.5 cm in diameter. Nevertheless, de Almeida and his colleagues[6] reported excellent late results even when the bile duct was 15 mm or less in diameter. We still prefer sphincteroplasty over choledochoduodenostomy for ducts this small, however.

Degenshein, in a study of 175 consecutive choledochoduodenostomies performed for a wide variety of malignant and benign disorders over an 18 year period, reported only two cases of late cholangitis.[7] Preoperatively, 112 of these patients were jaundiced, 21 were 80 years of age or older, and in 55 patients the procedure followed previous surgery on the biliary tract. Degensheim stated that a dilated common bile duct and a large anastomosis were essential for success, and he concluded that the fear of cholangitis following this procedure was not justified. Side-to-side choledochoduodenostomy was considered to be a safe and effective operation in a high-risk population.

Kraus and Wilson reported on a group of 68 patients who had choledochoduodenostomies for benign and malignant conditions from 1965 to 1975.[8] There were only two instances (3.6 per cent) of late cholangitis in the 56 patients who survived the operation and in whom follow-up data were available.

A study from England by Johnson and Rains strongly supported the use of choledochoduodenostomy for the treatment of recurrent common bile duct stones.[9] These investigators stated that the worldwide experience with follow-up periods of up to 20 years shows a late incidence of cholangitis of about 1 per cent "when the operation was performed correctly with an initial stoma size of at least 2.5 cm."

Two studies from Israel also report good results with choledochoduodenostomy. Berlatzky and Freund studied a group of 60 patients who had the operation for benign obstructive biliary tract disease.[10] The operations took place over a 15 year period ending in 1979, and the patients were followed for 1 to 15 years. All but one of the patients were free of abdominal complaints, recurrent cholangitis, or pancreatitis. One symptomatic patient developed the sump syndrome 6 years after operation; the symptoms were controlled by antibiotic therapy. Engelberg et al. reported on a group of 53 patients operated upon between 1965 and 1975 for benign disorders of the common bile duct.[11] Some of the operations were performed at the time of initial removal of stones from the common bile duct. Ninety-four per cent of the patients were free of pain, jaundice, or evidence of cholangitis 1 to 11 years after operation. Two patients (4 per cent) required reoperation for anastomotic strictures.

Several other authors have advocated choledochoduodenostomy as a supplementary procedure during removal of stones from the common bile duct. Schein et al. reported the results in 100 consecutive cases in which choledochoduodenostomy was performed at the time of choledocholithotomy when the common duct was at least 1.4 cm in diameter.[12] Among the 97 patients who survived the operation, there was not one readmission for cholangitis, nor was there any known instance of additional biliary surgery. Engin et al. support this view, stating that "lateral choledochoduodenostomy is the operation of choice after removal of common duct stones in the definitive treatment of choledocholithiasis."[13] Anderberg et al.[14] and Moesgaard et al.[15] reported the late results of side-to-side choledochoduodenostomy in 20 and 49 patients, respectively. The sump syndrome was not seen in any patient. Cholangitis in two patients was caused by anastomotic stricture in one and intermittent passage of intrahepatic stones in the other.

Papadimitriou et al.[16] used radionuclide scans of bile to study bile flow in 44 patients who had had side-to-side choledochoduodenostomies or sphincteroplasties 7 to 12 years previously. Bile flow was unimpeded in all cases, demonstrating that late function of the drainage procedures was uniformly excellent.

When cholangitis does occur as a late sequela of choledochoduodenostomy, endoscopic techniques are useful in diagnosis and treatment.[17, 18, 21] Osnes described the successful performance of "endoscopic choledochoduodenostomy" in six patients with obstruction of the terminal bile duct.[19] He specified that the distal bile duct protrude into the duodenum and suggested that in suitable circumstances, such as very poor risk patients, an endoscopic choledochoduodenostomy may be an appropriate alternative to a laparotomy. We advise caution in this approach.

PHYSICAL FACTORS AFFECTING CHOLEDOCHODUODENOSTOMY

Side-to-side choledochoduodenostomy should be performed only if the common bile duct is both dilated, which permits a generous stoma, and thick-walled, at a level low enough to be easily accessible to the duodenum. These factors render the anastomosis simple to perform and safe from the standpoint of possible leakage during healing. The procedure should not be performed if there is actual or threatened obstruction of the duodenum distal to the anastomosis, as may occur in carcinoma of the head of the pancreas.

An end-to-side choledochoduodenostomy[22] is preferable if the bile duct obstruction is high, if the duct is scarred (as in the usual iatrogenic stricture), or if the the caliber of the bile duct is small.

INDICATIONS

Malignant Obstructions of the Common Bile Duct

A surgically incurable malignant growth blocking the common duct and producing obstructive jaundice is a prime indication for a biliary bypass procedure. Although life will not be prolonged, its quality will be improved with the clearing of jaundice (a constant reminder to the patient of the disease), and itching will be relieved; the procedure is also bound to have a favorable effect on liver function. In patients without gallbladders, the common bile duct will invariably be found to be dilated and thick-walled and suitable for an anastomosis. Even when the gallbladder is present, however, if the growth threatens to block the cystic duct, it is preferable to remove the gallbladder and use the common bile duct.

If the neoplasm is potentially curable by a Whipple resection, and it is desired to perform a first-stage decompression to be followed later by a definitive resection, a side-to-side choledochoduodenostomy should be avoided, since it will complicate performance of the second stage. Instead, an anastomosis of jejunum to gallbladder or to the proximal end of the divided common bile duct will allow the second stage to be performed most readily.

Choledocholithiasis

If the operation is the first one for stones in the common bile duct, even if the gallbladder has been removed at a previous operation, most surgeons prefer to remove all calculi and avoid a drainage procedure if the sphincter of Oddi permits passage of a 12 or 14 catheter. If the sphincter of Oddi is stenosed, a transduodenal sphincteroplasty or a side-to-side choledochoduodenostomy should be considered. If the common bile duct is not dilated, we favor sphincteroplasty.

Recurrent Choledocholithiasis

If there is a proven *recurrence* of stones in the common bile duct (as opposed to *retention* of stones after presumed removal), even in the absence of jaundice or narrowing at the sphincter of Oddi, a biliary bypass procedure should probably be performed. One must presume that there is stasis of bile in the common bile duct as a result of functional, if not mechanical, obstruction.

Hepatic Duct or Common Duct Stones Retained at Operation

Occasionally, the surgeon is unable to remove all intrahepatic stones. On other occasions, there will be so many stones that the surgeon cannot be certain they have all been removed even after meticulous efforts have resulted in what appears to be a stone-free system. Under these circumstances, a side-to-side choledochoduodenostomy should be strongly considered if the duct is suitable.

Chronic Pancreatitis and Stenosis of the Sphincter of Oddi

Chronic pancreatitis may produce chronic obstruction of the common bile duct with jaundice, or it may be associated with a stenotic sphincter of Oddi, which produces intermittent symptoms resembling those of biliary colic, even in the absence of stones. If instruments will not pass into the duodenum and the common bile duct is dilated and thick-walled, a side-to-side choledochoduodenostomy is easier and often safer than transduodenal sphincteroplasty.

Side-to-side choledochoduodenostomy should not be regarded as a procedure competitive with transduodenal sphincteroplasty in operations for chronic pancreatitis or for stenosis of the distal common bile duct. Each procedure has its appropriate use, and surgeons who operate for these diseases should be adept at both. In general, transduodenal sphincteroplasty is preferred for dealing with a calculus impacted at the papilla of Vater, for patients who have obstruction of the pancreatic duct and who should have operative pancreatograms, and for patients who have narrowing or stenosis of the sphincter of Oddi but who have a thin-walled, normal-caliber common bile duct down to that point. Since the papilla of Vater may be difficult to find through a duodenotomy unless a catheter, bougie, or other instrument has been passed through it, a side-to-side choledochoduodenostomy may be easier to perform, provided that the common bile duct is dilated and thick-walled, and there is no reason to suspect the presence of a neoplasm that could result in early restenosis. To help exclude this possibility, a finger should be inserted through the dilated common bile duct or the duodenostomy to feel the papilla before making the anastomosis.

Neither a sphincteroplasty nor a biliary bypass will relieve symptoms of pancreatitis caused by obstruction of the pancreatic duct, which may require a separate pancreaticoenterostomy.

Extrahepatic Strictures of the Bile Duct

Management of stenosis of the sphincter of Oddi has already been discussed, and spontaneous benign strictures at other levels are rare. Iatrogenic strictures are almost always located proximal to the junction of the common bile duct and the cystic duct. A side-to-side choledochoduodenostomy is not usually feasible for iatrogenic strictures, but an end-to-side anastomosis, after resection of the stricture, is an excellent method of reconstruction if it can be performed without tension.

Summary

Allen and coworkers[20] reviewed the indications for drainage procedures in an article that is representative of the sentiment expressed by many of those who have had the greatest experience with choledochoduodenostomy. These authors recommended a drainage procedure in the following circumstances: (1) one or more previous choledochotomies for common duct stones; (2) large (>2 cm) duct; (3) multiple stones (e.g., ≥15) in the duct (because this so often reflects primary stone formation in the duct); (4) intrahepatic stones; (5) known or suspected residual stones in the duct; or (6) benign obstruction of the duct distal to the point where it passes behind the duodenum.

Choledochoduodenostomy was preferred over sphincteroplasty whenever the duct was suitable. The excellent late results of prophylactic drainage procedures support a policy of using them liberally when the foregoing indications exist.

TECHNIQUE

It has been emphasized that choledochoduodenostomy should be undertaken only if the common bile duct is dilated and thick-walled. It may be performed successfully in the infrequent situation in which the duct is not greatly enlarged (although an end-to-side anastomosis may be preferable), but it should not be attempted with a normal, thin-walled duct, irrespective of size. Experts on this subject also stress the importance of creating a wide anastomosis, since failure of the procedure can usually be attributed to stenosis of the anastomosis. The stoma should be at least 2 cm in diameter.

The surgeon should consider the possibility of performing a choledochoduodenostomy before making the choledochotomy used for exploring the duct. Exploration is usually performed through a longitudinal incision just distal to the junction of the cystic duct and the common bile duct. The best incision for a side-to-side choledochoduodenostomy, which may be transverse or longitudinal, is located more distally, adjacent to the duodenum.

Figure 23–1 shows a longitudinal opening in the common bile duct that will be pulled transversely and then approximated to the adjacent longitudinal opening in the duodenum, employing the Heineke-Mikulicz principle. It has been suggested that this technique helps to hold the anastomosis patent. Stay sutures are placed at the ends of the proposed anastomosis. Figure 23–2 shows the transverse incision in the duodenum and placement of the stay sutures. We use interrupted sutures of 3-0 silk, chromic catgut, or synthetic material for the entire anastomosis and do not believe that the kind of suture material is critical. Nonabsorbable suture material, such as fine silk, should not be used on the interior of the common bile duct when

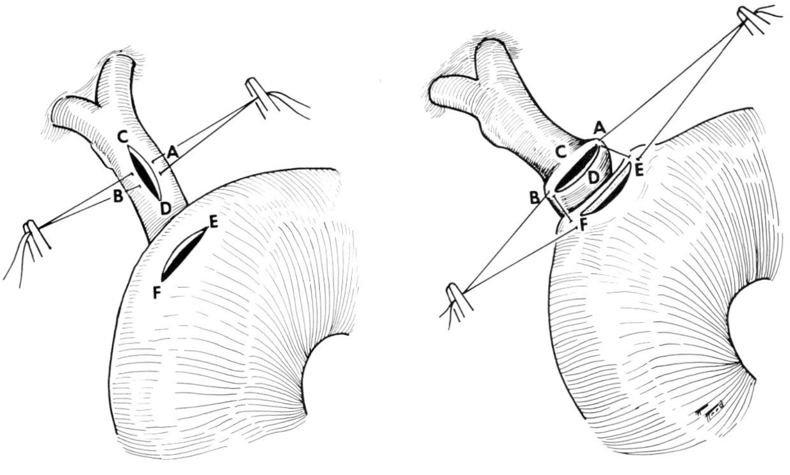

Figure 23–1. A longitudinal incision has been placed in the common bile duct close to the longitudinal incision in the duodenum. Two end sutures have approximated the incisions. (From Stuart M, Keo T, Hermann RE, Hoerr SO: Am J Surg *121*:555, 1971. Used by permission.)

it empties normally through the sphincter of Oddi, since silk can serve as the nidus for gallstone formation. This is a relatively unimportant consideration in a choledochoduodenostomy, in which any calculi formed at the anastomosis would pass readily into the duodenum.

The anastomosis may be constructed as a single layer of through-and-through interrupted sutures, particularly if the duct wall is thick and firm, or it may be constructed with a posterior inner layer of interrupted sutures through all layers, which is continued anteriorly and completed as a two-layer anastomosis. We usually prefer to place an outer layer posteriorly to anchor the anastomosis but omit the anterior outer layer or just place a few anterior outer sutures for additional support (Fig. 23–3). In some cases, excessive infolding of the anastomosis by two complete layers could predispose to late stenosis.

If the anastomosis is at least 2 cm in diameter and secure, we do not use a stent. If a T-tube is used as a stent, the long arm should not be brought through the anastomosis but through a proximal choledochotomy (Fig. 23–4) or a duodenotomy (Fig. 23–5), whichever is more convenient. If the stem of the T-tube is brought out through the duodenum, the duodenal exit should be secured by a pursestring suture to prevent leakage. The T-tube should be left in place for 10 days if brought out through the common bile duct, but it should be clamped and not removed for 3 to 4 weeks when it exits from the duodenum. A closed system, sump suction drain should be placed near the anastomosis at the conclusion of the operation.

Because they are often smaller, end-to-side choledochoduodenostomies should usually be stented with a short rubber catheter (Fig. 23–6). The catheter may be secured at the anastomosis by a single tight suture, which will hold the tube in place temporarily, allowing it to pass when the suture dissolves. The patient should be alerted to the fact that he may note the catheter in the stool at some time in the future.

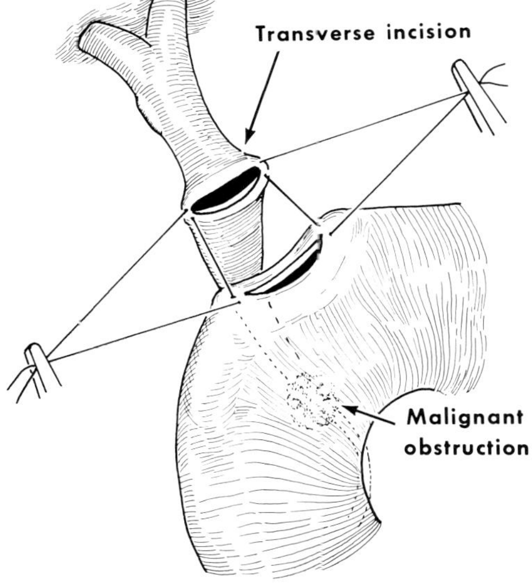

Figure 23–2. In this case, a transverse incision has been placed in the common bile duct instead of a longitudinal one. Two end stay sutures approximate the incisions. (From Stuart M, Keo T, Hermann RE, Hoerr SO: Am J Surg *121*:555, 1971. Used by permission.)

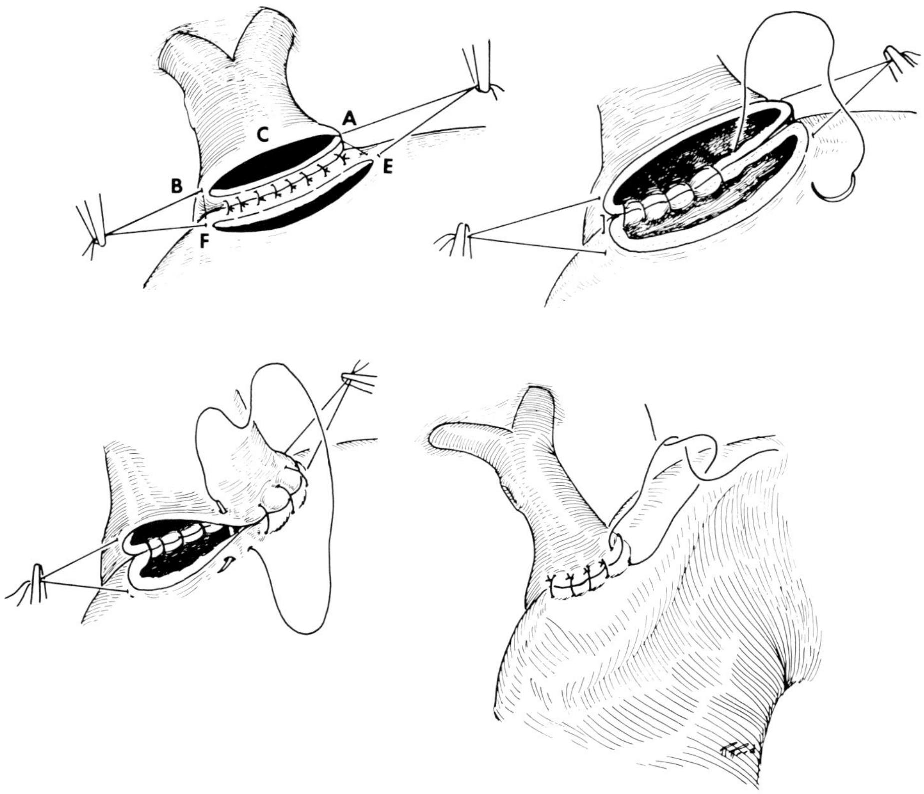

Figure 23–3. A posterior outer row of interrupted 3-0 sutures of silk, synthetic material, or chromic catgut has been placed through the seromuscular layers (upper left). A posterior continuous suture is being placed through all layers (upper right). An anterior continuous suture through all layers is half complete (lower left). An anterior outer row of interrupted 3-0 seromuscular sutures completes the anastomosis (lower right). *Note*: The anterior outer row of sutures is commonly omitted, and the entire anastomosis may be constructed of a single layer of through-and-through interrupted sutures. Although the illustration shows a continuous suture for the inner layer, we prefer interrupted sutures throughout (see text). (From Stuart M, Keo T, Hermann RE, Hoerr SO: Am J Surg *121*:555, 1971. Used by permission.)

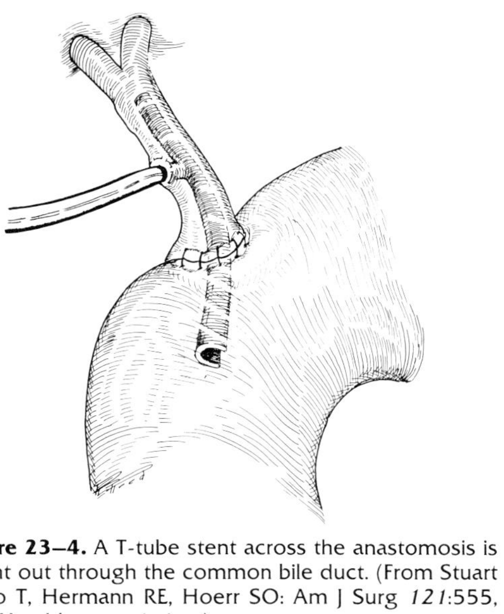

Figure 23–4. A T-tube stent across the anastomosis is brought out through the common bile duct. (From Stuart M, Keo T, Hermann RE, Hoerr SO: Am J Surg *121*:555, 1971. Used by permission.)

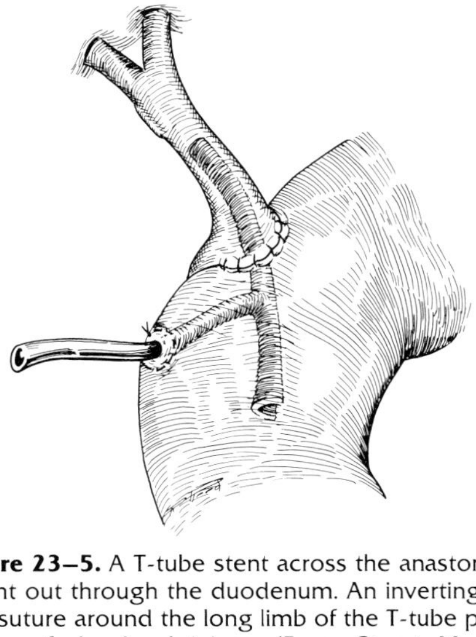

Figure 23–5. A T-tube stent across the anastomosis is brought out through the duodenum. An inverting purse-string suture around the long limb of the T-tube prevents leakage of duodenal juices. (From Stuart M, Keo T, Hermann RE, Hoerr SO: Am J Surg *121*:555, 1971. Used by permission.)

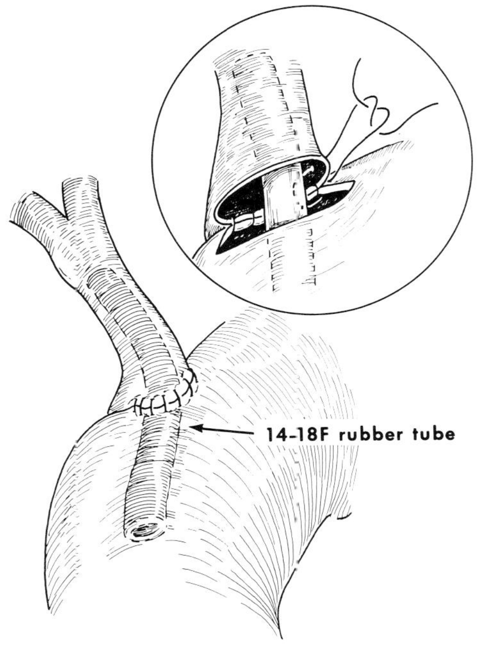

Figure 23–6. A shorter rubber tube is secured at the anastomosis by a tightly tied suture. It is designed to pass spontaneously. This technique is useful chiefly in end-to-side anastomoses. (From Stuart M, Keo T, Hermann RE, Hoerr SO: Am J Surg *121*:555, 1971. Used by permission.)

SUMMARY

Choledochoduodenostomy is a simple, safe, reliable method for creating an internal bypass of bile. A side-to-side anastomosis should be attempted only if the common bile duct is dilated and thick-walled, and the size of the anastomosis should be 2 cm or more. An end-to-side choledochoduodenostomy is useful for anastomoses close to the liver or when the duct is thick-walled but of normal caliber. Contrary to earlier beliefs, ascending cholangitis is an infrequent sequela and, when it does occur, usually signifies a strictured anastomosis, not the sump syndrome.

REFERENCES

1. Stuart M, Keo T, Hermann RE, et al: Palliation of malignant obstruction of the common bile duct by side-to-side choledochoduodenostomy. Am J Surg 1971;*121*:505.
2. Kaminski DL, Barner HB, Codd JE, et al: Evaluation of choledochoduodenostomy in the treatment of malignant obstruction of the biliary tree. Am J Surg 1976;*132*:565.
3. Stuart M, Hoerr SO: Late results of side-to-side choledochoduodenostomy and of transduodenal sphincterotomy for benign disorders. Am J Surg 1972;*123*:67.
4. Hertzer NR, Gray HW, Hoerr SO, et al: The use of T-tube splints in bile duct repairs. Surg Gynecol Obstet 1973;*137*:413.
5. Vogt DP, Hermann RE: Choledochoduodenostomy, choledochojejunostomy or sphincteroplasty for biliary and pancreatic disease. Ann Surg 1981; *193*:161.
6. de Almeida AM, Cruz AG, Aldeia FJ: Side-to-side choledochoduodenostomy in the management of choledocholithiasis and associated disease. Facts and fiction. Am J Surg 1984;*147*:253.
7. Degenshein GA: Choledochoduodenostomy: An 18 year study of 175 consecutive cases. Surgery 1974;*76*:319.
8. Kraus MA, Wilson SD: Choledochoduodenostomy. Importance of common duct size and occurrence of cholangitis. Arch Surg 1978;*115*:1212.
9. Johnson AG, Rains AJH: Prevention and treatment of recurrent bile duct stones by choledochoduodenostomy. World J Surg 1978;*2*:487.
10. Berlatzky Y, Freund H: Choledochoduodenostomy in the treatment of benign biliary tract disease. Am J Surg 1981;*141*:90.
11. Engelberg M, Avrahami I, Erdman S, et al: Choledochoduodenostomy—a useful procedure in the management of benign disorders of the biliary tract: a review of 53 cases. Am Surg 1980;*46*:344.
12. Schein CJ, Shapiro N, Gliedman ML: Choledochoduodenostomy as an adjunct to choledocholithotomy. Surg Gynecol Obstet 1978;*146*:25.
13. Engin A, Haberal M, Sanac Y: Side-to-side choledochoduodenostomy in the management of choledocholithiasis. Br J Surg 1978;*65*:99.
14. Anderberg B, Bolin S, Heuman R, et al: Choledochoduodenostomy for choledocholithiasis. Acta Chir Scand 1984;*150*:75.
15. Moesgaard F, Nielsen ML, Pedersen T, et al: Protective choledochoduodenostomy in multiple common duct stones in the aged. Surg Gynecol Obstet 1982;*154*:232.
16. Papadimitriou J, Fotopoulos A, Tsiftsis D, et al: Dynamic evaluation of long term patency of choledochoduodenostomy compared with sphincteroplasty. Surg Gynecol Obstet 1982;*155*:17.
17. Akiyama H, Ikezawa H, Kameya S, et al: Unexpected problems of external choledochoduodenostomy. Fiberscopic examination in 15 patients. Am J Surg 1980;*140*:680.
18. Barkin JS, Silvis S, Greenwald R: Endoscopic therapy of the "sump" syndrome. Dig Dis Sci 1980;*25*:597.
19. Osnes M: Endoscopic choledochoduodenostomy for common bile duct obstructions. Lancet 1979; *1*:1059.
20. Allen B, Shapiro H, Way LW: Management of recurrent and residual common duct stones. Am J Surg 1981;*142*:41.
21. Blair AJ III, Leung JWC, Cotton PB: Endoscopic treatment of stomal stenosis after choledochoduodenostomy: Preliminary report. Surgery 1985; *97*:487.
22. Cushieri A, Wood RAB, Metcalf MJ, Cumming JGR: Long-term experience with transection choledochoduodenostomy. World J Surg 1983;*7*:502.

S. AUSTIN JONES, M.D.

24

The Use of Transduodenal Sphincteroplasty in Biliary Tract Disease*

A sphincteroplasty is a transduodenal method of producing a choledochoduodenostomy between the distal end of the common duct and the side of the duodenum, with an opening as large as that of the supraduodenal common duct. The sphincters affecting the distal common and pancreatic ducts are rendered functionless. The stoma is noncontractile and permanently open. To achieve this result, the walls of the common duct and duodenum are serially divided between clamps and oversewn until the required ductal caliber is attained.

The resulting stoma differs both anatomically and physiologically from the one produced by a sphincterotomy, which leaves a large portion of the sphincter mechanism intact (Fig. 24–1). The inadequate stoma produced by sphincterotomy may allow trapping and retention of overlooked calculi. It may also cause intermittent bile stasis with eventual recurrent stone formation or cholangitis.

SPHINCTEROPLASTY VERSUS SPHINCTEROTOMY

Anatomic Considerations

The common and pancreatic ducts are in parallel as they pass obliquely through the duodenal wall. In the intramural course of the common duct its caliber markedly tapers, producing the terminal narrowing seen in a normal cholangiogram. Cadaver dissections demonstrate that the pancreatic duct is universally on the medial aspect of the common duct and usually enters the latter several millimeters above the papilla of Vater.[1]

Two important sphincters surround the ducts as they pass through the bowel wall. The first is made up of duodenal wall muscle. The second is a thin sheath of muscle encasing both ducts, which was originally described by Boyden. It develops 5 weeks later in fetal life than does the duodenal wall musculature.[2] In the diagram of normal anatomy (Fig. 24–2) the sphincter of Boyden is divided into three portions. The superior sphincter is produced by a blending of duodenal muscle and sheath fibers at the point where the duct enters the bowel. At the distal end the sheath combines with papillary fibers to form the inferior sphincter. Between these two the sheath is known as the middle or submucosal sphincter. The duodenal muscle and Boyden's sphincter can contract together or independently. An ampulla is often not found on dissection. It is clear that if one wishes to inactivate the constricting mechanism the incision must divide the superior as well as the other sphincters, and the apex of the incision will extend beyond the duodenal wall. Therefore, careful suture approximation, especially at the apex, is mandatory.

In Figure 24–3 one can see that the length of the intramural course of the duct varies in individuals.[1] This is of great importance surgically and is why the length of the sphincteroplasty incision does not determine its adequacy. We are frequently asked how long the incision should be. The answer is that it depends on the length of the sphincter; one must continue the incision upward until the

*Gratitude is expressed to previous coauthors George Gregory, M.D., Louis L. Smith, M.D., and Thomas B. Keller, M.D., for permission to use their cases in compiling this series.

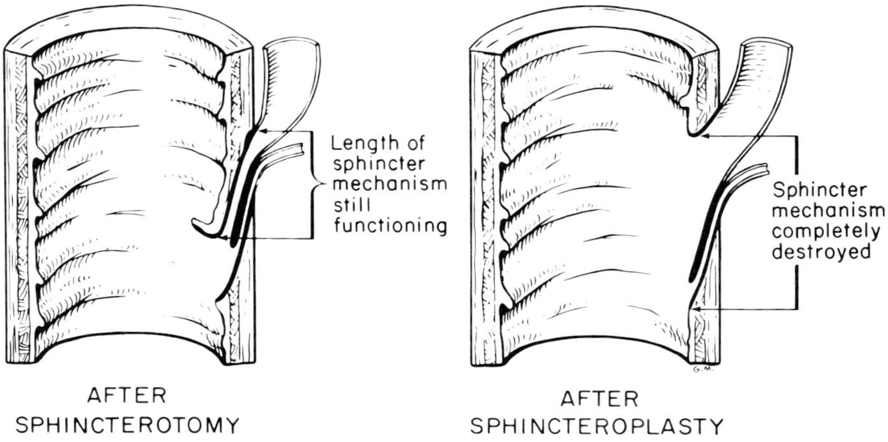

Figure 24–1. Sphincterotomy leaves a substantial amount of functioning sphincter behind. This is eliminated by sphincteroplasty.

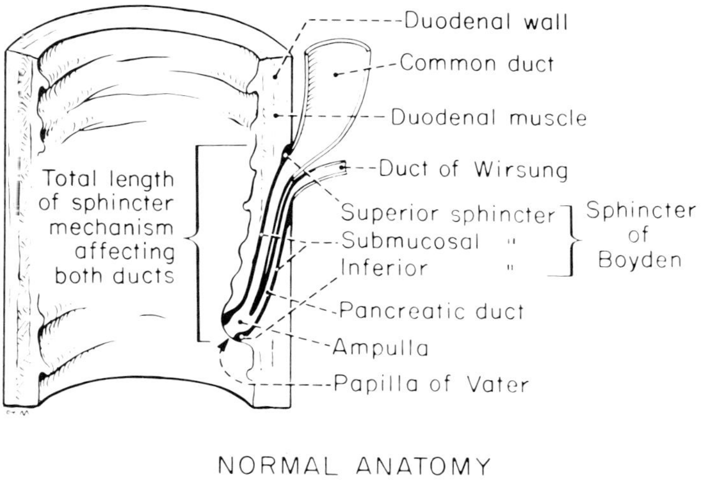

Figure 24–2. The common and pancreatic ducts can be compressed by duodenal muscle and Boyden's sphincter, working together or independently.

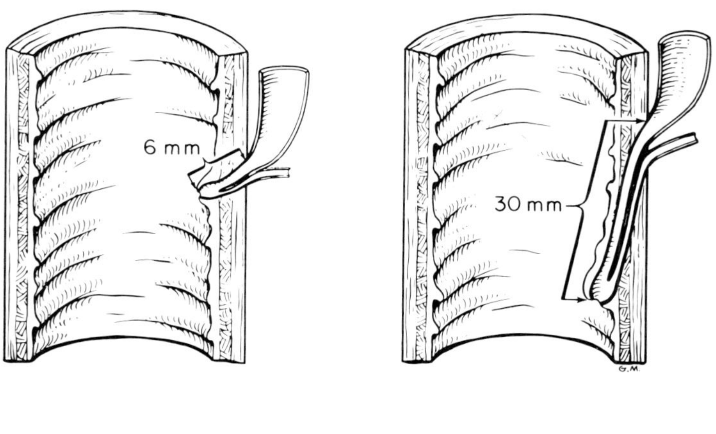

Figure 24–3. The length of the incision required to destroy the sphincters varies among individuals.

size of the opening equals that of the supraduodenal common duct. When this is accomplished, one can be confident that the entire sphincteric mechanism in that particular patient has been divided.[3]

Finally, it should be stressed that the pancreatic duct is always medial to the common duct. Therefore, the first pair of clamps is placed in the papilla in the 10 o'clock position. After the wall of the common duct and the duodenum is divided, the orifice of the pancreatic duct may be seen and avoided as subsequent pairs of clamps are placed directly anteriorly.

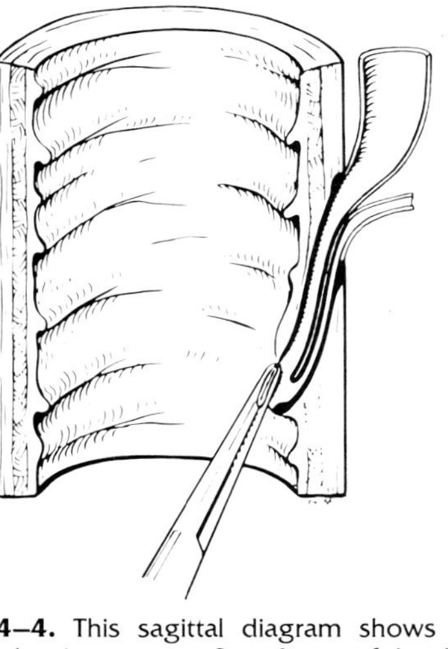

Figure 24–4. This sagittal diagram shows the first clamp placed to incorporate 3 to 4 mm of duodenal and common duct wall.

THE TECHNIQUE OF SPHINCTEROPLASTY

Sphincteroplasty can be performed by anyone familiar with biliary tract surgery, but we urge that the following steps be followed. They are the result of years of modification and have been used by others who have also obtained satisfactory results.[4, 5]

For purposes of orientation, a sagittal diagram of the intramural course of the common bile duct and the pancreatic duct is shown (Fig 24–4). The mosquito clamp, one of the first pair, is placed to include 3 to 4 mm of the wall of the duodenum and common duct. A second clamp is placed next to this one, the tissue between them is divided, and the clamps are oversewn with fine silk or Dexon.

Figure 24–5 shows the progressive steps of serial clamping, dividing, and suture approximation of the duodenal and common duct walls until the diameter of the opening is equal to that of the largest part of the supraduodenal common duct. At the upper end of the completed sphincteroplasty (at *D*) the operator has divided the superior sphincter, and therefore the incision has passed outside the duodenum at this point. The figure-of-8 apical stitch shown is needed to avoid a leak.

Having outlined the general conduct of a sphincteroplasty, we are now in a position to discuss the procedure step by step.

Antibiotics

Since most patients upon whom sphincteroplasty is performed have intermittent common duct obstruction, antibiotics should be started 2 hours preoperatively and continued for the first 24 hours postoperatively. Our regimen usually consists of an aminoglycoside and penicillin, but a cephalosporin is also adequate. At surgery a specimen of bile should be taken for culture and sensitivity studies.

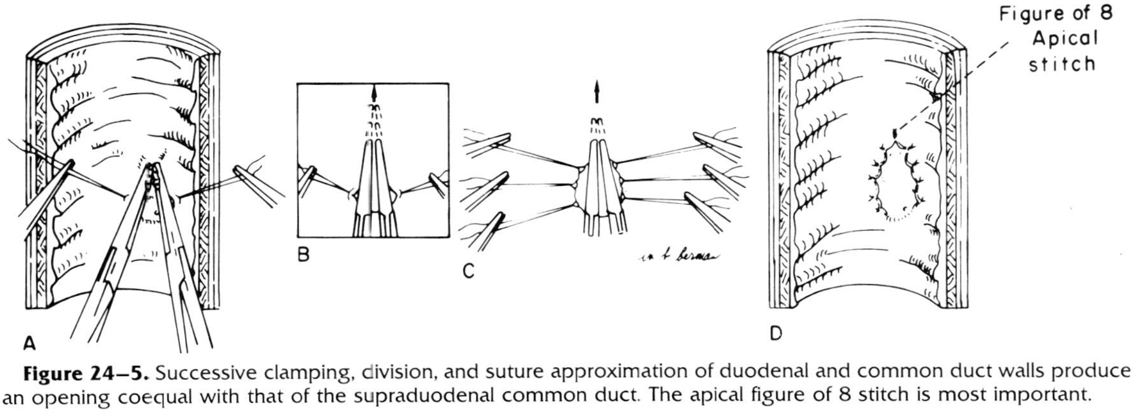

Figure 24–5. Successive clamping, division, and suture approximation of duodenal and common duct walls produce an opening coequal with that of the supraduodenal common duct. The apical figure of 8 stitch is most important.

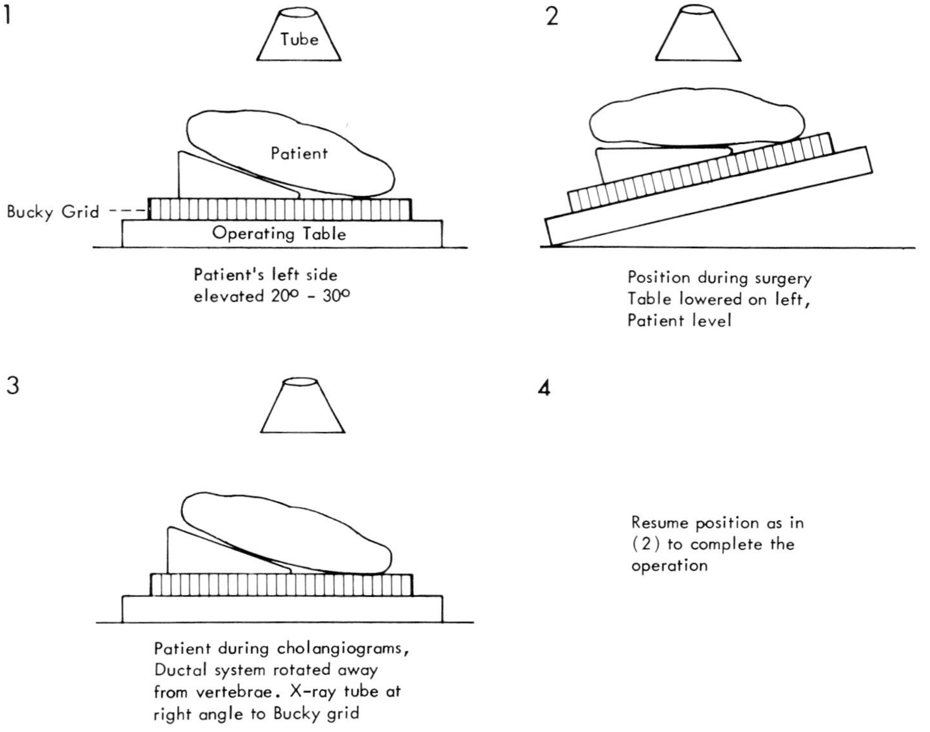

Figure 24–6. The patient is positioned so that rotation of the table avoids superimposition of ducts and vertebrae, and rays are at a right angle to the Bucky grid.

Position on the Operating Table

The patient's left side is elevated 25 to 30 degrees with a radiolucent plastic wedge as diagrammed in Figure 24–6(*1*). The table is rotated to the left, placing the patient in a supine position for the operation [Fig. 24–6(*2*)]. During cholangiography the table is returned to the position shown in Figure 24–6(*1*) in order to prevent superimposition of the ductal system and the vertebrae, and to place the Bucky grid at right angles, ensuring a sharp film.

Incision

A right subcostal incision is made at least three fingerbreadths below the costal margin, leaving a retractable upper flap. If the incision is placed more cephalad, the upper retractor blade will press upon an unyielding rib cage. If necessary, very wide exposure may be obtained by an upper midline extension of the subcostal incision.

Biliary Tract Dissection

All structures are inspected and the normal configuration established before any structure is tied, clamped, or divided.

Operative Cholangiography

After lowering of the left side of the table and removal of all radiopaque objects from the field, three injections of dilute Hypaque are made through a Cholangiocath catheter in the cystic duct (Fig. 24–7). The larger the ductal system, the greater the dilution should be. We use a 25 per cent solution for a 1 cm duct, a 15 per cent solution for a 2 cm duct, and so forth. The first injection is 2 ml; the second, 5 ml; and the third a larger amount depending on the size of the duct.

The surgeon should check all films with a radiologist. After the restraining suture is cut, the catheter is withdrawn and the cystic duct doubly ligated, the nearer tie being 5 mm from the common duct (Fig. 24–7).

A television monitor is of great value in observing and recording opening sphincter pressures, permitting a constant view of the entering dye, and making x-ray films possible when a questionable defect is observed.

Cholecystectomy

If at this point the operator has decided to do a sphincteroplasty, the gallbladder is removed. Regardless of the extent of disease in the gallbladder, it should be removed whenever a sphincteroplasty is performed.

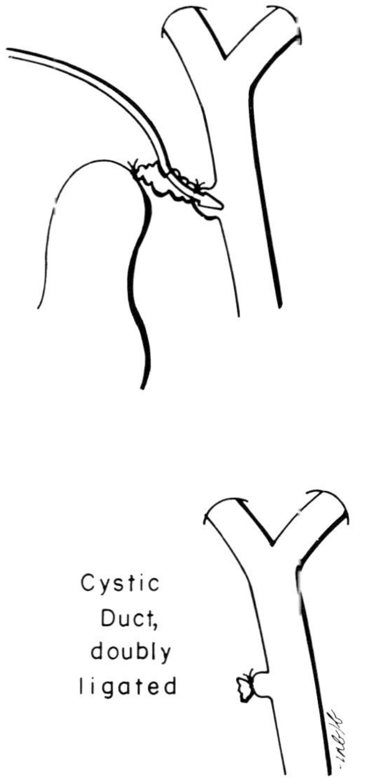

Figure 24–7. The Cholangiocath is held in the cystic duct by a temporary tie. The cystic duct is doubly ligated, the nearer tie 5 mm from the common duct.

The gallbladder cannot fill and function normally in the absence of the distal sphincters, and if it is left behind, stasis and infection may develop.

Mobilization of the Duodenum

This is accomplished by dividing the peritoneal reflection that covers the lateral portion of the second part of the duodenum and holds it in place. This important maneuver was first reported in 1895 by Maurice Jourdan as a method of better exposing the biliary tract. It was not until 8 years later that Kocher reported the same procedure, which has borne his name ever since, being universally known as the Kocher maneuver. It is interesting to note that Kocher's objective was to facilitate a Jaboulay gastroduodenostomy and that he did not use this maneuver in biliary tract surgery.[6]

It is important to divide the peritoneal reflection that forms the inferior border of the foramen of Winslow, as this adds greatly to the duodenal mobilization.

Common Duct Exploration

After the common duct is opened longitudinally between stay sutures, the ductal system is irrigated with saline and examined with delicate thumb and forefinger pressure, which not infrequently expresses stones. Scoops, forceps, Fogarty catheters, and a choledochoscope are then used. All manipulations must be done gently. When the ducts appear to be clear, a 10 F (3 mm) red rubber catheter is passed downward, guided with fingers behind the duct, and the point of catheter entry into the bowel selected as the site for the duodenotomy. If the rubber catheter does not pass into the duodenum, a biliary Fogarty catheter—slightly more rigid than the 10F catheter—may be used. We avoid using a metal probe unless the catheter technique is unsuccessful, fearing creation of a false passage. The papilla is never serially dilated, as hemorrhage or scarring with stenosis may follow this maneuver.

Duodenotomy

The duodenum is opened longitudinally, because one can never be absolutely certain of the location of the papilla. It always appears to be more distal in the second portion of the duodenum than one would expect. A longitudinal incision may be easily lengthened, and retraction on the delicate intestinal wall is minimized.

It must be emphasized that although the lateral duodenal wall can be freed, the medial border is in such intimate vascular relationship with the pancreas that it cannot be mobilized. Therefore, the Heineke-Mikulicz technique of longitudinal opening and transverse closure to maintain or enlarge the bowel lumen should not be applied here. Regardless of the axis of the duodenotomy, it must always be closed in the direction in which it is made.

If the duodenum is difficult to expose because of previous surgery or disease, it may be approached through the root of the transverse mesocolon[6] or by an extraperitoneal method.[7, 36]

Locating the Papilla of Vater

If the catheter can be passed from above, the papilla is clearly seen (Fig. 24–8). If the catheter cannot be advanced, a small Bakes dilator should be passed gently. If this fails, the duodenum should be opened and a search made for the papilla under direct vision and palpation. The latter is often rewarding, because the papilla resembles a small rubbery nodule on the posteromedial wall of the bowel. A small glass circle de-

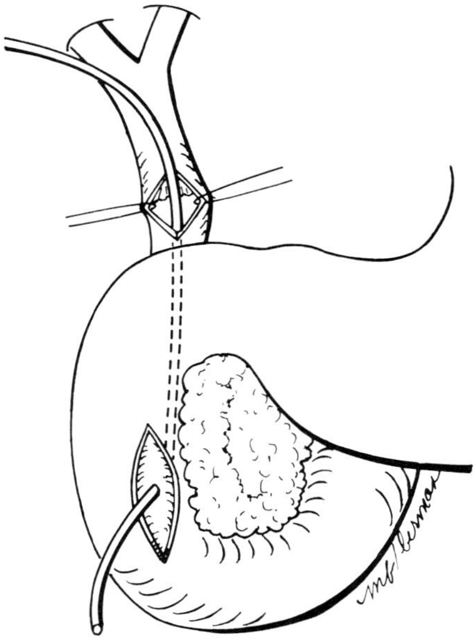

Figure 24–8. A 10 F (3 mm) red rubber catheter is passed downward through a choledochotomy into the duodenum. A duodenotomy will demonstrate the papilla.

signed to flatten the mucosal folds may show the small slitlike opening.[8] Careful observation with repeated suction and dabbing with a peanut sponge may help demonstrate bile and pancreatic juice issuing from the opening. Secretin may be used to stimulate pancreatic secretion.

Opening the Papilla

The First Pair of Clamps Applied. The papilla located, a pair of mosquito forceps is placed side by side at the 10 o'clock position to avoid injury to the pancreatic duct (Fig. 24–9). To aid in positioning the clamps, a stitch may be temporarily placed at the 10 o'clock position and put on tension (Fig. 24–10). If a biopsy is desired, the handles of the forceps are separated before they are applied, and the small wedge of tissue between the tips of the clamps is removed. The clamps are oversewn with sutures of 5-0 arterial silk, which are tied as each clamp is removed and used for traction.

Opening the papilla from below presents definite hazards. The operator may easily mistake the pancreatic duct for the common duct. After the papilla is incised, very gentle probing must be done to make certain that one is indeed in the common duct before proceeding.

Placement of Subsequent Pairs of Clamps. After the pancreatic duct has been identified, subsequent pairs of clamps are placed directly anteriorly (Fig. 24–11). The second pair of forceps (shown in b) are anterior, and the pancreatic duct may be seen at the 5 o'clock position.

Each successive pair of mosquito forceps is placed parallel to the last, but no more than 3 to 4 mm of common duct and duodenal wall are included at a time. This process of clamping, dividing, and oversewing is continued until the stoma equals the largest portion of the common bile duct (see Fig. 24–5[*c*]). When the full diameter of the duct is reached, the incision has passed through the duodenal wall, and the figure-of-8 apical stitch is placed to avoid a leak. Since we consider this operation to be a single-layer, side-to-side anastomosis, we feel more secure in using a nonabsorbable suture, and so far have seen no contraindication to its use.

The Importance of a Pancreatic Ductogram

A word is appropriate concerning those patients with acute recurrent pancreatitis. Sphincteroplasty is indicated only for recurrent attacks of pancreatitis when the pan-

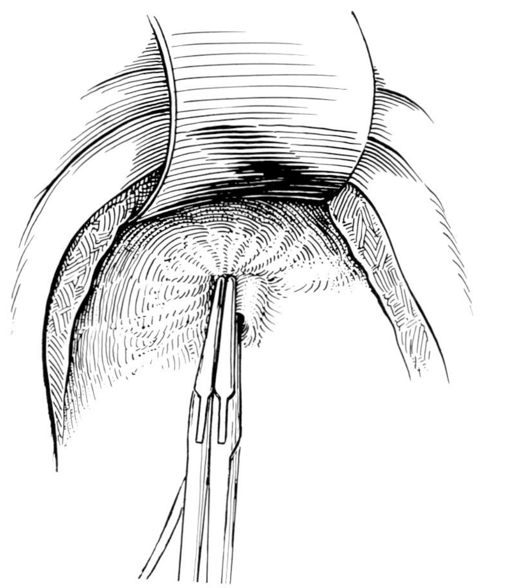

Figure 24–9. The first pair of clamps is placed at the 10 o'clock position to avoid damage to the pancreatic duct.

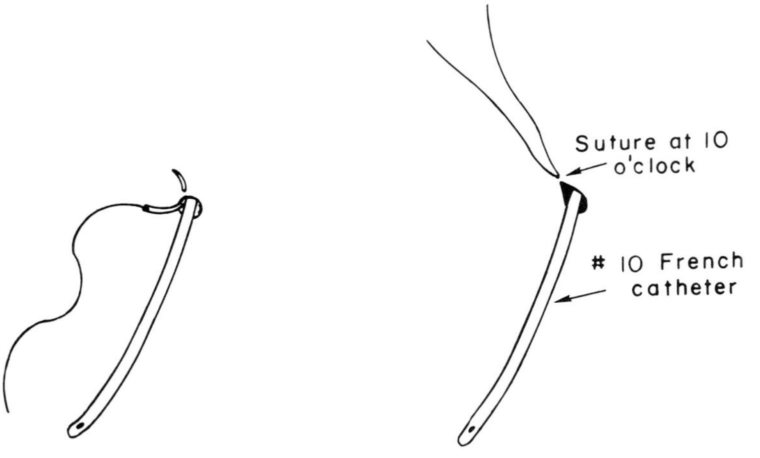

Figure 24–10. Traction on a temporary stitch at the 10 o'clock position is helpful in placing the first pair of clamps.

creatic ductogram shows no intrapancreatic ductal obstruction and when no gross pancreatic parenchymal disease is present. Thus, a pancreatogram is necessary to select the proper surgical procedure.[1] Most often this consists of preoperative endoscopic retrograde pancreatography (ERCP). If ERCP is unsuccessful, however, the surgeon can pass a small polyethylene tube upward through the papilla, and in most cases it will find its way into the pancreatic duct. If it does not, one must do a partial sphincteroplasty to locate the pancreatic duct. The sphincteroplasty should be completed, or the remaining sphincteric mechanism may contribute to postoperative pancreatitis. In performing an operative pancreatogram, only 1 to 3 ml of contrast medium is instilled under minimal pressure.

Division of the Septum Separating the Terminal Pancreatic and Common Duct Walls

When operating for acute recurrent pancreatitis without gross parenchymal disease or intrapancreatic ductal obstruction, one should divide the septum separating the terminal common and pancreatic ducts.[1] Division alone will suffice, as the septum is avascular.

Duodenal Wall Closure

The duodenum is closed in the direction in which it was opened. An inner row of continuous 3-0 chromic catgut or Dexon and an outer row of interrupted seromuscular 3-0 or 4-0 silk are employed.

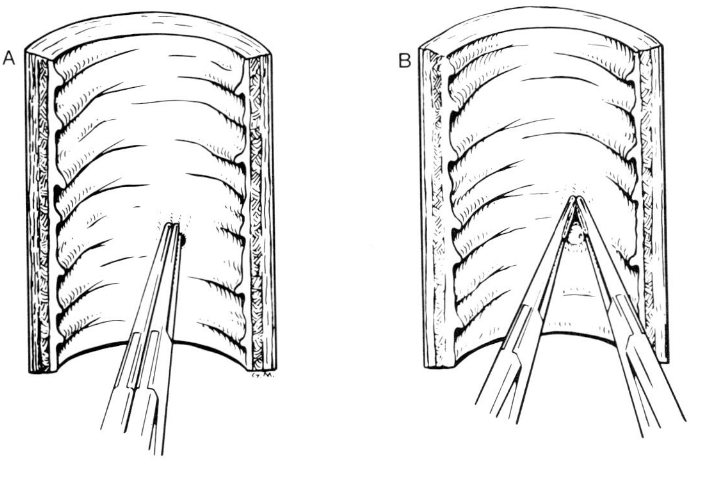

Figure 24–11. The first pair of clamps is shown at *A*. The second and succeeding pairs of clamps are placed directly anteriorly as in *B*. The pancreatic duct is diagrammed at the 5 o'clock position.

Use of the T-Tube

When a proximal choledochotomy has been performed, the common duct is closed around a 14F short-limbed T-tube. Completion cholangiograms may be obtained by injecting the contrast medium slowly, with the patient in the Trendelenburg position, or by occluding the distal duct with a small balloon catheter. If the common duct is not opened and the sphincteroplasty is done from below, we do not use a T-tube.

Drainage of the Gallbladder Bed

A Jackson-Pratt drain or some other closed-suction drain should be placed in the gallbladder bed. The drain and the T-tube are passed through small separate abdominal wall incisions and sutured to the skin.

Physiologic Considerations

From an anatomic standpoint, the wide opening resulting from a sphincteroplasty should permit any overlooked calculi to be flushed into the duodenum; it also eliminates bile stasis, which predisposes to recurrent stone formation. Does sphincteroplasty differ materially from sphincterotomy?

The muscular sphincters at the end of the bile duct are contracted by morphine sulphate. We compared the action of this drug on postsphincteroplasty and postsphincterotomy patients.[9–13] Figure 24–12 shows that morphine given to a postsphincterotomy patient produces a pressure rise that is maintained for almost an hour; the sphincters are still functioning. Following sphincteroplasty, morphine produces a sudden initial rise as the duodenum contracts and forces intestinal contents upward through the large opening. This is followed by a rapid fall to normal or subnormal pressures, which is sustained.

Following sphincterotomy, the administration of morphine produces complete occlusion of the distal duct (Fig. 24–13). The postsphincteroplasty patients show no change in ductal caliber or flow after morphine (Fig. 24–14).

Cineradiography before and after morphine administration in postsphincteroplasty and postsphincterotomy patients confirmed the foregoing findings and demonstrated both subjective and objective differences (Table 24–1).

Barium can be seen to reflux into the bile duct after sphincteroplasty, but this does not occur in all patients after sphincterotomy (Fig. 24–15). We consider failure of reflux to be evidence of an incomplete sphincteroplasty. With free flow of bile, cholangitis does not develop.

Eiseman demonstrated that sphincterotomy is followed by scar formation and a return of the caliber of the bile duct to its presphincterotomy size.[14] On the other hand, Vajcner demonstrated that sphincteroplasty, in contradistinction to sphincterotomy, permanently lowered the resistance of the sphincter of Oddi.[15]

The sphincteroplasties performed in our patients have remained open, as demonstrated by the absence of cholangitis, by late autopsy studies, and by demonstration of barium reflux on upper gastrointestinal se-

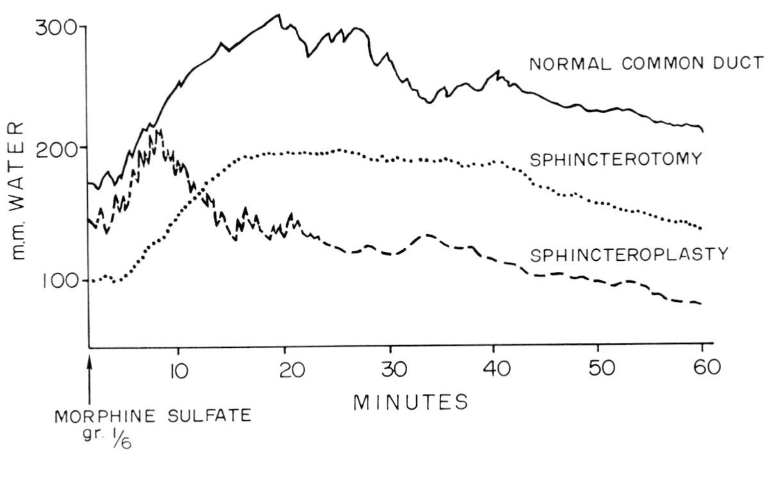

Figure 24–12. Morphine produces a pressure elevation of long duration after common duct exploration or sphincterotomy as the sphincters are still functioning. The transient rise seen in postsphincteroplasty patients is due to contraction of the duodenum with reflux of bowel content upward through the large stoma.

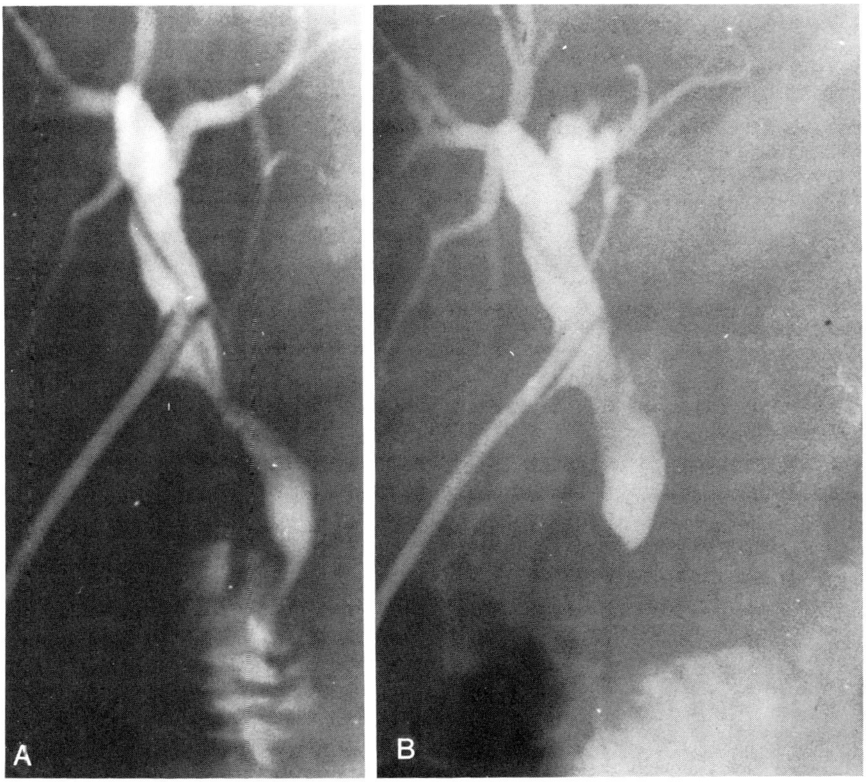

Figure 24–13. Postsphincterotomy T-tube cholangiograms before morphine (*A*) and after morphine (*B*). As the sphincters are not destroyed, they can contract and occlude the distal duct.

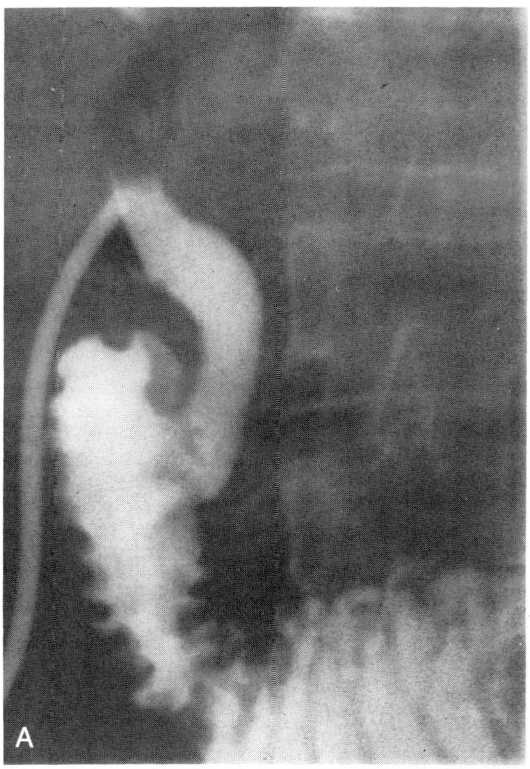

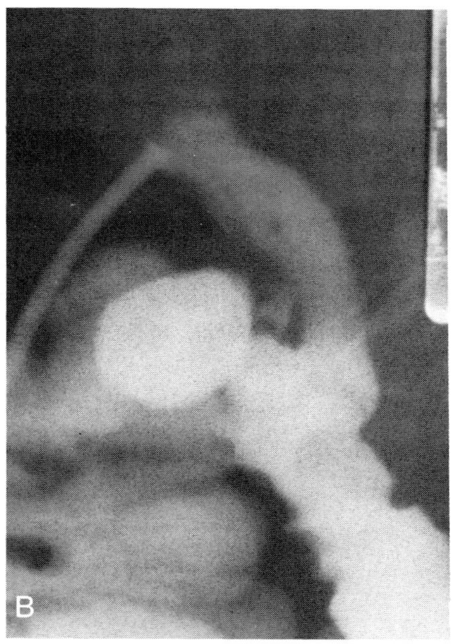

Figure 24–14. Postsphincteroplasty T-tube cholangiograms before morphine (*A*) and after morphine (*B*). As the sphincters have been destroyed, morphine cannot contract the distal duct. Note also that the flow of dye downward is so rapid that the hepatic radicles do not fill.

Table 24–1 POSTOPERATIVE T-TUBE CINERADIOGRAPHY

Factors to be Considered	After Sphincterotomy	After Sphincteroplasty
Position of patient	Supine	45 degree Trendelenburg
Rate of Hypaque infusion	15 to 30 drops/min	150 drops/min
Amount of Hypaque needed for study	30 to 60 ml	180 to 240 ml
Following intravenous morphine		
Distal duct	Occluded	Wide open
Proximal ducts	Dilated	Normal size
Pain	Marked	None
Nausea	Marked	None
Reflux from duodenum	None	In all cases

From Jones SA, Smith LL: Surgery 1972; *71*:565. Used by permission.

ries (Figure 24–15 shows a study performed 12½ years after sphincteroplasty).

Why should a sphincteroplasty remain patent while a standard end-to-side choledochoduodenostomy sometimes undergoes stricture formation? We believe this is because in the latter operation a circumferential suture line is necessary, whereas only the anterior portion of a sphincteroplasty must be sutured.

Residual Biliary Stones

Residual stones may be divided into two groups. The first includes calculi that originated in the gallbladder, passed into the ductal system, and were overlooked at the time of duct exploration. These stones are composed mainly of cholesterol and are firm and often faceted. The bile is clear. The second type is the stasis stone produced by chronic intermittent ductal obstruction. These calculi are soft and easy to crush in the fingers, conform roughly to the shape of the duct, and are associated with mud and sludge in the bile. Distal duct obstruction with proximal ductal dilatation is often demonstrable.

The overall incidence of residual bile duct stones averages 10 per cent after a positive, and 5 per cent after a negative, common duct exploration. Table 24–2 shows the results of some methods used to prevent residual calculi. Although more expert use of the choledochoscope, improved techniques of cholangiography, and so forth have decreased the incidence of this complication, some stones are still left behind.

Choice of a Bile Duct Drainage Procedure

There are numerous operations devised to obtain free drainage of the biliary ductal

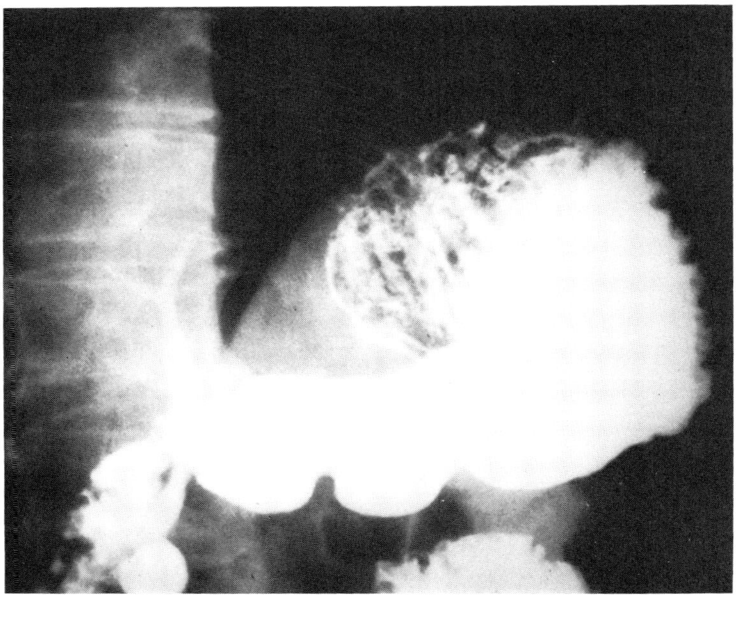

Figure 24–15. This demonstrates the desired postsphincteroplasty reflux as seen on upper gastrointestinal series. It also emphasizes permanence of the stoma, as this x-ray study was made 12½ years after sphincteroplasty.

Table 24–2 METHODS USED TO PREVENT RESIDUAL STONES

Technique	Author	Residual Stones (%) *Proven*	*Probable*	*Total*
Operative cholangiography	Jolley et al[22]	3.5	3.5	7.0
Sphincterotomy	Backer[23]	3.9	2.6	6.5
Ampullary dilatation	Chodoff[24]	7.0	–	7.0
Fogarty balloon	Fogarty et al[25]	7.6	–	7.6
Choledochoscope	Shore and Shore[26]	3.3	–	3.3
Sphincteroplasty	Present series	0	0	0

From Jones SA, Smith LL: Surgery 1972, *71*:565. Used by permission.

system, and sphincteroplasty is just one of them. These various procedures must not be considered as competitive, but rather as different ways of attaining the same goal. The operation selected should be chosen because it best suits the problem presented by the patient in question. Every approach has its advantages and disadvantages.

Lateral choledochoduodenostomy (between the side of the common duct and the first portion of the duodenum) was introduced by Riedel[16] and popularized in the United States by Madden.[17] The common duct must be at least 18 mm in diameter for a successful result. The ease and speed with which this operation can be accomplished make it useful in poor-risk patients. We have used it frequently to bypass a distal unresectable malignant obstruction in the absence of imminent duodenal obstruction. It is indicated for long distal strictures, such as those seen in chronic pancreatitis.

A disadvantage of the lateral anastomosis is the so-called sump syndrome (Fig. 24–16).

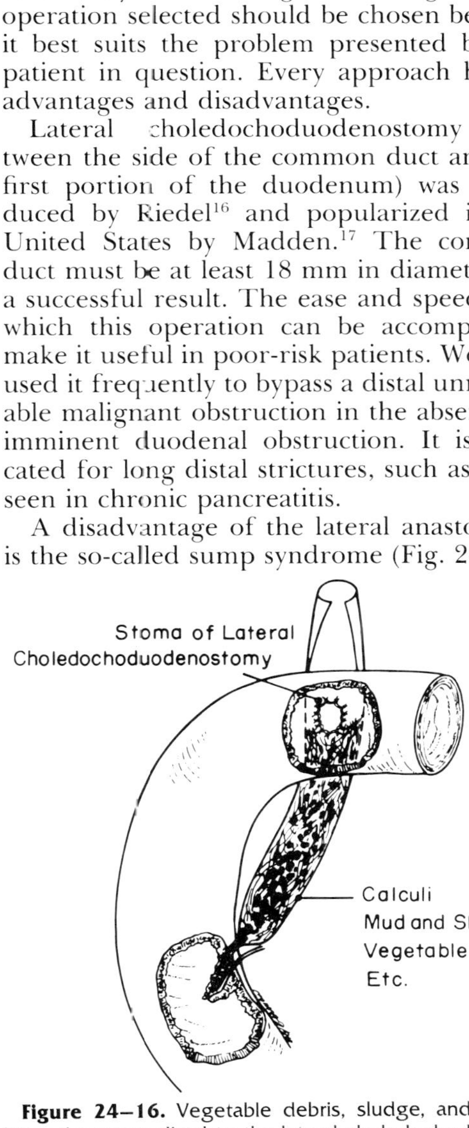

Figure 24–16. Vegetable debris, sludge, and calculi filling the sump distal to the lateral choledochoduodenostomy.

Because the distal intramural portion of the common duct becomes narrow, a blind pouch is created below the anastomosis. Vegetable debris may collect in this distal segment and eventually produce obstruction with cholangitis, jaundice, and pancreatitis. The incidence of the sump syndrome is difficult to determine. Madden reported no problems in over 100 patients. However, others have encountered this complication, and Lord Smith of Marlow has operated upon 25 patients with this syndrome, each of whom had had a side-to-side choledochoduodenostomy performed elsewhere.[18] All of his patients had cholangitis and an elevated alkaline phosphatase level, and some of them had associated jaundice and pancreatitis. All were relieved of biliary obstruction by transduodenal sphincteroplasty. Nowadays, endoscopic sphincterotomy would usually be the treatment of choice. Figure 24–17 shows an upper gastrointestinal series on a patient who developed obstruction and cholangitis following a lateral anastomosis. Thus, while the sump syndrome renders this a less than ideal operation for residual common duct stones, it may be the procedure of choice in a few selected patients.

Disadvantages besides the sump syndrome include lack of opportunity to inspect the papilla during the operation, with the chance that a tumor may be missed. The choledochoscope has not been infallible in this regard. Furthermore, the common duct must be enlarged before the procedure can be performed, and in some patients the duct is too small. In general, we have used lateral choledochoduodenostomy to drain a duct dilated as a result of malignant obstruction, occasionally for long distal strictures, and for treatment or prophylaxis of calculous disease in the aged and infirm, who cannot tolerate an operation of greater magnitude. It would appear to be most useful when long-term patency is not the primary objective.

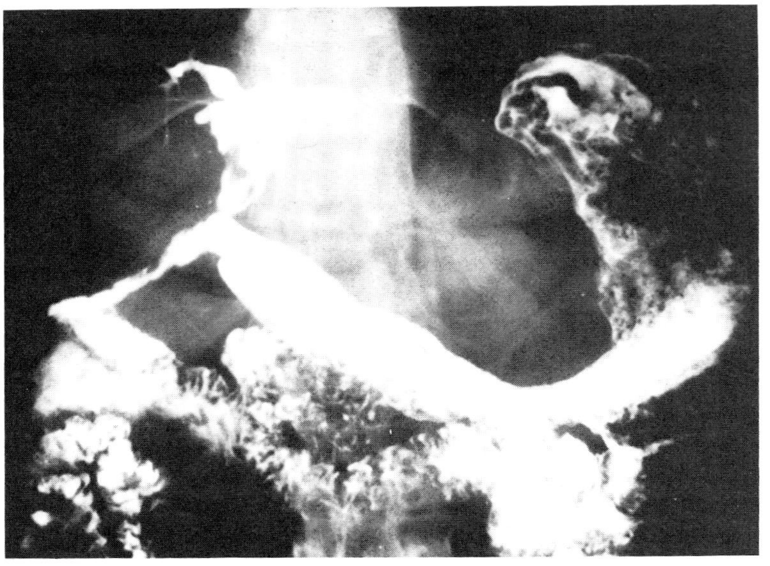

Figure 24–17. Upper gastrointestinal series after lateral choledochoduodenostomy. Note marked narrowing at anastomosis and dilated ductal tree.

With a grossly enlarged common duct and in patients with distal nonresectable malignant obstruction who can tolerate a more stressful procedure, a Roux-en-Y choledochojejunostomy may be considered. Some favor the use of the gallbladder for the bypass. In general, we do not.

Congenital cystic dilatation of the intrahepatic ductal system was described by Caroli in 1958.[19] The best treatment of this rare condition is lobectomy if the disease is confined to one lobe or segment. Unfortunately, most patients have bilobar involvement, and 60 per cent have extrahepatic bile duct dilatation, so internal drainage must be performed by Roux-en-Y choledochojejunostomy. External drainage is not advised.[20] Roux-en-Y choledochojejunostomy is also indicated for patients with large multiple intrahepatic calculi and infection and in those with a markedly enlarged bile duct packed with stones.

INDICATIONS FOR SPHINCTEROPLASTY

The most common indications for sphincteroplasty are impacted distal common duct stones; papillary stenosis (defined as being present when a 3 mm dilator cannot be passed); distal short benign common duct strictures; irremovable hepatic duct stones; mud, sludge, or stasis stones in the duct; or multiple ductal calculi when complete clearing of the ducts is doubtful.[27] Some have also recommended this operation for postcholecystectomy pain and recurrent idiopathic pancreatitis.[37] Until recent years we performed a sphincteroplasty whenever operating for residual stones, knowing that statistically an average of 25 per cent of patients operated upon for residual calculi will need another operation to clear the ducts.[9] The treatment of choice for most patients with postcholecystectomy choledocholithiasis today is endoscopic removal of the stones with a papillotomy.[29, 30] For those who come to operation, long-term results with this approach are similar to those obtained by drainage procedures.[33] The addition of a sphincteroplasty after choledocholithotomy is based on the type of stone, the character of the bile, and the caliber and configuration of the ductal system.[27] For example, if the common bile duct contains only one or a few stones of gallbladder origin and clean bile and if there is no mechanical obstruction and postexploratory cholangiography[15] is satisfactory, removal of the calculi should be adequate treatment and sphincteroplasty is not indicated. On the other hand, if the bile is muddy and contains sludge and stasis type stones, a sphincteroplasty may be indicated.[27]

It must be emphasized that ability to pass a dilator through the papilla does not prove that the flow of bile is unhindered. Figure 24–18 shows a distal stricture caused by pancreatitis. The patient had had four previous operations for biliary obstruction. At each procedure the duct reportedly contained

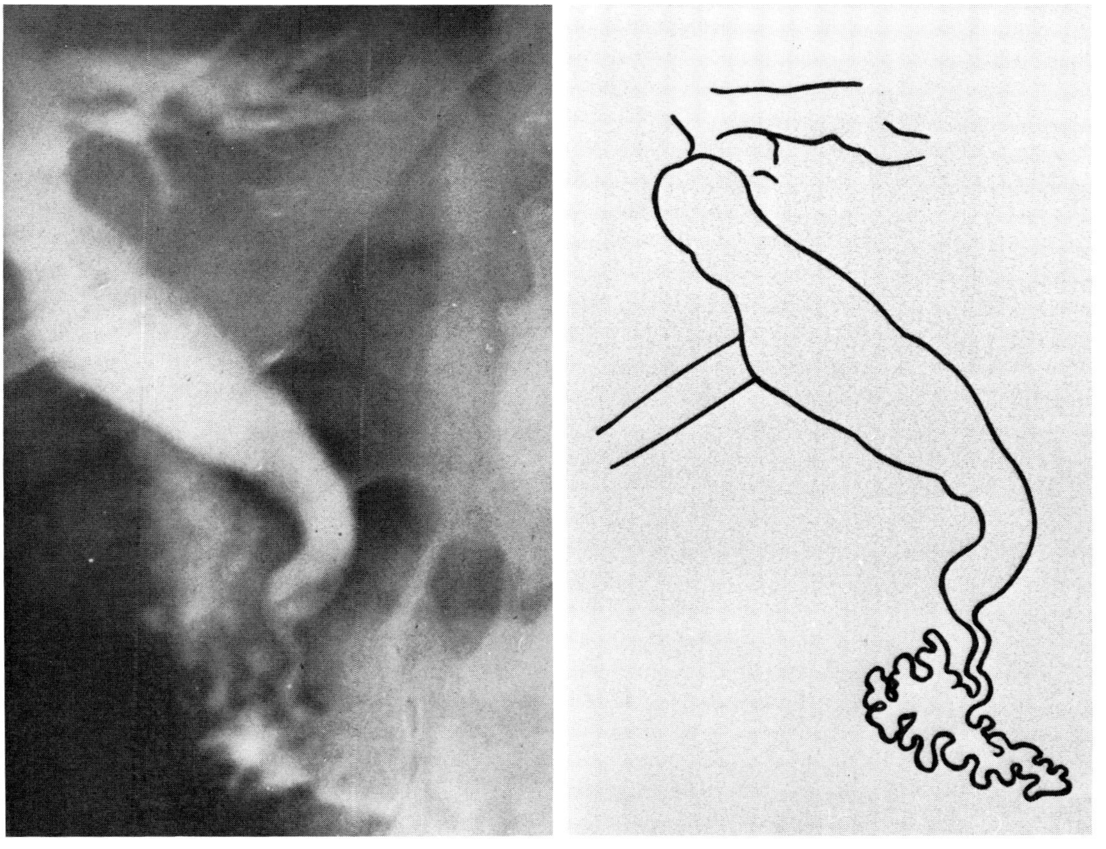

Figure 24–18. Distal stricture produced by pancreatitis. Dilated proximal ductal tree. Number 6 Bakes dilator could be passed from above into duodenum. Repeated episodes of cholangitis.

mud and sludge, and the proximal ducts were enlarged. As a No. 6 Bakes dilator could be passed into the duodenum at each procedure, it was believed that nothing further needed to be done. At each operation a T-tube was inserted, and in each instance cholangitis developed when it was withdrawn. Figure 24–19 shows the result following sphincteroplasty. After removal of the T-tube this time, the patient remained well.

Sphincteroplasty is *not* advised at either primary or secondary choledocholithotomy if only one or a few calculi of apparent gallbladder origin are present, if the bile is clear, if the papilla is 3 mm in diameter or larger, and if choledochoscopy and completion cholangiography show no residual abnormalities. Sphincteroplasty should not be considered in the presence of acute inflammation involving the distal duct, in particular acute pancreatitis. It should be avoided in patients with a peri-Vaterian diverticulum. It is not of value in treating Caroli's disease or a markedly dilated common bile duct.

RESULTS OF SPHINCTEROPLASTY

Our conclusions are based upon experience with 314 transduodenal sphincteroplasties performed over 27 years. There were three deaths in the 314 cases, a mortality rate of 0.96 per cent. In most other large series mortality varies between 1.9 and 4.2 per cent,[28, 32, 34, 35] although it was 11 per cent in one report.[31]

One of our patients developed a leak at the duodenotomy site, which was the only leak in the series. This patient survived but had a persistent fistula. There have been no deaths in the last 202 cases.

The overall morbidity of 4.7 per cent includes three patients with transient postoperative pancreatitis, six wound infections, and the single duodenal leak mentioned. Even though barium refluxes freely into the duct after sphincteroplasty, no patient has developed cholangitis, which underscores the fact that cholangitis does not develop in the absence of bile stasis.

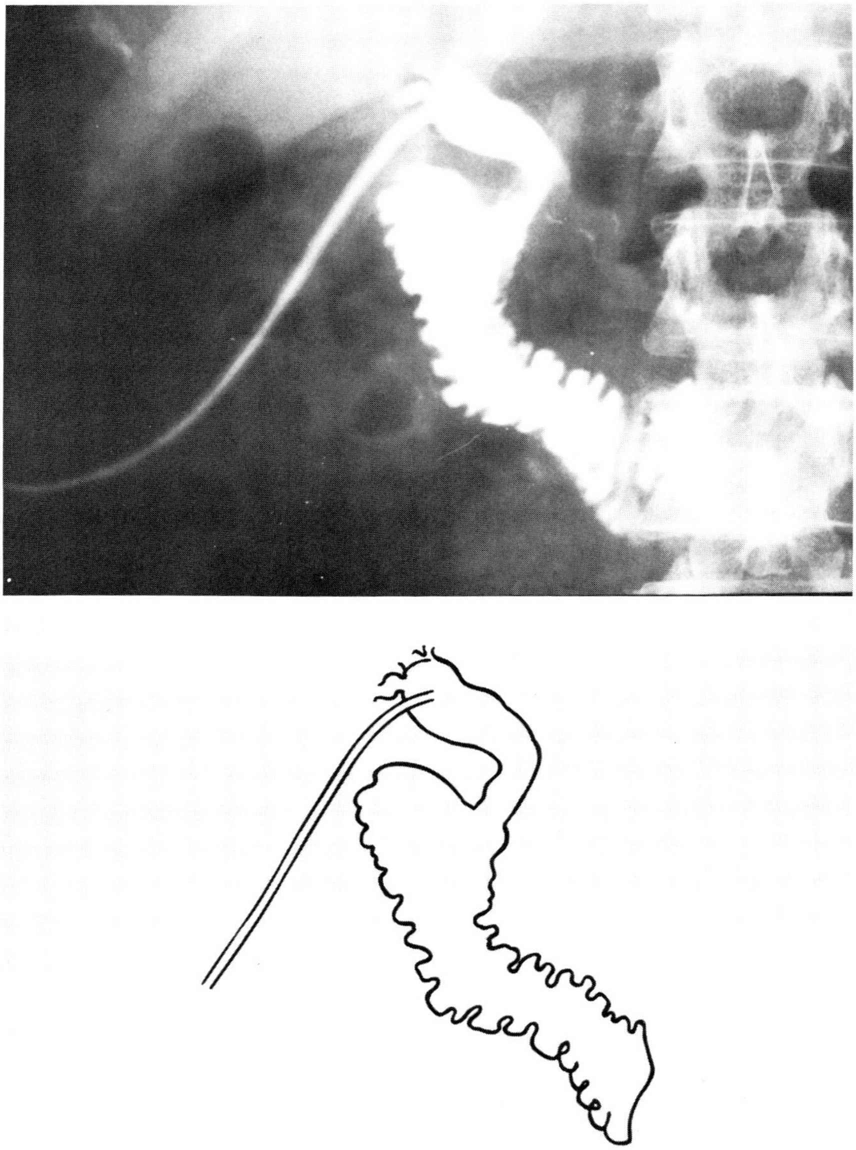

Figure 24–19. Short stricture eliminated by sphincteroplasty. Note insufficient back pressure to produce hepatic ductal filling. No recurrence of cholangitis at 2-year follow-up.

Of the 314 operations, 213 were performed for biliary tract obstruction and 101 for acute recurrent pancreatitis. Of those patients with obstruction, 189 had multiple common duct stones. Many of these patients had additional indications for the sphincteroplasty, including papillary stenosis, distal stricture, impacted calculi, mud, and sludge. Four had irremovable hepatic duct calculi. They were followed from 2 to 7 years after sphincteroplasty and remained asymptomatic. The indication for sphincteroplasty in 22 patients was residual stones.

All 213 patients were relieved of biliary tract obstruction. All had T-tube cholangiograms on about the ninth postoperative day. In five patients overlooked calculi were found. In each case the stones were immediately washed into the duodenum by T-tube irrigation as proved by another cholangiogram. It is possible that stones may have been overlooked in more than five cases, and they passed spontaneously from duct to bowel through the stoma during the interval between the sphincteroplasty and the time of postoperative T-tube cholangiography. In the practical sense, we have had no residual stones following sphincteroplasty.

REFERENCES

1. Jones SA, Smith LL, Gregory G: Sphincteroplasty for recurrent pancreatitis—A second report. Ann Surg 1958;*174:*180.
2. Boyden EA: The anatomy of the choledochal junction in man. Surg Gynecol Obstet 1957;*104:*641.
3. Jones SA, Steedman RA, Keller TB, Smith LL: Transduodenal sphincteroplasty (not sphincterotomy) for biliary and pancreatic disease—Indications, contraindications and results. Am J Surg 1969; *118:*292.
4. Lowery BD: Personal communication.
5. Rutledge RH: Sphincteroplasty and choledochoduodenostomy for benign biliary obstructions. Ann Surg 1976;*183:*476.
6. Discussion by Ponka JL: Reference to Kocher in inframesocolic transduodenal approach to the distal biliary-pancreatic ductal system. Villalba MR, Lucas RJ: Arch Surg 1978;*113:*496.
7. Ong G: Personal communication, 1978.
8. Jones SA: Instrument to aid in locating the papilla of Vater. Surgery 1963;*54:*480.
9. Jones SA, Smith LL, Keller TB, Joergenson EJ: Choledochoduodenostomy to prevent residual stones. Arch Surg 1963;*86:*1014.
10. Jones SA, Smith LL: Transduodenal sphincteroplasty for recurrent pancreatitis—A preliminary report. Ann Surg 1952;*136:*937.
11. Jones SA, Smith LL: A reappraisal of sphincteroplasty (not sphincterotomy). Surgery 1972;*71:*565.
12. Jones SA: Sphincteroplasty (not sphincterotomy) in the treatment of biliary tract disease. Surg Clin North Am 1973;*53:*1123.
13. Jones SA: Sphincteroplasty. *In* Controversy in Surgery.
14. Eiseman B, Brown WH, Virabutr S, Gattesfeld S: Sphincterotomy, an evaluation of its physiological rationale. Arch Surg 1959;*79:*140.
15. Vajcner A, Grossling S, Nicoloff DM: Physiologic evaluation of sphincteroplasty. Surgery 1967;*62:* 589.
16. Riedel BMCL: Erfahrungen uber die gallensteinkrankheit mit und ohne icterus. Berlin, Hirschwald, 1892, p 116.
17. Madden JL, Chun JY, Kandalaft S, Parekh M: Choledochoduodenostomy, an unjustly maligned surgical procedure? Am J Surg 1970;*119:*45.
18. Smith R: Personal communication, 1973.
19. Caroli J, Couinand C, Soupault R, et al: Une affection nouvelle des voies biliaires. La dilatation kystique unilobaire des canaux hépatiques. Sem Hop Paris 1958;*14:*496.
20. Watts DR, Lorenzo GA, Beal JM: Congenital dilation of the intrahepatic biliary ducts. Arch Surg 1974;*108:*592.
21. Way LW: Retained common duct stones. Surg Clin North Am 1973;*53:*1139.
22. Jolley PC, Baker JW, Schmidt HM, Walker JH, Holm JC: Operative cholangiography: A case for its routine use. Am Surg 1968;*163:*551.
23. Backer OG: Personal communication, 1970.
24. Chodoff RJ: Choledocholithiasis: Failure of routine operative cholangiography to improve results. J Einstein Med Cent 1960;*8:*215.
25. Fogarty TJ, Krippaehne WW, Dennis DL, Fletcher WS: Evaluation of an improved operative technique in common duct surgery. Am J Surg 1968;*116:*177.
26. Shore JM, Shore E: Operative biliary endoscopy. Ann Surg 1970;*171:*269.
27. Allen B, Shapiro H, Way LW: Management of recurrent and residual common duct stones. Am J Surg 1981;*142:*41.
28. Anderson TM, Pitt HA, Longmire WP: Experience with sphincteroplasty and sphincterotomy in pancreatobiliary surgery. Ann Surg 1985;*201:*399.
29. Leese T, Neoptolemos JP, Carr-Locke DL: Successes, failures, early complications and their management following endoscopic sphincterotomy: results in 394 consecutive patients from a single centre. Br J Surg 1985;*72:*215.
30. Staritz M, Poralla T, Dormeyer HH, Meyer KH, Buschenfelde Z: Endoscopic removal of common bile duct stones through the intact papilla after medical sphincter dilation. Gastroenterology 1985; *88:*1807.
31. Cave-Bigley DJ, Aukland P, Kane JF, Hardy EG: Transduodenal exploration of the common bile duct in a district general hospital. 1984;*66:*187.
32. Choi TK, Wong J, Lam KH, Lim TK, Ong GB: Late result of sphincteroplasty in the treatment of primary cholangitis. Arch Surg 1981;*116:*1173.
33. Broughan TA, Sivak MV, Hermann RE: The management of retained and recurrent bile duct stones. Surgery 1985;*98:*746.
34. Nardi GL, Michelassi F, Zannini P: Transduodenal sphincteroplasty. Ann Surg 1983;*198:*453.
35. Speranza V, Lezoche E, Minervini S, Careli F, Basso N, Simi M: Transduodenal papillostomy as a routine procedure in managing choledocholithiasis. Arch Surg 1982;*117:*875.
36. Choi TK, Lee NW, Wong J, Ong GB: Extraperitoneal sphincteroplasty for residual stones. Ann Surg 1982;*196:*26.
37. Moody FG, Becker JM, Potts JR: Transduodenal sphincteroplasty and transampullary septectomy for postcholecystectomy pain. Ann Surg 1983;*197:*627.

PETER COTTON, M.D.

25

Transendoscopic Therapeutic Techniques

Endoscopic access to the biliary tree can be obtained via the papilla of Vater through a duodenoscope; through a tract left by a T-tube following surgical exploration of the common bile duct; through the skin over the liver, having made a small fistula; through a laparoscope; and during surgical exploration using a choledochoscope. All these routes carry therapeutic as well as diagnostic potential; this chapter will be confined to the approach in which the duodenoscope is merely an extension of diagnostic endoscopic cholangiography[1] (see Diagnostic Endoscopic Cholangiography, Chapter 11). Diathermy sphincterotomy for removal of common bile duct stones is the main therapeutic technique. Other applications will be discussed.

DUODENOSCOPIC SPHINCTEROTOMY

Some early reports[2–5] of this technique refer to "papillotomy," but the effects are much more extensive than this term implies. The resulting orifice (as judged by endoscopy, radiology, and manometry) is more akin to surgical sphincteroplasty.

Equipment and Preparation

The most popular type of sphincterotomy "knife" originated in Erlangen;[2] it consists of standard duodenoscope cannulation tubing with a wire loop, of which 3.5 cm close to the tip is exposed (Fig. 25–1). This type has been referred to as the pull-type of knife, since traction on the wire forms a cutting bow (Fig. 25–2). Other knives in which the wire is pushed out to produce a cutting loop have been used.[5] Proximal connections allow injection of contrast agents through the catheter tip. The knife can be used through a standard duodenoscope, all the latest models of which are fully insulated. Sphincterotomy is usually performed with cutting current interspersed with coagulation when any bleeding occurs.

The precise indications for sphincterotomy are discussed further on. Contraindications include irreversible coagulation disorders and very large stones. Most patients selected for sphincterotomy are elderly and frail, and some are acutely ill (e.g., with septic cholangitis). Thus, careful medical assessment and treatment before and after the procedure are essential. Duodenoscopic sphincterotomy has certain complications (see later), and approximately 3 per cent of patients will require operative intervention within 24 hours of the procedure because of complications or sphincterotomy failure. Thus, the technique must be performed only in an institution with the appropriate specialized medical and surgical facilities. Those patients who are not already in the hospital are admitted on the day before the procedure for general clinical assessment and blood studies, including prothrombin time, platelet count, and blood grouping. The procedure and its possible consequences are explained in detail. Most patients with common bile duct stones have infected bile, and endoscopic instrumentation can aggravate or provoke clinical infection. Prophylactic antibiotics are often used, but their precise role remains conjectural.

Successful sphincterotomy provides excellent biliary drainage, and cholangitis probably occurs only when sphincterotomy attempts fail. Bile specimens can be taken for culture and antibiotic sensitivities, and antibiotic trials are in progress. Patients are fasted and sedated as for standard ERCP. We use a mixture of pethidine (Demerol)

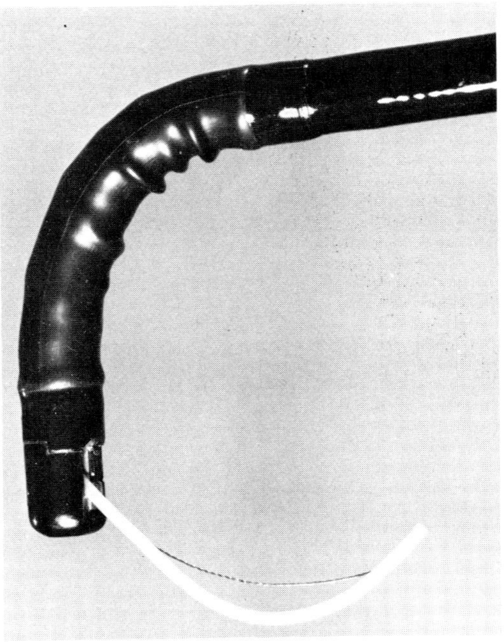

Figure 25–1. Tip of insulated duodenoscope with diathermy wire in "closed" position.

and diazepam (Valium), given intravenously immediately prior to the procedure. An anticholinergic agent or glucagon is required to ensure duodenal and sphincter relaxation. General anesthesia is unnecessary.

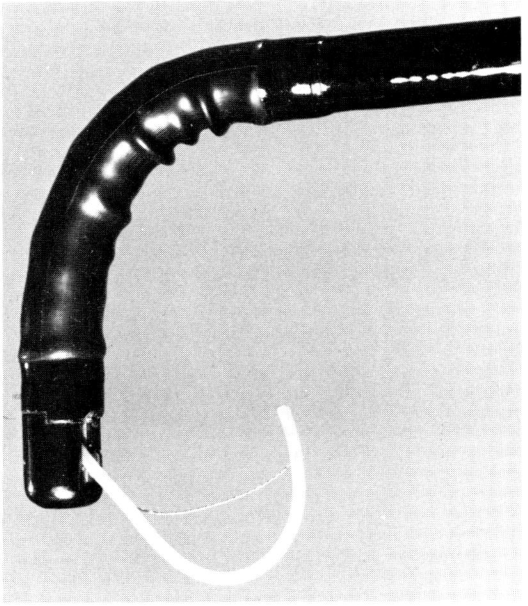

Figure 25–2. Traction on the wire produces a cutting bow.

Technique of Sphincterotomy

Successful sphincterotomy depends on correct equipment and patient preparation and on cooperation between a competent endoscopist and an interested radiologist. The duodenoscope is maneuvered to provide a face-on view of the papilla of Vater (Fig. 25–3); cannulation of the ampulla is then accomplished, and retrograde cholangiography is performed to confirm the indication for sphincterotomy (Fig. 25–4). A low-density contrast agent should be used to avoid obscuring small stones. The standard catheter is then replaced by a sphincterotomy knife, which is passed deep into the bile duct. It is crucial to establish (by further contrast injection, fluoroscopy, and radiography) that the knife is not in the pancreatic duct (Figs. 25–5 and 25–6). The knife is left deep in the bile duct while all electrical connections are checked and current settings are adjusted; it is then slowly withdrawn until half of the wire is exposed outside the papilla (Fig. 25–7), pointing at 11 or 12 o'clock. Slight traction

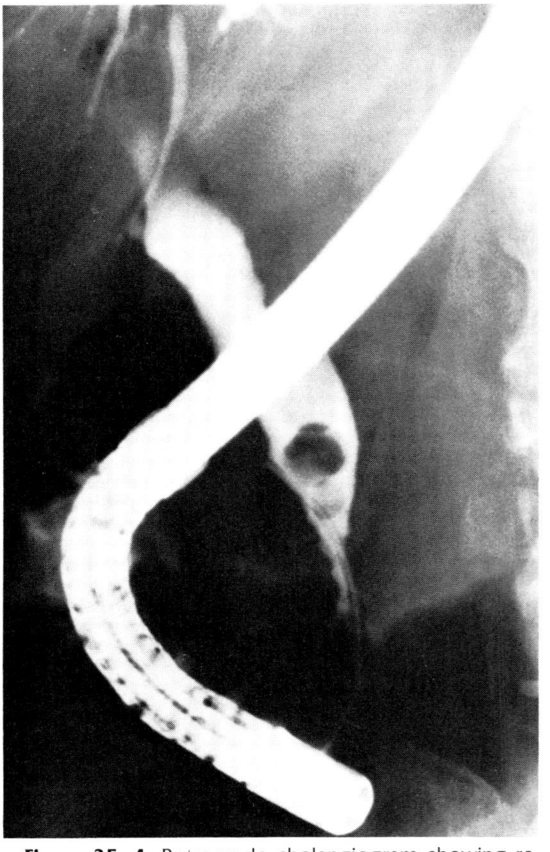

Figure 25–4. Retrograde cholangiogram showing retained stones.

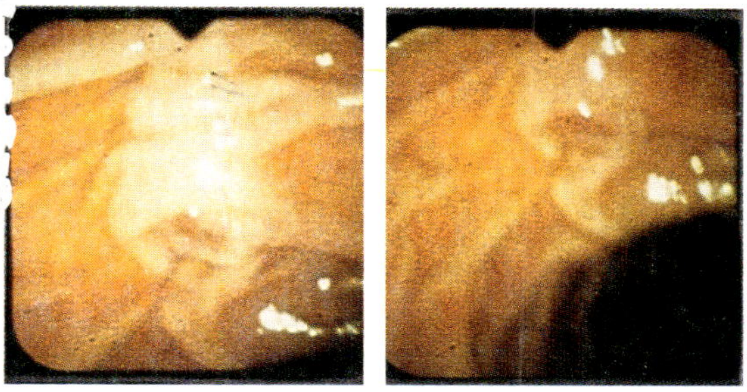

25–3

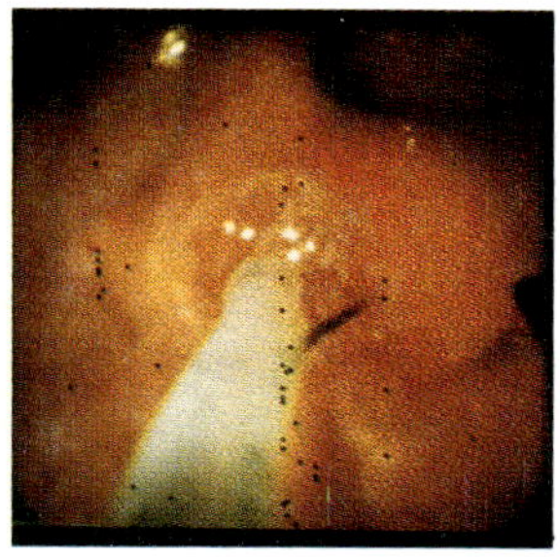

25–7

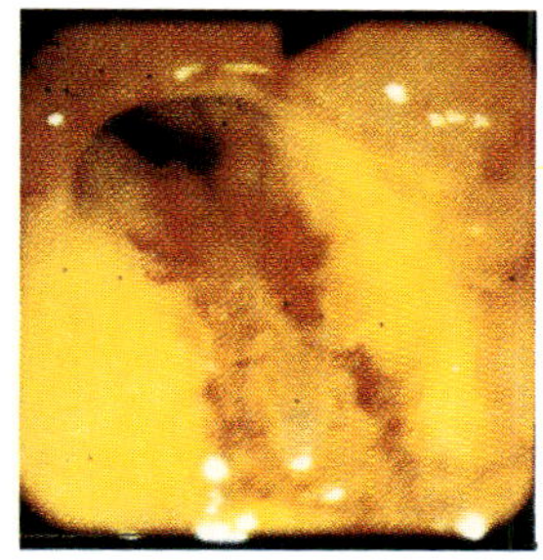

25–8

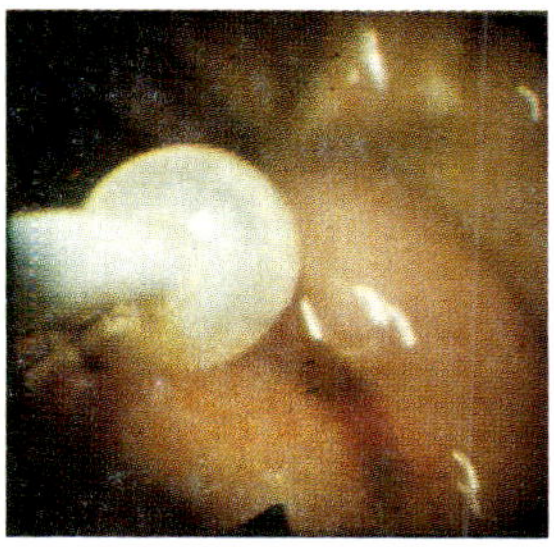

25–9

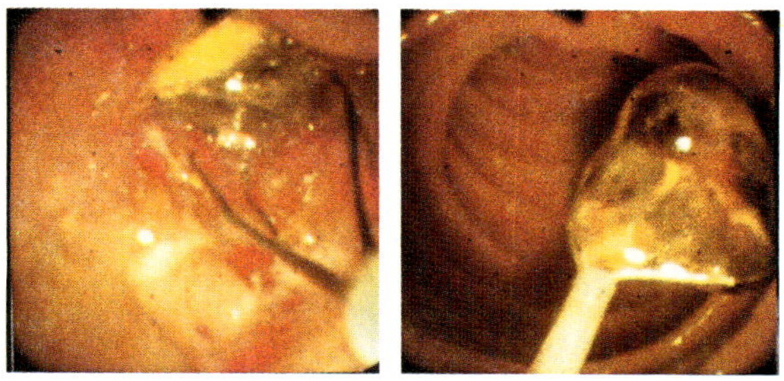

25–11

Figure 25–3. Face-on view of the papilla of Vater.

Figure 25–7. Diathermy knife withdrawn so that half of the wire is visible outside the papilla.

Figure 25–8. The papilla of Vater immediately after sphincterotomy.

Figure 25–9. Measurement of the orifice using a balloon catheter.

Figure 25–11. *A*, Basket extruding through the ampulla. *B*, Stone trapped in basket in the lumen of the duodenum.

on the wire produces a bow (Fig. 25–5), and short bursts of cutting current are applied while upward tension on the wire is maintained. Excess tension and current result in a rapid cut with little coagulation and considerable risk of bleeding. The cut should be made in three or four controlled increments, to a total length of about 15 mm. This unroofs the ampulla of Vater and exposes the distal bile duct (Fig. 25–8). There is usually a sudden efflux of bile, and the bowed knife should pass freely in and out of the orifice. In most patients no bleeding is seen; coagulation is applied when there is any oozing. The precise size of the sphincterotomy orifice is difficult to judge visually and is best documented with balloon-tipped catheters (Fig. 25–9). Our standard cut normally permits passage of a balloon inflated to 8 to 10 mm in diameter. The length of the cut in the individual patient is tailored somewhat to the size of any stone to be extracted, but the risks of bleeding and perforation increase as the cut encroaches on the transverse fold proximal to the papilla.

The total procedure from intubation to completion of sphincterotomy should take less than 30 minutes. Cannulation can prove more difficult, and occasionally impossible, in patients with large peripapillary diverticula or previous local surgery (which may narrow the duodenum) as well as after Billroth II partial gastrectomy. When approaching the papilla up the afferent loop, one may find a forward-viewing endoscope easier to use.

Patients are observed carefully in the hospital for at least 24 hours after the procedure; most patients are able to drink fluids on the same day and are ambulant and eating normally on the following day.

Stone Extraction

Endoscopic sphincterotomy is normally performed to remove stones from the com-

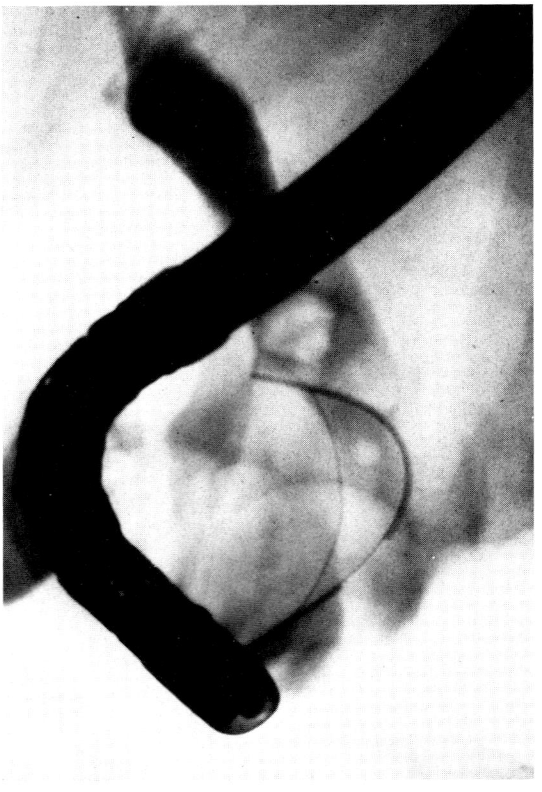

Figure 25–5. Diathermy wire correctly positioned in the terminal bile duct.

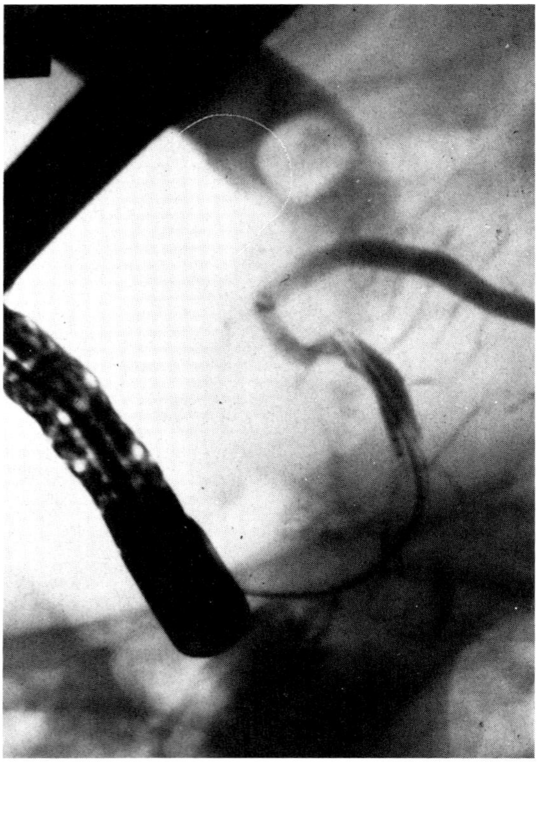

Figure 25–6. Diathermy wire in the pancreatic duct.

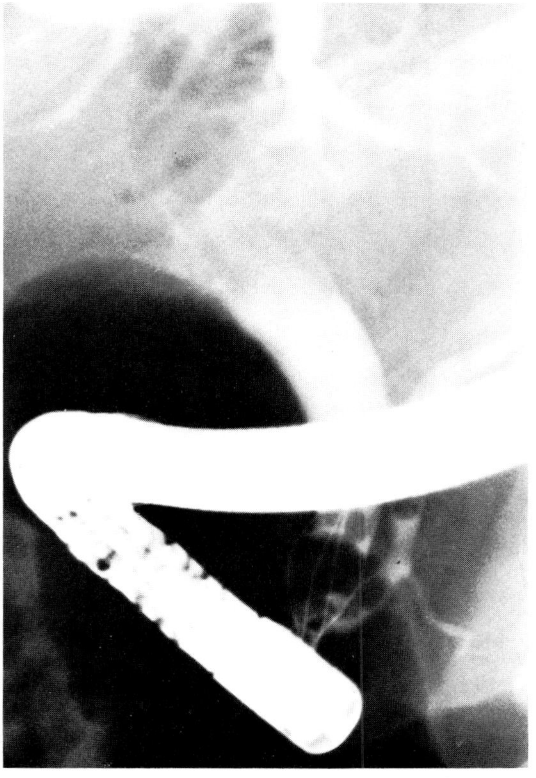

Figure 25–10. Endoscopic basket extraction of a stone.

mon bile duct. Most small stones pass spontaneously within a few days or weeks of an adequate sphincterotomy; further check cholangiography is then needed. Intravenous cholangiography is rarely diagnostic, since contrast matter leaves rapidly through the sphincterotomy. ERCP provides the best diagnostic method, but this means readmission to the hospital in case instrumental stone extraction is needed. Thus, one method of management is to discharge patients immediately after sphincterotomy, with a planned brief readmission in 4 to 6 weeks. This expectant policy is not appropriate in elderly and ill patients, especially those suffering from recurrent cholangitis, and there are often other pressures to complete the treatment quickly. Stones can be extracted at the time of sphincterotomy using balloon catheters or wire baskets. Balloons are effective with small stones and are also useful in confirming that the duct has been cleared, but they are fragile. Extraction baskets are available from endoscope manufacturers; most also allow contrast injection. Under radiographic control, the basket is passed beyond the stone, opened fully, and then withdrawn (Figs. 25–10 and 25–11). Several passes are often necessary, and success usually requires close radiologic cooperation; it may be necessary to tilt the x-ray table to move stones up and down the duct. Resistance is often felt at the sphincterotomy orifice when larger stones are extracted; in this situation, extra traction on the wire may simply drag the tip of the endoscope against the papilla. Use of a larger endoscope makes it possible to apply more tension and to use stronger baskets; however, there is a risk of impacting the basket and stone in the papilla. Relatively forceful extraction of stones immediately after sphincterotomy may also increase the risk of bleeding from the raw surface. Since this risk is greatest with large stones and basket extraction is superfluous for small stones, we have evolved another technique to facilitate and check on stone passage.

Transnasal Biliary Catheterization[6]

Unless all stones are removed immediately and convincingly (or the patient has a T-tube drain), it is now our practice to leave a catheter in the duct immediately after sphincterotomy. Standard Teflon tubing (2 mm diameter) is prepared in 3 m lengths. One such catheter is passed deep into the bile duct immediately after sphincterotomy and is preferably looped within the common hepatic duct. Looping is easier in dilated ducts and is facilitated by using a long guide wire or catheters with a preformed pigtail tip. The duodenoscope is removed, and the position of the catheter is checked radiologically (Fig. 25–12). The proximal end of the catheter is then rerouted from the mouth to the nose using temporary nasopharyngeal intubation. The catheter is taped to the cheek and drained into a bag. Bile cultures are taken. The indwelling tube is normally well tolerated, and patients eat and drink normally. A "transnasal cholangiogram" is performed via the catheter 1 or 2 days after sphincterotomy. In most patients the bile duct is clear of stones; the radiologist removes the tube, and the patient is discharged. If stones are still present, the duct is perfused via the tube for 2 or 3 days using dextrose saline (3 to 5 liters per day). If stones are still present when transnasal cholangiography is repeated 4 to 5 days after sphincterotomy, we usually repeat the endoscopy with a larger instrument for basket extraction. Transnasal biliary catheterization provides a route for the infusion

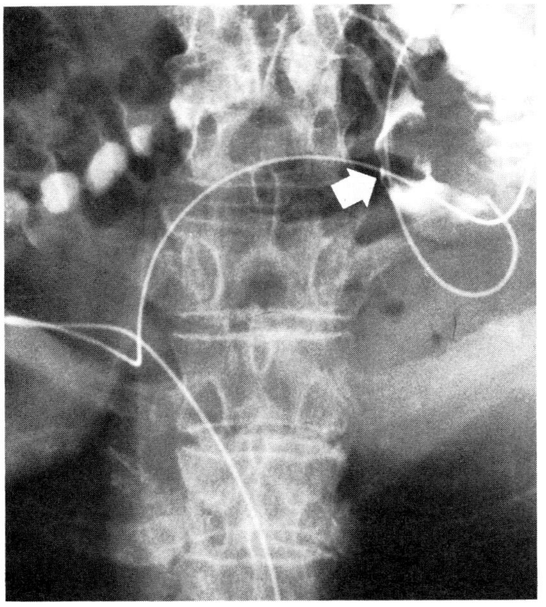

Figure 25–12. Transnasal cholangiogram showing the tip of the catheter looped in the common hepatic duct.

of chemicals to dissolve stones or reduce their size.

Results of Sphincterotomy and Stone Extraction

The length of hospital stay varies considerably depending upon the type of patient and the difficulty in stone extraction. The average stay for successful procedures is 3 days.

Results of the technique are consistent worldwide (Table 25–1).[7–13] Sphincterotomy fails in 5 to 10 per cent of attempts. The main indication is to remove stones, and this can be achieved in 80 to 90 per cent of cases.[14] The problems of particularly large stones are discussed further on.

Complications

In addition to its own risks, duodenoscopic sphincterotomy carries the usual risks of ERCP (Chapter 11), but these should be vanishingly small in the hands of experts. The short-term hazards of sphincterotomy itself are outlined in Table 25–1. The overall incidence is around 8 per cent, with fewer than half these patients requiring urgent surgical intervention.[14, 15] Bleeding is more likely with long cuts but is otherwise unpredictable and depends on local anatomic variations. Most large series report an incidence of bleeding of 2 to 5 per cent, but it was 9 per cent in one series.[16] The cause of severe bleeding in usually a retroduodenal artery that runs anterior to the common bile duct. Because of the rich collateral net of duodenopancreatic arteries, embolization is ineffective to control bleeding and direct operative control of the bleeding vessel is preferable. The incidence of retroperitoneal perforation is also related to the length of the cut. Most of these patients do not require surgery. Pancreatitis has been described when the pancreatic duct has been cut inadvertently, and it may occur during passage of stones. Cholangitis is most likely when sphincterotomy fails, or when calculi are retained for long periods thereafter; this risk may be minimized by the technique of transnasal biliary catheterization.[6, 17] Stone impaction can occur spontaneously or during basket extraction.

The mortality rate for endoscopic sphincterotomy is approximately 1.5 per cent.[7–12, 18] Deaths have followed all the complications listed in Table 25–1.

The Problem of Large Stones

Large stones are remarkably common and pose therapeutic problems. Their size influences the risk of complications and the like-

Table 25–1 RESULTS OF ENDOSCOPIC SPHINCTEROTOMY

Source		Total Patients	Sphincterotomy Success (%)	Complications: *Totals (%)*	*Deaths (%)*	*Bleed*	*Perforation*	*Pancreatitis*	*Cholangitis/impaction*
Surveys									
International	1978	3618	90.5	254(7.0)	50(1.4)	90	40	48	76
Great Britain	1979	679	87	58(8.5)	7(1.0)	17	5	20	16
USA	1980	1250	89	109(8.7)	15(1.2)	29	14	41	25

lihood of successful removal. With the standard cut of about 15 mm, all stones smaller than the duodenoscope on radiographic film (13 mm, representing 10 mm in reality) should pass spontaneously or be extractable. Stones up to 25 mm in diameter have been removed, but the likelihood of success is also dependent upon the shape of the distal bile duct.

Careful clinical assessment is essential in each patient to balance the risks of a larger sphincterotomy with those of exploratory surgery. It may be clinically justifiable to perform duodenoscopic sphincterotomy to provide emergency drainage (including a transnasal catheter) in severely ill patients even when the stones appear too large to be removed by endoscopic techniques. Some large stones are soft and can be fragmented.[19] This is easier to do with stronger baskets (used through a larger-channeled instrument), and balloon catheters are ideal for removal of small fragments and sludge. Even larger instruments allow the development of effective crushing forceps. Attempts have been made to fragment stones within the ductal system using electrohydrolysis[20] and an ultrasonic probe.[21] An alternative adjuvant method is to dissolve stones in situ[22] or reduce their size so that they can pass spontaneously. The technique of transnasal biliary catheterization allows biliary perfusion for days and weeks.[17, 23–25] The development of effective and safe chemicals will have a major therapeutic impact and may allow stone dissolution without sphincterotomy.

Potential Long-Term Complications

The short-term risks of endoscopic sphincterotomy are now established (Table 25–1). Final conclusions about the role of the technique will depend upon the long-term results, in particular, whether patients develop stenosis or cholangitis. Experience to date on relatively large numbers of patients followed for several years suggests that long-term complications are rare.[26, 31]

Although many centers have now reported follow-up of up to 5 years,[26–28] there are still no 10-year follow-up studies. Long-term results so far indicate that papillary stenosis following sphincterotomy is rare[27] but does occur.[29] Experience of surgical sphincter procedures and choledochoduodenostomy suggests that cholangitis occurs only if the orifice is too small; reflux of intestinal content up the bile duct does not cause problems if efflux is free. Thus, the important question appears to be whether or not the endoscopic sphincterotomy orifice remains widely patent. The duodenoscope provides an ideal tool for investigating this possibility. Patients can be examined at intervals by endoscopy, cholangiography, sphincter manometry,[30] and balloon catheter measurement of the orifice.

Indications[31]

Duodenoscopic Sphincterotomy for Stones

The technique is quick, cheap, acceptable to patients, and relatively safe. Its application depends upon the alternatives available to the individual patient and, particularly, upon their relative risks.

After Cholecystectomy. The prototype indication for sphincterotomy is removal of stones from the common bile duct of a patient who has undergone cholecystectomy previously (Fig. 25–13).[32, 66] Hitherto the only alternative to surgery has been oral treatment with bile salts, which appears relatively inef-

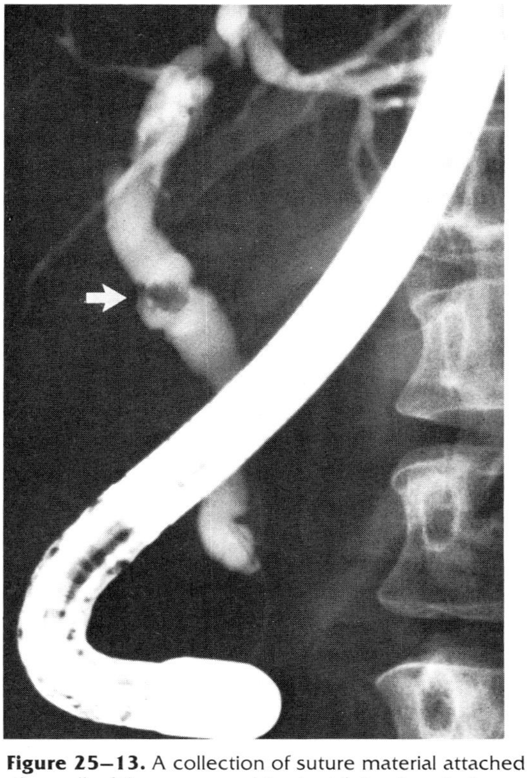

Figure 25–13. A collection of suture material attached to the wall of the common bile duct following cholecystectomy.

fective. The risks of biliary tract surgery depend upon several factors. Common duct exploration is more hazardous than simple cholecystectomy, and re-exploration may be even more difficult. Age has a crucial influence on the outcome. In patients aged less than 50 or 60 years, published mortality rates for common duct exploration average 1.5 per cent; in older persons the figure rises beyond 5 per cent.[33–35] The overall mortality for duodenoscope sphincterotomy is around 1.5 per cent, and most series largely concern elderly and frail patients; 75 per cent of our patients are more than 65 years old. Duodenoscopic sphincterotomy is thus clearly safer than surgery in elderly and high-risk patients and should now be considered their treatment of choice.[36] In younger patients the short-term risks of sphincterotomy and surgery are comparable; the potential long-term risks of sphincterotomy have to be weighed against the short-term advantage that it is easier, quicker, and cheaper for the patient. Our own results have so far encouraged us to use endoscopic sphincterotomy even in patients who have no medical or surgical contraindication to further operation; the wisdom of this decision has yet to be proved.

Patients With T-Tube Drainage Soon After Cholecystectomy. Several other therapeutic techniques can be considered when stones are discovered on a postoperative T-tube cholangiogram.[37] Perfusing the bile duct with chemicals to dissolve stones is time-consuming (and therefore expensive) and is often ineffective with current solvents; the situation would change quickly if more effective solvents were available. Stones can be extracted with forceps or steerable baskets[38] via the T-tube tract; the T-tube must be large and left in place for 4 to 6 weeks after surgery (see Chapter 10). A small fiberscope can be used by the same route.[61, 65] These T-tube tract techniques are preferred to sphincterotomy when conditions are right, since they do not compromise the sphincter of Oddi. However, sphincterotomy is an effective method when the T-tube is too small or incorrectly placed. If the stone lies below the T-tube, it will pass rapidly when contrast medium or saline is infused through the tube; when the stone lies in the common hepatic duct, it may be necessary to remove the tube to allow the stone to pass.

Patients With a Gallbladder. There are indications for sphincterotomy in patients who have not (yet) undergone cholecystectomy.

Acute Cholangitis and Choledocholithiasis. Sphincterotomy can provide emergency drainage in patients with severe cholangitis. Sphincterotomy and biliary catheterization can defuse the situation even if the stones are not immediately removed. The indwelling tube allows repeated cultures of the bile and infusion of antibiotics. Cholecystectomy can be performed after the acute illness has subsided. However, in some elderly patients in whom the common bile duct has been cleared of stones by sphincterotomy, it is justifiable not to proceed with cholecystectomy but to simply await events. For example, of 44 patients (mean age 75 years) discharged from our unit with the gallbladder in place after sphincterotomy, only five have so far required cholecystectomy for symptoms in a mean follow-up of 18 months.[39] There are now sizable groups of patients who have had sphincterotomy and in whom the gallbladder has not been removed who have been followed for more than 5 years. Between 10 and 20 per cent of these patients have required cholecystectomy.[14, 27, 40, 42] Many patients with common duct stones have a dilated cystic duct, through which relatively small gallbladder stones can pass spontaneously. Thus, sphincterotomy with transampullary choledocholithotomy leaving the gallbladder in situ appears to be a reasonable alternative in debilitated elderly patients who present with choledocholithiasis and who have no symptoms referable to the gallbladder.

It has been suggested that a similar approach should be extended to young and fit patients—that anyone known to have common duct stones should undergo endoscopic sphincterotomy prior to cholecystectomy. This speculation is based on the belief that the combined hazards of endoscopic sphincterotomy and simple cholecystectomy are less than those of cholecystectomy with duct exploration. There is very little proof in support of this speculation, and, for the average patient with choledocholithiasis who is going to have a cholecystectomy, preoperative ERCP or endoscopic papillotomy is not indicated.

Acute Pancreatitis. Endoscopic papillotomy may be indicated in patients with biliary pancreatitis during the acute phase or electively to treat residual choledocholithiasis. There has always been some reluctance to perform endoscopic cannulation and contrast injection of the bile duct in patients with pancreatitis. In 1980, Safrany reported the results of early endoscopic papillotomy (following diagnostic ERCP) for biliary pancreatitis in 15 patients. All patients became pain-free immediately after the procedure. Rapid and marked improvement was observed over the next 2 days in all 15 patients as amylase and bilirubin values became normal.[43] None of these patients appeared to have adverse reactions to the injection of hyperosmolar contrast into the duct of Wirsung. Several authors have since reported similar results.[44–48] Although it is still unclear whether urgent papillotomy will abort the pancreatitis and prevent the development of septic complications, this maneuver appears to be safe and restores ampullary patency without the need for an urgent operation. In the older patient, it may be all that is needed.

Endoscopic papillotomy with transampullary stone extraction is the treatment of choice in patients with previous cholecystectomy and recurrent choledocholithiasis.

Duodenoscopic Sphincterotomy for Papillary Stenosis

The concept of noncalculous "papillary stenosis" remains controversial.[49] It is mainly discussed in relation to postcholecystectomy symptoms. To some authors, papillary stenosis is a common diagnosis; others deny its existence. ERCP provides a new diagnostic method allowing examination of the papilla of Vater as well as detailed duct radiology, but there are still many problems. The radiologic appearance of the lower end of the bile duct varies considerably in health, and definitions of minor abnormalities are imprecise. Overall duct size is helpful only if previous radiographs are available for comparison. It is difficult to rely on bile duct emptying rates at ERCP, since they are affected by instrumentation and medication. Strict diagnostic criteria for papillary stenosis include histologic abnormalities in the papilla itself; unfortunately, endoscopic biopsies are not deep enough to provide adequate specimens. Duodenoscopy allows pressure measurements in and across the sphincter of Oddi.[30] It is simple to demonstrate that duodenoscopic sphincterotomy abolishes the gradient between the bile duct and duodenum, but we have not yet seen a convincing role for these measurements in the classification of patients with problems after cholecystectomy.

Like other groups,[7–12, 49] we have performed a small number of duodenoscopic sphincterotomies for "papillary stenosis" despite diagnostic and conceptual difficulties. The attempt seems justified in patients who are suffering from repeated and severe episodes of biliary type pain associated with biochemical evidence of cholestasis, particularly if the bile duct increases in size (as judged by repeated ERCP). Retrograde cholangiography often reproduces the pain in such patients. Good short-term results have been achieved in many patients subjected to sphincterotomy. However, Roberts-Thompson and Toouli obtained relief of biliary type pain in only 13 per cent of a group of 50 patients. They did not find the size of the common bile duct or the results of morphine-prostigmine test or endoscopic manometry to be of help in selecting patients who were likely to obtain good results.[50] Thus, sphincterotomy in this context remains experimental.

Malignant Stenosis of the Papilla

Duodenoscopy is the best method for diagnosing tumors of the papilla; it combines macroscopic examination and radiology with brush cytology and forceps biopsy.[1] Endoscopic drainage of malignant biliary obstruction can be accomplished by sphincterotomy in papillary tumors; it may be the only treatment indicated in elderly and frail patients[49] or as a method of preoperative biliary decompression.[40] Indeed, in some cases the tumor has become apparent only after sphincterotomy for "benign stenosis." The method is similar to that of standard sphincterotomy for stones when the biliary orifice of the ampulla can be identified. If this is not possible, the common bile duct may be punctured directly using diathermy through the duodenal wall above the papilla.[51] Higher strictures cannot be treated this way; however, flexible guide wires can be passed even in those that show a complete block to the passage of contrast. A nasobiliary tube or a biliary prosthesis can then be threaded over the wires and the obstructed duct drained (Fig. 25–14).[51, 52]

Endoscopic insertion of biliary prosthesis is successful in 80 to 90 per cent of cases, with few early complications. Current 10 French gauge prostheses block after 6 or 7 months but are easy to change.

Pancreatic Duct Stenosis

Surgical sphincterotomy or sphincteroplasty used to be a popular procedure in patients with recurrent pancreatitis. In some

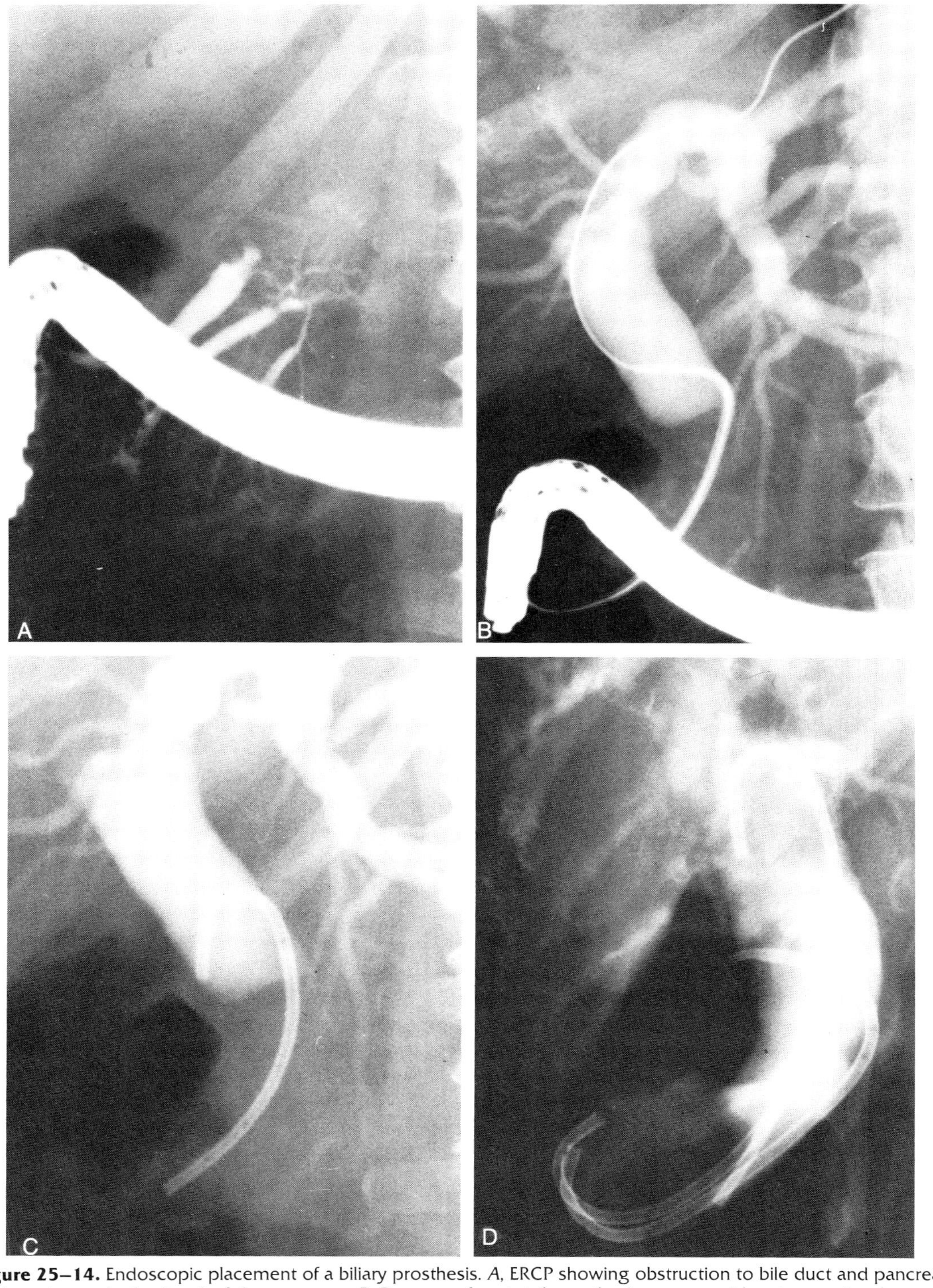

Figure 25–14. Endoscopic placement of a biliary prosthesis. *A*, ERCP showing obstruction to bile duct and pancreatic duct by a tumor in the head of the pancreas. *B*, Passage of a pigtail prosthesis over a guide wire previously passed through the malignant stricture. *C*, Single pigtail prosthesis in place. *D*, Same patient. Two further double-pigtail prostheses in place.

patients this may have helped by allowing small gallstones to pass. A large experience of endoscopic pancreatography indicates that stenosis of the pancreatic duct orifice itself is a very rare cause or association of pancreatitis. Thus, there can be few indications for endoscopic sphincterotomy at this orifice, even if its safety were established. Congenital stenosis at the accessory papilla may be important when Santorini's duct forms the main drainage channel for the pancreas; we have performed duodenoscopic sphincterotomy at the accessory papilla.[41]

Problems After Choledochoduodenostomy

A standard choledochoduodenostomy stoma is always easily visible in the roof of the distal duodenal bulb. Stomal stenosis may occasionally be associated with retained suture material, which can be removed endoscopically, and true stenosis can be treated by sphincterotomy or dilatation; so far, experience is limited. Following side-to-side choledochoduodenostomy, biliary sludge, stones, and food residue may accumulate in the bile duct between the stoma and the papilla and give rise to pain or pancreatitis, called the sump syndrome. Duodenoscopic sphincterotomy at the papilla is effective treatment.[56–58]

Occasionally surgeons produce choledochoduodenal fistulae just above the papilla of Vater when attempting to dilate it. This lesion is rarely clinically significant. When recurrent attacks of cholangitis occur, the bile duct orifice can be enlarged by connecting the fistula to the normal papillary orifice, using duodenoscopic sphincterotomy. Conversely, endoscopic diathermy puncture of the bile duct through the duodenal mucosa above the papilla has been suggested as a form of treatment for patients with papillary stenosis.

Other Therapeutic Techniques in the Bile Duct (and Gallbladder)

Noncalculous Filling Defects. Duodenoscopic sphincterotomy has been used for the removal of foreign bodies, such as worms and shrapnel, from the bile duct. Suture material occasionally compromises the bile duct lumen after cholecystectomy (Fig. 25–13). Removal by diathermy snare is safe only if performed under direct vision with a special instrument. Blood clot can accumulate in the bile duct after trauma to the liver or biliary tree and in patients with bile duct tumors. Blood usually passes spontaneously but can be flushed out with an endoscopic catheter.

Bile Duct Strictures. Endoscopic cholangiography provides good documentation of benign strictures of the bile duct, and attempts are now being made to dilate such strictures with balloon catheters (Fig. 25–15). In some cases it is desirable to leave a catheter through the stricture for several weeks; stones that are formed above it can be dissolved or fragmented.

Access to the Gallbladder. Currently it is difficult (but not impossible—Fig. 25–16) to manipulate instruments into the gallbladder endoscopically via the papilla; attempts are being made to place catheters in the gallbladder for infusion of chemicals (Fig. 25–17).

Combined Percutaneous and Duodenoscopic Approach. Duodenoscopic cannulation of the lower bile duct may fail in 5 to 10 per cent of attempts owing to difficult access (large diverticula) or sphincter stenosis. Cannulation and subsequent sphincterotomy can be facilitated by prior passage of a guide wire through the papilla from above (via the standard percutaneous transhepatic route or through any percutaneous fistula). The presence of a wire protruding through the papilla may be sufficient to allow duodenoscopic cannulation; in other cases it is necessary to pass a dilating balloon catheter over the guide wire.[62]

Peroral Choledochoscopy. Standard forward-viewing "pediatric" endoscopes can be passed via the mouth and into the bile duct directly through a sphincterotomy orifice, or through the stoma of a choledochoduodenostomy. The intact papilla will not accept an instrument larger than 3 mm in diameter. The first "baby" fiberscopes (3 mm in diameter) were designed to be used like cannulas, manipulated through "mother" instruments into the biliary or pancreatic duct system.[63]

These fiberscopes did not have controlled-tip deflection or channels for passing therapeutic devices. The latest prototype peroral choledochoscope is 5 mm in diameter, with controlled-tip deflection and an operating channel. The instrument allows therapeutic maneuvers, such as stone extraction and local diathermy in the bile duct, under direct vision.

Percutaneous Choledochoscopy. Small-caliber fiberscopes can be passed percutaneously into the bile duct through the tract

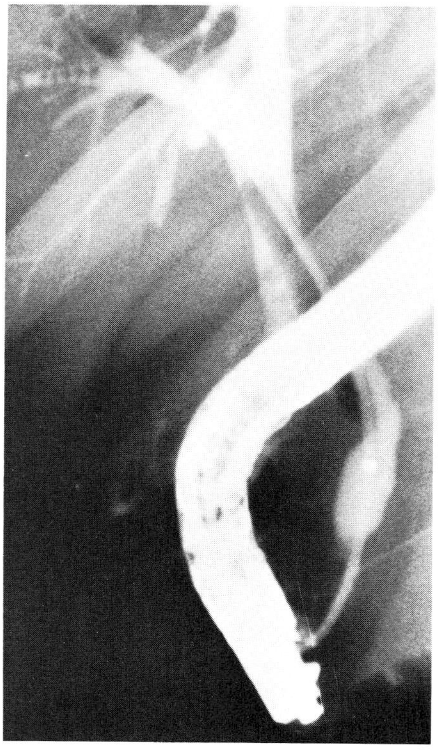

Figure 25–15. Use of dilating balloon catheter in the bile duct.

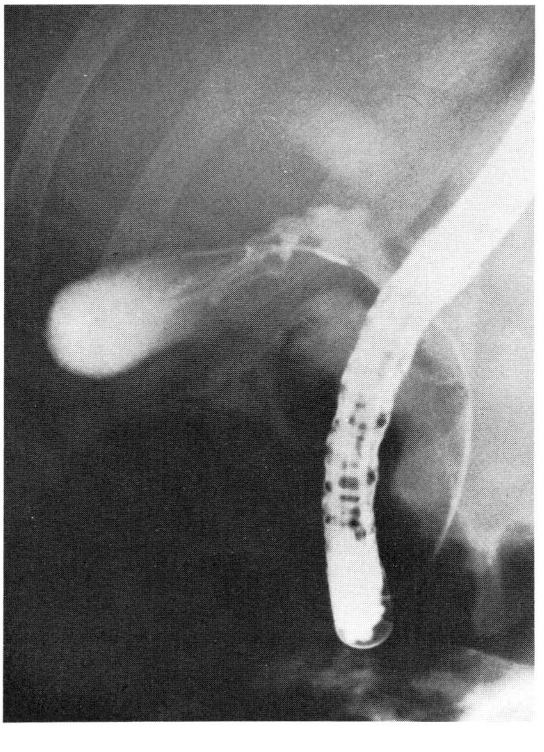

Figure 25–16. A stone basket has been passed into the gallbladder.

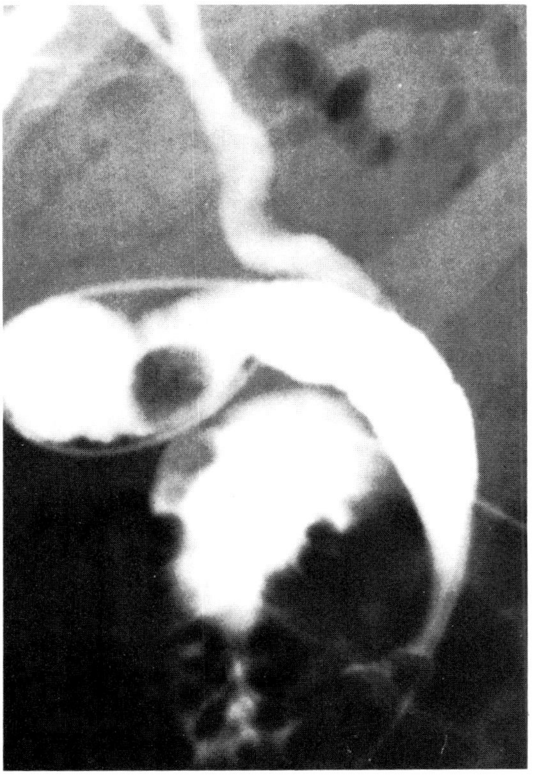

Figure 25–17. A pernasal tube looped in the gallbladder for infusion of chemicals around a gallbladder stone.

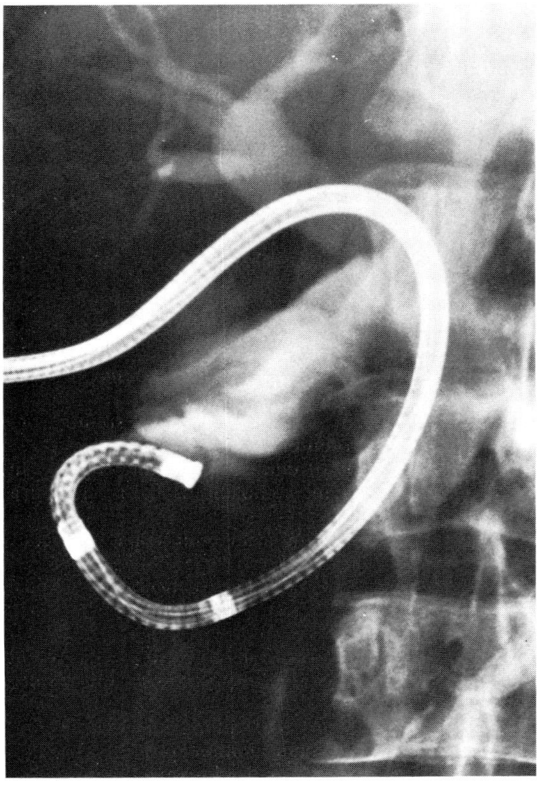

Figure 25–18. Choledochoscopy via the T-tube track; the tip of the instrument has been retroverted to provide a view of the papilla from within the duodenum.

left immediately after removal of a T-tube drain (Fig. 25–18).[64, 65] By this means, it is possible to extract retained stones under direct vision. The advantage of this method over the simpler steerable basket system is the great reduction in fluoroscopy time. The disadvantage, apart from the additional cost, is that because the instruments are larger it may be necessary to dilate the T-tube tract prior to intubation.

REFERENCES

1. Cotton PB: Progress report ERCP. Gut 1977;*18:*316.
2. Classen M, Demling L: Endoskopische sphincterotomie der papilla Vateri. Dtsch Med Wochenschr 1974;*99:*496.
3. Kawai K, Akasaka Y, Mirakami K, et al: Endoscopic sphincterotomy of the ampulla of Vater. Gastrointest Endosc 1974;*20:*148.
4. Cotton PB, Chapman M, Whiteside CG, et al: Duodenoscopic papillotomy and gallstone removal. Br J Surg 1976;*63:*709.
5. Sohma S, Matsuda T, Fujita R, et al: Endoscopic papillotomy: a new approach for extraction of residual stones. Gastrointest Endosc 1974;*16:*452.
6. Cotton PB, Burney PJG, Mason RR: Trans-nasal bile duct catheterization after endoscopic sphincterotomy. Gut 1979;*20:*285.
7. Reiter JJ, Bayer HB, Mennicken C, et al: Results of endoscopic papillotomy: a collective experience from nine endoscopic centres in West Germany. World J Surg 1978;*2:*505.
8. Geenan JE, Vennes JA, Silvis SE: Resume of a seminar on endoscopic retrograde sphincterotomy (ERS). Gastrointest Endosc 1981;*27:*31.
9. Cotton PB, Vallon AG: British experience with duodenal sphincterotomy for treatment of bile duct stones. Br J Surg 1981;*68:*373.
10. Safrany L: Duodenoscopic sphincterotomy and gallstone removal. Gastroenterology 1977;*72:*338.
11. Safrany L, Cotton PB: Endoscopic management of choledocholithiasis. Surg Clin North Am 1982;*62:*825.
12. Cotton PB: Non-operative removal of bile duct stones by duodenoscopic sphincterotomy. Br J Surg 1980;*67:*1.
13. Taylor BR, Ho CS: Nonsurgical treatment of common-bile-duct stones. Can J Surg 1984;*27:*28.
14. Silvis SE: Current status of endoscopic sphincterotomy. Am J Gastroenterol 1984;*79:*731.
15. Lam SK: A study of endoscopic sphincterotomy in recurrent pyogenic cholangitis. Br J Surg 1984;*71:*262.
16. Goodall RJR: Bleeding after endoscopic sphincterotomy. J R Coll Surg (Engl) 1985;*67:*87.
17. Kozarek RA: Transnasal pancreaticobiliary drains: indications and insertion technique. Am J Surg 1983;*146:*250.
18. Siegel JH: Endoscopic papillotomy in the treatment of biliary tract disease: 258 procedures and results. Dig Dis Sci 1981;*26:*1057.
19. Riemann JF, Seubert K, Demling L: Clinical application of a new mechanical lithotripter for smashing common bile duct stones. Endoscopy 1982;*14:*226.
20. Koch H, Stolte M, Walz V: Endoscopic lithotripsy in the common bile duct. Endoscopy 1977;*9:*95.
21. Davis H, Bean WJ, Barnes FS: Breaking up residual gallstones with an ultrasonic drill. Lancet 1977;*2:*226.
22. Way LW, Admirand WG, Dunphy JF: Management of choledocholithiasis. Ann Surg 1972;*176:*347.
23. Cotton PB, Vallon AG, Mason RR: Intraductal infusion of mono-octanoin for common duct stones. Lancet 1981;*1:*436.
24. Witzel L, Wiederholt J, Wolbert E: Dissolution of gallstones by perfusion with Capmul via a catheter introduced endoscopically into the bile duct. N Engl J Med 1980;*303:*465.
25. Siegel JH, Yatto RP: Biliary endoprostheses for the management of retained common bile duct stones. Am J Gastroenterol 1984;*79:*50.
26. Riemann JF, Lux G, Förster P, Altendorf A: Long-term results after endoscopic papillotomy. Endoscopy 1983;*15:*165.
27. Escourrou J, Cordova JA, Lazorthes F, Frexinos J, Ribet A: Early and late complications after endoscopic sphincterotomy for biliary lithiasis with and without the gall bladder 'in situ.' Gut 1984;*25:*598.
28. Rosch W, Riemann JF, Lux G, et al: Long term follow-up after endoscopic sphincterotomy. Endoscopy 1981;*13:*152.
29. Richieri JP, Pelissier G: Early papillary stenosis following successful endoscopic sphincterotomy for residual common bile duct stone. Endoscopy 1984;*16:*77.
30. Geenen JE, Hogan WJ, Schaffer RD, et al: Endoscopic electrosurgical papillotomy and manometry in biliary tract disease. JAMA 1977;*237:*2075.
31. Cotton PB: Endoscopic treatment of bile duct stones (apples and oranges). Gut 1984;*25:*587.
32. Demling L: Endoscopic papillotomy (EPT). Endoscopy 1983;*15:*162.
33. Glenn F, Hays DM: The age factor in the mortality rate of patients undergoing surgery of the biliary tract. Surg Gynecol Obstet 1955;*100:*11.
34. Haff RC, Butcher HR, Ballinger WF: Biliary tract operations. A review of 1000 patients. Arch Surg 1969;*98:*428.
35. Wenckert A, Robertson B: The natural course of gallstone disease. Gastroenterology 1977;*50:*376.
36. Mee AS, Vallon AG, Croker JR, et al: Non-operative removal of bile duct stones by duodenoscopic sphincterotomy in the elderly. Br Med J 1981;*3:*521.
37. Classen M, Ossenberg FW: The non-surgical removal of common bile duct stones. Gut 1977;*18:*760.
38. Burhenne HJ: Non-operative instrumental extraction of retained common bile duct stones. World J Surg 1978;*2:*439.
39. Cotton PB, Vallon AG: Duodenoscopic sphincterotomy for removal of bile duct stones in patients with gallbladders. Surgery 1982;*91:*628.
40. Alderson D, Lavelle MI, Venables CW: Endoscopic sphincterotomy before pancreatic-duodenectomy for ampullary carcinoma. Br Med J 1981;*282:*1109.
41. Cotton PB: Endoscopic sphincterotomy at the accessory papilla. Endosc Dig 1978;*3:*27.
42. Neoptolemos JP, Carr-Locke DL, Fraser I, et al: The management of common bile duct calculi by endoscopic sphincterotomy in patients with gallbladders in situ. Br J Surg 1984;*71:*69.
43. Safrany L, Neuhaus B, Krause S, Portocarrero G, Schott B: Endoskopische papillotomie bei akuter, biliar bedingter pankreatitis: Dtsch Med Wochenschr 1980;*105:*115.

44. Safrany L, Cotton PB: A preliminary report. Urgent duodenoscopic sphincterotomy for acute gallstone-related pancreatitis. Surgery 1981;*89*:424.
45. van der Spuy S: Endoscopic sphincterotomy in the management of gallstone pancreatitis. Endoscopy 1981;*13*:25.
46. Rosseland AR, Solhaug JH: Early or delayed endoscopic papillotomy (EPT) in gallstone pancreatitis. Ann Surg 1984;*199*:165.
47. Neoptolemos JP, London N, Slater N, Carr-Locke DL, Fossard DP, Moossa AR: A prospective study of ERCP and endoscopic sphincterotomy in the diagnosis and treatment of gallstone acute pancreatitis. Arch Surg, in press.
48. Roesch W, Demling L: Endoscopic management of pancreatitis. Surg Clin North Am 1982;*62*:845.
49. Classen M: Endoscopic approach to papillary stenosis. Endoscopy 1981;*13*:154.
50. Roberts-Thompson IC, Toouli J: Is endoscopic sphincterotomy for disabling biliary-type pain after cholecystectomy effective? Gastrointest Endosc 1985;*31*.370.
51. Cotton PB: Endoscopic methods for relief of malignant obstructive jaundice. World J Surg 1984;*8*:854.
52. Leung JWC, Emery R, Cotton PB, Russell RCG, Vallon AG, Mason RR: Management of malignant obstructive jaundice at The Middlesex Hospital. Br J Surg 1983;*70*:584.
53. Huibregtse K, Tytgat G: Palliative treatment of obstructive jaundice by a trans-papillary introduced large bore bile duct endoprosthesis. Experience in 45 patients. Gut 1982;*23*:371.
54. Riemann JF, Lux G, Rusch W, Beickert-Sterba A: Non-surgical biliary drainage. Technique, indication and results. Endoscopy 1981;*13*:157.
55. Zimmon DS, Clemett AR: Endoscopic stents and drains in the management of pancreatic bile duct obstruction. Surg Clin North Am 1982;*62*:837.
56. Siegel JH: Duodenoscopic sphincterotomy in the treatment of the "sump syndrome." Dig Dis Sci 1981;*26*:922.
57. Baker AR, Neoptolemos JP, Carr-Locke DL, Fossard DP: Sump syndrome following choledochoduodenostomy and its endoscopic treatment. Br J Surg 1985;*72*:433.
58. Tanaka M, Ikeda S, Yoshimoto H: Endoscopic sphincterotomy for the treatment of biliary sump syndrome. Surgery 1983;*93*:264.
59. Laurence BH, Cotton PB: Decompression of malignant biliary obstruction by duodenoscopic intubation of bile duct. Br Med J 1980;*1*:522.
60. Cotton PB: Duodenoscopic placement of biliary prostheses in malignant obstructive jaundice. Br J Surg 1982;*69*:501.
61. Berei G, Hamlin JA, Grundfest WS: Combined fluorendoscopic removal of retained biliary stones. Arch Surg 1983;*118*:1395.
62. Shorvon PJ, Cotton PB, Mason RR, et al: Percutaneous transhepatic assistance for duodenoscopic sphincterotomy. Gut 1985;*26*:1373.
63. Urakame Y: Per-oral cholangio-pancreatography (PTPS) and per-oral direct cholangioscopy (PDCS). Endoscopy 1980;*12*:30.
64. Himal HS: Endoscopic sphincterotomy. Can J Surg 1984;*27*:6.
65. Yamakawa T, Komaki F, Shikata J: Experience with routine postoperative choledoscopy via the T-tube sinus track. World J Surg 1978;*2*:379.

L. H. BLUMGART, M.D.,
R. F. McCLOY, M.D.

26

Postcholecystectomy Syndrome

ENDOSCOPIC TECHNIQUES AFTER CHOLECYSTECTOMY

The majority of patients with biliary calculi are cured following cholecystectomy and, when necessary, choledocholithotomy.[1–4] Indeed, of all patients who undergo cholecystectomy for gallstones, only 5 per cent have significant persistent or recurrent symptoms.[5] However, diagnosis of the cause of symptoms in these patients may be extremely difficult, and the need for further laparotomy may not be clear. While laparotomy performed on the basis of symptoms alone may result in an operative diagnosis, this is frequently not the case. Adhesions may hinder the exploration, and operative cholangiography may be difficult to perform in a patient who has previously had surgery. Abnormalities at the site of previously constructed surgical anastomoses are not readily diagnosed by external inspection at laparotomy. For these reasons, reoperation without an exact preoperative diagnosis frequently results in frustration for the surgeon and continued symptoms for the patient.[6] It is clear that the need for precise preoperative information in biliary tract surgery is nowhere more evident than in this group of patients.

In the past, intravenous cholangiography has been a mainstay in the diagnosis of patients who are symptomatic after cholecystectomy, and indeed it gives positive information in many cases. However, it is valueless in the presence of jaundice and inaccurate and imprecise in many nonjaundiced patients.[6] Even when the duct is adequately opacified, a definitive diagnosis may not be possible; stones may be present in a common bile duct thought to be normal (Fig. 26–1), or they may be absent from a dilated duct.

Recent years have seen extraordinary innovations in the imaging techniques available for diagnosis of biliary tract disorders. These developments have provided hitherto unforeseen possibilities in gathering exact information on which to base therapy and have resulted in the formation of new diagnostic approaches, especially for jaundiced patients. A major discussion has centered around the specific indications for these diagnostic procedures.[7,8] In our clinic, an integrated approach to the diagnosis of biliary tract obstruction has been established.[9,10] This relies on the initial use of ultrasonography and fine needle percutaneous transhepatic cholangiography (PTC), reserving endoscopic retrograde cholangiopancreatography (ERCP) for those patients in whom ductal anatomy is not outlined by fine needle PTC. This approach is *not* adhered to in the postcholecystectomy patient, in whom it is frequently important to perform not only cholangiography but also pancreatography,[11] cytology, and biopsy, and in whom inspection of the papilla of Vater or surgically created stomas are often essential for full diagnosis.[11–15]

Patients referred to our department with postcholecystectomy symptoms have usually already undergone many tests. Previous x-rays, including operative cholangiograms, T-tube cholangiograms, and intravenous cholangiograms, which may reveal a previously unsuspected diagnosis, are studied (Fig. 26–2). However, even if the biliary ductal system has been completely opacified and is considered normal, ERCP is performed, provided that there is clinical or biochemical evidence suggesting upper gastrointestinal disease, biliary obstruction, or pancreatitis. Endoscopy and ERCP are carried out in the x-ray department. The endoscopic and radiologic techniques have been previously described.[16,17] In all patients, an attempt is made to outline both the biliary and the pancreatic ductal systems; however, if an abnormality has been demonstrated in either the biliary or the pancreatic duct and the diagnosis is

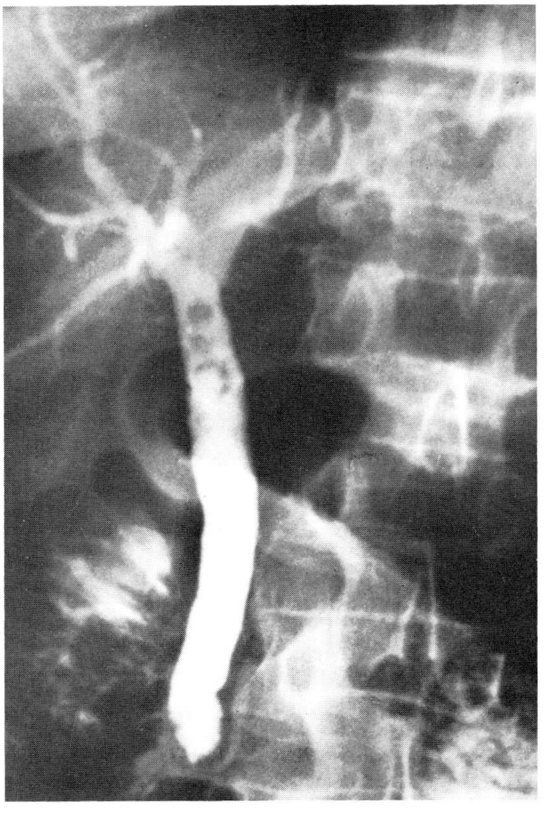

Figure 26–1. Stones within the common bile duct in a woman aged 52 years who was suffering from recurrent attacks of dyspeptic pain and ill health. Liver function tests showed no abnormality. Previous intravenous cholangiography was reported as normal. Note that the extrahepatic bile ducts are not grossly dilated. (From Blumgart LH, Carachi R, Imrie CW, et al: Br J Surg *64*:809, 1977.)

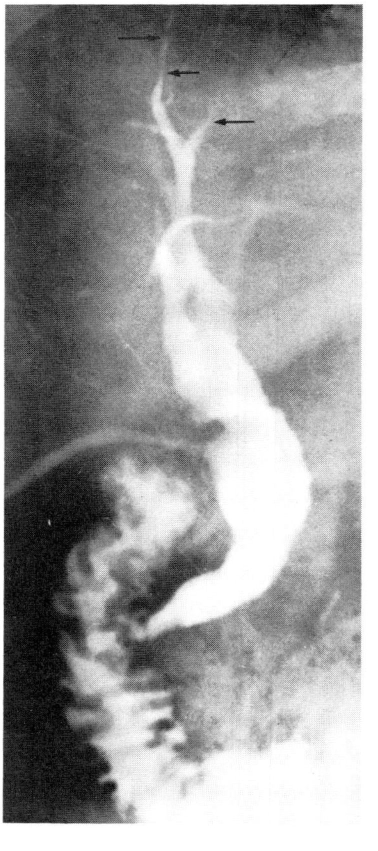

Figure 26–2. T-tube cholangiogram in a middle-aged woman who had recently undergone cholecystectomy for gallstones and exploration of the common bile duct for choledocholithiasis. Jaundice failed to subside. Examination of intrahepatic biliary radicles reveals irregular stricturing (*arrows*). Bile obtained from the T-tube and submitted to cytologic study revealed the presence of many malignant cells.

clear-cut, prolonged attempts to cannulate the remaining duct are not always made. During the examination, the duodenal cap and stomach are examined for associated lesions, such as duodenal or gastric ulceration. Following the examination, the patient is kept in the hospital overnight, serum amylase being measured within 3 hours of the procedure and again 15 hours later if pain or nausea is present. Complications are recorded.

The problems that may arise after cholecystectomy are considered in the following section, and the value of endoscopy and ERCP is evaluated. In addition, techniques allowing endoscopic papillotomy and removal of gallstones from the common bile duct are assessed.[18,19]

POSTCHOLECYSTECTOMY PROBLEMS

There is no such entity as a specific postcholecystectomy syndrome.[3] Although symptoms may arise as a result of abnormalities within the biliary tree or pancreas, they may be the result of associated disease, such as peptic ulceration, hiatus hernia, or diverticular disease of the colon. Furthermore, neuromuscular disorders associated with bile reflux into the stomach may occur in some patients with gallstones, and this may account for persistent flatulent dyspepsia. It has been proposed that many of these patients have a psychosomatic origin for their symptoms,[20] and indeed psychologic stress acting through the autonomic nervous system may be a factor in some cases.[21] It is thus most important in the diagnosis of postcholecystectomy symptoms to differentiate disorders arising in the biliary tree from associated diseases and, in particular, to try to ensure that the symptoms complained of are related to demonstrable abnormalities.

The symptom complex in the postcholecystectomy patient usually comprises dyspepsia or biliary pain, although presentation with jaundice, cholangitis, or pancreatitis is not infrequent. Symptoms may appear immediately after cholecystectomy, and this is especially likely if there has been iatrogenic damage to the biliary ductal system. In a study carried out in our clinic, patients were classified on admission according to their predominant symptom.[6] It was found that 21 of 52 patients suffered from upper abdominal pain, 18 from persistent or recurrent attacks of jaundice, 8 from recurring attacks of biochemically proven pancreatitis, and 5 from recurrent attacks of cholangitis. Many patients, of course, had a combination of these symptoms. The complexity of these cases is emphasized by the fact that no fewer than ten patients had already been submitted to at least one further laparotomy, and in five of these an additional operative procedure had been carried out. Despite this, all remained symptomatic. In a later study,[22] we assessed 157 patients who were symptomatic after cholecystectomy. The predominant problem leading to referral was recurrence of pain similar to that present before cholecystectomy in 57 individuals, development of a new pain considered on clinical grounds to be of biliary origin in 26, pain with raised amylase levels in 14, and jaundice in 57. One patient had rigor as a solitary problem, and in two the postoperative T-tube cholangiogram was equivocal.

We have updated previously published figures[22] for endoscopy and ERCP in this difficult group of patients. We have been able to define the diagnosis in 70 (93 per cent) of 75 patients undergoing ERCP for postcholecystectomy problems with only three (4 per cent) failed cannulations and two (3 per cent) complications. In patients presenting with biliary colic or dyspepsia, especially when their symptoms are similar to those that preceded the cholecystectomy, an abnormality is less often demonstrable than in those presenting with jaundice. In patients with cholangitis or pancreatitis, there was an abnormality on ERCP in every case. Coincidental upper gastrointestinal abnormalities are especially common in the dyspeptic group, and duodenal ulcer is often found even when one previous barium meal has been normal. It is important in such patients to show that the biliary tract and pancreas are normal and uninvolved.[11,12]

However, the majority of patients have abnormalities within the biliary or pancreatic ductal apparatus. Frequently, but by no means always, the symptoms arise as a result of residual common bile duct stones consequent on disease of the biliary tract. However, unsuspected pancreatic disease or a tumor may be present at the time of the original cholecystectomy and may pass unnoticed.[11] We have found persistence of jaundice after cholecystectomy and exploration of the common bile duct particularly sinister in this respect. In a series of 215 patients, we have found eight cases of carcinoma of the papilla of Vater, common bile duct, or pancreas. In other cases, however, symptoms result from complications of additional operative procedures carried out at the time of cholecystectomy.[13] This applies particularly to transduodenal exploration of the common bile duct.

Stones

In Western countries, most stones in the common bile duct come from the gallbladder, although occasionally they may arise primarily within the common bile duct on the basis of biliary stasis and infection. Careful and precise preoperative diagnosis helps to determine the presence of associated lesions and to reduce the frequency of errors in management in such cases. For instance, periampullary or bile duct carcinoma may coexist with common bile duct stones, and the tumor may be missed at initial exploration. We have now seen four patients in whom this sequence has occurred, the final diagnosis being made postoperatively by endoscopy. In jaundiced patients we now usually recommend duodenoscopy before operation, even if gallstones are known to be present. Similarly, common bile duct stones may be responsible for intermittent bouts of jaundice and yet be associated with coexistent hepatocellular disease, such as primary biliary cirrhosis or chronic active hepatitis. Such patients may remain jaundiced after choledocholithotomy.

The routine use of operative cholangiography during cholecystectomy, and in particular postexploratory cholangiography or choledochoscopy, has markedly reduced, but has not abolished, the incidence of residual bile duct stones.[24–30] In addition, information gleaned from operative cholangiography provides useful anatomic information that may prevent operative trauma. Common bile duct stones may remain after exploration of the duct and may be detected during postoperative T-tube cholangiography; furthermore, in some patients the common bile duct has never been explored and operative cholangiography never carried out. The presence of stones at operation has thus never been recognized.

There is a high rate of complications associated with residual common bile duct stones,[31] and since many are potentially serious, removal of the stones is usually advisable. Indeed, of 31 patients we have seen presenting with jaundice, cholangitis, or recurrent pancreatitis after cholecystectomy (in none of whom intravenous cholangiography had yielded the diagnosis), common bile duct stones or biliary mud were present and detected by ERCP in 16. Even in the absence of major complications, we found low-grade ill health and vague upper abdominal pain in three other patients who had no history of jaundice and in two of whom the liver function tests were normal.[6]

Complications of Surgery

Persistent symptoms may result from complications of operative procedures performed at the time of primary cholecystectomy and choledocholithotomy. Such complications arise from damage to the common bile duct, stenosis of surgical anastomoses, or technical errors made in the region of the papilla of Vater.

Supraduodenal choledochotomy is the preferred method of exploring the common bile duct at the primary operation. The procedure is simple in most instances, and there is only a small increase in the morbidity and mortality above that of cholecystectomy alone. It should be noted, however, that there should be no attempts to dilate the papilla of Vater by the passage of metal dilators from above. This is unnecessary, particularly if operative cholangiography has demonstrated free flow of contrast medium into the duodenum. Dilatation of the sphincter may produce acute postoperative pancreatitis or late papillary stenosis.[32,33] In addition, the instrument may perforate the bile duct proximal to the true papilla, producing a choledochoduodenal fistula (Fig. 26–3), which may be associated with late symptoms.[8,13] We have now seen 12 such fistulae, and five have been associated with previous exploration of the bile ducts. We refrain from instrumenting the papilla unless contrast medium fails to enter the duodenum during operative cholangiography. In such cases, a fine bougie or a Fogarty biliary catheter can be passed gently into the duodenum and palpated in the common bile duct behind the mobilized head of the pancreas.

Some surgeons advocate the use of transduodenal sphincterotomy or sphincteroplasty for *primary* exploration of the common bile duct,[34–39] but there seems to be no strong

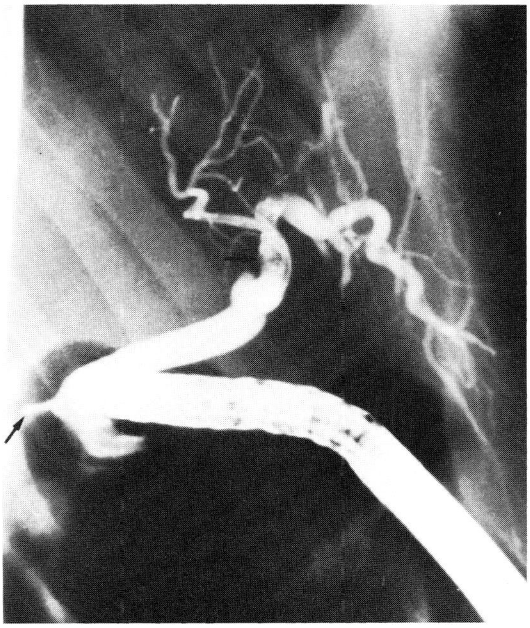

Figure 26–3. ERCP in a 37-year-old man who had previously undergone cholecystectomy and exploration of the common bile duct. The patient presented with recurrent episodes of abdominal pain with hyperamylasemia on several occasions. Note that the catheter inserted into the papilla has passed up the common bile duct to re-enter the duodenum through a choledochoduodenal fistula (lower arrow) well above the papilla of Vater. Within the right and left hepatic ducts and in the common hepatic duct are filling defects (upper arrow) thought to be due to inspissated collections of bile and not to air bubbles. Relief of symptoms followed performance of choledochojejunostomy Roux-en-Y.

argument for this approach unless there is an additional indication for improving biliary drainage. While the procedure is safe in some hands, particularly where widely practiced,[40,41] the morbidity is generally higher than for supraduodenal exploration of the common bile duct.[42–46] Furthermore, the late morbidity of sphincterotomy or sphincteroplasty is not inconsiderable. Restenosis occurs in some patients, and the occasional instance of damage to the orifice of the pancreatic duct may result in late pancreatitis. Even in the presence of a patent sphincteroplasty, the margins of the stoma may become rigid, producing peristomal inflammation and proximal retention of debris within a dilated ductal system.[8] In addition, when performing sphincteroplasty, some surgeons do a supraduodenal choledochotomy and pass a probe through the papilla from above, particularly if there is difficulty in identifying the papilla of Vater from below. The probe does not always pass readily,[41] and a false passage may be produced,[8] the probe or dilator being forced through the duodenal wall proximal to the papilla. Five of the 12 patients with choledochoduodenal fistulae we have seen had undergone an earlier surgical sphincterotomy or sphincteroplasty. The clinical manifestations of these cases may be vague upper abdominal pain and ill health, although jaundice, cholangitis, or recurrent acute pancreatitis may be present (Fig. 26–4).[13] Only endoscopy allows a precise diagnosis to be made.

Citing an otherwise high incidence of recurrent or residual stones, some authors recommend a drainage procedure of the common bile duct at primary operation as a regular concomitant of choledochotomy for gallstone disease.[47–50] Those who oppose this recommendation do so because of increased late morbidity from these procedures. This principally consists of cholangitis from reflux of duodenal contents into the bile duct, or the "sump syndrome" caused by food and bile debris trapped within the intrapancreatic

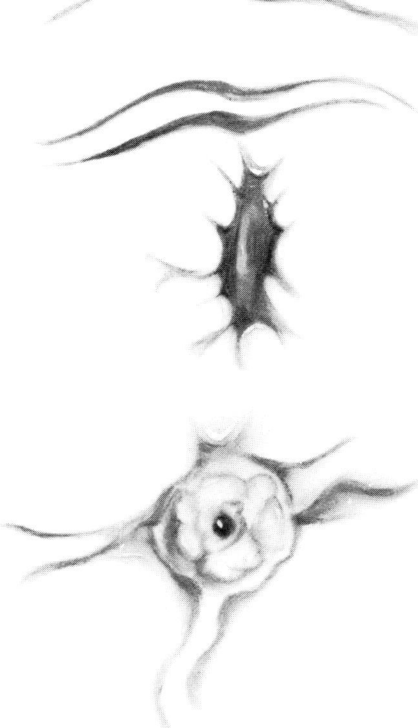

Figure 26–4. Artist's sketch of endoscopic appearance seen in a patient with a normal papilla of Vater and a choledochoduodenal fistula created in error proximal to the true papilla. The patient's operative records noted that sphincteroplasty had been performed.

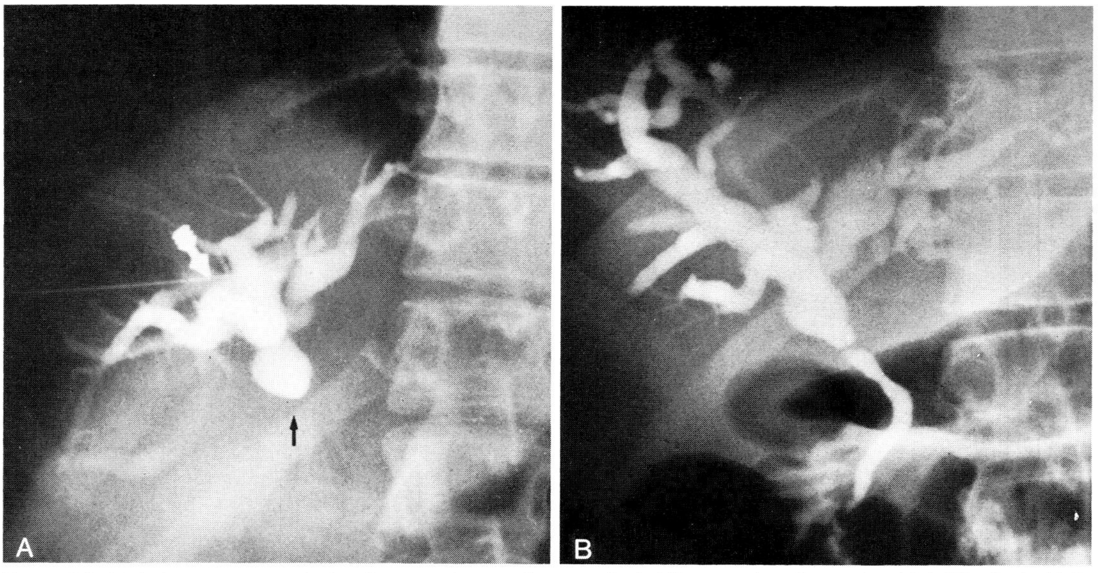

Figure 26–5. *A*, Percutaneous cholangiogram shows a fine needle (white arrow) and reveals a high bile duct stricture in a man presenting with jaundice after cholecystectomy. *B*, ERCP in the same patient reveals a normal common bile duct with a short stricture below the hilus of the liver.

portion of the bile duct after choledochoduodenostomy. We have performed side-to-side choledochoduodenostomy for benign conditions, using indications and techniques similar to those advocated by Madden,[51] Stuart and Hoerr,[52] and Allen and coworkers.[53] Provided that the anastomosis is 2 cm long and the common bile duct is no smaller than 15 mm in diameter, we have never encountered a case of ascending cholangitis. Similar results were reported by Lygidakis[54] and Schein and Gliedman.[55] Complications may occur, however, when a choledochoduodenostomy has been performed on a bile duct of normal caliber. The stomal orifice may be readily seen at endoscopy, and the surgical stoma and papilla may be individually catheterized. Chronic low-grade cholangitis is common following this operation, and we have noted infected inspissated bile aggregates in the common bile duct after ill-considered operations.[6]

Finally, postcholecystectomy symptoms (e.g. jaundice and cholangitis) may be associated with stenosis or stricture of the common bile duct as a result of operative trauma. Over 80 per cent of such injuries follow cholecystectomy, most often an operation that has been considered by the surgeon to be simple and without incident.[56] The majority of patients present within a month or two after surgery with jaundice or biliary fistula, and there is often a history of prolonged biliary drainage or a septic course. Occasionally, the immediate postoperative course is smooth, but the patient experiences late jaundice and cholangitis. Documentation of biliary stricture is usually possible with percutaneous cholangiography, sometimes combined with ERCP (Fig. 26–5).

Jaundice

While jaundice after cholecystectomy is most often the result of a residual common bile duct stone or biliary stricture, there are occasions when this is not so. Sometimes the patient is referred with a T-tube in situ draining freely despite the fact that the patient is still jaundiced (see Fig. 26–2). In others there is no T-tube; here again, endoscopic retrograde cholangiopancreatography is invaluable, since it may demonstrate retained stones, a normal biliary tree, or a residual carcinoma missed at initial laparotomy. The important point is that no patient who is jaundiced after cholecystectomy, and particularly after exploration of the common bile duct, should undergo another operation without preoperative direct cholangiography.

Pancreatic Disease

In many patients who remain symptomatic after cholecystectomy, there is associated dis-

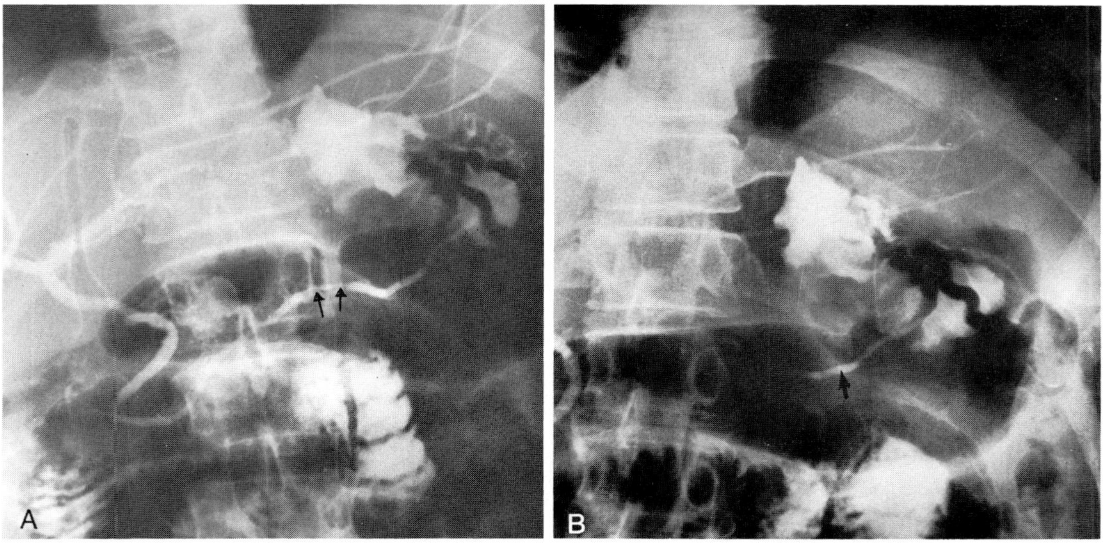

Figure 26–6. *A*, Choledochopancreatography in a 42-year-old woman who had undergone cholecystectomy 15 years earlier. She had experienced recurrent attacks of mild jaundice and at times severe upper abdominal pain. On several occasions a raised serum amylase value was noted in association with the pain. A second operation involved choledochotomy, but no cause for her symptoms was found. Note the normal extra- and intrahepatic bile ducts. The pancreatic duct is normal within the head and neck of the pancreas, but there are two strictures (*arrows*) of the duct in the proximal body with minimal distal dilatation. *B*, Delayed film reveals hold-up of contrast material (*arrow*) beyond the point of stricture 20 minutes after examination. Further investigations showed jaundice to be associated with the Dublin-Johnson syndrome. Distal pancreatectomy was performed, confirming the presence of the strictures and histologic changes of chronic pancreatitis in the distal pancreas. She now has complete relief of symptoms 2½ years after the operation.

ease of the pancreas.[6,11] Some cases involve recurrent acute pancreatitis consequent upon residual common bile duct stones, and the attacks always abate after the offending calculi have been removed. In others, a previous acute pancreatitis has produced a pancreatic ductal stricture or pancreatic cyst (Fig. 26–6). Such a stricture may cause chronic pancreatitis, which presents in due course with increasing pain. It is important to remember that a cholecystectomy may be performed for proven gallstones in a patient with upper abdominal pain, and coexisting chronic pancreatitis may be overlooked. We have seen several such patients who presented with persistent pain in the postoperative period (Fig. 26–7).

Endoscopic retrograde pancreatography has demonstrated chronic pancreatitis with a grossly abnormal duct in patients with biliary disease (not necessarily the cause of it) even in the absence of symptoms.[13] The changes are similar to those thought by Nardi to represent papillary stenosis.[57] The ductal abnormalities are not in themselves sufficient indication for surgery, and surgery should be considered only if the patient has symptoms and if the symptoms persist following abstinence from alcohol.

ENDOSCOPIC PAPILLOTOMY AND REMOVAL OF GALLSTONES

Residual stones can be removed from the common bile duct in a high proportion of patients by transendoscopic sphincterotomy. Cotton[58] reported the results in 134 patients referred for attempted removal of retained stones. Even this highly skilled endoscopist was unsuccessful in removing the stones in 11 per cent of patients, a figure similar to that reported by Safrany.[59] Ten patients, three of whom required emergency surgery, experienced complications, and there was one death. When the stones were 2 cm or more in diameter, the failure rate rose to 39 per cent. The results of endoscopic sphincteroplasty when performed by others are not so successful. Indeed, another series from the United Kingdom[60] showed that patients undergoing this procedure required a mean of 9.5 ± 5 days in the hospital; the duct could be cleared in only 70 per cent of patients, and the complication rate was 30 per cent. One patient of 37 died as a result of the procedure, and another, whose death would have been avoided if he had been treated surgically, died within a year.

A survey of British centers employing en-

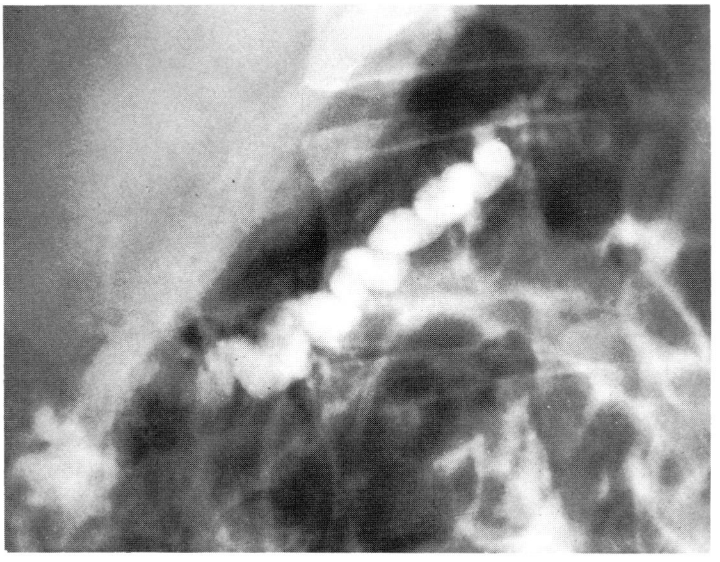

Figure 26–7. Endoscopic retrograde pancreatograpy in a middle-aged woman who admitted to a long history of heavy alcohol consumption. She had recently undergone cholecystectomy for cholelithiasis, and the presence of pancreatic damage had been missed. Note the grossly dilated and irregular pancreatic duct.

doscopic sphincterotomy for removal of common bile duct stones[61] revealed an overall success rate of 76 per cent. Nine deaths (1.2 per cent) were recorded in a total of 721 attempts (of which 590 were successful); the overall morbidity rate was 11 per cent. When complications arise, the majority are related to hemorrhage, pancreatitis, or cholangitis, and it is in this group that the mortality rate is highest. Indeed, of the first 58 patients with complications, 11 required an operation within hours or days, and 7 died.[62] The precise nature and extent of the operation required to achieve control are not detailed. The authors acknowledge, as do others experienced in this field, that the long-term results remain to be assessed.

The results of this and most other series describing endoscopic papillotomy for residual stones compare favorably with surgical series showing a higher mortality and morbidity rate. Indeed, of the 14 centers contributing to the survey,[62] 7 reported that they would always advise endoscopic sphincterotomy, even in low-risk postcholecystectomy cases. However, as pointed out by Girard and Legros,[63] the surgical mortality for reoperation on the common bile duct should be less than 2 per cent. In an analysis of six recent series of reoperations for retained or recurrent bile duct stones, these investigators found a mortality rate of 1.8 per cent in 498 operations, most deaths occurring in the elderly. Another series[64] reported 341 patients in whom choledocholithotomy was carried out for retained or recurrent calculi. Of these patients, 2.1 per cent died, but if patients with cholangitis and pancreatitis were excluded, only four patients (1.2 per cent) died after secondary choledocholithotomy.

There is no question that endoscopic sphincterotomy is ingenious and reasonably safe and can remove retained stones. There is good evidence that this may be the preferred approach in the elderly and in patients at high risk for surgery. On the other hand, there is no doubt that endoscopic sphincterotomy carries its own risks. The appropriateness of this technique in the young or the fit individual is questionable. Furthermore, in patients with large stones or a very large common bile duct, the failure rate is unacceptably high, and choledochoduodenostomy offers the best approach.[52,54,55] We have performed surgery for recurrent or residual bile duct stones or other biliary duct abnormalities occurring after cholecystectomy in 70 patients. Many of these had been elderly and ill, and many had undergone a previous surgical procedure. In a high proportion, biliary enteric bypass, either a side-to-side choledochoduodenostomy or a Roux-en-Y choledochojejunostomy, was necessary. There were no deaths. There is no doubt, however, that the operative mortality for surgical sphincteroplasty is higher.[42,43,57] The majority of the deaths in other series stem from acute pancreatitis.[65] Furthermore, sphincterotomy or sphincteroplasty has definite nonfatal complications.[6,13] Therefore, we prefer to avoid surgical interference with the ampulla of Vater and favor supraduodenal methods for exploration of the common bile duct (see earlier); we do not think, however, that the frequency of complications justifies the preferential use of endoscopic methods as suggested by Demling.[66]

Finally, experience of surgical interference with the sphincter of Oddi leads one to expect that endoscopic papillotomy may have a higher incidence of long-term effects and late stenosis than has been reported. Perhaps the most important fact, emphasized as a result of the development of endoscopic papillotomy, is the high incidence of retained or recurrent bile duct stones. This represents a fearful indictment of surgical approaches to the biliary tree and, in particular, of primary operations for gallstones. These problems are almost certainly associated with failure to perform pre- and postexploratory cholangiography or choledochoscopy and lack of a clear understanding of the indications for drainage procedures of the duct.[53]

REFERENCES

1. Burnett W, Shields R: Symptoms after cholecystectomy. Lancet 1958;*1*:923.
2. LeQuesne LP, Whiteside TG, Hand B: The common bile duct after cholecystectomy. Br Med J 1959; *1*:329.
3. Schofield GE, MacLeod RG: Sequelae of cholecystectomy. Br J Surg 1966;*53*:1042.
4. LeQuesne LP, Bolton JP: Postcholecystectomy symptoms. *In* Maingot R (ed): Abdominal Operations. 7th ed. New York, Appleton-Century-Crofts, 1980, p. 1103.
5. Bodvall B: The post-cholecystectomy syndrome. Clin Gastroenterol 1973;*2*:103.
6. Blumgart LH, Carachi R, Imrie CW, et al: Diagnosis and management of post-cholecystectomy symptoms: the place of endoscopy and retrograde choledochopancreatography. Br J Surg 1977;*64*:809.
7. Elias E, Hamlyn AN, Jain S, et al: Randomized trial of percutaneous transhepatic cholangiography with the Chiba needle versus endoscopic retrograde cholangiography for bile duct visualization in jaundice. Gastroenterology 1976;*71*:439.
8. Blumgart LH: Biliary tract obstruction—new approaches to old problems. Am J Surg 1978;*135*:19.
9. Benjamin IS, Allison MEM, Moule B, et al: The early use of fine needle percutaneous transhepatic cholangiography in an approach to the diagnosis of jaundice in a surgical unit. Br J Surg 1978;*65*:92.
10. Benjamin IS, Blumgart LH Biliary bypass and reconstructive surgery. *In* Liver and Biliary Disease: A Pathophysiological Approach. Wright R, Alberti G, Karran SR, Sadler HM (eds): Philadelphia, WB Saunders, 1978.
11. Ruddell WSJ, Ashton MG, Lintott DJ, et al: Endoscopic retrograde cholangiography and pancreatography in investigation of post-cholecystectomy patients. Lancet 1980;*1*:444.
12. Blumgart LH, Sokhi GS, Duncan JG: Endoscopy and retrograde choledochopancreatography in the diagnosis of post-cholecystectomy symptoms. Bull Soc Int Chir 1975;*6*:587.
13. Hunt DR, Blumgart LH: Iatrogenic choledochoduodenal fistula: an unsuspected cause of post-cholecystectomy symptoms. Br J Surg 1980;*67*:10.
14. Hunt DR: Investigation of post-cholecystectomy problems. Med J Aust 1982;*1*:214.
15. Cooperman M, Ferrara JJ, Carey LC, et al: Endoscopic retrograde cholangiopancreatography. Arch Surg 1981;*116*:606.
16. Burwood RJ, Davies GT, Lawrie BW: Endoscopic retrograde choledochopancreatography. A review with a report of a collaborative series. Clin Radiol 1973;*24*:397.
17. Blumgart LH, Salmon PR: Fiberduodenoscopy and transpapillary cholangiopancreatography. *In* Taylor S (ed): Recent Advances in Surgery. Edinburgh, Churchill Livingstone, 1973.
18. Classen M, Safrany L: Endoscopic papillotomy and removal of gall stones. Br Med J 1975;*4*:371.
19. Cotton PB, Chapman M, Whiteside CG, et al: Duodenoscopic papillotomy and gall stone removal. Br J Surg 1976;*63*:709.
20. Valberg LS, Jabbari M, Kerr JW, et al: Biliary pain in young women in the absence of gall stones. Gastroenterology 1971;*60*:1020.
21. Johnson AG: Cholecystectomy and gallstone dyspepsia. Ann R Coll Surg Engl 1975;*56*:69.
22. Hunt DR, Blumgart LH: Endoscopic abnormalities in patients with post-cholecystectomy symptoms. Surg Gastroenterol 1981;*1*:155.
23. Faris I, Thompson JPS, Grundy DJ, et al: Operative cholangiography. A re-appraisal based on a review of 400 cholangiograms. Br J Surg 1975;*62*:966.
24. Way LW, Admirand WH, Dunphy JE: Management of choledocholithiasis. Ann Surg 1972;*176*:347.
25. Rolfsmeyer ES, Bubrick MP, Kollitz PR, et al: The value of operative cholangiography. Surg Gynecol Obstet 1982;*154*:369.
26. Doyle PJ, Ward-McQuaid JN, Smith AM: The value of routine preoperative cholangiography—a report of 4000 cholecystectomies. Br J Surg 1982;*69*:617.
27. Levine SB, Lerner HJ, Leifer ED, et al: Intraoperative cholangiography. A review of indications and analysis of age-sex groups. Ann Surg 1983;*198*:692.
28. Kappes SK, Adams MB, Wilson SD: Intraoperative biliary endoscopy. Mandatory for all common duct operations. Arch Surg 1982;*117*:603.
29. Rattner DW, Warshaw AL: Impact of choledochoscopy on the management of choledocholithiasis. Experience with 499 common duct explorations at the Massachusetts General Hospital. Ann Surg 1981;*194*:76.
30. Escat J, Glucksman DL, Maigne C, et al: Choledochoscopy in surgery for choledocholithiasis. Six year experience in 380 consecutive patients. Am J Surg 1984;*147*:680.
31. Wenckert A, Robertson B: The natural course of gallstone disease: eleven-year review of 781 non-operated cases. Gastroenterology 1966;*50*:376.
32. Tondelli P, Gyr K, Stalder GA, et al: The biliary tract. Clin Gastroenterol 1979;*8*:487.
33. Heimbach DM, White TT: Immediate and long term effects of instrumental dilation of the sphincter of Oddi. Surg Gynecol Obstet 1979;*148*:79.
34. Wright AD: Surgery of the biliary tract. Ann R Coll Surg Engl 1960;*27*:373.
35. Hardy EG, Davenport TJ: The transduodenal approach to the common bile duct. Br J Surg 1969;*56*:667.

36. Hunter RR: Choledochotomy and transduodenal sphincterotomy. Ann R Coll Surg Engl 1972;*51*:250.
37. Carter AE: Kocher's periampullary approach for common bile duct calculi. Br J Surg 1973;*60*:117.
38. Peel ALG, Hermon-Taylor J, Ritchie HD: Technique of transduodenal exploration of the common bile duct. Ann R Coll Surg Engl 1974;*55*:237.
39. Jones SA: Sphincteroplasty (not sphincterotomy) in treatment of biliary tract disease. Surg Clin North Am 1973;*53*:1123.
40. Partington PF: 23 years of experience with sphincterotomy and sphincteroplasty for stenosis of the sphincter of Oddi. Surg Gynecol Obstet 1977; *145*:161.
41. Aubrey DA, Edwards JL: The selective use of combined supraduodenal and transduodenal exploration of the common bile duct. Br J Surg 1978; *65*:246.
42. Braasch JW, McCann JC Jr: Observations on single section of the sphincter of Oddi. Surg Gynecol Obstet 1967;*125*:355.
43. Colcock BP, Perry B: Exploration of the common bile duct. Surg Gynecol Obstet 1964;*118*:20.
44. Mahorner H, Browne ER: Results following transduodenal choledochoampulotomy. Ann Surg 1955; *141*:607.
45. Shieber W: Duodenotomy with common duct exploration. Arch Surg 1962;*85*:944.
46. Rothwell-Jackson RL: Sphincteroplasty in the treatment of biliary and pancreatic disease. Br J Surg 1968;*55*:616.
47. Rutledge RH: Sphincteroplasty and choledochoduodenostomy for benign biliary obstructions. Ann Surg 1976;*183*:476.
48. Aldrete J: In discussion of Saharia et al. Ann Surg 1977;*185*:598.
49. Saharia PC, Zuidema GD, Cameron JL: Primary common duct stones. Ann Surg 1977;*185*:598.
50. Schein CJ: Choledochal incontinence as a purposeful adjunct to choledocholithotomy. Surg Gynecol Obstet 1977;*144*:571.
51. Madden JL: Common duct stones: their origin and surgical management. Symposium on surgery of the biliary tree. Surg Clin North Am 1973;*53*:961.
52. Stuart M, Hoerr S: Late results of side-to-side choledochoduodenostomy and of transduodenal sphincterotomy for benign disorders. A twenty year comparative study. Am J Surg 1972;*123*:66.
53. Allen B, Shapiro H, Way LW: Management of recurrent and residual common duct stones. Am J Surg 1981;*142*:41.
54. Lygidakis NJ: Choledochoduodenostomy in biliary calculous diseases. Br J Surg 1981;*68*:762.
55. Schein CJ, Gliedman ML: Choledochoduodenostomy as an adjunct to choledocholithotomy. Surg Gynecol Obstet 1981;*152*:797.
56. Cattell RB, Braasch JW: General considerations in the management of benign strictures of the bile duct. N Engl J Med 1959;*261*:929.
57. Nardi GL, Michelassi F, Zannini P: Transduodenal sphincteroplasty. 5–25 year follow-up of 89 patients. Ann Surg 1983;*198*:453.
58. Cotton PB: Non-operative removal of bile duct stones by duodenoscopic sphincterotomy. Br J Surg 1980;*67*:1.
59. Safrany L: Endoscopic treatment of biliary tract disease. Lancet 1978;*2*:983.
60. Sloof M, Baker R, Lavelle MI, et al: What is involved in endoscopic sphincterotomy for gallstones? Br J Surg 1980;*67*:18.
61. Cotton PB: Endoscopic management of bile duct stones; (apples and oranges). Gut 1984;*25*:587.
62. Cotton PB, Vallon AG: British experience with duodenoscopic sphincterotomy for removal of bile duct stones. Br J Surg 1981;*68*:373.
63. Girard RM, Legros G: Retained and recurrent bile duct stones. Surgical or non-surgical removal? Ann Surg 1981;*193*:150.
64. McSherry CK, Glenn F: The incidence and cause of death following surgery for non-malignant biliary tract disease. Ann Surg 1980;*191*:271.
65. Imrie CW, McKay AJ, Benjamin IS, et al: Secondary acute pancreatitis: aetiology, prevention, diagnosis and management. Br J Surg 1978;*65*:399.
66. Demling L: Endoscopic papillotomy and removal of gall stones. J R Coll Surg Edinb 1977;*22*:385.

SECTION IV

BILIARY STRICTURES

LAWRENCE W. WAY, M.D.

27

Biliary Stricture

Benign strictures of the bile duct can result from surgical trauma, damage from common duct stones, toxic or ischemic damage from hepatic arterial infusions, primary infection (as in recurrent pyogenic cholangitis), external penetrating or blunt trauma, or sclerosing cholangitis.[1–9] The last three conditions are discussed in other chapters. The others will be covered here.

The morbidity from biliary strictures is high. The clinical manifestations consist predominantly of episodic cholangitis, but if the lesion is untreated for an extended period, secondary biliary cirrhosis may develop, which can progress to bleeding esophageal varices or hepatic failure.

CAUSE AND PREVENTION

The majority of bile duct strictures are caused by accidental injury of the duct during performance of a cholecystectomy. The injury is usually located in the segment of duct between the cystic duct junction and the bifurcation of the common hepatic duct.[5, 10] Although a number of pitfalls are recognized as potential causes of bile duct injuries, it is often difficult in retrospect to understand what happened in an individual case. Nevertheless, adhering to certain technical guidelines undoubtedly would minimize the occurrence of this serious problem.

Training and Supervision

Ductal injuries are related to the experience of the surgeon and probably to the method used in performing the cholecystectomy. Among cases seen over a 45-year period at our institution a disproportionate number followed cholecystectomies performed by surgeons who by today's standards would be considered inadequately trained.[8, 9] This factor is becoming progressively less prominent, however, as the number of such surgeons in practice decreases. A study from Scandinavia made a related observation, reporting that accidents involving the ducts were more common during operations performed by unsupervised residents than during those performed by surgeons who had completed their training.[1]

In many cases, the operative record demonstrates that the surgeon was confused in regard to the arrangement of the ducts. This can stem from distortion caused by disease, from variations in the anatomy, or from genuine anomalies. It is of interest, however, that most injuries do not occur during operations that the surgeon considered to be difficult and that injuries are uncommon during cholecystectomies that include a planned common duct exploration.[3, 8] Most often, operative cholangiography was not performed.[1, 3, 5]

Technique of Cholecystectomy

During cholecystectomy there are steps that are important in preventing injuries to the ducts. First, the operation is probably safer, particularly in difficult cases, if the dissection begins at the fundus and proceeds toward the duct, rather than the reverse. The plane of the dissection should at all times remain on the surface of the gallbladder. Second, before the cystic duct is divided, it should be dissected entirely free from neighboring structures. The junction between the cystic duct and common duct should be exposed, and a cholangiogram should usually be performed and inspected by the surgeon before the cystic duct is transected.[1,5] If these precepts were followed, confusion about the location of the common duct, the cause of many injuries, would be minimized.

Technical Miscues

A major cause of injuries is accidental placement of a ligature[3] or metal hemostasis clip on the common duct. In the case of clips, the diagnosis can be made by transhepatic or retrograde endoscopic cholangiograms when views from different angles show that the clip fails to rotate away from the duct. Prevention entails avoiding the placement of clips or sutures blindly in the hilus of the liver in pursuit of bleeding vessels. It is usually unnecessary for the dissection of the infundibulum to stray from the surface of the gallbladder into the fat and vessels in the triangle of Calot or into the hilus near the bifurcation of the common hepatic duct. The only safe place to use clips and sutures is where the vessels meet the gallbladder wall. If control of a vessel is lost, pressure should be applied for a few minutes and then gently removed. The exact site of bleeding will be apparent, and the vessel can be clamped precisely with a fine-tipped clamp.

In some patients with small mobile common bile ducts, traction on the cystic duct can tent the common duct far more than average, making it vulnerable to being caught by a clamp intended for the cystic duct. The duct can also be injured by attempts to separate an adherent cystic duct from the common duct. Both problems can be avoided by leaving a cystic duct stump of at least 5 to 10 mm. There is no need to divide the cystic duct close to the common duct, and one should not try to separate the two ducts when the cystic and common ducts share a common wall and run a parallel course. Furthermore, the cystic duct should be clamped only when the tissues have been allowed to relax (i.e., when they are not on traction).

A number of injuries involve laceration of the duct wall, as either a complete or an incomplete transaction. Complete transection most often involves the right lobar duct but may involve the common duct or common hepatic duct. Injury to the right lobar duct usually occurs when the confluence of the right and left ducts is low, an arrangement that places the right duct behind and close to the infundibulum of the gallbladder.

Unwise attempts at anastomosing an accessory duct to the main duct are among the miscellaneous causes of injury. If an accessory duct is encountered, this should be verified by an operative cholangiogram, preferably obtained before the accessory duct is divided. If the duct has already been divided, x-rays should be taken after contrast medium has been injected into both the divided duct and the common duct, making sure that the intrahepatic branches of each are completely opacified. A true accessory duct supplies only a small portion of liver tissue, whereas a lobar or major segmental duct supplies all or half of the lobe. An injured accessory duct is best managed by ligation, because an anastomosis with the main duct, which is usually small, runs a high risk of compromising the entire system. Ligation of the accessory duct results in atrophy of the segment of liver tissue that it drains but causes no significant change in hepatic function.

Anomalies and Anatomic Variations

Because surgeons have learned to anticipate anomalous bile ducts, there is a tendency when confronted with confusing anatomy to assume that anomalies are present. Until the evidence is conclusive, this interpretation should be resisted, because anomalies, including accessory ducts, are rare. It is more likely that a puzzling arrangement of ducts is really normal, perhaps distorted by inflammation, than that it is anomalous. Therefore, when attempting to unscramble the biliary anatomy one should be reluctant to postulate accessory ducts unless it is impossible to explain the pattern in any other way. An operative cholangiogram is essential in most such cases. We have seen many instances of biliary stricture in which the surgeon thought while performing cholecystectomy that an accessory duct or some other anomaly was present; after cholangiograms and re-exploration clarified the anatomy, however, it was evident that the arrangement of ducts was normal.

In the most usual configuration, the common duct bifurcates at its hepatic end into two lobar ducts, and the bifurcation nearly always lies outside the liver substance. As

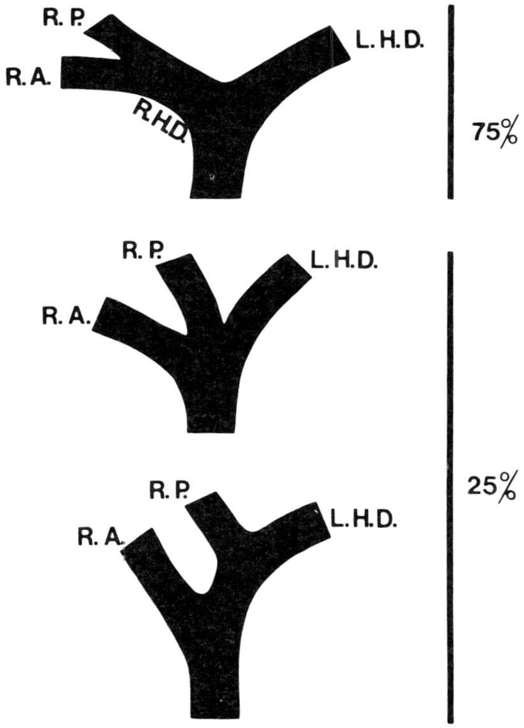

Figure 27–1. Common variations in the confluence of the lobar ducts (from Kune). R.A. = right anterior sequential duct; R.P. = right posterior segmental duct; R.H.D. = right hepatic duct; L.H.D. = left hepatic duct.

emphasized by Kune,[11] however, in 25 per cent of the population the duct branches as a trifurcation, with two segmental ducts going to the right lobe and a single lobar duct to the left lobe (Fig. 27–1). Because this arrangement is so common, it should be considered a normal variant, not an anomaly. A second common variation is a low union of the two lobar ducts.

With either of these arrangements the surgeon may fail to anticipate the presence of a major duct to the right lobe within a few millimeters of the infundibulum of the gallbladder. Assuming that the bifurcation has the classic shape, one may think that the left duct is, in fact, the common hepatic duct and that the area between it and the cystic duct contains no ductal structure. Another pitfall is to think that with either of these patterns the right duct represents an accessory duct instead of the principal right lobar or right anterior segmental duct. These considerations explain some injuries to the right duct or to a low-lying bifurcation.

CLINICAL FINDINGS

Presentation Early After Injury

The majority of bile duct injuries of significance become clinically manifest in the immediate postoperative period.[3, 5, 8, 9] It is less common for the postoperative period to be smooth and the first symptoms to appear months or years later. On the other hand, following an operation to repair the initial stricture, recurrent stricture formation ordinarily does not give rise to clinical findings for several months to years.[6, 12]

A rent in the duct will produce either bile drainage from abdominal drains or, if drains have not been used, bile ascites or bile peritonitis. Persistent drainage of bile after a biliary operation is never normal, and it cannot be eliminated by pulling the drains. If drainage continues for more than 5 to 7 days following a cholecystectomy, one should suspect the presence of a hole in one of the ducts, a leak from the cystic duct stump, or a severed accessory duct. If the bile is being evacuated adequately by the drains, investigative efforts can be postponed for a few more days, but if output continues, x-rays should be obtained. The most useful studies are a fistulogram through the drain tract and an ERCP. Usually, both are necessary to delineate the problem completely. The first test should be the fistulogram. Contrast medium can be injected directly through a closed drainage system (such as Jackson-Pratt drains), but if Penrose drains have been used, they should be removed and replaced by a catheter. A small hole may not be adequately outlined, and the main duct may not be completely filled. If questions remain, therefore, an ERCP should be performed. This will show the exact site of a leak from the main ductal system and whether or not it is associated with disruption of ductal continuity or the presence of obstruction.

Bile ascites has been an uncommon presentation in the past, but now that drainage of the gallbladder bed is used less often, it may become more common. The findings consist of jaundice and abdominal distention due to bile. The diagnosis is readily made by abdominal paracentesis. A HIDA scan usually demonstrates the bile leak, but ERCP or THC is necessary to provide more anatomic detail. Bile peritonitis gives similar findings plus sepsis.

Jaundice with or without cholangitis is another way that common duct injuries present in the immediate postoperative period. It may not be possible to distinguish clinically between obstruction due to gallstones or stricture if the jaundice is mild (i.e., bilirubin level < 6 mg/dl). Progressive jaundice that reaches higher levels over a few days usually means that a ligature is completely occluding the common duct. Postoperative jaundice, particularly if it persists for several weeks or is accompanied by fever and leukocytosis, should never be diagnosed as "hepatitis" unless that diagnosis has been supported by serum enzyme changes, liver biopsy, and normal cholangiograms.

The position of the right hepatic artery exposes it to injury in situations in which the duct is also injured. Hemobilia is the principal manifestation of clinically significant lesions. Therefore, patients with biliary strictures who present with evidence of gastrointestinal bleeding should be studied by selective angiography, which may demonstrate a hepatic artery aneurysm as the cause.[2, 3]

Presentation Late After Injury

Patients who present late after injury constitute the majority of cases. In those patients who have had only one previous biliary operation (cholecystectomy), the history most often consists of episodes of cholangitis dating back to a month or two from the time of the last operation.[8, 9] In patients with recurrent strictures, the symptoms may first appear any time in the subsequent 7 to 9 years after the previous stricture repair.[6, 12]

The attacks are generally mild and responsive to antibiotic therapy. Differentiation from common duct stones, the principal alternative diagnosis, should be made by direct cholangiography. In about 25 per cent of patients with recurrent strictures, gallstones are present on the hepatic side of the stricture; in fact, obstruction at the site of the stricture by hepatic stones may be responsible for the symptoms in some cases.[12] It is important to recognize that the stricture is usually the cause of the stones in such patients; removal of the stones alone is inadequate treatment.

A few patients present with painless jaundice without signs of infection. There is a greater risk in such cases that hepatic parenchymal disease, as opposed to an extrahepatic disorder, will be assumed to be responsible. It is important to keep in mind, therefore, that a benign post-traumatic biliary stricture can cause painless, steady jaundice; if the patient has previously had a cholecystectomy, cholangiography is indicated.

Chronic unrelieved obstruction for many years can lead to secondary biliary cirrhosis and its complications.[8] Most patients who develop cirrhosis have a history of disease more severe than average, including toxic cholangitis and several previous unsuccessful attempts at repairing the stricture.[9] Ascites or bleeding esophageal varices may be the reason for surgical consultation. Patients who have reached this stage may be divided into those who have treatable and the few who have untreatable strictures. The diagnosis of biliary stricture under these circumstances may be difficult, and pessimism about the outlook may be responsible for a general lack of investigative activity. Although there is certainly a basis for concern, the chances are still good that the patient will benefit from treatment of the stricture, so cholangiography is definitely indicated. We have seen dramatic, sustained resolution of ascites, encephalopathy, and malnutrition after dilatation of a chronic neglected bile duct stricture. Others have noted that resolution of portal hypertension and associated structural changes in the liver, including resorption of collagen, may follow relief of chronic biliary obstruction.[13]

LABORATORY FINDINGS

Elevated bilirubin and alkaline phosphatase levels are the rule when a biliary stricture becomes tight enough to cause symptoms. The bilirubin level usually fluctuates in concert with the symptoms over a few days, but the absolute level usually remains in the 2 to 6 mg/dl range, and levels above 10 mg/dl are uncommon unless cirrhosis has developed. Most often the bilirubin level returns to normal as the acute attack responds to antibiotics, and it may remain there until another attack occurs a month or so later. In the absence of treatment, jaundice and hyperbilirubinemia eventually become persistent.

The serum alkaline phosphatase level may fluctuate, but it often remains high even between attacks. In fact, when a stricture has been present for a year or more, the alkaline phosphatase level may be very slow to return to normal levels even after a completely successful operative repair. The absolute level of the alkaline phosphatase bears no relationship to the severity of the disease or other clinical variables.

A low albumin level is seen in the patients with most severe findings, including cirrhosis, and is associated with a worse prognosis.

The leukocyte count tends to parallel the severity of the cholangitis.

Other liver function tests, such as SGPT and SGOT, may be abnormal. An abnormal prothrombin time should be corrected before surgery.

RADIOLOGIC FINDINGS

Ultrasound and CT scans are nonspecific and of little clinical value. Dilatation of intrahepatic bile ducts may or may not be present. CT scans may demonstrate intrahepatic gallstones, which tend to have a relatively high calcium content.

Transhepatic cholangiography (THC) is the most valuable radiologic study, and it should be obtained in nearly every case, regardless of whether the intrahepatic bile ducts appear to be dilated on scans.[3, 8, 12] In most cases the stricture is short and close to the bifurcation of the common hepatic duct (Fig. 27–2). The special value of THC is its superior ability compared with ERCP to opacify the hepatic side of the stricture. Retrograde injections during ERCP may demonstrate the stricture, but the hepatic side is rarely opacified enough to portray the relationship of the stricture to the common hepatic duct and the lobar ducts. This is information of major importance to the surgeon when planning surgery and performing the dissection. If THC is performed cautiously, after cholangitis has subsided and under cover of antibiotics, the risk of sepsis is low.

HIDA scans may be of value in confirming the patency of ducts that are thought to be unobstructed.[3]

TREATMENT

Operative repair is indicated in all but a few cases of biliary stricture. The other treatment options include transhepatic or retrograde endoscopic dilatation, permanent stenting, and expectant management.

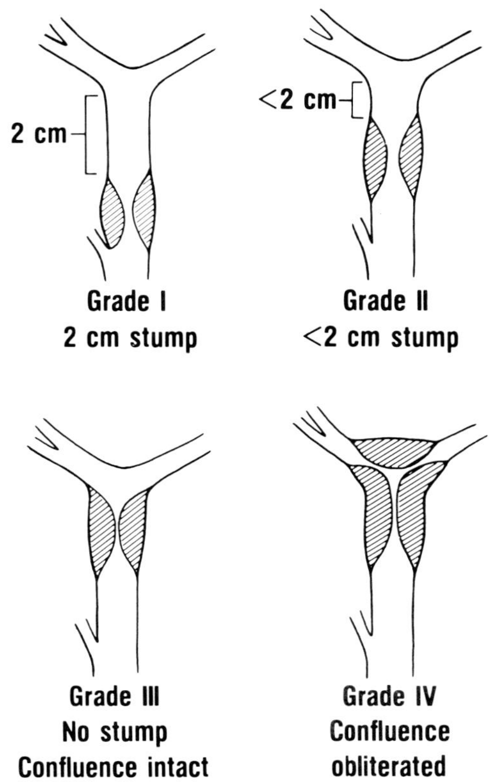

Figure 27–2. Classification of bile duct strictures. (After Bismuth H: *In* Blumgart LH [ed.]: The Biliary Tract, Vol. 5. New York, Churchill-Livingstone, 1982.)

Acute Injuries

Bile duct injuries discovered during surgery should be dealt with immediately.[14, 15] The nature of the injury and the anatomy of the biliary tree must be precisely determined. The surgeon must realize that what set out to be a 1½ hour operation may now require 3 to 4 hours or more. There is evidence that a well-done repair at the time of the original injury has a greater chance of success than later operations after a stricture has developed.[15]

To produce the best possible result one must select the reconstruction most likely to be definitive and carry through using meticulous surgical technique. If the common bile duct has been cleanly incised through part or all of its circumference, repair is best accomplished with fine (5-0 or 6-0) interrupted or running sutures of polyglycolic acid. Nonabsorbable suture material has a tendency to migrate into the lumen of the duct, where it can serve as a nidus for stone formation.[16] A running suture consisting of small stitches placed close together gives a precise closure that has the advantage of being watertight. If the tissues are distorted or if the duct is very small, however, interrupted sutures are preferable. Whichever method is used, one should attempt to construct an anastomosis that does not leak, for bile leakage contributes to periductular inflammation and further stricture formation.

When more than 1 cm of duct has been damaged (e.g., if it has been crushed by a clamp) or excised, the injured tissue should be debrided and a Roux-en-Y reconstruction performed. There may be reluctance to embark on a such lengthy and difficult operation, especially when the two ends of the damaged duct have been located and it appears as if they can be reapproximated. Nevertheless, a Roux-en-Y reconstruction is usually preferable under these circumstances, because even slight tension on the anastomosis can lead to late stricture formation. It may be difficult to anastomose a small bile duct to the jejunum, but the chances of achieving an unobstructed repair are better than with bringing the two ends of the duct together to span a long defect.

The problem is more complex when an injury is first detected in the immediate postoperative period. The manifestations at this point usually include a combination of cholangitis, jaundice, subhepatic infection, and external biliary fistula. In most cases, definitive repair must be postponed in favor of the more immediate objectives of eliminating infection and establishing unimpeded flow of bile. In particular, it is virtually impossible to perform a satisfactory bile duct repair in the presence of active hilar infection.

Therefore, the initial step usually consists of percutaneous or operative drainage of subhepatic collections. External biliary fistulae are best controlled by a catheter inserted by the radiologist percutaneously through the fistula into the duct. Complete obstruction of the duct is the only problem that requires reoperation at this point. Even this may be handled in some cases by percutaneous transhepatic intubation, however. Uncontrolled jaundice or sepsis may require an urgent operation, the main goal of which is to drain the bile duct or undrained abscesses. Reoperation can be scheduled 4 to 8 weeks after infection has been eliminated.

Elective Repair. Most biliary strictures can be scheduled for elective repair after infection and other aspects of the illness have been brought under control. Bismuth's classification of biliary strictures[2] is shown in Figure 27–2. The stage III and stage IV lesions are technically the most challenging.

Type of Reconstruction

The various techniques of reconstruction include Roux-en-Y hepaticojejunostomy, hepaticoduodenostomy, excision of the stricture and end-to-end repair, hepaticogastrostomy, insertion of a segment of jejunum between the duct and the duodenum, plastic repair of the stricture, Roux-en-Y mucosal grafting (the Rodney Smith procedure), and prosthetic replacement of the duct.[9]

Most cases are best treated by a Roux-en-Y hepaticojejunostomy or hepaticoduodenostomy.[2, 3, 5–8, 10, 12, 15, 17] Some of the aforementioned operations are associated with a high failure rate and have no current application. Others are useful only in specific circumstances.

The goal of the operation is to re-establish bile flow into the proximal gut by a tension-free anastomosis between two healthy tissues that are as free as possible of scar tissue. A Roux-en-Y limb of jejunum is the most mobile structure to which the duct can be joined, and for this reason a Roux-en-Y reconstruction is the procedure of choice in most cases. In general, one should approach the surgery with a plan to use a Roux-en-Y hepaticojejunostomy and switch to another method only if it seems able to meet the basic requirements of a good repair and is technically simpler. The stricture illustrated in Figure 27–3 was repaired with a Roux-en-Y hepaticojejunostomy. If the stricture is low on the duct, near the duodenum, a hepaticoduodenostomy is excellent. For proximal strictures, however, most surgeons consider hepaticoduodenostomy to be more difficult to perform and less likely to give a good result. Nevertheless, hepaticoduodenostomy is the method preferred by some.[18]

An end-to-end repair is rarely a good choice for established strictures. First, 1 cm or more of duct must be resected to remove most strictures, so bringing the ends of the duct together will inevitably produce tension, even following a good Kocher maneuver. Second, it is often difficult to find a good healthy duct below the stricture, and efforts to dissect it from surrounding tissues can be frustratingly slow and unrewarding. Finally, the obstructed proximal duct may be larger than the distal duct, which complicates the

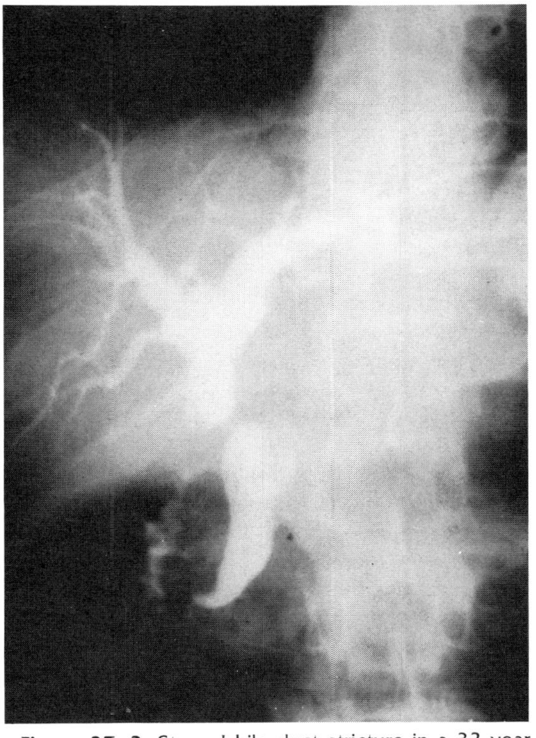

Figure 27–3. Stage I bile duct stricture in a 32-year-old woman. The chance of a successful repair in this kind of lesion exceeds 90 per cent. Transhepatic dilatation has no place in the treatment of this stricture.

anastomosis. Nevertheless, an occasional focal stricture with little surrounding scar tissue can be satisfactorily corrected by an end-to-end repair. One should not favor an end-to-end repair just because it seems to be more correct anatomically, for there are no functional advantages.

Peptic ulcer disease may be slightly less common if alkaline bile is routed into the duodenum instead of the jejunum,[19–20] but practically, this seems to be of little clinical importance.[22] There is no significant effect of the type of repair on liver function or the efficiency of digestion. Therefore, technical aspects of the repair should dominate over other considerations when deciding on the method of reconstruction.

The Roux-en-Y mucosal graft technique[23] is described in the accompanying section by Sir Rodney Smith. Although it can be performed quickly, in my opinion it is less precise than a direct anastomosis. Among the disadvantages of this technique are that the stricture is not usually excised and that the amount of tension on the tube supplying traction to the mucosal graft, its effects on blood supply of the mucosal graft, and the distance the graft is drawn into the duct are uncontrolled. Adjacent ducts may be blocked by the mucosal graft.[3]

Rarely, when resecting very high strictures, it may be impossible to perform an anastomosis between the end of the duct, deep in the hilar pocket, and the intestine. Cameron et al.[24] have shown that such patients can be managed by excision of the stricture, placement of transhepatic stents, and anastomosis of the gut to the hilus of the liver. The stents are left in place for about 12 months; when they are removed, the bile duct usually remains patent with no further treatment. Although the mucosa is not drawn into the ducts, in other respects this procedure resembles the one described by Sir Rodney Smith.

Hepaticogastrostomy has a poor record of success and is no longer used.[8]

Operative Technique

In addition to the type of reconstruction, the main determinants of success are surgical technique, amount of diffuse hilar fibrosis from previous infection, quality and caliber of the bile duct on the hepatic side of the stricture, location of the stricture, and presence of portal hypertension.[2, 3, 8, 10, 12, 17] The stricture must be dissected out cleanly and thoroughly. Most often the lesion is focal, occupying 5 to 8 mm of duct, with relatively normal duct on either side. The technical objective is to excise the lesion to a point where the proximal duct is soft and pliable and suitable for an anastomosis (i.e., above the scar tissue). This usually produces a specimen of duct that measures about 1 cm. To facilitate the anastomosis, about 5 mm of duct should be mobilized above the point of transection, but mobilization more extensive than this may jeopardize the ductal blood supply at the anastomosis.[17] The anastomosis is performed between the end of the duct and the side of the Roux-en-Y limb (or duodenum), as described previously. For established strictures in dilated thick-walled ducts the anastomosis is usually performed in two layers, an inner one of polyglycolic acid suture and an outer one of 4-0 or 5-0 silk or synthetic nonabsorbable suture material. The outer layer is meant to fold the gut up onto the duct, buttressing the initial layer. The nonabsorbable sutures should be placed so that they do not enter the lumen.

Some recurrent strictures at the site of a

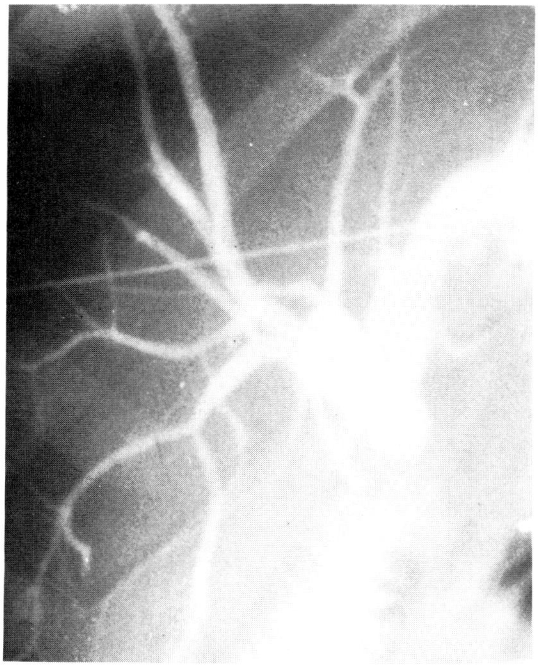

Figure 27–4. Recurrent stricture at the site of a hepaticojejunostomy. This very focal lesion can be repaired with an excellent chance of there being no recurrence.

previous hepaticojejunostomy are so focal that during their repair it is unnecessary to mobilize the posterior aspect of the duct or to excise the posterior 20 per cent of the circumference of the previous anastomosis (Fig. 27–4).[8] The anterolateral 80 per cent of the stricture can be excised and good tissue obtained for a reanastomosis on both the ductal and the intestinal side. The undisturbed posterior fixation may even contribute to healing of the new anastomosis because it helps immobilize the tissues. However, this method must not be used as a short cut in more difficult repairs.

Strictures that involve the bifurcation of the common hepatic duct (type IV strictures) may require separate anastomoses of the two lobar ducts.[2, 17] For type III strictures, however, the bifurcation can often be opened transversely[25] (especially onto the left duct) so that both orifices terminate in a single patch of suitable duct.

The technical problems presented by portal hypertension are often formidable.[3, 8, 9, 26] Blood loss during the dissection is often so great that the procedure must be aborted before the repair can be accomplished. A preliminary splenorenal shunt may correct the high portal pressure and facilitate a repair, but even so, the morbidity of the operation remains high because of the poor quality of liver function. For these reasons, transhepatic dilatation has a greater role in the treatment of strictures associated with cirrhosis and portal hypertension than of those without associated cirrhosis.

When the duct is 1.5 cm or less in diameter, the usual size, the anastomosis should be stented during healing. Larger ducts do not require a stent. Silastic tubing measuring 10F, 12F, or 14F is used most often. It is best to route the stent transhepatically, with the lower end either lying free in the lumen of the Roux-en-Y limb or passing through a Witzel tunnel in the Roux-en-Y limb to exit as a U-tube.

One method of inserting a transhepatic tube is as follows. The smallest Bakes dilator (3 mm) is inserted into the open end of the bile duct and passed into a peripheral branch of the right lobar ductal system until it will go no farther and is about 1 cm beneath the liver surface. It is then pushed through the wall of the duct and the liver substance until the olive tip comes to lie entirely outside the liver. A strand of 0-silk suture is tied around the tip of the dilator and the instrument is withdrawn, dragging the silk strand down through the ductal system and out the orifice of the common hepatic duct. The lower end of the 0-silk is then sutured to the end of the Silastic tube. Drawing on the hepatic end of the suture, the tube is pulled up through the ductal system and out the surface of the liver. The tube now has one end coming out of the orifice of the duct and the other from the liver surface. Holes are cut in the side walls of the tube over about a 10 cm span, and the tube is positioned so that the segment with holes in it straddles the anastomosis, making sure none of the holes is outside the liver or intestine. The hepatic side is brought out through a separate stab wound (not the incision), and the lower end is either allowed to lie within the lumen of the Roux-en-Y limb or brought out through a Witzel tunnel, as previously mentioned.

The transhepatic passage has become routine for stents in most institutions. The most common previous method involved inserting a tube through the wall of the Roux-en-Y limb of jejunum and threading it across the anastomosis into the duct. Often the ductal end would become dislodged, and the tube would coil in the Roux-en-Y limb of jejunum. Although inability to control this event was frustrating, it did contribute to our appreciation of the relative unimportance of stents.

Postoperative Care

How long to leave the stent in place postoperatively has been debated. Some advocate that the anastomosis be stented for 6 months or more in all patients.[6, 7] Others, including ourselves, recommend prolonged stenting only in a few selected cases.[2, 3, 10, 12, 27, 28]

The factors that govern the importance of stenting for more than a few weeks are (1) the quality of the anastomosis (i.e., whether a precise mucosa-to-mucosa apposition has been achieved), (2) the size of the duct, and (3) the amount of scar tissue in the wall of the remaining duct. There is no evidence that all biliary anastomoses require a stent. For example, the anastomosis of a large duct (e.g., greater than 1.5 cm) does not benefit from stenting, so stents are rarely used to support the bile duct anastomosis done as part of some common operations, such as a Whipple procedure. On the other hand, an anastomosis of a small thick-walled duct may have a better chance of long-term patency if it is stented for a prolonged period. After the majority of repairs, however, we remove the stents within 6 to 8 weeks.

Dilatation

Strictures can sometimes be dilated by balloon-tipped catheters passed transhepatically,[29–32] retrograde endoscopically,[33] or even following percutaneous puncture of the Roux-en-Y limb of a hepaticojejunostomy.[34] Experience has shown that the initial bile duct injury rarely responds to dilatation, so the use of dilatation is largely confined to treatment of strictured biliary-intestinal anastomoses following an earlier repair of the initial stricture.

Endoscopic dilatation can be repeated frequently with a low risk of complications, but this method is feasible only in patients who have had a hepaticoduodenostomy. Consequently, the endoscopic approach is often unavailable.

Transhepatic dilatation can usually be performed safely, but it should not be considered a minor procedure. All totalled, the time required for successful dilatation exceeds that of the average operation for biliary stricture. Complications include hepatic artery aneurysm with hemobilia and rupture of the strictured duct with bile peritonitis. Furthermore, even successful dilatation is often followed by restricturing, and additional dilatations are required months to years later.

Consequently, transhepatic dilatation should be used selectively in the management of biliary strictures, not as a first step for the average patient. From the surgical standpoint, the initial repair is usually the most difficult, but this is when dilatation is least useful. The results of surgery for recurrent stricture are generally good, and the cases in which a bad result is likely can usually be predicted preoperatively. The characteristics of lesions that have a high chance of being cured by surgery include the following: 5 mm or more of common hepatic duct remains; the proximal ductal system is dilated; the stricture is focal rather than diffuse; and cirrhosis and portal hypertension are absent. Patients who are poor operative risks in general (i.e., because of cardiac or pulmonary disease) or who have strictures that appear in the judgment of an expert to be unusually difficult to repair (especially those associated with portal hypertension) are the ones who should be selected for dilatation. For the remainder, who constitute about 90 per cent of the total, surgery can be performed more expeditiously than dilatation and carries lower risks and a higher chance of cure.

Bile Duct Prostheses

Many different types of material have been used in attempts to fashion a substitute conduit for bile, none of which has had appreciable success.[35, 36] Examples include metal (vitallium) tubes, vascular prosthetic grafts, prosthetic segments of vein or artery, various kinds of rubber tubing, and so forth. Stenosis regularly develops at the anastomosis between the bile duct and the prosthesis, and bile stasis leads to cholangitis.[36]

Bile Duct Regeneration

Belzer and Dunphy[35] found that after a portion of the wall of the bile duct was excised and the defect plugged with viable tissue, the remaining bile duct gradually grew in to fill the defect. Other than this, however, regeneration has not been observed. Belzer's technique has been used clinically with success,[37] but the opportunity to do so is rare.

In pigs, Cushieri et al.[38] used vein grafts to bridge defects in the duct, stenting the graft

Table 27–1 SUCCESS OF VARIOUS OPERATIVE PROCEDURES FOR REPAIR OF BILIARY STRICTURE*

	Hepatico-jejunostomy	Hepatico-duodenos-tomy	End-to-End Repair	Miscellaneous
All strictures	65/72(90%)	27/36(75%)	21/29(72%)	16/35(46%)
Recurrent strictures	34/46(72%)	6/9 (75%)	7/11(63%)	

*The two groups of patients span overlapping time periods.

with a Silastic tube for several months. At the end of this period, the vein had shrunk and the ends of the bile duct had migrated so that they were in direct apposition. There are no clinical reports on the use of this method.

PROGNOSIS

Some biliary strictures pose no special problems and are easily repaired. In many cases, however, technical aspects of the operation or other steps in management involve nuances recognizable only by those who have had considerable experience with this condition. It is usually wise, therefore, to handle biliary strictures as tertiary care, referring them to centers with the most experienced radiologic and surgical teams.

The operative mortality for stricture repair averages about 8 per cent.[2, 3] For repairs in patients without cirrhosis, the operative mortality is about 3 per cent. For those in patients with cirrhosis and portal hypertension, it is about 30 per cent.

The long-term results of surgical management of bile duct strictures at the University of California, San Francisco,[8, 9, 12] according to the type of repair are presented in Table 27–1. Similar results have been reported by others.[2, 3, 5, 6, 15, 17] In general, a permanent cure can be expected after surgical repair in 80 to 90 per cent of cases. In patients who develop recurrences, symptoms appear within 2 years in 70 per cent and within 7 years in 95 per cent. Delay in therapy in patients with abnormal liver function tests and episodic cholangitis exposes them to the risk of secondary biliary cirrhosis. Although a history of obstruction spanning 5 years or more antedates the development of cirrhosis in most cases, we have seen cases after 2 to 3 years of symptoms. Secondary biliary cirrhosis may lead to liver failure or portal hypertension, but progression to complications may be halted or reversed by treating the stricture.

REFERENCES

1. Andren-Sandberg A, Alinder G, Bengmark S: Accidental lesions of the common bile duct at cholecystectomy. Pre- and perioperative factors of importance. Ann Surg 1985;*201*:328.
2. Bismuth H: Postoperative strictures of the bile duct. *In* Blumgart LH (ed): The Biliary Tract, Vol. 5. New York, Churchill-Livingstone, 1982.
3. Blumgart LH, Kelley CJ, Benjamin IS: Benign bile duct stricture following cholecystectomy: critical factors in management. Br J Surg 1984;*71*:836.
4. Hillis TM, Westbrook KC, Caldwell FT, et al: Surgical injury of the common bile duct. Am J Surg 1977;*134*:712.
5. Kune GA: Bile duct injury during cholecystectomy: causes, prevention and surgical repair in 1979. Aust NZ J Surg 1979;*49*:35.
6. Pitt HA, Miyamoto T, Parapatis SK, et al: Factors influencing outcome in patients with postoperative biliary strictures. Am J Surg 1982;*144*:14.
7. Warren KW, Jefferson MF: Prevention and repair of strictures of the extrahepatic bile ducts. Surg Clin North Am 1973;*53*:1169.
8. Way LW, Bernhoft RA, Thomas MJ: Biliary stricture. Surg Clin North Am 1981;*61*:963.
9. Way LW, Dunphy JE: Biliary stricture. Am J Surg 1972;*124*:287.
10. Kalman PG, Taylor BR, Langer B: Iatrogenic bile-duct strictures. Can J Surg 1982;*25*:321.
11. Kune GA, Sali A: The Practice of Biliary Surgery, 2nd ed. Oxford, Blackwell Scientific Publications, 1980.
12. Pellegrini CA, Thomas MJ, Way LW: Recurrent biliary stricture. Patterns of recurrence and outcome of surgical therapy. Am J Surg 1984;*147*:175.
13. Weinbren K, Hadjis NS, Blumgart LH: Structural aspects of the liver in patients with biliary disease and portal hypertension. J Clin Pathol 1985;*38*:1013.
14. Longmire WP Jr: Early management of injury to the extrahepatic biliary tract. JAMA 1966;*195*:111.
15. Andren-Sandberg A, Johannson S, Bengmark S: Accidental lesions of the common bile duct at cholecystectomy. II. Results of treatment. Ann Surg 1985;*201*:452.
16. Galletti G, Ussia G, Bertoni R, et al: Comparison of the effects of polyglycolic acid and monofilament nylon sutures in the common bile duct of pigs. Ital J Surg Sci 1984;*14*:111.
17. Bolton JS, Braasch JW, Rossi RL: Management of benign biliary stricture. Surg Clin North Am 1980;*60*:313.
18. Hermann RE: Diagnosis and management of bile duct strictures. Am J Surg 1975;*130*:519.
19. McArthur MS, Longmire WP Jr: Peptic ulcer disease after choledochojejunostomy. Am J Surg 1971;*122*:155.

20. Nielsen ML, Jensen SL, Malmstrom J, et al: Gastrin and gastric acid secretion in hepaticojejunostomy Roux-en-Y. Surg Gynecol Obstet 1980;*150*:61.
21. Pappalardo G, Correnti S, Mobarhan S, et al: Long-term results of Roux-en-Y hepaticojejunostomy and hepaticojejunoduodenostomy. Ann Surg 1982;*196*:149.
22. Bismuth H, Franco D, Corlette MB, et al: Long term results of Roux-en-Y hepaticojejunostomy. Surg Gynecol Obstet 1978;*146*:161.
23. Wexler MJ, Smith R: Jejunal mucosal graft. A sutureless technic for repair of high bile duct strictures. Am J Surg 1975;*129*:204.
24. Cameron JL, Skinner DB, Zuidema GD: Long term transhepatic intubation for hilar hepatic duct strictures. Ann Surg 1976;*183*:488.
25. Stefanini P, Carboni M, Patrassi N, et al: Roux-en-Y hepaticojejunostomy: a reappraisal of its indications and results. Ann Surg 1975;*181*:213.
26. Sedgwick CE, Poulantzas JK, Kune GA: Management of portal hypertension secondary to bile duct strictures. Review of 18 cases with splenorenal shunt. Ann Surg 1966;*163*:949.
27. Hertzer NR, Gray HW, Hoerr SO, et al: The use of T-tube splints in bile duct repairs. Surg Gynecol Obstet 1973;*137*:413.
28. Braasch JW, Bolton JS, Rossi RL: A technique of biliary tract reconstruction with complete follow-up in 44 consecutive cases. Ann Surg 1981;*194*:635.
29. Molnar W, Stockum AE: Transhepatic dilatation of choledochoenterostomy strictures. Radiology 1978; *129*:59.
30. Teplick SK, Wolferth CC Jr, Hayes MF Jr, et al: Balloon dilatation of benign postsurgical biliary-enteric anastomosis strictures. Gastrointest Radiol 1982;*7*:307.
31. Salamonowitz E, Casteneda-Zuniga WR, Lund G, et al: Balloon dilatation of benign biliary strictures. Radiology 1984;*151*:613.
32. Vogel SB, Howard RJ, Caridi J, et al: Evaluation of percutaneous transhepatic balloon dilatation of benign biliary strictures in high-risk patients. Am J Surg 1985;*149*:73.
33. Foutch PG, Sivak MV Jr: Therapeutic endoscopic balloon dilatation of the extrahepatic biliary ducts. Am J Gastroenterol 1985;*80*:575.
34. Hutson DG, Russell E, Schiff E, et al: Balloon dilatation of biliary strictures through a choledocho-jejuno-cutaneous fistula. Ann Surg 1984;*199*:637.
35. Dunphy JE: Some observations, practical and impractical, on the function of the common bile duct. J R Coll Surg Edinb 1966;*2*:115.
36. Mendelowitz DS, Beal JM: Expanded polytetrafluoroethylene in reconstruction of the canine biliary system. Am J Surg 1982;*143*:221.
37. Rutledge RH: Methods of repair in noncircumferential bile duct defects. Surgery 1983;*93*:333.
38. Cushieri A, Baker PR, Anderson RJL, et al: Total and subtotal replacement of the common bile duct: effect of transhepatic silicone tube stenting. Gut 1983;*24*:756.

The Rodney Smith Method of Biliary Stricture Repair

SIR RODNEY SMITH, M.S., F.R.C.S.

The failure rate of operations to repair a bile duct stricture is 10 to 20 per cent. Many of the unsatisfactory results are the consequence of established secondary biliary cirrhosis. Another cause of failure is restenosis of the repair, be it bile duct to bile duct or bile duct to intestine. The aim of surgery is to construct a widely patent stoma that will remain widely patent and not contract down to produce another stricture. The anatomy of the biliary tree must be defined preoperatively by direct cholangiography (Fig. 27–5).

OPERATION UPON AN ESTABLISHED BILE DUCT STRICTURE

When operating to repair a long-standing stricture of the common hepatic or common bile duct, an ample incision giving good exposure is mandatory. Before approaching the porta hepatis, the surgeon should routinely mobilize both lobes of the liver and the hepatic flexure of the colon. The latter can then be removed completely from the right upper quadrant of the abdomen and packed away downward and to the left in order to secure

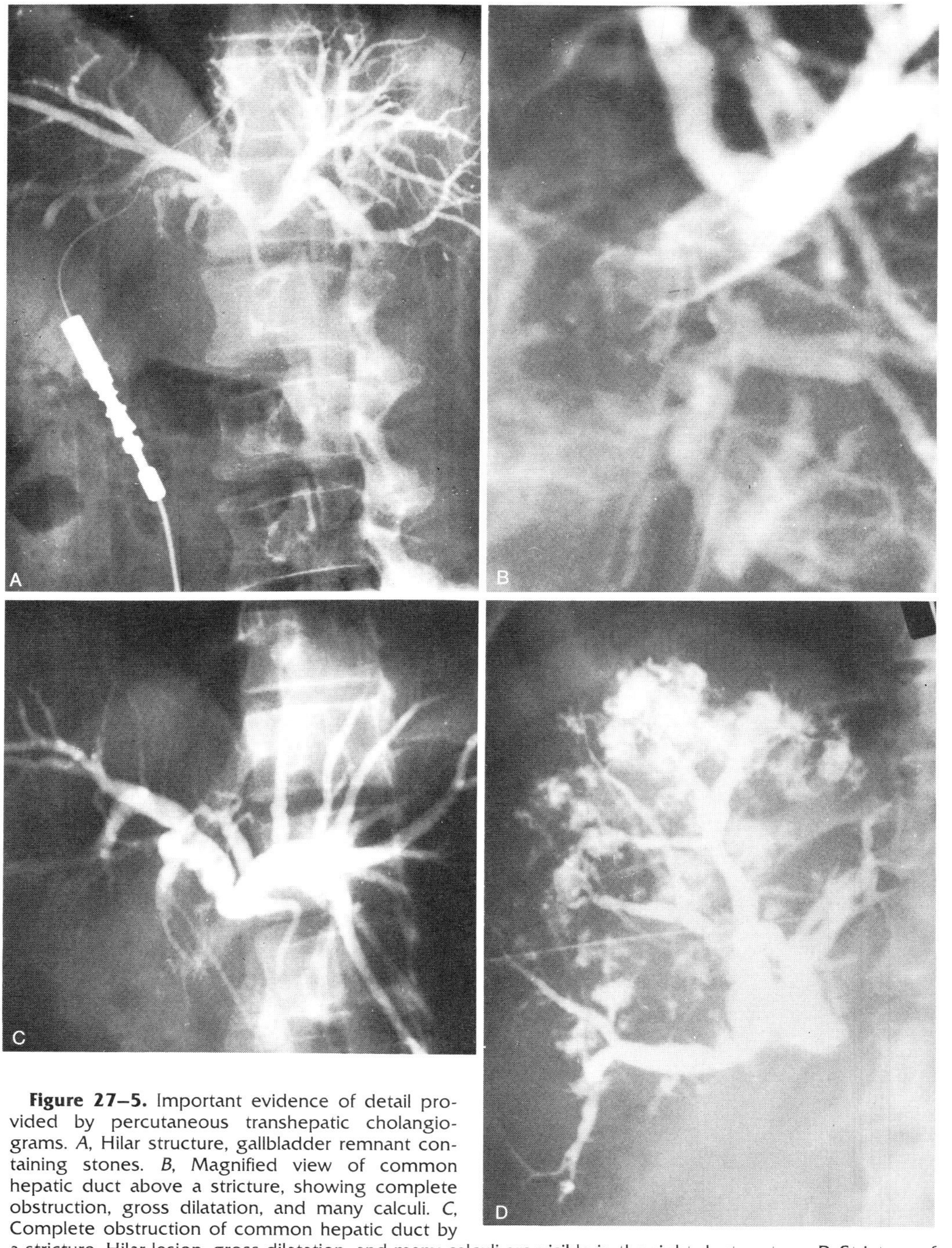

Figure 27–5. Important evidence of detail provided by percutaneous transhepatic cholangiograms. *A*, Hilar structure, gallbladder remnant containing stones. *B*, Magnified view of common hepatic duct above a stricture, showing complete obstruction, gross dilatation, and many calculi. *C*, Complete obstruction of common hepatic duct by a stricture. Hilar lesion, gross dilatation, and many calculi are visible in the right duct system. *D*, Stricture of common hepatic duct. Total obstruction. Gross sepsis producing "cherry-blossom duct," indicative of multiple cholangitic abscesses.

wide exposure of the area where the ductal damage has occurred.

The antrum, pylorus, and duodenum are carefully mobilized away from the liver. In dissecting the duodenum from the porta hepatis, a fistula between the common hepatic duct above the stricture and the lumen of the duodenum is often present, and this should be looked for. If found, it is divided, and the small opening into the duodenum is carefully closed. The dilated common hepatic duct above the stricture is sought in the dense scar tissue of the porta hepatis—if necessary, a needle and syringe may be used to identify the duct. Occasionally the injury is at such a high level that there is no common hepatic duct left, and in the scar tissue are discovered the ends of the right and left common hepatic ducts, opening independently. The duct or ducts are mobilized as far as possible and dissected free from scar tissue. With the use of probes and operative cholangiography the duct system above the stricture is displayed, and the interior of the duct is carefully inspected to determine the level at which the normal epithelial lining is visible. Bile from the intrahepatic ducts is taken for culture. Often the bile is dirty and contains a great deal of biliary mud and sometimes small stones as well. It is important to wash out the duct system before proceeding with the repair, and the most effective way of doing this is to insert a catheter that fits tightly into the opened duct and to distend the intrahepatic biliary system by injecting, slowly, up to 60 ml of sterile water or saline. The catheter is then pulled out; as this volume of fluid rushes out from the liver it brings with it solid debris, often lying high inside the smaller intrahepatic ducts. This procedure is repeated several times until the fluid returns clear. The operation can now continue.

The Anastomosis

The late Dr. Cattell of the Lahey Clinic recommended, even in late cases in which several unsuccessful attempts had been made at repair, that end-to-end anastomosis of the bile duct nevertheless be carried out.[1] Today most surgeons working in this field believe that a better long-term result is likely to be obtained with anastomosis of the common hepatic duct to the jejunum, and this is the most popular procedure at present.

In 30 years of endeavor I have changed my mind more than once in regard to the technique likely to yield the best results, and the stages through which my own thoughts have passed may be of interest.

On the face of it, one might well imagine that the repair of a divided hollow tube, such as a bile duct, would best be effected by end-to-end anastomosis, and as a young surgeon immediately after the Second World War I accepted without much further thought Dr. Cattell's assurance that this was, in fact, the case.

In my early cases, therefore, I relied upon an end-to-end anastomosis (Fig. 27–6) not only for a recently divided duct but also in the late case after excision of the resultant stricture. Like Cattell, I dissected out the contracted lower end of the duct and, mobilizing the head of the pancreas, shifted this up into the porta hepatis so that, even in the case of a hilar stricture, anastomosis could be performed without tension. And like Cattell, I found that far too many patients returned, having initially done well, with a recurrent stricture at the site of the anastomosis. By the late 1940s I had abandoned end-to-end anastomosis for an established stricture, particularly the high hilar stricture, in favor of hepaticojejunostomy employing a Roux loop. I continued to use a temporary indwelling

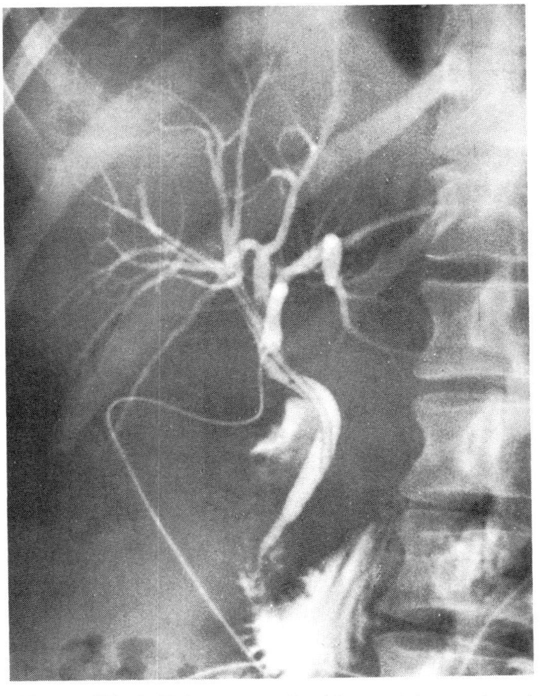

Figure 27–6. Stricture repaired by excision and end-to-end anastomosis. T-tube cholangiogram.

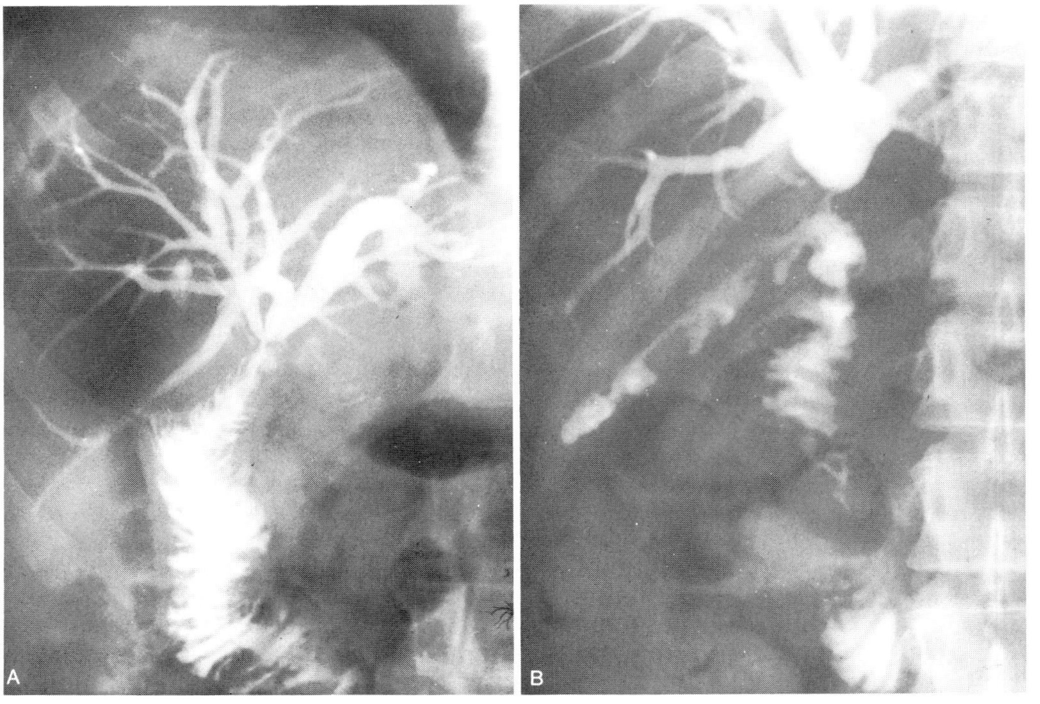

Figure 27–7. Restenosis after hepaticojejunostomy shown by percutaneous transhepatic cholangiography. *A*, Original Roux loop. *B*, Original Braun loop.

tube as a stent, and in 1949 for the first time I used, instead of a T-tube from below, a straight length of tube running transhepatically. I described 15 years' experience with the transhepatic tube in 1964, and quite soon it became apparent from publications that other surgeons favored a tube inserted in this way. Some of them had quite clearly come to this decision independently, in particular, Praderi of Montevideo, to whose thoughtful papers[2–4] in 1974 I would pay tribute.[4]

The results of hepaticojejunostomy splinted by a transhepatic tube were an improvement upon end-to-end anastomosis, but nevertheless I was disappointed to find that there were still too many failures for any degree of satisfaction. Those failures due to established biliary cirrhosis one could understand, but in patients in whom a favorable result was expected, some 25 per cent returned with evidence of restenosis at the site of the anastomosis (Fig. 27–7). Why, I asked myself, should the anastomosis restenose after removal of the transhepatic tube, even if this had been left in situ for 6 or even 12 months? I came to the conclusion that, at least in the very high recurrent hilar stricture, the reason probably lay in the impossibility of achieving, with a traditional sutured anastomosis, an adequate apposition of the bile duct epithelium and jejunal epithelium.[5–7]

As I wrote in 1972, trauma to the bile duct during cholecystectomy often occurs at a very high level.[8] Moreover, if the injury leaves, say, half a centimeter of common hepatic duct below the liver, this half-centimeter of usable common hepatic duct may disappear as a result of repeated unsuccessful attempts at repair. It is, thus, far more common for a surgeon to explore a stricture of the bile duct and find that the normal criteria for success cannot possibly be achieved. In particular, it does not appear possible to appose accurately the lining of the common hepatic duct above the stricture either to the lining of the distal duct below or to the epithelium of a loop of jejunum brought into the porta hepatis. It is of little use in these patients to core out of the thickened capsule of the liver a cylinder of scar tissue and call this a duct, for anastomosis of a cylinder of scar tissue without an epithelial lining to the jejunum, although it will serve for a while, is bound to restenose at a later date.[8]

It seemed to me that if access to the epithelial lining of the bile duct is so inadequate

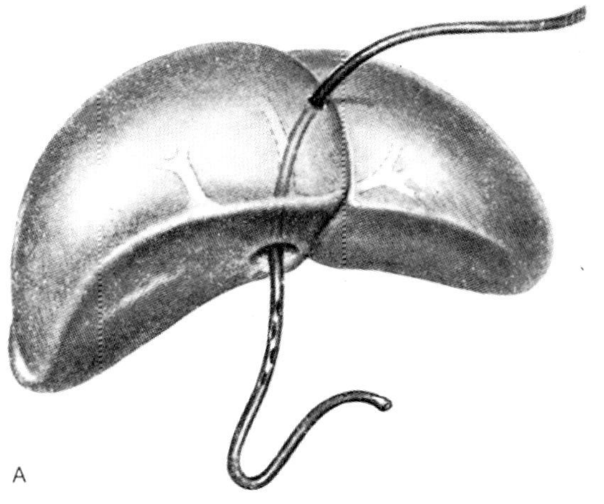

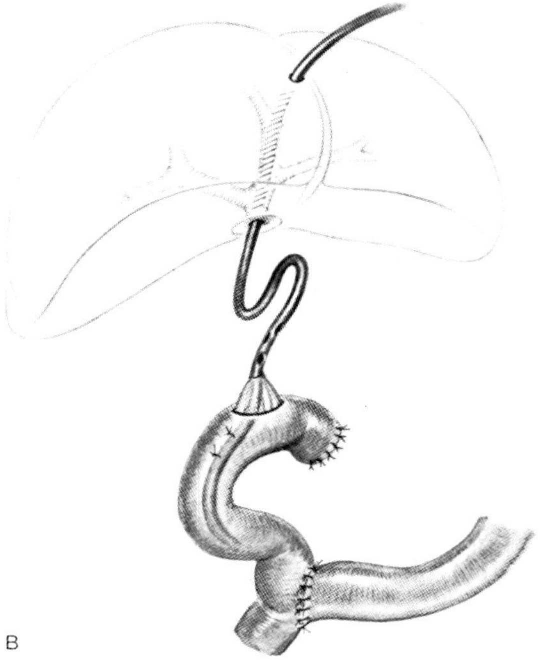

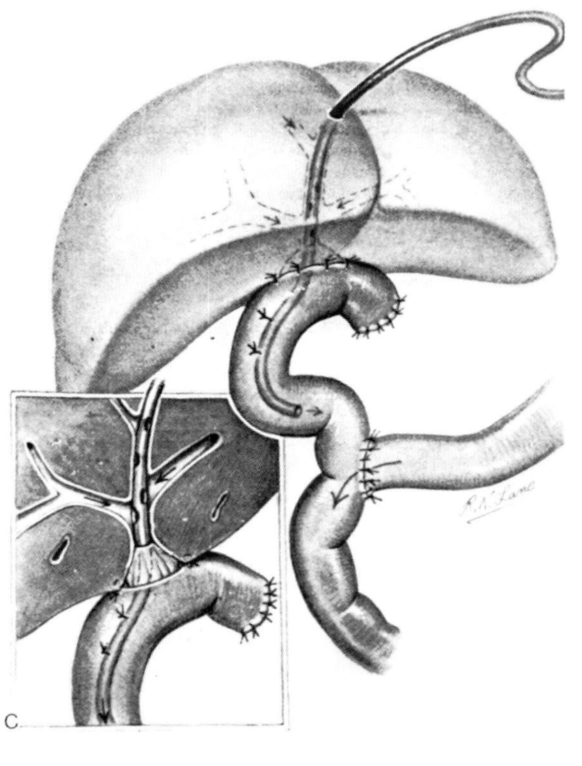

Figure 27–8. Mucosal graft operation. *A*, A transhepatic tube is placed as shown. The lateral holes will later be within the intrahepatic duct system. *B*, A Roux loop is constructed. Near the closed end of this a disc of muscle is cut away and a mucosal "diverticulum" fashioned. The tube is inserted via the apex of this into the jejunum and fixed by two sutures transfixing the tube. *C*, Traction on the tube draws the mucosal pocket well up into contact with the duct lining, however high the lesion, however dense the scar tissue.

through the mass of scar tissue in the porta hepatis that accurate suture to the epithelial lining of the jejunum appears to be impracticable, a successful repair could still be achieved if in some way the epithelial lining of the jejunum could be placed through the zone of fibrosis and in contact with the duct lining. This is the principle of the "mucosal graft" operation, which I introduced into my practice more than a decade ago. It is effected by cutting away a disc of the seromuscular coat of the jejunum in order to expose the mucosa and make a diverticulum that can be used as a mucosal graft to line the area where the epithelium is missing. A variety of methods have been employed to place this graft in situ.

Initially a specially constructed Y-tube was employed, which, with its two limbs inserted into right and left hepatic ducts, carries the jejunal mucosa up into contact with the epithelial lining of the hepatic duct system. (The tube later drops out into the jejunum and is passed per rectum.) This was a stage of transition and led to a technique employing both a mucosal graft and a transhepatic tube. The graft ensheathes and is attached to the tube, so that the sleeve of jejunal mucosa is drawn up through the scar tissue around the duct and well into the intrahepatic duct system (Fig. 27–8).

No sutures are used in the junction of hepatic duct epithelium and jejunal epithelium, but the weight of the Roux loop is supported by suturing it to the thickened capsule of the liver around the duct. A drain is placed below the liver adjacent to the anastomosis, and usually a second drain is placed below the diaphragm where the transhepatic tube emerges from the dome of the liver.

Postoperatively the transhepatic tube is attached to low suction. Suction is discontinued as soon as bile ceases to be recovered from the subhepatic drains, which are then removed. The transhepatic tube is then allowed to drain freely into a bag and after 7 to 10 days is spigotted. The patient is discharged after 12 to 14 days, having been taught to irrigate the tube once daily with sterile water or saline. Four months postoperatively the patient is readmitted to the hospital for 48 hours for a general assessment, including a tube-cholangiogram, bacteriologic examination of bile, and liver function tests, after which the tube is removed.

Results of the Mucosal Graft Operation

This is best divided into two parts: an evaluation of the immediate results in terms of technical difficulty, safety, complications, and success in relieving biliary obstruction; and late results, in particular the impact upon the problem of restenosis.

In regard to immediate results, the expectation that this technique would enable construction of a fully epithelialized channel between the hepatic duct system and the jejunum, however high the stricture and even if no duct epithelium outside the liver remained, have been fully realized (Fig. 27–9). Moreover, the facts that the epithelial apposition is sutureless and that bile is diverted from it by suction applied to the transhepatic tube should provide the best possible situation as regards healing of the new junction. The transhepatic tube is a safeguard against subhepatic or subphrenic leakage of bile and gives access to the intrahepatic duct system for bacteriology, radiology, and the topical use of antibiotics.

The technique is easier and swifter than suture techniques, and the immediate operative hazard is correspondingly lower. A personal unbroken series of 395 consecutive op-

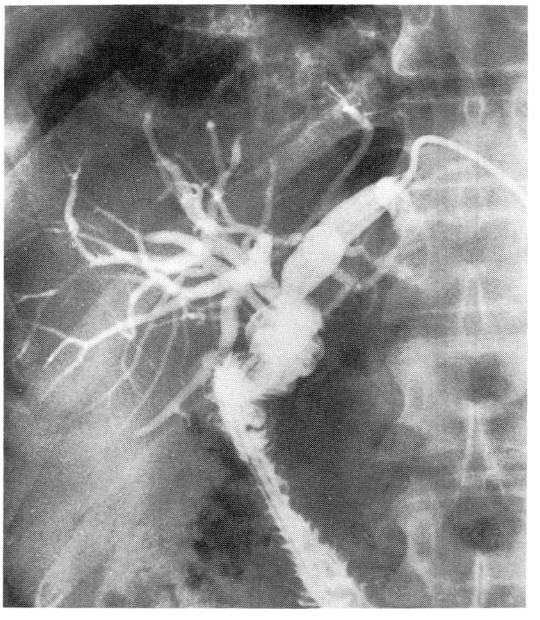

Figure 27–9. Mucosal graft operation. Mucosal pocket accurately apposed to very small residual stump of common hepatic duct. T-tube cholangiogram 1 week postoperatively. No bile leakage from day of operation. Ambulant patient ready to return home.

erations without mortality bears witness to this.

In regard to the late results, an analysis was made of all patients after a mucosal graft repair of a stricture on whom reliable records were available 2 years postoperatively. Although the selection of the 2-year point was arbitrary, the majority of patients who do develop a new stricture postoperatively present evidence of this during the first year, and almost all of them before 2 years have elapsed.

The number of patients available was 412. Of these, 85 per cent were anicteric and without symptoms, divided into 45 per cent with normal liver function tests, and 40 per cent still with a serum alkaline phosphatase value above normal. Eleven per cent had unsatisfactory results, which had, in fact, been anticipated at operation on account of (1) a long history and established biliary cirrhosis; or (2) a long history and secondary sclerosing cholangitis with multiple intrahepatic ductal strictures; or (3) a long history

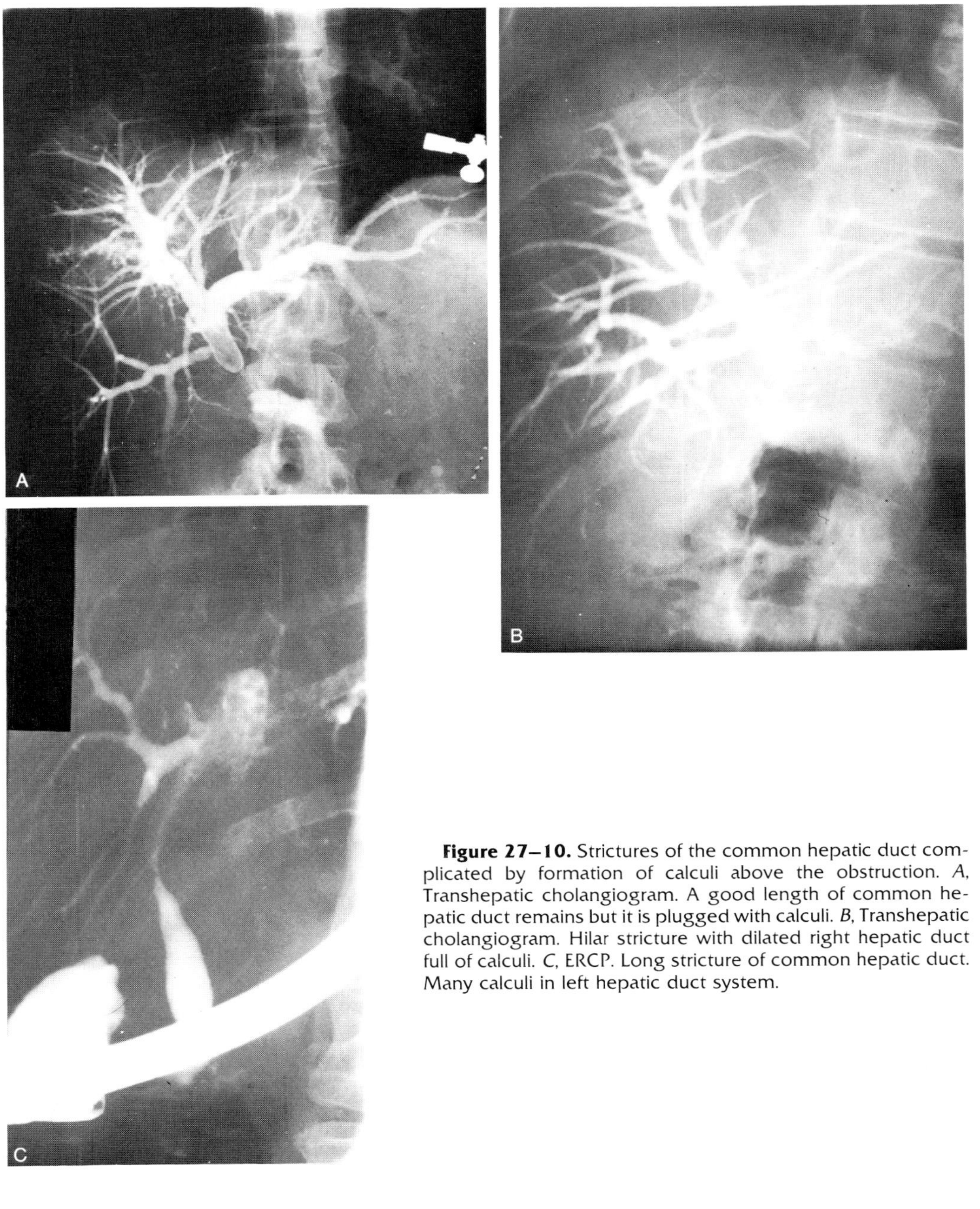

Figure 27–10. Strictures of the common hepatic duct complicated by formation of calculi above the obstruction. *A*, Transhepatic cholangiogram. A good length of common hepatic duct remains but it is plugged with calculi. *B*, Transhepatic cholangiogram. Hilar stricture with dilated right hepatic duct full of calculi. *C*, ERCP. Long stricture of common hepatic duct. Many calculi in left hepatic duct system.

and severe chronic purulent cholangitis with multiple intrahepatic calculi (Fig. 27–10).

Only 4 per cent had developed restenosis at the anastomosis when a favorable result had been anticipated. All of these have been reoperated upon.

Restenosis After a Mucosal Graft; Operative Findings

It is interesting and relevant that, when exposed, the type of restenosis after a mucosal graft is usually quite different from that after a sutured anastomosis. As already described, in the latter it is nearly always found that bile reaches the jejunum from the bile ducts via a contracted fibrous track with no epithelial lining. After a mucosal graft, if restenosis does occur, it is nearly always found that a fully epithelialized channel is still present but that a collar of scar tissue at the level of the capsule of the liver has closed in upon and compressed the grafted mucosal tunnel. Correction is simple. Without detaching the jejunum from the hilus of the liver and with access to the interior of the jejunum, graft, and biliary tree limited to a 1 cm incision in the jejunal loop itself, through which a Bakes dilator can be passed, the collar of scar tissue is excised. A temporary transhepatic tube is reinserted as a stent, and the jejunal loop is closed again with two or three fine seromuscular sutures of 3-0 catgut, a procedure taking some 20 to 30 minutes.

Conclusions

The early bile duct stricture with biliary obstruction but a relatively undamaged liver is a curable lesion and requires merely a widely patent and epithelialized channel through which bile can flow unimpeded. All patients in this group should be cured by surgery, although a few will need to be subjected to more than one operation before an acceptable result is achieved.

The late stricture with secondary biliary cirrhosis is largely incurable, although some clinical improvement will follow the provision of better biliary drainage by effective surgery. The more seriously incapacitated patients in this group with grossly damaged and deteriorating liver function should be seriously considered as candidates for hepatic transplantation. The risks are high, particularly if there is severe intrahepatic sepsis, but if the alternative is early death, a transplant should at least be considered.

REFERENCES

1. Cattell RB: Strictures of the biliary ducts. JAMA 1947;*134*:235.
2. Praderi R, Mazza M, Fossati CG, Estefan A: Le drainage trans-hepatique en seton. Nouv Presse Med 1974;*3*:2015.
3. Praderi RC, Delgado B, Mazza M, Fossati CG, Davidenko N: Drainages trans-hepatiques doubles. Lyon Chir 1974;*70*:294.
4. Praderi RC: Twelve years' experience with transhepatic intubation. Am Surg 1974;*179*:937.
5. Smith R: Injuries of the liver, biliary tree and pancreas. Br J Surg 1978; *65*:673.
6. Smith R: Obstructions of the bile duct. Br J Surg 1979;*66*:69.
7. Smith R: Strictures of the bile ducts. Proc R Soc Med 1969;*62*:131.
8. Smith R: Strictures of the bile ducts. *In* Badenoch J, Brook BN (eds): Recent Advances in Gastroenterology. Edinburgh, Churchill Livingstone, 1972, pp 331–342.

MAURICE MERCARDIER, M.D.

28

Intrahepatic Strictures and Malformations of the Bile Ducts in the Adult

This chapter deals with some aspects of the pathology of the intrahepatic bile ducts: benign and malignant strictures and congenital malformations, namely, congenital cystic dilatation of the intrahepatic ducts (Caroli's disease) and congenital hepatic fibrosis, a variant of Caroli's disease associated with fibrosis of the liver and portal hypertension.

STRICTURES OF THE INTRAHEPATIC BILE DUCTS

Strictures of the intrahepatic bile ducts are rare and in many cases unrecognized until autopsy. The most common cause of intrahepatic strictures is a carcinoma of the bile duct.[1–5] Strictures may, less commonly, be caused by inflammatory processes.[6] The stenosis may involve an intraparenchymatous hepatic duct or one of its segmental afferents. It results in proximal stasis, infection, stone formation, and biliary cirrhosis. The clinical characteristics are similar whether the stenosis was caused by an inflammatory process or a tumor. However, the prognosis and treatment of the lesion are determined by whether the stricture is inflammatory or neoplastic.

Carcinoma of the Intrahepatic Bile Ducts

Carcinomas of the intrahepatic bile ducts involve the segmental ducts or the right or left hepatic ducts during their intraparenchymatous course. Anatomically they are situated between carcinomas of the bile canaliculi (malignant cholangiomas, which take the form of a massive hepatic tumor) and carcinomas of the extraparenchymatous hepatic duct.

The first cases were published by Billington in 1952,[6] and Altemeier in 1957,[2] while a number of authors such as Sanes and MacCallum,[1] and Meyerowitz and Aird in 1962[4] had described them in publications devoted to carcinomas of the bile ducts in general.

Carcinomas of the intrahepatic bile ducts are rare. They should be suspected whenever peroperative cholangiograms show obstruction of one of the two hepatic ducts or of one of their segmental branches. These tumors are seen usually after age 40 and are twice as common in men as in women. The etiology is unknown.

Pathology

The lesion arises from the wall of the duct. It usually measures about 2 cm in diameter but may reach 10 cm in some cases. The pattern may be that of a scirrhous adenocarcinoma with resulting stenosis or of a papillary adenocarcinoma with polyp formation within the lumen of the dilated duct.[7]

The tumor spreads locally along the wall of the duct and from one duct to another at the convergence of the hepatic ducts. It most often occurs in the parenchyma as a single mass or multiple nodules. The tumor is often accompanied by metastases in segments of the liver remote from the primary lesion. Polypoid tumors may fragment and free pieces migrate through the extrahepatic duct, producing the same clinical manifestations as gallstones.

Whether it is a scirrhous or a polypoid adenocarcinoma, the tumor obstructs the bile flow. Biliary stasis leads to infection, precipitation of pigment and formation of calculi, benign adenomatous proliferation of the duct mucosa, and development of biliary cirrhosis proximal to the lesion. The liver in the obstructed zone first appears to be enlarged and green, and the ducts are distended. This is followed by atrophy of the parenchyma, which retracts around ducts filled with white bile.

Histologically, the lesion appears either as a scirrhous adenocarcinoma, with sparse neoplastic acini contained within a dense fibrous stroma, or as a papillary adenocarcinoma, rich in neoplastic proliferation.[7] The liver itself shows signs of stasis (bile duct plugs and centrilobular precipitation of pigment), infection (duct and periportal inflammation), and cirrhosis (periportal fibrosis).

Clinical and Laboratory Characteristics

The clinical and laboratory findings are not specific. They give no precise indication as to the diagnosis before operation, and the tumor is discovered only as a result of operative exploration, radiologic examination, or autopsy.

Clinical findings may be limited to a progressive change in the patient's general condition accompanied by episodes of fever that vary in severity and duration.[13] The patient is anxious, sleeps poorly, has a poor appetite, loses weight, becomes dehydrated and anemic and finally cachectic. He may die before investigations have revealed the cause of his illness.

In most cases, the tumor eventually results in hepatobiliary manifestations, but these are nonspecific. For example, patients may complain of intermittent, dull, aching pain in the right upper quadrant that radiates to the right shoulder. Jaundice may develop and may have the characteristics of neoplastic processes: It worsens progressively and is accompanied by neither pain nor fever, but by pruritus. Occasionally, the jaundice initially resembles that caused by gallstones: It is preceded by pain, it is accompanied by fever, and it fluctuates.

In most cases, the liver is normal on physical examination, but it may be enlarged, with a smooth surface and firm consistency. The tumor may also result in isolated hypertrophy of one hepatic lobe or segment, which is due to biliary retention proximal to the obstruction and, later, to the development of localized cirrhosis. This kind of limited hepatomegaly should suggest the correct diagnosis, although this rarely happens. When present, hepatomegaly is not accompanied by other physical findings. The gallbladder is not palpable, there is no local subcostal tenderness, and Murphy's sign is negative. In most cases, the symptoms and signs merely indicate biliary obstruction and infection.

Laboratory examinations confirm the foregoing findings. Obstruction is manifested by a marked increase in levels of bilirubin, alkaline phosphatase, and cholesterol. Laboratory signs of infection include leukocytosis, with an increased proportion of polynuclear cells on differential count.

Special Investigations

Many techniques are available.[8–12] Each should be considered in order to decide how best to determine the diagnosis, site, and nature of the lesion responsible for biliary obstruction or infection.

Oral cholecystography outlines the gallbladder and sometimes the extrahepatic bile ducts, but it does not opacify the intrahepatic bile ducts.

An ultrasound scan of the gallbladder and liver, which is often obtained early in the evaluation, may show dilated ducts proximal to the site of obstruction.[9, 10] CT scans would also demonstrate dilatation of the ducts, and if it were large enough, the primary tumor or a metastasis might be seen. This is uncommon, however.[11]

The most important test is direct cholangiography, whether obtained by the transhepatic or the retrograde approach. Retrograde cholangiography (ERCP) may fail to opacify the intraheptic ducts adequately, and it would not be expected to fill the obstructed ducts. Transhepatic cholangiography (THC) is the only means of opacifying the latter. It may be that both tests would be required to depict the abnormalities completely. (See Chapters 10 and 13 for further details in direct cholangiography and the work-up of patients with obstructive jaundice.)

Selective arteriography of the hepatic and superior mesenteric arteries is essential whenever surgical exploration is planned. This may define the tumor, indicated by a basket-like vascular arrangement around a filling defect, and may show local displacement and compression.

Diagnosis

All the major causes of obstructive jaundice or cholangitis must be considered. When the site of the disorder has been localized to one of the intrahepatic ducts, other causes of intrahepatic duct obstruction must be thought of: gallstones, benign tumor, and inflammatory stricture. In reality, the data are difficult to interpret and the diagnosis is usually made only at operation. In the course of surgical exploration, the following should arouse suspicion of an intrahepatic cholangiocarcinoma:

1. Cirrhosis of the liver limited to one lobe or segment, the green color and firm consistency of the involved segment contrasting with the brown color and suppleness of the neighboring parenchyma.
2. Distention of the bile ducts, which is sometimes visible on external inspection by surface changes, or, more often, by palpation with the detection of one or more fluid collections under pressure.
3. Tumor infiltration along the inferior aspect of the liver toward the hilus, which would indicate extension from the intrahepatic segment to the extrahepatic segment along one of the bile ducts.

These findings are especially significant when exploration of the extrahepatic bile ducts shows them to be normal or merely the site of cholelithiasis. Good operative cholangiograms that provide a complete picture of the entire biliary tree should be obtained. In order to achieve this, the contrast medium may have to be introduced under pressure directly into the common duct. The presence of a tumor may be inferred from (1) sudden complete block with amputation of a segment of the intrahepatic biliary tree, and (2) stenosis of a large duct with proximal dilatation, which may contain calculi as a result of stasis. Such an image indicates intrahepatic lithiasis or a benign tumor. In general, inflammatory stenosis produces localized and regular narrowing of the duct. Slight differences are difficult to interpret, however, and the most difficult diagnosis lies between malignant stricture and benign, fibrous, or inflammatory stricture.

Instrumental exploration of the intrahepatic bile ducts is the best way of making an exact diagnosis. The ducts are first explored using a probe or a catheter, which localizes the obstruction when it meets the narrowing. A fragment of tissue at the site of the obstruction should then be obtained by curettage or swabbing of the narrowed area with atraumatic instruments. A biopsy may also be obtained externally by puncture aspiration when the lesion is deep-seated or by a biopsy needle when it is close to the surface of the liver.

The histologic differentiation between inflammatory and neoplastic stenosis is particularly difficult. Both types may display fibrosis as well as proliferation in the glandular acini that may simulate a well-differentiated adenocarcinoma;[2] an excess of fibrous tissue that may mask a carcinoma;[2, 14] and proliferation of the accessory canalicular glands in association with inflammatory stricture, in particular since this proliferation may represent a premalignant state.[3]

Benign Stricture of the Intrahepatic Bile Ducts

Benign stricture of the intrahepatic bile ducts is a rare condition. Its existence should nevertheless be borne in mind, since it may be responsible for unexplained episodes of cholangitis. It should be considered whenever the cause of cholangitis is not found in the extrahepatic bile ducts.

In the strict sense, the stricture involves the intraparenchymatous segment of the hepatic ducts or their segmental branches. It should be distinguished from hilar stricture, if for no other reason than that the therapeutic methods differ for each.

The cause of benign stricture of the intrahepatic bile ducts is unknown. Some may be congenital,[15, 16] whereas others may be the result of bacterial infection. Rarely, it may represent focal intrahepatic sclerosing cholangitis. This possibility should come to mind especially when the patient is suffering from ulcerative colitis, since these two conditions are so often found together.

Benign stricture takes the form of a short ringlike stenosis as shown by radiologic studies. It consists of fibrous proliferation involving the wall of the duct. Proximally, there is stasis and biliary infection, while the rest of the unobstructed parenchyma remains healthy.[17] Microscopically, the obstructed segment of liver contains bile pigment in the hepatocytes and Kupffer cells and numerous lymphohistiocytic and polynuclear infiltrates around the bile canaliculi.

The clinical findings consist of pain, fever, and jaundice. Pain, frequently the presenting feature, may precede other manifestations by several months. It is located in the upper abdomen and is dull, vague, and intermittent and sometimes accompanied by poor appetite and vomiting. Fever is irregular, occurring first as intermittent exacerbations and later becoming permanent and in the form of a plateau. It is accompanied by rigors and may precede jaundice. The jaundice is generally moderate and variable.

The whole picture is that of incomplete obstruction of the bile ducts. The finding of increased bilirubin and alkaline phosphatase supports the clinical suspicions. It is then necessary to confirm the obstruction, localize its site, and attempt to ascertain its nature by ERCP or THC and CT scans.[8-12]

Preoperative cholangiography may fail to reveal the stricture because it is so limited. Surgery is indicated, however, to determine the cause of the cholangitis. Careful radiologic studies during surgery make it possible to detect the lesion if the intrahepatic biliary system is completely filled. The lesion may be seen as a sudden block of the contrast medium and absence of a segmental duct of the biliary tree. It may also appear as a localized stenosis with distention of the proximal ducts. As a general rule, benign stricture differs from malignant stricture in being less extensive; it is quite focal instead of being fusiform with irregular borders, but such differences may be difficult to appreciate. In any event, the operative method is the same: drainage or excision of the involved segment of the liver in order to protect the patient from the persistence of cholangitis and its possible complications.

The course of benign stricture of the intrahepatic bile ducts is dominated by stasis and biliary infection. It may extend to involve the whole biliary tree and be responsible for bacteremia or even septicemia. Thus, benign stricture of the intrahepatic bile ducts is treated by the same surgical methods as malignant stricture, the only difference being that the outcome is more favorable.

Treatment of Intrahepatic Biliary Stricture

The treatment of intrahepatic biliary stricture is mostly surgical, although a distinction must be drawn between palliative and curative methods. The first are aimed at relieving the patient from the manifestations of obstruction and biliary infection by ensuring permanent drainage of the obstructed bile. The second seek to eradicate the stenosis, in particular neoplastic stenosis, but involve resection of all parenchyma drained by the involved duct. Antibiotic therapy is merely an adjuvant for treating cholangitis before and after surgery.

Numerous operations of varying difficulty are available.[18-32] Selection should be made bearing in mind the patient's age, general condition, and severity of cholangitis and remembering that the long-term results of radical methods are scarcely better than those of palliative methods, while the operative mortality of the former is much greater.

Palliative Operations. *Short-term palliative operations* should be reserved for patients with malignant lesions who are in precarious condition with a limited life expectancy. Percutaneous transhepatic catheter drainage is the simplest technique. The catheter is left in place, firmly fixed to the abdominal wall. It ensures biliary drainage proximal to the stricture and relief of biliary obstruction and cholangitis. This method may be employed following laparotomy when surgical exploration has revealed the presence of metastases. It carries some risk of intraperitoneal biliary leak along the tube.[33]

Long-term palliative operations are aimed at the establishment of a wide anastomosis between the obstructed bile ducts and the digestive tract. This approach is confined to patients in good general condition, since the operation is relatively long and stressful. These procedures may be used for curing the rare patient with benign stenosis and for palliation in the more common patient with malignant stenosis. The anastomosis must be made using an intrahepatic duct of adequate size. The duct selected should be sought in a peripheral segment in a safe zone close to the lateral and anterior border of the lobe of the liver in which the stenosis is located.

In the left lobe of the liver, the duct of segment III is the most suitable. It may be reached by performing a limited section of the left lobe (Longmire procedure);[23, 30] by limited anterolateral resection of segment III (Hepp procedure),[22] or by a wedge-shaped limited resection of the latter; or by just opening the parenchyma of the liver following the umbilical cord remnant.[20]

In the right lobe of the liver, reaching the

dilated duct is much more difficult in view of the absence of any precise anatomic landmark and the frequent variations in the vascular-biliary relations. The best technique is resection of the tip of the right lobe of the liver[22] or hepatotomy of the anterior edge in the direction of the duct detected by puncture.

The best part of the digestive tract to use for draining the obstructed duct is an excluded jejunal loop (Roux-en-Y), at least 50 cm long. The anastomosis to the fragile walls of the duct is difficult to perform at the base of a narrow incision in hypertrophied parenchyma. In order to be effective in the long term it should be wide, with careful mucosal apposition. Ideal conditions eliminate the need for draining the anastomosis, but if the duct is very small and the anastomosis difficult or tenuous, a drain should be inserted.

In fact, the results of these operations, even when performed by the most experienced surgeons, are not fully satisfactory. Mortality rates vary from 15 to 25 per cent, which is intolerable for an operation for a benign stenosis. The morbidity rate is also prohibitive, biliary fistula being the most common complication. For these reasons, it is preferable to use percutaneous intubation of the obstructed duct and dilatation of the stricture.

Intrastenotic intubation, described in 1961 by Praderi,[24, 25] is less risky than hepaticointestinal anastomosis. Its use is confined to patients who are in a precarious general condition. It poses few technical problems. After a choledochotomy is performed, an instrument (e.g., a dilator or calculus forceps) is passed carefully through the stenosis from below upward into the biliary tract. It is gently pushed along the involved hepatic duct to pass through the stenosis and then beyond the stricture to bring it as close as possible to the surface of the liver. The liver capsule is incised at this point, and the hepatic tissue is broken down with a finger in order to reach and exteriorize the tip of the guide. A tube is then fixed to its extremity, with lateral orifices in the segment that will remain within the liver. By drawing the guide downward, the drainage tube is pulled into position.

Drainage may then be established in an antegrade or descending manner. In the latter, the upper extremity of the tube is exteriorized through the surface of the liver and the abdominal wall, being solidly fixed to the peritoneum, aponeurosis, and skin. In the former, the lower extremity of the drain is left in the common bile duct, which is closed,[25] or it is brought through a Roux-en-Y jejunal loop or the duodenum after passing through the papilla, the latter being widely opened. However, the best technique is to exteriorize both ends of the tube through the abdominal wall, making a U-tube.[27] This last procedure eliminates the risk of a biliary leak and allows the ducts to be irrigated and the tube to be changed if it becomes obstructed by bile deposits. Some have advocated bringing the closed end of the Roux-en-Y to the abdominal wall. The advantage of this procedure is that one may then remove all tubes from the biliary tract but the surgeon or the interventional radiologist still has easy access to the ducts by percutaneous puncture of the blind end of the Roux-en-Y loop of jejunum attached to the abdominal wall. This allows frequent access to the bile ducts to clear the debris and stones from ducts proximal to the stricture.[32, 33]

Curative Operations. While palliative operations are used in patients in poor general condition or with neoplastic stenoses accompanied by metastases, it is appropriate in other patients to perform a radical resection, with the aim of obtaining cure by removing the lesion and the obstructed hepatic parenchyma. Rather than performing a limited excision of parenchyma, an operation that is always delicate, we feel it is preferable to remove the half of the liver in which the stenosis is situated. In the case of a neoplastic stenosis, such a wide excision fulfills the criteria of curative cancer surgery. In the presence of a benign inflammatory stenosis, it may appear to be excessive, but in fact it prevents any possibility of recurrence while minimizing technical complications. Thus, left lobectomy is carried out when the stenosis is situated in the left hepatic duct, always a relatively easy procedure. Similarly, right hepatectomy is performed when the lesion involves the right hepatic duct or its large afferent ducts (right paramedian hepatic duct, lateral hepatic duct). Right lobectomy is more difficult, but the technique has become standardized, and even in patients with malignant tumors the postoperative mortality rate should be around 5 per cent.[87]

CAROLI'S DISEASE

Described in 1958, Caroli's disease is characterized by congenital cystic dilatations of the intrahepatic bile ducts.[34, 35] Sometimes it remains limited to one segment or to a section of hepatic parenchyma, whereas in other cases it involves half or all of the liver.[36–40] The cysts are most frequently multiple. They are spherical or ovoid and always communicate with the biliary ducts, which differentiates them from single or multiple biliary cysts. This congenital malformation is often associated with a renal malformation—precalyceal canalicular ectasia or nephrospongiosis.[41–43]

Caroli's disease is rare: Approximately 40 to 50 authentic cases have been reported,[34, 35, 39, 41–51] four of them by the author.[38, 39] It affects both males and females. It may present in the first years of life (the first case described by Caroli was a 2-year-old child[35]) or later in the young adult. The disease is transmitted by heredity, falling within the context of autosomal recessive diseases.

Pathology

Ectasia of the bile ducts takes the form of round or oval dilatation separated by ductal segments of approximately normal caliber. The size of the ducts ranges from 2 to 10 cm. The largest are often found in or near Spiegel's lobe. The hepatic parenchyma surrounding the ectatic ducts is of normal color and consistency.

Histologic examination confirms the absence of abnormalities in the hepatic lobules as well as the presence of small portal spaces containing only a single bile duct, one or two veins, and one or two arteries. The characteristic lesions are to be found in large portal spaces; i.e., the disorder affects only the segmental bile ducts. At the site of the ectasia and of the afferent bile ducts leading to it, the wall is thickened by fibrous infiltration and contains distended canaliculi, although the epithelium has a papillomatous appearance resembling a normal gallbladder. These appearances of active hyperplasia, more marked at the actual site of dilatation, favor a congenital lesion.

It is particularly striking to note that these dilatations have no effect on the portal system: There is never any portal hypertension or splenomegaly. The major complication is intraductal lithiasis. It is invariably present, being secondary to stasis and consisting of numerous calculi of varying sizes, which may migrate into the extrahepatic bile ducts.[39, 52–55, 59] Blackish, they consist of calcium bilirubinate. The intrahepatic stones are responsible for the majority of complications, usually infections: liver abscess, subphrenic abscess, septicemia—complications that often result in death. This emphasizes the need for early recognition of the condition in order to prevent the development of infection and intervene surgically so as to eradicate the lesions when they are limited to one segment of the liver. There is some evidence that Caroli's disease may be associated with a higher incidence of cholangiocarcinoma.[49, 56–58]

Clinical Findings

Congenital dilatation of the intrahepatic bile ducts produces its most important consequences at a more or less advanced age, but the initial manifestations usually appear in childhood or adolescence.[39]

The disease is marked by recurrent episodes of unexplained fever of a pseudomalarial type, with the usual repercussion in the patient's general condition. Pain is not invariably present but often develops later in association with fever. The pain is located in the right hypochondrium and is dull in character.

Jaundice is rare and results from obstruction of the common bile duct by a stone that has migrated from an area of dilatation. This disease may thus be summarized as consisting of episodes of pain and fever, which are capricious in their course, and the patient may pass through asymptomatic periods lasting several years during which the general condition is perfectly normal.

Physical examination is normal, even during acute attacks. There is neither hepatomegaly nor splenomegaly. There are no signs of portal hypertension; at the very most, percussion over the liver may elicit tenderness.

Liver function tests are virtually unaltered even after the disease has progressed for several years. Leukocytosis with an increased differential polynuclear count is seen only during episodes of acute cholangitis.

The diagnosis is made by radiologic examination of the biliary system as well as the urinary tract in a patient with an intermittent unexplained febrile syndrome. The abnormalities of the intrahepatic bile ducts are seen, while the frequently associated precalyceal malformations of the kidneys are demonstrated by intravenous urography.

Radiologic Study

Transhepatic cholangiography is the examination of choice. It reveals round or oblong, unequal-sized cysts of the intrahepatic ducts, which are frequently predominant at the periphery of the liver.

The extrahepatic bile ducts are often normal, although dilatation of the common bile duct or the gallbladder may be seen. There may be calculi in the common bile duct that have migrated from the areas of dilatation. Echotomography and CT scanning clearly demonstrate the ductal dilatations and the calculi that they contain.[61, 62]

Selective arteriography of the hepatic artery not only reveals the duct dilatations in the form of a checkerboard of circular or oval cavities but also provides information concerning the vasculature of the liver, which is of help during surgery. It is important information, and the examination is relatively free of risk in skilled hands.

Intravenous urography should be performed routinely to look for the frequently associated nephrospongiosis, which may be clinically latent.

Radiologic studies not only confirm the diagnosis but also determine the extent of the lesion and make it possible to recognize diffuse forms that are unsuitable for surgical treatment and localized forms that may be treated by excision.

Course

The spontaneous course of Caroli's disease is dominated by biliary infection. This may result in liver abscess formation, which in turn may progress to the formation of subphrenic abscesses. The latter may, on the right, open into the pleura and, on the left, into the pericardium. The picture is sometimes that of septicemia of considerable gravity. Long-term suppuration may lead to amyloidosis and to malignant change in the mucosa of the areas of congenital ectasia in the form of cholangiocarcinomas.[49, 56–58] The latter are not rare, above all, when the malformations of the intraheptic ducts are accompanied by "cysts" of the common bile duct.[55, 60, 63]

Operative Findings

Exact assessment of the lesion is possible only at the time of surgical exploration.

The external appearance of the liver is usually normal. Its surface is smooth and regular, and the dilatations of the bile ducts are not usually perceived. The site and extent of the dilatations may be recognized by feeling the parenchyma with the tip of the index finger. Palpation with pressure leaves an abnormal depression, which persists in the form of a pit over the site of a cystic duct. Opening one of the most superficial dilatations reveals cavities that vary in size and contain stagnant bile and a variable number of black calculi of different sizes.

The cysts should not be opened, however, but should instead be examined by operative cholangiography by direct puncture of one of the cavities or by injection into the gallbladder or common bile duct. During cholangiography it is useful to clamp the common bile duct in order to obtain maximum reflux of contrast medium into the intrahepatic bile ducts to fill the dilated ducts. This gives accurate information concerning the extent of the lesions and their topography in relation to the hepatic parenchyma, and it offers the best possibility to select adequate treatment.

Operative cholangiography also has the merit of demonstrating the absence of any obstruction at the level of the sphincter of Oddi, of detecting the presence of any stones that may be in the process of migration into the hepatic ducts or common bile duct, and of confirming the always possible association of saclike or fusiform ectasia of the common bile duct, since cystic changes here are frequently found in the presence of intrahepatic cysts.[55, 60, 63]

Treatment

There is a difference between limited forms, fortunately the most common, and diffuse forms of Caroli's disease. Localized forms that, at the most, involve one entire lobe of the liver (usually the left), are curable by surgery. They should be treated by hemihepatectomy, associated or not with the treatment of any problem affecting the common duct.[39, 64–69] When calculi have migrated into the extrahepatic bile duct, removal of calculi or sphincterotomy, or both, may be needed. Ectasia of the extrahepatic ducts, when it is associated with the congenital malformations of the intrahepatic bile ducts, may be helped by sphincteroplasty. Too often, appropriate surgery is performed only after one or more previous operations, because the existence of Caroli's disease either was unknown at the time of the first operation or was recognized but inappropriately treated. Although more difficult, reoperations should be undertaken without hesitation. The patients should receive perioperative antibiotics.

Forms of the disease that involve both

halves of the liver pose particularly difficult therapeutic problems. A number of approaches have been suggested. Sphincterotomy has given poor results because of association with reflux cholangitis. The same applies to choledochoduodenostomy. Hepaticojejunostomy using a Roux-en-Y jejunal loop 50 cm long should minimize the risks of reflux but does nothing to facilitate the evacuation of pigment stones contained within the dilated ducts. In one such patient we performed an extended left hepatectomy plus removal of all calculi from the bile ducts of the right side of the liver, bypassing the right ductal system into a jejunal loop brought up as a Y. The immediate result was satisfactory but was followed by a recurrence that resulted in the patient's death 3 years later. Nevertheless, the potential value of this method should be borne in mind.

The same outlook applies to lithotomy and Roux-en-Y drainage of the ducts of both halves of the liver. This consists of approaching the biliary tree via the common bile duct, with removal of intrahepatic stones under cholangiographic control using scoops, curettes, Dormia baskets, and Fogarty balloon catheters; washing of the bile ducts under pressure; and, finally, the establishment of permanent drainage of the latter. Two drains with perforations in their midparts are introduced from below, one into the left hepatic duct and the other into the right hepatic duct. The upper extremity emerges at the convexity of the liver after having passed through the area of dilatation, while the lower extremity passes into a jejunal loop brought up as a Y and anastomosed to the common bile duct. Both extremities of each drain are exteriorized through the abdominal wall. Such an arrangement permits not only return of the bile into the digestive tract but also lavage of the areas of dilatation. The latter is performed periodically using isotonic solutions containing appropriate antibiotics and chenodeoxycholic acid. Several variations of this procedure have been described.[32, 39, 70] The purpose is to have relatively easy access to the biliary ducts postoperatively.

Medical treatment consists, first, of antibiotics, of stone-dissolving agents, and of biliary intubation; and second, of analgesics and antispasmodics. It is usually possible to deal with infection, at least, for a long period, permitting normal growth and weight development in children suffering from the condition.

Prognosis

The prognosis of Caroli's disease is dependent on the extent of the lesions. Forms limited to one segment or to one half of the liver may be cured by excision. Forms involving the duct system of the entire liver are associated with a grave prognosis, regardless of the method of therapy. The only hope for cure lies in the possible discovery of an agent that might be capable of dissolving pigment lithiasis, the calculi responsible for the obstruction that produces biliary infection and its consequences.

CONGENITAL DILATATION OF THE INTRAHEPATIC BILE DUCTS AND ASSOCIATED FIBROCHOLANGIOMATOSIS

Congenital dilatation of the intrahepatic bile ducts may be associated with fibrocholangiomatosis (congenital hepatic fibrosis).[16, 51, 71–81] More common than Caroli's disease, the association of these two lesions was described in 1954 by Grumbach et al. under the name of fibrocystic disease of the liver with portal hypertension in the child.[82] The disorder, in general, affects children and adolescents. It is characterized by (1) congenital dilatation of the segmental bile ducts, (2) proliferation at a lobular level of biliary canaliculi, and (3) the existence of an extensive fibrous reaction that extends from the portal spaces to the periphery of the hepatic lobules.

This last lesion produces cirrhosis, which results in marked portal hypertension,[82–85] esophageal varices, and splenomegaly, while dilatation of the segmental bile ducts results in cholangitis.[86] It is these two complications that may be lethal: portal hypertension resulting in hemorrhage and cholangitis as a source of sepsis. The patients may also have nephrospongiosis, as in Caroli's disease. The two disorders are thus closely related, however, while patients with pure segmental congenital dilatation usually live to adult life, most patients with associated fibrosis die in childhood or adolescence because of the complications of portal hypertension.

In patients with fibrocholangiomatosis, the liver is hard and often very large, weighing as much as 2.5 kg. The appearance is identical to that of cirrhosis but without large regenerating nodules. Hepatomegaly is invariably accompanied by portal hypertension and splenomegaly with gastroesophageal varices. On section, the hepatic parenchyma shows fibrous tissue containing vast cavities—the dilated bile ducts.

In most cases, the disease presents in childhood as a form of congenital cirrhosis.[82–84] The initial manifestation is gastrointestinal hemorrhage, anemia, or signs of hypersplenism. Examination reveals hepatomegaly and splenomegaly, and an upper gastrointestinal series demonstrates gastroesophageal varices. Dilatation of the segmental bile ducts often produces no manifestations, or what manifestations do appear may be attributed to the hepatic parenchymal disease.

Sometimes the patient presents with signs of cholangitis, but it is rare for the correct diagnosis of bile duct abnormalities to be made from the outset as an explanation for the acute febrile episodes. The special investigations described in the section on Caroli's disease are those most likely to result in the correct diagnosis. In the majority of cases congenital dilatation of the segmental bile ducts goes unrecognized, even at surgery, since in the presence of fibrosis the characteristic "fitting" sign of the disorder is absent. Only routine cholangiography with complete filling of the biliary tree is capable of demonstrating the characteristic abnormalities. Now that endoscopic retrograde cholangiography is readily available, the diagnosis is more often made preoperatively, whereas in the past it either was a serendipitous finding on operative cholangiograms or was recognized only at autopsy, often after portal bypass that resulted in a fatal attack of cholangitis.

Thus the prognosis of segmental congenital dilatation of the bile ducts associated with fibrocholangiomatosis is most unfavorable. Death may result either from the consequences of portal hypertension or from biliary infection. It should nevertheless be borne in mind that there is a hope of transient remission if portal stasis is treated by portacaval anastomosis and an attempt is made to control attacks of cholangitis by selective antibiotic therapy. In any event, the prognosis of congenital dilatation of the segmental bile ducts associated with hepatic fibrosis is gloomier than for the pure form, at least for those cases of the latter with localized changes that can be treated effectively by hepatic resection. Hepatic transplantation may provide a cure for some of these patients.

REFERENCES

1. Sanes S, MacCallum JD: Primary carcinoma of the liver. Cholangioma in hepatolithiasis. Am J Pathol 1972;*18:*675.
2. Altemeier WA, Gall EA, Zinninger MM, et al: Sclerosing carcinoma of the major intra-hepatic bile ducts. Arch Surg 1957;*75:*450.
3. Hess R, Werthemann A: Primary stenosing cholangitis: its relation to carcinoma. Gastroenterology 1957;*88:*305.
4. Meyerowitz BR, Aird L: Carcinoma of the hepatic ducts within the liver. Br J Surg 1962;*50:*178.
5. Mistilis S, Schiff A: A case of jaundice due to unilateral hepatic duct obstruction with relief after hepatic lobectomy. Gut 1963;*4:*13.
6. Billington BP: Intra-hepatic obstructive jaundice. Med J Aust 1952;*39:*663.
7. Qualman SJ, Haupt HM, Bauer TW, et al: Adenocarcinoma of the hepatic duct junction. A reappraisal of the histologic criteria of malignancy. Cancer 1984;*53:*1545.
8. O'Connor KW, Snodgrass PJ, Swonder JE, et al: A blinded prospective study comparing four current noninvasive approaches in the differential diagnosis of medical versus surgical jaundice. Gastroenterology 1983;*84:*1498.
9. Matzen P, Malchw-Moller A, Brun B, et al: Ultrasonography, computed tomography and cholescintigraphy in suspected obstructive jaundice—a prospective comparative study. Gastroenterology 1983; *84:*1492.
10. Eyre-Brook IA, Ross B, Johnson AG: Should surgeons operate on the evidence of ultrasound alone in jaundiced patients? Br J Surg 1983;*70:*587.
11. Thorsen MK, Quiroz F, Lawson TL, et al: Body computed tomography. Primary biliary carcinoma: CT evaluation. Radiology 1984;*152:*479.
12. Subramanyam BR, Raghavendra BN, Balthazar EJ, et al: Ultrasonic features of cholangiocarcinoma. J Ultrasound Med 1984;*3:*405.
13. Wanebo HJ, Grimes OF: Cancer of the bile ducts. The occult malignancy. Am J Surg 1975;*130:*262.
14. Thornjarnarson B: Carcinoma of the intra-hepatic bile ducts. Arch Surg 1958;*71:*906.
15. Cohen MM: Congenital disease of the liver and biliary tract in adults. Can J Surg 1984;*27:*211.
16. Barros JL, Polo JR, Sanabia J, et al: Congenital cystic dilatation of the intrahepatic bile ducts (Caroli's disease): Report of a case and review of the literature. Surgery 1979;*85:*589.
17. Schanmugaratnam KI: Primary carcinoma of the liver and biliary tract. Br J Cancer 1956;*10:*232.
18. Alexandres JM, Roge D, Germain M, et al: Les possibilités de la chirurgie dans les cancers des canaux intra-hepatiques. Ann Chir 1973;*27:*547.
19. Cady B, Fortner JC: Surgical resection of intrahepatic bile duct cancer. Am J Surg 1969;*118:*104.
20. Campeau M, Meillere D: Les anastomoses biliodigestives intra-hepatiques. Techniques et indications. J Chir 1965;*89:*281.

21. Dogliotti AM: Traitement chirurgical des retrecissements cicatriciels des voies biliaries. Lyon Chir 1957;*53*:563.
22. Hepp J, Moreaux J, Lechaux JP: Les anastomoses bilio-digestives intra-hepatiques dans les cancers des voies biliaries. Presse Med 1973;*27*:1829.
23. Longmire WP, Sandord M: Intra-hepatic cholangiojejunostomy with partial hepatectomy for biliary obstruction. Surgery 1948;*24*:264.
24. Praderi R: Coledocostomia transhepatica. Bol Soc Cir Urug 1961:*32*:237.
25. Praderi R: Twelve years' experiences with transhepatic intubation. Ann Surg 1974;*170*:937.
26. Ross AP, Braasch JW, Warren KW: Carcinoma of the proximal bile ducts. Surg Gynecol Obstet 1973;*136*:923.
27. Terblanche J: Is carcinoma of the main hepatic duct junction an indication for liver transplantation or palliative surgery? A plea for the U-tube palliative procedure. Surgery 1976;*79*:127.
28. Longmire WP, Tompkins RK: Lesions of the segmental and lobar hepatic ducts. Ann Surg 1975;*182*:478.
29. Blumgart LH, Kelley CJ: Hepaticojejunostomy in benign and malignant high bile duct stricture: approaches to the left hepatic ducts. Br J Surg 1984;*71*:257.
30. Cameron JL, Gayler BW, Harrington DP: Modification of the Longmire procedure. Ann Surg 1978;*187*:379.
31. Hutson DG, Russell E, Schiff E, et al: Balloon dilatation of biliary strictures through a choledochojejuno-cutaneous fistula. Ann Surg 1984;*199*:637.
32. Barker EM, Winkler M: Permanent-access hepaticojejunostomy. Br J Surg 1984;*71*:188.
33. Carrasco CH, Zornoza J, Bechtel WJ: Malignant biliary obstruction: Complications of percutaneous biliary drainage. Radiology 1984;*152*:343.
34. Caroli J, Soupault R, Kossakowski J, et al: La dilatation polykystique congenitale des voies biliaires intra-hepatiques. Essai de classification. Sem Hop Paris 1958;*14*:128.
35. Caroli J, Couinaud C, Soupault R, et al: Une affection nouvelle, sans doute congenitale, des voies biliaires. La dilatation kystique unilobaire des canaux hepatiques. Sem Hop Paris 1958;*14*:136.
36. Glenn F, McSherry CK: Congenital segmental cystic dilatation of the biliary duct system. Ann Surg 1973;*177*:705.
37. Hunter FM, Akdamar K, Sparks RD, et al: Congenital dilatation of intrahepatic bile ducts. Am J Med 1966;*40*:188.
38. Mercardier M, Clot JP, Melliere D, et al: Nouvelles observations de dilatation congenitale des voies biliaires intra-hepatiques (Maladie de Caroli). Sem Hop Paris 1968;*44*:283.
39. Mercadier M, Chigot JP, Clot JP, et al: Caroli's disease. World J Surg 1984;*8*:22.
40. Rosenwarne MD: Cystic dilatation of the intrahepatic bile ducts. Br J Radiol 1972;*45*:845.
41. Gilbertini G, Lode R, Torricelli A: Communicating cavernous ectasia of intrahepatic bile ducts associated with multiple cysts of the renal medulla. Panminerva Med 1965;*7*:227.
42. Lamy M, Nezolof C, Jammet ML, et al: La maladie polykystique hepatorenale. Arch Fr Pediatr 1961; *18*:293.
43. Nakanuma Y, Terada T, Ohta G, et al: Caroli's disease in congenital hepatic fibrosis and infantile polycystic disease. Liver 1982;*2*:346.
44. Beau A, Prevot J, Manciaus M, et al: Un nouveau cas de malformation polykystique congenitale des voies biliaires. J Chir 1960;*80*:442.
45. Belloli G, Vianello A, Campobasso P, et al: Sulla dilatazione congenita segmentaria della vie biliari intraepatiche o mallattia di Caroli. Minerva Pediatr 1972;*24*:2133.
46. Benitendi B, Bressan G: Contributo alla conoscenza della dilatazione cistica congenita segmentaria delle vie biliari intrahepatiche. Acta Chir Ital 1968; *29*:501.
47. Berenguer J, Olaso V, Rayon M, et al: Dilatacion congenita no obstructiva de los conductos biliares intrahepaticos segmentarios (enfermedad de Caroli). Presentacion de una observation y revision de la literatura. Clin Espanol 1976;*140*:567.
48. Caroli J: Congenital dilatations of the segmental intrahepatic biliary tree. Clin Gastroenterol 1973; *2*:148.
49. Dayton MT, Longmire WP, Tompkins RK: Caroli's disease: A premalignant condition? Am J Surg 1983;*145*:41.
50. Chaumerliac H, Barrier JA, Barrier JP, et al: Dilatation kystique congenitale du choledoque associée à une maladie de Caroli. Bordeaux Med 1969; *2*:1448.
51. Dusol M Jr, Levi JU, Glasser K, et al: Congenital hepatic fibrosis with dilation of intrahepatic bile ducts. A therapeutic approach. Gastroenterology 1976;*71*:839.
52. Farach M, Helou E, Nasser W, et al: Un nouveau cas de maladie de Caroli avec dilatations geantes bilobaires segmentaires, compliquée de lithiase et guerie chirurgicalement. Rev Med Chir Mal Foie 1966;*41*:305.
53. Hamyln AH, James OFW, Douglas AP, et al: Caroli's disease with intrahepatic gallstones and Salmonella infection. Postgrad Med J 1976;*52*:656.
54. Murray-Lyon IM, Shilikin KB, Laws JW, et al: Nonobstructive dilatation of the intrahepatic biliary tree with cholangitis. Q J Med 1972;*41*:477.
55. Paris JC, Quandalle P, Houcke M, et al: Un cas de maladie de Caroli associée à un kyste congenita du choledoque et compliquée d'une lithiase biliaire intra-hepatique. Lille Med 1977;*22*:226.
56. Gallagher PJ, Millis RR, Mitchinson MJ: Congenital dilatation of the intrahepatic bile ducts with cholangiocarcinoma. J Clin Pathol 1972;*25*:804.
57. Jones AW, Shreeve DR: Congenital dilatation of intrahepatic biliary ducts with cholangiocarcinoma. Br Med J 1970;*2*:277.
58. Taylor CO, Ellis JG: Fatal complications of Caroli's disease. Am J Gastroenterol 1982;*77*:75.
59. Sahel J, Bourry J, Sarles H: Maladie de Caroli avec pancreatite aigue et angiocholite. Nouv Presse Med 1976;*32*:2067.
60. Meeker WR, Nighbert EJ: Association of cystic dilatation of intrahepatic and common bile ducts with Laurence Moon Biedl Bardet syndrome. Am J Surg 1971;*22*:822.
61. Moreno AJ, Parker AL, Spicer DO, et al: Scintigraphic and radiographic findings in Caroli's disease. Am J Gastroenterol 1984;*79*:299.
62. Levy VG, Darnis F: Dilatation kystique des voies biliaires intra-hepatiques (Maladie de Caroli). A propos d'un cas ratent devouvert par cholangiographie orale. Med Chir Dig 1976;*5*:5.
63. Gots RE, Zuidema GD: Dilatation of the intrahepatic biliary duct in a patient with a choledocal cyst. Ann Surg 1970;*119*:726.

64. Watts DR, Lorenzo GA, Beal JM: Congenital dilatation of the intrahepatic biliary ducts. Arch Surg 1974;*108*:592.
65. Zer M, Chaimoff C, Dintsman M: Cystic dilatation of intrahepatic bile ducts. Arch Surg 1973;*106*:225.
66. Schrumpf E, Bergan A, Blomhoff JP: Partial hepatectomy in Caroli's disease. Scand J Gastroenterol 1981;*16*:581.
67. Ramond MJ, Huguet C, Danan G, et al: Partial hepatectomy in the treatment of Caroli's disease. Report of a case and review of the literature. Dig Dis Sci 1984;*29*:367.
68. Nagasue N: Successful treatment of Caroli's disease by hepatic resection. Report of six patients. Ann Surg 1984;*200*:718.
69. Martin F, Corcos V, Albano O: La dilatation congenitale des voies biliaires intra-hepatiques segmentaires (maladie de J Caroli). Presse Med 1965; *73*:2565.
70. Witlin LT, Gadacz TR, Zuidema GD: Transhepatic decompression of the biliary tree in Caroli's disease. Surgery 1982;*91*:205.
71. Foulk WT: Congenital malformations of the intrahepatic biliary tree in the adult. Gastroenterology 1970;*58*:253.
72. Tsuchiya R, Nishimura R, Koshiya I: Congenital cystic dilatation of the bile ducts associated with Laurence-Moon-Biedl-Bardet Syndrome. Arch Surg 1977;*112*:82.
73. Boquien Y, Leger L, Guyet P: Deux cas de dilatation congenitale des canaux biliaires intra-hepatiques associée à une cirrhose du foie et à des malformations diverses. Rev Med Chir Mal Foie 1958;*33*:73.
74. Boquien Y, Delumeau G, Lenne Y, et al: Fibroadenomatose biliaire et dilatation congenitale des voies biliaires intra-hepatiques. Rev Med Chir Mal Foie 1967;*42*:265.
75. Caroli J, Corcos V: La dilatation congenitale des voies biliaires intra-hepatique. Rev Med Chir Mal Foie 1964;*39*:1.
76. Erlinger S, Sakellardis A, Maillard JN, et al: Les formes angiocholitiques de la fibrose hepatique congenitale. Presse Med 1969;*77*:1189.
77. Feverly J, Tanghe W, Kerremans R, et al: Congenital dilatation of the intrahepatic bile ducts. Gut 1972;*13*:604.
78. Guenin P, Vinnalou J, Benhamou JP, et al: Dilatation kystique des voies biliaires intra-hepatiques et fibrose hepatique congenitale. Rev Med Chir Mal Foie 1963;*38*:149.
79. Levy VC, De Saint-Maur PP: Les maladies kystiques et fibrokystiques du foie (hamartomes biliaries). Essai de classification anatomoclinique. Med Chir Dig 1976;*5*:2.
80. Mall JC, Chahremant GG, Boyer LL: Caroli's disease associated with congenital hepatic fibrosis and renal tubular ectasia. Gastroenterology 1974;*66*:1029.
81. Murray Lyon LM, Ockenden BG, Williams R: Congenital hepatic fibrosis—is it a single entity? Gastroenterology 1973;*64*:653.
82. Grumbach R, Bourillon J, Auvert JP: Maladie fibrokystique du foie avec hypertension portale chez l'enfant. Sem Hop Arch Anta Pathol 1974;*30*:74.
83. Auvert J: Les cirrhoses de l'enfant avec hypertension portale. Analyse de 5 cas, dont 4 traités par derivation splenomenale. Rev Int Hepat 1955;*5*:1243.
84. De Ferron A, Gordeed A, De Ferron C, et al: La fibroangio-adenomatose du foie avec hypertension portale chez l'enfant. Presse Med 1961;*69*:1147.
85. Saubier E, Viard M, Partensky C, et al: Kyste de l'hepatocholedoque avec dilatation segmentaire congenitale des voies biliaires intra-hepatiques (maladie de Caroli) et hypertension portale. Lyon Chir 1971;*64*:299.
86. Pridgen JA, Bradley A, McInnis D: Primary intrahepatic gallstones. Arch Surg 1977;*112*:1037.
87. Stimpson R, Pellegrini CA, Way LW: Factors affecting the morbidity and mortality of elective liver disections. Am J Surg. In press.

SEYMOUR I. SCHWARTZ, M.D.

29

Sclerosing Cholangitis

Sclerosing cholangitis, also referred to as stenosing cholangitis, obliterative cholangitis, and fibrosing cholangitis, is a rare inflammatory disease causing fibrous narrowing of all or parts of the bile duct system. The disorder may be an isolated pathologic process, having been designated as primary sclerosing cholangitis, or may be associated with a wide variety of inflammatory, vascular, and fibrosing disorders.

The criteria for assigning a diagnosis of sclerosing cholangitis are thickening and fibrosis of the extrahepatic bile duct system or intrahepatic cholangioles, or both, absence of choledocholithiasis, absence of previous bile duct operation, and absence of drug-induced or viral hepatitis. It is now felt that "sclerosing cholangitis" should include all patients with the affliction, regardless of the presence or absence of associated diseases, and that the nomenclature of "primary sclerosing cholangitis" is no longer appropriate.

Sclerosing cholangitis was first described by Delbert[1] in 1924, and a second case appeared in the same journal a year later.[2] Miller[3] recorded the first case in the English literature in 1927. The first review and large personal series was reported by Schwartz and Dale in 1958.[4] Since then, personal series have been reported by Holubitsky and McKenzie,[5] Warren et al.,[6] Thorpe et al.,[7] Oviedo et al.,[8] Cutler and Donaldson,[9] Myers et al.,[10] Thompson et al.,[11] Schwartz,[12] Danzi et al.,[13] Fee et al.,[14] Cameron et al.,[37] and Thompson et al.[39]

ETIOLOGY

The etiology of sclerosing cholangitis remains obscure. The two categories of causes that have received the greatest attention have been bacterial infection and hypersensitivity or immune responses. In some patients, *E. coli* organisms have grown from bile cultures. Although there is no question that some patients with ulcerative colitis have portal bacteremia, this cannot be defined as leading to the development of cholangitis.[15] *Strongyloides* larvae were noted in the common bile duct of one patient with sclerosing cholangitis.[13] Those who would like to implicate an immunologic factor confront the fact that serologic analyses have uncovered no substantiating findings in most cases. Eosinophilia in the blood and tissues of some patients with sclerosing cholangitis and diffuse retroperitonitis[16] is somewhat suggestive of hypersensitivity. The association of sclerosing cholangitis with chronic pancreatitis, and sicca complex in two siblings with demonstrated leukocyte migration inhibition in the presence of bile antigen, have been suggestive of an immune mechanism.[17] Record et al.[18] reported an example of familial sclerosing cholangitis associated with immune deficiency. Also, mitochondrial antibodies have been demonstrated in a few cases,[7] and nonspecific vasculitis[19] and generalized lymphadenopathy with hypergammaglobulinemia[42] have been seen in others. It has been shown experimentally that chronic inflammation of the bile ducts can be induced by the Shwartzman reaction.[20] Leukocyte migration inhibition tests to determine the cellular immune response to antigens in a protein fraction of bile have demonstrated a positive response in patients with this disease.

PATHOLOGY

Grossly there is diffuse thickening of the bile ducts. Sclerosing cholangitis may encompass the entire extrahepatic ductal system or just a segment of the biliary tree. Most patients with sclerosing cholangitis have diffuse extra- and intrahepatic involvement. The disease tends to be particularly severe at or near the bifurcation of the common hepatic duct.[37]

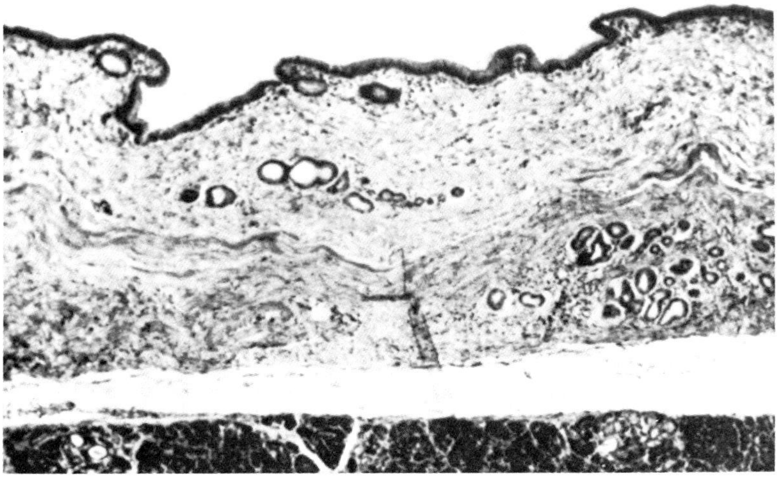

Figure 29–1. Distal common bile duct. The mucosa is intact, and there is marked fibrous thickening with glandular hyperplasia and minimal round cell infiltration. Masson stain; original magnification × 50. (From Thompson BW, Read RC: Am J Surg 1977; *128*:177. Used by permission.)

In a few patients, involvement is limited to the distal portion of the bile duct and the response to a biliary bypass in these individuals is excellent.[39] An occasional patient may have segmental involvement of the bifurcation of the common hepatic duct only.[43] However, in general, a focal stricture at the confluence of the right and left hepatic ducts only should be considered a sclerosing carcinoma until proven otherwise, since the segmental forms of sclerosing cholangitis are very rare.

The bile duct wall is markedly thickened, with consequent narrowing of the lumen. However, obstruction is not complete, and a thin probe or radiopaque contrast medium can be shown to enter the duodenum. The gallbladder is usually normal but may be involved in the process.

Surrounding the ducts there is a dense inflammatory reaction in the region of the gastrohepatic ligament, at times making identification of the duct extremely difficult. Large succulent nodes are present in this area. The bile within the extrahepatic ducts varies from a clear yellow to a thick sludge.

Biopsy of the involved extrahepatic bile duct reveals an intact mucosa with submucosal inflammation, fibrosis, glandular hyperplasia, and distortion (Fig. 29–1).[40] Rarely, eosinophilia has been noted in the duct wall. The gallbladder wall may show round cell infiltrates and aggregates. The regional lymph nodes demonstrate nonspecific hyperplasia. The liver biopsy is characterized by bile stasis. Proliferation of the small bile canaliculi is uncommon, but there may be an obliterative intimal proliferation of the hepatic arterioles. In some patients the sclerosing process is mainly intrahepatic, in which case the pathologic changes are indistinguishable from those of primary biliary cirrhosis.[21, 22] In these situations there is concentric periductal fibrosis and the small and medium-sized ducts are reduced to fibrous cords (Fig. 29–2).

A broad spectrum of disorders has been associated with sclerosing cholangitis. Ulcerative colitis is the most common. It is present in 20 to 35 per cent of patients with sclerosing cholangitis[6, 7, 23, 24, 39] and was found in up to 50 per cent of the patients in one report.[37] However, only approximately 1 per cent of patients with ulcerative colitis develop sclerosing cholangitis.[40] The etiologic relationship of sclerosing cholangitis to ulcerative colitis is not known, but some have found regression of sclerosing cholangitis following total colectomy.[44] Crohn's disease and proctosigmoiditis[13] have also been noted. Retroperitoneal fibrosis (Ormond's disease),[16] retractile mesenteritis,[19] Riedel's thyroiditis,[16] Weber-Christian disease,[25] pancreatitis,[17] xanthomatosis,[14] vasculitis,[26] porphyria cutanea tarda,[13] and sicca complex[17] have all occurred in association with sclerosing cholangitis.

CLINICAL MANIFESTATIONS

Unlike other inflammatory disorders of the biliary tract, males are affected more often than females. A review of the literature revealed that the patients were between 17 and 74 years of age, with a median of 38 years.[27] Patients with sclerosing cholangitis associated with other disorders are generally younger.

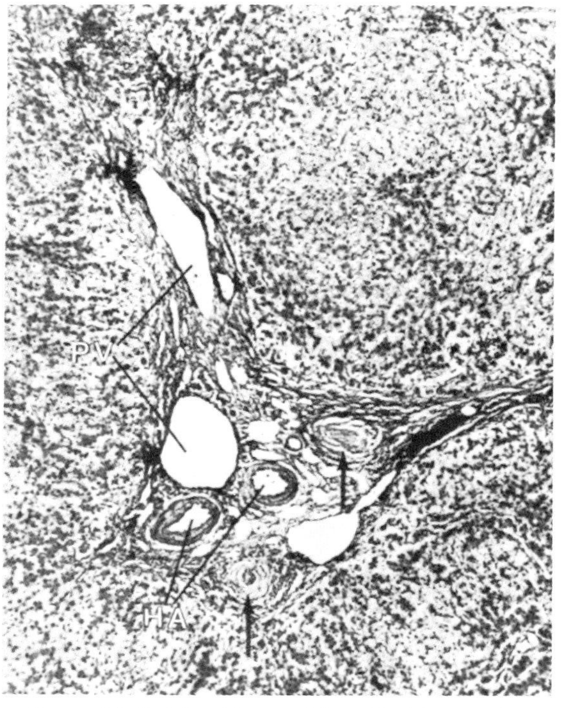

Figure 29–2. Edge biopsy of liver. Portal zone shows sclerosed interlobular duct (*upper arrow*) and interlobular duct with periductal fibrosis (*lower arrow*). The patient was a 64-year-old male. PV, portal vein branches, HA, hepatic artery branches. Verhoeff Van Gieson stain × 40.

The onset of symptoms is usually insidious, and patients frequently recall that epigastric or right upper quadrant pain had occurred intermittently for years. Malaise, nausea, and weight loss may accompany the abdominal discomfort. Pruritus and jaundice are frequently intermittent for a variable period before becoming persistent. The stool may be acholic or very pale.

The physical examination is unrevealing. In the absence of manifestations of associated diseases, only mild upper abdominal tenderness and minimal to moderate hepatomegaly may be noted.

LABORATORY AND RADIOLOGIC FINDINGS

Eosinophilia is present in about one quarter to one third of patients. The blood chemistries reflect an obstructive jaundice. The alkaline phosphatase value is increased, often markedly, and is frequently out of proportion to the serum bilirubin elevation. The serum cholesterol is usually increased and may exceed 300 mg/dl. The increases in the SGOT and SGPT are moderate and more compatible with a diagnosis of biliary obstruction than with that of hepatocellular disease. Antimitochondrial antibodies have been noted in an occasional patient, but the titers are low, much below the level seen in patients with primary biliary cirrhosis.

The major diagnostic advances have occurred in the field of radiology, and it is only recently that a precise preoperative diagnosis has been possible. Oral cholecystography and intravenous cholangiography are rarely feasible, since the serum bilirubin value is generally elevated above the critical 3.0 mg/dl level. In an occasional patient with minimal jaundice, the diagnosis has been suggested by intravenous cholangiography, but the opacification is generally poor. In the past, percutaneous transhepatic cholangiography (PTC) failed to opacify the extrahepatic duct system in most cases, particularly when the intrahepatic duct was involved, since it was difficult to aspirate bile and determine if the

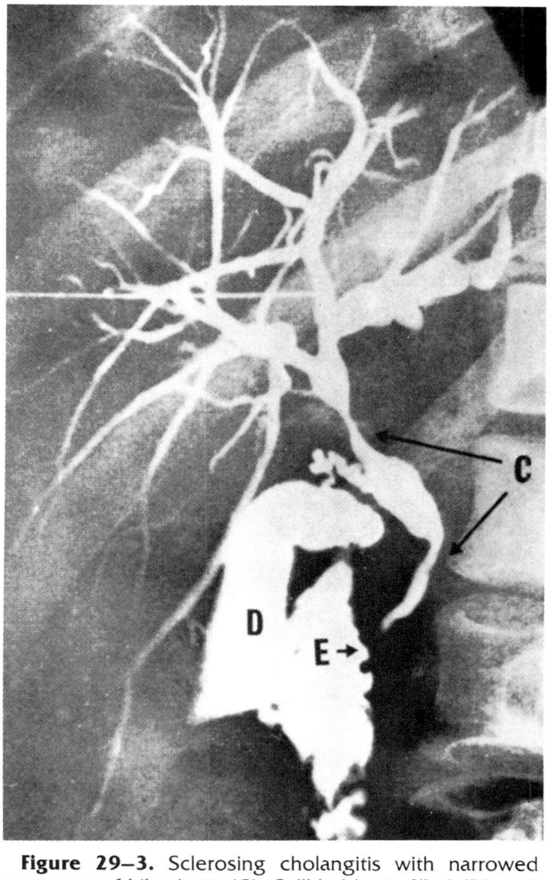

Figure 29–3. Sclerosing cholangitis with narrowed segments of bile ducts (C). Gallbladder is filled (D), and contrast medium flows into duodenum unobstructed (E). (From Jain S, Long RG, Scott J, et al: Br J Radiol 1977; *50*:175. Used by permission.)

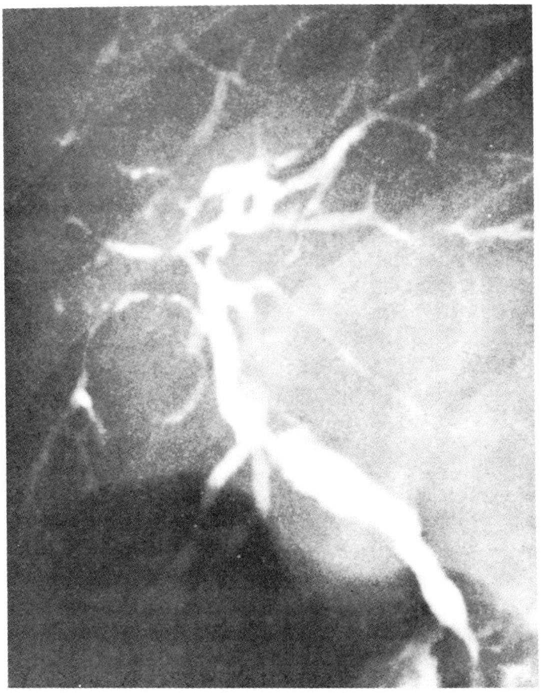

Figure 29–4. Sclerosing cholangitis. Cholangiogram showing focal stenoses and ectasia of intra- and extrahepatic ducts. (From Rohrmann CA, Ansel HJ, Ayoola EA, et al: AJR 1977; *128*:45. Used by permission.)

needle was in a hepatic duct. However, using the skinny Chiba needle, Jain et al.[28] successfully demonstrated the process in three of five patients with sclerosing cholangitis (Fig. 29–3).

Endoscopic retrograde cholangiopancreatography (ERCP) is uniquely suited to the initial evaluation of these patients and also provides a method of following patients who do not have T-tubes in place. The cholangiographic findings consist of intra- or extrahepatic ductal stenosis, ectasia, and beading and pruning of the extrahepatic ducts (Fig. 29–4).[24] Marked diffuse narrowing of the common bile duct may be accompanied by pruning and beading of the intrahepatic ducts (Fig. 29–5).[30] Cholescintigraphy, using Tc-99m DISIDA has been of help in some cases.[38]

DIFFERENTIAL DIAGNOSIS

Sclerosing cholangitis must be differentiated from other lesions that present with obstructive jaundice. Choledocholithiasis, carcinoma of the pancreas or ampulla of Vater, chronic pancreatitis causing bile duct obstruction, and recurrent nonsuppurative cholangitis must all be excluded. Primary biliary cirrhosis can generally be distinguished by demonstration of antimitochondrial antibodies, and also it is not characterized by eosinophilia.

Congenital cystic disease may affect the entire biliary tract and is manifested by recurrent attacks of jaundice and cholangitis during childhood. The age of the patient helps differentiate this lesion from sclerosing cholangitis, and the characteristic ductal thickening of sclerosing cholangitis is not present.

The lesion that is most difficult to differentiate is a sclerosing bile duct carcinoma. The clinical manifestations and laboratory findings are identical to those in patients with sclerosing cholangitis. Even the cholangiographic findings cannot completely exclude the possibility of carcinoma. The diagnosis may be established at operation by cytopathologic analysis of the bile or bile duct wall scrapings or biopsy of a bile duct lesion. However, frequently these maneuvers do not provide a definitive diagnosis, and the ultimate differentiation between sclerosing cholangitis and carcinoma of the bile duct must be resolved by the patient's course or by autopsy findings.

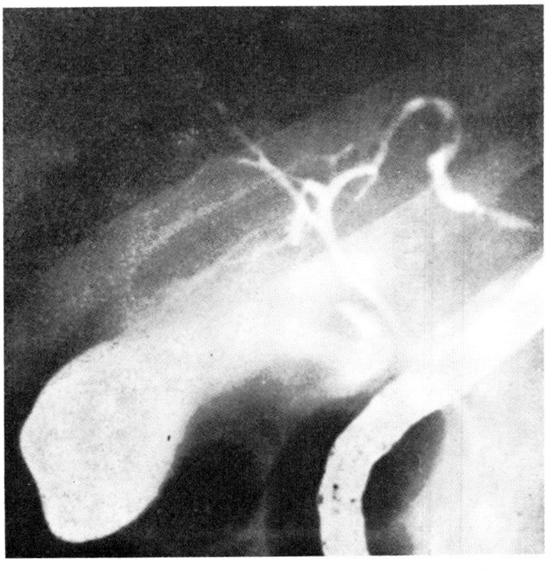

Figure 29–5. A markedly narrowed common bile duct is noted. There is beading of the left intrahepatic biliary tree. The right intrahepatic system has a "pruned tree" appearance.

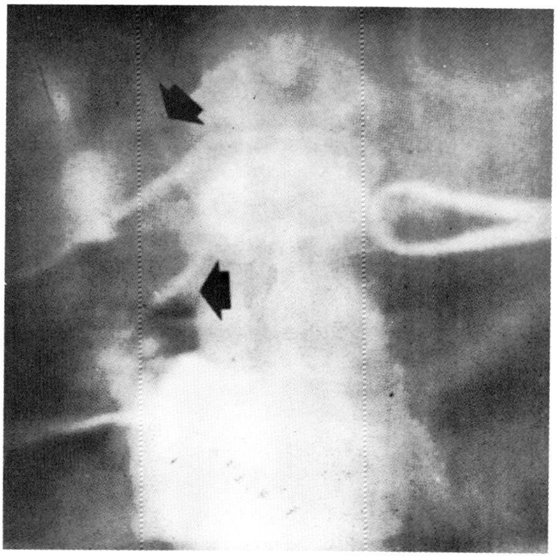

Figure 29–6. Intraoperative cholangiogram. Note common bile duct and passage of radiopaque medium into duodenum (*arrowheads*).

MANAGEMENT

The diagnosis is usually made or strongly suspected during surgical exploration. The presence of a dense inflammatory reaction in the region of the gastrohepatic ligament, particularly if the patient had not had surgery in this region, should suggest the possibility of sclerosing cholangitis. Palpation of the common bile duct and the common hepatic duct gives the sensation of a cordlike structure of normal diameter. The wall of the involved duct is incised with difficulty; after the lumen is entered the edges of the incision characteristically pout out, and the wall is noted to be markedly thickened. Generally, only a fine probe or Bakes' dilator can be inserted into the lumen. Operative cholangiography (Fig. 29–6) demonstrates an extensively narrowed lumen but passage of radiopaque medium into the duodenum. The bile should be sent for cytopathologic evaluation, and a biopsy should be made from representative portions of the diseased duct.

The insertion of a T-tube usually provides the most adequate drainage. It is a palliative procedure and has the advantage of allowing sequential cholangiograms in order to determine the effect of therapy and the general course of the disease. A small-diameter, short-limbed T-tube is preferred, and it is maintained in place until a normal lumen evolves or until no progress in luminal dilatation occurs over a 1-month period. Others advocate prolonged biliary stenting using Silastic tubes.[37, 44] After exploration and dilatation of the lobar ducts, a small (No. 3) Bakes' dilator is passed into one of the lobar ducts and gently pushed through the parenchyma of the liver until it traverses Glisson's capsule. A string is then attached to the end of the dilator, and the dilator and string are brought back through the ducts and through the choledochotomy. The string is attached to the end of the Silastic tube and serves as a guide to thread the Silastic tube through the stricture ducts, through the parenchyma of the liver, and ultimately outside the abdomen through a stab wound. The procedure is then repeated in the other major duct, and the lower ends of the Silastic tube are left within the ductal system or are brought out as a U through an additional stab wound. For further details on the technique of biliary stenting, refer to Chapter 33.

Pitt et al. recommend a more aggressive approach to patients with sclerosing cholangitis. They used biliary stenting and a choledochoenteric anastomosis in 75 per cent of their patients. In a group of 17 patients in whom this technique was used they obtained good to excellent results in 13 (75 per cent). Their series is unique, however, in that it includes several patients with disease limited to the very distal portion of the common bile duct.[41] Resection of a portion of the biliary tract and hepaticojejunostomy may also be successful in the rare patient with segmental disease limited to the common hepatic duct or the bifurcation.[43]

Cholecystojejunostomy is applicable only if the stenotic lesion is limited to an area of the common duct distal to a patent cystic duct. This is rare. If the gallbladder is normal, it is preferable not to remove it, since a distal stenotic lesion may progress and obstruct the common duct. This also is rare.

Corticosteroids have been widely used. Prednisone, 40 to 60 mg daily for weeks to months, has achieved good results,[10, 12] as evidenced by return of the duct lumen to a normal caliber (Fig. 29–7) and correction of the jaundice. Steroids act directly on the ductal disease in their role as anti-inflammatory agents and reduce the hyperbilirubinemia in their capacity as direct choleretic agents. In patients who have been treated successfully with T-tube drainage and corticosteroids, if jaundice recurs after the T-tube has been removed, another course of steroids

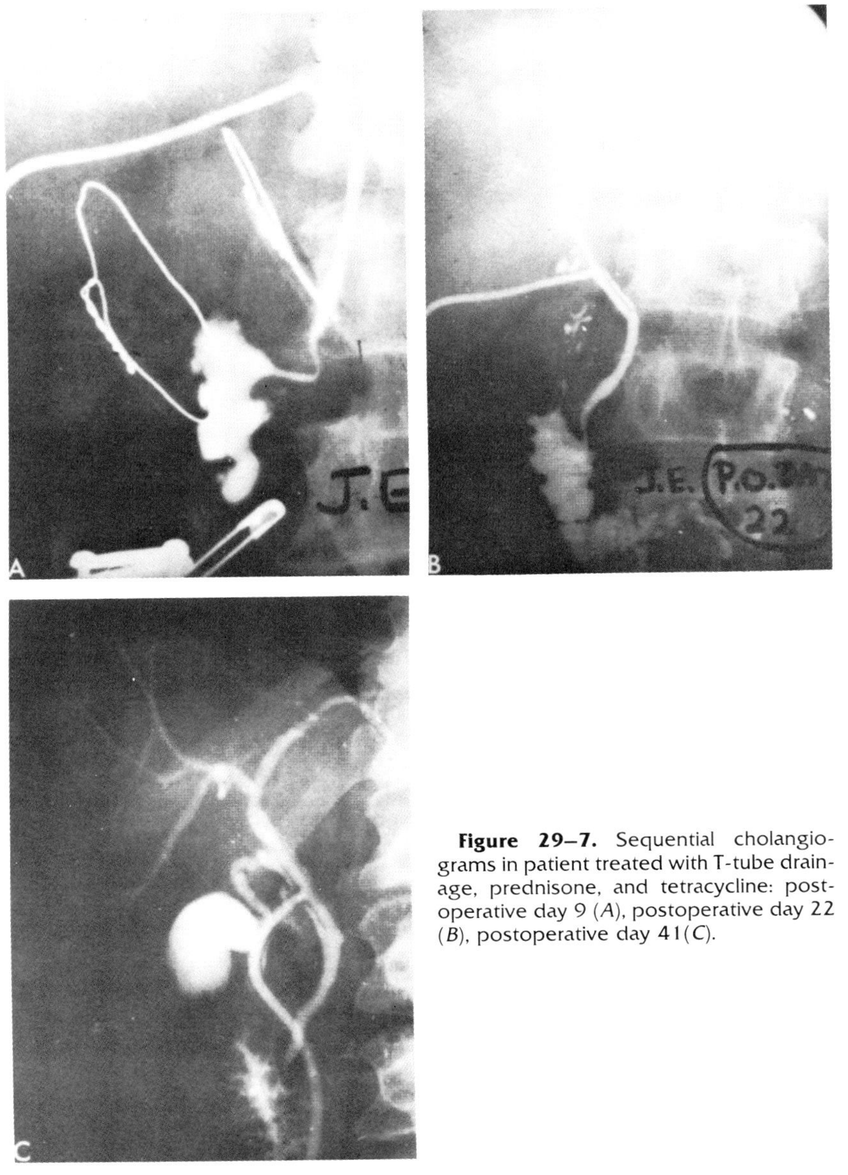

Figure 29–7. Sequential cholangiograms in patient treated with T-tube drainage, prednisone, and tetracycline: postoperative day 9 (*A*), postoperative day 22 (*B*), postoperative day 41(*C*).

may result in another, at times permanent, remission.

Favorable results have been reported with the administration of corticosteroids in combination with azathioprine.[32] However, death from liver abscesses in a patient with sclerosing cholangitis has been attributed to this combination of drugs.[33] Favorable results have been reported in several patients treated with drainage alone, unassociated with either steroid or immunosuppressive therapy.

Antibiotics that achieve therapeutic levels in bile should be used for 5 to 6 days after insertion of a T-tube. Long-term therapy is not advisable, but reinstitution may be required for treatment of ascending cholangitis. Dehydrocholic acid may be employed to increase the fluidity of bile. If a reduction of bile flow into the intestine is associated with malabsorption, a fat-free diet with 40 gm of medium-chain triglyceride fat-soluble vitamins (100,000 units vitamin A, 100,000 units vitamin D, and 10 mg vitamin K) plus calcium should be administered daily.[34] Cholestyramine has been used, with successful resolution of jaundice.[35] It has been proposed that since hepatic copper overload is present in both sclerosing cholangitis and primary biliary cirrhosis, and promising results have been reported in the management of the latter, penacillamine might be applicable for the management of patients with sclerosing cholangitis.[36]

PROGNOSIS

Reports regarding the prognosis have been inconclusive. In most instances the course has been one of progressive liver failure, biliary cirrhosis, and death. In the initial review,[4] 43 per cent of previously reported patients had died, whereas most of our own patients were doing well at the time of publication. We have now followed one patient for over 19 years and another for over 21 years. Oviedo et al.[8] reported three patients alive and well 14, 5, and 1½ years after T-tube drainage alone. Fee et al.[14] followed 18 patients, in whom steroids had been employed, for at least 1 year after T-tube drainage. Five died of their disease, two died of unrelated causes, and 11 showed evidence of slow deterioration. No patient experienced a complete remission. The results reported by Thompson et al., in which six of nine patients died of progressive disease, is in keeping with many reports.[11] In the Wiesner and LaRusso series, 26 of 39 patients (67 per cent) were alive at the time of follow-up, for a mean duration from diagnosis to follow-up of 57 months.[36] Pitt et al. reported that 18 of 22 patients (82 per cent) were alive 52 months after the operation, and 65 months after the diagnosis of sclerosing cholangitis. Two thirds of these patients had biliary stenting combined with a choledochoenterostomy.[41]

REFERENCES

1. Delbert P: Retrecissement du choledoque; cholecystoduodenostomie. Bull Mem Soc Nat Chir 1924; *50*:1144.
2. Lafourcade J: Deux observations d'obliteration cicatricelle du choledoque. Anastomose laterale entre le choledoque et le duodenum dans le second. Bull Mem Soc Nat Chir 1925;*51*:828.
3. Miller RT: Benign stricture of bile ducts. Ann Surg 1927;*86*:296.
4. Schwartz SI, Dale WA: Primary sclerosing cholangitis; review and report of six cases. Arch Surg 1958;*77*:439.
5. Holubitsky IB, McKenzie AD: Primary sclerosing cholangitis of the extrahepatic bile ducts. Can J Surg 1964;*7*:277.
6. Warren KW, Athanassiades S, Mong JI: Primary sclerosing cholangitis: a study of forty-two cases. Am J Surg 1966;*3*:23.
7. Thorpe MEC, Scheuer PJ, Sherlock S: Primary sclerosing cholangitis, the biliary tree, and ulcerative colitis. Gut 1967;*8*:435.
8. Oviedo MA, Volkmer D, Scanlon EF: Primary sclerosing cholangitis. Arch Surg 1974;*109*:747.
9. Cutler B, Donaldson GA: Primary sclerosing cholangitis and obliterative cholangitis. Am J Surg 1969;*117*:502.
10. Myers RN, Cooper JH, Padis N: Primary sclerosing cholangitis. Am J Gastroenterol 1970;*53*:527.
11. Thompson BW, Read RC, White JH: Sclerosing cholangitis. Arch Surg 1972;*104*:460.
12. Schwartz SI: Primary sclerosing cholangitis: A diseased revisited. Surg Clin North Am 1973;*53*:1161.
13. Danzi JT, Makipour H, Farmer RG: Primary sclerosing cholangitis. A report of nine cases and clinical review. Am J Gastroenterol 1976;*65*:109.
14. Fee HJ, Gewirtz H, Schiller J, et al: Sclerosing cholangitis and primary biliary cirrhosis—a disease spectrum? Ann Surg 1977;*186*:589.
15. Brooke BN, Slaney G: Portal bacteremia in ulcerative colitis. Lancet 1958;*1*:1206.
16. Bartholomew LG, Cain JC, Wollner LB, et al: Sclerosing cholangitis. N Engl J Med 1963;*269*:8.
17. Waldram R, Kopelman H, Tsantoulas D, et al: Chronic pancreatitis, sclerosing cholangitis, and sicca complex in two siblings. Lancet 1975;*1*:550.
18. Record CO, Shilkin KB, Eddleston AL, et al: Intrahepatic sclerosing cholangitis associated with a familial immunodeficiency syndrome. Lancet 1973; *2*:18.
19. Thompson BW, Read RC: Sclerosing cholangitis and other intra-abdominal fibroses. Am J Surg 1974;*128*:777.

20. Roberts S: Cited in the discussion by Dr. Warren H. Cole in Schwartz SI, Dale WA: Primary sclerosing cholangitis: review and report of six cases. Arch Surg 1958;*77*:439.
21. Longmire WP Jr: When is cholangitis sclerosing? Am J Surg 1978;*135*:312.
22. Blathal PS, Powell LW: Primary intrahepatic obliterative cholangitis: a possible variant of sclerosing cholangitis. Gut 1969;*10*:886.
23. Goldgraber MB, Kirsner JB: Chronic granulomatous cholecystitis and chronic fibrosing choledochitis associated with chronic ulcerative colitis: a case report. Gastroenterology 1960;*38*:821.
24. Smith MP, Loe RH: Sclerosing cholangitis: a review of recent case reports and associated diseases and four new cases. Am J Surg 1965;*110*:239.
25. Mitchinson MJ: Systemic idiopathic fibrosis: systemic Weber-Christian disease. J Clin Pathol 1965;*18*:645.
26. Heilstrom HR, Perrezstable EC: Retroperitoneal fibrosis with disseminated vasculitis and intrahepatic sclerosing cholangitis. Am J Med 1966;*40*:184.
27. Brantigan CO, Brantigan OC: Primary sclerosing cholangitis: case report and review of the literature. Am Surg 1973;*39*:191.
28. Jain S, Long RG, Scott J, et al: Percutaneous transhepatic cholangiography using the "Chiba" needle—80 cases. Br J Radiol 1977;*50*:175.
29. Rohrmann CA, Ansel HJ, Ayoola EA, et al: Endoscopic retrograde intrahepatic cholangiogram: radiologic findings in intrahepatic disease. AJR 1977;*128*:45.
30. Ackert J, Tobias H: The endoscopy corner. Am J Gastroenterol 1977;*68*:498.
31. Altemeier WA, Gall EA, Culbertson WR, et al: Sclerosing carcinoma of the intrahepatic (hilar) bile ducts. Surgery 1966;*60*:191.
32. Javett SL: Azathioprine in primary sclerosing cholangitis. Lancet 1971;*1*:810.
33. Wagner A: Azathioprine treatment in primary sclerosing cholangitis. Lancet 1971;*2*:662.
34. Whelton MJ: Sclerosing cholangitis. Clin Gastroenterol 1973;*2*:163.
35. Polter DE, Gruhl V, Eigenbrodt EH, et al: Beneficial effect of cholestyramine in sclerosing cholangitis. Gastroenterology 1980;*79*:326.
36. Wiesner RH, LaRusso NP: Clinicopathologic features of the syndrome of primary sclerosing cholangitis. Gastroenterology 1980;*79*:200.
37. Cameron JL, Gayler BW, Sanfey H, et al: Sclerosing cholangitis. Anatomical distribution of obstructive lesions. Ann Surg 1984;*200*:54.
38. Ament AE, Bick RJ, Mirald GD, et al: Sclerosing cholangitis: Cholescintigraphy with Tc-99m–labeled DISIDA. Radiology 1984;*151*:197.
39. Thompson HH, Pitt HA, Tompkins RK, Longmire WP: Primary sclerosing cholangitis. A heterogenous disease. Ann Surg 1982;*196*:127.
40. Williams LF, Schoetz DJ: Primary sclerosing cholangitis. Surg Clin North Am 1981;*61*:951.
41. Pitt HA, Thompson HH, Tompkins RK, Longmire WP: Primary sclerosing cholangitis: Results of an aggressive surgical approach. Ann Surg 1982; *196*:259.
42. Bass NM, Chapman RW, O'Reilly A, Sherlock S: Primary sclerosing cholangitis associated with angioimmunoblastic lymphadenopathy. Gastroenterology 1083;*85*:420.
43. Smadja C, Roxley NB, Benjamin IR, Blumgart LH: Idiopathic localized bile duct strictures: Relationship to primary sclerosing cholangitis. Am J Surg 1983; *146*:404.
44. Wood RAB, Cuschieri A: Is sclerosing cholangitis complicating ulcerative colitis a reversible condition? Lancet 1980;*4*:716.

SECTION V

BENIGN AND MALIGNANT TUMORS

DAVID L. NAHRWOLD, M. D.

30

Benign Tumors and Pseudotumors of the Biliary Tract

INTRODUCTION

Knowledge about benign tumors and pseudotumors of the gallbladder and the biliary duct system is limited because these lesions are encountered so infrequently. Few institutions or individuals have had enough experience to study the clinical manifestations and methods of diagnosis and therapy in a comprehensive manner. Current concepts must be gleaned from individual case reports or studies of small groups of cases; in many instances the terminology used to describe these tumors is confusing, and in others, conclusions have been based on insufficient information.

These difficulties have been recognized, and we can look forward to a more accurate and detailed understanding of benign tumors and pseudotumors of the biliary tract in the future. Thus, some of the conclusions in the present review must be tentative, and we can expect them to change as the gaps in knowledge are filled.

BENIGN TUMORS AND PSEUDOTUMORS OF THE GALLBLADDER

Estimates of the frequency of benign tumors of the gallbladder range up to 8.5 per cent of surgical specimens.[1] The reported figures vary widely according to the method of computation and the criteria used to designate lesions as tumors. For example, 21 benign gallbladder tumors were found in the course of 4000 consecutive biliary tract operations at The Bowman Gray School of Medicine (0.5 per cent).[2] The incidence was six times higher in the experience of Ochsner, who found 45 tumors among 1523 cholecystectomy specimens (3.0 per cent).[3] Thus, the true incidence is not known, but available data suggest that it is less than 3 per cent in patients who have cholecystectomy. The incidence in the general population is probably much lower.

Pathology

The collection of 180 benign gallbladder tumors and pseudotumors at the Armed Forces Institute of Pathology (AFIP) was reviewed by Christensen and Ishak in 1970.[4] They proposed a classification (Table 30–1)

Table 30–1 CLASSIFICATION OF BENIGN TUMORS AND PSEUDOTUMORS OF THE GALLBLADDER

I. Benign Tumors
  A. Epithelial
    1. Adenoma, papillary
    2. Adenoma, nonpapillary
  B. Supporting tissue
    1. Hemangioma
    2. Lipoma
    3. Leiomyoma
    4. Granular cell tumor
    5. Carcinoid
II. Benign pseudotumors
  A. Hyperplasia
    1. Adenomatous
    2. Adenomyomatous
  B. Heterotopia
    1. Gastric mucosa
    2. Intestinal mucosa
    3. Pancreas
    4. Liver
  C. Polyp
    1. Inflammatory
    2. Cholesterol
  D. Miscellaneous
    1. Fibroxanthogranulomatous inflammation
    2. Parasitic infection

Modified from Christensen AH, Ishak KG: Arch Pathol 1970; *90*:423.

that has helped clarify the terminology used to describe these tumors and that should be used as a frame of reference in the future.

Benign Tumors

True tumors may arise from the columnar epithelium of the gallbladder or from the supporting tissue exclusive of the epithelium. Adenomas are true epithelial neoplasms. They may be sessile or, more commonly, pedunculated. The terms *papilloma, adenomatous polyp,* and *benign polyp,* all of which have been used to describe adenomas, should be dropped to avoid further confusion. Papillary adenomas consist of a branching vascular tissue forming villous projections covered by a single layer of columnar or cuboidal epithelium. Nonpapillary adenomas are rounded lesions covered by columnar epithelium. Histologically, the body of the tumor consists of multiple acini lined with columnar cells. Sometimes there is cystic dilatation of the glands.

Some adenomas have both papillary and nonpapillary elements. Christensen and Ishak[4] chose to classify them according to the predominant features. They found 51 adenomas in the AFIP collection of 180 benign tumors and pseudotumors; about 43 per cent were papillary and 57 per cent nonpapillary. Adenomas may occur in any portion of the gallbladder. Frequently, more than one is present.

The possibility that gallbladder adenomas are premalignant has been raised because carcinoma in situ has been found in a small number of adenomas,[5,6] of both the papillary[7] and the nonpapillary[4] types. Cholelithiasis was common among the reported cases of adenomas that harbored in situ carcinoma, and the frequent association of cholelithiasis and gallbladder cancer has been cited to support the thesis that adenomas may be premalignant.[7] The problem with this argument is that adenomas that do not contain in situ carcinoma frequently are found in gallbladders that contain stones. This association was present in one third of cases from the AFIP series. The number of reported cases is simply too small to calculate a statistical relationship between cholelithiasis and benign adenoma with or without in situ carcinoma. Kozuka et al.[6] have reported finding invasive carcinoma in several adenomas and adenomatous residue in several gallbladder adenocarcinomas. Thus, the entire spectrum from benign to malignant has been observed, which strongly supports the notion that adenomas are premalignant.

Benign neoplasms of the supporting tissues of the gallbladder are extremely rare. Cases of hemangioma, fibroma, neurofibroma, leiomyoma, lipoma, and paraganglioma have been reported; in most instances the tumors have been incidental findings, and no specific clinical manifestations could be ascribed to them. The exception to this statement is granular cell myoblastoma, of which several examples have been reported.[4, 8, 9] These lesions tend to occur in the cystic duct and cause obstruction, which results in symptomatic hydrops of the gallbladder. The gallbladder does not opacify on oral cholecystography, because contrast media cannot pass through the cystic duct. The reported cases of granular cell myoblastoma of the cystic duct have occurred in females, most of whom have not had concomitant cholelithiasis.

Carcinoid tumors may occur in the gallbladder, but there have been no reported cases of the carcinoid syndrome.[11] The lesions may metastasize, although the majority have been isolated tumors. One case was reported in which a carcinoid tumor was associated with adenocarcinoma of the gallbladder.[12] There is no typical symptomatology, and most gallbladder carcinoids have been incidental findings at surgery or autopsy.

Benign Pseudotumors

Pseudotumors are masses of tissue that are not true neoplasms. The most common are the hyperplastic lesions, which are categorized as adenomatous or adenomyomatous hyperplasia. Adenomatous hyperplasia is a distinct lesion histologically; that it may be symptomatic has received too little recognition. In the experience of Elfving and associates,[13] 6.5 per cent of 871 gallbladders removed at surgery had no gross or microscopic evidence of cholelithiasis, inflammation, tumor, or cholesterolosis. In 50 patients (5.9 per cent), there was microscopic evidence of adenomatous hyperplasia, which occurred in two forms. The villous type is characterized by a thickened mucosa with long, irregular, ramifying folds that give the appearance of villi projecting into the gallbladder lumen. In the spongy type, the villous projections appear to have coalesced, forming a network of thickened mucosa with the appearance of a sponge. Either type of adenomatous hyperplasia may be focal or diffuse. Clinically, the patients were symptomatic, and the majority had abnormalities on oral cholecystography, including nonopacification, poor filling, and poor contraction. About three fourths of the patients became asymptomatic after cholecystectomy. Clearly, additional documentation and study of adenomatous hyperplasia are warranted to determine its pathogenesis and clinical significance.

Adenomyomatous hyperplasia is the most common of the benign pseudotumors of the gallbladder.[4, 13–17] There has been confusion about this lesion, in part because of the many terms that have been used to describe it, including adenoma, adenomyoma, adenomyomatosis, cystadenoma, myoepithelial anomaly, intramural cholecystitis cystica, and fibromyoadenoma. Adenomyomatous hyperplasia may be diffuse, segmental, or localized. The localized form is by far the most common and usually occurs in the fundus. Grossly, this pseudotumor presents as a nodule in the fundus with central umbilication on the mucosal side. Histologically, there is proliferation of epithelial and smooth muscle elements surrounded by dilated mucus-filled glands. These glands are actually mucosal diverticula, or Rokitansky-Aschoff sinuses, which have the microscopic appearance of branched tubular projections into or through the hyperplastic muscle of the gallbladder wall. There is no capsule or sharp delineation of the margin of an area of adenomyomatous hyperplasia (Fig. 30–1).

There has been speculation that the lesion results from incomplete canalization of the fetal gallbladder or that it represents an embryonic rest or hamartoma. There are no reports of adenomyomatous hyperplasia in children, which argues against these possibilities. Gallstones and histologic evidence of cholecystitis are present in about half the cases, but there is no convincing evidence that adenomyomatous hyperplasia is caused by, or predisposes to, inflammation. There is no reason to suspect that the lesion is associated with the development of gallbladder carcinoma.

Jutras and his associates[14] proposed that adenomyomatous hyperplasia, cholesterolosis, and neuromatosis are all hyperplastic lesions and include them under the generic title of "hyperplastic cholecystoses." These authors believe that these conditions are associated with radiologically determined functional abnormalities of the gallbladder, including hyperconcentration, hyperexcitability, and hyperexcretion. This thesis has not been adequately tested, but other examples of hyperconcentration and hyperexcretion of contrast material in patients with adenomyomatous hyperplasia or cholesterolosis have been reported.[18]

Woodard[16] postulated an injury-repair sequence for the etiology of adenomyomatous hyperplasia, believing that this would best explain the histologic appearance of the lesions.

Benign pseudotumors composed of heterotopic tissue occasionally are found within the gallbladder. Gastric and pancreatic heterotopias are the most frequent, but intramural pseudotumors of intestinal mucosa and hepatic and thyroid tissue have been reported as well. The heterotopic gastric mucosa does not produce ulceration or bleeding,

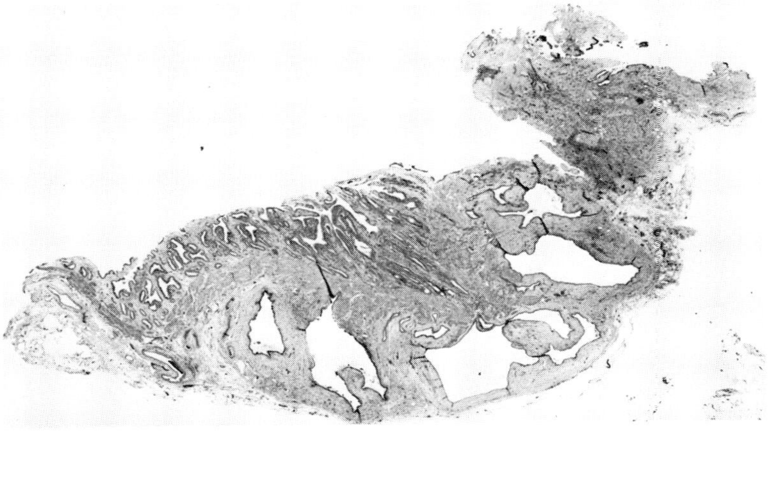

Figure 30–1. Histologic section of an area of adenomyomatous hyperplasia in the fundus of the gallbladder. On the mucosal side (*top*) there is epithelial proliferation extending into the hyperplastic muscular layer. Large Rokitansky-Aschoff sinuses are present near the serosal side.

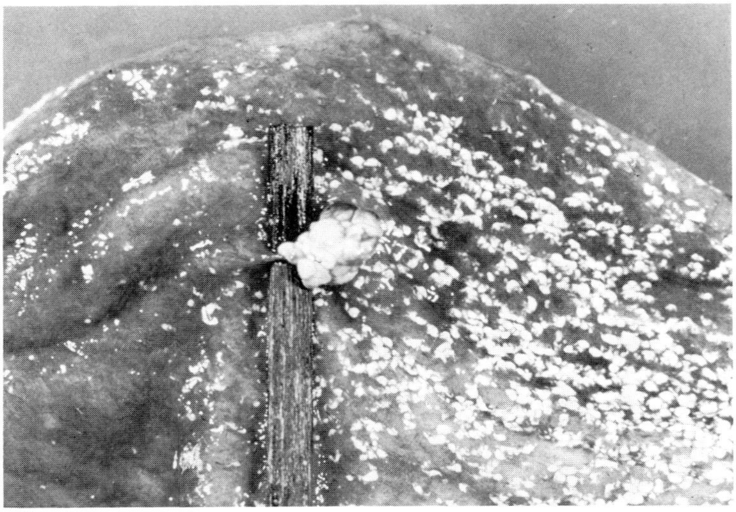

Figure 30–2. Mucosal surface of an opened gallbladder, which shows cholesterolosis and a cholesterol polyp attached by a delicate pedicle.

but the lesion is sometimes associated with cholecystitis because it tends to be located in the neck of the gallbladder, where it can cause obstruction.[19]

When used in the context of benign gallbladder tumors and pseudotumors, the term "polyp" is reserved for two specific entities, inflammatory polyps and cholesterol polyps. Inflammatory polyps are small projections from the mucosa that consist of glandular epithelial elements proliferating within a connective tissue stroma. The stroma is heavily infiltrated with inflammatory cells, and the adjacent mucosa shows the typical microscopic findings of chronic cholecystitis. Gallbladder calculi may be absent. Inflammatory polyps may be multiple.

Cholesterol polyps are much more frequent.[14, 15] They are a localized form of cholesterolosis composed of aggregations of cholesterol-laden histiocytes, called foam cells, covered by a single layer of normal columnar epithelium. They are lobulated and attached to the mucosa by a delicate pedicle, which may break and permit the polyp to float freely in the gallbladder lumen (Figs. 30–2 and 30–3). Surprisingly, neither cholelithiasis nor cholesterolosis of the mucosa is frequently associated with cholesterol polyps. Cholesterol polyps are often multiple.

Christensen and Ishak[4] also described tumor-like nodules of the gallbladder wall in seven patients with acute or chronic cholecystitis, six of whom also had cholelithiasis. These nodules, which they called fibroxanthogranulomatous inflammation, consisted of foamy histiocytes admixed with inflammatory cells and sometimes giant cells, surrounded by a vascular fibroblastic reaction. The mucosa over these pseudotumors was invariably ulcerated. There is no additional information about this lesion, which appears to be asso-

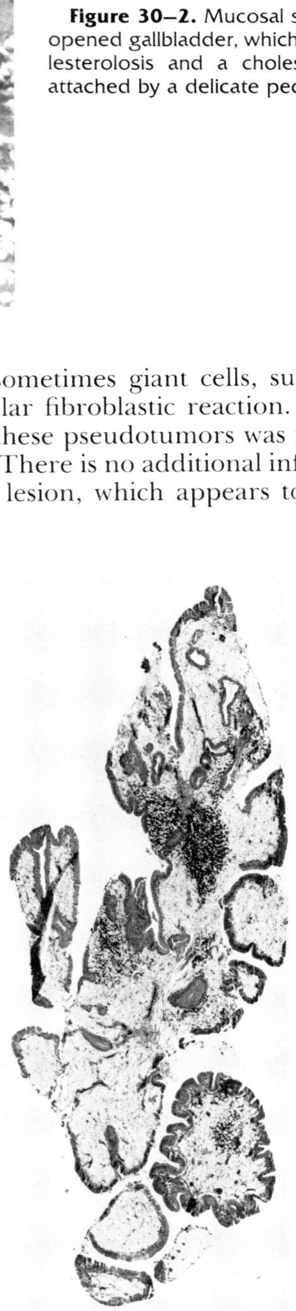

Figure 30–3. Histologic section of the cholesterol polyp shown in Figure 30–2, showing lobulated collections of foamy histiocytes covered by a single layer of epithelium.

ciated with cholelithiasis and the development of cholecystitis.

Two pseudotumors representing chronic granulomatous inflammation of the gallbladder from parasitic infections also were included in the AFIP collection.

Clinical Findings

Certain benign tumors and pseudotumors are more likely to cause symptoms than others, but whether the symptoms in a given patient can be ascribed to the presence of the tumor is problematic. Gallbladder tumors, as pointed out earlier, may be associated with cholecystitis and cholelithiasis. In the AFIP collection of 180 cases, 93, or about one half, had microscopic evidence of cholecystitis, and 49, or about one fourth, had associated cholelithiasis. If a patient with a benign tumor also has cholecystitis or cholelithiasis (or both), it is not possible to attribute the symptoms to the tumor. The symptoms in patients with tumors unassociated with calculi or inflammation are right upper quadrant or epigastric pain and discomfort, flatulence, intolerance of fatty foods, nausea, vomiting, and other dyspeptic complaints. The high incidence of indigestion and nonspecific upper gastrointestinal complaints in the general population who have no known organic disease adds to the confusion.

Whatever the pathophysiologic mechanism, it is clear that some patients with papillary or nonpapillary adenomas have symptoms referable to the gallbladder. Lesions located near the outlet of the gallbladder or those on a pedicle long enough to reach the outlet can produce symptoms by restricting the flow of bile during gallbladder contraction. In one case, acute cholecystitis resulted when a pedunculated adenoma passed into the cystic duct.[20] Rarely, papillary adenomas become detached from the mucosa and presumably cause obstruction, or they may bleed and cause hemobilia with symptoms from passage of blood clots.[21] The presence of in situ carcinoma within an adenoma has not been associated with specific symptoms.

In general, the rare tumors of supporting tissue have not caused symptoms and have been incidental findings at surgery or autopsy. The exception is granular cell myoblastoma, which by virtue of its location in the cystic duct, causes obstruction and hydrops of the gallbladder in the absence of stones. The symptoms include right upper quadrant pain, nausea, vomiting, and occasionally jaundice.

The patients with adenomatous hyperplasia studied by Elfving and associates,[13] none of whom had calculi, experienced right upper quadrant pain, intolerance to certain foods, and a variety of other nonspecific gastrointestinal complaints. Because three fourths of them became asymptomatic after cholecystectomy, the adenomatous hyperplasia probably produced the symptoms, but it is impossible to gauge the possible psychologic benefits of surgery under such circumstances.

Adenomyomatous hyperplasia is frequently associated with cholecystitis and calculi, but there is no question that even in the absence of calculi these lesions can cause right upper quadrant pain and other biliary symptoms.[15–17] Jutras et al.[14] suggest that some patients with the hyperplastic cholecystoses, including adenomyomatous hyperplasia, cholesterolosis, and neuromatosis (proliferation of autonomic nerve fibers), develop pain because of excessive gallbladder contraction.

Heterotopic gastric mucosa frequently is associated with cholecystitis. The symptoms manifested by the patients in the AFIP series included right upper quadrant pain, epigastric distress, nausea, and vomiting. In some cases the clinical manifestations may be related to the location of the lesion in the neck of the gallbladder.

In summary, the symptoms of benign tumors and pseudotumors resemble those of gallstone disease. It would be impossible to identify the specific lesion responsible for the complaints on the basis of the history and physical examination.

Diagnosis

The preoperative diagnosis of benign tumors and pseudotumors can be made by cholecystography, ultrasound, and CT scans (see Chapters 7 to 9). The symptoms are indicative of gallbladder disease, so an oral cholecystogram is usually the first study ordered. The roentgenologic features of benign tumors include one or more rounded radiolucent filling defects next to the mucosa, which are usually less than 1 cm in diameter and which do not change location on repeated examination or changes in the position of the patient. These findings are best seen in a well-opacified gallbladder and on films made after ingestion of a fatty meal.

A notch in the contour of the gallbladder on a tangential view where the lesion meets the gallbladder wall is characteristic of a sessile adenoma. Unfortunately, a gallstone may become attached to the gallbladder wall or embedded within it, so that differentiation between a sessile adenoma and a stone may be difficult. The stalk of a pedunculated adenoma, when visible, is a helpful diagnostic sign. However, a slender stalk may be obscured by densely concentrated opaque media. Inflammatory and cholesterol polyps may have the same roentgenographic characteristics as adenomas and may be impossible to differentiate from them. The delicate stalk of a cholesterol polyp is almost never demonstrated (Fig. 30–4). Cholesterol polyps may also be detected by ultrasonography.[15, 22]

Obviously, granular cell myoblastoma, which occurs in the cystic duct, and gastric heterotopias, which occur in the infundibulum, cannot be diagnosed roentgenographically when they produce obstruction and nonopacification of the gallbladder.

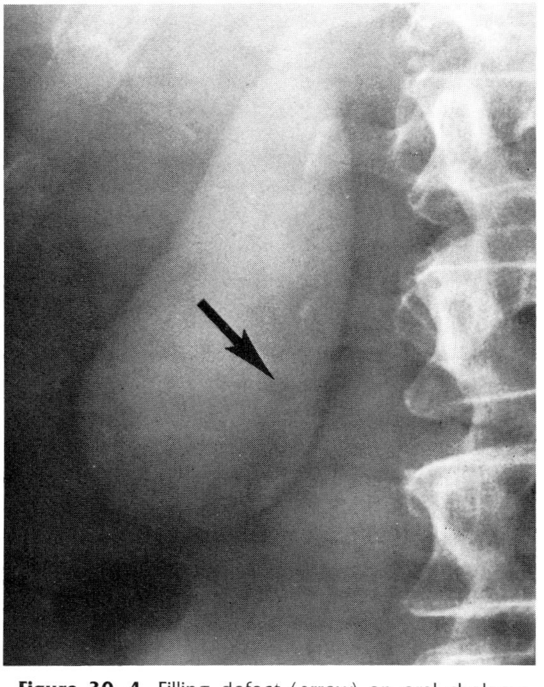

Figure 30–4. Filling defect (*arrow*) on oral cholecystogram. The location of the defect did not change on repeated examination or when the position of the patient was changed. The lesion is the cholesterol polyp shown in Figure 30–2. The pedicle is not visible.

Adenomyomatous hyperplasia has the most characteristic appearance on oral cholecystography.[14, 23] The localized type, which occurs in the fundus, appears as a sessile filling defect with a central opaque indentation. The lesion is surrounded by a ring of opaque dots, which represent filling of the small diverticula (Rokitansky-Aschoff sinuses) at the periphery of the lesion. The segmental and generalized types are characterized by thickening of the gallbladder and an irregular contour in the area of involvement. Occasionally, the thickening is marked enough to produce a waist-like configuration, resulting in compartmentalization of the gallbladder. As mentioned, the presence of intramural diverticula is a key diagnostic sign. The roentgenographic appearance of adenomyomatous hyperplasia varies with the degree of gallbladder distention, the angle of projection, and various other technical factors.[14] Adenomyomatosis may sometimes be diagnosed from the sonographic findings of focal mural thickening associated with small anechoic cystic spaces.[24]

The frequency of an accurate diagnosis by oral cholecystography obviously will vary with the quality of the radiographs and the ability of the surgeon and the radiologist to interpret them correctly. Tinsley and his associates[22] analyzed 35 cases of polypoid lesions of the gallbladder in patients without associated cholelithiasis. The radiographs were interpreted as definitely demonstrating papilloma or polyp in 63 per cent. A definitive diagnosis could not be made in 28 per cent, and other diagnoses were made in 9 per cent. The frequent presence of calculi in gallbladders that harbor benign (or malignant) tumors reduces the possibility of a preoperative diagnosis even further. Thus, it is incumbent upon the surgeon and the pathologist to open and examine gallbladders carefully at the time of cholecystectomy. While there may be no practical value in diagnosing a benign gallbladder tumor or pseudotumor at the operating table, it is important to determine whether or not a tumor is malignant lest the abdomen be closed without the appropriate dissection for a potentially curable cancer of the gallbladder.

Treatment

It is generally accepted that cholecystectomy should be performed in patients who have symptoms referable to the gallbladder and either gallstones or nonopacification of the gallbladder on oral cholecystography. Approximately one third to one half of individuals who harbor known or unknown benign tumors of the gallbladder fall into this category, and the decision in favor of surgical therapy is not difficult in these cases. Under these circumstances the presence of the tumor often is discovered by the pathologist after the procedure has been completed. Surgeons should acquire the habit of opening the gallbladder in the operating room for the reasons cited previously. This is especially important when stones are not palpable, particularly in the case of a hydrops of the gallbladder, which may be due to an obstructing tumor.

Cholecystectomy should be performed in patients who have symptoms referable to the gallbladder and the roentgenographic finding of a tumor in a gallbladder that does not contain stones. Given the low mortality rate for simple cholecystectomy, there is no justification for patients' having to endure protracted discomfort from a condition for which there is no nonsurgical remedy. In elderly patients and those with serious concurrent disease who have minimal or vague symptoms, the risk of operation must be balanced against the unlikely risk of the development of carcinoma in an adenoma and the small risk that the lesion is actually a gallbladder carcinoma. The specific radiographic features of the tumor may be helpful in this regard.

Patients who have clear-cut radiographic evidence of adenomyomatous hyperplasia should have a cholecystectomy if they have symptoms referable to the gallbladder. However, when the diagnosis is certain and symptoms are absent or vague, there is no need for surgical therapy, because this lesion is not premalignant.

The experience with benign gallbladder tumors and pseudotumors is too limited to draw conclusions about the long-term results of cholecystectomy. Tinsley and associates[22] followed 35 patients after cholecystectomy; all but three had cholesterol polyps. Excellent results were obtained in 66 per cent, but 23 per cent had only moderate improvement with persistence of some preoperative complaints, and 11 per cent had little or no improvement. A similar rate of good results has been reported by others.[17] Their experience confirms that it is difficult to ascribe specific abdominal complaints to gallbladder disease and reinforces the principle that surgeons should openly discuss this difficulty with patients during the decision-making process.

BENIGN TUMORS AND PSEUDOTUMORS OF THE EXTRAHEPATIC BILE DUCTS

Benign bile duct tumors are even more rare than benign gallbladder tumors. Burhans and Meyers,[2] who reviewed the 88 cases reported as of 1970, found 21 benign gallbladder tumors and only 4 benign tumors of the extrahepatic ducts during the course of 4000 consecutive biliary tract operations at The Bowman Gray School of Medicine (0.1 per cent). Only four benign bile duct tumors were found during 20,000 consecutive biliary tract operations at the Mayo Clinic (0.02 per cent).[26]

Pathology

There is no accepted pathologic classification of benign tumors and pseudotumors of the bile ducts, probably because of the paucity of cases. Many case reports do not adequately describe the gross and microscopic findings, and a heterogeneous group of terms have been applied to the various growths that have been observed. Chu[27] reviewed the 54 cases reported up to 1950 and found only 29 in which adequate information was available for histologic categorization. There is a need for a central repository for specimens from the bile ducts so that the material can be analyzed and categorized in detail. Thus, the classification given in Table 30–2 is based on sketchy information and

Table 30–2 PROPOSED CLASSIFICATION OF BENIGN TUMORS AND PSEUDOTUMORS OF THE EXTRAHEPATIC BILE DUCTS

- I. Benign tumors
  - A. Epithelial
    1. Adenoma
    2. Cystadenoma
    3. Papilloma
  - B. Supporting tissue
    1. Fibroma
    2. Leiomyoma
    3. Neurinoma
    4. Granular cell myoblastoma
    5. Carcinoid
- II. Benign pseudotumors
  - A. Hyperplasia
  - B. Heterotopia
    1. Gastric mucosa

must be viewed as tentative and possibly simplistic.

Benign Tumors

The extrahepatic bile ducts are lined by columnar epithelium. The walls of the ducts contain tubular glands that are also lined with columnar epithelial cells and that communicate with the lumen and apparently secrete mucus. Whether benign epithelial tumors arise from the bile duct epithelium, from the intramural glands, or from both is unknown. Adenomas may occur within the walls of bile ducts and may be found throughout the extrahepatic duct system. They are usually single and consist of acini lined with columnar cells in a connective tissue stroma. The stroma may have fibrous tissue elements or smooth muscle in varying proportions, which has led to the designation of some tumors as fibroadenoma or adenomyoma.[28] When located near the ampulla of Vater, some adenomas assume a polypoid configuration with a pedicle that allows the tumor to prolapse through the ampulla or, rarely, into the pancreatic duct.[29] It is not clear whether these pedunculated tumors should be designated as "polyps" to distinquish them from other kinds of adenoma, or whether they are simply adenomas that have grown into the lumen and have acquired a pedicle because of chronic traction. The malignant potential of adenomas has not been established, but cellular atypia has been reported in some cases. The glandular spaces in adenomas, which are lined by columnar or cuboidal epithelium, may become very large and multicystic.

Cystadenomas occur most commonly within the liver, but they have been found within the extrahepatic ductal system as well.[30–37] They consist of multilocular cysts lined by columnar or cuboidal epithelium, which is sometimes thrown into papillary folds. Surrounding the loculated mucin is a dense, cellular, fibrous stroma that may contain cholesterol-laden foam cells and areas of hyalinization. Cystadenocarcinoma, a tumor with similar characteristics, is also found in the liver and the extrahepatic ductal system. The fact that cystadenocarcinomas may contain areas characteristic of benign cystadenoma supports the thesis that cystadenoma may undergo malignant transformation.[33] Certain characteristics of cystadenomas resemble those of adenomas that contain large cystic spaces. It is not known, nor has it previously been proposed, that there is any relationship between these two tumors.

Papillomas have a connective tissue stroma with frondlike branches. They are covered by a single layer of columnar epithelium and may contain glandular structures lined with columnar epithelium. Single papillomas tend to occur more frequently in the distal portion of the common duct.[28] Cellular atypia, thought possibly to represent a premalignant change, may be present, and the development of adenocarcinoma has been documented.[38] When more than one papilloma is present, the condition is referred to as papillomatosis. Papillomatosis has a tendency to recur and to undergo transition to epithelial dysplasia, carcinoma in situ, and invasive carcinoma.[42] Thus, single and multiple papillomas are premalignant lesions.

Adenomas of various types, cystadenomas, and papillomas constitute the majority of benign tumors and pseudotumors. Tumors of supporting tissue, including fibroma,[27] leiomyoma,[43] angioleiomyoma,[44] neurinoma,[45] schwannoma,[46] carcinoid,[47] and apudoma,[48] are rare. Granular cell myoblastoma, which accounts for less than 10 per cent of benign tumors of the extrahepatic bile ducts, has been found only in the common bile duct.[49, 52] It occurs most commonly in black females.

Benign Pseudotumors

Adenomatoid hyperplasia is a poorly understood proliferation of the glands underlying the epithelium of the ampulla of Vater, which may cause the mucosa to be thrown into folds and to prolapse through the ampulla. In some cases the glands are dilated and cystic.[53] Varying degrees of inflammation may be present.[54] There has been speculation that this process, about which little is known, may lead to stenosis of the sphincter of Oddi or to the development of an adenoma.[55] Heterotopic gastric mucosa has been found in the common duct, where on frozen section it may be mistaken for adenocarcinoma.[56, 57]

The average age of the 43 patients with benign bile duct tumors in the series of Dowdy et al.[28] was 50 years. There were 22 males and 21 females. In contrast to the high incidence of cholelithiasis in benign gallbladder tumors, only 12 per cent of the patients in this collected series had associated biliary tract calculi. About three fourths of the tumors were located in the ampullary region or the common bile duct.

Clinical Findings

Most patients with benign tumors or pseudotumors of the extrahepatic bile ducts present with jaundice, which is intermittent in about one half the cases. Pain, usually not severe, is another frequent symptom. About one fourth of the patients reviewed by Dowdy[58] had chills and fever, presumably from cholangitis. Hemobilia is uncommon. Nonspecific symptoms, such as dyspepsia and weight loss, may be present. Pancreatitis may occur if the lesion obstructs the orifice of the pancreatic duct.[29]

The physical findings are nonspecific. A palpable gallbladder or enlarged liver may be present when there is sufficient bile duct obstruction. Obviously, an enlarged gallbladder indicates that the tumor is located distal to the entrance of the cystic duct. Liver function tests are indicative of obstructive jaundice.

Diagnosis

Most of the reported cases were accumulated before the widespread use of ultrasonography, percutaneous transhepatic cholangiography (PTC), and endoscopic retrograde cholangiopancreatography (ERCP). Some cases were suspected from findings of intravenous cholangiography, but most were diagnosed after the common duct was opened during an exploration for obstructive jaundice. Direct cholangiography now often permits the diagnosis of benign tumor to be suspected preoperatively. This was the case in one patient with an adenoma of the distal common duct[28] and in another with biliary papillomatosis,[40] both conditions being demonstrated by ERCP.

Because most patients with benign bile duct tumors present with obstructive jaundice, diagnostic studies are directed toward the more common causes of obstruction, such as common duct stones and carcinoma of the head of the pancreas. Fortunately, these studies are also appropriate for obstruction due to benign tumors. At present, when the history, physical examination, and liver function tests show clear evidence of obstructive jaundice, ultrasonography is usually performed to determine the presence or absence of dilated bile ducts. Transhepatic cholangiography is done when the bile ducts are dilated, and ERCP when they are not. Thus, roentgenographic examination of the entire biliary tract is performed in most patients with obstructive jaundice. Endoscopic examination of the papilla, and biopsy when indicated, are carried out when transhepatic cholangiography shows a distal common duct or ampullary lesion. In some patients, endoscopic examination and biopsy are performed when a barium contrast study suggests an ampullary or duodenal lesion. Except for benign tumors that are accessible to forceps biopsy through the endoscope, these diagnostic studies will not establish the histologic diagnosis of benign tumor, but they will localize the site of the tumor and help the surgeon plan the operation. One can expect that certain radiographic characteristics of benign tumors will become more evident as experience with these diagnostic modalities accumulates. The diagnosis of biliary papillomatosis, for example, is strongly suggested when multiple fixed filling defects are evident on cholangiography.

Treatment

The principles of surgical treatment are to establish the diagnosis, completely excise the tumor, and reconstruct the biliary tract. After the location and extent of the lesion have been determined, biopsy and frozen section are essential, because palpation and direct observation are inadequate to rule out malignant tumors of the extrahepatic duct system, the ampulla, or the head of the pancreas. When the diagnosis has been established, a benign tumor in the common hepatic or common bile duct should be treated by excision of the appropriate portion of the duct. End-to-end reconstruction over a T-tube splint is preferred, but when this is not possible, the proximal end of the bile duct should be anastomosed to the duodenum or to a Roux-en-Y loop of jejunum. We prefer the latter method.

Tumors in the ampullary area or the vaterian segment of the common duct usually are amenable to local excision through a duodenotomy, and they may be excised widely in conjunction with a sphincteroplasty. The surgical decision may be difficult when the tumor is located in the intrapancreatic portion of the common bile duct, where it is not amenable to sleeve resection of the duct or excision through a duodenotomy. Complete excision may be possible only by a pancreaticoduodenectomy (Whipple procedure). An alternative is to leave the tumor in place and perform a biliary-enteric anastomosis to relieve the obstruction. The latter option would be appropriate for elderly patients or those with serious concurrent disease, but the decision to perform a Whipple procedure in other patients must be based on factors pertinent to the case at hand. Tumors in the hepatic ducts must be treated by hepatic lobectomy if an alternative reconstructive procedure cannot be carried out.

The treatment of patients with biliary papillomatosis is a special problem for which there is no satisfactory solution. Most of the patients have been treated by curettage, with uniformly poor results because of the propensity for recurrence and the development of invasive cancer. When possible, these lesions should be treated by radical excision of the involved portion of the duct system.

The case for radical excision of benign tumors is emphasized by the results in 88 benign bile duct tumors collected by Burhans and Meyers in 1971.[2] There were recurrences in 11 of 49 (22 per cent) patients who had curettage or excision of the duct wall. In contrast, there was only one recurrence in 18 patients (6 per cent) who had radical procedures ranging from sleeve resection of the bile duct to hepatic lobectomy. The mortality rate for local excision was 8 per cent, and it was only slightly higher (11 per cent) for radical excision.

The high recurrence rate and the premalignant nature of some of the benign tumors of the extrahepatic ductal system support the use of a relatively aggressive approach.

REFERENCES

1. Kirklin BR: Cholecystographic diagnosis of papillomas of the gallbladder. Am J Roentgenol 1931;*25*:46.
2. Burhans SR, Meyers RT: Benign neoplasms of the extrahepatic biliary ducts. Am Surg 1971;*37*:161.
3. Ochsner SF, Ochsner A: Benign neoplasms of the gallbladder: Diagnosis and surgical implications. Ann Surg 1960;*151*:630.
4. Christensen AH, Ishak KG: Benign tumors and pseudotumors of the gallbladder. Report of 180 cases. Arch Pathol 1970;*90*:423.
5. Tabah EJ, McNeer G: Papilloma of the gallbladder with in-situ carcinoma. Surgery 1953;*34*:57.
6. Kozuka S, Tsubone M, Yasui A, et al: Relation of adenoma to carcinoma in the gallbladder. Cancer 1982;*50*:2226.
7. Hulten J, Johansson H, Olding L: Adenoma of the gallbladder and extrahepatic bile ducts. Acta Chir Scand 1970;*136*:203.
8. Sawyer KC: The unrecognized significance of papillomas, polyps and adenomas of the gallbladder. Am J Surg 1970;*120*:570.
9. Reul GJ Jr, Rubio PA, Berkman NL: Granular cell myoblastoma of the cystic duct. Am J Surg 1975;*129*:583.
10. Abt AB, Feinberg E, Kunita S: Granular cell myoblastoma of the extrahepatic biliary tract. Mt Sinai J Med 1971;*38*:457.
11. Bergdahl L: Carcinoid tumors of the biliary tract. Aust N Z J Surg 1976;*46*:136.
12. Wada A, Ishiguro S, Tateishi R, et al: Carcinoid tumor of the gallbladder associated with adenocarcinoma. Cancer 1983;*51*:1911.
13. Elfving G, Lehtonen T, Teir H: Clinical significance of primary hyperplasia of gallbladder mucosa. Ann Surg 1967;*165*:61.
14. Jutras JA, Longtin JM, Levesque HP: Hyperplastic cholecystoses. Am J Roentgenol Radium Ther Nucl Med 1960;*83*:795.
15. Berk RN, van der Vegt JH, Lichtenstein JE: The hyperplastic cholecystoses: Cholesterolosis and adenomyomatosis. Radiology 1983;*146*:593.
16. Woodard BH: Adenomyomatous hyperplasia of the human gallbladder. South Med J 1982;*75*:533.
17. Meguid MM, Aun F, Bradford ML: Adenomyomatosis of the gallbladder. Am J Surg 1984;*147*:260.
18. Jacobs LA, DeMeester TR, Eggleston JC, et al: Hyperplastic cholecystoses. Arch Surg 1972;*104*:193.
19. Bentivegna S, Hirschl S: Heterotopic gastric mucosa in the gallbladder presenting as a symptom-producing tumor. Am J Gastroenterol 1972;*57*:423.
20. Lund NM, Burman CEL: Case of acute cholecystitis and obstruction due to pedunculated papilloma, identical with attack of acute cholecystitis and gallstones. Br J Surg 1951;*38*:390.
21. Akoi Y, Okamura T, Kurimoto H, et al: Papilloma of the gallbladder. Am J Surg 1976;*131*:614.
22. Tinsley AR, Mulkerin LE, Van der Luide JM, et al: Polypoid lesions of the acalculous gallbladder. South Med J 1975;*68*:958.
23. Price RJ, Stewart ET, Foley WD, et al: Sonography of polypoid cholesterolosis. Am J Roentgenol 1982;*139*:1197.
24. Colosimo C Jr, Vecchioli A, Colagrande C: Hyperplastic cholecystosis: Study by ceruletide-assisted cholecystography. Gastrointest Radiol 1983;*8*:255.
25. Raghavendra BN, Subramanyam BR, Balthazar EJ, et al: Sonography of adenomyomatosis of the gallbladder: Radiologic-pathologic correlation. Radiology 1983;*146*:747.
26. Marshall JM: Tumors of the bile ducts. Surg Gynecol Obstet 1932;*54*:6.
27. Chu PT: Benign neoplasms of the extrahepatic biliary ducts. Arch Pathol 1950;*50*:84.
28. Dowdy GS Jr, Olin WG Jr, Shelton EL Jr, et al: Benign tumors of the extrahepatic bile ducts. Arch Surg 1962;*85*:165.
29. Ohmori K, Kinoshita H, Shiraha Y, et al: Pancreatic duct obstruction by a benign polypoid adenoma of the ampulla of Vater. Am J Surg 1976;*132*:662.
30. Short WF, Nedwich A, Levy HA, et al: Biliary cystadenoma. Report of a case and review of the literature. Arch Surg 1971;*102*:78.

31. Marsh JL, Dahms B, Longmire WP Jr: Cystadenoma and cystadenocarcinoma of the biliary system. Arch Surg 1974;*109*:41.
33. Ishak KG, Willis GW, Cummins SD, et al: Biliary cystadenoma and cystadenocarcinoma. Cancer 1977;*39*:322.
34. Rutledge JN, Pratt MC, Taupmann RE: Biliary cystadenoma mistaken for an echincoccal cyst. South Med J 1983;*76*:1575.
35. Nagorney DM, LeSage GD, Charboneau JW, et al: Cystadenoma of the proximal common hepatic duct: The use of abdominal ultrasonography and transhepatic cholangiography in diagnosis. Mayo Clin Proc 1984;*59*:118.
36. Stanley J, Vujic I, Schabel SI, et al: Evaluation of biliary cystadenoma and cystadenocarcinoma. Gastrointest Radiol 1983;*8*:245.
37. Organ B, Petrek J: Biliary cystadenoma. South Med J 1984;*77*:262.
38. Cattell RB, Braasch JW, Kahn F: Polypoid epithelial tumors of the bile ducts. N Engl J Med 1962;*266*:57.
39. Gouma DJ, Mutum SS, Benjamin IS, et al: Intrahepatic biliary papillomatosis. Br J Surg 1984;*71*:72.
40. Mercadier M, Bodard M, Fingerhut A, et al: Papillomatosis of the intrahepatic bile ducts. World J Surg 1984;*8*:30.
41. Veloso FT, Ribeiro T, Teixeira AA, et al: Biliary papillomatosis: Report of a case with a 5-year follow-up. Am J Gastroenterol 1983;*78*:645.
42. Neumann RD, LiVolsi VA, Rosenthal NS, et al: Adenocarcinoma in biliary papillomatosis. Gastroenterology 1976;*70*:779.
43. Kane GA, Polgar V: Leiomyoma of the common bile duct causing obstructive jaundice. Med J Aust 1976;*1*:698.
44. Ponka A, Laasonen L, Strengell-Usanov L: Angioleiomyoma of the common bile duct. Acta Med Scand 1983;*213*:407.
45. Oden B: Neurinoma of the common bile duct. Acta Chir Scand 1955;*108*:393.
46. Balart LA, Hines C Jr, Mitchell W: Granular cell schwannoma of the extrahepatic biliary system. Am J Gastroenterol 1983;*78*:297.
47. Little JM, Gibson AAM, Kay AW: Primary common bile duct carcinoid. Br J Surg 1968;*55*:147.
48. Van Steenbergen W, Fevery J, Vanstapel MJ, et al: Case report: Fourteen-year follow-up of an apudoma of the bile ducts at the hilum of the liver. Gastroenterology 1983;*84*:1585.
49. Dewar J, Dooley JS, Lindsay I, et al: Granular cell myoblastoma of the common bile duct treated by biliary drainage and surgery. Gut 1981;*22*:70.
50. Dursi JF, Hirschl S, Gomez R, et al: Granular cell myoblastoma of the common bile duct: Report of a case and review of the literature. Rev Surg 1975; *32*:305.
51. Manstein ME, McBrearty FX, Pellechia PE, et al: Granular cell tumor of the common bile duct. Dig Dis Sci 1981;*26*:938.
52. Chandrasoma P, Fitzgibbons P: Granular cell tumor of the intrapancreatic common bile duct. Cancer 1984;*53*:2178.
53. Baggenstoss AH: Major duodenal papilla: Variations of pathologic interest and lesions of the mucosa. Arch Pathol 1938;*26*:853.
54. Dardinski VJ: Inflammatory adenomatoid hyperplasia of major duodenal papilla in man. Am J Pathol 1931;*7*:519.
55. Barber KW Jr, ReMine WH, Harrison EJ Jr, et al: Benign neoplasms of the extrahepatic bile ducts, including papilla of Vater. Arch Surg 1960;*81*:479.
56. Blundell CR, Kanun CS, Earnest DL: Biliary obstruction by heterotopic gastric mucosa at the ampulla of Vater. Am J Gastroenterol 1982;*77*:111.
57. Welling RE, Krause RJ, Alamin K: Heterotopic gastric mucosa in the common duct. Arch Surg 1970;*101*:626.
58. Dowdy GS Jr: The Biliary Tract. Philadelphia, Lea & Febiger, 1969, p 163.

JAMES FOSTER, M. D.

31

Carcinoma of the Gallbladder

INTRODUCTION

Most surgeons believe that removal of the entire gross lesion and a margin of normal tissue will cure or palliate the gastrointestinal cancers of the largest number of patients. However, there is a widespread fatalism about gallbladder cancer, which can briefly be summarized as follows: "If the disease has caused symptoms or is clinically obvious at the bedside or at operation, the patient will succumb, whatever is done. Only if an unsuspected cancer is found incidentally, usually by the pathologist after cholecystectomy for presumed benign disease, will the patient have a chance for long-term survival."

Do the facts support this pessimism? Can the disease be diagnosed at an earlier stage? Is there justification for more than cholecystectomy in selected cases? Will operative measures short of resection provide palliation, and is chemotherapy or radiotherapy of any use?

This chapter will cover what is known about gallbladder carcinoma in order to address some of these questions and provide guidelines for therapy. Unfortunately, the overall picture remains grim.

HISTORY

In 1777, Maximillian de Stoll, Professor of the Practice of Medicine in Vienna, described in *Pars Prima Rationis Medendi* the autopsy findings of three patients who probably died of gallbladder carcinoma. By 1889 Musser was able to collect 100 cases, and in 1894 Aimes published a comprehensive and detailed review of the natural history, clinical features, and lethal nature of this disease.[79] The first cholecystectomy for carcinoma was performed by Bardenheuer in 1887, but the patient died postoperatively. Hochenegg probably performed the first successful cholecystectomy for carcinoma in 1890. No recurrence was evident during an 8-month follow-up.[87]

In Keen's classic third paper on liver resection for tumor (1899), 6 of 76 cases were operations for gallbladder carcinoma.[44] In 1932 Finsterer reported a patient who survived for 5 years after cholecystectomy and resection of adjacent liver, although in 1947 Sheinfield found no other long-term survivors among 36 similarly treated patients.[77] In 1949 Arminski noted that more than 3000 cases of gallbladder carcinoma had been reported in the literature. Among 417 cases that he studied, there were 16 five-year survivors after 284 operations, most of which were simple cholecystectomies.[6]

In 1954 Glenn and Hayes recommended that gallbladder carcinoma be treated by wide cholecystectomy and regional lymphadenectomy and a wedge resection of liver comprising the gallbladder bed.[30] However, Pack et al.[65] advocated hepatic lobectomy in addition to cholecystectomy, and in 1961 Brasfield described a woman who survived for more than 5 years after right hemihepatectomy for a papillary tumor with minimal invasion of the gallbladder bed.[15]

Four comprehensive reports, each about a decade apart, help put this disease in perspective. Thomas Arminski, in the report noted earlier, collected 1388 cases from the literature and added 25 new ones. In 1960, Gerald Strauch reported 70 cases and reviewed the previous 10 years' experience (1061 cases) reported in the American literature.[80] Vaittinen of Finland, in an encyclopedic 81-page report published in 1970, summarized the total world experience, which comprised 4658 patients with gallbladder carcinoma, 3911 of whom were operated upon.[87] Finally, Piehler and Crichlow in 1978 reviewed 6222 patients with gallbladder carcinoma reported in the English literature.[69] Unfortunately, these reports show little improvement in the results of therapy from one decade to the next. In fact, there has been hardly any progress in diagnosis and therapy in the entire 80-year period that clinicians have dealt with this disease.

EPIDEMIOLOGY

Gallbladder cancer (GBC) is the fifth most common gastrointestinal cancer in the United States (after rectum, colon, pancreas, and stomach). Because many cases are first diagnosed at autopsy, the frequency of this lesion may not be apparent to many surgeons. The annual incidence of carcinoma of the gallbladder is 2.5 per 100,000 population, and about 6500 patients die with this disease every year in the United States.[80] Cancer is found in 1 to 3 per cent of cholecystectomy specimens and in 8 to 10 per cent of specimens from patients over 70 years of age. GBC constitutes about 3 to 4 per cent of carcinomas of the gastrointestinal tract and about 8 to 10 per cent of gastrointestinal tract cancers in women.[57] It represents about two thirds of carcinomas of the extrahepatic biliary tree and 2 to 3 per cent of all cancers.

Gallbladder cancer is a disease of older people; the age of most patients is between 55 and 70 years, with most being in their late sixties and early seventies. Females predominate by a ratio of 3 to 4.5:1. There is no difference in the age incidence between males and females.[87] The incidence of GBC in Caucasian women is higher than in black women.[51] The incidence of GBC is six to ten fold higher in Mexican, American Indian, and Alaskan natives.[13,51] Although the prevalence of gallstones is high in these groups, the incidence of GBC is even greater.[13, 74, 91] Blacks have a low incidence of gallbladder carcinoma but a high incidence of hepatocellular carcinoma. Automotive, textile, and metal fabricating workers are also prone to the disease.[14, 51] Although GBC has been found in siblings,[85] there appears to be no hereditary or familial predisposition.[87]

GBC has been reported to arise in gallbladders that have been infected with typhoid bacilli many years previously,[10, 92] but the most common association is with cholelithiasis. The clinical evidence relating gallstones to GBC is circumstantial but impressive. GBC is more common among females than males in approximately the same proportion as gallstone disease.[10, 54, 87] From 70 to 80 per cent of patients with GBC have gallstones. Thorbjarnarson and Vaittinen both reported that among patients with GBC the incidence of gallstones is much higher in women than in men.[82, 87] In both sexes there is no difference in the composition of the gallstones in cancerous or noncancerous gallbladders. However, the risk of cancer appears to increase with increasing size of gallstones, so that patients with gallstones larger than 3 cm have a tenfold greater chance to develop cancer than do those with gallstones less than 1 cm.[23]

Although the incidence of GBC in patients with gallstones is low, the incidence increases with age.[91] Ross and Hickok reported a 7 per cent incidence of cancer in surgically removed gallbladders in patients over age 70 years,[75] yet there are other data suggesting that the risk of cancer, even in the elderly, is very low. Lund followed patients with known gallstones without operation for many years and noted an incidence of GBC of only 1 per cent.[55]

Polk and others have emphasized the high risk of carcinoma developing in "porcelain" (i.e., calcified) gallbladders. He cites Etala, who found 16 primary carcinomas in 26 patients with porcelain gallbladders and only 62 cases of GBC in 1760 non-porcelain gallbladders. Polk collected reports of 100 patients with porcelain gallbladders in the literature and found 22 cancers.[70]

Whether there is a relationship between cholecystostomy and GBC is not clear, but gallbladder carcinoma may develop months or years after cholecystostomy.[87] For example, Castle et al. reported that 7 per cent of patients with GBC had had a previous cholecystostomy. In some, there was an interval of several years between the cholecystostomy and the finding of GBC; in the majority, no gallstones were found at the time of operation for GBC.[18]

Most patients with GBC have had symptoms—presumably from benign gallbladder disease—for more than 5 years before diagnosis. Whether the prolonged irritation by the gallstones causes the neoplastic change in the gallbladder epithelium, or whether biochemical events associated with gallstone formation also predispose to malignant epithelial change remains to be determined. Some stone-containing gallbladders have greatly increased cell turnover and mitotic activity, paralleling changes seen in the premalignant stages of epithelium in other parts of the gastrointestinal tract.[71] Dysplasia is frequently observed in the bordering region of gallbladder carcinomas, and it coexisted with metaplasia in 80 per cent of the specimens in one study.[53] The relationship between dysplasia and metaplasia—thought to develop as a consequence of the chronic inflammatory changes induced by gallstones—is not clear, but some believe that gallbladder metaplasia is a precursor of gallbladder dysplasia and cancer.[7, 52] Others believe that cholelithiasis leads to epithelial hyperplasia, which in some patients becomes atypical hyperplasia, which may progress to carcinoma in situ.[2] An alternative (but less likely) hypothesis is that gallstones form as a result of the cancer. Gallbladder cancer has also been found in a patient 5 years after he started chenodeoxycholic acid therapy for gallstone dissolution.[41] The fact that 10 to 30 per cent of patients with GBC do not have gallstones or chronic cholecystitis indicates that the etiology is probably multifactorial.

Many investigators have attempted to produce GBC in experimental animals. Carcinoma developed in 5 of 51 quinea pigs after sterile glass rods had been implanted into their gallbladders.[57] Fortner and others induced gallbladder carcinoma in cats (but not in dogs) by introducing into the gallbladder pellets soaked in methylcholanthrene, a known carcinogen structurally related to bile acids.[10] Similar tumors were produced in dogs after the administration of o-aminoazotoluene. Kowalewski and Todd (1971) produced dysplasia throughout the biliary system in hamsters by feeding them dimethylnitrosamine (DMN).[95] GBC developed in 68 per cent of DMN-treated hamsters that also had cholesterol pellets placed in their gallbladders, but in only one animal without cholesterol pellets.[95] It is tempting to assume that mechanical factors may also lower the threshold to chemical carcinogenesis in humans, but Willis has warned of the dangers of making such conclusions from animal experiments.[93]

PATHOLOGY

Benign tumors of the gallbladder are rare, are usually small, and almost always are incidental findings on a cholecystogram or at an operation performed for some other condition. Cholesterol and inflammatory polyps, adenomyosis, adenoma, or heterotopic tissue may appear as filling defects on oral cholecystograms. Since most gallbladders that harbor a malignant tumor do not opacify on oral cholecystography, most filling defects on oral cholecystograms are caused by benign lesions. Lipomas, leiomyomas, and other benign neoplasms as well as pseudotumors have been described, but they are exceedingly rare and of little clinical significance.

Are any of these lesions premalignant? With the possible exception of adenomas, they probably are not. For example, Kozuka et al. found carcinoma in 7 of 18 gallbladder adenomas. None of the adenomas smaller than 10 mm had malignant changes, whereas carcinoma was found in all adenomas greater than 15 mm.[50]

Peison and Rabin collected eight cases of primary melanoma of the gallbladder.[66] Rare cases of primary lymphoma, sarcoma, carcinosarcoma, and carcinoid tumors have also been reported.[12, 87] However, most malignant primary tumors of the gallbladder are carcinomas, 90 per cent being adenocarcinoma. Most are scirrhous, but mucus-secreting and papillary forms are also seen. Pure squamous tumors and mixed adenoepidermoid tumors (adenoacanthoma) constitute about 5 per cent of gallbladder carcinomas. In view of the clinical aggressiveness of primary carcinomas, a surprisingly high majority of tumors are histologically well differentiated, less than 10 per cent being anaplastic.

GBC is usually staged by histologic criteria, but Beltz and Condon[8] proposed the following clinical staging classification:

Stage A—Unrecognized at operation, discovered later by a pathologist.

Stage B—Recognized at operation; localized, curative operation possible.

Stage C—Incurable at operation, but palliative operation possible.

Stage D—Incurable disease, biopsy only or post mortem diagnosis.

Histologic staging is usually done retrospectively. Four categories are generally used (adapted from Nevin et al.[60]).

Stage I—Intramucosal only; in situ carcinoma.

Stage II—Invasion into gallbladder muscle only; microinvasive.

Stage III—Invasion through all layers of gallbladder wall with or without involvement of cystic duct node; localized invasive.

Stage IV—Extension into liver or other viscera, or metastases to lymph nodes beyond the bile duct area and to other distant sites.

Stratification of patients by a combined staging grading is useful in predicting the outcome of therapy.[8, 28, 60] The tumor may occur anywhere in the gallbladder, although the site of origin may be difficult to determine because most cancers have grown beyond the limits of resectability before they are discovered. In most series a majority of the lesions have been thought to originate in the fundus.[6, 10, 87] Appleman's retrospective analysis of 21 five-year survivors from the Mayo Clinic allowed an unusual opportunity to study the pathologic features of early disease. In 12 of the 21 cases there was a multicentric origin of cancer, and in four gallbladders there was diffuse, benign mucosal hyperplasia.[5]

The gallbladder may be contracted and thickened by a scirrhous carcinoma or enlarged and filled with mucus by a mucoid adenocarcinoma. In advanced cases it may be difficult to find any remnant of normal gallbladder wall. Perforation of the cancerous gallbladder, which has been seen in up to 10 per cent of cases, may be into an adjacent hollow viscus or into the free peritoneal cavity.[6] Localized perforation may result in a pericholecystic abscess. Many of the complications of gallstone disease mimic carcinoma, and vice versa. Whenever there are firm adhesions between the surface of the gallbladder and neighboring structures, or whenever it is difficult to dissect the gallbladder from the liver surface because of extensive scarring, the surgeon should suspect cancer and obtain a biopsy for frozen section.

Fahim thoroughly described the modes of spread of GBC. The tumors are locally aggressive, but they spread to distant sites late in the course of the disease. Lymphatic spread is first to the cystic duct and common duct nodes, next to the pancreaticoduodenal nodes behind the duodenum, and then to the nodes around the celiac axis and the superior mesenteric artery.[25] There are no lymph nodes in the true hilum of the liver; therefore, skeletonization of the structures of the porta hepatis makes little sense for patients with gallbladder carcinoma. Lymph node spread is present at the time of diagnosis in 45 to 80 per cent of patients.[6, 73, 84, 87]

Two papers in 1932 from Germany and Scandinavia described the existence of a plexus of cholecystic veins that drains into the capillary bed of the quadrate lobe and from there into the hepatic veins.[25] Portal vein communications to the gallbladder were said not to exist, and the tributaries connecting with the hepatic veins were stated to provide a pathway for venous spread of tumor. I take issue with this description, which has been repeated in the literature without challenge by many authors. I injected the portal and hepatic venous systems of more than 50 cadaver livers with colored vinyl acetate plastic, and after acid corrosion of the specimen, I uniformly found the gallbladder outlined by portal venous radicles (unpublished results). In no case was a branch of the hepatic veins demonstrated to drain the gallbladder. The observed distribution of metastases (common in the liver and rare in the lungs) also is more consistent with portal venous than with hepatic venous spread.

Direct extension of infiltrating tumor into the liver is common (52 per cent, according to Vaittinen[87]), and invasion of the bile duct, duodenum, stomach, colon, and retroperitoneal structures is not rare. Intraductal spread is uncommon and usually is associated with papillary tumors. This may be a manifestation of multifocal origin, but Appleman et al. described one patient who was apparently cured after cholecystectomy with extraction of free pieces of tumor from the common bile duct.[5] Diffuse peritoneal seeding is rare, and widespread dissemination to lung, bone, and brain is a late manifestation seen in a minority of patients.

PRESENTATION AND DIFFERENTIAL DIAGNOSIS

Most articles on gallbladder carcinoma contain an extensive description of the patient's presenting complaints and the laboratory and radiographic abnormalities. At the bedside, however, knowledge of the most common findings is of little value if one is concerned with curing the disease. If cholecystectomy is performed for gallstone disease and the gallbladder contains a small carcinoma, the patient may be helped. If the carcinoma itself has grown large enough to cause symptoms, the surgeon rarely has much to offer except biopsy confirmation of diagnosis.

The usual symptoms and signs are listed in Table 31–1. Thirty to 50 per cent of patients with gallbladder carcinoma give a history of right upper quadrant distress for 6 to 30 years before diagnosis.[87] A recent change in the pattern of pain is often noted

Table 31–1 PRESENTING SIGNS AND SYMPTOMS OF GALLBLADDER CARCINOMA

	Per Cent With Finding						
Author	*Pain*	*Weight Loss*	*Jaundice*	*Mass*	*Tenderness*	*Hepatomegaly*	*Ascites*
Arminski (1949)	76	64	58	53	64	49	21
Burdette (1957)	82	47	50	54	55	53	7
Strauch (1960)	66	59	51	40	—	—	—
Hardy and Volk (1970)	19	34	61	52	44	86	—
Vaittinen (literature review, 1970)	79	56	48	49	51	46	17
Vaittinen (Finnish experience, 1970)	81	42	41	50	40	46	6
Weiskopf and Esselstyn (1976)	67	62	32	8	—	—	—

retrospectively, and advanced age should raise the index of suspicion. Some patients with GBC present with acute cholecystitis manifested by fever, leukocytosis, and localized pain and tenderness.

The serum alkaline phosphatase and bilirubin levels are the laboratory values most often elevated in patients with gallbladder carcinoma, but they do not help in differentiating benign from malignant disease. The oral cholecystogram does not opacify in 90 per cent of patients with gallbladder cancer, and intravenous cholangiography is unsuccessful in 93 per cent.[87] Barium contrast studies of the gastrointestinal tract are abnormal in about one third of cases, usually owing to invasion or compression of the duodenum, distal stomach, or transverse colon.[8]

Endoscopic retrograde cholangiopancreatography (ERCP) may suggest the diagnosis.[58, 61] Of 45 cases examined by ERCP, the bile duct did not opacify in 8 cases, there were 4 false negative studies, and a filling defect was demonstrated in 3 of 33 cases. The gallbladder could not be filled in 18 patients, and infiltration of the common bile duct was seen in 8 patients.[61]

Angiography is not helpful in detecting early lesions, but it may help demonstrate the extent of advanced disease.[57] Gothlin and Pettersson compared angiographic findings in 18 patients with gallbladder carcinoma and 17 patients with cholecystitis and found no reliable differentiating features.[31] Ultrasound or CT scans may show localized thickening of the gallbladder wall in patients who have gallstones or a locally invasive neoplasm,[4, 20, 42, 94] but they are unable to detect curable carcinoma. Laparoscopy has been able to diagnose late disease,[87] and it may be useful in avoiding laparotomy for diagnosis. The presence and pattern of distribution of carcinoembryonic antigen (CEA) in the normal and the neoplastic gallbladder epithelium closely resemble those in other gastrointestinal epithelia.[3] Thus, elevated CEA values may occur in patients with GBC. Duodenal cytology is usually unrewarding.[87] Biopsy specimens of obviously unresectable mass lesions may be obtained by percutaneous needle aspiration.

Even with all the new diagnostic techniques, a preoperative diagnosis can only be made in 5 to 18 per cent of patients.[39, 67, 68, 73, 79, 87] The diagnosis of resectable carcinoma of the gallbladder is almost always made at laparotomy by the surgeon or postoperatively when the pathologist inspects the specimen.

OPERATION FOR GALLBLADDER CANCER

Indications

The arguments for removing a diseased or stone-containing gallbladder are covered in other chapters. Although Evarts Graham advocated cholecystectomy for prophylaxis against the development of gallbladder carcinoma as long ago as 1931,[33] careful analysis does not support this approach. Calculation of risks versus benefits shows that cholecystectomy cannot be recommended for the principal purpose of preventing GBC.[62, 73, 79, 90] Even in elderly women, the risk of the operation exceeds the risk of carcinoma.

A more difficult question is whether any

Table 31–2 EXTENT OF SPREAD OF TUMOR AT OPERATION*

Lymph Nodes	Per Cent	Direct Infiltration	Per Cent	Embolic Spread	Per Cent
Regional	42	Liver	52	Liver	51
Retroperitoneal	23	Bile duct	25	Peritoneum	19
Mesenteric	14	Hepatic duct	17	Lungs	8
		Pancreas	11	Bone	5
		Stomach	10	Adrenals	4
		Duodenum	8		
		Colon	5		

*1611 patients with gallbladder carcinoma.
Adapted from Vaittinen (1970); percentages rounded off.

resection beyond cholecystectomy is warranted when GBC is diagnosed at laparotomy or postoperatively. Although the disease is very aggressive locally, distant spread occurs late. At least on theoretical grounds, a rationale can be presented for removal of regional nodes and a margin of adjacent liver. In fact, there is a general acceptance of this approach, even though the data in support of it are inconclusive.[35, 45, 46, 76, 88]

Most often the surgeon finds that the gallbladder carcinoma has grown beyond the limits of resection. Table 31–2 documents the extent of spread of tumor at the time of primary diagnosis. Resection "for cure" (removal of all gross disease) is possible only about 25 per cent of the time.[1,87] Most patients have involvement of celiac or other distant lymph nodes, retroperitoneal fixation, or direct invasion of the hilar structures. Diffuse embolic hepatic metastases are rare, but satellite nodules near the gallbladder fossa are common with aggressive infiltrating tumors. Ten to 65 per cent of patients with advanced disease never leave the hospital, and the mean survival is only 4 months. Over 90 per cent of patients die within 1 year.

Choice of Operation

Cholecystectomy is the operation most often done for resectable gallbladder carcinoma. However, the surgeon can extend the resection by performing a dissection of the regional lymph nodes, by liver resection, or by en bloc removal of viscera involved by direct extension.

Lymphadenectomy has been performed by limited removal of the tissues around the cystic duct–common bile duct junction, by skeletonization of all the structures of the porta hepatis, and even by pancreaticoduodenectomy (Whipple procedure), which removes all the lymph nodes behind and above the head of the pancreas. The careful studies of Fahim[25] suggest that the dissection should remove the nodes in Calot's triangle and along the right lateral and posterior surfaces of the common bile duct, extending behind the duodenum and head of the pancreas. A Kocher maneuver mobilizes the duodenum enough to allow a safe dissection of the lymphatics along the common bile duct. There is no need to skeletonize all the structures of the porta hepatis, and circumferential dissection of the common bile duct may jeopardize its blood supply. The right lateral border of the portal vein is the deep limit of the dissection, and the common duct nodes can be adequately removed by a dissection that proceeds inferiorly only as far as the entrance of the common bile duct into the duodenal wall in the pancreaticoduodenal groove posteriorly.

Recommendations for liver resection have varied from a wedge resection of a few grams of tissue from the gallbladder bed to removal of the right lobe and the medial segment of the left lobe. Because the gallbladder lies in the plane between the anatomic right and left lobes of the liver, there is no anatomic rationale for a right hepatic lobectomy for gallbladder carcinoma. However, wedge resection of the tissue forming the gallbladder bed may be appropriate in some cases, particularly when the cancer appears to be confined to the fundus or when the pathologist reports that a small tumor has limited extension through the wall. In most instances the wedge resection should consist of a 1.5 to 2 cm rim of normal tissue teased out, with blunt dissection and metal clips used to secure the blood vessels. Hilar control of the major vessels is usually unnecessary but can be achieved by a Pringle maneuver. A larger wedge of liver can be safely removed by bluntly dissecting the common hepatic duct beyond the confluence of the major lobar ducts, pushing the confluence posteriorly while proceeding up into the liver hilum. Because the arteries and the portal vein lie behind the bile duct, the surgeon can dissect through liver substance anterior to the duct, using blunt technique or even mattress sutures to remove as large a piece of the quadrate lobe as is necessary to encompass the entire gallbladder bed and a generous margin of uninvolved liver (see Chapter 11, Foster and Berman[26] for technical details). Portions of the stomach, duodenum, transverse colon, and even common bile duct may be resected if invaded by localized gallbladder carcinoma.

Are any of these extended procedures supported by results? The answer is difficult to determine because details of the pathologic findings and operative technique are lacking in most reports, and no trial has been conducted to systematically compare the different operations.

Results of Operation

Any comparison of different modes of treatment must take into account the stage of the disease. In some cases a gallbladder removed for presumed benign disease has been found later to contain an invasive cancer. Re-exploration within a few weeks to perform an extended resection often reveals extensive lymph node and regional involvement that was overlooked by the unsuspecting surgeon at the first operation. Consequently, data reported on the clinical stage of occult tumors are of questionable accuracy.

Table 31–3 lists the operations performed on the 3911 patients reviewed by Vaittinen, and Table 31–4 summarizes the reports since Vaittinen's paper, adding 2509 cases. An operation was performed in 82 per cent of patients. In 38 per cent (2257/5923) of the operated patients, the gallbladder was resected, and three quarters of these resections encompassed all visible tumor. Thus, in 30 per cent of all patients who were explored, a "curative" resection was possible. Of the 1486 patients resected for cure and followed for 5 years or until death, 214 (14.5 per cent) survived for 5 years.

Table 31–3 OPERATIONS PERFORMED FOR GALLBLADDER CARCINOMA*

Procedure	Per Cent
Cholecystectomy alone	33.4
Curative	27.0
Palliative	6.4
Cholecystectomy plus liver resection	3.0
Cholecystectomy, liver resection, and lymphadenectomy	1.2
Other radical operations	18.1
Palliative operations	18.1
Exploration and biopsy	43.7

*Literature review of 3911 patients.
From Vaittinen (1970).

Ninety-two per cent of the 5-year survivals in Vaittinen's report had been treated by cholecystectomy alone. In the more recent reports, 72 (95 per cent) of 76 five-year survivors had cholecystectomy alone. All ten patients in Adson's series who had disease limited to the gallbladder wall (Stages I and II) were alive from 3 to 10 years after operation. Seven patients (five with occult tumors, and two known to have cancer at operation) had cholecystectomy alone, and three others had cholecystectomy, wedge excision of the liver, and regional lymphadenectomy. Retrospectively, the lymph nodes and liver of the latter three patients were negative for tumor. All are free of disease, one at 5 years and two at less than 1 year after operation.[1]

Only 3 of the 31 patients not included in Vaittinen's literature review[87] who had extended resections lived as long as 5 years (all reported by Adson[1]). One of these three died with recurrent disease at 6 years. Thus, 3.7 per cent of all operated patients survived for 5 years, and at least nine of the 5-year survivors eventually died with recurrent disease.

Long-Term Survival

Vaittinen lists 138 "permanent cures" in his 1970 review,[87] but whether this was defined as survival for 5 years is unclear. Table 31–5 lists reports of 108 other patients who survived for 5 years after cholecystectomy for gallbladder carcinoma. Accurate information about therapy is known for all but 14 of these patients. Eighty-nine (95 per cent) of 94 patients had cholecystectomy alone, three had extended resections, and two received radiotherapy after cholecystectomy. In 48 (87 per cent) of the 55 patients about whom there was sufficient information, the GBC was not recognized by the surgeon at operation.

Factors that correlate most closely with

Table 31–4 TREATMENT OF GALLBLADDER CARCINOMA—PUBLISHED REPORTS

			Resections				
Author	***Patients***	***Operations***	***Number***	***Curative***	***Extended Operations***	***Unresectable***	***5-Year Survivors***
Vaittinen (1970) (literature review)	4658	3911	1493	1243	16	2418	128
Vaittinen (1970) (Finland)	390	300	123	31	6	177	10
Gradisar and Kelly (1970)	41	36	19	—	0	17	1
Hardy and Volk (1970)	59	43	14	—	0	29	1
Solan and Jackson (1971)	57	45	18	10	3	27	0
Holmes and Mark (1971)	72	44	22	—	2	22	1
Pemberton et al. (1971)	100	85	40	—	2	45	2
Ram (1971)	47	41	31	—	0	10	1
Hart and Modan (1972)	334	242	85	—	?	157	14
Adson (1973)	112	112	50	26	7	62	6*
Beltz and Condon (1974)	117	103	28	18	2	75	2
Ohlsson and Aronsen (1974)	181	101	40	38	2	61	1
Donaldson and Busuttil (1975)	68	53	14	14	0	39	1
Moossa et al. (1975)	82	30	—	—	3	—	4
Treadwell and Hardin (1976)	43	43	28	21	3	15	7
Richard and Cantin (1976)	108	93	41	21	0	52	7
Weiskopf and Esselstyn (1976)	48	48	18	18	3	30	2
Nevin et al. (1976)	66	66	57	—	0	9	14
Piehler and Crichlow (1977)	48	43	19	11	2	24	1
Oswalt and Cruz (1977)	33	32	17	5	0	15	3
Perpetuo et al. (1978)	75	61	50	4	0	265	6
Gupta et al. (1980)	328	307	42	—	10	58	2
Koo et al. (1981)	100	84	36	20	6	58	2
Totals	7167	5923	38%	30%	1%	61%	216 (3.7%)

*Five other patients alive and well from 3 to 10 years after cholecystectomy.

long-term survival are occult carcinoma and the histologic type, stage, and grade of the carcinoma. Hart and Modan found that 33 per cent of patients whose tumor was localized to the gallbladder were alive after *5* years, in contrast to only 2 per cent who were alive at *1* year when regional spread was grossly obvious. Thirty-four per cent of patients with papillary adenocarcinoma were alive at *5* years, whereas less than 10 per cent of patients with other histologic types survived *1* year. In fact, the median survival of 15 patients with localized papillary carcinoma was 5 years![38] Nevin et al. analyzed 399 cases about which there was accurate histologic information concerning depth of tumor invasion and found that 100 per cent of 40 patients with Stages I and II disease who survived operation lived for 5 years or more. The outcome in Nevin's 17 patients with Stages I and II disease was as follows: 3 operative deaths, 3 patients followed less than five years, and 11 five-year survivors.[60] Clearly, an "occult" papillary tumor that does not extend beyond the muscularis of the gallbladder wall has an excellent chance of being cured permanently by cholecystectomy alone.

All three patients who survived 5 years after an extended operation were reported by Adson, whose operation combined wedge liver resection with lymph node dissection and cholecystectomy. In one of these patients the disease was limited to the gallbladder wall, and in the other two there was either hepatic invasion or lymph node involvement of an unstated degree. One of the latter two patients died with recurrent tumor after 6 years.[1]

Two patients survived for prolonged periods after radiotherapy in addition to cholecystectomy. One had a Stage II squamous cell tumor that might have been cured by cholecystectomy alone,[78] but the other had an invasive lesion involving the blood vessels of the gallbladder bed.[22]

Extended Operation

Vaittinen's review included seven 5-year survivors after 187 extended operations, defined as removal of the gallbladder together with adjacent liver, lymph nodes, or involved adjacent viscera.[87] Included were the Sheinfeld series, which contained one 5-year survivor among 36 cases of combined resection

Table 31–5 GALLBLADDER CARCINOMA: 5-YEAR SURVIVAL

Author	Number of Patients	Per Cent of Curative Operations	Occult Tumors	Operation	Comment
Vaittinen (1970)	10	32	?	10 GB	5 papillary tumors 4 patients DWD after 5 years
Gradisar and Kelly (1970)	1	—	1	GB	
Hardy and Volk (1970)	1	—	1	GB	patient DWD at 62 months
Holmes and Mark (1971)	1	—	1	GB	suicide at 5 years NED
Pemberton et al. (1971)	2	—	1	GB	
Ram (1971)	1	—	1	GB	DWD after 5 years
Hart and Modan (1972)	14	—	?	?	7 papillary, 7 nonpapillary tumors
Adson (1973)	11*	29	5	8 GB 3 GB + L + LN	2 DWD at 6 years
Beltz and Condon (1974)	2	11	2	GB	both papillary tumors
Ohlsson and Aronsen (1974)	1	3	1	GB	in situ carcinoma
Thorbjarnarson (1975)	3	—	—	GB	
Bivins et al. (1975)	4	—	4	GB	3 in situ, 1 microinvasive
Donaldson and Busuttil (1975)	1	7	1	GB	
Moossa et al. (1975)	4	—	4	GB	
Nevin et al (1976)	14	—	?	GB	13 limited to gallbladder wall, 1 with involved cystic duct node.
Treadwell and Hardin (1976)	7	33	?	GB	3 papillary, 4 infiltrating
Richard and Cantin (1976)	7	33	7	GB	
Weiskopf and Esselstyn (1976)	2	7	2	GB	3 other patients alive less than 5 years
Piehler and Crichlow (1977)	1	9	1	GB	papillary tumor
Oswalt and Cruz (1977)	3	60	3	GB	2 in situ, 1 microinvasive
Smoron (1977)	1	—	1	GB + RAD Rx + 5-FU	Stage II squamous tumor
Del Regato and Spjut (1977)	1	—	—	GB + RAD Rx	
Perpetuo et al. (1978)	1	25	1	GB	in situ cancer
Bergdahl (1980)	7	—	7	7 GB	all Stage I or II
Gupta et al. (1980)	6	—	4	6 GB	
Koo et al. (1981)	2	10	—	2 GB	
Totals	108		48/55		9 Patients died after 5 years

*Five patients with occult cancer alive 3–10 years, all counted as 5-year survivors.
GB = Cholecystectomy; L = liver resection; LN = lymphadenectomy; DWD = dead with disease; NED = no evidence of disease.

of the liver and gallbladder[77]; the Glenn and Hayes series of 19 extended operations with two 5-year survivors[30]; and the Pack and Brasfield series with one 5-year survivor after seven hepatic lobectomies (with four operative deaths).[64] Table 31–6 lists 89 cases reported since 1970. Three patients had a lymph node dissection in addition to cholecystectomy; in one a segment of the common bile duct was also resected.[86, 90] The other 86 patients had resection of a portion of liver, which in seven cases included a lymphadenectomy. Twenty-one per cent of these patients died after operation, while only 5 per cent of those at risk (4 out of 80) lived 5 years. Two of the 5-year survivors were dead 6 and 15 years after operation of recurrent (or new) carcinoma. In a recent survey of the Japanese experience, which included 100 hospitals, Tashiro et al. found that survival correlated well with the stage of the tumor. When they compared the results of cholecystectomy alone with those of more extensive operations according to stage, they found no difference in survival for Stages I and II lesions. Although the proportion of patients alive at 2 and 3 years for Stage III lesions was larger among those receiving more extensive operations, the 5-year survival was the same for both groups.[81]

Adson makes a persuasive case for wedge resection of adjacent liver combined with cholecystectomy and regional lymphadenectomy. However, review of his data reveals that of 26 patients with grossly curable disease, microscopic examination showed disease limited to the gallbladder wall in ten (five of these tumors were occult and five

Table 31–6 EXTENDED OPERATIONS*

	Liver Resection		Lymphadenectomy Without Liver Resection	Total
	Wedge	*Lobectomy*		
Patients	62	24	3	89
Operative deaths	10	9	0	19 (21%)
DWD less than 3½ years	41	13	3	
AFD less than 5 years	4	1	0	
AWD less than 1 year	3	0	0	
Lost to follow-up	1	0	0	
5-Year survivors	3†	1†	0	4(5%)

*Recent experience (14 series).
†One patient after wedge resection and one patient after lobectomy died with disease after 5 years.
DWD = dead with disease; AWD = alive with disease; AFD = alive free of disease.
References: 8, 9, 26, 31–35, 37, 39, 42, 47, 57–59, 62, 63, 67, 68, 79, 86, 87, 90.

were apparent at operation). Seven of these patients had cholecystectomy alone, and three had the extended procedure. All ten are alive and without evident disease from 3 to 10 years after operation. Sixteen other patients had microscopic disease outside the gallbladder wall. Of the 12 who had cholecystectomy alone, 11 died of their disease in less than 15 months. The twelfth patient died of recurrent papillary tumor 6 years after her first operation. Four patients had the extended operation: Two were dead with disease at 3½ years and 6 years, and two were alive and apparently free of disease, one at less than a year after surgery and one at 13 years.[1]

Foster[26] collected 35 cases of liver resection for GBC in a nationwide survey and found only one 5-year survivor—the same patient reported by Brasfield in 1961.[15] Careful study of that case raises doubt about the extent of the disease at the time of liver resection. A photomicrograph said to show tumor in the liver appears instead to show a single nest of carcinoma in a lymphatic lying in the inflamed areolar tissue of the gallbladder bed. Extended right hepatic lobectomy and a lymph node dissection were performed 3 days after cholecystectomy. The primary tumor was a 1.5 cm papillary adenocarcinoma of the gallbladder fundus without regional lymph node involvement.[15] Although this patient was probably cured of gallbladder carcinoma by surgery, she died 15 years later of a carcinoma of the bile duct.[26]

Therefore, the evidence does not support the use of right hepatic lobectomy for gallbladder carcinoma. Extension of right lobectomy to include the quadrate lobe (medial segment of the left lobe) can be argued theoretically, but there has never been a case in which long-term survival followed a major hepatic lobectomy in which disease was present in the liver at any distance from the gallbladder bed. Lobectomy has no advantage over wedge resection, and for grossly curable lesions the postoperative morbidity will be greater with the larger operation. Table 31–6 contains the collected experience from the literature. Major hepatic resection for GBC was followed by a 35 per cent mortality rate.

A wedge resection of the liver bed can be done safely, and the addition of a local lymphadenectomy should not increase the operative risk. This procedure deserves consideration for patients with Stage III and perhaps for those with limited Stage IV disease. Unfortunately, most tumors are more advanced when discovered, and the smaller lesions are found by the pathologist rather than by the surgeon.

Occult Lesions

Table 31–7 summarizes the data on 267 patients whose gallbladder carcinomas were unsuspected by the surgeon at the time of cholecystectomy. These are not necessarily all small lesions at an early stage, because in some instances a difficult dissection of a tumor invading the liver was interpreted by the surgeon to be a manifestation of chronic inflammation. The tumor was grossly occult in 18 per cent of operations for GBC. These cases constitute the majority of the curable lesions.

The 5-year survival was 23 per cent in patients with clinically occult GBC and was higher if only patients with histologic Stages I and II disease are considered. Nevertheless, more than three quarters of patients with

Table 31–7 CLINICALLY OCCULT CARCINOMAS

Author	Operated Patients	Occult Tumors	5-Year Survivors	AFD Less Than 5 Years	Dead with Disease
Burdette (1957)	61	11	2	1	8
Strauch (1960)	64	9	1	2	6
Gerst (1961)	132	21	6	1	14
Chandler and Fletcher (1963)	49	9	2	0	7
Frank and Spjut (1967)	—	16	2	1	13
Hardy and Volk (1970)	43	6	1*	0	5
Gradisar and Kelly (1970)	36	5	1	0	4
Ram (1971)	41	10	1*	0	9
Holmes and Mark (1971)	44	7	1	2	0
Beltz and Condon (1974)	103	14	2	0	12
Kott and Urca (1974)	—	9	2*	3	4
Ohlsson and Aronsen (1974)	116	23	1	2	20
Moossa et al. (1975)	30	6	4	1	1
Bivins et al. (1975)	—	9	4	3	2
Donaldson and Busuttil (1975)	53	10	1	0	9
Weiskopf and Esselstyn (1976)	48	14	2	0	6
Richard and Cantin (1976)	93	21	7	0	14
Nevins et al. (1976)†	—	17	11	2	0
Oswalt and Cruz (1977)†	—	2	2	—	0
Piehler and Crichlow (1977)	43	8	1	1	6
Hanna and Rider (1978)	51	9	0	0	9
Bergdahl (1980)	120	32	7	0	23
Totals		268	61	19	

*One patient dead with disease after 5 years.
†Pathologic stages I and II basis for inclusion (nonclinical series).
AFD = Alive free of disease.

lesions not recognized by the surgeon died of their disease, usually within 2 years. Furthermore, 4 of 62 patients with occult tumors died with recurrent cancer after 5 years, two in the sixth year, one in the seventh year, and one in the eighth year after cholecystectomy (Table 31–7).

Would a routine policy of opening every gallbladder and searching for signs of neoplastic change make a difference in the outcome? It would not for Stages I and II lesions, but perhaps it would for early Stage III lesions. At least, diagnosis during surgery would stimulate a more thorough search for evidence of spread.

Palliative Operations

The very short survival of patients with advanced disease limits the surgeon's ability to palliate when resection is not possible. Dissection in the liver hilum is often impossible because of direct extension of tumor or massive lymph node involvement. Cholecystostomy may invite growth of tumor through the abdominal wall. Pain is almost never relieved unless it is due to biliary obstruction, and debulking has no place because chemotherapy and immunotherapy have little effect on even small amounts of residual disease.

Often the patient's interests will be best served by biopsy alone if the lesion is unresectable, but occasionally some relief can be provided by biliary decompression or by bypass of an obstruction of the gastrointestinal tract. If technically possible, an attempt should be made to insert a tube stent through the site of an obstructed bile duct. Passage of Bakes dilators will often open the duct enough to allow insertion of a transhepatic tube, a T-tube, or a U-tube.

NONOPERATIVE THERAPY

Radiotherapy

Radiotherapy would seem to be indicated in the treatment of an unresectable tumor that often kills before widespread dissemination has occurred. Enthusiasm for irradiation of adenocarcinomas has increased in recent years, and therapists have learned much about the ability of the liver to tolerate radiation. Yet there is little in the literature about the effects of radiation on GBC.

Hanna and Rider treated 35 of 51 GBC patients with radiotherapy, 10 with curative doses averaging 4000 rads, and 25 with palliative doses of 2600 rads. There were nine patients with occult tumors in this series, but it is not clear whether they were among those treated with radiotherapy. No patient survived for 5 years, but those receiving radical or palliative radiotherapy lived an average of 10.4 months compared with 5.3 months for 16 patients who did not receive radiotherapy.[36] Vaittinen found no benefit from radiotherapy given after "curative" surgery in seven patients.[87]

Smoron gave 4000 rads to a woman with a fungating bleeding adenocarcinoma that was growing through the abdominal wall 18 months after cholecystectomy. The mass disappeared, and the patient was apparently well 16 months later. He noted no response to radiotherapy in four other patients with advanced GBC. He also reported one patient with Stage II squamous cell carcinoma of the gallbladder treated prophylactically with radiotherapy and 5-FU who was alive and well 6 years later.[78] Del Regato and Spjut reported the only other 5-year survival after radiotherapy in a patient with Stage III disease.[22]

Moossa et al. reported little success in three patients with radiation therapy without surgery, five patients given chemotherapy, and four who received a combination of radiotherapy and chemotherapy. However, one patient lived 30 months after surgery and palliative radiotherapy, and another was alive and well 2 years after radiation for an occult Stage III lesion.[57] Weiskopf and Esselstyn reported a short remission in "several" of four patients with advanced disease who received cobalt teletherapy.[90]

Iwasaki et al. delivered a single intraoperative dose of 3000 rads through a special cone to four patients with GBC.[43] Todoroki et al. used this approach in six patients, several of whom experienced both relief of biliary obstruction and other signs of palliation.[83] There has been increasing attention to the use of intraoperative radiation therapy in recent years. The main advantage of this method is the possibility of delivering a relatively high dose to the tumor bed while protecting the adjacent structures and moving the bowel out of the field. Recanalization of an obstructed bile duct may be achieved by this method.[48] The presence of transhepatic catheters for biliary decompression affords an opportunity for the temporary insertion of intracavitary radiation sources, such as iridium, cesium, or radium, to boost the radiation dose. In some series, these techniques have been used as the only radiation source with encouraging preliminary results.[48]

Overall, the data in support of radiotherapy are meager but hopeful. The curative potential of operation may be enhanced by postoperative radiotherapy, and palliation, including relief from jaundice, may be achieved for short periods in patients with more advanced disease.

Chemotherapy

Vaittinen,[87] Pemberton et al.,[67] and Weiskopf and Esselstyn[90] reported little or no response to chemotherapy in patients with GBC. Moertel treated 31 patients with 30 different chemotherapeutic regimens and noted five transient objective responses.[56] Oswalt and Cruz reported a median survival of 20 weeks for 13 patients given chemotherapy compared with 8 weeks for untreated patients. Eight patients were treated with 5-FU and five with a four-drug regimen. There was no difference in the response to these two regimens. One patient with a "tumor that had extended locally" was treated with 5-FU and survived for 6 years, but the nature of the operation and stage of the tumor were not reported.[63]

Treadwell and Hardin noted increased survival 1 year after operation in patients with advanced disease (2 of 9 treated patients versus none of 16 untreated patients) who received a combination of chemotherapy and radiotherapy. However, none of the untreated patients who survived for at least 1 year developed recurrence, whereas four of five who received chemotherapy and radiotherapy who survived for at least one year died of tumor.[86] It seems likely that patient selection affected these results, and the data could even be interpreted as showing an adverse effect of systemic chemotherapy on long-term survival.

Davis et al. treated 39 patients with fluoropyrimidines. Of 23 receiving systemic therapy, the median survival was 4 months and the longest survival was 15 months. Six patients received intra-arterial therapy, and none lived as long as 1 year.[21] Watkins et al. reported two favorable responses (at least 3 months) in six patients undergoing hepatic artery catheterization and perfusion for gallbladder carcinoma.[89] Piehler and Crichlow perfused two patients with 5-FU, and both were dead from their disease within 3 months.[68]

Thus, currently available chemotherapeutic agents seem to have little influence on GBC.

CONCLUSIONS AND RECOMMENDATIONS

After reviewing this evidence, one is tempted to agree with John Homans, who wrote in 1931, "The cancerous gallbladder can seldom be removed and removal almost never prevents recurrence of the cancer."[40] The following summary is based on the evidence presented previously.

When the diagnosis of GBC is evident preoperatively, there is nothing that can be accomplished by operating unless biliary or gastrointestinal obstruction is present. Even in these situations, vigorous attempts at bypassing the obstruction may result in complications that shorten the patient's life. A biopsy specimen may be obtained by percutaneous techniques.

If, at operation, the tumor is found to extend beyond the bile duct nodes or gallbladder bed and immediately adjacent liver, no attempt at resection should be made. Biliary decompression or relief of gastrointestinal obstruction may be possible in a few patients. Radiotherapy will provide temporary control of tumor growth in a minority of such patients, whereas currently available chemotherapeutic agents have little to offer. More information is needed before hepatic artery ligation or cannulation for perfusion can be recommended.

If the presence of a localized GBC is recognized at operation before a cholecystectomy is performed, and the diagnosis is confirmed by biopsy, an en bloc resection of gallbladder and a wedge of adjacent liver is recommended. In addition, an in-continuity dissection of the cystic and common bile duct lymph nodes should be performed. Most of these patients will have advanced disease.

If GBC is not clinically obvious but is discovered after the gallbladder is opened during surgery, a careful examination should be made to determine the gross and microscopic extent of disease. If no spread is evident beyond the gallbladder wall, and if the pathologist reports that the tumor does not invade beyond the gallbladder muscularis, nothing more should be done. If neither gross nor microscopic spread beyond the gallbladder wall is evident, but the disease is apparently localized to the gallbladder fossa or to the bile duct nodes, a wedge resection of the gallbladder bed and a dissection of the ductal nodes should be performed. Unresectable localized disease should be treated by radiotherapy.

If the diagnosis of cancer is unsuspected at operation and is made 1 to 2 days later by the pathologist, no further surgery is indicated if the disease is limited to the gallbladder wall (Stage I or II), particularly if the tumor is papillary. There is an excellent chance in this situation that the patient will be cured. If the tumor has invaded beyond the muscularis, one of three courses can be recommended: (1) immediate reoperation and extended resection if spread is not obvious; (2) reoperation in 2 to 3 months, an interval that may allow separation of the very aggressive (and probably incurable) tumors from the less aggressive (and perhaps curable) ones; or (3) postoperative radiotherapy with curative doses. My preference is for the second option, but it cannot be defended with data.

THE FUTURE

More extensive operations will not cure more patients with carcinoma of the gallbladder. A policy of prophylactic removal of all stone-containing gallbladders provides an effective but impractical remedy, whose risks seem to outweigh its benefits. No dramatic progress in radiotherapy or chemotherapy is likely in the near future. What is really needed is discovery of a tumor marker that will signal an early change from inflamed to neoplastic epithelium: a radioactive or radiopaque marker that the liver can excrete in bile and that the neoplastic epithelium of the gallbladder will concentrate, or a biochemical marker that can be measured in blood. Only then will it be possible to diagnose carcinoma of the gallbladder early enough to improve the outcome of therapy.

REFERENCES

1. Adson MA: Carcinoma of the gallbladder. Surg Clin North Am 1973;53:1202.
2. Albores-Saavedra J, Alcantra-Vazquez A, Cruz-Ortiz H, Herrera-Goepfert R: The precursor lesions of

invasive gallbladder carcinoma. Hyperplasia, atypical hyperplasia and carcinoma in situ. Cancer 1980;*45*:919.
3. Albores-Saavedra J, Morales AR, Henson DE: Carcinoembryonic antigen in normal, preneoplastic and neoplastic gallbladder epithelium. Cancer 1983;*52*:1069.
4. Allibone GW, Fagan CJ, Porter SC: Sonographic features of carcinoma of the gallbladder. Gastrointest Radiol 1981;*6*:169.
5. Appleman RM, Morlock CC, Dahlin DC, et al: Long term survival in carcinoma of the gall-bladder. Surg Gynecol Obstet 1963;*117*:459.
6. Arminski TC: Primary carcinoma of the gallbladder. Cancer 1949;*2*:379.
7. Azadeh B, Parai SK: Argentaffin cells, intestinal metaplasia and antral metaplasia in carcinoma of the gall bladder. Histopathology 1980;*4*:653.
8. Beltz WR, Condon RE: Primary carcinoma of the gallbladder. Ann Surg 1974;*108*:108.
9. Bergdahl L: Gallbladder carcinoma first diagnosed at microscopic examination of gallbladders removed for presumed benign disease. Ann Surg 1980; *191*:19.
10. Bevan G: Tumours of the gallbladder. Clin Gastroenterol 1973;*2*:175.
11. Bivins BA, Meeker WR Jr, Weiss DL, et al: Carcinoma in situ of the gallbladder: a dilemma. South Med J 1975;*68*:297.
12. Born MW, Ramey WG, Ryan SF, Gordon PE: Carcinosarcoma and carcinoma of the gallbladder. Cancer 1984;*53*:2171.
13. Boss P, Lanier AP, Dohan PH, Bender TR: Cancers of the gallbladder and biliary tract in Alaskan natives: 1970–1979. J Natl Cancer Inst 1982;*69*:1005.
14. Brandt-Rauf PW, Branwood AW: Case report. An unusual case of gallbladder cancer in an automotive worker. Cancer 1980;*30*:333.
15. Brasfield RD: Right hepatic lobectomy for carcinoma of the gallbladder: a five-year cure. Ann Surg 1961;*153*:563.
16. Burdette WJ: Carcinoma of the gallbladder. Ann Surg 1957;*145*:832
17. Carmo M, Perpetuo MO, Valdivieso M, et al: Natural history study of gallbladder cancer. A review of 36 years' experience at M. D. Anderson Hospital and Tumor Institute. Cancer 1978;*42*:330.
18. Castle WN, Wanebo HJ, Fechner RE: Carcinoma of the gallbladder and cholecystostomy. Arch Surg 1982;*117*:946.
19. Chandler JJ, Fletcher WS: A clinical study of primary carcinoma of the gallbladder. Surg Gynecol Obstet 1963;*117*:297.
20. Crade M, Taylor KJW, Rosenfield AT, Ulreich S, Simeone J, Sommer G, Viscomi GN: The varied ultrasonic character of gallbladder tumor. JAMA 1979;*241*:2195.
21. Davis HL, Ramirez G, Ansfield FJ: Adenocarcinomas of the stomach, pancreas, liver and biliary tracts. Cancer 1974;*33*:193.
22. Del Regato JA, Spjut HJ: Cancer; Diagnosis, Treatment, and Prognosis. 5th ed. St. Louis, CV Mosby, 1977.
23. Diehl AK: Gallstone size and the risk of gallbladder cancer. JAMA 1983;*250*:2323.
24. Donaldson LA, Busuttil A: A clinicopathological review of 68 carcinomas of the gallbladder. Br J Surg 1975;*62*:26.
25. Fahim RB, McDonald JR, Richards JC, et al: Carcinoma of the gallbladder. Ann Surg 1962;*156*:114.
26. Foster JH, Berman MM: Solid Liver Tumors. Philadelphia, WB Saunders, 1977.
27. Frank SA, Spjut HJ: Inapparent carcinoma of the gallbladder. Am Surg 1967;*33*:367.
28. Friedman RB, Anderson RE, Gilchrist KW, Carbone PP: Prognostic factors in invasive gallbladder carcinoma. J Surg Oncol 1983;*23*:189.
29. Gerst PH: Primary carcinoma of the gallbladder. A thirty-year summary. Ann Surg 1961;*153*:369.
30. Glenn F, Hayes DM: The scope of radical surgery in the treatment of malignant tumors of the extrahepatic biliary tract. Surg Gynecol Obstet 1954; *99*:529.
31. Gothlin J, Pettersson H: Angiography in malignant and chronic inflammatory lesions of the gallbladder. Acta Radiol (Diagn) 1976;*17*:343.
32. Gradisar IA, Kelly TR: Primary carcinoma of the gallbladder. Arch Surg 1970;*100*:232.
33. Graham EA: The prevention of carcinoma of the gallbladder. Ann Surg 1931;*93*:317.
34. Gupta S, Udupa KN, Gupta S: Primary carcinoma of the gallbladder: A review of 328 cases. J Surg Oncol 1980;*14*:35.
35. Hamrick RE, Liner FJ, Hastings PR, Cohn I Jr: Primary carcinoma of the gallbladder. Ann Surg 1982;*195*:270.
36. Hanna SS, Rider WD: Carcinoma of the gallbladder or extrahepatic bile ducts: the role of radiotherapy. Can Med Assoc J 1978;*118*:59.
37. Hardy MA, Volk H: Primary carcinoma of the gallbladder. Am J Surg 1970;*120*:800.
38. Hart J, Modan B: Factors affecting survival of patients with gallbladder neoplasms. Arch Intern Med 1972;*129*:931.
39. Holmes SL, Mark JBD: Carcinoma of the gallbladder. Surg Gynecol Obstet 1971;*133*:561.
40. Homans J: A Textbook of Surgery. Springfield, IL, CC Thomas, 1931, p 891.
41. Irving AD: Carcinoma of the gall-bladder in a patient on long-term chenodeoxycholic acid therapy. Clin Oncol 1981;*7*:245.
42. Itai Y, Araki T, Yoshikawa K, Furui S, Yakhiro N, Tasaka A: Computed tomography of gallbladder carcinoma. Radiology 1980;*137*:713.
43. Iwasaki Y, Ohto M, Todoroki T, et al: Treatment of carcinoma of the biliary system. Surg Gynecol Obstet 1977;*144*:219.
44. Keen WW: Report of a case of resection of the liver for the removal of a neoplasm with a table of seventy-six cases of resection of the liver for hepatic tumors. Ann Surg 1899;*30*:267.
45. Kelly TR, Chamberlain TR: Carcinoma of the gallbladder. Am J Surg 1982;*143*:737.
46. Klamer TW, Max MH: Carcinoma of the gallbladder. Surg Gynecol Obstet 1983;*156*:641.
47. Koo J, Wong J, Cheng FC, et al: Carcinoma of the gallbladder. Br J Surg 1981;*68*:161.
48. Kopelson G, Gunderson LL: Primary and adjuvant radiation therapy in gallbladder and extrahepatic biliary tract carcinoma. J Clin Gastroenterol 1983;*5*:43.
49. Kott I, Urca I: Carcinoma in situ of the gallbladder. Med Chir Dig 1974;*3*:181.
50. Kozuka S, Tsubone M, Yasui I, Hachisuka K: Relation of adenoma to carcinoma of the gallbladder. Cancer 1982;*50*:2226.

51. Krain LS: Gallbladder and extrahepatic bile duct carcinoma. Geriatrics 1972;*27*:111.
52. Laitio M: Histogenesis of epithelial neoplasms of human gallbladder I. Dysplasia. Pathol Res Pract 1983;*178*:51.
53. Laitio M: Histogenesis of epithelial neoplasms of human gallbladder II. Classification of carcinoma on the basis of morphological features. Pathol Res Pract 1983;*178*:57.
54. Lowenfels AB: Gallstones and the risk of cancer. Gut 1980;*21*:1090.
55. Lund J: Surgical indications in cholelithiasis: prophylactic cholecystectomy elucidated on the basis of long-term follow-up on 526 nonoperated cases. Ann Surg 1960;*151*:153.
56. Moertel CG: The gallbladder. In Holland JF, Frei E (eds): Cancer Medicine. Philadelphia, Lea & Febiger, 1973.
57. Moossa AR, Anagnost M, Hall AW, et al: The continuing challenge of gallbladder cancer. Am J Surg 1975;*130*:57.
58. Musher DR, Madayag MA, Tobias H: Carcinoma of the gallbladder: a diagnosis aided by endoscopic retrograde and percutaneous hepatic cholangiography. Am J Gastroenterol 1976;*66*:79.
59. Nagashima HJ, Watanabe AW, Hayashi S, Takei N, Sakatra T, Takata S, Mano K: Primary carcinoma of the gallbladder and the extrahepatic bile duct. Gastroenterol Jpn 1982;*17*:245.
60. Nevin JE, Moran TJ, Kay S, et al: Carcinoma of the gallbladder. Cancer 1976;*37*:141.
61. Ogoshi K, Niwa M: The diagnostic evaluation of ERCP in pancreatic and biliary carcinoma. Gastroenterol Jpn 1977;*12*:218.
62. Ohlsson EG, Aronsen KF: Carcinoma of the gallbladder. Acta Chir Scand 1974;*140*:475.
63. Oswalt CE, Cruz AB Jr: Effectiveness of chemotherapy in addition to surgery in treating carcinoma of the gallbladder. Rev Surg 1977;*34*:436.
64. Pack GT, Brasfield RD: Right hepatic lobectomy for cancer of the gallbladder. *In* Pack GI, Ariel IM (eds): Treatment of Cancer and Allied Diseases. 2nd ed. New York, Paul B. Hoeber, 1962.
65. Pack GT, Miller TR, Brasfield RD: Total right hepatic lobectomy for cancer of the gallbladder: report of three cases. Ann Surg 1955;*142*:6.
66. Peison B, Rabin L: Malignant melanoma of the gallbladder. Cancer 1976;*37*:2448.
67. Pemberton LB, Diffenbaugh WF, Strohl EL: The surgical significance of carcinoma of the gallbladder. Am J Surg 1971;*122*:381.
68. Piehler JM, Crichlow RW: Primary carcinoma of the gallbladder. Arch Surg 1977;*122*:26.
69. Piehler JM, Crichlow RW: Primary carcinoma of the gallbladder. Surg Gynecol Obstet 1978;*147*:929.
70. Polk HC: Carcinoma and the calcified gallbladder. Gastroenterology 1966;*50*:582.
71. Putz P, Willems G: Proliferative changes in the epithelium of the human lithiasic gallbladder. J Natl Cancer Inst 1978;*60*:283.
72. Ram MD: Carcinoma of the gallbladder. Surg Gynecol Obstet 1971;*132*:1044.
73. Richard PF, Cantin J: Primary carcinoma of the gallbladder. Study of 108 cases. Can J Surg 1976;*19*:27.
74. Rios-Dalenz J, Takabayashi A, Henson DE, Strom BL, Soloway RD: The epidemiology of cancer of the extra-hepatic biliary tract in Bolivia. Int J Epidemiol 1983;*12*:156.
75. Ross FP, Hickok DF: Hernia and gallbladder surgery in patients over seventy. N Engl J Med 1960;*262*:501.
76. Sato T, Koyama K, Yamauchi H, Matsuno S: Early carcinoma of the gallbladder. Gastroenterol Jpn 1981;*16*:459.
77. Sheinfeld W: Cholecystectomy and partial hepatectomy for carcinoma of the gallbladder with local liver extension. Surgery 1947;*22*:48.
78. Smoron GL: Radiation therapy of carcinoma of the gallbladder and biliary tract. Cancer 1977;*40*:1422.
79. Solan MJ, Jackson BT: Carcinoma of the gallbladder. Br J Surg 1971;*58*:593.
80. Strauch GO: Primary carcinoma of the gallbladder. Surgery 1960;*47*:368.
81. Tashiro S, Konno T, Mochinaga M, Nakakuma K, Murath E, Yokoyama I: Treatment of gallbladder carcinoma in Japan. Jpn J Surg 1982;*12*:98.
82. Thorbjarnarson B, Glenn F: Carcinoma of the gallbladder. Cancer 1959;*12*:1009.
83. Todoroki T, Iwasaki Y, Okamura T, et al: Intraoperative radiotherapy for advanced carcinoma of the biliary system. Cancer 1980;*46*:2179.
84. Tragerman LJ: Primary carcinoma of the gallbladder. Review of 173 cases. Calif Med 1953;*78*:431.
85. Trajber HJ, Szego T, de Camargo HSA Jr, Mester M, Marujo WC, Roll S: Adenocarcinoma of the gallbladder in two siblings. Cancer 1982;*50*:1200.
86. Treadwell TA, Hardin WJ: Primary carcinoma of the gallbladder: the role of adjunctive therapy in its treatment. Am J Surg 1976;*132*:703.
87. Vaittinen E: Carcinoma of the gallbladder. A study of 390 cases diagnosed in Finland 1953–1967. Ann Chir Gynaecol (Suppl) 1970;*168*:7,
88. Wanebo HJ, Castle WN, Fechner RE: Is carcinoma of the gallbladder a curable lesion? Ann Surg 1982;*195*:270.
89. Watkins E Jr, Khazei AM, Nahra KS: Surgical basis for arterial infusion chemotherapy of disseminated carcinoma of the liver. Surg Gynecol Obstet 1970;*130*:581.
90. Weiskopf J, Esselstyn CB: Carcinoma of the gallbladder. A twenty-six year review. Am J Gastroenterol 1976;*65*:522.
91. Weiss KM, Hanis CL: All "silent" gallstones are not silent. N Engl J Med 1984;*310*:657.
92. Welton JC, Marr JS, Friedman SM: Clues concerning the etiology of carcinoma of the gallbladder. Lancet 1979;*1*:791.
93. Willis RA: Pathology of Tumours. 4th ed. Chapter 25. London, Butterworths, 1967.
94. Yum HY, Fink AH: Sonographic findings in primary carcinoma of the gallbladder. Radiology 1980;*134*:693.
95. Kowalewski K, Todd EF: Carcinoma of the gallbladder induced in hamsters by insertion of cholesterol pellets and feeding dimethylnitrosamine (35293). Proc Soc Exp Biol Med 1971;*136*:482.
96. Perpetuo MD, Valdivieso M, Heilbrun LK, Nelson RS, Connor T, Bodey JP: Natural history study of gallbladder cancer: a review of 36-year experience at M.D. Anderson Hospital and Tumor Institute. Cancer 1978;*42*:330.

MAURICE MERCARDIER, M.D.

32

Carcinoma of the Bile Duct: Surgical Therapy

Carcinoma of the bile duct is relatively rare, but it is of special interest in view of its insidious onset, the difficulty of making the diagnosis early enough for successful treatment, and the technical problems in removing it. The tumors discussed in this chapter involve those of the extrahepatic biliary system, i.e., the segment extending from the distal centimeter of the hepatic lobar ducts to the ampulla of Vater. This includes carcinomas of the bifurcation of the common hepatic duct and carcinomas of the common bile duct. Tumors of the intrahepatic ducts are discussed in Chapter 28 and tumors of the ampulla of Vater in Chapter 34.

The first case of carcinoma of the common bile duct was reported by Fardel in 1840, according to Renshaw.[1] Braasch et al. in 1967 reported a series of 146 cases of carcinoma of the extrahepatic bile ducts, including 57 cases of carcinoma of the hepatic ducts, 27 cases of carcinoma of the midportion of the common bile duct, and 62 cases of carcinoma of the distal segment.[2] Longmire et al. in 1973 reported a series of 63 cases, including 34 of carcinoma of the upper third of the extrahepatic bile ducts, 13 of carcinoma of the middle third, and 16 of carcinoma of the distal segment (Table 32–1).[3] Our experience currently amounts to 32 cases of carcinoma of the common hepatic duct, 12 cases of proximal carcinoma of the common bile duct, and 22 cases of distal carcinoma of the common bile duct.

Table 32–1 LOCATION OF CARCINOMA OF THE MAIN BILE DUCT

Location	Author			
	Braasch[2]	*Longmire*[3]	*Mercadier*[11]	*Sako*[14]
Common hepatic duct	57	34	32	297
Common bile duct				203
Proximal	27	13	12	
Distal	62	15	22	

Predisposing factors, if they exist, are little known.[4–7] The coexistence of carcinoma and cholelithiasis is not rare,[4] but it appears likely that stones most often form as a result of stasis proximal to the lesion. It is unlikely that they precede or have an etiologic relationship to the tumor. By contrast, a malignancy may develop in a papilloma or in the presence of papillomatosis of the common duct. Braasch et al. have reported a number of cases strongly supporting such a hypothesis.[2]

Tumor is seen more frequently during the third to the seventh decade of life, with the highest frequency being between the fifth and seventh decades. Gender does not appear to play an etiologic role even though carcinoma of the common bile duct is slightly more common in men than in women in a proportion of 3 to 2.

PATHOLOGY AND HISTOLOGY[5, 6]

Carcinoma of the common bile duct may be of three types: (1) nodular scirrhous tumor, the most common; (2) infiltrating scirrhous tumor, uncommon; and (3) papillary tumor, extremely rare. The first two types cause progressive biliary obstruction, with proximal dilatation. The papillary form generally presents as partial biliary obstruction complicated by cholangitis. From a histologic standpoint, the lesion usually has the appearance of an adenocarcinoma or anaplastic carcinoma and, more rarely, of a papillary tumor.[8, 9] Mucinous and scirrhous forms are variants of adenocarcinoma. Squamous, carcinoid, and sarcomatous tumors are rare.[10]

The method of spread of the tumor is of considerable practical importance. The tumors extend through the submucosa both proximally and distally and in depth from the center to the periphery. There may be multifocal patches of tumor or a continuous layer associated with marked fibroblastic proliferation that resembles sclerosing cholangitis. In addition to spread along the duct, the tumor may directly invade adjacent tissues. For distal carcinomas, this means that the pancreas may be invaded, and in such cases the histologic distinction between clear cell biliary carcinoma and carcinoma of the pancreatic excretory ducts may be difficult.[11] Vascular invasion (i.e., along the axis of the portal vein and the hepatic artery) is rare, but when it occurs, a curative excision is not possible.

Distant spread occurs through veins and lymphatics. Invasion of the regional venules and perinervous lymph channels is common. Perineural invasion explains the frequency and severity of pain. In order of decreasing frequency the involved lymph nodes are retropancreatic and hepatic nodes, subpyloric nodes, and preaortic nodes. The nodes of the superior mesenteric group are rarely invaded, but when they are, excision is impossible. Lymph nodes are involved in about 50 per cent of cases, more commonly when the primary lesion is larger.[12–16] Even though it may appear to be localized, carcinoma of the bile duct diffuses readily, although visceral metastases are rare and late. This explains why wide excision is required if there is to be any hope for cure or prolonged survival.

Slow and progressive obstruction of the bile duct occurs in the stenosing nodular scirrhous form. This results in complete biliary obstruction, which produces distention of the entire biliary tree proximally. The end result is fibrosis of the portal spaces and then biliary cirrhosis, which may be complicated by portal hypertension with all its consequences—hepatomegaly, splenomegaly, ascites, and esophageal varices. Incomplete obstruction is seen in the diffuse scirrhous form and the papillary form. This causes partial biliary obstruction and infection, with resulting cholangitis, which may finally result in septicemia and hepatic abscess formation. The cause of death is, in fact, more often related to infection or to severe hepatic insufficiency than to progression of the carcinoma.[12]

CLINICAL CHARACTERISTICS

Carcinoma of the bile duct develops late in life, often after age 50 or 60. The patient presents with obstructive jaundice, which most often is typical of neoplastic disease, although it sometimes resembles that due to choledocholithiasis. The true onset of the disorder occurs far earlier than its first clinical manifestations.[15] The earliest symptoms attract little attention, but they may be elucidated by a careful history: dull vague pain in the upper part of the abdomen or the dorsolumbar region, transient subicteric episodes, unexplained fatigue and weight loss, poor appetite (in particular for meat and fats), nausea, diarrhea, and so forth.

In most cases, the jaundice is typical of that caused by neoplasms. It develops progressively, and its course is inexorable. It is accompanied by neither pain nor fever but is associated with pruritus, which may be severe, leading to an inability to sleep and rest and the production of skin lesions from scratching. The patient loses his appetite, complains of nausea, and loses weight. On examination, the liver is generally enlarged, smooth, firm, and nontender, while the gallbladder may be distended (in the absence of associated fibrosis) when the tumors are located below the junction of the common bile duct and the cystic duct. These two findings are indicative of cholestasis. The diagnosis of neoplastic jaundice may be easily made at this stage, but the differential diagnosis includes carcinoma of the common bile duct, carcinoma of the head of the pancreas, chronic fibrosing pancreatitis affecting the head of the pancreas, a stone impacted in the common bile duct, and even a penetrating posterior duodenal ulcer. It is now rare to see patients at such a late stage, when biliary cirrhosis has developed and produced manifestations of portal hypertension—hepatomegaly, splenomegaly, ascites, or esophageal varices with gastrointestinal hemorrhage.

The clinical presentation of carcinoma of the bile duct may resemble gallstone obstruction when it includes moderate jaundice, preceded by pain in the right upper quadrant, and accompanied by fever and chills. The liver may be of normal size and the gallbladder not distended. These are the manifestations of incomplete obstruction of the common bile duct complicated by stasis and infection. They are most often seen in patients with papillary neoplasms, which may shed vegetations down the bile duct, or of the diffuse infiltrating form, which makes the duct a rigid tube, hampering the easy flow of bile.

LABORATORY INVESTIGATIONS

The laboratory findings reflect the degree of biliary obstruction and infection. Increased bilirubin and alkaline phosphatase levels are common, while levels of transaminases, albumin, and globulin are close to normal. This pattern reflects the absence of liver cell damage, a rare complication at the time of initial diagnosis.

Increased levels of alpha-2 globulins are common. When the tumor obstructs only a portion of the biliary tract (i.e., predominantly the left or the right duct), a dissociation between a markedly increased alkaline phophatase value and a slight increase in bilirubin occurs. When the carcinoma is relatively advanced, the hematocrit may be less than 40 per cent, the leukocyte count is often increased, and the prothrombin level may be less than 80 per cent.

SPECIAL INVESTIGATIONS

Special investigations should contribute to the diagnosis of carcinoma of the common bile duct if they are well selected and carefully studied.

Ultrasonography and CT scanning are helpful in determining the approximate level of obstruction.[17, 18] They frequently show dilated intrahepatic ducts. The extrahepatic biliary tract and the gallbladder may be dilated in low common bile duct lesions. Ultrasonography is useful in ruling out other causes of biliary obstruction (i.e., gallstones), and CT scan may show lymph node or liver metastasis in late stages.

Transhepatic (THC) and retrograde endoscopic cholangiography (ERCP) are the most useful tests, and one of them should be performed in every patient suspected of having a bile duct neoplasm. Transhepatic cholangiography is best able to demonstrate the ductal system on the hepatic side of the obstruction, which is important for determining the feasibility of resection and selecting the best procedure. In addition, some form of percutaneous biliary drainage may be left in place following THC. With a catheter in place, brush cytology and even biopsy of high lesions can be performed.[19]

Retrograde cholangiography may be slightly safer than THC.[20] It defines the inferior limits of the lesion, and although the duct on the hepatic side can usually be opacified, the anatomy in this area is not as well defined as by THC. Retrograde cholangiography has the additional virtue, however, of providing information about the duodenum and the ampulla of Vater. In general, the choice between THC and ERCP is based on the level of the lesion as estimated by ultrasound or CT scans. The more proximal lesions are best studied by THC and the more distal ones (those closer to the duodenum) by ERCP. For further details in the diagnostic work-up of this lesion, refer to Chapters 10 and 13.

Arteriography is a very helpful examination. Studies of the arterial and venous phases reveal any spread of tumor along the vascular axes and give a precise picture of the vascularization of the entire operative region. Obstruction of the portal vein and obvious encasement of the hepatic artery are usually considered signs of unresectability.[21, 22]

Upper gastrointestinal series, which is invariably performed in patients with obstructive jaundice or cholangitis, may show deformation of the medial wall of the second part of the duodenum when a carcinoma of the common bile duct has invaded the pancreas and duodenum.[2, 13]

Duodenal intubation for obtaining bile samples after the stimulation of biliary secretion is not commonly used. Some authors feel that it helps by providing samples for cytologic studies. This test may be useful when a trained cytologist is available for interpretation of the samples.

SURGICAL THERAPY

Operative Diagnosis

The special investigations mentioned earlier are not always essential, since surgery is frequently indicated when the clinical picture is typical of complete or incomplete obstruction of the common bile duct.[23, 24] However, using the methods available today, the precise cause of the obstruction is often identified before the operation.[21–24]

Surgical exploration reveals distention of the gallbladder and hepatic ducts in lower lesions. The tumor is sometimes situated in the hepatic pedicle and takes the form of a swelling of variable size. Sometimes it is found in the distal segment of the common bile duct and then takes the form of a mass difficult to distinguish from a pancreatic lesion.

Cholangiographic studies are required when such lesions are found and preoperative cholangiography has not been performed. The contrast medium is injected by direct puncture of the distended gallbladder or dilated common hepatic duct. Its progression is followed under fluoroscopic control, preferably with image intensification, x-ray films being taken as required. The study will show distention of the biliary system proximal to an obstruction. Common duct cancer appears as a straight or curved block, regular or irregular, which resembles that seen in carcinoma of the pancreas but located higher along the course of the bile duct. With partial obstruction, the contrast medium defines a long narrow area similar to that seen in chronic pancreatitis or fibrosing cholangitis, although the borders of the neoplastic lesions are notched and irregular, a fine difference that is often overlooked.

A definitive diagnosis may be made only by frozen-section histologic examination. While the presence of hepatic or lymph node metastases indicates a malignant tumor, only examination of the lesion itself confirms its biliary origin. For this purpose, it is possible to perform lavage of the bile duct in the region of the tumor and look for neoplastic cells on immediate examination, to collect a sample by swabbing the tumor itself, or to perform an immediate examination of a fragment of tumor. The best method is to obtain a small slice or core needle biopsy specimen involving the full thickness of the duct wall.

Once the diagnosis has been established, a choice of the appropriate operation must be made in view of the patient's general health, the presence or absence of lymph node or hepatic metastases, the local spread of the lesion, and above all, the site of the lesion.

Operative Techniques

The indications for wide excision procedures, aimed at obtaining a cure, have increased through the years. Excision should be attempted in all reasonably fit patients when the tumor is limited, when it does not extend to the vascular elements of the hepatic pedicle, and when it is not accompanied by metastases.[28] Resection is the only curative treatment and offers the best form of palliation for those in whom cure is not possible. The approach differs for tumors of the hilus (Klatskin tumors), tumors of the suprapancreatic segment of the bile duct, and tumors involving the distal segment of the common bile duct.[23–25]

Tumors of the common hepatic duct or the bifurcation of the right and left lobar ducts are not immediately evident upon examination of the extrahepatic bile ducts. Exposure of the tumor, to assess its resectability, is gained by opening the peritoneum overlying the hepatic duct just as it meets the capsule of Glisson. In fact, dissection of the anterior aspect of the bifurcation of the hepatic ducts can be best achieved by entering the capsule of Glisson and carefully separating the parenchyma of the liver from the anterior surface of the ducts. The next step involves surrounding the right and left hepatic ducts individually. Care must be taken not to injure the branches of the portal vein or the hepatic artery that are immediately behind and closely attached to these ducts. Dissection should then proceed following the anterior aspect of the right and left lobar duct walls as far as is needed to encompass the tumor or as far proximally as is possible. Once the hepatic duct bifurcation has been exposed and both right and left ducts have been isolated, a decision must be made as to whether to proceed with the resection. If it appears that the ducts can be divided proximal to the tumor, and if the hepatic ducts have been successfully mobilized and isolated from the adjacent vascular structures, the tumor is resectable. At this point, it is preferable to look for the distal end of the tumor, dissect the bile duct below it, and divide it. The distal end of the duct is then closed, and a clamp is applied to the proximal end just below the tumor. With the proximal end of the divided duct used as a handle, the dissection can proceed upward, separating the posterior aspect of the hepatic duct and the tumor from the portal vein and the right hepatic artery. The dissection is carried upward as far as possible or until normal ducts above the tumor have been found and the biliary duct transected.

At this time, transhepatic catheters are

placed through the right and left ducts (or its branches) as described in Chapter 33. These catheters are useful to orient the reconstruction, to stent the anastomosis, and to study the cholangiojejunostomy in the immediate postoperative period. They are well tolerated by the patient and can be used to thread radioactive iridium wires to provide radiation therapy to the tumor bed later in the postoperative course.[26–28]

If the transection has been done on the hepatic duct bifurcation or in the right and left ducts near the bifurcation, the biliary tract can be reconstructed using a Roux-en-Y cholangiojejunostomy. When the transection of the biliary duct is more proximal, involving secondary branches of the left and the right ducts, one must bring a Roux-en-Y loop to the hilus of the liver and anastomose it, using the anterior aspect of the portal vein as the posterior wall of the anastomosis and Glisson's capsule as the anterior wall.

Tumors of the supraduodenal segment of the common bile duct should be removed by wide resection, which involves transecting the common hepatic duct just below the junction of the left and right hepatic ducts and the common bile duct as low as possible, i.e., in the pancreatic segment. The gallbladder is also removed. The operation is completed either by re-establishment of biliary continuity or by a biliointestinal anastomosis, preferably the latter. In the first case, in view of the wide distance separating the common hepatic duct from the common bile duct, it is useful to free and widely mobilize the duodenopancreatic unit in order to reduce anastomotic tension. A T-tube is placed to support the anastomosis and to drain bile. In the second case, an intestinal anastomosis between the hepatic duct and a jejunal loop brought up either as a Y or inverted U avoids anastomotic tension. We prefer an end-to-side anastomosis suspending the jejunal loop from Glisson's capsule. Hepaticoduodenostomy may be attempted, but in addition to the risk of tension at the anastomosis, it is associated with the reflux of duodenal contents into the dilated biliary tree.

Tumors of the distal segment of the common bile duct require a duodenopancreatectomy (Whipple procedure). This operation allows not only for a wide excision of the lesion but also for a satisfactory lymph node dissection. The bile duct is divided at the level of the common hepatic duct in order to be at a distance from the tumor, which necessitates excision of the gallbladder. The lower two thirds of the stomach are also resected, and a truncal vagotomy is performed to avoid subsequent development of a peptic ulcer. The entire duodenum and all of the right part of the pancreas (i.e., the head and isthmus) are removed. Re-establishment of intestinal continuity involves three anastomoses to the jejunum: (1) end-to-end pancreaticojejunostomy, (2) end-to-side hepaticojejunostomy, and (3) end-to-side gastrojejunostomy, about 40 cm from the hepaticojejunostomy.

Therefore, this is a wide, satisfactory cancer operation. It has worked so well that although we initially reserved it for tumors of the distal common duct, we now use it also for lesions of the supraduodenal segment and, more generally, for infiltrating neoplasms in this area regardless of their origin. This is because of the difficulty of determining the exact limits of tumor extension in most cases.

Pancreaticoduodenectomy may be performed in patients in poor general condition with marked jaundice if the patient is prepared appropriately. For example, in some cases it may be wise to drain the biliary tract percutaneously before proceeding with the operation to allow the jaundice to clear and adequate liver function to be restored. The general condition of the patient can also be improved by hyperalimentation during this time.

When a bile duct tumor is unresectable, there are several alternatives that can be considered. Tumors of the bifurcation or lobar ducts that are not resectable may be treated by percutaneous drainage or endoprosthesis (see Chapters 10 and 33). For all other lesions, biliointestinal bypass procedures offer a better palliation than does percutaneous drainage or endoprosthesis. Depending on the location of the tumor, either the gallbladder or the common hepatic duct can be used.

Whenever it is technically feasible, *hepaticojejunostomy* should be performed, as it is the best method of internal biliary bypass. Hepaticojejunostomy is the ideal palliative procedure for low-lying tumors, since the anastomosis is situated a distance from the tumor when the latter is located above or behind the pancreas. It is performed using a jejunal loop brought up as a U or Y. It may be carried out in a side-to-side fashion, retaining the gallbladder, or it may be performed in an end-to-side fashion after transecting the common hepatic duct below the junction of the left and right hepatic ducts with removal of the gallbladder. The distal segment of the common bile duct is sutured in such cases. Although this is the best of the palliative techniques, it is relatively complicated. Therefore, it should be reserved for lesions that are impossible to excise or that are complicated by metastases, whenever the patient's general condition permits a relatively long surgical procedure.

Cholecystoduodenostomy establishes a connection between the base of the gallbladder and the second part of the duodenum, its principal merit being its simplicity. Cholecystojejunostomy to a loop or Roux-en-Y limb of jejunum is more complex but more satisfactory, since it avoids reflux of digestive contents into the gallbladder. Use of the gallbladder, however, is justified only when patency of the cystic duct is not threatened by extension of the tumor. Thus, it is used only when dealing with lesions of the retropancreatic segment of the common bile duct.

We have performed *external bypass of bile* in the past, but we now feel it is contraindicated. It ensures regression of jaundice and the lessening of infection but is associated with the risk of metabolic complications as a result of fluid and electrolyte depletion.

Transtumoral intubation by a T-tube of small caliber, though relatively rigid, does not have the same dangers, since biliary loss is avoided as soon as the long horizontal branch of the tube is clamped. The tube may be inserted at the site of the tumor or above it. The vertical branch must re-establish flow of bile from the dilated ducts into the duodenum, passing through the tumor. It is possible to insert such a drain when obstruction is incomplete, i.e., when the carcinoma is of the diffuse scirrhous or papillary type, but this is more difficult when obstruction is complete, when the lesion is of a nodular type. In the latter case the tumor is difficult to dilate and the tube may be introduced only by force, which is hazardous.

PROGNOSIS

Carcinoma of the bile duct is rapidly fatal in the absence of surgical treatment. The mean survival scarcely exceeds 3 to 6 months. Thus, surgery should be used in all fit patients who appear to have resectable lesions, with the aid, if necessary, of short but intensive preoperative preparation. It is, in fact, almost always possible to perform at least a palliative operation in tumors that arise below the common hepatic duct. This ensures bypass of bile into the digestive tract and regression of jaundice, disappearance of pruritus, and improvement in the patient's condition. Survival averages 6 to 9 months, but the palliation is real. In certain cases, usually in patients with nodular infiltrating scirrhous tumor, palliation may last for 3 years or more.

A better prognosis follows excision, especially duodenopancreatectomy. Longmire reported that out of 11 patients with tumors of the distal segment, 10 survived for more than 1 year, and five of the nine patients treated by pancreaticoduodenectomy were living 1 to 15 years after surgery. Among 13 cases of carcinoma of the mid-duct, only four were suitable for segmental resection, the other nine being inoperable because of involvement of the hepatic artery or portal vein. The survival here was, respectively, of 1, 4, 5, and 11 years.[3] Warren's experience confirmed the value of pancreaticoduodenectomy: 36 per cent of 26 patients who had distal lesions were alive 5 years postoperatively.[16]

REFERENCES

1. Renshaw K: Malignant neoplasm of extra-hepatic biliary ducts. Ann Surg 1922;*76:*205.
2. Braasch JW, Warren KW, Kune CA: Malignant neoplasms of the bile ducts. Surg Clin North Am 1967;*47:*627.
3. Longmire WP, McArthur MS, Bastounis EA, et al: Carcinoma of the extra-hepatic biliary tract. Ann Surg 1973;*178:*333.
4. Chen PH, Lo HW, Wang CS, et al: Cholangiocarcinoma in hepatolithiasis. J Clin Gastroenterol 1984;*6:*539.
5. Kozuka S, Tsubone M, Hachisuka K: Evolution of carcinoma in the extrahepatic bile ducts. Cancer 1984;*54:*65.
6. Qualman SJ, Haupt HM, Bauer TW, et al: Adenocarcinoma of the hepatic duct junction. A reappraisal of the histologic criteria of malignancy. Cancer 1984;*53:*1545.
7. Juttijudata P, Prichanond S, Churnratanakul S, et al: Hilar intrahepatic cholangiocarcinoma and its etiology. J Clin Gastroenterol 1984;*6:*503.
8. Brown BB: Primary carcinoma of the extra hepatic bile duct. Br J Surg 1960;*49:*22.
9. Hepp J, Mercadier M, Balansa [no init]: Les cancers des voies biliaires extra-hepatiques. Arch Mal App Dig 1954;*43:*1041.
10. Horn RC, Yakovac WC, Kaye R, et al: Rhabdomyosarcoma of the common bile duct: report of a case. Cancer 1955;*8:*469.
11. Mercadier M, Clot JP, Grillot C: Les cancers du choledoque retropancreatique. Ann Chir 1968; *22:*1255.

12. Altemeier WA, Gall EA, Zinninger MM, et al: Sclerosing carcinoma of the major intra-hepatic bile ducts. Arch Surg 1957;*75*:450.
13. Goldenberg IS: Carcinoma of the biliary tract. Am J Surg 1953;*86*:292.
14. Sako S, Seitzinger GL, Garside E: Carcinoma of the extra-hepatic bile ducts. Review of the literature and report of six cases. Surgery 1957;*41*:416.
15. Wanebo HJ, Grimes OF: Cancer of the bile duct. The occult malignancy. Am J Surg 1975;*130*:262.
16. Warren KW, Mountain JC, Lloyd-Jones W: Malignant tumors of the bile ducts. Br J Surg 1972; *59*:501.
17. Thorsen MK, Quiroz F, Lawson TL, et al: Primary biliary carcinoma: CT evaluation. Radiology 1984; *152*:479.
18. Subramanyam BR, Raghavendra BN, Balthazar EJ, et al: Ultrasonic features of cholangiocarcinoma. J Ultrasound Med 1984;*3*:405
19. Evander A, Ihse I, Lunderquist A, et al: Percutaneous cytodiagnosis of carcinoma of the pancreas and bile duct. Ann Surg 1978;*188*:90.
20. Carrasco CH, Zornoza J, Bechtel WJ: Malignant biliary obstruction: Complications of percutaneous biliary drainage. Radiology 1984;*152*:343.
21. Voyles CR, Bowley NJ, Allison DJ, et al: Carcinoma of the proximal extrahepatic biliary tree: radiologic assessment and therapeutic alternatives. Ann Surg 1983;*197*:188.
22. Chitwood WR, Meyers WC, Heaston DK, et al: Diagnosis and treatment of primary extrahepatic bile duct tumors. Am J Surg 1982;*143*:99.
23. Launois B, Campion JP, Brissot P, et al: Carcinoma of the hepatic hilus. Surgical management and the case for resection. Ann Surg 1979;*190*:151.
24. Ottow RT, August DA, Sugarbaker PH: Treatment of proximal biliary tract carcinoma: An overview of techniques and results. Surgery 1985;*97*:251.
25. Lamy J, Michotey C, Bricot R, et al: Tumeurs malignes de la voie biliaire principale. Ann Chir 1965;*19*:1035.
26. Fletcher MS, Brinkley D, Dawson JL, et al: Treatment of hilar carcinoma by bile drainage combined with internal radiotherapy using ^{192}iridium wire. Br J Surg 1983;*70*:733.
27. Mornex F, Ardiet JM, Bret P, et al: Radiotherapy of high bile duct carcinoma using intracatheter iridium 192 wire. Cancer 1984;*54*:2069.
28. Rossi RL, Heiss FW, Beckmann CF, Braasch JW: Management of cancer of the bile duct. Surg Clin North Am 1985;*65*:59.

J. TERBLANCHE, Ch.M., F.R.C.S.

33

*Tumors of the Hepatic Duct Bifurcation: Stent Therapy**

The clinical presentation, treatment, and results of therapy of carcinoma arising in different parts of the biliary tree vary considerably. Imprecise definition of the site of lesions, as reported in the literature, makes the true incidence in different regions difficult to determine. To overcome this difficulty, the following classification, which divides the extrahepatic biliary tree into five regions, was suggested:[1] These are (1) carcinoma of the main hepatic duct junction, (2) carcinoma of the common hepatic duct and supraduodenal common bile duct, (3) carcinoma of the intrapancreatic bile duct and ampulla, (4) diffuse carcinoma of the bile duct (involving more than one region), and (5) carcinoma of the gallbladder. Carcinoma localized to the cystic duct alone is very rare but could be considered a sixth region.

Only carcinoma in region 1, carcinoma of the main hepatic duct junction, will be considered in this section. Region 1 lesions include carcinoma of the upper common hepatic duct and the main right and left hepatic ducts at their confluence. Although this portion of the biliary tree is extrahepatic, its close relationship to the portal vein and hepatic artery branches makes treatment of lesions in this region particularly challenging. On the other hand, the high incidence of scirrhous lesions in this region may improve the prognosis because they grow slowly.

Although an analysis of earlier publications on bile duct carcinoma leaves the impression that region 1 lesions are uncommon, recent evidence suggests that they are more common than previously suspected, the diagnosis frequently having been missed in the past, even at operation. Altemeier[2] suggested this possibility in 1957, and it has been confirmed by more recent reports.[1, 3–6]

The results of treatment have been disappointing, although some early reports did indicate that prolonged survival occasionally occurred.[7, 8] Recent papers have emphasized that good palliation can be achieved in many of these patients as long as the diagnosis is made.[1, 6, 9–12]

ETIOLOGY

Gallstones

Although there is a clear relationship between cholelithiasis and carcinoma of the gallbladder (region 5), the evidence for a relationship between cholelithiasis and carcinoma in other regions of the biliary tree is less compelling. Most authorities accept an associated incidence of between 30 and 40 per cent,[2, 13–15] but it is unclear whether this incidence is higher than expected in the general population of the same age and sex distribution.[16]

Most reports do not define in which regions of the biliary tree neoplasms associated with cholelithiasis were situated, but the incidence in reports dealing only with region 1 has been low.[3, 4] None of our 26 reported cases was associated with gallstones.[1, 5] Whether or not there is an etiologic relationship between gallstones, a common condition, and carcinoma of the main hepatic duct junction (region 1), therefore, remains an open question.

Ulcerative Colitis

Although none of our patients had ulcerative colitis, the evidence suggesting a link,

*This work was supported by the South African Medical Research Council and the Staff Research Fund, University of Cape Town. Dr. H. R. Sanders, Chief Medical Superintendent, Groote Schuur Hospital, is thanked for permission to publish patient data.

albeit relatively uncommon, is convincing.[1] It has been suggested that tumors of the extrahepatic bile ducts are approximately ten times more frequent in patients with ulcerative colitis,[17] and many of the reported patients have had lesions in region 1.[17, 18]

Other Tumors

Although reported, a definite association with other tumors[1, 14, 19, 20] and other diseases[60] is yet to be proved.

PATHOLOGY

Carcinoma of the main hepatic duct junction usually presents macroscopically as a small, firm, intramural, scarlike collar or nodule. Histologically these lesions are well-differentiated scirrhous carcinomas with islands of relatively well-differentiated adenocarcinoma (consisting of clusters of acini or ducts) embedded in a dense connective tissue stroma.[3] The lesions tend to be slow-growing and remain localized until late in the course of the disease. Although metastases were previously thought to be relatively uncommon, more are being seen in patients after palliative bypass procedures.[21]

Less commonly, a large, bulky, hard mass is present in the porta hepatis. This is the more common form of adenocarcinoma that contains less stroma. Intraluminal papillary carcinomas occasionally occur in this region. If portions of the lesion break off, they may give rise to symptoms suggestive of choledocholithiasis or may be associated with fluctuating jaundice, which may be confusing.[5]

A report from Japan proposed a classification based on the gross appearance: polypoid, nodular, scirrhous constricting, and diffusely infiltrating. Four (17 per cent) of 23 patients had the polypoid type. Histologically these tumors had a papillary and tubular pattern. All four patients were apparently cured by resection and were alive at 2 1/2 to 5 years.[22]

Poorly differentiated carcinoma localized to region 1 is distinctly rare. Poorly differentiated diffuse carcinoma of the bile duct (region 4) may involve the common hepatic duct junction, but this lesion is not under consideration in this chapter. Both the prognosis and the treatment of the latter lesion are quite different from localized region 1 lesions.

CLINICAL PRESENTATION

Sex and Age

In contradistinction to carcinoma of the gallbladder, which occurs predominantly in women, there is a slight male preponderance in carcinoma of the extrahepatic biliary tree, which also applies to lesions at the main hepatic duct junction.[1, 3–5, 12, 22]

A wide age distribution has been noted, varying from the young to the very old, with the majority of cases occurring in patients in their 50s and 60s. When considering the differential diagnosis of obstructive jaundice, it is important to remember that this lesion may occur in young patients.[1, 2, 5, 15, 19] One of the author's patients was 24 years old at the time of diagnosis.[5] He had a papillary growth with fluctuating jaundice, which in association with his young age was responsible for a delay of almost a year before the correct diagnosis was made.

Symptoms and Signs[3–6, 12]

The patient usually presents with typical extrahepatic biliary obstruction. The presentation is similar to that of lesions localized to region 2, except that the gallbladder may be distended in patients with low growths in region 2 (supraduodenal common bile duct).

Jaundice. The classic presentation is progressive obstructive jaundice with bilirubin levels frequently in excess of 20 mg/dl (> 340 S.I. units). The jaundice is usually of recent onset,[1, 3–5] and it may occasionally fluctuate, which tends to confuse the diagnosis.[16, 23] Fluctuating jaundice may occur in scirrhous lesions and is not confined to the papillary lesions mentioned earlier. An occasional patient presents before the onset of jaundice. In this case the lesion is usually an incidental finding during an investigation performed for other reasons during the phase of partial obstruction.

Pruritus. This is often an early and prominent feature and may even precede the onset of jaundice.[3] It tends to become particularly troublesome in the later stages of the disease if the obstruction is not relieved.

Pain. Pain is usually absent or mild.[3, 5] When present, it is at most a dull right upper quadrant ache. Pain has tended to be featured more prominently in retrospective reviews of extrahepatic bile duct carcinoma and has been uncommon in reviews of lesions localized to the main hepatic duct junction.[3–5] Other than colic associated with dislodgment of part of a papillary growth, absence of pain is a useful diagnostic feature.[5, 21]

Vague Digestive Complaints. These occur fairly frequently and include indigestion, diarrhea, and occasional nausea and vomiting.

Anorexia and Weight Loss. Anorexia and weight loss are prominent features in carcinoma of the main hepatic duct junction and are frequently out of proportion to the duration and level of jaundice.[1, 3–5]

Hepatomegaly. Patients with the typical lesion invariably have a firm, smooth hepatomegaly that is palpable 5 to 10 fingerbreadths below the costal margin by the time of presentation.[3–5] Hepatomegaly has even been noted in patients presenting before the onset of jaundice.[3, 4]

Gallbladder. An enlarged palpable gallbladder does not occur with these high lesions. When the gallbladder is clearly palpable, the lesion is either in region 2 or diffuse (region 4).

Fecal Occult Blood. This has been positive, when tested, in about 50 per cent of patients.

Rigors and Fever. Manifestations of cholangitis are rare unless an invasive procedure has been performed on the biliary tract. The bile is almost invariably sterile on culture before the duct has been subjected to instrumentation.[4]

Natural History

The classic scirrhous lesion is slow-growing and remains localized until late in the course of the disease. Even early reports contained references to patients who had prolonged survival without specific treatment. Death is usually due to liver failure as a result of obstruction of the bile duct and, less commonly in late cases, obstruction of the portal vein, with the associated features of portal hypertension. Now that patients are living longer as a result of palliative procedures, extrahepatic metastases are being observed more frequently.

LABORATORY FINDINGS

Laboratory tests are not particularly helpful in making the diagnosis. The patients typically have the classic findings of extrahepatic biliary obstruction. The bilirubin is frequently in excess of 20 mg/dl (> 340 S.I. units). The alkaline phosphatase value is always raised and often is very high. In the early phase before complete obstruction, it may be the only abnormal biochemical finding. Other alterations in liver function tests occur after obstruction has been present for some time and are not helpful in diagnosis. Immunologic tests (mitochondrial antibody titers) are useful in ruling out primary biliary cirrhosis.

Radiology

As would be expected, upper gastrointestinal contrast studies are rarely abnormal in carcinoma of the main hepatic duct junction, in contradistinction to carcinoma of the ampulla or the pancreas, in which these investigations may be useful.

Conventional oral cholecystograms and intravenous cholangiograms are contraindicated in these markedly jaundiced patients.[1]

Since the advent of ultrasound and CT scanning, misdiagnosis has become rare.[6] Dilated intrahepatic ducts in the absence of dilated extrahepatic ducts are a definitive indication for direct cholangiography.

The vitally important diagnostic aids are preoperative percutaneous transhepatic cholangiography (PTC) and endoscopic retrograde cholangiopancreatography (ERCP). I believe that it is better for the surgeon to see the top of the lesion, rather than the bottom, on the x-ray, as the lower extent can easily be delineated at operation. Therefore, PTC is favored over ERCP when investigating patients with obstructive jaundice suspected to be secondary to a hepatic duct carcinoma. In some cases both investigations are indicated. ERCP may be of use in the diagnosis of carcinoma of the pancreas.[24]

Reports over the past 15 years have emphasized that in most cases it is possible to make a firm diagnosis of this lesion preoperatively using PTC.[1, 4–6, 12, 21, 25, 26, 58, 59] Under these circumstances, misdiagnosis should be a thing of the past.[1] The only errors in diagnosis with PTC should be with a diffuse lesion (region 4) when this is misdiagnosed as a localized carcinoma in region 1.[1]

The interesting phenomenon frequently noted on PTC is a small irregular tract through the lesion with filling of the distal common bile duct (Fig. 33–1*A*). In Figure 33–1*A*, dilated lymphatics are also seen in

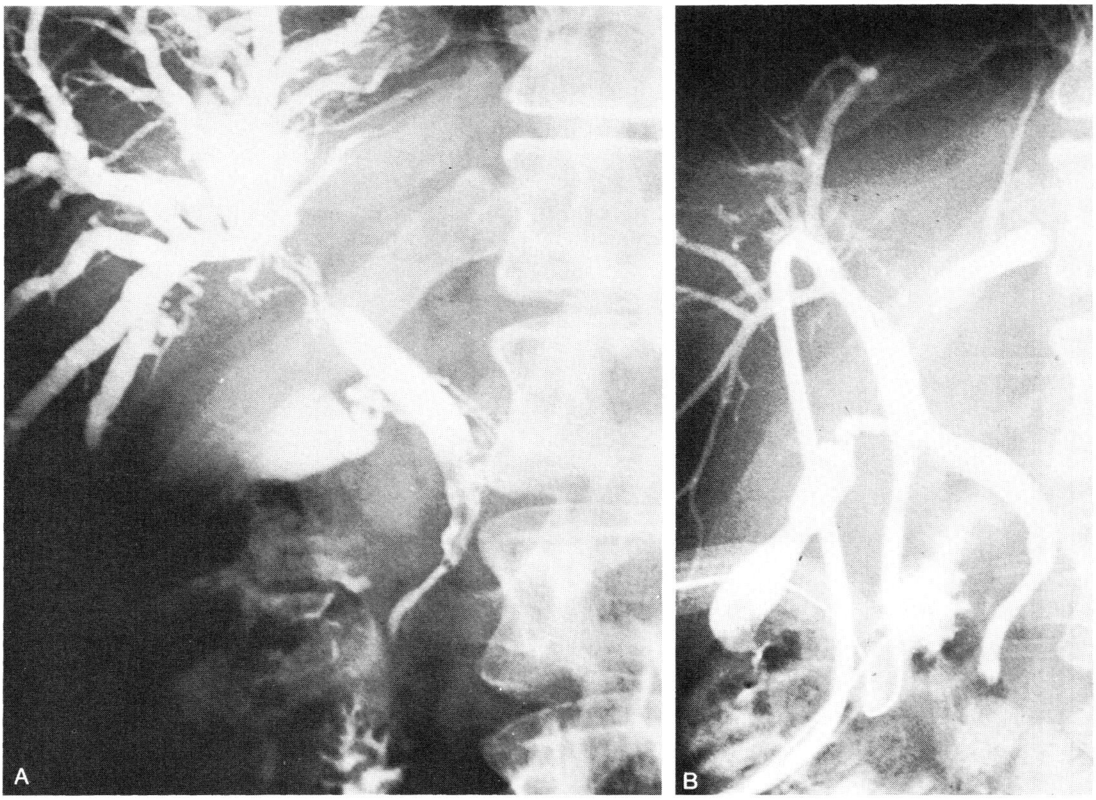

Figure 33–1. *A,* Preoperative percutaneous transhepatic cholangiogram in patient 12 (H.D.) performed immediately before his first reoperation in our institution, showing the classic lesion of carcinoma of the main hepatic duct junction. *B,* U-tubogram 2 weeks postoperatively, showing the rapid collapse of the decompressed right hepatic duct system and the typical narrow lesion in the lower portion of the main left hepatic duct. (From Terblanche J, Louw JH: Surg Clin North Am 1973;*53*:1245.)

the region of the lesion, which have filled owing to an interstitial injection.

The value of combined arteriography and venography in assessing resectability preoperatively has been stressed.[27]

DIAGNOSIS AND DIFFERENTIAL DIAGNOSIS

Preoperative Diagnosis

It is usually possible to make a firm diagnosis preoperatively, but this requires an awareness of the condition, as the clinical features and biochemistry do not differentiate the lesion from other causes of extrahepatic biliary obstruction. Ultrasound and CT scanning are usually suggestive, while PTC with or without ERCP is necessary for definitive preoperative diagnosis and to localize the lesion to a particular region of the biliary tract.

Benign strictures of the bile duct occur only after previous surgery. Other neoplastic obstructions of this portion of the bile duct may be the result of local extension of a primary carcinoma of the gallbladder or a metastatic deposit in the hilus of the liver. In the patient who has not had a previous biliary tract operation, the main differential diagnoses to be considered are sclerosing cholangitis, primary biliary cirrhosis, and intrahepatic cholestatic jaundice. A normal biliary tree on ultrasound, with or without confirmation on PTC and ERCP, will suggest one of the last two diagnoses. Cholangiography should also differentiate carcinoma from sclerosing cholangitis.[1, 2]

Although the rare benign lesions of the bile duct may be suspected on PTC, they require operative evaluation for confirmation.

Operative Diagnosis

Because of its scarlike appearance and high location in the porta hepatis (the lesion may be difficult to see and feel), coupled with the finding of a collapsed or normal-sized gallbladder and common bile duct, this lesion understandably has often been missed at operation. This will continue to occur if the possibility of a Klatskin tumor is not considered and if preoperative ultrasonography followed by PTC or ERCP is not performed. If these studies are employed routinely in jaundiced patients, carcinoma of the main hepatic duct junction will not be missed.[1, 5, 6, 12] Operative cholangiography can also be used to establish the diagnosis,[5] but better definition is achieved in the radiology department preoperatively.

On exploration of the common bile duct, the lesion has a typical appearance when viewed through the choledochoscope, consisting of a tapering stenosis in the upper common hepatic duct. There is a characteristic gritty feel when it is probed with Bakes dilators. Having dilated the lesion, it is usually possible to obtain a suitable biopsy for histologic diagnosis using the biopsy attachment of the rigid Storz choledochoscope.[1] Our group has previously emphasized that the diagnosis can—and must—be made, even in the absence of histologic proof, as worthwhile palliation can frequently be achieved without repeated laparotomies.[21] However, using the aforementioned apparatus, it is possible to obtain suitable biopsies.

The rare benign lesions will be confirmed by visualization through the choledochoscope. Frozen sections must be studied to establish a firm diagnosis and to ensure that treatment is appropriate.[1]

TREATMENT

Dilatation, U-Tube Splintage, and Radiotherapy

Unless the lesion is easily resectable, our group believes that the best treatment is a combination of dilatation, U-tube splintage, and radiotherapy.[1, 9, 28, 29]

Historical Aspects

Altemeier first drew attention to the prolonged palliation that could be achieved by dilating the lesion from within the bile duct at operation, with or without splintage by intubation.[2] This has been confirmed by many subsequent investigators.[1] However, encrustation and blockage or dislodgment of the tube stent with restenosis by the growth have resulted in repeated operations in many patients. Unsatisfactory results in one patient who required repeated operations in 1968 led our group to evolve the U-tube replaceable stent technique to avoid this problem. Although it was unsuccessful for technical reasons when attempted in the first patient treated in early 1969, the technique was successfully employed in two other patients in that year.[1, 5, 21, 30] Praderi independently used a similar technique, which was reported in the South American literature.[31, 32] A U-tube replaceable stent has also been developed by several workers for use in treating bile duct strictures,[1] with the first report appearing in the German literature in 1951.[33]

Insertion of the U-Tube

The lesion is best exposed through an upper midline or right paramedian incision.[1] The diagnosis should have been established preoperatively by ultrasound followed by PTC or ERCP, but if not, an operative cholangiogram is essential. The lesion is confirmed by inspection and palpation, and the abdomen is explored for signs of spread, which is unusual. The lesion is assessed for resectability, which has rarely been possible in our cases. The visible and palpable extent of the tumor should be marked with metal clips to assist with subsequent radiotherapy planning.

The collapsed common bile duct is opened longitudinally above the duodenum. A 3 mm Bakes dilator is passed upward and the typical firm lesion felt. Choledochoscopy is essential, the short-limbed rigid Storz choledochoscope being preferred.[1, 34] Using this instrument, the lesion may be noted to have the characteristic appearance of a smooth constriction in the upper common hepatic duct. The rare papillary growth with its frondlike appearance will also be obvious.[21]

The choledochoscope is removed and the lesion carefully dilated using graduated Bakes dilators. A 3 mm Bakes dilator is gently forced through the lesion into one or both main hepatic ducts. In most of our cases, it has been possible to enter only the right duct system. However, drainage of one lobar duct has proved perfectly adequate[1, 35] as long as the other duct is uninfected. The dilatation must be undertaken with care to avoid splitting the lesion or creating a false passage.[1] After removal of the 3 mm dilator, white bile gushes forth. Thereafter, 4 mm and 5 mm dilators are gently forced through the lesion, which has a firm and typically gritty feel. Occasionally the 6 mm dilator can also be passed, but it should not be forced, in order to avoid splitting the tumor. Recently, dilatation using a Gruntzig balloon catheter under intraoperative radiologic control has superseded the use of the metal Bakes dilators.

The rigid choledochoscope is reinserted, and the intrahepatic bile ducts on one or both sides are inspected for the presence of multifocal lesions. The instrument is also passed downward to the ampulla for the same reason.[34] The choledochoscope is removed and the biopsy apparatus attached. Using this setup, we have been able to obtain suitable biopsy material from within the dilated tumor in most patients.

The second largest dilator used (usually 4 mm) or a flexible catheter is manipulated into a dilated major hepatic duct near the lower anterior surface of the liver, where it can easily be seen and felt. A small 1 cm incision is made in Glisson's capsule, and the dilator is gently pushed out through the thin overlying liver tissue. A strong thread is attached to the dilator, which is extracted through the lesion and out the lower common bile duct. The U-tube is firmly sutured to the thread and gently pulled via the opening in the common bile duct through the lesion and out through the surface of the liver (Fig. 33–2*B*). An instrument to simplify insertion of the U-tube has been described.[36]

A long, firm-walled, plastic, Levin-type Argyle gastric tube is used at the time of the initial intubation (Sherwood Medical Industries Ltd., United Kingdom). The first Silastic tubing used by our group was soft-walled and proved unsatisfactory,[1, 21] but firm Silastic tubes are now available.[37] The largest diameter tube that will pass (usually 16) is used. A long tube is preferred, as it is easier to handle and replace. A Silastic tube is preferred for prolonged intubation and is used to replace the polyethylene tube after radiotherapy is completed.

The tube is partly withdrawn through the opening in the lower common bile duct, and two single side holes are cut so that one will be sited immediately above and one immediately below the tumor (Fig. 33–2*B*). Each hole is oval, with the long axis parallel to the axis of the tube, is approximately 1 cm long, and is made so that part of the radiopaque marker line on the tube is excised. Big holes are preferable, and multiple small holes are not required. The distance between the holes can be accurately judged by assessing the length of the lesion using the choledochoscope. The holes must be sited near one another, usually 2 to 3 cm apart; if they are too far from the lesion, one may lie outside the liver or bile duct, which would allow bile to leak and require the tube to be replaced.[1] It is usually possible to judge the correct position of the tube at operation without radiologic control. After the tube is carefully positioned, the choledochotomy is snugly repaired around it. Each limb of the tube is brought out through the abdominal wall via a separate stab incision. Fixation of the two limbs without intra-abdominal slack is best achieved by attaching them to a cross-piece cut from one end of the tube. This prevents movement or dislodgment of the tube (Fig. 33–3). The U-tube should not be sutured to the skin. Two separate Penrose drains are inserted and placed adjacent to each limb of the U-tube, as early bile leakage is not uncom-

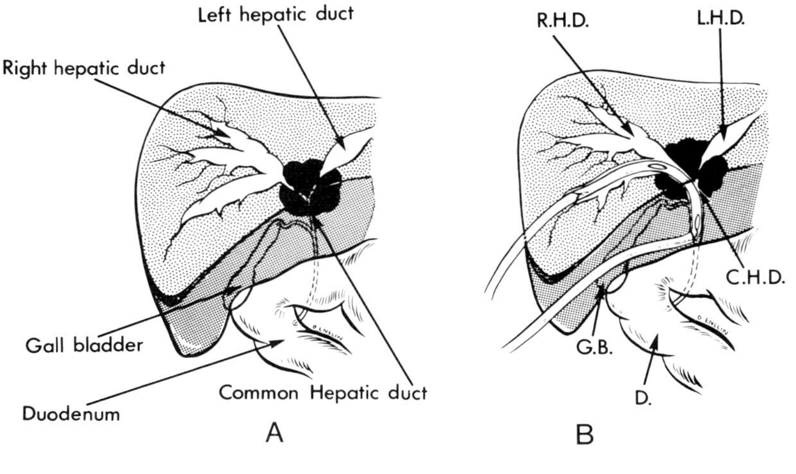

Figure 33–2. The U-tube procedure. *A*, The carcinoma situated at the main hepatic duct junction. *B*, The U-tube in situ after dilatation. (From Terblanche J, Saunders SJ, Louw JH: Surgery 1972;*71*: 720. Used by permission.)

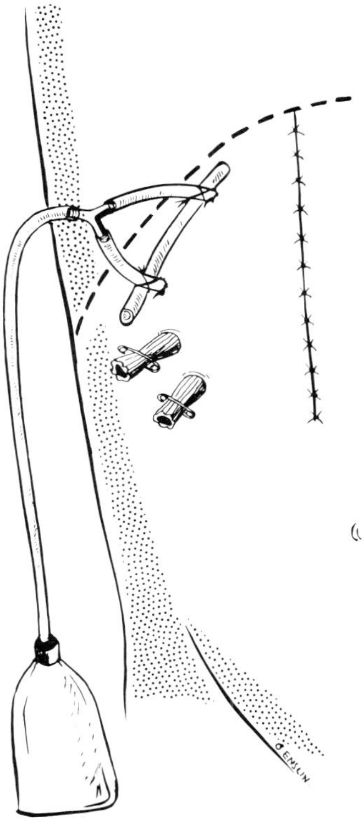

Figure 33–3. The U-tube draining into a collecting bag, showing the method of fixation. (From Terblanche J, Saunders SJ, Louw JH: Surgery 1972;*71*:720. Used by permission.)

mon and the plastic U-tube does not form a satisfactory tract. The abdomen is closed after finally checking that the tube has not become displaced.

The ends of the U-tube are left long and attached to one another by a large rubber T-tube, which drains into a closed sterile plastic bag. The Y-connector and short limbs of the tube shown in Figure 33–3 are no longer used.

The U-tube system allows bile to drain from the distended intrahepatic bile ducts via the tube, past the lesion into the lower common bile duct, and then into the duodenum (see Fig. 33–1*B*). Therefore, bile flows normally into the gastrointestinal tract, and an external biliary fistula is avoided.

Care of the U-Tube and Conversion to a Circle or O-Tube

As soon as the patient is stable postoperatively, the U-tube is converted to a circle or O-tube by connecting the two ends of the U-tube together with a short length of rubber tubing (cut from the original T-tube that was used to join the ends of the U-tube to the drainage bag). This is preferable to clamping the tube, which was previously recommended. Any bile flowing around the outer limb of the O-tube will return to the lower common bile duct and into the duodenum.

The liver shrinks postoperatively once the obstruction is relieved (see Fig. 33–1*B*). Therefore, the tube frequently loosens and requires refixing; this is easily accomplished on the ward, as the tube is secured by fixation to the crosspiece and not to the patient. If the tube becomes displaced, this is heralded by bile leakage around the upper or lower limb of the tube or through the Penrose drain. It can usually be repositioned on the ward by pushing inward the end of the tube around which the leakage is occurring. Repositioning in the radiology department (see Fig. 33–1*B*) is required if this is unsuccessful.

The patient is given a three-dose broad-spectrum antibiotic cover, and cholangitis has been an uncommon problem. The tube is flushed twice daily with saline in the early postoperative period.

Before discharge from the hospital, the Penrose drains are removed, and the patient is taught to irrigate and care for the U-tube. Sterile saline irrigations are continued once a day indefinitely, in the hope that this will slow down encrustation and lessen the frequency with which the tube will have to be changed. Each patient becomes an expert in handling his own tube. Paraffin gauze or dry dressings are used around the site where the tubes emerge from the abdomen. Sometime later, granulation tissue occasionally accumulates at these sites, but it is simple to remove or cauterize.

In the rare case in which cholangitis has been a problem, broad spectrum-antibiotics have been used with success in most instances.

Replacement of the U-Tube

The U-tube must be replaced when it becomes blocked, which occurs on the average at 6- to 18-month intervals. Blockage is heralded by difficulty with irrigation, jaundice, or cholangitis. We currently replace the rigid plastic tube with a Silastic tube after radiotherapy is completed.

The tube is replaced by railroading a new tube into position. This is simple and can be performed with parenteral analgesia. The new long tube is firmly sutured to the old one and pulled through the preformed tract. The lower limb of the new tube is brought partly out of the abdomen, and holes are cut in the same sites as in the old tube, using the old tube as a template. The new tube is then accurately repositioned by measurement against the old tube and is fixed as before (see Fig. 33–3). The position is checked the next day by U-tubogram before the patient is discharged from the hospital.

Radiotherapy

The long-term survival achieved in our patients suggests that radiotherapy in combination with the U-tube technique may possibly cure this condition.[1] Thus, unless contraindicated, the patients have received 6000 rads administered to the local tumor area postoperatively. Marking the tumor site at operation with metal clips, and the position of the holes cut in the radiopaque line in the tube and sited immediately above and below the lesion, assist with radiotherapy planning. We currently prefer not to administer cytotoxic drugs in addition to radiotherapy. Internal radiotherapy using iridium-192 wire has also yielded promising results.[38]

Results

Our group has published the results in 26 patients.[1] The last 15 consecutive cases constituted a prospective study of the treatment of carcinoma of the main hepatic duct junction. These individuals were operated on between 1968 and 1973 and have been followed until the present time or death. The survival data have been updated on several occasions.[1, 28, 29] The results as of November 1979 are presented in Tables 33–1 and 33–2. Two patients were alive and well at over 8 years. Both had the U-tube procedure combined with radiotherapy. Good palliation was achieved in the other long-surviving patients. The U-tube procedure was performed in eight patients and combined with radiotherapy in the last four. The last two patients, both of whom ultimately died of their disease, had a course of cytotoxic therapy first, and radiotherapy was delayed until the cytotoxic therapy had been completed.

Other workers have also reported satisfactory results with the U-tube,[31, 37, 39] although most investigators have not combined this with early high-dose radiotherapy, which we believe to be an important part of the treatment.[1, 38, 40]

Other Forms of Treatment

Other forms of treatment for carcinoma of the main hepatic duct junction have been reviewed.[1]

Dilatation and Intubation

Prolonged palliation can be achieved by dilatation of the lesion and intubation using stents other than the U-tube,[1, 3, 4, 6, 12, 37] but really prolonged survival has been rare. However, one of our patients survived for 5 years after dilatation and T-tube intubation fol-

Table 33–1 UPDATED DATA ON THE 15 PATIENTS IN THE PROSPECTIVE STUDY OF CARCINOMA OF THE MAIN HEPATIC DUCT JUNCTION OPERATED UPON BETWEEN 1968 AND 1973[21]

Case	Patient	Age	Sex	Procedure	Survival
1.	B.S.	42	M	Incorrect diagnosis—dilated only—cholecystoduodenostomy	Died: 1 yr, 7 mos
2.	J.B.	46	M	Nil	Died: 1 yr, 7 mos
3.	E.V.	71	F	Dilated—T-tube, radiotherapy	Died: 5 yrs
4.	D.H.	24	M	Dilated—T-tube	Died: 1 yr, 2 mos
5.	D.v.S.	34	F	Dilated–T-tube	Died: 3 yrs
6.	S.D.	53	M	Dilated—T-tube, *U-tube*	Died: 2¾ yrs
7.	N.M.	72	F	Dilated—catheter, *U-tube*	Died: 4½ mos
8.	F.S.	78	F	Nil	Died: 1 wk
9.	E.S.	75	F	Dilated—*U-tube*	Died: 2 wks
10.	M.Mc.K.	87	F	Dilated—*U-tube*	Died: 5 wks
11.	P.S.	83	M	Nil	Died: 24 hrs
12.	H.D.	63	M	Incorrect diagnosis—cholecystojejunostomy; dilated—*U-tube*, radiotherapy	Died: > 8 yrs
13.	M.N.	30	M	Dilated—*U-tube*	Alive and well: > 14 yrs
14.	A.G.	70	F	Dilated—*U-tube*, Endoxan, radiotherapy	Died: 3 yrs
15.	M.M.	70	M	Dilated—*U-tube*, Endoxan, radiotherapy	Died: 2½ yrs

Table 33–2 UPDATED SURVIVAL DATA IN THE 15 PROSPECTIVE STUDY PATIENTS (1968–1973)[21, 28]

Number of Patients		Survival in Years
Alive:	1	14 years
Dead:	14	
	9	> 1 year Longest: 8, 5, 3, 3, 2¾, 2¾, 2¼
	5	< 1 year Average age, 79 years

lowed by radiotherapy.[28] The technique of dilatation is the same as described in the section on the U-tube.

If local stents or T-tubes are used, they unfortunately become blocked or displaced in time. This has necessitated multiple, difficult operations to replace the stents and to achieve prolonged survival.[1, 14, 41] The use of a potentially replaceable transhepatic stent was first reported by Praderi in Uruguay,[42] but this author and others have found this more difficult to replace than the U-tube. A transhepatic stent differs from the U-tube in that only one end is brought out through the skin. The tube, therefore, runs from the skin through the liver and the lesion, into the distal common bile duct or through the ampulla into the bowel. On the other hand, Cameron et al. have found transhepatic stents relatively easy to replace.[37]

Radical Resection

Although resection should be the ultimate treatment, the majority of patients reported in the literature have had unresectable lesions, and even in patients undergoing supposedly curative resections, long-term survival has been rare.[1, 54, 61–64] Iwasaki et al., however, reported 14 resections among 23 patients with carcinoma of the hepatic duct junction.[11] Local resection of the bile duct junction was performed in 12 of these 14 patients. These authors consider the lesion resectable if proximal extension is limited to below the second bifurcation of the intrahepatic bile ducts in both the right and the left lobes, if distal extension of the lesion is limited, and if neither the hepatic artery nor the portal vein has been invaded by the tumor. Their technique includes excision of the intrahepatic bile ducts beyond the second bifurcation together with the hepatic tissue at the hilus of the liver. Reconstruction is by hepaticojejunostomy. Nine of the 14 patients had grossly complete resections, which have been termed "curative" resections. Six of these patients were alive and well 5 to 25 months postoperatively.[11] Other authors have presented the results of resection, and although follow-up has usually been short,[43, 44] a few long-term survivors have been reported.[22, 45] Although these results are remarkable, a longer follow-up is required, and these results must be compared with those that can be achieved with the U-tube procedure plus radiotherapy.

Unlike carcinoma of the main hepatic duct junction, carcinoma of the bile duct in region 2 should be resected whenever possible. The author is currently following a 20-year survivor.[1]

Bypass Using Intrahepatic Duct to Bowel Anastomosis

The results of palliative bypass procedures using intrahepatic bile ducts anastomosed to the gastrointestinal tract have been disappointing in general.[1] However, Bismuth and Corlette published 80 cases of carcinoma in the hilar region with cholangioenteric anastomosis in 45.[10] They prefer the round ligament technique, in which the left anterolateral segment duct is exposed and anastomosed to bowel. Three patients were alive at the time of reporting (two at 8 months and one at 50 months), and 39 were followed until death, with an average survival of 13 months (range 2 to 49 months).[10] These results have stimulated others to evaluate the procedure.[46, 47] Although these results are of interest, they must be compared with those achieved using the less traumatic U-tube procedure. An alternative technique has also been developed.[48]

Percutaneous Transhepatic Catheterization

Percutaneous transhepatic catheterization can be used for two purposes:[55] first, as an external biliary fistula for proximal drainage, as a temporary procedure while the patient is made fit for major surgery;[49] and second, as a permanent external biliary fistula in an unfit elderly patient.[38, 50–53] Percutaneous catheterization through a biliary tumor may also allow the placement of radioactive iridium wire to deliver local radiotherapy.[57, 64–66]

It is also possible to dilate and intubate the lesion under local anesthesia using the percutaneous route under radiologic control. Burcharth reported the use of this technique to insert an endoprosthesis. Most of his cases were periampullary lesions (region 3), but there were two cholangiocarcinomas.[50] Unfortunately, this stent is more difficult to replace than a U-tube. Burcharth has, however, reported its replacement in three patients with cholangiocarcinoma.[51] For further details on percutaneous transhepatic catheterization, refer to Chapter 10.

Radiotherapy Alone

Although the use of radiotherapy alone has been advocated, it should be used in conjunction with a replaceable stent.[1, 65]

Liver Transplantation

The controversy regarding hepatic transplantation for this lesion has been fully reviewed.[1, 28, 29, 67] The author does not consider hepatic transplantation to be a justifiable form of treatment for this condition at present.

No Treatment

In assessing the results of different methods of treatment, it is important to remember that a number of patients with this slow-growing lesion have survived for prolonged periods with no treatment at all, or after laparotomy and biopsy only. Survival of over 1 year after biopsy proof of diagnosis has been reported.[1]

REFERENCES

1. Terblanche J: Carcinoma of the proximal extrahepatic biliary tree—definitive and palliative treatment. Surg Ann 1978;*11*:249.
2. Altemeier WA, Gall EA, Zinninger MM, et al: Sclerosing carcinoma of the major intrahepatic bile ducts. Arch Surg 1957;*75*:450.
3. Klatskin G: Adenocarcinoma of the hepatic duct at its bifurcation within the porta hepatis. An unusual tumor with distinctive clinical and pathological features. Am J Med 1956;*38*:241.
4. Whelton MJ, Petrelli M, George P, et al: Carcinoma at the junction of the main hepatic ducts. Q J Med 1969;*38*:211.
5. Terblanche J, Saunders SJ, Louw JH: Prolonged palliation in carcinoma of the main hepatic duct junction. Surgery 1972;*71*:720.
6. George PA, Brown C, Foley RTE: Carcinoma of the hepatic duct junction. Br J Surg 1981;*68*:14.
7. Meyerowitz BR, Aird I: Carcinoma of the hepatic ducts within the liver. Br J Surg 1962;*50*:178.
8. Glenn F, Hays DM: The scope of radical surgery in the treatment of malignant tumors of the extrahepatic biliary tract. Surg Gynecol Obstet 1954;*99*:529.
9. Terblanche J: [In discussion] Cameron JL, Gayler BW, Zuidema GD: The use of silastic transhepatic stents in benign and malignant biliary strictures. Ann Surg 1978;*188*:552.
10. Bismuth H, Corlette MB: Intrahepatic cholangioenteric anastomosis in carcinoma of the hilus of the liver. Surg Gynecol Obstet 1975;*140*:170.
11. Iwasaki Y, Ohto M, Todoroki T, et al: Treatment of carcinoma of the biliary system. Surg Gynecol Obstet 1977;*144*:219.
12. Lees CD, Zapolanski A, Cooperman AM, et al: Carcinoma of the bile ducts. Surg Gynecol Obstet 1980;*151*:193.
13. Strohl EL, Reed WH, Diffenbaugh WG, et al: Carcinoma of the bile ducts. Arch Surg 1963;*87*:567.
14. Ross AP, Braasch JW, Warren KW: Carcinoma of the proximal bile ducts. Surg Gynecol Obstet 1973;*136*:923.
15. Andersson A, Bergdahl L, van der Linden W: Malignant tumors of the extrahepatic bile ducts. Surgery 1977;*81*:198.
16. Brown DB, Strang R, Gordon J, et al: Primary carcinoma of the extrahepatic bile ducts. Br J Surg 1961;*49*:22.
17. Ritchie JK, Allan RN, Macartney J, et al: Biliary tract carcinoma associated with ulcerative colitis. Q J Med 1974;*63*:263.
18. Akwari OE, van Heerden JA, Foulk WT, et al: Cancer of the bile ducts associated with ulcerative colitis. Ann Surg 1975;*181*:303.
19. van Heerden JA, Judd ES, Dockerty MB: Carcinoma of the extrahepatic bile ducts. A clinicopathologic study. Am J Surg 1967;*113*:49.
20. Lees CD, Hermann RE: Familial polyposis coli associated with bile duct cancer. Am J Surg 1981;*141*:378.
21. Terblanche J, Louw JH: U-tube drainage in the palliative therapy of carcinoma of the main hepatic duct junction. Surg Clin North Am 1973;*53*:1245.
22. Todoroki T, Okamura T, Fukao K, et al: Gross appearance of carcinoma of the main hepatic duct and its prognosis. Surg Gynecol Obstet 1980;*150*:33.
23. Pelleya-Kouri R, Dusol M, Orta D, et al: Bile duct carcinoma mimicking chronic liver disease. Arch Intern Med 1976;*136*:1051.
24. Conn HO, Redeker AG, Zimmon DS: PTC versus ERC—An editor's dream. Gastroenterology 1976; *71*:520.
25. Longmire WP, McArthur MS, Bastounis EA, et al: Carcinoma of the extrahepatic biliary tract. Ann Surg 1973;*178*:333.
26. Wanebo HJ, Grimes OF: Cancer of the bile duct: the occult malignancy. Am J Surg 1975;*130*:262.
27. Williamson BWA, Blumgart LH, McKellar NJ: Management of tumors of the liver. Combined use of arteriography and venography in the assessment of resectability, especially in hilar tumors. Am J Surg 1980;*139*:210.
28. Terblanche J: Is carcinoma of the main hepatic duct junction an indication for liver transplantation or palliative surgery? A plea for the U tube palliative procedure. Surgery 1976;*79*:127.
29. Terblanche J: Hepatic transplantation: replay. (Letter.) Surgery 1976;*79*:727.
30. Terblanche J: Progress in liver transplantation and the treatment of bile duct carcinoma. S Afr Med J 1971;*45*:1149.

31. Praderi RC: Twelve years' experience with transhepatic intubation. Ann Surg 1974;*179*:937.
32. Praderi RC: Obstruccion neoplasica de los hepaticos. Rev Argent Cirug 1971;*20*:115.
33. Goetze O: Die transhepatische dauerdrainage bei der hohen gallengangsstenose. Langenbecks Arch Klin Chir 1951;*270*:97.
34. Tompkins RK, Johnson J, Storm FK, et al: Operative endoscopy in the management of biliary tract neoplasms. Am J Surg 1976;*132*:174.
35. Longmire WP, Tompkins RK: Lesions of the segmental and lobar hepatic ducts. Ann Surg 1975;*182*:478.
36. Tatarchuk TW, White TT: A new instrument for inserting a U tube. Am J Surg 1979;*137*:425.
37. Cameron JL, Broe P, Zuidema GD: Proximal bile duct tumors. Surgical management with stents. Ann Surg 1982;*196*:412.
38. Fletcher MS, Brinkley D, Dawson JL, et al: Treatment of high bile duct carcinoma by internal radiotherapy with iridium-192 wire. Lancet 1981;*2*:172.
39. Smith R: Personal communication, 1976.
40. Blumgart LH: Biliary tract obstruction: new approaches to old problems. Am J Surg 1978;*135*:19.
41. Fortner JG, Kallum BO, Kim DK: Surgical management of carcinoma of the junction of the main hepatic ducts. Ann Surg 1976;*184*:68.
42. Praderi R: Coledocostomia transhepatica. Bol Soc Cir Urug 1961;*32*:237.
43. Evander A, Fredlund P, Hoevels J, et al: Evaluation of aggressive surgery for carcinoma of the extrahepatic bile ducts. Ann Surg 1980;*191*:23.
44. Hart MJ, White TT: Central hepatic resection and anastomosis for stricture or carcinoma at the hepatic bifurcation. Ann Surg 1980;*192*:299.
45. Launois B, Campion JP, Brissot P, et al: Carcinoma of the hepatic hilus. Surgical management and the case for resection. Ann Surg 1979;*190*:151.
46. Dudley SE, Edis AJ, Adson MA: Biliary decompression in hilar obstruction. Round ligament approach. Arch Surg 1979;*114*:519.
47. Malt RA, Warshaw AL, Jamieson CG, et al: Left intrahepatic cholangiojejunostomy for proximal obstruction of the biliary tract. Surg Gynecol Obstet 1980;*150*:193.
48. Cahow CE: Intrahepatic cholangiojejunostomy: a new simplified approach. Am J Surg 1979;*137*:443.
49. Mori K, Misumi A, Sugiyama M, et al: Percutaneous transhepatic bile drainage. Ann Surg 1977;*185*:111.
50. Burcharth F: A new endoprosthesis for nonoperative intubation of the biliary tract in malignant obstructive jaundice. Surg Gynecol Obstet 1978; *146*:76.
51. Burcharth F, Jensen LI, Olesen K: Endoprosthesis for internal drainage of the biliary tract. Technique and results in 48 cases. Gastroenterology 1979; *77*:133.
52. Dooley JS, Dick R, Olney J, et al: Non-surgical treatment of biliary obstruction. Lancet 1979; *2*:1040.
53. Pollock TW, Ring ER, Oleaga JA, et al: Percutaneous decompression of benign and malignant biliary obstruction. Arch Surg 1979;*114*:148.
54. Blumgart LH, Benjamin IS, Hadis NS, et al: Surgical approaches to cholangiocarcinoma at confluence of hepatic ducts. Lancet 1984;*1*:66.
55. Clouse ME, Evans D, Costello P, et al: Percutaneous transhepatic biliary drainage. Complications due to multiple duct obstructions. Ann Surg 1983;*198*:25.
56. Siegel JH, Daniel SJ: Endoscopic and fluoroscopic transpapillary placement of a large caliber biliary endoprosthesis. Am J Gastroenterol 1984;*79*:461.
57. Mornex F, Ardiet JM, Bret P, et al: Radiotherapy of high bile duct carcinoma using intracatheter Iridium 192 wire. Cancer 1984;*54*:2069.
58. Voyles CR, Bowley NJ, Allison DJ, et al: Carcinoma of the proximal extrahepatic biliary tree. Radiologic assessment and therapeutic alternatives. Ann Surg 1983;*197*:188.
59. Kozuka S, Tsubone M, Hachisuka K: Evolution of carcinoma in the extrahepatic bile ducts. Cancer 1984;*54*:65.
60. Juttijudata P, Prichanond S, Churnratanakul S, et al: Hilar intrahepatic cholangiocarcinoma and its etiology. J Clin Gastroenterol 1984;*6*:503.
61. Alexander F, Ross RL, O'Bryan M, et al: Biliary carcinoma. A review of 109 cases. Am J Surg 1984;*147*:503.
62. Beazley RM, Hadjis N, Benjamine IS, et al: Clinicopathological aspects of high bile duct cancer. Experience with resection and bypass surgical treatments. Ann Surg 1984;*199*:623.
63. Vioegeku DR, Crummy AB, Weese JL: Percutaneous transhepatic cholangiography, drainage, and biopsy in patients with malignant biliary obstruction. An alternative to surgery. Am J Surg 1985;*150*:243.
64. Ottow RT, August DA, Sugarbaker PH: Treatment of proximal biliary tract carcinoma: An overview of techniques and results. Surgery 1985:*97*:251.
65. Hishikawa Y, Shimada T, Miura T, et al: Radiation therapy of carcinoma of the extrahepatic bile ducts. Radiology 1983;*146*:787.
66. Conroy RM, Shahbazian AA, Edwards KC, et al: A new method for treating carcinomatous biliary obstruction with intracatheter radium. Cancer 1982; *49*:1321.
67. Starzl TE, Shunzaburo I, Shaw BW, Van Thiel DH, Gartner JC, et al: Analysis of liver transplantation. Hepatology 1984;*4*:475.

LESLIE WISE, M.D.
MARTIN TINDEL, M.D.

34

Carcinoma of the Ampulla of Vater

INTRODUCTION

The so-called carcinomas of the ampulla of Vater include carcinomas of the terminal common bile duct and terminal pancreatic duct as well as those carcinomas of the duodenum that are located in or just around the ampulla of Vater. In most instances, it is impossible to localize precisely the site of origin of these tumors either macroscopically or microscopically. Whatever their origin, ampullary tumors produce a firm localized mass that tends to obstruct the terminal common bile duct and the main pancreatic duct.

In most adults, the main duct of the pancreas (duct of Wirsung) enters the ampulla of Vater, the result of the common embryologic origin of the common bile duct and the ventral pancreas. However, the two ducts may empty into the duodenum through separate openings. The ampulla of Vater is situated on the posteromedial aspect of the lower part of the second portion of the duodenum.

Cancer of the pancreas, once a rare disease, has been steadily increasing in the United States for the past 35 years.[1] It is now the eighth most common cancer and the fifth most common cause of cancer death. Compared with 1930, the incidence has roughly doubled in women and tripled in men. In both men and women, 3 per cent of all cancers originate in the pancreas, and 5 per cent of all cancer deaths are due to a primary pancreatic tumor. Based on the estimates of the American Cancer Society, there were 25,000 newly diagnosed cases and 22,600 recorded deaths from pancreatic tumors in the United States in 1982.[2] In a review of 15,000 patients with pancreatic cancer, the absolute 5-year survival rate was only 0.4 per cent,[3] certainly a dismal prognosis. The most common location of pancreatic cancer varies in different series; the head is the most frequent site in clinical series, but in autopsy studies, cancers of the body and tail predominate.[4] Periampullary tumors are relatively rare. They are slightly more common in men than in women. Carcinomas of the head of the pancreas are three to four times as frequent as periampullary carcinomas.[5,6]

The average length of survival of all patients diagnosed as having cancer of the pancreas is 3 to 4 months, with over 90 per cent of patients being dead in less than 1 year.[7,8] The 5-year survival even for localized lesions (i.e., without local or distant metastases) is less than 5 per cent.[9] Seidman et al. estimate that in the United States there is approximately a 1 per cent probability at birth of eventually developing cancer of the pancreas.[10]

There are four risk factors that have been extensively studied and linked with the increased incidence of pancreatic neoplasms: diabetes mellitus, cigarette smoking, diet, and occupational exposure. The link between diabetes and pancreatic cancer may have been overestimated in the past because many patients develop diabetes just several months before the diagnosis is made. Wynder, however, showed a significant relationship between pancreatic cancer and early-onset diabetes in females but not in males.[11] Another study showed the risk of pancreatic cancer to be twofold in diabetic females compared with nondiabetic females.[12] Clark and Mitchell[13] examined a population of 400,000, seeking an association between diabetes and pancreatic cancer. During a 5-year period, 65 cases of pancreatic cancer and 729 cases of diabetes were diagnosed. Fifty-two of the diabetics were considered to be unstable, as defined by low body weight and a tendency to ketosis and ketonuria. Twenty-one of these diabetic patients were over 60 years of age, and in this subgroup, 10 patients (48 per cent) subsequently developed cancer of the pancreas during the period of observation.

Cigarette smoking has been shown to impart a two- to threefold increased risk for the development of pancreatic cancer.[11] This does not apply to pipe and cigar smoking.[14] Wynder proposed that carcinogens from cigarette smoke reach the pancreas after being concentrated in the gallbladder and the common duct.[14] Cigarette smoking may account for the male to female predominance of pancreatic cancer, as there is no sex difference when one examines nonsmokers.[15] Also, pancreatic cancer appears 10 years earlier, on the average, in smokers as compared with nonsmokers.

In a Japanese study, patients who developed pancreatic cancer had a higher consumption of meat and lower consumption of vegetables when compared with controls.[16] High-fat diets have been shown to enhance tumor production in experimental animals. Nitrites, used in meat preservation, are converted to nitrosamines in the body. Nitrosamines have been shown to induce pancreatic cancer in animals.[17]

MacMahon et al.[18] showed an increased risk of pancreatic cancer associated with consumption of coffee but not tea or alcohol. Of interest was that this study excluded periampullary lesions. There is no convincing evidence that chronic pancreatitis predisposes to cancer of the pancreas.[19]

Epidemiologic studies have identified occupational factors that have been linked with an increased incidence of pancreatic cancer. Higher levels were noted among members of the American Chemical Society[20] (although specific chemical inducers were not identified) and, in á small series, among workers exposed to β-naphthylamine and benzidine.[21] In most of the studies cited, the authors did not distinguish between periampullary and head of pancreas lesions.

PATHOLOGY

The exact origin of carcinomas of the periampullary region is usually impossible to determine, either macroscopically or microscopically. Grossly they are all located at the ampulla, and microscopically they are all adenocarcinomas with various degrees of differentiation. The reason for the intermittent jaundice and occult gastrointestinal bleeding that occurs in these patients is recurrent sloughing of the central portion of the tumor.

When a carcinoma arises in the periampullary region, the resulting obstruction causes dilatation of the bile ducts and gallbladder. It may also cause obstruction of the duct of Wirsung, which can result in secondary pancreatic changes.

Grossly, a periampullary tumor can be best palpated after mobilization of the second part of the duodenum by compressing the lateral wall of the duodenum against the medial wall; ampullary tumors are felt as hard projections at the level of the papilla. On opening of the duodenum they appear as a papillary mass. A summary of the pathologic features found in our series of 62 patients is summarized in Table 34–1. All true periampullary carcinomas are ductal or duodenal in origin. The cells may have a papillary arrangement or may appear to be in solid sheets. Variations include squamous carcinomas (adenoacanthomas), mucinous carcinomas, and ciliated adenocarcinomas. Carcinoids of the ampulla of Vater have also been reported. Surrounding the malignant lesion there is often a zone of pancreatitis. Of the pancreatic tumors, approximately 90 per cent arise from the ductal system and 10 per cent from the acini.

A periampullary carcinoma may spread by direct extension along the common bile duct, the duct of Wirsung, the duodenum, or the head of the pancreas. Lymphatic spread is to the regional peripancreatic lymph nodes. Cubilla et al.[22] found that adenocarcinomas of the head of the pancreas often metastasize to lymph nodes not usually removed during

Table 34–1 PATHOLOGIC FEATURES OF PERIAMPULLARY TUMORS

Lesion	Percentage
Well-differentiated adenocarcinoma	29.0
Poorly differentiated adenocarcinoma	14.5
Well-differentiated papillary adenocarcinoma	4.8
Poorly differentiated papillary adenocarcinoma	37.1
Papillary mucinous adenocarcinoma	1.6
Nonpapillary mucinous adenocarcinoma	4.8
Other	8.0
Inflammatory Infiltrate Accompanying Tumor	
Insignificant	52.0
Mild to moderate	43.0
Prominent	5.0
Greatest Dimension of Tumor (47 Resected Cases)	
1 to 2 cm	25.5
2.0 to 3.0 cm	27.6
3.1 to 4.0 cm	23.4
More than 4.0 cm	23.5

From Wise L, Pizzimbono C, Dehner L: Am J Surg 1976; *131*:141.

Table 34–2 PRESENTING FEATURES OF PERIAMPULLARY CARCINOMA*

Symptoms	Number of Patients	Percentage of 62 Patients
Weight loss	56	90
Anorexia	45	73
Jaundice	42	68
Dark urine	39	63
Pale feces	35	56
Abdominal pain	33	53
Nausea	32	52
Hepatomegaly	25	40
Vomiting	22	35
Fever	21	34
Constipation	19	31
Pruritus	17	27
Palpable gallbladder	15	24
Chills	14	23
Charcot's triad (chills, fever, jaundice)	11	18
Diarrhea	8	13
Splenomegaly	5	8
Ascites	4	6
Aluminum-colored feces	2	3
Incidental Finding†	1	1.6

*Not mutually exclusive.

†This patient had multiple polyposis of the colon. During exploration for further polyps, a carcinoma of the ampulla was found incidentally.

From Wise L, Pizzimbono C, Dehner L: Am J Surg 1976: *131*:141.

the routine Whipple procedure; periampullary tumors, in contrast, tend to metastasize only to the periampullary lymph nodes that are removed during the Whipple procedure. Ampullary tumors are usually diagnosed prior to the appearance of obvious vascular metastases; the latter, if they occur, usually are found in the liver and the lung.

CLINICAL FEATURES

Periampullary carcinomas are slightly more common in men than in women, and most patients are over age 50 years.[23,24] Weight loss, anorexia, and obstructive jaundice, with pale stools and dark urine, are the usual clinical features. The presenting manifestations in our 62 patients are shown in Table 34–2. The duration of symptoms before hospital admission varied from less than a month (37 per cent) to 2 years (3 per cent).

Jaundice is usually progressive, but in about 10 per cent of patients it may be fluctuating, probably owing to necrosis and periodic sloughing of the central portion of the ampullary tumor.

Pain was a significant feature in 53 per cent of our cases; in the series of Warren and Jefferson[25] the incidence was 41 per cent. It used to be said that ampullary carcinomas are characterized by "painless jaundice," but this is not typical. In fact, abdominal pain usually precedes the jaundice.[24] It has also been stated that pain associated with pancreatic cancer is usually alleviated by sitting in a flexed position; this was *not* true in our patients, however.

Hepatomegaly is a fairly common feature and was present in 40 per cent of patients in our series. It is almost always due to biliary obstruction, not to secondary malignant involvement of the liver. Sawai and Talvalkar,[23] in a review of 22 patients with periampullary carcinoma, found that on exploration the liver was enlarged in 70 per cent but that metastases to the liver were present in only 41 per cent. An enlarged liver does not imply unresectability.

A *palpable gallbladder* is present in about 25 per cent of patients.[25] In 1890, Courvoisier[26] observed that a palpable gallbladder in the presence of jaundice is unlikely to be due to a stone and most likely reflects obstruction by an ampullary or pancreatic head carcinoma. The pathophysiologic explanation is that calculous obstruction is less complete and is associated with fibrosis of the gallbladder wall, which limits its ability to distend.

Cholangitis has been noted in approximately 20 per cent of patients with periampullary tumors; this syndrome is more common, however, in choledocholithiasis.

The combination of the pale stool of obstructive jaundice and the presence of small amounts of blood (due to blood loss from an ulcerating ampullary lesion) may lead to the so-called silvery (aluminum) stool.

In one of our patients, the periampullary tumor was noted as an incidental finding during a routine exploration for multiple polyposis of the colon. Clarke et al.,[27] Cooke,[28] Suzanne et al.,[29] Turner,[30] Qizilbash,[31] and Mir-Madjlessi et al.[32] have also described the association of polyposis coli with periampullary carcinoma; it has been suggested that endoscopy and hypotonic duodenography be considered in patients with colonic polyps who present with noncolonic alimentary symptoms.

LABORATORY INVESTIGATIONS

The most important laboratory study is the confirmation of *obstructive jaundice* and the presence of *guaiac-positive stools*. Anemia is present in about 50 per cent of these patients, but it is usually mild.

Liver Function Tests

Liver function tests usually show an obstructive picture with relatively little disturbance of hepatocellular function. Serum alkaline phosphatase is usually elevated, even before the onset of jaundice. The serum transaminase values are usually normal or only slightly elevated as opposed to hepatitis, in which they often rise to more than 1000 IU. In mechanical common bile duct obstruction, the transaminase values are usually below 500.

Upper Gastrointestinal Series

A periampullary carcinoma may produce a variety of effects on the upper gastrointestinal series: (1) a localized indentation on the concave border of the duodenum; (2) a characteristic double indentation of the concave border of the second part of the duodenum, known as the reversed-3 sign of Frostberg; (3) the enlarged gallbladder, which is secondary to the periampullary obstruction, may cause an indentation on the convex border of the duodenum near the junction of the first and second parts.

Upper gastrointestinal series suggested an ampullary lesion in 72 per cent of our patients; in 28 per cent, however, this test was false negative.[24] The most typical finding was a mass distorting the periampullary region (33 per cent), but in 22 per cent the typical reversed-3 sign could be seen. Others have reported that the upper gastrointestinal series was abnormal in only one third of patients with carcinoma of the ampulla of Vater.[33,34]

Hypotonic Duodenography

This technique is a refinement of the conventional upper gastrointestinal series, in which relaxation of the duodenum is obtained with the use of Pro-Banthine[35]; it may provide a more accurate assessment of the ampullary region in some instances. Periampullary lesions may lead to alterations in the mucosal pattern, rose thorn projections, and, in more advanced cases, filling defects; however, false negative results occur in about 40 per cent of cases.

Intravenous Cholangiography

Intravenous cholangiography may reveal a dilated common bile duct, but this examination is not applicable in patients with a serum bilirubin of over 4 mg/dl.

Percutaneous Transhepatic Cholangiography (PTC)

PTC is useful in jaundiced patients. Using the skinny (Chiba) needle the complications are minimal. This test may show tapered obstruction of the terminal common duct. PTC provides little or no information about the pancreas itself but is useful in preliminary decompression of the biliary tree. Current indications for PTC include: (1) as a preoperative adjunct if the serum bilirubin is over 20 mg/dl, (2) as a means of avoiding surgery in a deeply jaundiced patient with obvious metastases, and (3) as a temporary measure if a period of hyperalimentation is needed prior to surgery.[36] Recent evidence, however, suggests that preoperative decompression in jaundiced patients may not be necessary. When the complications of PTC are taken into consideration, patients do no better after 2 to 3 weeks of drainage than if they are explored without decompression.[37]

Selective Angiography

Lesions of the head of the pancreas may displace the gastroduodenal artery laterally or stretch the anterior and posterior pancreaticoduodenal arcade. Abnormal tumor vessels or specific tumor vessels with a characteristic tumor blush are rarely found. Demonstration of vascular irregularity ("encasement") in the region of the tumor may also be seen in chronic pancreatitis and is, therefore, nondiagnostic.

Invasion of the portal or superior mesenteric veins or encasement of the celiac axis, superior mesenteric artery, or hepatic artery is a sign of surgical unresectability. For optimal diagnostic value, superselective injection into the dorsal pancreatic, inferior pancreaticoduodenal, and gastroduodenal arteries should be performed.[38] Venous changes are best demonstrated in the late phase of selective angiography.

Herlinger and Finlay[39] performed angiography on 103 patients, of whom 35 were shown to have carcinoma of the pancreas at laparotomy. Thirty-two such lesions were correctly diagnosed as cancer, resulting in a 91.4 per cent accuracy rate. Prospective exclusion of pancreatic carcinoma was made on 61 of 68 patients (accuracy rate of 89.7 per cent). Of the 35 carcinomas of the pancreas, five were truly periampullary; these tended to be smaller avascular lesions, with less obvious signs of vascular encasement. The authors concluded that selective angiography could consistently identify lesions as small as 1 to 2 cm in diameter. In an earlier study (1973), Herlinger[40] compared ultrasound with arteriography in 20 cases of pancreatic cancer. He found both to be of equal value in the diagnosis of lesions greater than 4 cm in diameter but angiography to be more accurate in identifying smaller lesions. Herlinger concluded that angiography was more likely to demonstrate small, early lesions than either CT scan or ultrasound and that early referral of patients for angiography might identify lesions while they were smaller and potentially curable.

Suzuki et al.[41] studied the arteriographic findings in 87 patients with periampullary cancer. The arteries visualized were classified as those confined to the pancreas, those adjacent to the pancreas, and those of extrapancreatic organs. In this study, the lesions most amenable to cure were correlated with no vascular encasement or encasement confined to the anterior pancreaticoduodenal arcade (Group I). In this group of 20 patients, the resectability rate was 78 per cent. Of the lesions in 24 patients with evidence of vascular involvement outside the pancreas (Group III), only one was found to be resectable at exploration. Patients in Group I had a mean survival of over 2 years. Once the lesion involved the posterior pancreaticoduodenal arcade or extended outside the pancreas, survival after resection abruptly declined. Angiography identified liver metastases in 11 of 17 patients, for a 64 per cent accuracy rate. Based on their results, the authors concluded that angiography could reliably identify those patients in whom major resection would be appropriate and likewise identify lesions most likely to be unresectable.

We feel that angiography in the appropriate hands can consistently identify small (2 cm) lesions in the periampullary region and can reliably predict resectability. Importantly, it outlines the vasculature of the upper abdomen and alerts the surgeon to variations from normal anatomy, such as a right hepatic artery or main hepatic artery arising from the superior mesenteric artery. It should routinely be performed before exploring a patient in whom the possibility exists for major resection.

Ultrasound and CT Scan

Ultrasonographic signs of pancreatic cancer consist of enlargement of the gland, encroachment of the common bile duct and pancreatic duct, and changes in the internal character of the gland.[42] These include a loss of intensity and a decrease in the number of internal echoes. Since these findings are also seen in chronic pancreatitis, it may be difficult to distinguish between an inflammatory mass and a periampullary tumor. At present, the lower limit of size at which a pancreatic carcinoma can be diagnosed on ultrasonography is 2 cm.[43] However, in about 20 per cent of patients the studies are technically inadequate.[45,46] When only technically adequate studies are examined, a sensitivity for the detection of pancreatic cancer of between 75 and 90 per cent has been reported.[44] These studies include pancreatic tumors of all sizes and in all locations. The absence of cholelithiasis in jaundiced patients with a dilated common bile duct should be interpreted as indirect evidence of a periampullary lesion.

Tumors that markedly alter the size or contour of the pancreas can be detected by CT scanning, but small neoplasms easily may be missed by this method.[43] In addition, metastases 1 cm or larger to the liver or peritoneum may be recognized.

Using the fast scanners, the accuracy rate for CT scan in the detection of pancreatic cancer has been approximately 90 per cent.[47,48] The size and location of these tumors are not described in the reports. It is widely accepted, however, that small intrapancreatic tumors cannot be detected by CT scan except by the presence of indirect signs, such as hepatobiliary dilatation.

It is not clear whether CT scan or ultrasound is the more accurate method for identifying early lesions of the ampulla or the head of the pancreas. Taylor et al.[43] prospectively evaluated ultrasound in 83 patients with symptoms suggestive of pancreatic cancer. Ultrasound correctly diagnosed as positive 16 of 17 patients later proven to have cancer of the pancreas (sensitivity of 94 per cent). It likewise showed 65 to 66 patients negative for cancer, for a specificity of 99 per cent. Refined techniques of imaging resulted in complete visualization of the pancreas in 90 per cent of cases studied, a figure higher than is usually reported. The advantages of ultrasonography over CT scan include lower cost, avoidance of radiation exposure, and better resolution of small lesions, especially those in the region of the head of the pancreas. Based on these data, Taylor advocates ultrasound as the initial diagnostic test in patients whose clinical history is suspect for periampullary and pancreatic neoplasms.

Kamin et al.[49] directly compared CT scan with ultrasound in the diagnosis of pancreatic lesions in 102 patients. Only 64 of 102 patients had technically adequate ultrasound examinations, compared with 100 of 102 adequate CT scans. When ultrasound was technically adequate, its accuracy (84 per cent) was not statistically different from CT scan (96 per cent). Owing to the high numbers of technically inadequate ultrasound studies, the authors recommended CT scan as the preferred initial noninvasive diagnostic test in patients suspected of having periampullary lesions.

In interpreting the literature it is our opinion that with increasing refinement of ultrasonic scanning techniques, the percentage of technically satisfactory tests should be equal to that of CT scan. In addition, small lesions that do not disrupt the pancreatic capsule, such as ampullary lesions, are more likely to be missed on CT scan. For these reasons, and the facts that ultrasound is less expensive than CT scanning and does not expose the patient to ionizing radiation, we recommend that ultrasound be the initial diagnostic test in the directed work-up for periampullary cancer. CT scanning can be utilized when the ultrasound examination is technically inadequate or when additional information concerning surrounding structures is required.

Fiberoptic Gastroduodenoscopy and Biopsy

ERCP (endoscopic retrograde cholangiopancreatography) is performed with the use of a lateral viewing duodenoscope. After entering the duodenum, the examiner identifies the main papilla or papilla of Vater, does a biopsy if it is abnormal, and cannulates it with a Teflon ERCP catheter. Contrast studies are performed next with diluted Renografin. The principal complications of ERCP are injection pancreatitis and sepsis.

Ampullary lesions are diagnosed by the presence of an ulcerating tumor mass replacing the ampulla of Vater. Duodenal lesions adjacent to the papilla as well as carcinomas arising in the distal common bile duct will also be identified and may undergo biopsy. In patients with very small ampullary tumors, a biopsy forceps may be passed into the ampulla. Endoscopic papillotomy may be needed in these cases in order to approach the lesion directly.[150,153] In addition, endoscopic papillotomy may temporarily relieve biliary obstruction in some patients with relatively small tumors that have produced complete biliary obstruction.[151]

In a prospective study of patients with periampullary cancer, Hall et al.[50] found that ERCP could be performed successfully in 78 per cent of 112 examinations. Technical failures were due to gastric outlet obstruction in four patients and an inability to cannulate the ampulla of Vater in 21 patients. Successfully performed ERCP had a 92 per cent accuracy (34/37) in diagnosing periampullary cancer.

Harada et al.[51] found that endoscopic aspiration cytology was diagnostic in 100 per cent of patients with ampullary cancer. This is advantageous because it allows the surgeon to proceed to definitive operative therapy without opening the duodenum during surgery or performing transduodenal biopsy.

Fiberoptic gastroduodenoscopy is probably the most valuable preoperative diagnostic tool for periampullary carcinoma. Not only does it allow direct visualization of the lesion but it also enables a tissue diagnosis to be made at this time.

Pancreatic Scan

The use of selenomethionine (^{75}Se), which is picked up selectively by the pancreas, has been popularized in recent years. The greatest deficiency of this method is that its resolution is such that lesions smaller than 2 to 3 cm in diameter cannot be detected. Wood et al.[52] found that pancreatic scan correctly diagnosed 57 per cent of those patients with pancreatic carcinoma with a false positive rate of 13 per cent and a false negative rate of 30 per cent. Because of the failure to make the correct diagnosis in 43 per cent of patients, this test has not achieved major clinical importance as a diagnostic tool.

In evaluation of the usefulness of ultrasound, CT scan, ERCP, and angiography, attempts have been made to identify which test is most accurate in diagnosing periampullary lesions and what sequence of tests should be used when more than one is necessary. Wood et al.[52] prospectively analyzed ultrasound, CT scan, ERCP with biopsy, and angiography in 89 patients suspected of having pancreatic cancer. Ultrasound was found to be more accurate than CT scan or angiography in the detection of a periampullary mass, while ERCP with biopsy achieved the highest rate of correct diagnosis. Based on their findings, the authors concluded that ultrasound should be the first investigation in patients suspected of having pancreatic or periampullary lesions and that ERCP with biopsy was the procedure most likely to provide a definitive diagnosis. This study, however, did not evaluate the CT scan.

We agree that in a patient suspected of harboring a periampullary cancer, ultrasound should be the first diagnostic test in the work-up. If the results are positive for a lesion, the next test should be ERCP with biopsy and/or aspiration cytology. Selective celiac and superior mesenteric angiography should be performed next to delineate the foregut vasculature and assess resectability in preparation for exploratory laparotomy. CT scan may be utilized if the initial ultrasound study is technically inadequate or if additional information concerning surrounding organs is desired.

Tumor Markers

Because of the poor survival rates for cancer of the pancreas and periampullary lesions, a screening test for these neoplasms would be highly desirable to potentially improve survival rates. Significant work to date has been done on three fetal antigens, namely carcinoembryonic antigen (CEA), alpha fetoprotein (AFP), pancreatic oncofetal antigen (POA), as well as the enzyme pancreatic ribonuclease. Thus far, no agent has been found to be a definitive marker for cancer of the pancreas.

Carcinoembryonic Antigen (CEA)

CEA was first identified by Gold and Freedman in 1965.[53] Although now known to be unsuitable for mass screening to detect occult colon cancer, it has been shown to be useful in monitoring selected patients who have been resected for cure and are at risk to develop recurrent or metastatic disease. In this setting, a rising CEA level may be the first indication of metastases and can appear before any other objective evidence.

CEA values are elevated in approximately 80 per cent of patients with pancreatic cancer if all stages of disease are considered.[54,55] The precise role of CEA in the diagnosis and management of pancreatic and periampullary lesions remains to be defined. Although produced by some pancreatic cancers, it is not produced by all. In addition, CEA is produced by many other neoplastic and nonneoplastic abdominal conditions.

Ona et al.[55] found serum CEA levels to be elevated in 85 per cent (23/27) of patients with pancreatic malignancy; values greater than 2.5 ng/ml were considered elevated. Eighteen of the 27 patients had CEA values greater than 5 ng/ml. In Ona's study, CEA determinations were found to be superior to upper gastrointestinal series, hypotonic duodenography, celiac arteriography, percutaneous transhepatic cholangiography, and liver scanning in making the diagnosis of pancreatic cancer. Most patients in this study, however, had advanced disease. This confirmed the findings of others, i.e., that patients with advanced pancreatic cancer will have elevated CEA levels, but this in no way allows for improved earlier diagnosis.

Kalser et al.[54] studied 102 patients with histologically proven pancreatic and periampullary lesions. He showed that circulating CEA levels were increased in 80 per cent of patients (81/102) if levels above 5 ng/ml were considered abnormal. Patients with localized, resectable disease (Group I) had the lowest levels of CEA, followed by those with locally invasive, nonresectable disease (Group II). The highest levels were found in patients with distant metastatic disease (Group III). In each group, however, approximately 20 per cent had normal (<5 ng/ml) CEA levels. Jaundiced patients had higher levels of CEA than did nonicteric patients in each group. In Groups II and III, those patients who had CEA levels less than 5 ng/ml survived significantly longer than those with CEA levels greater than 5 ng/ml. The authors concluded that CEA could be helpful in two respects: (1) In nonjaundiced patients with known pancreatic disease, CEA levels greater than 9.0 ng/ml were highly suggestive of malignant rather than inflammatory disease; and (2) in patients with unresectable lesions, survival time was significantly longer when the CEA level was less than 5 ng/ml (9.5 versus 4.5 months in Group II, and 5.3 versus 2.5 months in Group III). CEA was thus a prognostic indicator in these patients.

Fitzgerald et al.[56] evaluated the accuracy of various diagnostic techniques in 184 patients suspected of having cancer of the pancreas. If CEA levels greater than 2.5 ng/ml were considered abnormal, 83 per cent (75/90) had positive values and 17 per cent (15/90) had normal levels and thus had false negative studies; there were 49 per cent false positive results (18/37). If abnormal levels were raised to 5 ng/ml, only 57 per cent of patients had elevated values (51/90). False negative findings occurred in 43 per cent (39/90) and false positive findings in 11 per cent (4/37) of patients. CEA thus appeared to be relatively unreliable as a diagnostic test.

The CEA elevations in pancreatic secretions are higher (and occur earlier) than the simultaneous serum determinations. Brandstatter et al.[57] combined ERCP, aspiration cytology, and CEA levels in aspirated pancreatic secretions. They achieved a 100 per cent diagnostic accuracy in 47 patients studied, nine of whom had pancreatic cancer.

CEA levels are influenced in pancreatic malignancy by the degree of cellular differentiation; undifferentiated lesions produce the highest levels of CEA.[54] They are also affected by the extent of local disease and the presence of hepatic metastases. In addition, biliary obstruction will raise CEA levels further.[58]

According to Zamcheck and Martin,[59] CEA is not elevated in early pancreatic cancer because the lesions are ductal and much of the antigen is secreted into the duodenum, so that little or no CEA may enter the circulation. In addition, the normal liver has a high ability to clear CEA from the blood stream. In periampullary lesions, the level of CEA reaching the blood stream may be too small to be detected in the absence of jaundice. Following resection, however, CEA may be a useful tool to assess disease-free state or progression of disease.

In summary, although CEA values are often elevated in patients with pancreatic and periampullary cancer, elevations are most common with advanced, unresectable disease. Also, many other abdominal neoplastic and non-neoplastic diseases, such as chronic pancreatitis, nonmalignant obstructive jaundice, and cirrhosis of the liver, produce elevations of CEA. It is thus unlikely that CEA will prove to be particularly useful either as a screening agent or as a diagnostic test for pancreatic and periampullary cancer.[60]

Pancreatic Oncofetal Antigen (POA)

A new fetal antigen, separate from CEA, was reported in 1974 by Banwo et al.,[61] who termed it pancreatic oncofetal antigen (POA). Wood and Moossa[62] investigated the value of CEA, POA, and AFP in 38 patients with proven pancreatic cancer. The sensitivity of POA was 91 per cent compared with 57 per cent for CEA and 3 per cent for AFP. True positive results were 60 per cent for POA versus 48 per cent for CEA. True negative results were 94 per cent for POA versus 75 per cent for CEA. In this study, a negative result essentially ruled out pancreatic cancer. When *both* CEA and POA were elevated, true positivity rose to 73 per cent. Most of these patients had advanced disease, however. The authors concluded that although POA was superior to either CEA or AFP, it could not stand alone as a diagnostic screening test for pancreatic cancer. A negative test, however, excluded the presence of pancreatic cancer with an error rate of only 6 per cent. In a subsequent study,[63] Moossa examined over 750 patients suspected of having pancreatic cancer. The highest levels of POA were found in the sera of patients with pancreatic cancer; increased levels of POA were also found in the sera of patients with cancer of the lung, stomach, colon, biliary tract, and breast. Elevated values of POA were found in some patients with benign conditions. POA, unlike CEA, was more apt to be elevated in patients with well-differentiated carcinomas. The authors showed in eight patients with high preoperative POA values, an abrupt fall following resection, with rising postoperative levels paralleling tumor recurrence. Those with initially low levels showed no response either to resection or to subsequent development of metastases. The authors felt that although not diagnostic, an elevated POA taken in conjunction with other symptoms should lead to a more comprehensive work-up of the pancreas to rule out malignancy. A negative POA in this study essentially excluded pancreatic cancer.

Alpha Fetoprotein (AFP)

Alpha fetoprotein (AFP) was measured *prospectively* in 38 patients with proven pancreatic cancer.[62] Of these, only 3 per cent had a positive test for AFP (>40 ng/ml). AFP was inferior to both CEA and POA as a tumor marker in this study; it probably has no use as a diagnostic tool or screening agent in pancreatic cancer.

Pancreatic Ribonuclease (RNase)

In 1976, Reddi and Holland[64] evaluated serum ribonuclease (RNase) as a possible tumor marker for cancer of the pancreas. Of 30 patients with pancreatic cancer, 90 per cent had RNase levels in excess of 250 units/ml, whereas 90 per cent of 69 patients with other forms of cancer (breast, colon, lung, and stomach) had levels below this value. Elevations were also seen in patients with severe renal insufficiency, so proper interpretation depended on normal renal function. The authors concluded that serum RNase could serve as a biochemical marker for carcinoma of the pancreas, with values greater than 250 units/ml necessitating appropriate clinical examination to establish the diagnosis. Other studies evaluating RNase as a biochemical marker for pancreatic cancer, however, have not been as encouraging.[65, 66] Elevations of RNase have been found in cancers of the ovary[67] and the colon,[68] in myelogenous leukemia,[69] and in nonmalignant conditions such as hepatocellular necrosis, acute cholecystitis, and acute pancreatitis.[68] Therefore, the clinical usefulness of serum RNase as a specific tumor marker for cancer of the pancreas is, at best, questionable. One reason for the discrepancy between the findings of Reddi and Holland[64] and those of subsequent studies is that differing methods to assay RNase were used. Warshaw et al.,[70] using biochemical assays identical to those of Reddi and Holland, found that 20 of 29 patients with biopsy-proven cancer of the pancreas had serum RNase levels above the upper limit of normal. No patient (0/12) with chronic pancreatitis had an abnormal serum RNase value. The sensitivity of RNase was 69 per cent, while the specificity of elevated RNase was 90 per cent. The authors felt that the relatively low sensitivity (69 per cent) constituted a serious limitation to the value of serum RNase as a screening test. They thought, however, that the finding of elevated serum RNase levels might be particularly helpful in distinguishing carcinoma from other causes of biliary obstruction, including chronic pancreatitis, and in selecting those patients who require more invasive studies. Despite initial enthusiasm, RNase, as CEA and POA before it, has been found to be too nonspecific to serve as a biochemical marker for pancreatic cancer. It may eventually prove useful, however, to distinguish pancreatic cancer from other conditions such as chronic pancreatitis in the context of a comprehensive diagnostic work-up.

In conclusion, none of the markers described have the sensitivity or specificity required to serve as a diagnostic or screening agent for pancreatic cancer. POA is the only marker that has been shown to be of some value in monitoring the effectiveness of surgery and in predicting recurrence in selected patients with resectable pancreatic and periampullary cancer.

TREATMENT

The problem the surgeon faces with periampullary tumors may be summarized as follows:

A. Preoperative and operative diagnosis
B. What to do when the diagnosis of periampullary carcinoma is made
   1. Pancreaticoduodenectomy (Whipple procedure)
   2. Total pancreatectomy
   3. Pylorus-preserving pancreaticoduodenectomy
   4. Transduodenal local resection
   5. Palliative bypass procedure

Preoperative and Operative Diagnosis

In our series, the preoperative diagnosis of ampullary carcinoma was made in only 26 per cent of the patients. However, in another 34 per cent the preoperative diagnosis was carcinoma of the head of the pancreas. It should be noted that many of our patients presented before the advent of ERCP, ultrasonography, and skinny needle transhepatic cholangiography. *With current techniques a periampullary carcinoma should be diagnosed preoperatively in over 90 per cent of cases.*

The differentiation between periampullary carcinoma and carcinoma of the head of the pancreas is by no means clear. In fact, although it is commonly stated that carcinoma of the head of the pancreas has a much worse prognosis than does ampullary carcinoma, it is usually not clear on what criteria the differentiation between these two entities is made. Periampullary carcinomas include tumors having their primary origin from the terminal part of the duct of Wirsung, from smaller ducts near the ampulla, and from surrounding duodenal mucosa. In other words, some of the ampullary tumors really arise from the head of the pancreas, and, in our view, the diagnosis of periampullary carcinoma versus carcinoma of the head of the pancreas is a macroscopic topographic rather than a histologic diagnosis. The typical ampullary tumor has a fungating or ulcerating surface seen from the duodenal aspect. With larger tumors arising in the head of the pancreas, it is usually difficult to state the primary site of origin. The better prognosis ascribed to ampullary tumors may reflect a smaller and less advanced tumor rather than a tumor with a biologic potential different from that of a cancer of the head of the pancreas. In a large series, Warren et al.[71] reported that the operative mortality was less and the chances of long-term survival higher with periampullary cancers than with cancers of the head of the pancreas. In a multi-institutional study in Japan by Nakase et al.,[72] however, only 17 of 330 patients with cancer of the ampulla survived for 5 years.

Ampullary tumors can be felt by compressing the lateral wall of the duodenum against the medial wall. If the presence of a periampullary tumor is suspected and if a biopsy-proven diagnosis has not been made preoperatively, we feel that duodenotomy should be performed at the level of the ampulla, followed by biopsy under direct vision.

The accuracy and risk of pancreatic biopsy has been evaluated by Lightwood et al.,[73] who retrospectively analyzed 177 pancreatic biopsies at their institution. Of these, 153 were wedge biopsies and 24 were needle core biopsies with the Vim-Silverman needle. Wedge biopsies had a false negative rate of 14 per cent, and core biopsies had a false negative rate of 50 per cent. Direct wedge biopsy had a serious complication rate of 3 per cent, but there were no deaths; needle biopsy resulted in three complications (14 per cent) with two deaths (9 per cent). There were five transections of a major pancreatic duct with wedge biopsy(5/153 = 3 per cent) and one transection with needle core biopsy (1/24 = 4 per cent). No false positive results were noted with either technique. This study suggests that open wedge biopsy, in general, is safer and more reliable than needle core biopsy. This is due, in part, to the fact that open biopsy allows for visualization of damage (i.e., transected pancreatic duct).

An alternative technique to wedge biopsy and needle core biopsy is the fine or *skinny needle aspiration*. This consists of aspiration of tissue with a 23-gauge needle and staining of the contents on a slide by the Papanicolaou method. The cross-sectional area of this needle is 14 times less than that of the Vim-Silverman needle. It is a technique that dates from the 1930s[74] but until recently had not enjoyed widespread popularity in the United States. Its efficacy and safety, however, have been confirmed by a number of studies in the European literature. Because of the known complications of open biopsy of the pancreas either by wedge or by needle core biopsy, needle aspiration is an attractive alternative technique for intraoperative use. Several studies have indicated its high accuracy and safety for intraoperative evaluation of suspicious pancreatic lesions.[75, 76] Christoffersen and Paul,[75] confirmed 66 of 68 cases of pancreatic cancer with a fine needle aspiration biopsy. Other studies have shown a similarly high accuracy rate with this technique.[77] The needle used in aspiration biopsy is shorter than the core biopsy needle and more easily manipulated; because of the thin diameter, the tract seals without difficulty. Percutaneous preoperative aspiration biopsy, whereby the needle is guided via ultrasound[77, 78] or CT scan in localizing the tumor, is gaining favor in many centers. This technique allows for a diagnosis to be made preoperatively and may in certain situations obviate the need for a laparotomy (such as in a jaundiced patient with obvious metastases).

One disadvantage of the skinny needle biopsy is the lack of sufficient numbers of trained personnel to read the slide after biopsy.[79] Tumor seeding through percutaneous tracts is another theoretical complication. Needle tract implantation has been reported with the use of core type needles in several cases.[80] Kline and Neal,[81] however, reviewed more than 3000 skinny needle aspirations and failed to document a single instance of implantation. Similarly, Ho et al.[82] reported more than 1500 abdominal percutaneous aspirations without an implantation.

Pancreatic biopsy with confirmation of malignancy should usually precede pancreatoduodenectomy in most cases of suspected cancer. In our series of pancreatoduodenectomies, in 9 per cent of patients there was no evidence of carcinoma on frozen tissue section.[24] Similarly, in the series of Crile et al.,[83] of 29 biopsies with carcinoma of the ampulla, 10 per cent were false negative. An impacted stone in the ampulla may mimic an ampullary tumor. It is clear that it is impossible to obtain positive tissue diagnosis for periampullary cancer 100 per cent of the time. In the few cases in which the clinical suspicion of a surgeon with extensive experience in pancreatic tumors remains high, based on diagnostic work-up and operative findings, and repeated attempts at biopsy fail to confirm malignancy, we believe it is permissible to proceed with radical resection. The patient must be carefully prepared for such an event and must understand the possible untoward metabolic consequences of pancreaticoduodenectomy versus the chance of losing the opportunity for cure through resection of a small occult periampullary lesion. We do not believe that surgeons without special training and experience in pancreatic neoplasms should undertake Whipple resection without tissue confirmation.

What to do When the Diagnosis of Periampullary Carcinoma is Made

The results of pancreatoduodenectomy for carcinomas of the head of the pancreas, in general, have been disappointing. The results with periampullary carcinomas, however, have been reported to be much better. Pancreatoduodenectomy should be avoided in the presence of metastases or lesions that extend into the bile ducts beyond the limits of resection.[84]

Pancreatoduodenectomy (Whipple Procedure)

Pancreatoduodenectomy is usually carried out as a one-stage procedure, but in extremely poor-risk patients with high serum bilirubin levels, T-tube choledochostomy has sometimes been used as a first-stage procedure to relieve the jaundice.[6] The technique of percutaneous transhepatic biliary drainage has rendered the need for preliminary T-tube choledochostomy unnecessary to achieve biliary decompression before performing a pancreatoduodenectomy.

Fish and Cleveland,[85] in a review of the literature up to 1964, collected 1169 cases of pancreatoduodenectomy for periampullary cancer with 19.9 per cent operative mortality. Since 1964, more than 2000 additional cases have been reported. The collected results of pancreatoduodenectomy for periampullary cancers have been summarized in Table 34–3. Our results with pancreatoduodenectomy, local excision, and palliative bypass procedures for periampullary carcinomas are shown in Tables 34–4 to 34–6.

The complications of pancreatoduodenectomy have been reviewed by Warren and Jefferson[25] and Braasch and Fray.[86] Since most of the morbidity and mortality after pancreatoduodenectomy results from leakage at the site of pancreatojejunostomy,[25] since malignant cells have been found within the ductal system at operation,[87] since transection may lead to seeding, and since ductal carcinoma may be multicentric,[88] total pancreatectomy has also been advised for periampullary cancer.[89]

Total Pancreatectomy

Although multicentricity and the potential for performing a more complete lymph node dissection argue in favor of total pancreatectomy, no clear-cut advantage either in increased survival or in decreased morbidity has been shown in the literature when comparing total pancreatectomy with the Whipple resection. Whereas Brooks and Culebras[90] reported a longer survival time for total pancreatectomy in a small series, Piorkowski et al.[91] showed no difference in length of survival or postoperative complications between the two operations. When considering truly periampullary lesions, i.e., ampulla of Vater, distal common bile duct, or duodenum, the question of multicentricity is probably not applicable; we therefore recommend the Whipple procedure for all operable lesions of the periampullary region.

Pylorus-Preserving Pancreaticoduodenectomy

The pylorus-preserving pancreaticoduodenal resection retains the entire stomach,

Table 34–3 PANCREATODUODENECTOMY FOR PERIAMPULLARY CARCINOMA

Author	Year	Number of Patients	Operative Mortality (%)	3-Year Survival Rate (%)*	5-Year Survival Rate (%)*
Fish and Cleveland[85] (collected series)	1964	1169	19.9	—	—
Fish and Cleveland[85]	1964	38	23.7	10.3	3.4
Buckwalter et al.[112]	1964	53†	22.6	—	—
Jordan[113]	1964	28	21.4	40.0	35.7
Judd[114]	1964	28	21.4	—	—
Monge et al.[115]	1964	120	17.5	48.1	35.3
Monge et al.[116]	1964	37	10.8	—	27.3
Moody and Thorbjarnarson[117]	1964	24	25.0	61.1	33.3
Child and Frey[118]	1966	21	33.3	—	25.0
Longmire and Shafey[119]	1966	13	15.4	36.4	27.3
Maki et al.[120]	1966	42	31.0	—	—
Sako[121]	1966	11	0.0	27.3	27.3
Salmon[122]	1966	35	16.0	48.3	37.9
Warren et al.[71]	1967	156	14.7	—	32.6
Howard[123]	1968	14	0.0	—	—
Sato et al.[124]	1968	48	29.2	—	—
Beall et al.[125]	1970	14	21.4	—	9.1
Crile et al.[126]	1970	29	20.0	—	13.0
Ponka and Uthappa[127]	1971	11	0.0	—	36.4
Dencker[128]	1972	39	28.0	27.0	23.0
Lansing et al.[129]	1972	22	45.4	—	41.6
Baker et al.[130]	1973	15	26.7	45.5	36.4
Crane et al.[131]	1973	26	23.0	—	42.0
Gilsdorf and Spanos[132]	1973	88†	23.0	—	17.4
Longmire[133]	1973	26	13.8	—	33.2
Smith[134]	1973	180	4.4	47.1	30.8
Aston and Longmire[135]	1974	26	13.8	—	—
Gatti et al.[136]	1974	11	27.3	—	37.5
Wilson and Block[137]	1974	13	23.0	—	30.0
Hoffman and Donegan[138]	1975	14	14.3	—	54.0
Wise et al.[24]	1975	39	15.3	45.5	24.2
Warren et al.[139]	1975	198	15.0	42.0	32.0
Makipour et al.[140]	1976	23	8.0	—	17.0
Akwari et al.[99]	1977	87	12.6	—	34.0
Coutsoftides et al.[141]	1977	12	17.0	—	40.0
Sato et al.[142]	1977	46	7.0	33.0	26.0
Nakase et al.[72] (57 institutions)	1977	351	16.0	9.0	6.0
Stephenson et al.[143]	1977	53	17.0	—	12.0
Schlippert et al.[95]	1978	31	22.6	—	12.5
Forrest and Longmire[144]	1979	34	11.0	—	21.0
Williams et al.[145]	1979	27	11.0	—	27.0
Herter et al.[146]	1982	45	—	—	27.8
Piorkowski et al.[91]	1982	19	11.0	15.0	5.0
Walsh et al.[147]	1982	44	15.9	—	11.0
Cohen et al.[148]	1982	49	2.4	—	28.0
Combined data		3409	18.4	‡	‡
Data since 1964		2240	17.7	‡	23.4

*These survival figures are corrected and include only those patients who survived the operation; reports of fewer than 10 cases are excluded.

†Includes head of pancreas.

‡Not determinable based on available information.

Dashed line indicates data not stated in article.

Table 34–4 SURVIVAL DATA ACCORDING TO PROCEDURE

Procedure	Percentage
Pancreatoduodenectomy (39 patients)	
Operative mortality (died within 1 month)	15.3 (6/39)
3-Year crude survival	38.4 (15/39)
5-Year crude survival	20.5 (8/39)
Local Excision (8 patients)	
Operative mortality	12.5 (1/8)
3-Year survival	50.0 (4/8)
5-Year survival	37.5 (3/8)
Palliative Procedures (15 patients)	
Operative mortality	6.6 (1/15)
Survival (not corrected for operative mortality)	
4.7 months	75.0
12.0 months	50.0
22.9 months	25.0

From Wise L, Pizzimbono C, Dehner L: Am J Surg 1976; *131*:141.

Table 34–5 PANCREATODUODENECTOMY SURVIVAL RATES (CRUDE) ACCORDING TO NODE INVOLVEMENT (FINAL PATHOLOGY SPECIMEN)

Interval	Positive Nodes (17)	Negative Nodes (22)	P Value
3 Years	29.4%	47.6%	$p < 0.05$
5 Years	11.7%	25.8%	$p < 0.05$

From Wise L, Pizzimbono C, Dehner L: Am J Surg 1976; *131*:141.

Table 34–6 SURGICAL COMPLICATIONS

Complication	Pancreato-duodenectomy	Local Excision	Palliative
Operative Mortality	6/39 (15.3%)	1/8 (12.5%)	2/15 (13.3%)
Complications	24/39 (62.0%)	2/8 (25.0%)	3/15 (20.0%)
Significant Complications*			
Pancreatic fistula	4	1	0
Biliary fistula	4	0	0
Fecal fistula	1	0	0
Wound infection	9	1	1
Wound dehiscence	0	0	0
Pelvic abscess	3	0	1
Subphrenic abscess	3	1	0
Gastrointestinal hemorrhage	2	0	0
Pulmonary complications	11	1	0
Renal failure	3	0	0
Intestinal obstruction	1†	0	0
Septicemia	4	1	0

*Not mutually exclusive.
†Fourteen days postoperatively, requiring bowel resection.
From Wise L, Pizzimbono C, Dehner L: Am J Surg 1976; *131*:141.

pylorus, and first part of the duodenum. It was developed by Traverso and Longmire[92] to minimize the undesirable gastrointestinal sequelae of the Whipple procedure. They subsequently advocated this technique for periampullary lesions of the head of the pancreas without lymph node metastases. It is probably not an adequate cancer operation for larger lesions of the head of the pancreas or distal common bile duct. The advantages of this technique are that the stomach is preserved intact and the patient does not have to modify the size of his meals. Long-term results comparing this operation with the standard pancreaticoduodenectomy are not yet available.[93]

Transduodenal Local Resection

Another alternative to pancreaticoduodenectomy is local resection of the periampullary tumor with reimplantation of the pancreatic and biliary ducts. As early as 1899, Halsted[94] reported a successful local resection for ampullary cancer. Whipple et al. summarized the results of transduodenal resection in 1935.[149] The operative mortality was 34 per cent. Of those who survived, 10 to 15 per cent lived for 3 years or longer. Since then, approximately 150 cases of transduodenal local excision have been reported by various authors. The mean operative mortality is around 25 per cent. However, most of these cases were reported before the antibiotic era. Although in most of these reports long-term follow-up data were not included, the results indicate that with the use of local excision for periampullary cancer, at least 37 patients survived from 2 to 22 years.

Schlippert et al.[95] reported on seven patients (mean age of 69 years) who underwent local resection; one died postoperatively; two of six subsequently required Whipple resection for recurrent disease. The mean survival for the group was 29.3 months. This compared with a 27.3 month survival for those patients undergoing Whipple resection at their institution. Others have reported similar experience.[152] In our study,[24] eight patients underwent local resection; 50 per cent survived for three years (4/8) and 38 per cent survived for five years (3/8). We suggest that local resection with reimplantation of the common bile and pancreatic ducts into the duodenum is an acceptable alternative procedure to pancreatoduodenectomy in elderly, poor-risk patients with small tumors.[24, 96] In the event of recurrence, the patient may require bypass surgery.

Palliative Bypass Procedure

If a periampullary carcinoma is unresectable, a palliative biliary drainage procedure should be considered, either by cholecystojejunostomy or by choledochojejunostomy, each with a diverting enteroenterostomy. It is also advisable to construct a gastroenterostomy simultaneously as a prophylactic measure against duodenal obstruction. Blievernicht et al.[97] reviewed 115 patients undergoing palliative bypass for unresectable periampullary carcinoma; of 93 patients presenting with biliary obstruction, 42 underwent biliary bypass alone and 51 underwent biliary bypass with prophylactic gastrojejunostomy. Of those patients who underwent only biliary diversion, 42 per cent (13/42) required a subsequent operation for gastroduodenal obstruction. Based on these results, the authors concluded that for most patients with unresectable periampullary tumors who develop biliary obstruction, a gastrojejunostomy should be constructed to avoid the need for further surgery. In another study from the Mayo Clinic, Sarr et al.[98] studied patients with unresectable pancreatic lesions. One hundred and seven patients who underwent biliary drainage alone were compared with 107 patients who underwent both biliary and gastric bypass. Of 53 patients in the biliary bypass group for whom adequate follow-up was available, eight (15 per cent) required reoperation for duodenal obstruction within 9 months. Only one patient who received a double bypass required reoperation for obstruction of the gastroenterostomy, which occurred 3 years after the initial operation. In our opinion, prophylactic gastric bypass should be performed in all patients with unresectable disease who have biliary obstruction and who are expected to live more than one or two months. The minimal morbidity of gastrojejunostomy is more than negated by the major morbidity of a second operation when gastroduodenal obstruction occurs.

FACTORS INFLUENCING SURVIVAL

Factors that have been shown to increase survival in ampullary cancer include negative regional lymph nodes, papillary as opposed to ulcerating lesions, and a high degree of histologic differentiation (Broder's Grades 1 and 2).[99] The mean survival of patients with positive nodes is only one-half to one-third that of patients with negative nodes. The ratio of positive to negative involvement has been approximately 1:4 with periampullary lesions in several recent studies. Some authors consider involved lymph nodes to be a contraindication to pancreaticoduodenectomy. In our study,[24] of 17 patients with positive nodes who underwent resection, 30 per cent lived three years and 12 per cent lived five years. This may be compared with 15 patients whose lesions were deemed unresectable for cure and who had bypass procedures; none of these patients survived for five years.

Warren et al. analyzed the survival of 348 patients with periampullary tumors operated on at the Lahey Clinic from 1942 to 1971.[100] Of 23 patients with ampullary lesions and positive nodes, only 9.5 per cent survived five years, as opposed to a 40 per cent five-year survival of patients with negative nodes (24/60). Involved lymph nodes outside the area of resection were considered a contraindication to pancreaticoduodenectomy for periampullary lesions.

CHEMOTHERAPY

Virtually all patients diagnosed as having cancer of the pancreas or periampullary region will succumb to their disease. Although on initial exploration many of the periampullary lesions will appear resectable, lymph node metastases will render many of these patients incurable by surgery alone. Therefore, chemotherapy and/or radiotherapy has been sought both for advanced disease not suitable for resection and as an adjuvant in those patients in whom pancreaticoduodenectomy has been performed. Historically, these tumors were thought to be unresponsive to both chemotherapy and radiotherapy. This was, in part, based on the fact that patients in earlier clinical trials were often severely debilitated, malnourished, or jaundiced. Such patients are not good candidates for chemotherapy. More recently, with proper patient selection based on performance status guides, single-agent and multiple-drug regimens have shown some effect on the course of advanced pancreatic cancer.

5-Fluorouracil (5-FU) has been the most widely used single agent. Partial response rates (shrinkage of measurable tumor up to 50 per cent) vary from 15 to 30 per cent if the drug is given intravenously.[101] Mitomycin C and streptozocin[102] have been used as single-agent drugs and have achieved partial response rates equal to those of 5-FU in several small series. Median survival has not changed with any single agent.

Multiple-drug regimens, combining several agents each known to have some effect on pancreatic cancer, have also been evaluated. Those with the highest response rate to date are the SMF regimen (streptozocin, mitomycin C and 5-FU) with a 43 per cent partial response rate (10/23)[103]; the FAM regimen (5-FU, Adriamycin, and mitomycin C) with a 37 per cent response rate (10/27);[104] and, most recently, FAM-S (5-FU, Adriamycin, mitomycin C, and streptozocin) with a 48 per cent response rate (12/25).[105] In the SMF study, Wiggins et al.[103] defined a partial response as a 50 per cent or greater decrease in measurable tumor mass 6 weeks after initiation of therapy. A complete remission represented the disappearance of all measurable lesions 6 weeks after initiation of therapy. In their study, 39 per cent of patients achieved a partial response (9/23) and one patient achieved a complete response. Median survival of responders was over 7 months, while nonresponders had a median survival of 3 months. Toxicity of the regimen included nausea and vomiting, myelosuppression, and nephrotoxicity (30 per cent of cases). The authors felt that these side effects were relatively well tolerated and easily manageable. Although in this study responders lived longer than did nonresponders, the authors concluded that this was not conclusively shown to be a direct result of the chemotherapy. Median survival for all patients was 6 months. In addition, there was no arm in this study to show the survival pattern of untreated controls.

Smith et al.,[104] using the FAM regimen, treated 39 patients with advanced metastatic adenocarcinoma of the pancreas; 27 of these patients had measurable disease; 37 per cent (10/27) achieved a partial response and three others had stabilization of disease. Median survival of responders was 12 months, compared with 3.5 months for nonresponders ($p<0.01$). Median survival for all patients was 6 months; toxicity consisted of mild to moderate gastrointestinal symptoms and myelosuppression. Unlike the SMF regimen, there was no nephrotoxicity. In general, the toxic side effects of FAM regimen appeared less severe than those of SMF regimen. Both studies were conducted in the same institution (Georgetown University). A study of Bitran et al.[106] with a modification of the FAM regimen reported a partial response in 40 per cent of patients treated (6/15), with a median survival in excess of 12 months. Although somewhat encouraging, all four studies were Phase II trials without patient randomization and without untreated controls, and hence without proof for increased survival. Such trials are necessary before combination chemotherapy can be recommended for the treatment of metastatic or unresectable pancreatic or periampullary lesions. There is no evidence that chemotherapy is of any value as an adjuvant following resection for periampullary or pancreatic carcinoma.

CURRENT RADIOTHERAPEUTIC APPROACHES TO PANCREATIC CANCER

The deep location of the pancreas and its relationship to the liver, the kidneys, and the spinal cord precluded delivery of large doses of external-beam radiation prior to the development of megavoltage techniques. Cancer of the pancreas was, therefore, thought to be radioresistant. This concept is changing, however, as the result of experience with the new modes of radiotherapy. Recently, increased effectiveness has been shown with the following modalities: implantation of radioisotopes,[107] precision high-dose radiotherapy,[108] intraoperative radiotherapy,[109] and combination radiotherapy and chemotherapy for unresectable or metastatic disease.[110]

Interstitial therapy with radioactive implants was one of the earliest modes of radiotherapy used in the treatment of periampullary and pancreatic lesions, but it was largely abandoned after the 1920s.[111] Shipley et al.[107] found no significant difference in survival patterns between a group of 12 patients treated with permanent I-125 implants together with 4000 to 5000 rads of external-beam irradiation and a group of 10 patients who underwent resection for cure at the same institution during the same time period.

Precision high-dose therapy refers to the delivery of up to 7000 rads of external radiotherapy to the pancreas while sparing the surrounding spinal cord, kidneys, and liver. At the Thomas Jefferson University Hospital, 41 patients with biopsy-proven unresectable pancreatic cancer were treated with this modality.[108] Their survival was comparable to that of 31 patients who had resection for cure at the Massachusetts General Hospital in a separate study that was used as a historical control.

The Gastrointestinal Tumor Study Group has completed a randomized prospective clinical trial comparing high-dose radiotherapy (6000 R) alone to 6000 R with 5-FU and 4000 R with 5-FU[110] for unresectable pancreatic carcinoma. The survival of the radiated group without chemotherapy (17 weeks) was significantly inferior to the other two groups (28 and 35 weeks), and this arm was dropped from the study. High-dose radiotherapy combined with chemotherapy offered improved survival (44 weeks) compared with either radiotherapy alone or moderate radiotherapy with chemotherapy (32 weeks).

One Japanese group reported improved palliation in 21 patients with unresectable pancreatic carcinoma who received a single intraoperative dose of 3000 to 4000 rads.[109] There was, however, no increased survival. This technique is currently being evaluated in trials at the National Cancer Institute, Howard University, and the Massachusetts General Hospital.

In conclusion, radiotherapy, once thought to be virtually useless in pancreatic cancer, may offer significant palliation in unresectable lesions. In fact, there are occasional long-term survivors.

REFERENCES

1. Silverberg E: Cancer statistics, 1983. CA 1983;*33*:16.
2. American Cancer Society: 1983 Cancer Facts & Figures. New York, American Cancer Society, 1983.
3. Gudjonsson B, Livstone EM, Spiro HM: Cancer of the pancreas: diagnostic accuracy and survival statistics. Cancer 1978;*42*:2492.
4. Duff GL: Clinical and pathological features of carcinoma of the body and tail of the pancreas. Bull Johns Hopkins Hosp 1939;*65*:69.
5. Aston SJ, Longmire WD: Pancreaticoduodenal resection. Arch Surg 1973;*106*:813.
6. Wilson SM, Block GE: Periampullary carcinoma. Arch Surg 1974;*108*:539.
7. Cancer Incidence and Mortality in the United States. SEER 1973–1976; Bethesda, MD, US Department of Health, Education, and Welfare. NIH Publication No. 78, 1978, p 1837.
8. Gray LW Jr, Crook NJ, Cohn I Jr: Carcinoma of

the pancreas. *In* Seventh National Cancer Conference Proceedings. Philadelphia, JB Lippincott Co, 1973, p 503.
9. Herter FP, Cooperman AM, Ahlborn TN, et al: Surgical experience with pancreatic and periampullary cancer. Ann Surg 1982;*195*:274.
10. Seidman H, Silverberg E, Bodden A: Probabilities of eventually developing and dying of cancer. CA 1978;*23*:33.
11. Wynder EL, Mabuchi K, Maruchi N, et al: Epidemiology of cancer of the pancreas. J Natl Cancer Inst 1973;*50*:645.
12. Kessler II: Cancer mortality among diabetics. J Natl Cancer Inst 1970;*44*:673.
13. Clark CC, Mitchell PEG: Diabetes mellitus and primary carcinoma of the pancreas. Br Med J 1961;*2*:1259.
14. Wynder EL: An epidemiologic evaluation of the causes of cancer of the pancreas. Cancer Res 1975;*35*:2228.
15. Hammond EC: Smoking in relation to the death rates of one million men and women. Natl Cancer Inst Monogr 1966;*19*:1.
16. Ishii K, Nakamura K, Ozaki H, et al: Epidemiological problems of pancreatic cancer (in Japanese). Jpn J Clin Med 1968;*26*:1839.
17. Pour PM, Runge RG, Birt D, et al: Current knowledge of pancreatic carcinogenesis in the hamster and its relevance to human disease. Cancer 1981;*47*:1573.
18. MacMahon B, Yen S, Trichopoulos D, et al: Coffee and cancer of the pancreas. N Engl J Med 1981;*304*:630.
19. Buncher CR: Epidemiology of pancreatic cancer. *In* Moosa AR (ed): Tumors of the pancreas. Baltimore, Williams & Wilkins, 1980, p 422.
20. Li FP, Fraumeni JF, Mantel N, et al: Cancer mortality among chemists. J Natl Cancer Inst 1969;*43*:1159.
21. Mancuso TF, El-Attar AA: Cohort study of workers exposed to beta naphthylamine and benzidine. J Occup Med 1967,*9*:277.
22. Cubilla AL, Fortner J, Fitzgerald PJ: Lymph node involvement in carcinoma of the head of the pancreas area. Cancer 1978;*41*:880.
23. Sawai M, Talvalkar GV: Periampullary carcinoma—a clinicopathologic study of twenty-two cases. Indian J Cancer 1977;*14*:325.
24. Wise L, Pizzimbono C, Dehner L: Periampullary cancer: a clinicopathologic study of sixty-two patients. Am J Surg 1976;*131*:141.
25. Warren KW, Jefferson MF: Carcinoma of the exocrine pancreas. *In* Carey LC (ed): The Pancreas. St. Louis, CV Mosby Co, 1973.
26. Courvoisier LG: Kasuistisch-statistische Beitrage zur Pathologie und Chirurgie der Gellenwege. Leipzig FCV, Vogel, 1890.
27. Clarke CN, Normal NJ, Smith JA, et al: Pancreatitis and duodenal obstruction due to periampullary carcinoma associated with familial polyposis coli. Postgrad Med J 1978;*54*:418.
28. Cooke SA: Polyposis coli. The clinical spectrum in adults. S Afr Med J 1978;*53*:454.
29. Suzanne J, Camelot G, Miguet JP, et al: Gardner's syndrome and duodenal adenocarcinoma. Study of a case and literature review. Gastroenterol Clin Biol 1977;*1*:455.
30. Turner AG: The importance of upper gastrointestinal tract assessment in Gardner's syndrome. Dr J Clin Pract 1976;*30*:178.
31. Qizilbash AH: Familial polyposis coli and periampullary carcinoma. Can J Surg 1976;*19*:166.
32. Mir-Madjlessi SH, Farmer RG, Hawk WA, et al: Adenocarcinoma of the ampulla of Vater associated with familial polyposis coli: report of a case. Dis Colon Rectum 1973;*16*:542.
33. Dreiling DA, Grenstein A: Diagnosis of pancreatic disease. *In* Carey LC (ed): The Pancreas. St. Louis, CV Mosby Co, 1973.
34. Crane JM, Gobbel WG, Scott HW: Surgical experience with malignant tumors of the ampulla of Vater and duodenum. Surg Gynecol Obstet 1973;*37*:937.
35. Mallet G, Jacquemet P: Results of 500 cases of hypotonic duodenography. J Radiol Electrol 1963;*44*:249.
36. Nakayama T, Ikeda A, Okuda K: Percutaneous transhepatic drainage of the biliary tract: technique and results in 104 cases. Gastroenterology 1978;*74*:554.
37. Norlander A, Kalin B, Sunblad R: Effect of percutaneous transhepatic drainage upon liver function and postoperative mortality. Surg Gynecol Obstet 1982;*155*:161.
38. MacGregor A, Hawkins IF: Selective pharmacodynamic angiography in the diagnosis of carcinoma of the pancreas. Surg Gynecol Obstet 1973; *137*:917.
39. Herlinger H, Finlay DB: Evaluation and follow-up of pancreatic arteriograms. A new role for angiography in the diagnosis of carcinoma of the pancreas. Clin Radiol 1978;*29*:277.
40. Herlinger H: Comparison of ultrasound and arteriography in the diagnosis of pancreatic carcinoma. Proceedings of the 13th International Congress of Radiology, Madrid. 1973;*2*:372.
41. Suzuki T, Tani T, Honjo I: Appraisal of arteriography for assessment of operability in periampullary cancer. Ann Surg 1975;*182*:66.
42. Doust BD: The use of ultrasound in the diagnosis of gastrointestinal disease. Gastroenterology 1976;*70*:602.
43. Taylor KJW, Buchin PJ, Viscomi GN, et al: Ultrasonographic scanning of the pancreas. Radiology 1981;*138*:211.
44. DiMagno EP: Pancreatic cancer: a continuing diagnostic dilemma. Ann Intern Med 1979;*90*:847.
45. Levitt RG, Geisse GG, Sagel SS, et al: Complementary use of ultrasound and computed tomography in studies of the pancreas and kidney. Radiology 1978;*126*:149.
46. Moss AA, Kressel HY: Computed tomography of the pancreas. Am J Dig Dis 1977;*22*:1018.
47. Fawcitt RA, Forbes WHC, Isherwood K, et al: Computed tomography in pancreatic disease. Br J Radiol 1978;*51*:1.
48. Haaga JR, Alfidi RJ, Harrilla TR, et al: Definitive role of CAT scanning of the pancreas. Radiology 1977;*124*:723.
49. Kamin DD, Bernardino ME, Wallace S, et al: Comparison of ultrasound and computed tomography in the detection of pancreatic malignancy. Cancer 1980;*46*:2410.
50. Hall TJ, Blackstone MO, Cooper MJ, et al: Prospective evaluation of endoscopic retrograde cholangiopancreatography in the diagnosis of periampullary cancers. Ann Surg 1978;*187*:313.
51. Harada H, Sasaki T, Yamamoto N, et al: Assessment of endoscopic aspiration cytology and endoscopic retrograde cholangiopancreatography in pa-

tients with cancer of the hepato-biliary tract. Part II. Gastroenterol Jpn 1977;*12*:59.
52. Wood RA, Moossa AR, Cushieri A: The prospective analysis of four methods of investigating the pancreas for carcinoma. Clin Oncol 1977;*3*:395.
53. Gold P, Freedman SO: Determination of tumor specific antigens in human carcinoma by immunologic tolerance and absorption techniques. J Exp Med 1965;*14*:439.
54. Kalser M, Barkin J, Redlhammer R, et al: Circulating carcinoembryonic antigen in pancreatic carcinoma. Cancer 1978;*42*:1468.
55. Ona FU, Zamcheck N, Dhar P, et al: Carcinoembryonic antigen (CEA) in the diagnosis of pancreatic cancer. Cancer 1973;*31*:324.
56. Fitzgerald PJ, Fortner JG, Watson RC, et al: The value of diagnostic aids in detecting pancreas cancer. Cancer 1978;*41*:868.
57. Brandstatter G, Kratochuil P, Wiedner F, et al: The diagnosis of pancreatic carcinoma by combined endoscopic retrograde pancreatography, aspiration cytology, and carcinoembryonic antigen determination in pancreatic secretions. Wien Klin Wochenschr 1978;*90*:347.
58. Barkin JS, Kalser MH, Kaplan R, et al: Initial levels of CEA and their rate of change in pancreatic carcinoma following surgery, chemotherapy, and radiation therapy. Cancer 1978;*42*:1472.
59. Zamcheck N, Martin EW: Factors controlling the circulating CEA levels in pancreatic cancer—some clinical correlations. Cancer 1981;*47*:1620.
60. Holyoke ED, Douglass HO, Goldrusen MH, et al: Tumor markers in pancreatic cancer. Semin Oncol 1979;*6*:347.
61. Banwo O, Versey J, Hoggs JR: A new oncofetal antigen for human pancreas. Lancet 1974;*1*:643.
62. Wood RAB, Moossa AR: The prospective evaluation of tumor associated antigens for the early diagnosis of pancreatic cancer. Cancer 1978; *42*:1620.
63. Moossa AR, Levin B: The diagnosis of "early" pancreatic cancer. Cancer 1981;*47*:1688.
64. Reddi KK, Holland JF: Elevated serum ribonuclease in patients with pancreatic cancer. Proc Natl Acad Sci 1976;*73*:2308.
65. Chretin PB, Mathews W Jr, Twomey PL: Serum ribonucleases in cancer: relation to tumor histology. Cancer 1973;*31*:175.
66. Kottel RH, Hoch SO, Parsons RG, et al: Serum ribonuclease activity in cancer patients. Br J Cancer 1978;*38*:280.
67. Sheid B, Lu T, Pedrinan L, et al: Plasma ribonuclease. A marker for the detection of ovarian cancer. Cancer 1977;*39*:2204.
68. Doran G, Allen-Mersh TG, Reynolds KW: Ribonuclease as a tumor marker for pancreatic cancer. J Clin Pathol 1980;*33*:1212.
69. Akagi K, Yamanaka M, Murai K, et al: Serum acid ribonuclease in myelogenous leukemia. Cancer Res 1978;*38*:2168.
70. Warshaw AL, Lee KH, Wood WC, et al: Sensitivity and specificity of serum ribonuclease in the diagnosis of pancreatic cancer. Am J Surg 1980;*139*:27.
71. Warren KW, Veidenheimer MC, Pratt HS: Pancreatoduodenectomy for periampullary cancer. Surg Clin North Am 1967;*47*:639.
72. Nakase A, Matsumoro Y, Urchida K, et al: Surgical treatment of cancer of the pancreas and the periampullary region: cumulative results in 57 institutions in Japan. Ann Surg 1977;*185*:52.
73. Lightwood R, Reber HW, Way LW: The risk and accuracy of pancreatic biopsy. Am J Surg 1976;*132*:189.
74. Martin HE, Ellis EB: Aspiration biopsy. Surg Gynecol Obstet 1939;*59*:578.
75. Christoffersen P, Paul P: Preoperative pancreas aspiration biopsies. Acta Pathol Microbiol Scand (Suppl) 1970;*212*:28.
76. Fosgren L, Orell S: Aspiration cytology in carcinoma of the pancreas. Surgery 1973;*73*:38.
77. Hancke S, Holm HH, Koch F: Ultrasonically guided percutaneous fine needle biopsy of pancreas. Surg Gynecol Obstet 1975;*140*:361.
78. Smith EH, Barton RJ, Young CC, et al: Percutaneous aspiration biopsy of the pancreas under ultrasonic guidance. N Engl J Med 1975;*292*:825.
79. Beazley RM: Percutaneous needle biopsy for diagnosis of pancreatic cancer. Semin Oncol 1979;*6*:344.
80. Burkholder GV, Kaufman JJ: Local implantation of carcinoma of the prostate with percutaneous needle biopsy. J Urol 1966;*95*:801.
81. Kline TE, Neal HS: Needle aspiration biopsy—A safe diagnostic procedure for lesions of the pancreas. Am J Clin Pathol 1975;*63*:16.
82. Ho CS, McLoughlin MJ, McHattie JD, et al: Percutaneous fine needle aspiration biopsy of the pancreas following endoscopic retrograde cholangiopancreatography. Radiology 1977;*125*:351.
83. Crile G Jr, Isbiter WH, Hawk WA: Carcinoma of the ampulla of Vater and the terminal bile and pancreatic ducts. Surg Gynecol Obstet 1970; *131*:1052.
84. Tompkins RK, Johnson J, Storm FK, et al: Operative endoscopy in the management of biliary tract neoplasms. Am J Surg 1976;*132*:174.
85. Fish JC, Cleveland BR: Pancreaticoduodenectomy for periampullary carcinoma. Analysis of 38 cases. Ann Surg 1964;*159*:469.
86. Braasch JW, Fray BN: Technique of radical pancreaticoduodenectomy with consideration of hepatic arterial relationships. Surg Clin North Am 1976;*56*:631.
87. Ron DE: Cancer of the pancreas: plea for total pancreatectomy. Am J Surg 1964;*159*:469.
88. Collins JJ, Craighead JE, Brooks JR: Rationale for total pancreatectomy for carcinoma of the pancreatic head. N Engl J Med 1966;*274*:599.
89. Phiam MB, ReMine WH: Further evaluation of total pancreatectomy. Arch Surg 1975;*110*:506.
90. Brooks JR, Culebras JM: Cancer of the pancreas. Palliative operation, Whipple procedure or total pancreatectomy? Am J Surg 1976;*131*:516.
91. Piorkowski RJ, Blievernicht SW, Way LW, et al: Pancreatic and periampullary carcinoma: experience with 200 patients over a 12-year period. Am J Surg 1982;*143*:189.
92. Traverso LW, Longmire WP Jr: Preservation of the pylorus in pancreaticoduodenectomy. Surg Gynecol Obstet 1978;*146*:959.
93. Longmire WP Jr, Traverso W: The Whipple procedure and other standard operative approaches to pancreatic cancer. Cancer 1981;*47*:1706.
94. Halsted WS: Contributions to the surgery of the bile passages, especially the common bile duct. Br Med Surg J 1899;*141*:645.
95. Schlippert W, Lucke D, Amuras S, et al: Carcinoma of the papilla of Vater: a review of fifty-seven cases. Am J Surg 1978;*135*:763.
96. Thorbjarnarson B: Carcinoma of the biliary tract:

III. Carcinoma of the ampulla of Vater. NY State J Med 1975;*75*:860.
97. Blievernicht SW, Neifeld JP, Terz JS, et al: The role of prophylactic gastrojejunostomy for unresectable periampullary carcinoma. Surg Gynecol Obstet 1980;*151*:794.
98. Sarr MG, Gladen HE, Beart RW, et al: Role of gastroenterostomy in patients with unresectable carcinoma of the pancreas. Surg Gynecol Obstet 1981;*152*:797.
99. Akwari OE, Van Heerden JA, Adson MA, et al: Radical pancreaticoduodenectomy for cancer of the ampulla of Vater. Arch Surg 1977;*112*:457.
100. Warren KW, Choe DS, Plaza J, et al: Results of radical resection for periampullary cancer. Ann Surg 1974;*181*:534.
101. Carter SK, Lomis SL: The integration of chemotherapy into a combined modality approach for cancer treatment. VI. Pancreatic adenocarcinoma. Cancer Treat Rev 1975;*2*:193.
102. Stolinsky NS, Sadoff L, Braunwald J, et al: Streptozotocin in the treatment of cancer: a phase II study. Cancer 1972;*30*:61.
103. Wiggins RG, Woolly PV, MacDonald JS, et al: Phase II trial of streptozotocin, mitomycin C, and 5-fluorouracil (SMF) in the treatment of advanced pancreatic cancer. Cancer 1978;*41*:387.
104. Smith FP, Hoth DF, Levin B, et al: 5-Fluorouracil, Adriamycin, and mitomycin C (FAM) chemotherapy for advanced adenocarcinoma of the pancreas. Cancer 1980;*46*:2014.
105. Bukowski RM, Schacter LP, Groppe CW, et al: Phase II trial of 5-fluorouracil, Adriamycin, mitomycin C, and streptozotocin (FAM-S) in pancreatic carcinoma. Cancer 1982;*50*:197.
106. Bitran JD, Desser RK, Kurloff MF, et al: Treatment of metastatic pancreatic and gastric adenocarcinomas with 5-fluorouracil, Adriamycin, and mitomycin C (FAM). Cancer Treat Rep 1979; *63*:11.
107. Shipley WU, Cohen AM, Nardi GL: A comparative study of surgery vs. radioactive iodine-125 implantation in the treatment of pancreatic cancer (Abstract). Int J Radiat Oncol 1978 (Suppl 2);117:1.
108. Dobelbower RR Jr, Strubler KA, Kutcher G, et al: Precision radiotherapy for cancer of the pancreas: techniques and results. Int J Radiat Oncol 1980;*6*:1127.
109. Hiroaka T, Nakagawa I, Tashiso S, et al: Intraoperative irradiation therapy for unresectable pancreatic cancer. Nippon Gan Ghiryo Gakki Shi 1975;*13*:146.
110. The Gastrointestinal Study Group: A multi-institutional comparative trial of radiation therapy alone and in combination with 5-fluorouracil for locally unresectable pancreatic cancer. Ann Surg 1979;*189*:205.
111. Fortner JG, D'Angelo GJ, Hilaris BS, et al: Iodine 125 implantation for unresectable cancer of the pancreas. Postgrad Med J 1970;*47*:226.
112. Buckwalter JA, Lawton RL, Tidrick RT: Pancreatoduodenectomy. Arch Surg 1964;*89*:331.
113. Jordan GL: Surgical management of carcinoma of the pancreas and periampullary region. Am J Surg 1964;*107*:313.
114. Judd ES: Surgery of the biliary tract and pancreas. Mayo Clinic Proc 1964;*39*:927.
115. Monge JJ, Dockerty MB, Wollaeger EE, et al: Clinicopathologic observations on radical pancreatoduodenal resection for periampullary carcinoma. Surg Gynecol Obstet 1964;*118*:275.
116. Monge JJ, Judd ES, Gage RP: Radical pancreatoduodenectomy. A 22-year experience with the complications, mortality rate and survival rate. Ann Surg 1964;*160*:711.
117. Moody F, Thorbjarnarson B: Carcinoma of the ampulla of Vater. Am J Surg 1964;*107*:572.
118. Child CG, Frey CF: Pancreaticoduodenectomy. Surg Clin North Am 1966;*46*:1201.
119. Longmire WP, Shafey OA: Certain factors influencing survival after pancreaticoduodenal resection for carcinoma. Am J Surg 1966;*3*:8.
120. Maki T, Sato T, Kakizaki G: Pancreatoduodenectomy for periampullary cancer. Arch Surg 1966;*92*:825.
121. Sako Y: Surgical experience with carcinoma of the pancreas and ampulla of Vater. Prog Clin Cancer 1966;*2*:309.
122. Salmon PA: Carcinoma of the pancreas and extrahepatic biliary system. Surgery 1966;*60*:554.
123. Howard JM: Pancreaticoduodenectomy: forty-one consecutive Whipple resections without an operative mortality. Ann Surg 1968;*168*:629.
124. Sato T, Saitoh Y, Koyama K, et al: Preoperative determination of operability in carcinomas of the pancreas and the periampullary region. Ann Surg 1968;*168*:876.
125. Beall MS, Dyer GA, Stephenson HE Jr: Disappointments in the management of patients with malignancy of pancreas, duodenum, and common bile duct. Arch Surg 1970;*101*:461.
126. Crile G, Isbister WH, Hawk WA: Carcinoma of the ampulla of Vater and the terminal bile and pancreatic ducts. Surg Gynecol Obstet 1970; *131*:1052.
127. Ponka JL, Uthappa NS: Carcinoma of the ampulla of Vater. Am J Surg 1970;*121*:263.
128. Dencker H: Pancreaticoduodenectomy for periampullary tumors. Acta Chir Scand 1972;*138*:293.
129. Lansing PB, Blalock JB, Ochsner JL: Pancreatoduodenectomy: a retrospective review from 1949 to 1969. Am J Surg 1972;*38*:79.
130. Baker RR, Pio Roda CA, Lee JM: Carcinoma of the head of the pancreas and periampullary region. Johns Hopkins Med J 1973;*132*:212.
131. Crane JM, Gobbel WG, Scott HW: Surgical experience with malignant tumors of the ampulla of Vater and duodenum. Surg Gynecol Obstet 1973;*137*:937.
132. Gilsdorf RB, Spanos P: Factors influencing morbidity and mortality in pancreatoduodenectomy. Ann Surg 1973;*177*:332.
133. Longmire WP: Periampullary tumors. J R Coll Surg Edinb 1973;*18*:131.
134. Smith R: Progress in the surgical treatment of pancreatic disease. Am J Surg 1973;*125*:143.
135. Aston SJ, Longmire WP: Management of the pancreas after pancreaticoduodenectomy. Ann Surg 1974;*179*:322.
136. Gatti DJ, O'Brien PH, Grooms GA: Analysis of pancreatoduodenectomy. South Med J 1974; *67*:278.
137. Wilson SM, Block GE: Periampullary carcinoma. Arch Surg 1974;*108*:539.
138. Hoffman RE, Donegan WL: Experience with pancreatoduodenectomy in a cancer hospital. Am J Surg 1975;*129*:292.
139. Warren KW, Choe DS, Plaza J, et al: Results of radical resection for periampullary cancer. Ann Surg 1975;*181*:534.
140. Makipour H, Cooperman A, Danzi J, et al: Carcinoma of the ampulla of Vater: review of 38 cases

with emphasis on treatment and prognostic factors. Ann Surg 1976;*183*:341.
141. Coutsoftides T, MacDonald J, Shibata HR: Carcinoma of the pancreas and periampullary region. A 41-year experience. Ann Surg 1977;*186*:730.
142. Sato T, Saitoh Y, Noto N, et al: Follow-up studies of radical resection for pancreaticoduodenal cancer. Ann Surg 1977;*186*:581.
143. Stephenson LW, Blackstone EH, Alderete JS: Radical resection for periampullary carcinomas: results in 53 patients. Arch Surg 1977; *112*:245.
144. Forrest JF, Longmire WP: Carcinoma of the pancreas and periampullary region—a study of 279 patients. Ann Surg 1979;*189*:129.
145. Williams JA, Cubilla A, Maclean B, et al: Twenty-two year experience with periampullary carcinoma at Memorial Sloan-Kettering Cancer Center. Am J Surg 1979;*138*:662.
146. Herter FD, Cooperman AM, Ahiborn TJ, et al: Surgical experience with pancreatic and periampullary cancer. Ann Surg 1982;*195*:274.
147. Walsh DB, Eckhauser FE, Cronenwett JL, et al: Adenocarcinoma of the ampulla of Vater. Ann Surg 1982;*195*:152.
148. Cohen JR, Kuaka N, Geller W, et al: Pancreaticoduodenectomy—a 40-year experience. Ann Surg 1982;*195*:608.
149. Whipple AO, Parsons WB, Mullins CR: Treatment of carcinoma of the ampulla of Vater. Ann Surg 1935;*102*:763.
150. Nako NL, Siegel JH, Stenger RJ, et al: Tumors of the ampulla of Vater—early diagnosis by intraampullary biopsy during endoscopic cannulation. Gastroenterology 1982;*83*:459.
151. Alderson D, Lavelle MI, Venables CW: Endoscopic sphincterotomy before pancreaticoduodenectomy for ampullary carcinoma. Br Med J 1981;*282*:1109.
152. Isaksson G, Ihse J, Andren-Sandberg A, et al: Local excision for ampullary carcinoma. Acta Chir Scand 1982;*148*:163.
153. Siegel JH, Yatto RP: Endoscopic evaluation and therapy of periampullary adenoma. Am J Gastroenterol 1983;*78*:225.

SECTION VI

OTHER ASPECTS OF BILIARY TRACT DISEASE

G. B. ONG, D.Sc.

35

Recurrent Pyogenic Cholangitis

Recurrent pyogenic cholangitis, a term coined by Cook et al.,[1] is a condition characterized by episodic attacks of Charcot's intermittent fever. It is a pancholangitis resulting from obstruction by gallstones in the intra- or extrahepatic biliary tract. In addition, the gallbladder may contain stones. It is one of the most common conditions seen in developing countries in Eastern and Southern Asia and is found principally in areas of lower economic development. The patient is usually acutely ill and may have had several previous attacks. In the beginning the attacks may be mild, and spontaneous remission usually occurs. Repeated attacks, however, may lead to acute liver failure or, gradually, to biliary cirrhosis.

INCIDENCE

Recurrent pyogenic cholangitis is the most common abdominal emergency hospital admission in Hong Kong.[2] It is also found in other areas in Southeast Asia, including Malaysia, Vietnam, Taiwan, and the Philippines. It is widespread among Chinese throughout China. On the North American continent and in other Caucasian countries, the disease is also encountered among Chinese immigrants, and it may first appear years after they have settled in the new country. It is still prevalent in Japan and Korea, although the distribution in these countries is now mostly confined to rural areas.

Sex Incidence. Distribution is equal in both sexes, similar to the incidence of intrahepatic stones described by Rufanov[3] in Russia. It is most common in the third, fourth, and fifth decades of life but is also seen in extremes of age, and even children may be affected.[1, 4–6]

PATHOLOGY

Recurrent pyogenic cholangitis involves the entire hepatobiliary system.[6] The changes are most marked in the intrahepatic ducts. Generally, the liver is enlarged and edematous, and after many attacks it may be scarred and distorted. The intrahepatic ducts may be stenosed, with proximal dilatation and sometimes sacculation. The liver parenchyma may become thin and the duct walls thickened. The ducts may contain myriad stones with infected bile or mucus. Occasionally, the junction between the right and left hepatic ducts may be strictured while the caliber of the common bile duct remains normal (Fig. 35–1).

Liver

Microscopically, the lesion in the liver is confined mainly to the portal tracts.[6] There is extensive infiltration by polymorphonuclear leukocytes, which diminishes toward the central vein. In severe cases, thrombosis of the portal radicles and even suppuration may occur. There is proliferation of the bile ducts, which in time become fibrotic. In chronic cases, with repeated infection, biliary cirrhosis may develop.

Extrahepatic Bile Duct

The extrahepatic duct may undergo marked dilatation as well as fibrosis, resulting in a huge, thick, and rigid duct. The dilatation may extend all the way to the sphincter of Oddi, or it may stop just above the first part of the duodenum, leaving the intrapancreatic part of the common bile duct of nor-

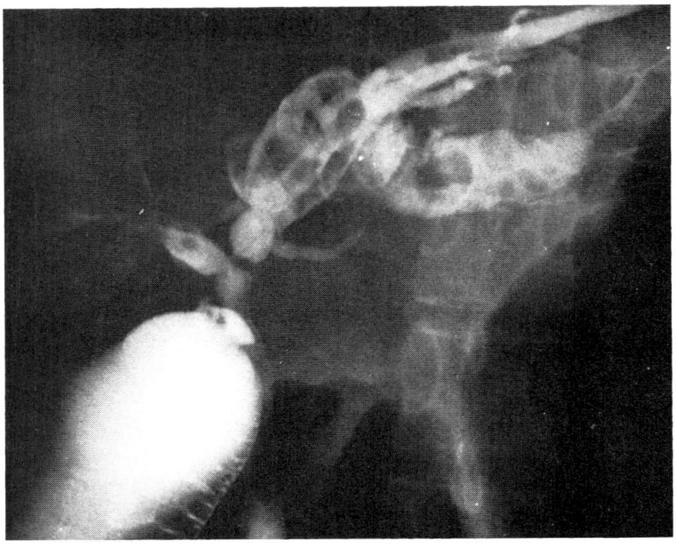

Figure 35–1. Cholangiogram showing stricture at the junction of the right and left hepatic ducts. The ducts proximal to the strictures are dilated and contain stones.

mal caliber. The sphincter of Oddi may be normal, especially in cases in which the dilatation starts above the duodenum. In other cases the sphincter may be edematous, especially during an acute episode. Stricture formation may occur, and there may be pseudopolyps or even adenoma formation. The dilated duct usually contains stones.

Gallbladder

The gallbladder may be contracted, containing the usual calcium bilirubinate stones. It is much more common, however, for the gallbladder to be markedly distended, with or without stones. The gallbladder contains stones in about one third of cases. The bile is invariably infected. When the gallbladder is distended, there is usually obstruction at the lower end of the common bile duct. The distention may be so great that the blood supply becomes compromised, and the gallbladder becomes gangrenous, ruptures, and causes peritonitis.

COMPLICATIONS

Liver Abscess

Single or multiple small liver abscesses may be present. The abscess cavities usually contain stones, which obstruct the bile duct. The abscesses may rupture through the diaphragm into the pleural cavity or into the pericardium. In the former situation, rupture of an abscess into a bronchus results in the formation of a biliary-bronchial fistula.

Rupture of the Gallbladder

This is a serious complication, as a tense gallbladder discharges its infected contents into the general peritoneal cavity.

Biliary Enteric Fistula

Occasionally, the gallbladder may rupture into the colon or the small bowel.[7] However, it is much more common for a fistula to occur between the common bile duct and the second part of the duodenum. Air in the biliary tract may be shown by plain x-rays of the abdomen, but the fistula can be demonstrated only by barium meal or by opening the second part of the duodenum during surgery.[8]

Gram-negative Septicemia

This is a serious condition and may end fatally. It occurs commonly in jaundiced patients with recurrent pyogenic cholangitis, indicating an impacted stone at the lower end of the common bile duct. Occasionally, it may occur with severe infection secondary to infestation with *Clonorchis sinensis*.[9]

Pancreatitis

Acute pancreatitis is found in 12.2 per cent of patients. The pancreatitis is usually mild and is caused by the passage of stones through the sphincter of Oddi. If there is obstruction to the lower end of the common bile duct, biliary tract drainage is essential for recovery.[10]

Thrombophlebitis

Thrombophlebitis of the hepatic vein, a direct consequence of the biliary sepsis, is rare. Septic emboli may be thrown into the pulmonary arterioles, giving rise to pulmonary hypertension.[11]

Analysis of Stones

The stones in recurrent pyogenic cholangitis are friable and flake off easily. On cross section some of them may be laminated, but most are amorphous, yellow, and powdery. On microscopic section through the center of the stone, remnants of parasites, such as *Ascaris lumbricoides* or *Clonorchis sinensis*, are occasionally found.[9] Cultures taken from the center of the stones may produce both aerobic and anaerobic enteric organisms.

PATHOGENESIS

Parasitic infestation has been suggested as the cause of this disease. That parasites or their remnants are associated with stone formation is not open to doubt. Teoh[9] examined 42 stones from both the intrahepatic ducts and the common bile duct, and in 24 he found parasites or their remnants. Of these, 16 were remnants of *Ascaris* and 8 were remnants of *Clonorchis sinensis*. Similar findings have been reported more recently by Wang.[12]

Earlier studies of the stones in this disease showed that they are mainly of calcium bilirubinate.[1,4] Recently, however, chemical analysis of stones from Chinese patients revealed that the cholesterol content, even of the intrahepatic stones, is higher than previously found. The majority of stones are of mixed composition, while pure calcium bilirubinate stones are less common. This is probably due to the better nutritional state of the population.

It has been shown that aerobic and anaerobic enteric organisms may reach the biliary tract via the portal system. Microscopic studies of the liver demonstrate destruction of the liver parenchyma, which is most obvious at the confluence of the small bile ducts.[2] With necrosis of the liver cells, support for the bile ducts is diminished. This leads to dilatation proximal to the confluence of the ducts, followed by stasis of the infected bile in the dilated portion of the duct. Because of this, the bile components precipitate, and primary liver stones form (Fig. 35–2).

Escherichia coli, which is the chief organism cultured, produces β-glucuronidase. This enzyme causes hydrolysis of the water-soluble bilirubin glucuronide into free bilirubin, which, when combined with calcium, precipitates and forms stones. However, not all infected bile results in stone formation. This is because normal bile contains glucaro-1,4 lactone, which inhibits the hydrolysis of bilirubin glucuronide even in the presence of β-glucuronidase. However, if there is a diminished concentration of glucaro-1,4 lactone, β-glucuronidase will cause a perceptible increase of bilirubin, which reacts with calcium to form calcium bilirubinate stones.[13] Foreign bodies, such as dead parasites or ova, may serve as nidi for stone formation. The discovery of parasitic remnants in the stones examined by Teoh[9] and Wang[12] does not necessarily mean that the stones were caused by the presence of parasites.

If the anatomic changes in the intrahepatic ducts are not marked, no stasis occurs, and the infection can be controlled by antibiotics. Bile composition remains normal, and stones will not form. Inflammatory changes can oc-

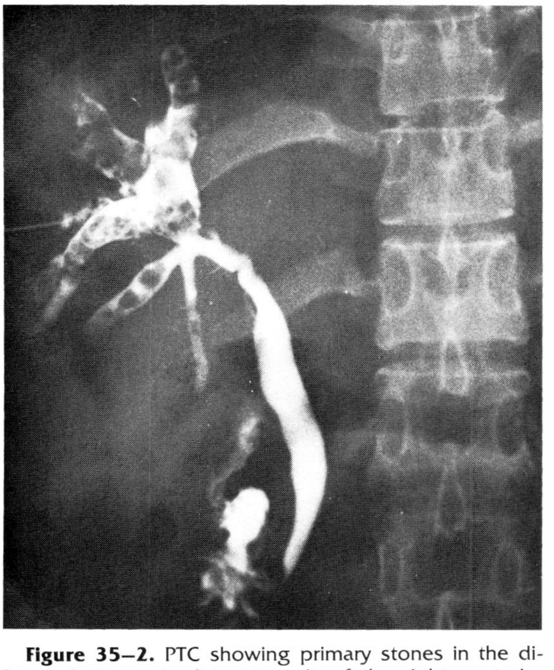

Figure 35–2. PTC showing primary stones in the dilated duct proximal to stenosis of the right posterior segmental duct.

cur in the gallbladder, common bile duct, and sphincter of Oddi. If obstruction of the sphincter of Oddi produces stasis, stones may form in the gallbladder or common bile duct. Gallbladder stones may drop into the common bile duct and then migrate into the intrahepatic ducts. Should these stones be caught in the liver, secondary stones will form (Fig. 35–3). Because of chronic obstruction and persistent infection, the common bile duct becomes dilated and, with fibrosis, permanently thickened.

The gallbladder may be contracted if the whole thickness of its wall is infected. On the other hand, it may become distended if the obstruction is in the lower end of the common bile duct and infection is confined to the mucosa and bile.

CLINICAL FEATURES

The usual presenting symptoms are chills or rigor, fever, and jaundice. There may have been previous such attacks; if so, they have usually been mild. Jaundice may be hardly noticeable and is confined to the sclerae. The pain is distending in character. The fever seldom exceeds 38°C. The symptoms may subside spontaneously, and the next episode may occur as long as 2 years after the first attack. The second attack may be slightly more severe, but, again, it may subside spontaneously with or without the administration of antibiotics. There may be several such episodes before the interval between attacks becomes shorter, the symptoms become more severe, and the patient seeks hospital admission. Pain now takes a different character and is described as distending or lancinating. It is confined to the right upper quadrant but may radiate to the back and is sometimes referred to the shoulders. In some instances, the pain may be colicky and followed by fever. Jaundice may not appear until one or two days after the onset of pain.

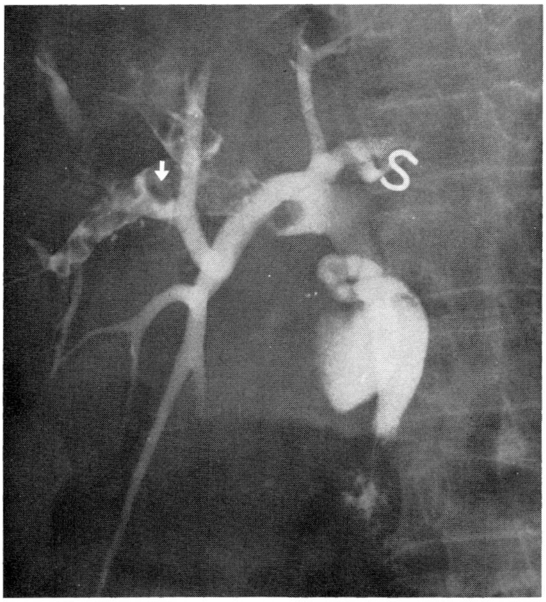

Figure 35–3. Migratory stone (*arrow*) in the right hepatic duct with secondary stones proximal to it.

After several attacks, the jaundice may be deep and the fever as high as 40°C. The pulse rate is increased, but the blood pressure is normal. However, after repeated attacks of colic and high fever, shock may develop.

Physical examination will usually reveal an ill patient who is in pain. The physical signs are most obvious in the abdomen. The liver may be palpable and tender. The gallbladder may occasionally be felt as a globular mass that moves with respiration. The spleen is enlarged in about 25 per cent of patients, often reflecting portal venous thrombosis.[6]

Laboratory Findings

Blood examination may reveal a mild anemia in some patients. There is usually leukocytosis, but the white blood cell count is not exceptionally high, except in some patients who have fulminating infection accompanying infestation by *Clonorchis sinensis.*[11]

The alkaline phosphatase level is usually raised but the transaminase level is usually normal, except in very severe cases with septicemia and total obstruction of the bile duct. The alkaline phosphatase level may not revert to normal for months after relief of the obstruction.

In the acute phase, urine examination may reveal decreased output of urobilinogen and the presence of bile pigments. Examination of the stool may yield parasites or ova, but the rate of positive examinations is not much greater than in the general hospital population.[4]

Bacteriology

Bile cultures are usually positive. In one series the incidence was 88 per cent. Both aerobic and anaerobic bacteria can be cultured, and the predominant species are enteric organisms, such as *E. coli*. Bacteroides are present in a smaller proportion of cases. Clostridia are seldom found in the bile but may occasionally be isolated from nearby lymph nodes. During the acute stage, organisms have been grown from the portal blood in 44 per cent of patients.[4]

Radiology

Plain x-ray films of the abdomen seldom help, as most of the calculi are radiolucent. Air in the biliary tract may be demonstrated on plain x-ray films of the abdomen, indicating a biliary enteric fistula. In such patients, there may be a history of sudden relief of pain after a very severe attack.

Percutaneous Transhepatic Cholangiogram (PTC)

Transhepatic cholangiograms are helpful in demonstrating the bile ducts and stones. PTC is relatively safe and allows for adequate preoperative planning. PTC should be performed under antibiotic coverage. Surgery should usually be performed shortly after the study is completed.

Endoscopic Retrograde Cholangiography (ERCP)

Endoscopic retrograde cholangiography is useful in demonstrating the nature of the lesions, especially in patients who have had previous operations.[14] However, ERCP must be performed with care, because overdistention of the bile ducts may lead to septicemia. ERCP permits simultaneous performance of an endoscopic sphincterotomy,[15] if this is thought to be indicated.

Other Tests

Radioisotope scan of the liver is not helpful in this disease, except when a large abscess has formed (Fig. 35–4). Ultrasound may be useful in demonstrating the large bile ducts and may reveal the presence of stones. Computerized axial tomography may demonstrate a grossly dilated duct with intrahepatic stones (Fig. 35–5). None of these investigations is superior to transhepatic or retrograde cholangiography, however.

DIAGNOSIS

In endemic areas, diagnosis can usually be made on clinical grounds from the typical history of Charcot's intermittent fever and recurrent attacks. Examination may reveal an enlarged, tender liver. The urine may show bile with decreased urobilinogen concentrations. Liver function tests show increased alkaline phosphatase levels. During remissions, endoscopic retrograde cholangiography usually reveals the obstruction and stones in the biliary system. Intravenous cholangiography may occasionally show a dilated duct, but in most instances the study fails to image the biliary tract.

Recurrent pyogenic cholangitis may be mistaken for chronic active renal disease or hepatitis. The demonstration of the viral hepatitis B surface antigen is useful in differential diagnosis.

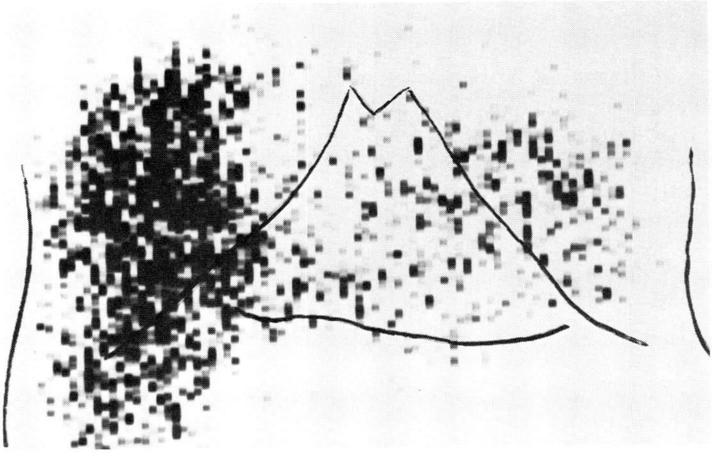

Figure 35–4. Radioactive technetium 99m scan showing no uptake of the abscess in the left lobe of the liver.

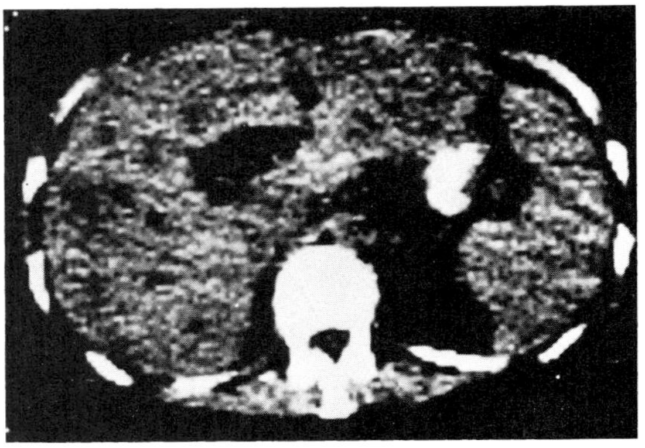

Figure 35–5. CT scan showing dilated intrahepatic bile ducts in recurrent pyogenic cholangitis.

Ruptured hepatoma is another condition that is occasionally confused with recurrent pyogenic cholangitis. If there is a history of sudden pain in the right upper quadrant followed by shock and rapid loss of blood, an abdominal paracentesis should be performed. In areas where this disease is prevalent, hepatoma can be diagnosed if pure blood is obtained on paracentesis.

When the jaundice in recurrent pyogenic cholangitis is mild, the presentation may occasionally be mistaken for a perforated peptic ulcer. The presence or absence of free air in the abdominal cavity should settle the diagnosis.

A ruptured appendix is occasionally thought to be recurrent pyogenic cholangitis, but there really should seldom be much confusion; with ruptured appendicitis the liver or the gallbladder is not palpable.

A ruptured liver abscess may be mistaken for ruptured gallbladder. However, a ruptured abscess seldom gives rise to jaundice, unless it is associated with cholangitis.

Pancreatitis is associated with recurrent pyogenic cholangitis in 12.5 per cent of cases. The diagnosis is usually made only at operation.

Whenever there is doubt, it is safer to perform a laparotomy, for the gallbladder may rupture, giving rise to severe peritonitis.

TREATMENT

Nonsurgical Treatment

Most patients with recurrent pyogenic cholangitis improve with a course of conservative treatment. Nasogastric suction should be instituted to relieve abdominal distention and vomiting and the hemodynamic status of the patient should be monitored closely.

Intravenous fluids, analgesics, and broad-spectrum antibiotics should be administered. With this treatment, fever usually subsides. The pain is relieved, and the abdominal distention and jaundice also gradually subside. Further investigations and preparations may then be carried out. The usual plan is to prepare the patient for operation within a week or two after the attack. However, conservative measures must be abandoned when (1) the pain is not controlled with analgesics; (2) there are signs of spreading peritonitis, an indication the gallbladder has ruptured or is about to rupture; and (3) the pulse rate and temperature are rising, indications of impending septicemia.

Operative Treatment

The kind of operation to be performed depends on the findings and on the general state of the patient. If there is empyema of the gallbladder, with or without rupture, and the general condition of the patient warrants it, a cholecystectomy should be carried out. Cholecystostomy may be necessary if the condition of the patient is poor.

If the common bile duct is dilated, a choledochotomy should be performed and biliary stones or mud should be extracted. A T-tube is then inserted and the abdomen drained. If the condition of the patient is critical, however, it may only be possible to do a choledochotomy to establish T-tube drainage, leaving impacted stones at the lower end of the common bile duct for later removal. However, one must be reasonably certain that adequate decompression of the proximal biliary tract has been accomplished. When gram-negative septicemia has developed, relief of the obstruction, even under local anesthesia, is the only hope to save the patient. This may be accomplished percutaneously. Relieving the obstruction enables the patient to recover from a critical condition, following which further definitive treatment can be planned. When the operation is done electively, more time may be taken to explore the abdomen and to institute definitive treatment.

Cholecystectomy should be performed (1) when the gallbladder is contracted, (2) when there are multiple stones in the gallbladder and the common bile duct and the intrahepatic ducts contain no calculi, and (3) when gallbladder empyema is present.

Operative cholangiography should be performed to determine whether there are residual stones in the common bile duct and whether there is free drainage through the sphincter of Oddi. If the contrast medium trickles into the duodenum and there is no evidence of stones in the common bile duct, a T-tube should be inserted without further exploration. Slow flow of contrast medium into the duodenum may be due to edema of the sphincter of Oddi, and in a week or two another cholangiogram will show no obstruction. If a stone is suspected, a Kocher maneuver is performed and the back of the head of the pancreas is palpated. If a stone is dislodged from the lower end of the common bile duct into the supraduodenal duct, a choledochotomy is performed, and the stone is extracted. Often, there are residual stones. The use of the choledochoscope is helpful in their removal.

Sphincteroplasty

This is a suitable operation when chronic obstruction and infection have produced marked thickening and rigidity of the common duct. In the presence of advanced ductal changes, choledochostomy with choledocholithotomy and T-tube drainage leads to recurrence of stones in the common bile duct. If the dilatation of the common bile duct extends to the ampulla, a transduodenal sphincteroplasty[16] is the operation of choice.

The hepatic flexure is mobilized and packed away from the operative field, exposing the second portion of the duodenum. A duodenotomy is made and the duodenal papilla identified. Should there be difficulty in identifying the papilla, manipulation of the gallbladder will cause bile to be discharged into the duodenum, which will serve as a guide. When the papilla is identified, two stitches are placed on its border, and the papilla is incised between them into the common duct. The sphincter is cut, and an anastomosis between the wall of the common bile duct and the duodenum is made with interrupted nonabsorbable sutures. The incision is extended, and more sutures are applied until the opening in the duct is as large as the greatest diameter of the duct, which may be as much as 1.5 cm. The lateral anastomosis in the duodenum results in an oblique opening that will prevent reflux of duodenal contents into the bile duct in about 50 per cent of patients.

In cutting the lower end of the common bile duct, a branch of the pancreaticoduodenal artery may be cut and brisk bleeding may occur. However, this can be easily controlled with sutures.

Jones[17] applies two hemostats to the opening of the sphincter. The wall of the common bile duct is then cut between the hemostats, and interrupted sutures are applied. The duodenum is closed vertically in two layers. In some cases, the sphincteroplasty can be simplified by inserting a rubber catheter through a supraduodenal choledochotomy into the second part of the duodenum. The second part of the duodenum is incised transversely and the catheter pulled out through this opening. The sphincter is then easily identified, and a sphincteroplasty can be performed over the bougie. However, this maneuver is not easily performed when the bile duct is markedly dilated, because the tip of the bougie may coil within the dilated bile duct and may not get through the sphincter of Oddi.

The results of sphincteroplasty in the treatment of recurrent pyogenic cholangitis are very satisfactory, provided that there are no intrahepatic stones and no strictures in the intrahepatic ducts.[16] In a follow-up study of 271 patients with an average of 7.3 years, 83.4 per cent were in excellent health, while another 8.5 per cent had only mild symptoms. In 22 patients (8.1 per cent) the symptoms were severe enough to warrant admission to hospital. Seventeen were operated upon, and stones were found to have recurred in eight patients. These stones could have dropped down from the liver. The sphincteroplasty strictured in four patients; two patients, whose gallbladders were not removed previously, developed empyema, and two developed liver abscess.

Development of liver abscess in such patients is most probably due to reflux of duodenal contents into a stenotic intrahepatic duct. This leads to severe infection of the proximal duct, resulting in the formation of liver abscesses. In one patient who had no evidence of stenosis or stricture, the bile was infected. In retrospect, it is possible that this patient would have recovered without a further operation.

The overall mortality of sphincteroplasty

performed on 342 patients over a 13 year period was 4.7 per cent.

Choledochojejunostomy

A Roux-en-Y choledochojejunostomy[18] was performed on 128 patients with recurrent pyogenic cholangitis. The indication for this operation is dilatation of the common bile duct above the duodenum. The duct must be irreversibly dilated, thickened, and rigid. When the bile duct is thin-walled but dilated, choledochojejunostomy is contraindicated. Strictures invariably develop after such an anastomosis.[4]

The vertical limb of the Roux loop should be at least 45 cm long to prevent reflux of enteric contents into the biliary tract. Reflux of intestinal contents into the stenotic intrahepatic ducts produces stagnation of infected material that may lead to abscess formation and septicemia.

The anastomosis between the common bile duct and the jejunum should be performed end-to-end with one layer of interrupted sutures. It should be accurate without any strangulation.

Of the 128 patients who had this operation, 79 had had previous operative procedures, including cholecystectomy and sphincteroplasty; in 49 patients, choledochojejunostomy was the primary procedure. The operative mortality among these 128 patients was 2.3 per cent. Follow-up over a median period of 8 years in 106 of them revealed that 73.6 per cent had excellent results, 13.2 per cent had fair results, and 14 per cent had recurrent symptoms requiring reoperation. The findings at reoperation were recurrent stones in the intrahepatic ducts. In four of these patients, the anastomoses had strictured; in two patients, infected bile subsequently caused liver abscesses. In a further two patients, liver abscesses were found.

The results of choledochojejunostomy, as compared with sphincteroplasty in the treatment of recurrent pyogenic cholangitis, may appear to be inferior, but if account is taken of the fact that choledochojejunostomy was performed on the patients who had poor results after previous operations, the results are superior. Nevertheless, choledochojejunostomy is a more difficult operation to perform, and in the hands of an inexperienced surgeon the mortality rate is probably higher.

Endoscopic Sphincterotomy

The role of endoscopic sphincterotomy is still unclear, although promising results have been reported.[15] This procedure may be particularly useful in patients who present special risks for laparotomy. Endoscopic sphincterotomy is not without its own complications in this disease, however. Major complications were experienced in 7.5 per cent of patients, which led to emergency surgery in 3 per cent and death in 1.5 per cent.[15]

It is dangerous to perform this operation in cases of recurrent pyogenic cholangitis because in order to remove some of these big stones, which are not necessarily impacted at the sphincter of Oddi but are found higher up in the common bile duct, a long sphincteroplasty is needed. This may necessitate cutting through the head of the pancreas, and the pancreaticoduodenal artery may be damaged, giving rise to severe bleeding. However, passage of small stones may be facilitated by endoscopic sphincterotomy.

Management of Intrahepatic Stones

In our series of 634 patients with recurrent pyogenic cholangitis, 164 (25.8 per cent) had stones in the intrahepatic ducts,[19] which often were associated with stones in the common bile duct or in the gallbladder. The presence of intrahepatic stones poses special problems in management.[19–21] The majority of the stones are confined to the left intrahepatic duct, and, fortunately, this is much more amenable to treatment. When there is destruction of the lateral segment of the left lobe, a hepatic resection is the best form of treatment (Fig. 35–6). This was done in 26 patients.

The operation is performed by first mobilizing the left lateral segment of the liver until the left lateral segmental vein is exposed. This vein usually joins the medial segmental vein to form the left hepatic vein, which drains into the inferior vena cava. A little dissection into the substance of the liver exposes the lateral segmental vein. After the coronary ligament is divided, the left lateral segment of the left lobe of the liver is depressed inferiorly. When division and suture ligation of the lateral segmental vein have been done, the lateral segment of the left lobe of the liver is rotated and brought forward toward the abdominal wound. By doing this, the segmental artery, portal vein, and

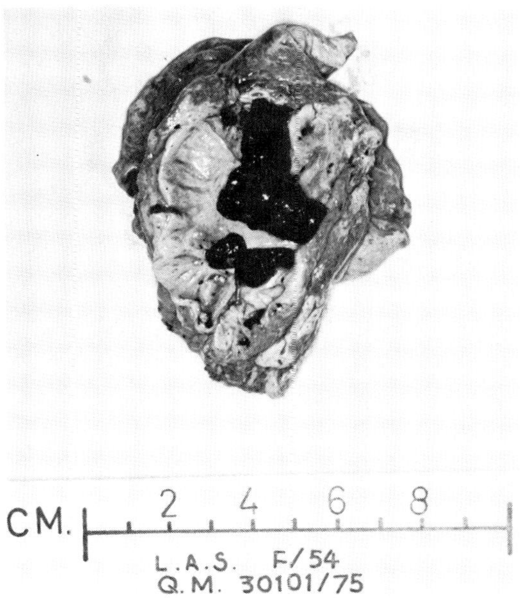

Figure 35–6. Lateral segmentectomy specimen showing stones in a sacculated and thickened left lateral segment of the liver. Note the thinned-out liver tissue.

hepatic duct can be individually divided between clamps and ligated. Now the lateral segment of the left lobe of the liver is ready for division, and the demarcation line is quite clear. After division and removal of the segment, points of oozing at the raw surface of the liver are suture ligated. The raw surface can be covered with the falciform ligament, which is freed from the anterior abdominal wall and stitched to the capsule of the liver.

Of the 26 patients treated by partial hepatectomy, there was one death. The remaining 25 have been followed for a median of 7 years and 8 months.[19] They are in excellent health.

When there is no stricture but the entire ductal system is markedly dilated, the best treatment is to make a high choledochotomy and remove the stones from the right and left hepatic ducts with scoops and by flushing. A flexible choledochoscope helps in finding stones in the smaller bile ducts, which can then be scooped out. After flushing, a T-tube is inserted for drainage of the bile ducts.

Stones that form in the right intrahepatic ducts proximal to a stenosis present greater problems, for hepatotomy through the periphery of the liver is difficult and often accompanied by substantial blood loss. Furthermore, removal of the stones through the liver substance is not satisfactory. However, by splitting the liver along the plane that divides the right and left lobes, the bifurcation of the common hepatic duct may be exposed. There is minimal blood loss if the dissection is made to the right of the middle hepatic vein. If there is bleeding from the middle hepatic vein, it may be sutured or ligated. Inside the liver, the duct, which is markedly dilated, is situated anterior to the corresponding artery and vein. The duct is incised between stay-sutures, and stones and sludge are removed.

The opening of the right posterior division and the anteroposterior subsegmental duct can be seen, and further clearance of stones can be carried out. The stenotic duct is then excised and reanastomosed. A small T-tube or transhepatic tube may be inserted, and the incision in the right hepatic duct closed with nonabsorbable sutures. The incised edges of the liver are then brought together with interrupted catgut sutures. The results in these patients are still uncertain, as there has been insufficient experience to gauge the outcome.

Management of Retained Stones

After surgery, almost 30 per cent of patients with recurrent pyogenic cholangitis have retained stones. Many of these cannot be detected during the operation because they are in the intrahepatic ducts. Subsequently, they begin to drop into the common bile duct. These stones can be removed through the T-tube tract.[22]

An alternative is to perform an extraperitoneal sphincteroplasty.[23] This operation is done with the patient in the supine position. The incision is similar to that for extraperitoneal lumbar sympathetectomy and is made from the tip of the eleventh rib toward the midline, just above the umbilicus. The oblique and transverse muscles are cut in line with the incision. In obese patients, the rectus sheath may be opened transversely and the rectus muscle retracted medially. By dissecting extraperitoneally, the anterior surface of the right kidney comes into view, and, on further dissection medially, the second part of the duodenum is exposed. The anterior surface of the head of the pancreas serves as a landmark. The duodenum is cleared and four stay-sutures are placed on the anterior surface of the second part of the duodenum. A transverse or vertical incision is made. The sphincter of Oddi is identified and a sphincteroplasty carried out.

Residual stones can then be scooped out through the sphincteroplasty opening. This operation avoids the need to dissect into dense adhesions in the peritoneal cavity. Since we began removing residual stones through the T-tube tract, we have performed this operation less frequently. However, it is an alternative method when T-tube tract removal is not possible.

PROGNOSIS

The prognosis is good, provided that obstruction is eliminated and an internal drainage procedure is done. Failure is usually due to strictures with stones proximally in the intrahepatic ducts, which may be impossible to remove.

Recurrent symptoms may be caused by failure to provide proper drainage in patients whose disease is advanced and irreversible.

REFERENCES

1. Cook J, Hou PC, Ho HC, et al: Recurrent pyogenic cholangitis. Br J Surg 1954;*42*:188.
2. Ong GB: Recurrent pyogenic cholangitis. Medical Annual 1968, pp 25–36.
3. Rufanov IG: Liver stones. Ann Surg 1936;*103*:580.
4. Ong GB: A study of recurrent pyogenic cholangitis. Arch Surg 1962;*84*:199.
5. Yue PCK: Recurrent pyogenic cholangitis in children. Aust NZ J Surg 1974;*44*:53.
6. Chou ST, Chan CW: Recurrent pyogenic cholangitis: a necropsy study. Pathology 1980;*12*:415.
7. Shiu MH: An unusual case of spontaneous internal biliary fistulae. Br J Surg 1967;*54*:969.
8. Ong GB, Lee TC, Low G, et al: Air in the biliary passage of choledochoduodenal origin. Br J Surg 1962;*50*:172.
9. Teoh TB: A study of gall-stones and included worms in recurrent pyogenic cholangitis. J Pathol Bacteriol 1963;*86*:123.
10. Ong GB, Adisehiah M, Leong CH: Acute pancreatitis associated with recurrent pyogenic cholangitis. Br J Surg 1971;*58*:891.
11. Lai KS, McFadzean AJS, Yeung R: Microembolic pulmonary hypertension in pyogenic cholangitis. Br Med J 1968;*1*:22.
12. Wang HK: Oriental choledocholithiasis. Surg Gastroenterol 1982;*1*:317.
13. Maki T: Pathogenesis of calcium bilirubinate gallstones: role of *E. coli*, β-glucuronidase and coagulation of inorganic ions, polyelectrolytes and agitation. Ann Surg 1966;*164*:90.
14. Lam SK, Wong KP, Chan PKW, et al: Recurrent pyogenic cholangitis: a study by endoscopic retrograde cholangiography. Gastroenterology 1978; *74*:1196.
15. Lam SK: A study of endoscopic sphincterotomy in recurrent pyogenic cholangitis. Br J Surg 1984;*71*:262.
16. Choi TK, Wong J, Lam KH, et al: Late result of sphincteroplasty in the treatment of primary cholangitis. Arch Surg 1981;*116*:1173.
17. Jones SA: Sphincteroplasty (not sphincterotomy) in the treatment of biliary tract disease. Surg Clin North Am 1973;*53*:1123.
18. Choi TK, Wong J, Ong GB: Choledochojejunostomy in the treatment of primary cholangitis. Surg Gynecol Obstet 1982;*155*:43.
19. Choi TK, Wong J, Ong GB: The surgical management of primary intrahepatic stones. Br J Surg 1982;*69*:86.
20. Nakayama F, Koga A: Hepatolithiasis: present status. World J Surg 1984;*8*:9.
21. Koga A, Miyazaki K, Ichimiya H, et al: Choice of treatment for hepatolithiasis based on pathological findings. World J Surg 1984;*8*:36.
22. Burhenne HJ: Percutaneous extraction of retained biliary tract stones: 661 patients. AJR 1980;*134*:889.
23. Choi TK, Lee NW, Wong J, et al: Extraperitoneal sphincteroplasty for residual stones. An update. Ann Surg 1982;*196*:26.

JAN H. LOUW, CH.M.
HEINZ RODE, M.MED.

36

Ascariasis

INTRODUCTION

Human ascariasis is almost always caused by the giant roundworm *Ascaris lumbricoides*, which owes its specific name to its resemblance to the common earthworm. It has been recognized since ancient times, and references to it are found in texts from Mesopotamia, Greece, Rome, and China.[1] The female measures from 20 to 35 cm in length and 3 to 6 mm in width: the male is smaller, with a length of 15 to 31 cm and a diameter of 2 to 4 mm.[2]

The normal habitat of the adult parasite is the human small intestine, where it obtains its nourishment from the semidigested food of the host and possibly from the epithelial cells of the intestinal mucosa.[3] A female worm has a productive capacity of about 27 million eggs with an average daily output of 200,000.[3] Its life span in the human intestine is about 1 year, and it is capable of surviving outside the body for nearly a month in nonnutritive media.[3]

Both fertilized and unfertilized ova are passed in the stools of the host and under favorable conditions in water and soil, fully developed infective embryos are formed in 2 to 3 weeks. The optimal temperature for development is about 25°C. Low temperatures retard development but favor survival of the ova, which remain viable for long periods on the soil or in manure heaps throughout the winter months when subjected to freezing temperatures. A moist, loose soil with moderate shade is favorable for survival, and, in temperate climates, invasive *Ascaris* ova can survive for up to 6 years.[4] However, the embryonated ova cannot withstand drying or direct sunlight.

The human host is infected by ingestion of contaminated food. The infection is acquired as soon as a child begins to crawl and to place his fingers or toys contaminated with ova into the mouth. As a result, children are more commonly and more severely infected than are adults. Lack of sanitary facilities and poor child care promote the continuous pollution of the soil by fecal matter from parasitized individuals. In most areas the highest incidence of infection occurs in children under 16 years of age. The ingested ova hatch in the small intestine, and the larvae, penetrating the intestinal wall, migrate via the liver, lungs, bronchi, trachea, glottis, and pharynx to return to the intestine, where they become mature worms.[3] This migration usually terminates within 14 days after infection.[4] Almost 90 per cent of the adults reside in the jejunum and less than 1 per cent in the duodenum. The average worm load per person is 12 parasites, but among individuals living under primitive conditions it is often as high as 500 to 700 and may exceed 2000.[2] Occasionally the worms may migrate into the stomach, or they may descend into the rectum and be passed in the feces, but they do not normally reside in the stomach or colon.

EPIDEMIOLOGY

Ascariasis is a worldwide problem. The infection is prevalent in areas where sanitation and personal hygiene are poor, and fresh human feces are used as fertilizer. Infestation is particularly common in rural areas owing to overcrowding and unsanitary conditions (shantytowns). Monroe,[5] extrapolating from the estimates of Stoll[6] in 1947 in order to take into account the expanding world population, estimated that in 1976, on the basis of a world population of 3.5 billion, the prevalence of *Ascaris* infections was 1.3 billion. Of those afflicted, 4.8 million resided in North America, 67 million in Central and South America, 96 million in Africa, and 536 million in China.

In the Far East, about 90 per cent of the population is infected. In mainland China, ascariasis is prevalent everywhere.[7] The literature also contains reports from Malaysia,[8] Korea,[8] India,[9] Pakistan,[10] the Philippines,[11] Israel,[13] and Iran.[14] In Japan, the incidence in 1949 was 63 per cent but fell to 0.7 per cent in 1971.[12] Epidemics have been observed in Central Europe, but in recent years the incidence has decreased because of improved standards of living and hygiene in rural areas.[5]

In the United States, ascariasis is more prevalent in the southern than in the northern states and also more common in rural than in urban areas.[2] The incidence has decreased in Georgia,[15] but in 1975 infection was still present in 8 to 28 per cent of the population, especially in rural areas.[16] It is still relatively common in South Carolina,[17] Florida,[18] Virginia,[19] and other southeastern states, where the infestation in rural areas has been estimated at 50 per cent.[20] In these areas, infected persons are often clustered in families.[19] In South America, heavy infestation has been reported from Brazil, Colombia, Mexico, Peru, and Venezuela.[5]

On the African continent the overall prevalence is almost 50 per cent,[5] but in tropical and subtropical areas it rises to 90 per cent.[21, 22] In zones with extremely cold or hot and dry climates the incidence is lower than in regions where more humid, warm, and even temperatures prevail. In Cape Town, which has a temperate climate, over 70 per cent of children attending the Red Cross Children's Hospital harbor the worm. The problem, however, is not confined to endemic areas, because in these days of international travel there is ample opportunity for the parasites to have free rides around the world in the bodies of their hosts. Today many a physician far from the Orient and tropical areas may be called upon to deal with the complications caused by the worm.

PATHOLOGY

The phase of larval migration of the ascaris is not relevant to this review, nor are the nutritional and toxic effects of adult *Ascaris* infection. The local effects of adult *Ascaris* infection depend on the location of the parasite, the number of worms present, and death of the worms. The factors responsible are mechanical, owing to the presence and movements of the worms; chemical, owing to the metabolic products of the ascaris; and irritative, owing to the presence of disintegrating parasites and their ova. Other local complications arise from the renowned wanderlust of the parasite and its tendency to explore orifices, ducts, and cavities that communicate with the gastrointestinal tract. One of the openings that seems to attract the worm is the ampulla of Vater, leading to biliary ascariasis.

In areas where ascariasis is prevalent, local complications account for a significant number of admissions to children's wards. For example, at the Red Cross Children's Hospital in Cape Town, ascariasis accounts for 10 to 15 per cent of all acute abdominal emergencies admitted to the surgical service. Intestinal complications such as obstruction, perforation, necrosis, and even gangrene are the most frequent. During the period 1958 through 1977 we dealt with 1100 acute abdominal emergencies complicating ascariasis at the Red Cross Children's Hospital; of these, 632 (57 per cent) were intestinal and 424 (38.5 per cent) were biliary (Table 36–1).

The children with biliary ascariasis were all under 13 years of age, with the peak incidence in the age group 4 to 10 years, only one being under the age of 1 year (Fig. 36–1). Boys and girls were affected equally. During the same period we encountered 54 cases of biliary ascariasis at our other teaching hospitals (Groote Schuur and Somerset). Of these, 24 were teenagers (13 to 19 years), 14 were in the third decade (20 to 29 years), and the remaining 16 were evenly spread over the fourth to seventh decades, the oldest being 65 years (Fig. 36–1). In the United States the peak incidence of biliary ascariasis is also in young children.[15, 16, 19, 20] In the Far East, on the other hand, most of the large series reported consist of adults,[23–26] but Chang and Han[27] published a series of 788

Table 36–1 ACUTE ABDOMINAL COMPLICATIONS OF ASCARIASIS
(Red Cross Children's Hospital, 1958–1977)

	Number	Per Cent
Intestinal lesions	623	56.6
Biliary lesions	424	38.5
Pancreatitis	43	4.0
Appendicitis	2	0.2
Peritonitis	8	0.7
Total	1100	

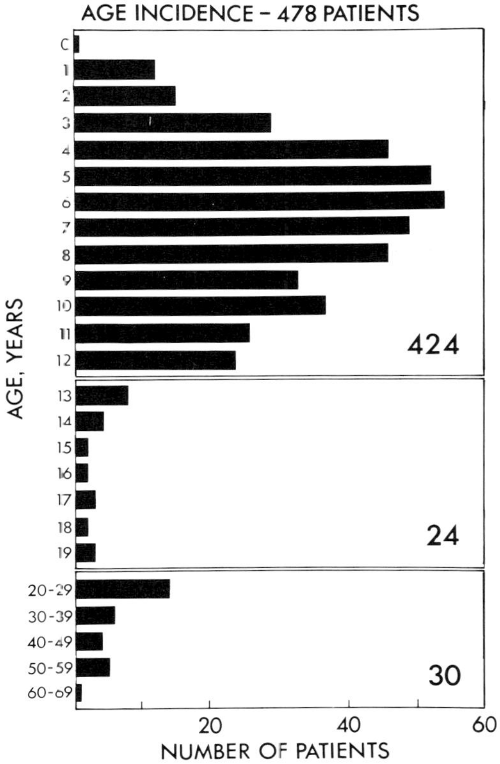

Figure 36–1. Distribution of patients with biliary ascariasis according to age.

children encountered at the Peking Children's Hospital over a period of 5 years. In Europe, biliary ascariasis is also more frequent in adults.[4]

PATHOGENESIS

The *Ascaris* is capable of reaching the duodenum against peristalsis by means of its own writhing movements. This is liable to occur with heavy infestations when the worms choke the jejunum. Migration is also promoted by anesthesia, fever, improper anthelmintic treatment, ingestion of drugs, and a peppery diet.[4] Overcrowding in the duodenum predisposes to invasion of the ampulla of Vater, and biliary ascariasis not infrequently occurs as a postoperative complication when infected patients are not dewormed before surgery.[4]

Having found its way into the ampulla, the worm passes some distance up the common bile duct, leaving its tail and about half of its body in the duodenum.[13,24,27] Sometimes it negotiates the pancreatic duct instead. As a rule, only a single worm enters the common bile duct, but we have encountered up to 80, and as many as 200 have been reported.[25] Irritation by the movements of the worm or its excretory products results in spasm of the choledochal and ampullary sphincters with partial biliary obstruction.[9] Sometimes there is concomitant obstruction of the pancreatic duct, and in 81 (17 per cent) of our 478 cases the serum amylase value was raised without clinical evidence of pancreatitis. During the same period we treated an additional 46 patients in whom the worm entered the pancreatic duct and caused severe acute pancreatitis. In patients who have been operated upon during the acute attack, pancreatic edema has often been observed in association with biliary ascariasis.[2]

Biliary obstruction tends to last as long as a live worm remains in situ, and apparent survival of the ascaris in the bile duct for up to 3 months has been recorded.[2] On the other hand, worms have been observed to survive for only up to 12 days in pure bile;[2] it should be remembered, however, that they can live outside the body in non-nutritive media for almost a month.[3] On balance, it is reasonable to assume that they may survive in the common bile duct for 4 weeks. Fortunately, the vast majority retreat into the duodenum. Exactly how the ascaris manages to extricate itself is not known. Chang and Han[27] have suggested the following mechanisms: (1) Spasm of the ductal sphincters causes vigorous movements of the untrapped body and tail of the worm, which may enable it to retract its head; (2) flushing of the bile duct promoted by antispasmodics and gallbladder contraction may force the worm out of the duct; or (3) when the whole of the worm has entered the duct, the head may turn backward on itself. Usually, only live worms return to the intestine, but dead and decayed worms may occasionally be discharged from the bile duct.[27] However, once the intrahepatic ducts and liver are infested with large numbers of worms, they are usually there to stay.

Persistence of the worm in the bile ducts may result in serious complications (Table 36–2). De and Sinha[9] have shown that ascarides excrete products of anaerobic metabolism that contain various polypeptides capable of producing allergic manifestations. In high concentration these act as chemical irritants, causing muscular spasm and mucosal necrosis. Chang and Han[27] reported necrosis

Table 36–2 BILIARY COMPLICATIONS (RED CROSS CHILDREN'S HOSPITAL, 1958–1977)

	Children (Under 20 Years) (448)	Adults (Over 20 Years) (30)	Total
Perforation of common bile duct	2	—	2
Acute cholecystitis	1	1	2
Stricture	2	2	4
Stones	—	3	3
Stricture plus stones	1	6	7
Granulomatous hepatitis	16	4	20

of the bile ducts in 11 of 18 patients who came to surgery, and we have had two such cases with perforation of the common duct. Acute cholecystitis with necrosis or gangrene may occur in a similar way, but it is rare. Wang et al.[23] reported an incidence of 5 per cent in 141 cases, and we have had two cases. Chang and Han[27] have also reported the occurrence of hemobilia.

The formation of biliary strictures is usually associated with death of the worm in the common bile duct. The presence of nonviable and disintegrating ascarides causes destruction of the ductal mucosa, exudation with abundant eosinophils, and a fibromatous reaction. In such cases, dense fibrous tissue forms, with heavy infiltration by round cells and plasma cells as well as foreign body giant cells, with foci of calcification surrounding *Ascaris* ova and disintegrated worm segments.[28] Once a stricture has developed, calculus formation with superadded infection and suppurative cholangitis may occur. These complications are more frequent in adults; in our series, only 3 of the 448 children developed strictures, one of them complicated by stones, whereas 8 of the 30 adults had strictures, 6 of them complicated by stones. In addition, three of the adults developed primary pigment stones, which is a relatively common complication of biliary ascariasis in the Orient.[13, 29] The ascarides produce β-glucuronidase, which hydrolyzes water-soluble bilirubin diglucuronide to form insoluble free bilirubin, which, in turn, precipitates as calcium bilirubinate.[29] Wang et al.[23] found that one third of the stones recovered from their patients with ascariasis contained debris of dead ascarides. The high incidence of ascariasis in the East no doubt plays a role in the frequency of primary hepatic duct pigment stones in that part of the world.[30, 31]

Hepatic granulomata constituted the most frequent complication in our series, but, seen in perspective, the condition is still unusual, accounting for only 20 (4.2 per cent) of the 478 cases. The rarity of hepatic ascariasis in the East has been stressed by Saw et al.[8] and Muazzam et al.[10] but the condition is apparently common in Singapore.[22] The worms may find their way into the ramifications of the intrahepatic ducts, especially those of the left lobe of the liver. They usually die but may deposit ova before doing so. The ova perish, but in two of our cases there was segmentation and even embryonation.[32] Both viable and dead ova as well as the disintegrating worms provoke a nonspecific foreign body reaction, with the formation of chronic granulomatous foci in the liver parenchyma. These tend to be studded throughout the liver as hard, sometimes umbilicated, grayish white to pale yellow nodules of 0.5 to 2 cm (Fig. 36–2). Occasionally, confluence of the nodules results in extensive replacement of the liver parenchyma with adherence of the omentum, which may contain similar nodules.[2] Histologically the lesions are characterized by a chronic granulomatous process surrounding ascaris eggs and disintegrated worms. Eventually the lesions are transformed into hyalinized scars without evidence of ova.

In many cases the outcome is not so favorable. Secondary infection of the granulomata with the development of hepatic abscesses occurs about 50 per cent of the time. These abscesses are particularly serious because they may rupture into the peritoneal cavity or even through the diaphragm into the pleural cavity and lung, often with a lethal outcome.[33] The infecting bacteria are both aerobic *(E. coli, Klebsiella*, and *Proteus)* and anaerobic *(Bacteroides* and *Clostridium)*, and gas formation is not uncommon. When large numbers of parasites are trapped in the intrahepatic bile ducts, thousands of eggs are released upon disintegration of the worms, with resultant acute and chronic suppurative cholangitis. In such cases the liver becomes greatly enlarged and its surface bosselated with patches of grayish discoloration. Within the liver there are multiple irregular cavities

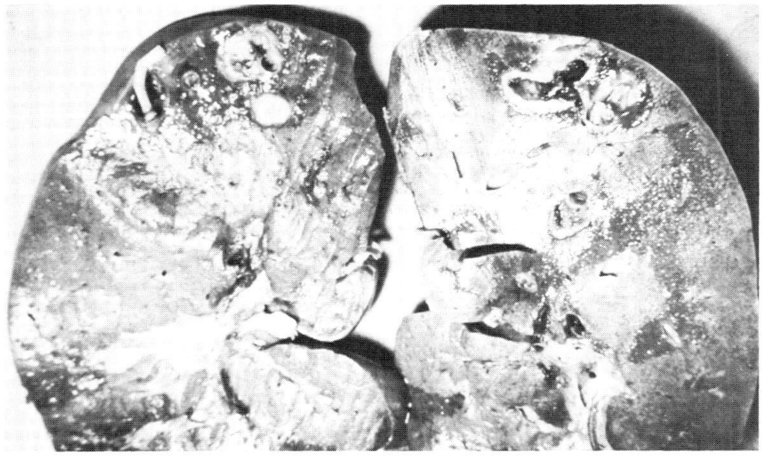

Figure 36–2. Multiple hepatic granulomata due to *Ascaris*.

filled with foul-smelling purulent material as well as disintegrating worms. Many patients with this complication die as a result of the infection. One of the most severe complications of ascaridic cholangitis is extension of the inflammatory process to the hepatic or portal veins, with the development of pylephlebitis; this was responsible for the only death in our series, that of our oldest patient, aged 65 years. Arean and Crandall[2] mention that worms may enter the lumen of the hepatic veins and so find their way into the vena cava, the right side of the heart, and the lungs, producing fatal pulmonary emboli. They quote a remarkable case reported by Phuoc and Schmauss,[34] in which a worm embolus passed through a patent foramen ovale to lodge in the left popliteal artery.

CLINICAL PRESENTATION (Table 36–3)

The clinical presentation depends on the presence or absence of complications. There is a striking difference in the incidence of complications between children and teenagers on the one hand, and adults on the other. For example, only 5 per cent of the children in our series presented with complications, whereas complications were present in 60 per cent of the adults (Table 36–4). The reason for this is probably that fresh infestation is uncommon in adults. Most adult cases, therefore, represent long-standing ascariasis, and these patients are likely to suffer from the complications of chronic infestation.

Fifty per cent of the children under 13 years in our series were anemic, 17 per cent severely so. The anemia was of the microcytic normochromic type in two thirds and of the microcytic hypochromic type in one third. In addition, 56 per cent of the children under 13 years were at or below the third percentile for weight. These findings applied to both uncomplicated and complicated cases and were attributed to a combination of protein-calorie malnutrition, infection, and chronic blood loss caused by associated parasites. The teenagers and adults were neither anemic nor undernourished. According to the clinical presentation, patients with biliary ascariasis can be divided into uncomplicated and complicated cases.

Table 36–3 CLINICAL PRESENTATION OF BILIARY ASCARIASIS

Clinical Finding	Uncomplicated (440)	Complicated (38)
Acute right upper quadrant pain	437	34
Vomiting	398	20
History of worms	247	28
Worms in stool/vomitus	210	23
Pyrexia	121	32
Jaundice	10	18
Right upper quadrant tenderness	422	37
Enlarged liver	71	24
Palpable gallbladder	50	6

Uncomplicated Biliary Acariasis

The clinical presentation in all our uncomplicated cases was that of a short, sharp illness

Table 36–4 COMPLICATIONS OF BILIARY ASCARIASIS IN RELATION TO AGE

	Patients Under 20 Years (448)	Patient Over 20 Years (30)
Uncomplicated	428 (95%)	12 (40%)
Complicated	20 (5%)	18 (60%)

commencing with the sudden onset of severe right upper quadrant abdominal colic associated with vomiting and marked tenderness in the right subcostal region, especially just to the right and slightly below the xyphoid. These symptoms and signs lasted for 2 to 5 days, on an average. In two thirds of the patients there was a previous history of worms and/or worms in the stools or vomitus. So characteristic is the presentation that on these criteria alone a clinical diagnosis of worms in the common duct is justifiable, and very many such cases have been successfully treated on an outpatient basis.

It should be noted that pyrexia (up to 39°C) is not a common feature and that clinical jaundice is distinctly rare. Moderate hepatomegaly is present in some patients (mostly children), but this is due to coincident malnutrition and is unrelated to the worms. On the other hand, the presence of a palpable gallbladder in 56 (11.4 per cent) of the patients was regarded as a positive sign of biliary ascariasis.

Leukocytosis is observed in nearly half the patients with biliary ascariasis, but counts above 20,000/cu mm are rare. Eosinophilia exceeding 6 per cent was present in one third of the patients in our series and a sedimentation rate exceeding 20 mm/hour in two thirds of them.

Complicated Biliary Ascariasis

The clinical presentation depends on the complication. Patients with acute perforation of the common bile duct or gangrenous cholecystitis are severely ill, with signs and symptoms of acute peritonitis. Those with strictures present with jaundice and a previous history of attacks of right upper quadrant pain. Patients with stones present with right upper quadrant pain and jaundice with or without fever and chills. Those with hepatic granulomata without secondary infection present with chronic ill health and a nodular hepatomegaly with or without mild jaundice and a low-grade fever. With the onset of secondary infection, however, they become acutely ill, and as bona fide hepatic abscesses develop they manifest a high, swinging pyrexia and, often, secondary pulmonary signs at the lung bases. The one patient in our series with pylephlebitis complicating suppurative cholangitis was admitted in extremis with a high fever and deep jaundice. He succumbed soon afterward from severe toxemia and hepatorenal failure.

In contrast to the uncomplicated cases, right upper quadrant colic and vomiting are not prominent features, whereas fever, nodular hepatomegaly, and jaundice are relatively common. Indeed, we have come to regard persistent fever and jaundice in a patient with suspected biliary ascariasis as evidence of the presence of complications.

LABORATORY TESTS (Table 36–5)

Uncomplicated Biliary Ascariasis

A striking feature of the uncomplicated cases among our patients was the infrequency of cholestasis. Only about 10 per cent had abnormal liver function tests, and only 2 per cent were jaundiced. An abnormal serum amylase value was found in 81 (17 per cent) of our patients, but none of them had clinical evidence of acute pancreatitis.

Examination of the feces may reveal the presence of fertilized and unfertilized ova in the stools. Sopranova's test, based on the presence of volatile fatty acids in feces and urine, as well as various immunologic tests, have been reviewed by Pawlowski, who concluded that the tests are not very specific.[4] Chang and Han[27] have found that the recovery of ova in duodenal fluid obtained by aspiration is of diagnostic value.

Complicated Biliary Ascariasis

In contrast to the uncomplicated cases there is evidence of deranged liver function in well over 50 per cent of patients with complicated biliary ascariasis. Any patient with suspected biliary ascariasis who has abnormal liver function tests should be considered a complicated case. Indeed, we have found that elevation of the serum bilirubin

Table 36–5 BIOCHEMICAL DATA IN BILIARY ASCARIASIS

Finding	Uncomplicated (440)	Complicated (38)
Bilirubinuria	19	20
Raised serum bilirubin	46	21
Raised alkaline phosphatase	41	16
Raised transaminase	43	10
Raised amylase	77	4

Table 36–6 RADIOLOGIC DATA IN BILIARY ASCARIASIS

Finding	Uncomplicated (440)	Complicated (38)
Worms in small intestine (plain x-ray)	130	8
Gas in common bile duct	4	3
Worms in duodenum (barium meal)	25	3
Worm in common bile duct	325	7
Dilated common bile duct	23	5

above 4 mg/dl (70 μ mol/L) almost invariably denotes the presence of a complication. Only four of the 38 patients in our series had a raised serum amylase—two had perforation of the common bile duct and two had biliary strictures.

DIAGNOSTIC IMAGING (Table 36–6)

Plain x-rays, barium meal examination, oral and intravenous cholangiography, ultrasonography, and transhepatic, endoscopic retrograde, or operative cholangiography may be of great value in establishing the diagnosis of ascariasis.

Uncomplicated Biliary Ascariasis

In about one third of our uncomplicated cases, worms were demonstrated in the small bowel on plain x-rays. The whirlpool appearance of massive infestation[35] (Fig. 36–3) is important in patients with suggestive symptoms and signs. In four of our patients, gas was noted in the biliary system on plain radiographs (Fig. 36–4), which we regard as highly suspicious. In one of our patients with uncomplicated biliary ascariasis, there was calcification in the pancreas (Fig. 36–5).

Barium meal demonstrated worms in the duodenum in 25 cases (6 per cent), and this finding, coupled with the typical history, was regarded as very suggestive of biliary ascariasis (Fig. 36–6). In none was it possible to demonstrate a worm protruding from the ampulla of Vater, although this has been reported by others.[27]

Oral cholecystography is of little help, but intravenous cholangiography is of great value.[36] For example, in 325 (74 per cent) of the patients in our series, the typical linear defect in a dilated duct, which is highly characteristic of ascariasis, could be demonstrated

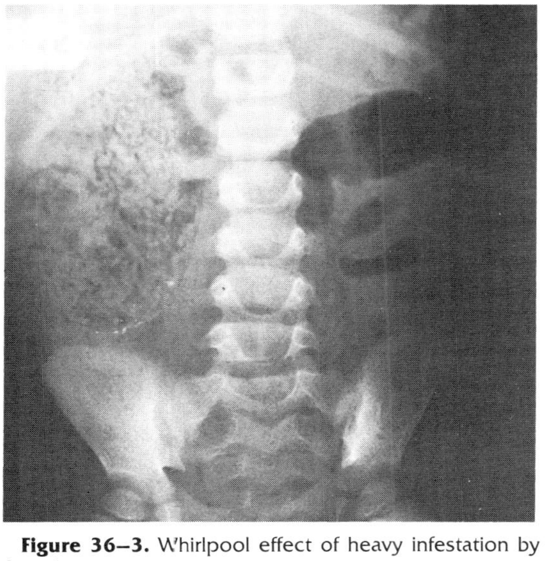

Figure 36–3. Whirlpool effect of heavy infestation by *Ascaris.*

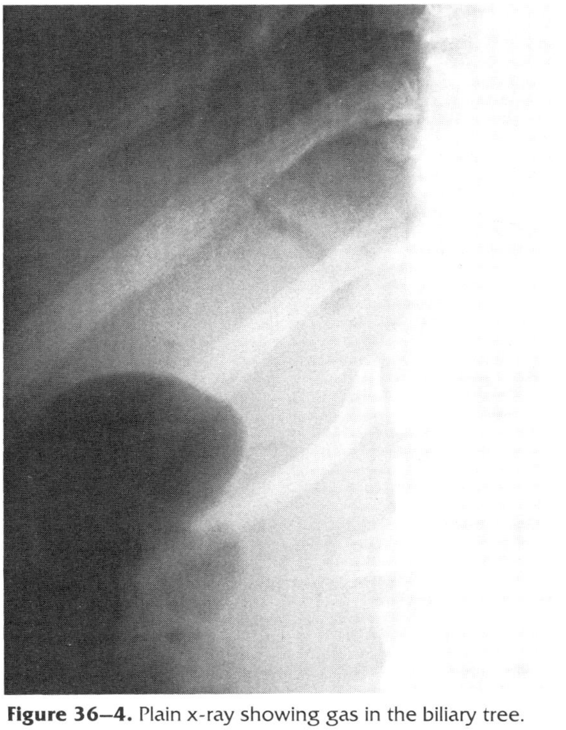

Figure 36–4. Plain x-ray showing gas in the biliary tree.

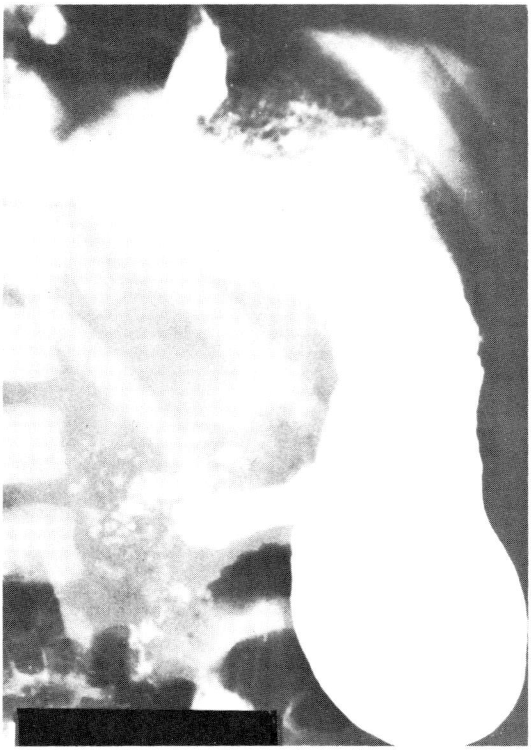

Figure 36–5. Pancreatic calcification and barium in the stomach of a child with biliary ascariasis.

(Fig. 36–7). In 23 (5 per cent) of our patients, the common duct was simply dilated. The significance of this finding per se is debatable because it is difficult to assess in children, and at best it can only be regarded as presumptive evidence of biliary ascariasis. In most patients with biliary ascariasis the duct is dilated, and in several of them the dilatation persisted for a week or more after disappearance of the worm.[36] We therefore regard the presence of a dilated duct in a child with a typical history as suggestive of an attack of biliary ascariasis but not necessarily as indicative of the presence of a worm in the duct. This attitude is illustrated by our experience in five patients in whom the dilatation was gross and persisted for 2 weeks. Laparotomy was performed in all patients, but worms were recovered from two patients only.

In many patients with biliary ascariasis, intravenous cholangiography fails to opacify the bile duct even though the serum bilirubin and alkaline phosphatase levels are normal. In such patients, as well as in those who are jaundiced, ultrasonography may be of particular value.[37–42] With ultrasonography, impacted worms may be seen in a dilated biliary duct. Distention of the gallbladder or swelling of the pancreas can occasionally be observed. This was well demonstrated in a boy aged 14 years who presented with the typical clinical features of right upper quadrant colic, vomiting, right subcostal tenderness, and mild jaundice. Intravenous cholangiography

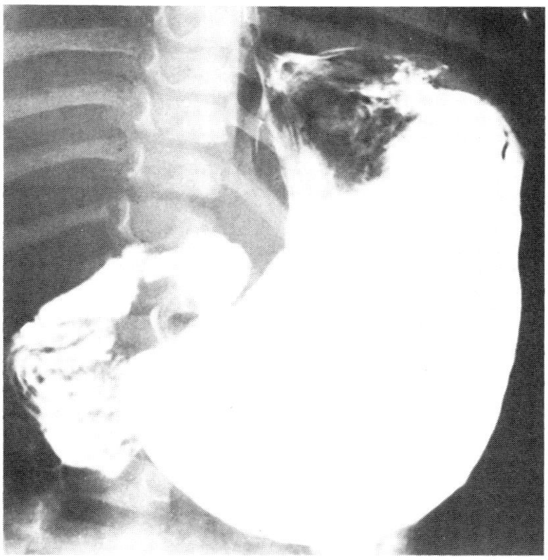

Figure 36–6. Barium meal showing worms in the duodenum.

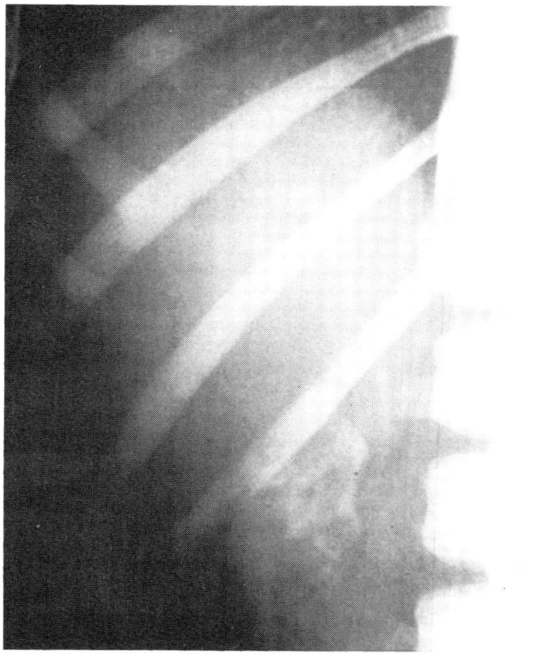

Figure 36–7. Intravenous cholangiogram, 20-minute roentgenogram, showing linear defect due to *Ascaris* in a dilated common bile duct.

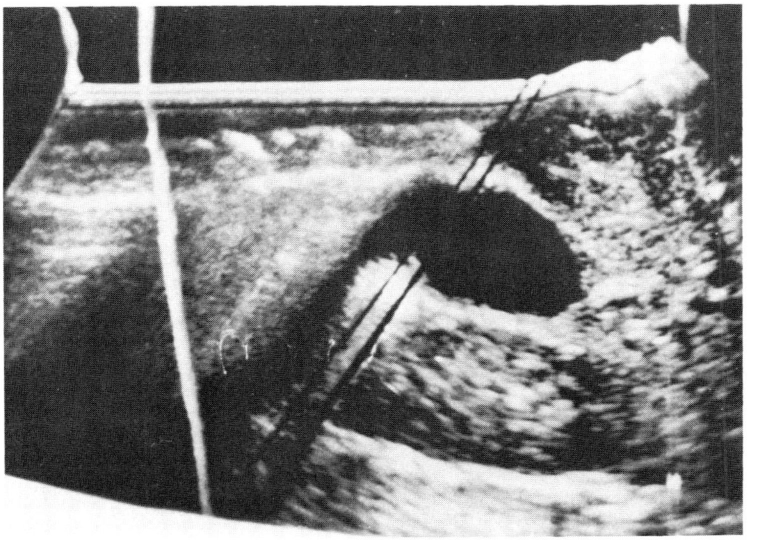

Figure 36–8. Ultrasonogram showing a dilated gallbladder.

failed to demonstrate the bile ducts. Ultrasonography showed gross dilatation of the gallbladder, common bile duct, and intrahepatic ducts, with obstruction of the distal common bile duct (Fig. 36–8). After 5 days of treatment, his condition had subsided sufficiently to allow a barium meal, which demonstrated worms in the duodenum. During the next week he was dewormed and his serum bilirubin level and liver function tests returned to normal. Repeat ultrasonography 2 weeks after admission showed that the gallbladder and bile ducts had returned to normal. Using real-time ultrasonography it is also possible to identify ascarides within the bile ducts. The worm produces a long, thin linear echo without a distal acoustic shadow, the so-called inner tube sign.[37, 39] In transverse sections the parasite produces a central, bright, specular echo within the dilated duct, causing a "bullseye" appearance.[38]

Another investigation of value in patients in whom intravenous cholangiography fails and indirect signs of biliary ascariasis are indeterminate is endoscopic retrograde cholangiopancreatography (ERCP). Van der Spuy[43] reported on three children, aged 3, 4, and 7 years, in whom the diagnosis was made on ERCP (Fig. 36–9). All three cases were uncomplicated, but in each child the alkaline phosphatase level was raised (in one the serum bilirubin value was marginally elevated), and in none did intravenous cholangiography opacify the ducts. The examination is made easier if a vermifuge is given the day before to eliminate the duodenal worms. Biliary ascarides may be seen protruding from the ampulla of Vater.[44]

Percutaneous transhepatic cholangiography (PTC) is not indicated in uncomplicated cases. The absence of significant dilatation of the ducts makes the test difficult. Intraoperative cholangiography, however, is helpful in patients suspected of having biliary ascariasis.

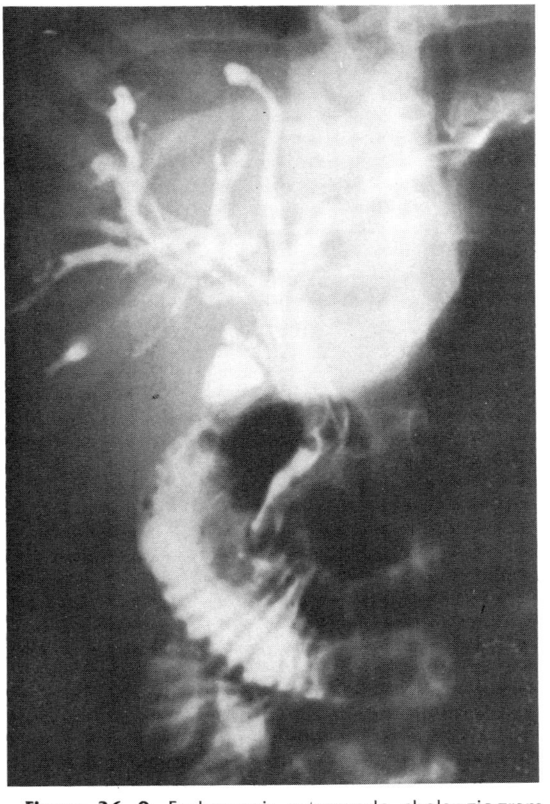

Figure 36–9. Endoscopic retrograde cholangiogram showing at least five linear filling defects in a dilated common bile duct and intrahepatic ducts.

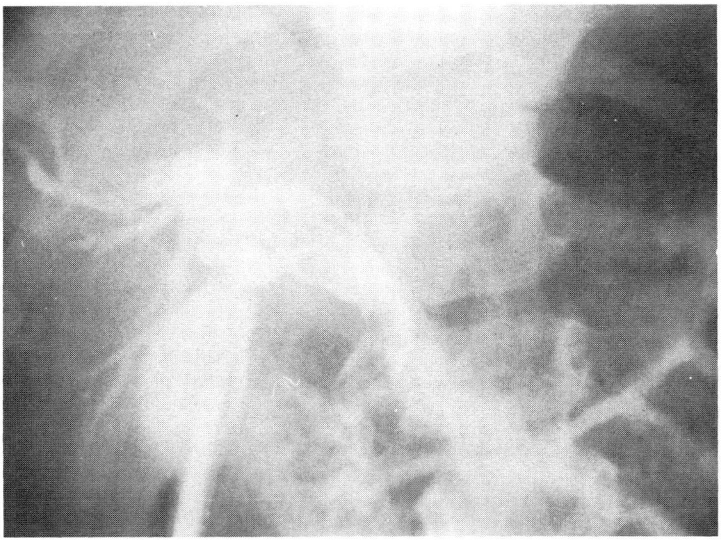

Figure 36–10. Postoperative cholangiogram (after previous cholecystostomy) showing a worm in the common duct.

In this regard, the following case is of interest. A 4½ year old boy presented with abdominal colic, vomiting, and a suspected mass in the right upper quadrant but no jaundice. Intussusception complicating ascariasis was suspected, and laparotomy was undertaken. The gallbladder was tensely distended but not inflamed, and cholecystostomy was performed. There were no worms in the gallbladder. Postoperative cholangiography revealed a greatly dilated common duct containing a worm (Fig. 36–10). A second cholangiogram done a week later showed no change, but despite this the boy was well and not clinically jaundiced, although the serum bilirubin value remained mildly elevated. Two weeks after the cholecystostomy the patient was re-explored, and a dead worm was removed from the bile duct. Subsequent T-tube cholangiography showed that the common bile duct had returned to normal caliber and the T-tube was removed 3 weeks postoperatively. Thereafter, recovery was uneventful, but the total period of hospitalization was 7 weeks. This period could have been reduced to 10 days if an intraoperative cholangiogram had been done at the time of the first laparotomy.

Complicated Biliary Ascariasis

In complicated cases, worms may also be demonstrated in the small bowel on plain x-rays (8 out of our 38 cases). In two of our complicated cases there was also pancreatic calcification. Worms in the duodenum may be demonstrated on barium meal. For example, in one of our patients with a previous choledochoduodenostomy for a common duct stricture, barium entered the biliary tract and demonstrated the presence of worms in the ducts (Fig. 36–11). Intravenous cholangiography is of little value because of the frequent presence of jaundice or the critical condition of the patient. In only one of our patients did the intravenous cholangiogram demonstrate a dilated duct with a stricture and a linear filling defect. In another, dilated ducts containing stones were demonstrated, and, at subsequent surgery, stones and worm debris were found. In three who had had previous biliary-intestinal short-circuiting procedures, *gas was present in the bile ducts,* while in two patients, gas in hepatic abscesses was demonstrated (Fig. 36–12).

ERCP should obviously play an important role in patients who present with jaundice. Pillay et al.[45] have reported on three adults in whom a diagnosis of biliary ascariasis complicated by calculi and strictures was made on ERCP. PTC should also be used in the work-up of jaundiced patients, although the presence of cholangitis may render the investigation risky.[42, 46] Figure 36–13 shows dilated bile ducts due to stricture of the common bile duct in one of our patients. Subsequent histologic studies of the strictured area revealed dense fibrous tissue with cellular infiltration and foci of calcification surrounding *Ascaris* ova and disintegrated worm segments.

Where preoperative cholangiography has failed, operative cholangiography becomes

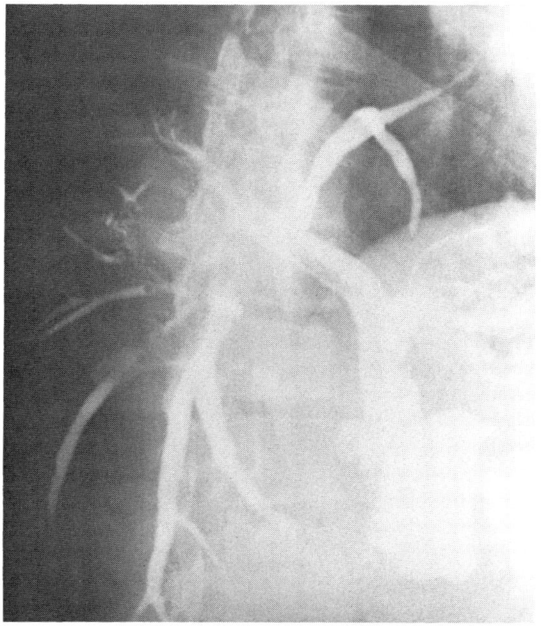

Figure 36–11. Barium meal in a patient who had a previous choledochoduodenostomy. Barium entered the biliary system and outlined an *Ascaris* parasite in the common duct and right hepatic duct.

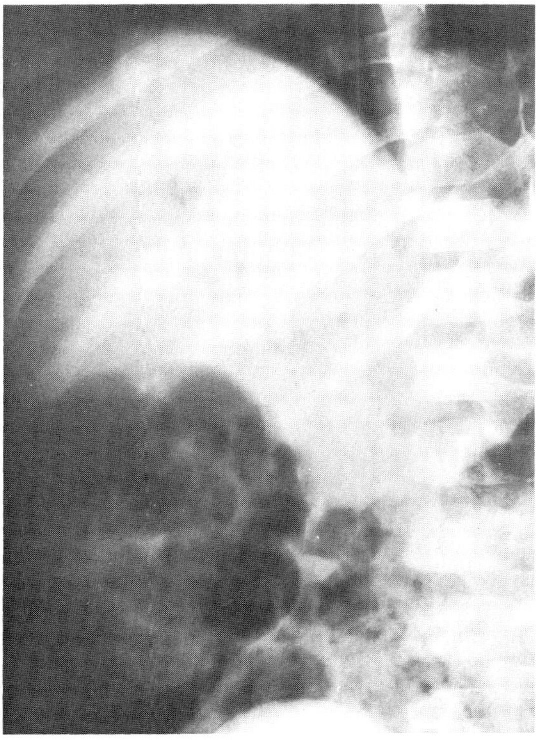

Figure 36–12. Plain x-ray showing gas in a hepatic abscess due to ascarides.

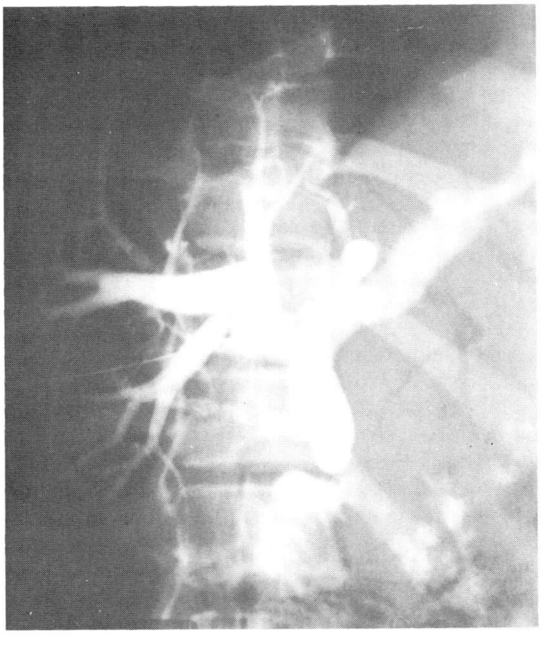

Figure 36–13. Percutaneous transhepatic cholangiogram showing a stricture of the common bile duct due to fibrosis secondary to *Ascaris* infection.

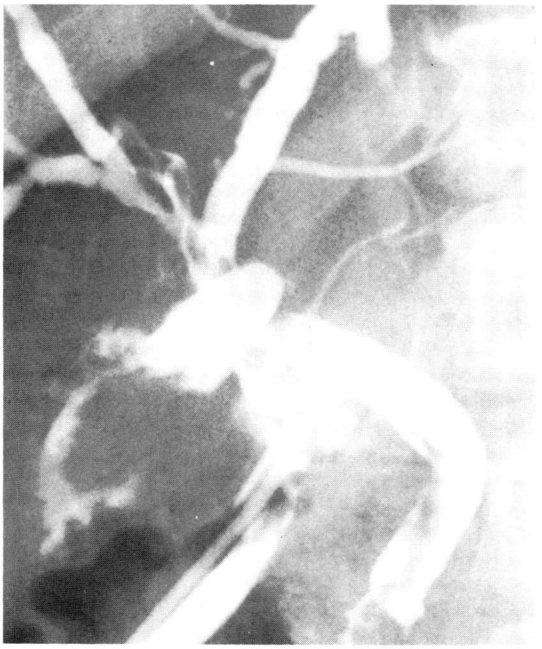

Figure 36–14. Operative cholangiogram showing an *Ascaris* parasite in the common bile duct.

essential. In six of our patients this investigation revealed worms in dilated common ducts (Fig. 36–14); in two, a stricture of the duct with proximal dilatation (Fig. 36–15); and in three, stones and worm debris in dilated ducts (Fig. 36–16).

Radioisotope scanning of the liver may be of some value in detecting hepatic granulomata (Fig. 36–17), particularly those complicated by secondary infection and abscess formation (Fig. 36–18). Ultrasonography is also useful for the detection of a mass (Fig. 36–19), and, occasionally, arteriography may be required to determine that such a mass is not neoplastic (Fig. 36–20).

TREATMENT

Uncomplicated Biliary Ascariasis

We believe that uncomplicated cases of biliary ascariasis should be treated conservatively, and we resort to operative treatment only when complications are suspected. Despite reports, mainly from the Far East, that recommended early surgical removal of the worms from the bile duct,[23–25] as early as 1966 we made a strong plea for a conservative approach in children.[47] Based on our good results, we again recommended a conservative approach in 1974, when our series stood at 148 patients.[28] From our experience it is clear that conservative management of uncomplicated biliary ascariasis is entirely satisfactory—most cases will subside within 24 to 48 hours, and most patients are well within 3 to 8 days.[47]

Indeed, operative intervention more than doubles the period of hospitalization and carries the risk of worms escaping into the peritoneal cavity. A conservative approach is particularly rewarding in young patients (under 20 years) because of the rarity of complications in this age group. Our experience parallels that of Chang and Han,[27] who, in their series of 788 children treated over a 5 year period at the Peking Children's Hospital, found that 97.7 per cent responded to medical treatment. On the other hand, others recommend early surgical removal of the worms from the common bile duct in all cases.[23–25, 48] It should be noted, however, that almost all these reports are based on experience in older patients, about 60 per cent of whom have complications requiring surgical intervention. Whether this justifies such an aggressive approach in every case is debatable, because we found that adults with uncomplicated biliary ascariasis responded to conservative measures as well as the children did.

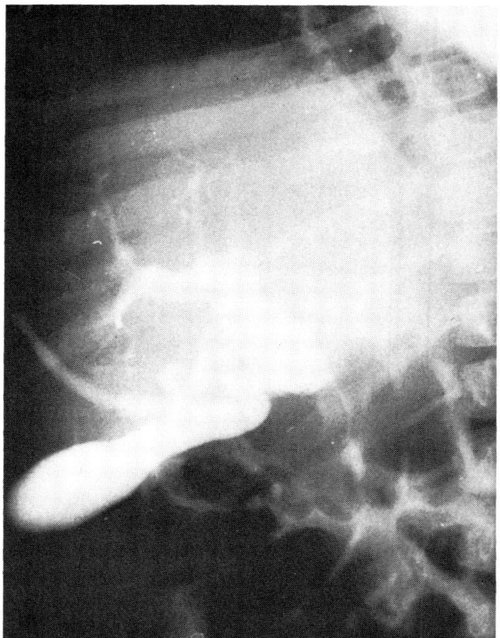

Figure 36–15. Operative cholangiogram showing a stricture of the common bile duct and gross dilatation of the biliary tree.

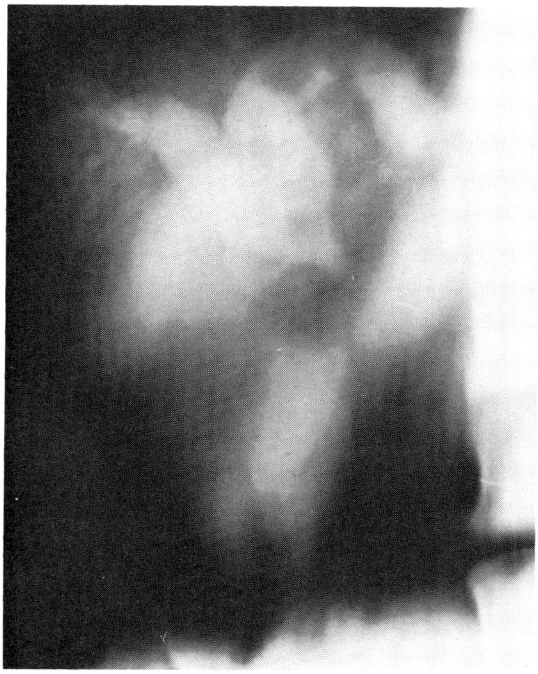

Figure 36–16. Operative cholangiogram showing gallstones secondary to *Ascaris* infection.

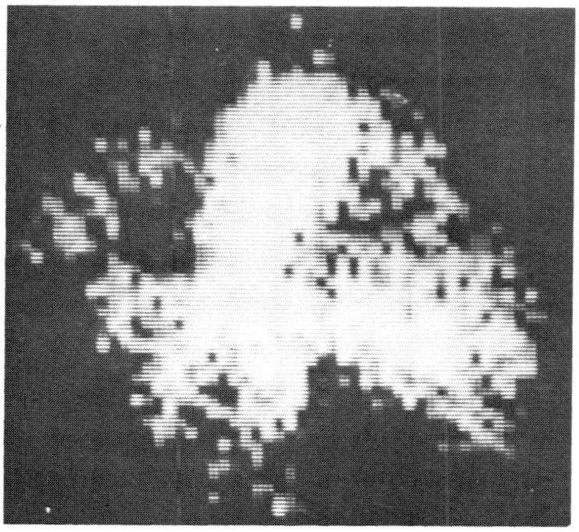

Figure 36–17. Liver scan showing multiple granulomata.

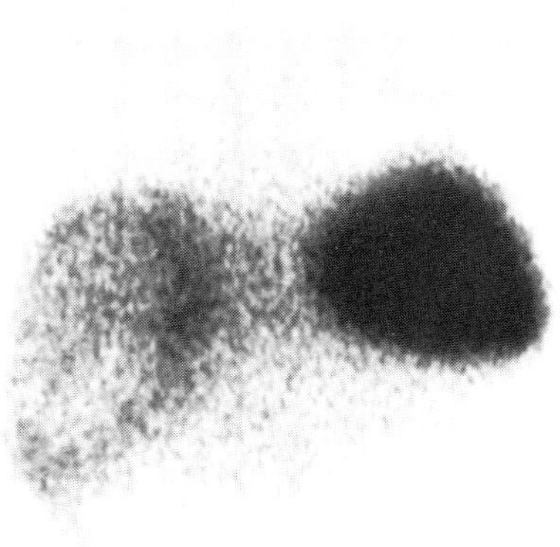

Figure 36–18. Isotope scan showing liver and spleen with an abscess in the liver.

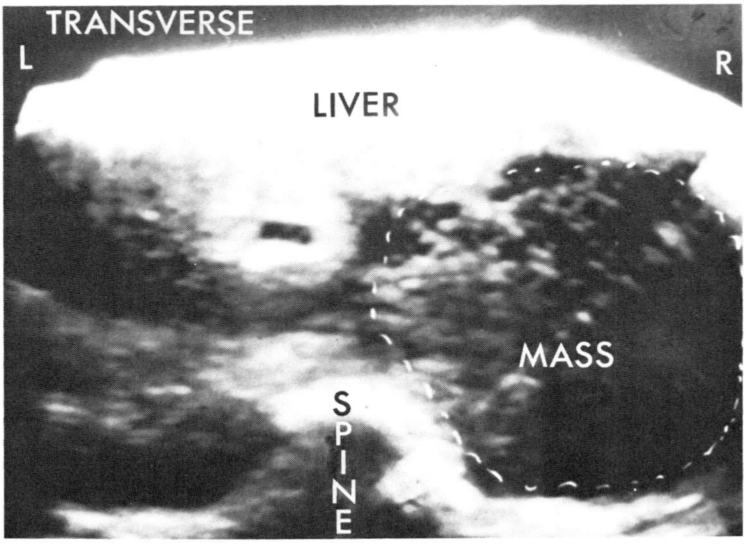

Figure 36–19. Ultrasonogram showing a liver mass compatible with an abscess containing worm debris.

The initial treatment consists of gastrointestinal decompression, intravenous fluids, antispasmodics, and sedation until the acute symptoms subside, usually within 3 days. The patient is then given a vermifuge. It is wise to wait until the acute symptoms have resolved prior to anthelmintic therapy to avoid killing the worms in the biliary tree. Intravenous cholangiography or ERCP can be used to check the biliary tree after therapy, and endoscopic papillotomy may be needed if additional parasites are found in the bile ducts at this time.[42] At first we used piperazine citrate (Antepar), but in recent years we have changed to mebendazole (Vermox). Piperazine adipate or Entacyl and diethyl carbamazine thiabendazole have been used by others.[20, 22] Following the administration of vermifuge, large numbers of worms are passed in the stools and the symptoms cease. For example, 90 per cent of 427 patients with uncomplicated biliary ascariasis treated conservatively by us became entirely asymptomatic within 5 days. In the remaining 10 per cent there was a slight recrudescence of pain shortly after administration of the anthelmintic, but all but one patient settled down within 10 days; the mean period of hospitalization was 7 days. Some individuals returned later, however, with reinfestation.

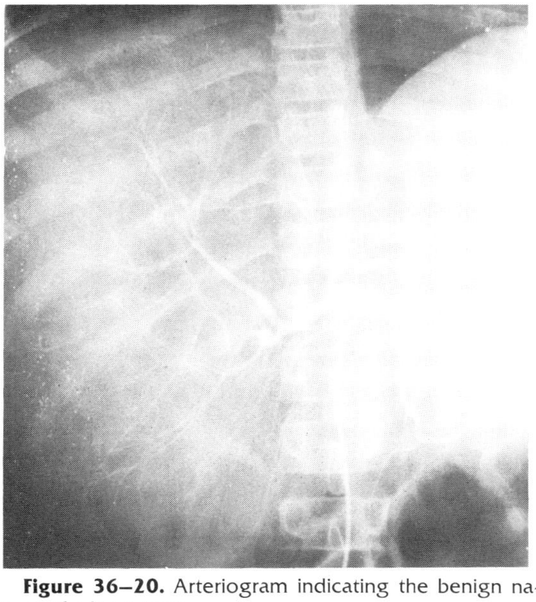

Figure 36–20. Arteriogram indicating the benign nature of a liver mass.

In our series of 440 uncomplicated cases of biliary ascariasis, only 13 patients were operated upon. A discussion of the management of these patients highlights several aspects of the operative treatment of uncomplicated biliary ascariasis.

1. *Mistaken diagnosis* (four patients). In three individuals, acute subhepatic appendicitis was suspected, and in one, acute intussusception. In all of them the gallbladder was distended and tense, and worms were palpable in the common duct. Further surgery was withheld in all but one patient, in whom choledochotomy was performed and five worms removed. On the eighth postoperative day, worms emerged alongside the T-tube without apparent ill effect, and tube cholangiography demonstrated additional worms in the common duct. Further x-rays on the tenth day showed a clear and patent common duct, and the T-tube was removed. The child

recovered rapidly after a vermifuge, but his period of hospitalization was 3 weeks. The others were well enough to be discharged within 10 days.

2. *Persistent linear filling defects in the ducts for 2 to 3 weeks* (five patients). In one, already referred to, a dead worm was retrieved from the common duct after 2 weeks; in another, live worms were removed from the common bile duct; in the remaining three, no worms were found. Two of these patients, however, discharged worms via and beside the T-tube afterwards. The mean period of hospitalization was 3 weeks. Fortunately, none of these patients discharged worms into the peritoneal cavity.

3. *Persistent dilatation of the common duct for 2 to 3 weeks* (four patients). A worm was retrieved from the common duct of only one of these patients. The others underwent unnecessary choledochotomy, and, although they recovered without complications, they had to spend an additional 10 days in the hospital.

In regard to persistent presence of worms in the duct as judged by linear defects or dilatation of the common bile duct, it would appear that we were too hasty in resorting to surgery after 2 to 3 weeks. The risk of leaving worms in the common bile duct is related to the death of the worm, which may result in stricture and/or stone formation. Therefore, much depends upon how long the worm can survive in the biliary system. From our experience, it appears to be fallacious to assume death of the worm within 3 weeks; perhaps it should be assumed that ascarides can survive and therefore get out of the bile duct for 4 to 6 weeks. Had this been our guideline it is possible that at least eight of our patients would have been saved an unnecessary operation and 10 additional days of hospitalization. It has now become clear that patients with persistent filling defects in the common duct on follow-up cholangiography should be given a further trial of medical therapy, including anthelmintics, unless they have developed cholangitis. When medical therapy fails or severe infection is present, endoscopic removal or surgery may be needed.

Complicated Biliary Ascariasis

Operative treatment is required in addition to anthelmintic therapy in most cases of complicated biliary ascariasis. Complications were present in 5 per cent of the patients under 20 years of age in our series and in 60 per cent of patients over 20 years. All of them required surgical intervention either as an emergency or electively.

Operation may also be indicated, as discussed earlier, for patients with persistent filling defects on follow-up cholangiography or those with persistent symptoms after anthelmintic therapy. Some of these patients, however, may be treated by endoscopic sphincterotomy. Persistent biliary worms may be removed by endoscopy. If the worm is protruding from the ampulla of Vater, extraction is relatively easy.[42] If the worm is completely within the common bile duct, evacuation may be achieved by irrigating the common bile duct with saline solution and administering intravenously an antispasmodic to relax the sphincter of Oddi.[44]

At the time of surgery, worms are usually palpable as thickened cords in the bile duct. When in doubt, operative cholangiography through the gallbladder or the cystic duct is helpful. Biliary worms should be removed through a longitudinal choledochotomy with ring forceps. The biliary tree should then be carefully inspected (aided by compression of the liver surface), thoroughly irrigated, and drained through a T-tube. Some recommend flushing of the biliary system and duodenum with vermifuges.[13, 20, 25] Piperazine citrate and 2 per cent santonin in alcohol have been used, injecting a quarter of the solution into the gallbladder, a quarter into the common duct, and half into the duodenum, and clamping the T-tube for 8 to 24 hours thereafter.

The bile ducts should be checked postoperatively with T-tube cholangiography to ascertain the absence of worms. If postoperative infestation has occurred, the T-tube should be irrigated with saline solution to flush the parasites into the intestine. Parasites that persist after 4 weeks can be removed through the T-tube tract or endoscopically.

Emergency surgery was necessary in 12 of 38 patients with complicated biliary ascariasis treated by us. Two had perforation of the common bile duct and required laparotomy and drainage, two had acute cholecystitis and required cholecystectomy, and eight had abscesses complicating hepatic granulomata and required drainage. All of them had stormy postoperative courses but recovered completely.

When biliary strictures or stones are present, they require independent treatment. For example, in our series, 14 patients with strictures and/or stones required elective operations. Only three of these patients were children, and two of them responded to dilatation of the stricture and prolonged T-tube drainage. The third, who had a stricture and stones, required a cholecystojejunostomy, which subsequently had to be revised twice, and he now has biliary cirrhosis. Three of the adults with primary pigment stones were treated by choledochostomy and have remained well. Two of the adults had strictures without stones, and both had undergone previous cholecystectomy. They were treated by choledochoduodenostomy and have done well. The remaining six adults had strictures complicated by stones. Of these, one had a previous cholecystectomy and three had previous biliary-intestinal anastomoses. All had histories of *Ascaris* infestation dating back to childhood. They were all treated by choledochojejunostomy with removal of stones and have remained well since. For further details on the treatment of biliary strictures, refer to Chapter 27.

Liver granulomata or abscesses may require exploration. Occasionally, worms are seen under the capsule of the nodule. Prominent nodules should be explored by unroofing them, extracting the worms, and lavaging the cavity. We have operated on 12 patients with hepatic granulomata, essentially to establish the diagnosis. Biopsy and drainage were all that was done to these patients, and all have remained reasonably well. Others, however, advocate routine biliary decompression through a T-tube to avoid leakage from the cavity.[42] It is hoped that the granulomata will gradually fibrose and become inactive.

There is little doubt that the complications of biliary ascariasis require surgical treatment and that the results of surgery, particularly in those patients with strictures of the bile ducts, are not very encouraging. In some patients, emergency surgery may be lifesaving, and this is probably why some surgeons have become so aggressive in their approach to biliary ascariasis on the whole. However, it is important to realize that these complications are extremely rare in children.

SUMMARY AND CONCLUSIONS

Ascariasis is a worldwide problem. It is particularly prevalent in the Far East, Africa, and tropical zones, but in these days of international air travel may be encountered anywhere.

Biliary obstruction is a surprisingly common complication of ascariasis and occurred in almost 40 per cent of patients with acute abdominal problems due to the worm who were admitted to a children's hospital in Cape Town.

The diagnosis is made on a history of worms in vomitus or stools, severe biliary colic, right upper quadrant tenderness, and sometimes a palpable gallbladder and positive radiographic findings, especially a linear filling defect in a dilated common bile duct on intravenous cholangiography.

In children, 95 per cent of the cases are uncomplicated and present with a short, transient illness. In adults, on the other hand, complications such as strictures of the bile ducts, gallstones, hepatic granulomata, liver abscesses, and even pylephlebitis occur in 60 per cent of the cases.

Conservative treatment is recommended for uncomplicated cases, but laparotomy should be performed and appropriate surgery carried out in the following circumstances: (1) marked jaundice with a serum bilirubin above 4 mg/dl (70 μ mol/L); (2) gross or irregular hepatic enlargement, (3) associated local or generalized peritonitis, (4) failure of response to conservative therapy, (5) persistence of a linear shadow in the common bile duct for more than 4 weeks, and (6) persistent dilatation of the common duct for more than 6 weeks.

In the majority of patients operated upon, exploration of the duct with removal of worms and flushing of the biliary system with a vermifuge is all that is required. Cholecystectomy is only rarely indicated, but choledochojejunostomy or choledochoduodenostomy is sometimes necessary, and hepatic abscesses may require drainage.

REFERENCES

1. Hoppli R: Parasites and Parasitic Infections in Early Medicine and Science. Singapore, University of Malaya Press, 1959.
2. Arean VM, Crandall CA: Ascariasis. *In* Marcial-Rojas PA (ed): Pathology and Protozoal and Helminthic Diseases with Clinical Correlation. Baltimore, Williams & Wilkins, 1971, p 769.
3. Belding DL: Textbook of Parasitology. 3rd ed. New York, Appleton-Century-Crofts, 1965, p 1374.
4. Pawlowski ZS: Ascariasis. Clin Gastroenterol 1978; 7:157.
5. Monroe LS: Gastrointestinal parasites of man. *In* Bockus HL (ed): Gastroenterology. Philadelphia, WB Saunders, 1976, p 133.
6. Stoll NR: This wormy world. J Parasitol 1947;*33*:1.
7. WHO. Control of Ascariasis. A Report of a WHO

Expert Committee. WHO Technical Rep Ser No. 379, Geneva, 1967.
8. Saw HS, Somasundaram K, Kamatti R: Hepatic ascariasis. Arch Surg 1974;*108*:733.
9. De AK, Sinha P: Surgical complications of ascaris infestation in the gastrointestinal tract in man, their pathogenesis (a histopathological study) and clinical significance. Third International Congress of Parasitology—Proceedings, 1974; *2*:791.
10. Muazzam MG, Khaleque KA, Ibrahim M: Hepatic ascariasis. J Trop Med Hyg 1960;*63*:95.
11. Warner FS, Healy JD: Fatal ascariasis in a Negrito child. JAMA 1961;*176*:949.
12. Morishita K, Yokogawa M: Recent Status of Ascariasis Control in Japan: A Progress Report. Abstracts of the International Congress on Tropical Medicine and Malaria. 9th ed. Athens, 1973, p 176.
13. Pfefferman R, Floman Y, Rozin RR: Ascariasis of the biliary system. Arch Surg 1972;*105*:118.
14. Boulvin R: Les incidences chirurgicales de l'ascaridiose in Iran. Acta Chir Belg 1959;*58*:161.
15. Martin LK: Hookworm in Georgia. Am J Trop Med Hyg 1972;*21*:919.
16. Blumenthal DS, Schultz MG: Incidence of intestinal obstruction in children affected with *Ascaris lumbricoides*. Am J Trop Med Hyg 1975;*24*:801.
17. Waller CE, Othersen HB Jr: Ascariasis. Surgical complications in children. Am J Surg 1970;*120*:50.
18. Turley K, Sherman RT: Biliary ascariasis. Am Surg 1976;*42*:166.
19. Williams D, Burke G, Hendley JO: Ascariasis: a family disease. J Pediatr 1974;*84*:853.
20. Sauer PE, Murdock CE, Erwin JH, et al: The surgeon and the worm. Arch Surg 1968;*97*:595.
21. Jung RC Jelliffe DB: Intestinal helminths. *In* Trowell HC, Jelliffe DB (eds): Diseases of Children in the Subtropics and Tropics. London, Edward Arnold Ltd, 1958, p 402.
22. Manson P: Ascariasis. *In* Manson-Bahr PH (ed): Manson's Tropical Diseases. 15th ed. London, Bailliere, Tindall and Cassell, 1960, p 786.
23. Wang HC, Tang C, Liu HH, et al: Biliary ascariasis: an analysis of 141 cases. Chin Med J 1956;*74*:445.
24. Liang SF, Wang HC, Wang TH, et al: Parasitic invasion of the biliary tract: a report of 140 surgically treated cases. Chin Med J 1957;*75*:418.
25. Wright RM, Dorrough RL, Ditmore HB: Ascariasis of the biliary system. Arch Surg 1963;*86*:402.
26. Yang SCH, Laube PJ: Biliary ascariasis. Report of 19 cases. Ann Surg 1946;*123*:299.
27. Chang CC, Han CT: Biliary ascariasis in childhood. A clinical analysis of 788 cases. Clin Med J 1966;*85*:167.
28. Louw JH: Biliary ascariasis in childhood. S Afr J Surg 1974;*12*:219.
29. Orloff MJ: The biliary system. *In* Sabiston DC (ed): Davis-Christopher Textbook of Surgery. 11th ed. Philadelphia, WB Saunders, 1977, p 1236.
30. Small DM: Cholelithiasis. *In* Bockus HL (ed): Gastroenterology, Vol IV. Philadelphia, WB Saunders, 1976, p 740.
31. Maki T: Cholelithiasis in Japanese. Arch Surg 1961;*82*:599.
32. Anstey L: Granulomatous ascaris hepatitis. S Afr Med J 1966;*40*:13.
33. Ochsner A, DeBakey EG, Dixon JL: Complications of ascariasis requiring surgical treatment. Am J Dis Child 1949;*77*:389.
34. Phuoc HH, Schmauss AK: Embolie eines ausgewachsenen ascaris lumbricoides in die arteria femoralis. Munch Med Wochenschr 1955;*107*:1482.
35. Issacs I: Roentgenographic demonstration of intestinal ascariasis in children without using barium. Am J Roentgenol Rad Ther Nucl Med 1956;*24*:215.
36. Cremin BJ, Fisher RM: Biliary ascariasis in children. Am J Roentgenol Rad Ther Nucl Med 1976;*126*:352.
37. Schulman A, Roman T, Dalrymple R, et al: Sonography of biliary worms (ascariasis). J Clin Ultrasound 1982;*10*:77.
38. Cremin BJ: Ultrasonic diagnosis of biliary ascariasis: "a bull's eye in the triple O." Br J Radiol 1982;*55*:683.
39. Schulman A, Loxton AJ, Heydenrych JJ, et al: Sonographic diagnosis of biliary ascariasis. AJR 1982;*139*:485.
40. Uflacker R, Wholey MH, Amaral NM, et al: Parasitic and mycotic causes of biliary obstruction. Gastrointest Radiol 1982;*7*:173.
41. Cerri GG, Leite GJ, Simoes JB, et al: Ultrasonographic evaluation of ascaris in the biliary tract. Radiology 1983;*146*:753.
42. Lloyd DA: Hepatobiliary ascariasis in children. Surg Annu 1982;*14*:277.
43. Van der Spuy S: Biliary ascariasis: endoscopic aspects. S Afr Med J 1978;*53*:1030.
44. Spitaels JM, Lloyd DA, Boultbee JE: Biliary ascariasis. S Afr Med J 1978;*54*:1044.
45. Pillay SP, Baker LW, Angorn IB: *Ascaris lumbricoides* producing obstructive jaundice. J R Coll Surg Edinb 1978;*23*:25.
46. Messer J, Solano C, Romeu J, et al: An unusual case of obstructive jaundice. Am J Gastroenterol 1984;*79*:152.
47. Louw JH: Abdominal complications of *Ascaris lumbricoides* infestation in children. Br J Surg 1966;*53*:510.
48. Phillips RD, Yune HY: Surgical helminthiasis of the biliary tract. Ann Surg 1960;*152*:905.

JOHN LOEWENTHAL, M.B.
LAWRENCE W. WAY, M.D.

37

Echinococcosis

Echinococcosis, a cestode infection, is one of the zoonoses, which have been defined as "those diseases and infections which are naturally transmitted between animals and man." While it occurs principally in sheep-raising countries, it is now widespread, as the dog, a definitive host, is a common animal in all latitudes. Also, increasing migration, the high mobility of troops, and the greater incidence of world travel among all people suggest that this complaint may be more frequently encountered in the future.[22]

HISTORY

The word *echinococcosis* is of Greek origin and means "hedgehog berry." *Hydatid* is, of course, also of Greek origin and means "a drop of water" or a "watery vesicle." This name was first used in 1808 by Rudolphi.[9] The disease has been known since earliest times; it was noted in the Talmud and was also known to Hippocrates, who speaks in his fifty-fifth aphorism of "livers full of water." The first North American case was observed by Low in 1808 and reported in 1822.[9]

EPIDEMIOLOGY[34]

This disease is a major cause of human morbidity and mortality in many parts of the world. The parasite produces the disease not only in humans but also in many other species. While it occurs in most of the sheep-raising areas of the world, in some of them it falls particularly heavily. The disease has long been endemic in Australia and New Zealand, Greece, Siberia, Turkistan, Mongolia, North China, Japan, the Philippines, the Middle East, and South America. In Iceland there was a particular problem in the nineteenth century. The disease was very prevalent, but owing to proper education of the population and implementation of the simple public health measures necessary to control the spread of the infection, it has been largely wiped out.

There is a spectrum of virulence of the infestation. In Canada and Alaska, a benign sylvatic form of *Echinococcus granulosus* occurs, the intermediate hosts being the moose and caribou and the definitive host being the wolf. In central Europe, Siberia, Canada, and Alaska, infection with a related species, *E. multilocularis*, occurs. The natural definitive and intermediate hosts of this species are foxes and small cricetid rodents (e.g., voles), respectively. In man this infestation forms a dense honeycomb of small cystic spaces, which infiltrates the host organ widely like a local malignancy.[23, 38] It can be treated only by major organ resection and despite treatment is highly lethal.[17]

BIOLOGY OF THE PARASITE[9, 34]

In man and grazing animals—the intermediate hosts—it is the cystic larval stage of the small cestode worm, *E. granulosus*, that is responsible for hydatid disease. The adult worm normally inhabits the ileum of the dog, which is its common definitive host. The complete life cycle of the worm requires the involvement of both a carnivorous and a herbivorous or omnivorous mammal. The most common domestic linkage is dog/sheep, but the cystic stage of this domestic cycle can also occur in cattle, swine, goats, horses, camels, and man (Fig. 37–1). The sylvatic cycle involves carnivores such as wolves, jackals, dingoes, and jaguars and, as intermediate hosts, elk, moose, reindeer, wallaby, and kangaroo. The domestic cycle is the one of greater clinical significance and is largely confined to sheep-raising areas, where a close

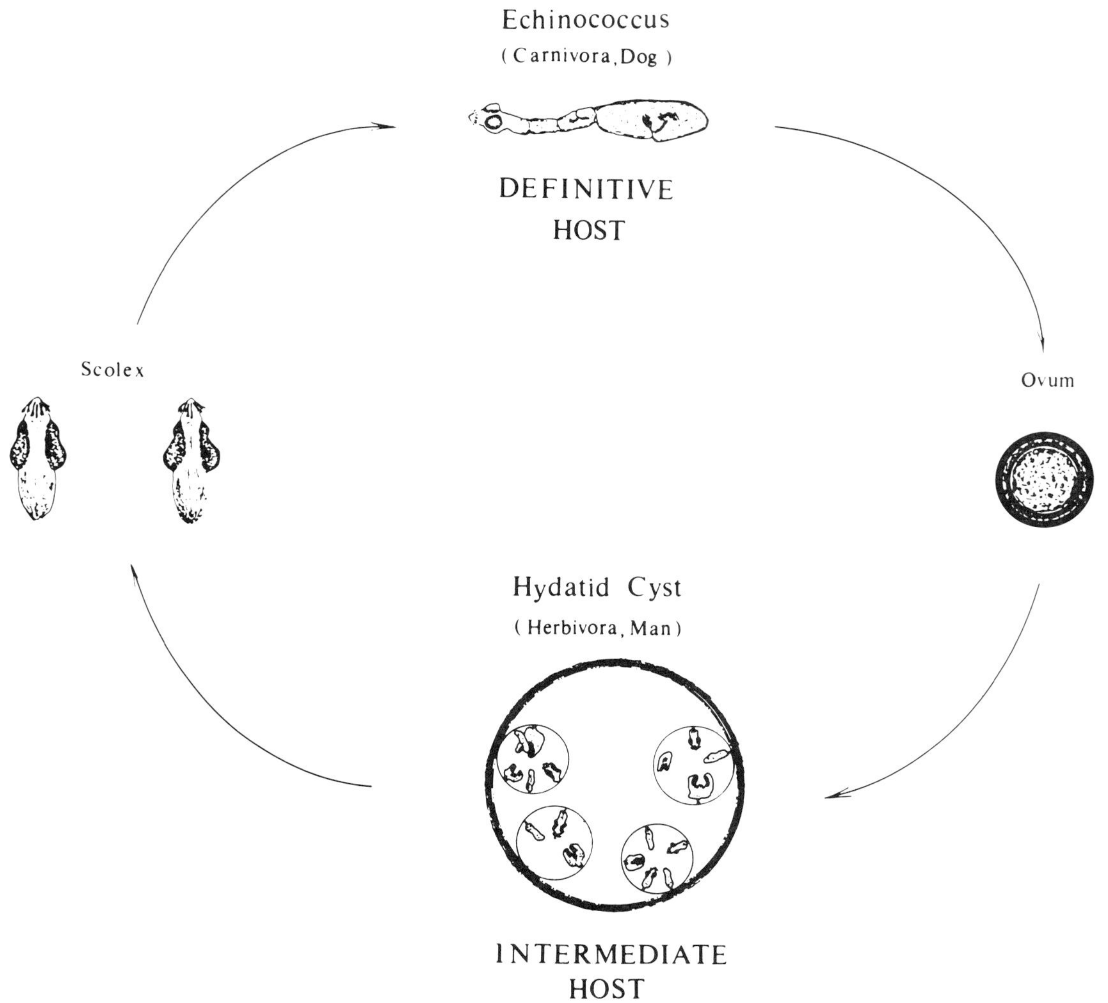

Figure 37–1. Life cycle of *Echinococcus granulosus.*

and intimate relationship exists between men and their dogs.

The worm, as seen in the small intestine of the dog, is made up of a head and three other segments measuring in all 3 to 6 mm in length (Fig. 37–2). The head is small (0.3 to 0.5 mm transverse diameter) and at its end is a retractile rostellum. Around the rostellum is a double row of chitinous hooklets in each row. These vary in shape and undoubtedly assist in the fixation of the worm to the mucosa of the host ileum. Behind this row are four suckers (0.16 mm in diameter), and behind this is a neck. The next segment is ill defined and slightly longer than it is broad, whereas the third segment is bigger and broader. When fully developed, this terminal segment measures 0.6 mm and as a result is substantially as large as the aggregate of the other three segments. It contains male and female gonads.

The ova are small (30 to 36 μ) and very resistant to physical agents. In the fresh state, they have a semi-glutinous capsule outside a firm chitinous shell, which, in turn, closely surrounds the ovarian cell and its yolk. Segmentation proceeds while the ovum is still in the terminal segment of the worm, and a

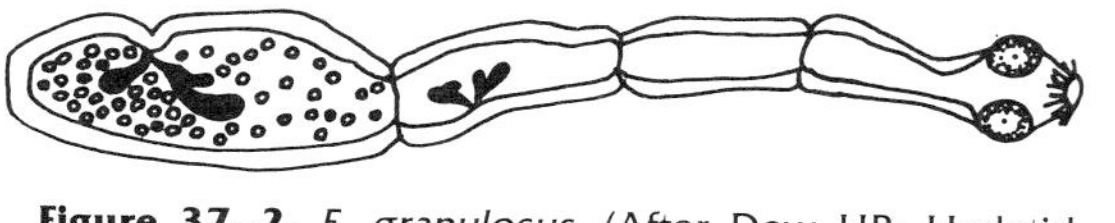

Figure 37–2. *E. granulosus.* (After Dew HR: Hydatid Disease: Its Pathology, Diagnosis and Treatment. Sydney, Australasian Medical Publishing Co., 1928.)

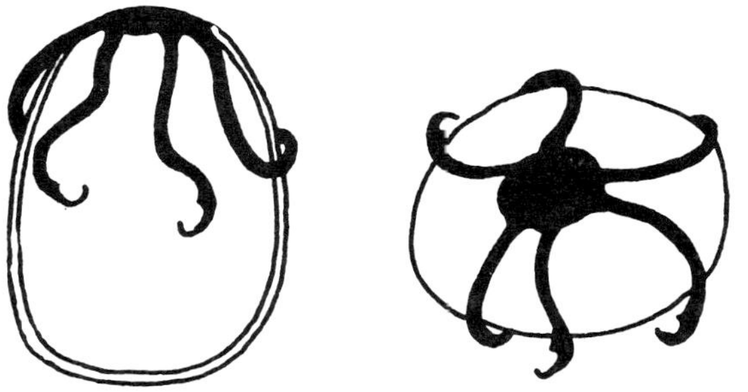

Figure 37–3. *E. granulosus*: the hexacanth or "boring" embryo. (After Dew HR: Hydatid Disease: Its Pathology, Diagnosis and Treatment. Sydney, Australasian Medical Publishing Co., 1928.)

cellular six-hooked embryo is thus developed (Fig. 37–3). This is known as the oncosphere or hexacanth ("boring") embryo. The ripe segments, crowded with ova, are discharged from the bowel of the dog, which may pass many thousands of ova daily; the ova may then be ingested by man and by herbivora such as sheep and cattle. In these animals the parasite passes through the metacestode (cystic) stage, but it can return to the dog only if the dog eats the infected organs or carcass of such an animal. As dogs these days have little access to human viscera, man represents an end stage to the parasite.

DEVELOPMENT IN THE INTERMEDIATE HOST

Implantation

The hexacanth embryo is rapidly hatched in the stomach or upper small bowel of the intermediate host and becomes very active, boring through the wall of the bowel, making its way into a tributary of the portal vein, and thence being carried to the liver. Dew[9] demonstrated the presence of the embryo in the portal vein within 8 hours of feeding ova to young pigs. In the liver the embryo may come to rest anywhere in the liver lobules. It may, however, pass through the liver filter and enter the inferior vena cava, whence it is carried to the lungs, which in humans and most animals is the second most frequent location of cysts. Lung and liver cysts may coexist. Clearly, the organism may, in a few instances, escape the meshes of the pulmonary filter and so infect bones, brain, heart, kidney, muscle, or other tissues.

Early Cystic Development

The hydatid follicle may be recognized in the liver within 12 hours of infestation as an accumulation of mononuclear cells, with abnormal staining reactions in the surrounding liver cells indicating, even at this early stage, that a diffusible toxin is being elaborated. At the end of 7 days the parasite is more distinctly demarcated from the surrounding liver cells, the vascular reaction is more intense, and some local hemorrhagic extravasation may be seen. It appears that up to this stage the parasite may be overwhelmed and that phagocytosis may occur. If it survives, by the end of 3 weeks the follicle is much larger and contains a cyst visible to the naked eye. Growth is now usually even, and a perfectly spherical shape is the rule. However, the line of least resistance may be followed, with consequent variations in shape.

At 3 months the follicle may be 40 to 50 mm in diameter; it has an inner nucleated and one outer laminated layer with elasticity appearing in its laminations, so that rupture of the adventitia may allow the cyst to slip out readily. By 5 months the main adventitious capsule, which is produced from the host tissues, is much more fibrous and may appear white and avascular to the naked eye. It is largely acellular, but there are spaces within it that enclose blood vessels and sometimes small bile ducts with intact epithelium. The persistence of small biliary channels in the adventitia is a characteristic feature, and patent ducts may be discovered close to the parasite itself. The larger ducts and blood vessels may act as points of resistance and lead to distortion of the cyst. Large patent veins may persist in the adventitia, and the cyst may even project into their lumen.

As late as 5 months there may be signs of retrogression of the cyst. As this proceeds the fluid is absorbed, the laminated membrane becomes folded and degenerated, and the adventitia contracts and thickens. A wrinkled fibrotic sac results, which may become the site of calcareous deposits, or the whole cyst may be absorbed and replaced by a fibrous nodule.

Fully Developed Cyst

Survival of the cyst is the rule, with steady increase in size by the deposition of laminated hyaline material. A large unilocular cyst results, which in man may contain many liters of fluid. The laminated membrane may reach 0.5 cm in thickness and is usually white; since it is elastic and loosely attached to the adventitia, it readily collapses and separates from the adventitia when intracystic pressure is lowered by puncture or rupture. When collapsed, it may be withdrawn complete from the adventitious capsule. The elasticity of the laminated membrane ensures loosening and dissemination of the scolices when the cyst ruptures—a factor of great biologic significance. Its thickness also ensures a certain degree of rigidity of the cyst wall, giving protection to the thin germinal layer and the developing brood capsules.

The thin germinal layer (endocyst) of 10 to 25 μ thickness is attached very lightly to the laminated membrane. It gives rise to the brood capsules, which contain the scolices, and also the hydatid fluid and the laminated membrane itself. The colorless crystal-clear hydatid fluid (specific gravity 1.008 to 1.015) acts as a protective buffer and nutritive medium to the developing scolex and has antigenic properties. Anaphylaxis can result from its injection into sensitized subjects.

Development of Brood Capsules and Scolices

Completed biologic development of the cyst is attained with the development from the germinal layer of brood capsules, in which the scolices or future worm heads develop. This usually occurs after 6 months of growth. The brood capsule develops as a small cellular mass in the germinal layer, which becomes vacuolated as it grows. The scolex in due course repeats the process in the wall of the brood capsule and goes on to full differentiation and maturation with a tenuous attachment by a fine pedicle to the capsule wall. Slight trauma may set the capsule free and also rupture it, releasing the scolices. As they may be present in thousands and are just barely visible, they have been referred to as hydatid sand.[9] It has been estimated that 1 ml of this hydatid sand contains 400,000 scolices. This larval stage, the scolex, is remarkable for being capable of differentiating in two directions. In the dog, the scolex develops into adult tapeworms. In the intermediate host (sheep, man, and so forth), each of the released scolices is capable of differentiating into a new hydatid cyst. Thus, a scolex has the potential of developing either into a tapeworm in an intestinal site or into a hydatid cyst in a tissue site, a degree of heterogeneous morphogenesis unusual for a metazoan organism.

Daughter Cyst Formation

Daughter cyst formation is regarded as a defense reaction to some noxious stimulus. Because the cyst may exist for long periods in man, the consequent liability of the parasite to some type of damage makes daughter cyst formation common in human infection.

The daughter cysts are true replicas of the mother cyst, being composed of an outer laminated and an inner nuclear layer and usually containing brood capsules and scolices. Their size and number vary enormously, and they may be seen either floating freely (Fig. 37–4) or so tightly packed that they mold and distort each other and thereby produce multivesicular cysts (Fig. 37–5). This development may be initiated by trauma from a direct blow, muscle contraction, or operation. Growth of the enlarging cyst along a natural channel, with a weakening and perforation of the hydatid membranes through lack of support and consequent leakage of hydatid fluid, has a similar effect. Such a point of perforation may allow ingress of blood, serum, bile, secretions, or infecting microorganisms with consequent damage to the simple cyst, leading to daughter cyst formation. Such a change is frequently and typically seen in hydatid cysts in the liver of adults, where the daughter cysts are usually

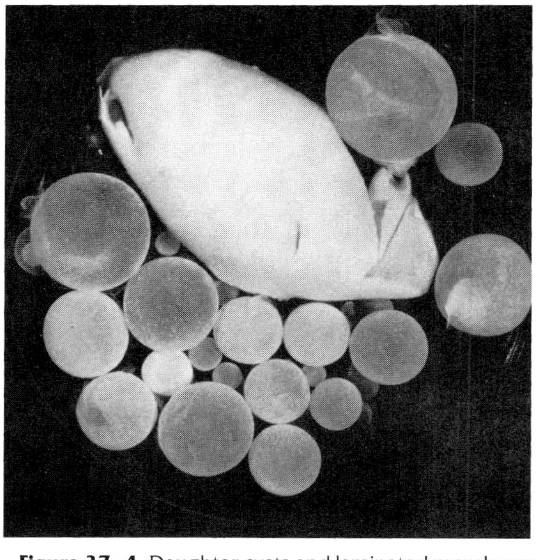

Figure 37–4. Daughter cysts and laminated membrane. Operative specimen.

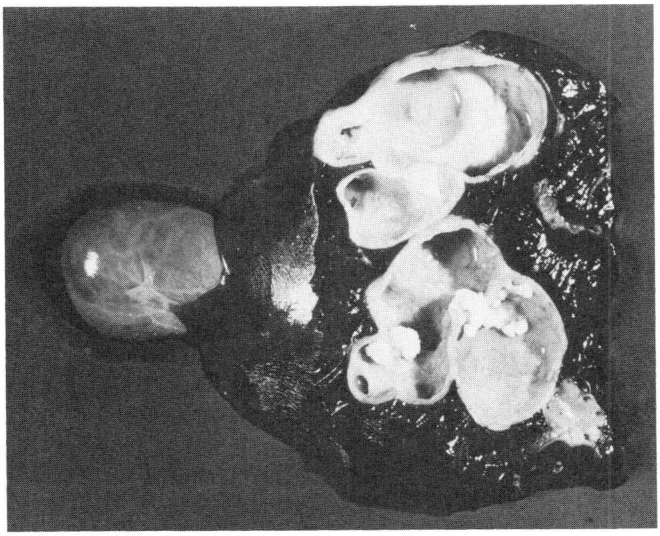

Figure 37–5. Multivesicular cysts.

bile-stained. In children, on the other hand, univesicular cysts are the rule. At the extreme, granddaughter cysts may arise within daughter cysts.

CLINICAL FEATURES

Latency

The outstanding feature of simple uncomplicated cysts is their extraordinary clinical latency. From the available evidence it would appear that many infestations are contracted during childhood, so that in the absence of complications, the cyst may be nearly as old as the patient. The host has usually accommodated to it with remarkable indifference, and his development and well-being are rarely impaired in any significant way. Any organ in the body may be affected, and symptomless, unsuspected cysts may be detected on routine examinations. Occasionally, a child harboring a large infestation becomes cachectic ("hydatid cachexia") and improves remarkably when the parasite is removed. Not all infections are of childhood onset, however, for there is good epidemiologic evidence that the disease may be contracted by adults, with the appearance of clinical manifestations within a few years.

Pressure Effects

Sooner or later, pressure effects appear, and bizarre symptoms may result from direct pressure or distortion of neighboring viscera. In confined areas, such as the central nervous system, the effect of quite small cysts may be serious. In less restricted areas, such as the liver, the cysts may occupy the greater part of the right lobe, and this can lead to compensatory hypertrophy of the left lobe, which, in turn, can lead to distortion of the costal margin and bulging of the chest or abdominal wall. It is remarkable that, in man, cysts may reach a size much greater than in any other animal. Pain, varying from local discomfort to a heavy dragging sensation, is a common effect of such pressure.

Death of the Parasite

Death of the parasite may take place at any time, though cysts have been known to remain alive for as long as 40 years. In the case of multiple infestation, some cysts may contain an active living parasite and others may be dead and degenerated. Death usually results from leakage or from a type of senility. Calcification in the wall of a dead cyst is common (Fig. 37–6).

Rupture

As the cyst enlarges, it comes into intimate contact with natural channels, such as bronchi, bile ducts, or any hollow viscus, and at the point of contact the cyst wall weakens, so that rupture of the cyst may occur.

The effect on the cyst of rupture may be

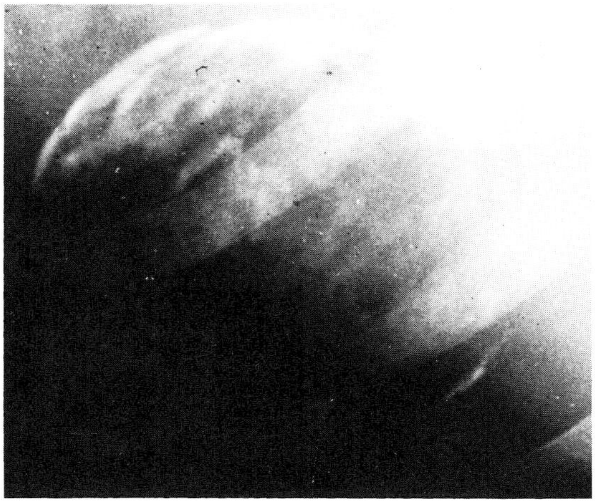

Figure 37–6. Calcified dead cyst.

twofold. Rupture into a large channel may allow more or less complete emptying of the fluid and laminated membrane and lead to spontaneous cure. Rupture into the biliary tract occurs in 5 to 10 per cent of patients with hydatid disease of the liver.[21, 45] In the biliary tract, discharge of the cyst contents in this way may cause severe colic and/or partial, intermittent, or complete ductal obstruction with cholangitis[1, 12, 21, 25, 27, 40, 45] or pancreatitis.[28] There may be associated anaphylaxis from the sudden absorption of the hydatid antigen in the sensitized patient; pruritus or an urticarial rash is the external manifestation. Episodes of asthma may occur. More commonly, however, the evacuation of cyst contents is incomplete, and secondary infection develops. The infecting organism is usually a fecal one, and this results in severe toxic and systemic upset. Occasionally the patient presents urgently with spontaneous or post-traumatic rupture.

The release of brood capsules, scolices, and even daughter cysts from a hepatic cyst into the peritoneal cavity may produce more sinister late results. It has long been recognized that young daughter cysts can implant and develop independently outside the original cyst. It has not always been realized, however, that scolices and brood capsules may behave similarly. The process constitutes a secondary smaller life cycle for the parasite, which occurs in the intermediate host alone, and which possesses the peculiarity that it can return at any time to the normal cycle. This phenomenon is known as secondary echinococcosis. A period of several years usually elapses between the original rupture and the onset of symptoms from secondary implantation. In some cases, 12 to 15 years may elapse. Implantation is not infrequently seen in operation scars, and secondary cysts arising in such wounds result from scolices liberated at the original operation.[24]

Suppuration

The laminated membrane is a potent antibacterial barrier, and leakage of the cyst is an essential preliminary to suppuration. The entry of serum into the cyst makes it an excellent medium for bacterial growth. In the liver, infected cysts are invariably bile-stained, so that leakage into the biliary tree is a constant accompaniment of suppuration in this situation. Infection of the parenchyma of the host tissue, however, may leave uncontaminated cysts unaffected; hydatid cysts of the lung may remain uncontaminated and apparently indifferent to a pneumonic infection around them. Once infection becomes established in the cyst, however, a pyogenic membrane develops on the inner surface of the adventitia. As a result, the walls of the cavity become increasingly rigid, and collapse and obliteration become progressively less likely. Rupture of an infected cyst may be through the diaphragm and pleura into a bronchus, producing a bronchobiliary fistula.[29, 39] This complication is said to occur in from 3.6 to 22 per cent of cases of liver hydatid cysts.[9] It invariably causes pain in the chest and upper abdomen, fever, cough, and bile-stained sputum, which may also contain recognizable hydatid elements.

Distribution of Cysts in the Body

Classic earlier descriptions reported 75 per cent of cysts occurring in the liver, 10 per cent in the lungs, and the remainder throughout the body. Recent evidence indicates that a larger proportion occurs in the lungs, the proportions being on the order of a 50 to 60 per cent incidence in the liver, 30 to 40 per cent in the lungs, 13 per cent in other areas of the abdomen, and 7 per cent in other sites. Liver cysts are multiple in 45 per cent of cases. Forty per cent of patients with cysts in the lung also have cysts in the liver, and 25 per cent of those with cysts in the liver have simultaneous pulmonary cysts.

SPECIAL INVESTIGATIONS

Standard x-ray examination readily reveals calcification in senile cysts (Fig. 37–6), but x-ray is of limited value with uncomplicated cysts.

Organ imaging has added another dimension to the diagnosis of hydatid disease. The liver scan will show a typical rounded defect, most frequently in the dome of the right lobe of the liver. Obviously, other lesions, such as benign nonparasitic cysts, will produce a similar appearance. Ultrasound has been useful in demonstrating the cystic nature of the lesion and will sometimes show the presence of unmistakable daughter cysts within the main cyst cavity.[14, 16] Ultrasonography is particularly useful in the work-up of patients who have hydatid cysts ruptured into the biliary ducts,[25, 27] as it is possible to differentiate daughter cysts from gallstones in many of these patients.[6, 37] Computerized axial tomography will show the cystic nature of the lesion as well as daughter cysts and other unsuspected small cysts.[15] Retrograde endoscopic cholangiography may be useful to demonstrate communication between the bile ducts and the cyst.[8, 27] Percutaneous transhepatic cholangiography with conventional sheathed needle may aid in the diagnosis of intrabiliary rupture of hydatid cyst, as daughter cysts may be identified in the common bile duct.[13, 36, 37]

IMMUNOLOGIC DIAGNOSIS

The antigenic nature of hydatid fluid is the basis of several immunologic tests.[4, 19, 35] Since the intensity of the immune reactions depends on the degree of absorption of antigen, they are not positive in all cases. Infected children often have negative tests; adults whose cyst shows the results of trauma (i.e., the presence of multiple daughter cysts) are more likely to have been exposed to hydatid antigen and usually give positive reactions to serologic testing.

The Casoni intradermal test is based on cutaneous hypersensitivity in response to intradermal injection of hydatid fluid. An urticarial reaction develops in 60 to 70 per cent of cases, but the test may also be positive in carcinomatosis, leishmaniasis, and teniasis.[7, 29] The high frequency of false positive reactions due to the presence of nonspecific antigens in hydatid fluid limits the diagnostic usefulness of skin testing.

Many serologic tests have been evaluated, including the indirect hemagglutination (IHA), immunofluorescent (IF), immunoelectrophoresis (IEP), bentonite fixation (BF), complement fixation (CF), latex agglutination (LA), double diffusion (DD), enzyme-linked immunosorbent assay (ELISA), and so forth.

A high-titer IHA reaction usually indicates active infection but is absent (i.e., false negative) in about 10 per cent of cases. Viable liver infection is more likely to be associated with a high titer than is lung infection or the presence of a senescent or dead parasite in the liver. Intermediate titers have been observed in serum from patients with collagen disease, cirrhosis of the liver, and schistosomiasis. A strong cross reaction occurs only with cysticercosis. Although they usually fall, titers may remain high after successful surgery.

Most laboratories perform the IHA test in combination with the IEP, IF, CF, BF, LA, or DD test.[19, 29] The strategy recommended by Schantz and Kagan consists of performing an initial screening with the IHA or LA test, followed by the IEP test if the first test is positive.[35] A positive IEP result is highly specific for active infection; only patients with *Taenia solium* cysticercosis have been observed to give a cross reaction. If the IHA or LA test is positive and the IEP test is negative, the serologic diagnosis is inconclusive.

Following successful surgery or spontaneous death of the parasite, the IEP test becomes negative within 6 to 12 months. Unless a preoperative specimen has been tested, however, interpretation of the reaction of convalescent sera may be difficult.

TREATMENT[2, 4, 10, 11, 26, 29–32, 39, 40]

The aims of treatment are (1) to remove the parasite completely, (2) to prevent contamination of the field by active scolices, and (3) to allow for healing of the residual cavity.

Cysts presenting on the lower surface of the liver are best exposed by an abdominal incision. Cysts located on the dome of the right lobe are best approached by a thoracotomy through the eighth intercostal space.

At operation, when the liver is exposed, the white adventitia of the cyst can usually be recognized (Fig. 37–7), and the area must be carefully isolated with meticulous tech-

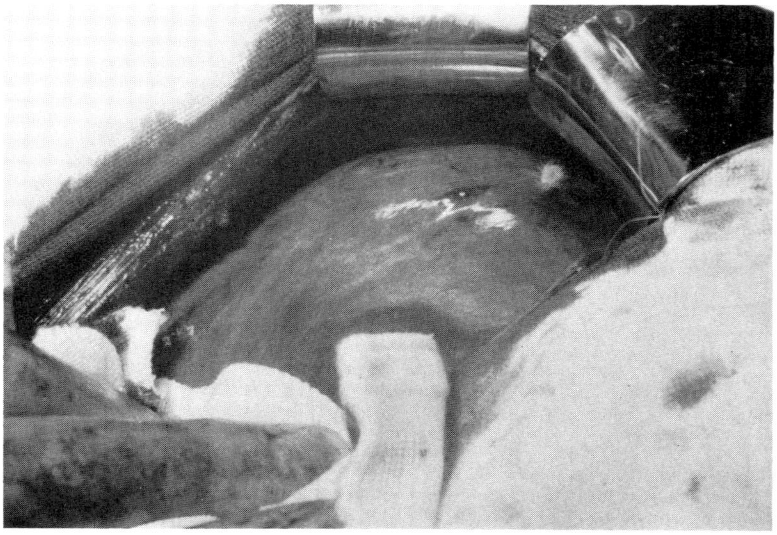

Figure 37–7. Hydatid cyst of liver: appearance on surface.

nique to avoid spillage and consequent dissemination. Drapes and packs colored blue or black are of advantage, as they contrast with the whitish color of laminated membrane and daughter cysts so that spillage is more easily detected. It should be remembered that more than one cyst is present in about half the cases, so that exploration must be thorough. A logical first step is to try to sterilize the cyst and its contents. The isolated cyst is partially aspirated, and hypertonic (20 per cent) NaCl solution or 0.5 per cent silver nitrate solution is injected. This is best accomplished using a large trocar connected to a three-way system. (A large-bore T-tube can be used instead of a three-way stopcock.) This system allows the surgeon to aspirate the cyst and intermittently inject NaCl solution to clear the tubing from membranes. Scolicidal agents are also used in multivesicular cysts to kill any scolices spilt from ruptured daughter cysts, but they cannot penetrate intact daughter cysts unless in contact with them for many hours.

The use of formalin as a scolicidal agent is best avoided if the cyst aspirate is bile-stained, as there is a risk of the formalin entering the bile ducts in such cases.

After most of the cyst contents have been aspirated, the cyst can be opened and carefully evacuated with a strong sucker (Fig. 37–8). The laminated membrane can be best managed with ring forceps. When removal is completed, the inside of the cyst should be

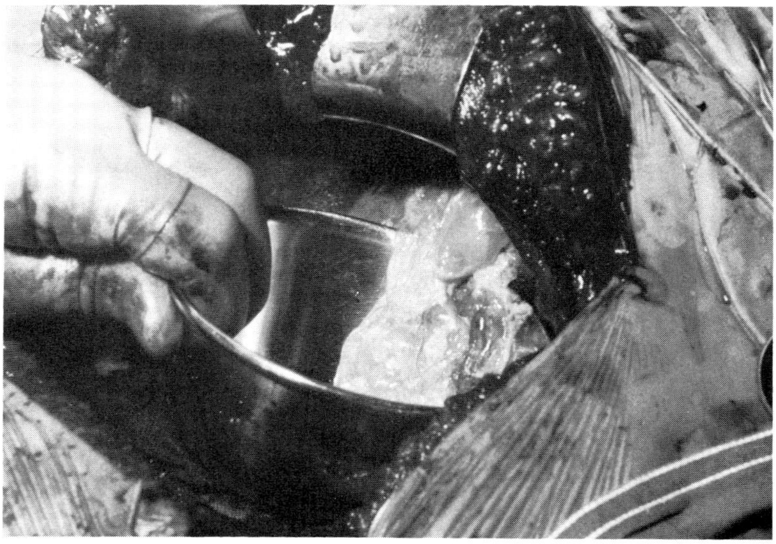

Figure 37–8. Emptying the cyst.

examined for pouches or the presence of another cyst that may be bulging into the cavity. Very commonly, small bile leaks may be detected in the adventitia wall, and these should be closed by oversewing with nonabsorbable suture. The adventitia of the cyst may be removed completely in superficial cysts, but in most cysts the deep parts of the adventitia are in close contact with large vessels and ducts and should be left undisturbed. The cavity (Fig. 37–9) may then be filled with warm saline solution and closed with a running catgut suture without drainage. If in doubt about the presence of infection, a drain may be left down to the area of closure.

Saidi[31, 32] has recommended management of the main cyst by freezing with a cryoprobe. This technique seems to be safe and effective, but the special equipment required has not made it popular. He also advises instillation of aqueous silver nitrate solution (0.5 per cent) for 2 minutes after removal of the parasite; this is then washed out with normal saline.

Multivesicular cysts, which typically are of long standing and comparatively large, usually have a thicker, irregular adventitia and perhaps some peritoneal adhesions. The presence of daughter cysts may be inferred from the repeated stoppage of the flow on aspiration. After such cysts are opened, evacuation is slow and may be difficult, the contents often being thick and turbid. These cavities, after being completely emptied, may also be filled with saline solution and closed unless there is gross bile contamination, obvious infection, or doubt as to the completeness of evacuation. Under these circumstances, when closure of the cavity is contraindicated, the cavity may be closed around a large tube, or it may be marsupialized by Lindemann's procedure.

Lindemann's operation consists of suturing the adventitia to the parietes, thereby allowing free and direct drainage of the cavity to the exterior. This process is comparatively safe, but the convalescence is slow, drainage may persist for months or years, and the technique is rarely used today. To avoid such a prolonged and tedious resolution, good results have been reported from the introduction of omentum into the cavity after fashioning a broad-based pedicle of it. In multiple cysts, two or three pedicles have been used; in cysts of the diaphragmatic surface, it has been introduced through a counteropening on the inferior surface of the cyst wall. Papadimitriou and Mandrekas[26] have reported a striking reduction in hospital stay when this was the preferred method for obliterating the cystic cavity. Over the past 15 years, obliteration of the cavity by internal suturing ("capitonnage") has been recommended, and this method of infolding the cyst walls may still be useful for small cysts.

Rupture of a liver hydatid into the biliary tree requires relief of the resulting obstructive jaundice, usually by exploration and drainage of the common bile duct as well as treatment of the primary cyst or cysts.[1, 38] When complete evacuation of membranes

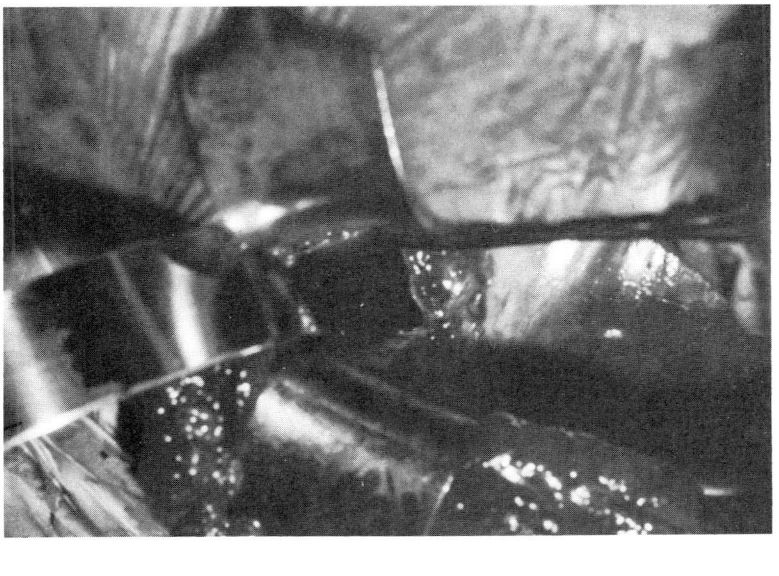

Figure 37–9. Opening of the residual cavity.

from the biliary tract is not possible, a sphincterotomy may be required. However, in most cases T-tube drainage of the common bile duct suffices. Unless the gallbladder is involved by the parasite, the gallbladder should be preserved whenever possible. Lygidakis advocates total cystectomy with enucleation between the false capsule of the host and the chitinous outer layer of the cyst for small and moderate-sized cysts. For large cysts, he performs either a lobectomy or a partial cystectomy with internal drainage by Roux-en-Y pericystojejunostomy. According to Lygidakis, drainage of the cyst into a Roux-en-Y loop eliminates the possibility of persistent biliary drainage, fistulae, hemorrhage, and residual disease. In a series of 39 patients with intrabiliary rupture of hydatid cysts treated according to this strategy, he reported an overall mortality of 2.6 per cent, morbidity of 5.8 per cent, and a hospital stay of only 10 days.[21]

The management of patients who have developed a bronchobiliary fistula as the result of penetration of the diaphragm by the liver cyst and consequent destruction of lung parenchyma with superimposed infection can tax the ingenuity of the surgeon.[29, 38] The majority of such patients require thoracotomy, resection of affected tissue, and drainage of the primary liver cyst.

The simplest and most commonly used method of handling the cyst cavity after evacuating the parasite is to fill it with saline solution and to close the edges with running absorbable sutures.

Complications of Surgery

In a review of 87 patients who underwent operation between 1964 and 1974, Little[20] reported that none suffered a severe allergic response to the removal of a hydatid cyst. Nineteen (24 per cent of those operated on) suffered chest infection postoperatively. Thirteen per cent of those having removal of abdominal hydatids developed a subphrenic abscess. Prolonged drainage from a cyst for more than 21 days was recorded in 27 per cent of those who had surgery. Other major complications, such as wound infection, occurred. Over a mean period of 5 years, 5 per cent of this group developed a proven recurrence requiring further surgical intervention. Only two patients died as a direct result of their hydatid disease. A similar experience with recurrent cyst formation has been reported by Mottaghian and Saidi.[24] These authors found that recurrence correlated with the presence of multiple cysts and with technical problems during surgery that resulted in spillage of cyst contents into the peritoneal cavity.

Indication for Operation

The decision to operate on a patient with hydatid disease is not always straightforward. There is little question about what should be done with a fit patient who has a large, trauma-prone hydatid cyst in the liver, while cysts in bone, the spine, the heart, or the brain will demand surgery for the preservation of life or function. It is equally clear that an elderly unfit patient with an asymptomatic calcified cyst should not generally be considered for surgery. The problem really arises in the middle-aged patient with an asymptomatic cyst in the liver. Since the natural history of hydatid cysts is one of growth and potential complications, we believe that asymptomatic cysts in healthy patients should be removed. When there is calcification of the cyst, one may take a more conservative approach. While it is true that such a cyst may be viable and that it may rupture or become infected, these events are rare.

It is probably a reasonable rule to operate on pulmonary hydatids if they coexist with liver cysts and if the patient is capable of withstanding surgery. Because of the poorly developed adventitial reaction and the almost uniform occurrence of bronchial communications, the chance of rupture of the hydatid with intrapulmonary dissemination of hydatid materials is ever present. In the liver, however, or the spleen, the presence of a relatively small hydatid—up to about 7 cm in diameter—should not necessarily indicate surgery. The morbidity in Little's series among the elderly was related largely to surgery, not to spontaneous complications caused by the hydatid.[20] It has been shown that very few hydatids are viable in patients older than 60 years, and advanced age should certainly make one lean toward conservatism unless the cyst is symptomatic. The chances of major complications from the presence of the cyst would seem to be much less than the very real risks of severe postoperative chest infection, subphrenic abscess, secondary cyst infection after surgery, and prolonged drainage from the cyst following operative intervention.

Drug Therapy

The drug mebendazole (-methyl 5-benzoyl benzimidazol-2-carbonate) or albendazole[5, 18, 41–44] is effective against the cystic form of *E. granulosus* infestation in experimental animals and has also been shown to reduce the size of experimental alveolar hydatid. Preliminary trials in humans[42, 44] suggest that the drug may have a role as an adjunct to surgical treatment, but the results of therapy are somewhat unpredictable and side effects are common.[41] It is most effective for pulmonary hydatids, less so for liver infections, and essentially ineffective for disease of the bone, brain, eye, and other sites. Mebendazole is certainly worth trying in those unfortunate patients with widely disseminated hydatid disease whose problems are not amenable to surgery, or in those with localized disease who are poor surgical risks for other reasons.

REFERENCES

1. Al-Hashimi HM: Intrabiliary rupture of hydatid cyst of the liver. Br J Surg 1971;*58*:228.
2. Amir-Jahed AK, Fardin R, Farzad A, et al: Clinical echinococcosis. Ann Surg 1975;*182*:541.
3. Apt W, Knierim F: An evaluation of tests for hydatid disease. Am J Trop Med Hyg 1970;*19*:943.
4. Barros JL: Hydatid disease of the liver. Am J Surg 1978;*135*, 597.
5. Bekhti A, Nizet M, Capron M, et al: Chemotherapy of human hydatid disease with mebendazole. Follow-up of 16 cases. Acta Gastroenterol Belg 1980;*43*:48.
6. Biggi E, Derchi L, Cicio GR, et al: Sonographic findings of hydatid cyst of the liver ruptured into the biliary ducts. J Clin Ultrasound 1979;*7*:381.
7. Castagnari L, Sorice F: Immunoprecipitation tests in the diagnosis of human hydatidosis. Folia Allergol 1971;*18*:511.
8. Cottone M, Amuso M, Cotton PB: Endoscopic retrograde cholangiography in hepatic hydatid disease. Br J Surg 1978;*65*:107.
9. Dew HR: Hydatid Disease: Its Pathology, Diagnosis and Treatment. Sydney, Australasian Medical Publishing Company, 1928.
10. Dugalic D, Djukic V, Milicevic M, et al: Operative procedures in the management of liver hydatidoses. World J Surg 1982;*6*:115.
11. Ekrami Y: Surgical treatment of hydatid disease of the liver. Arch Surg 1976;*111*:1350.
12. Ertan A, Sahin B, Kandilci V, et al: The mechanism of cholestasis from hepatic hydatid cysts. J Clin Gastroenterol 1983;*5*:437.
13. Farrelly C, Lawrie BW: Diagnosis of intrabiliary rupture of hydatid cyst of the liver by fine-needle percutaneous transhepatic cholangiography. Br J Radiol 1982;*55*:372.
14. Hadidi A: Ultrasound findings in liver hydatid cysts. J Clin Ultrasound 1979;*7*:365.
15. Ismail MA, Al-Dabagh MA, Al-Janabi TA, et al: The use of computerised axial tomography (CAT) in the diagnosis of hydatid cysts. Clin Radiol 1980;*31*:287.
16. Itzchak Y, Rubinstein Z, Heyman Z, et al: Role of ultrasound in the diagnosis of abdominal hydatid disease. J Clin Ultrasound 1980;*8*:341.
17. Kasai Y, Koshino I, Kawanishi N, et al: Alveolar echinococcosis of the liver. Studies on 60 operated cases. Ann Surg 1980;*191*:145.
18. Kayser HJS: Treatment of hydatid disease with mebendazole at Frere Hospital, East London. A preliminary report. S Afr Med J 1980;*58*:560.
19. Kertesz V, Robertson PW, Sharp P: Evaluation of three serological tests for the diagnosis of hydatid disease. Med J Aust 1979;*2*:678.
20. Little JM: Hydatid disease at Royal Prince Alfred Hospital 1964 to 1974. Med J Aust 1976;*1*:903.
21. Lygidakis NJ: Diagnosis and treatment of intrabiliary rupture of hydatid cyst of the liver. Arch Surg 1983;*118*:1186.
22. Matossian RM, Rickard MD, Smyth JD: Hydatidosis: a global problem of increasing importance. Bull WHO 1977;*55*:499.
23. Mosimann F: Is alveolar hydatid disease of the liver incurable? Ann Surg 1980;*192*:118.
24. Mottaghian H, Saidi F: Postoperative recurrence of hydatid disease. Br J Surg 1978;*65*:237.
25. Ovnat A, Peiser J, Avinoah E, et al: Acute cholangitis caused by ruptured hydatid cyst. Surgery 1984; *95*:497.
26. Papadimitriou J, Mandrekas A: The surgical treatment of hydatid disease of the liver. Br J Surg 1970;*57*:431.
27. Papadimitriou J, Tsiftis D, Tountas C: Hydatid cyst of the liver ruptured into the biliary tract. Curr Surg 1983;*40*:339.
28. Pellegrini CA, Paloyan D, Acosta JM, et al: Acute pancreatitis of rare causation. Surg Gynecol Obstet 1977;*144*:899.
29. Reventos J, Nogueras FM, Rius X, et al: Hydatid disease of the liver with thoracic involvement. Surg Gynecol Obstet 1976;*143*:570.
30. Romero-Torres R, Campbell JR: An interpretive review of the surgical treatment of hydatid disease. Surg Gynecol Obstet 1965;*121*:851.
31. Saidi F: Surgery of Hydatid Disease. 1st ed. Philadelphia, WB Saunders, 1976.
32. Saidi F, Nazarian I: Surgical treatment of hydatid cysts by freezing of cyst wall and instillation of 0.5 per cent silver nitrate solution. N Engl J Med 1971;*284*:1346.
33. Sayek I, Yalin R, Sanac Y: Surgical treatment of hydatid disease of the liver. Arch Surg 1980; *115*:847.
34. Schantz PM: Echinococcosis. *In* Steele JS, Arambulo P (eds): Handbook of Zoonoses, Vol III. Boca Raton, CRC Press, 1981.
35. Schantz PM, Kagan IG: Echinococcosis (Hydatidosis). *In* Houba V (ed): Immunological Investiga-

tion of Tropical Parasitic Diseases. New York, Churchill Livingstone, 1980.

36. Tuttle RJ: Cause of recurring obstructive jaundice revealed by percutaneous transhepatic cholangiography—hydatid cyst. N Engl J Med 1970;*283*:805.
37. Uflacker R, Wholey MH, Amaral NM, et al: Parasitic and mycotic causes of biliary obstruction. Gastrointest Radiol 1982;*7*:173.
38. Wilson JF, Rausch RL: Alveolar hydatid disease. A review of clinical features of 33 indigenous cases of *Echinococcus multilocularis*. Am J Trop Med Hyg 1980;*29*:1340.
39. Yacoubian HD: Thoracic problems associated with hydatid cyst of the dome of the liver. Surgery 1976;*79*:544.
40. Zielinski VE, Elmslie RG: Jaundice and hydatid disease of the liver. Med J Aust 1969;*1*:839.
41. Albendazole: worms and hydatid disease (Editorial). Lancet 1984;*2*:675.
42. Kammerer WS, Schantz PM: Long-term follow-up of human hydatid disease (*Echinococcus granulosus*) treated with a high dose mebendazole regimen. Am J Trop Med Hyg 1984;*33*:132.
43. Langer JC, Rose DB, Keystone JS, Taylor BR, Langer B: Diagnosis and management of hydatid disease of the liver: A 15-year North American experience. Ann Surg 1984;*199*:412.
44. Morris DL, Dykes PW, Marriner S, Bogan J, Burrows F, Skeene-Smith H, Clarkson MJ: Albendazole: Objective evidence of response in human hydatid disease. JAMA 1985;*253*:2053.
45. Xu Ming-gian: Complications of the hydatid disease of the liver. J Nippon Med Sch 1984;*51*:113.

GERALD W. PESKIN, M.D.

38

Biliary Fistula

A biliary fistula is, with occasional exceptions, a complication of long-standing and advanced biliary tract disease. Unless created intentionally to divert stagnant bile, it represents a clinical problem potentially encompassing fluid and electrolyte disturbances, dehydration and malnutrition, acid-base imbalance, infection (both local and systemic), intestinal obstruction, hemorrhage, and death. The relative rarity of this condition in any individual practice coupled with the strong possibility of inflicting harm with inappropriate therapy may explain the bewilderment of clinicians as they approach the management of this complication.

DEFINITION

A biliary fistula is an established, unnatural communication between any portion of the biliary tree and another area or surface. *Congenital* biliary fistulae are rare connections between the ductal system and the gastrointestinal and respiratory tracts. Far more common are the *acquired* fistulae, which are of two principal types—*spontaneous* and *iatrogenic* or *traumatic* (internal or external). Fistulae have been described as arising from intra- or extrahepatic bile ducts and/or the gallbladder and terminating in the stomach; small or large intestine; another portion or duct of the biliary system; the urogenital organs, including kidney, ureter, bladder, uterus, and vagina as well as ovarian cysts; the thoracic viscera, including bronchi, pleura, and pericardium; the portal vein; the hepatic artery; and the peritoneum as well as on the skin. Two or more fistulae may coexist.

INCIDENCE

The frequency with which biliary fistulae occur is difficult to determine because many produce minimal symptoms and are never diagnosed, while others heal once the obstructing gallstone has moved on, leaving little evidence of their previous existence.

Puig-Sureda,[1] using a sample of 66,340 autopsies in which gallstones were found, calculated an overall incidence of spontaneous biliary fistula of 0.22 per cent. In relation to clinical practice, Epperson and Walters[2] of the Mayo Clinic reported an incidence of 0.88 per cent among 9716 cases of biliary tract surgery; Glenn and Mannix[3] noted a 0.9 per cent rate in more than 4500 patients treated surgically for biliary disease at the New York Hospital–Cornell Medical Center; Hicken and Coray[4] at the University of Utah and Latter Day Saints Hospital represented the other end of the spectrum, with an incidence of 4.2 per cent in more than 3500 patients undergoing biliary surgery. Thus, 1 of every 25 to 100 patients seeking surgical therapy for biliary tract disorders will possess some type of biliary fistula.

It is difficult to predict any radical change in the incidence of this complication, since it is caused predominantly by gallstone disease. While the increasing prevalence of biliary calculi and the ever increasing longevity of our population cannot be denied, the more aggressive and earlier approach to cholelithiasis appears to balance the scale. Those fistulae associated with trauma undoubtedly will multiply over the years but represent such a small segment of the overall picture that they cannot of themselves change the totals significantly.

PATHOGENESIS

Inflammation

In most patients, a lengthy history of biliary tract disease is evident.[5, 42] Often there have been frank attacks of right upper quadrant pain due to acute obstructive cholecystitis. During these episodes, the serosal surfaces of the gallbladder and/or the common duct involved in the inflammatory reaction become densely adherent to the serosa of the intestinal viscera that rest in close approximation. As the process continues, adhesions form that tend to maintain their respective relationships so that when another attack occurs, the same surfaces are involved.

Glenn and Mannix[3] have outlined the sequence of events that occur in acute obstructive cholecystitis to explain fistula development through the agglutinated area. First, a stone impacts in the gallbladder ampulla, causing reaction in the adjacent wall where the cystic artery enters, thus reducing arterial blood supply. At about the same time, venous and lymphatic drainage is diminished by the inflammatory compression. As decreased vascular and lymphatic competence is experienced, the absorption of water by the gallbladder mucosa ceases. Thus, a vicious cycle is created, with the increased intraluminal fluid creating greater wall tension, further reducing blood supply and causing wall edema, which, in turn, depresses the absorptive potential of the mucosa. The eventual loss of vascularity to areas of the gallbladder causes these areas to become ischemic and gangrenous. The nearby and adherent visceral serosa becomes irritated. As the ischemic area in the wall of the gallbladder becomes gangrenous, the increased pressure within results in its contents first penetrating its own necrotic wall, and then causing a thrombosis and congestion of the wall of the adjacent organ. Thrombosis of the intestinal wall vessels causes necrosis with a resultant defect, the beginning of the biliary fistula.

The decompression of the tense gallbladder by discharge of its contents into an adjacent segment of the intestinal tract is followed by dislodgment of the obstructing stone(s), which may then pass into the intestine. If small, the stone is carried onward and evacuated through the rectum. If large, it may cause obstruction. The terminal ileum, because of its small diameter, is the most frequent site at which such a stone becomes wedged (see Chapter 17).

The duration of symptoms of biliary tract disease prior to identification, if not actually formation, of a biliary fistula has ranged in different series from 8 to 20 years.

Just as the biliary tract may be the primary site of the inflammatory process and create a fistula by burrowing outward, so also may a fistula develop with the primary focus of inflammation outside the biliary tract, pressing inward. This mechanism is exemplified by the fistula created when a duodenal ulcer perforates into the common bile duct. Again, the inflammatory response associated with ulcer penetration and perforation causes an adherence of the ulcer site to the choledochus or gallbladder. The necrotizing characteristics of the inflammatory response as well as the acidity of the upper gastrointestinal tract contents create the communication. The usual posterior duodenal ulcer is more likely to penetrate into the bile ducts, while those ulcers more anterior or lateral may perforate directly into the gallbladder.

Fistulization may also evolve from the presence of an abscess, generally in the subhepatic space or within the lesser sac. The inflammatory response evoked by the abscess, plus the pressure that may be generated as a result of its increasing content or bacterial activity, may cause its adherence to the bile ducts or gallbladder and eventually produce sloughing and the formation of a passage. Thus, one may have an indirect type of fistula with the communication from the biliary tract through the bed of an abscess cavity into an adjacent viscus.

In occasional cases, fistula formation has been attributed to the presence of echinococcic, amebic, or tuberculous disease.

Finally, the inflammatory nature of acute obstructive cholecystitis may produce adherence of the gallbladder to the abdominal wall; with neglect, generally on the part of the patient, this results in spontaneous fistulization of the bile flow to the skin surface. Although the right upper quadrant of the abdomen is the most common site for the external orifice, the falciform and round ligaments may direct the suppuration toward the umbilical region (phlegmon of Jean Louis Petit).

Neoplasia

Intra-abdominal malignant disease is a less common cause of biliary fistulae, accounting for 0.3 per cent to 4 per cent of cases in varying series. The primary lesions most often are found in the biliary passages, pancreas, colon, and stomach. The cancer generally produces degenerative necrosis of contiguous viscera as a result of the pressure of its growth and its interference with local blood supply.

Congenital Defect

Communications between the biliary tract and the tracheobronchial tree may be of a congenital nature and are rare malformations. Fewer than ten cases have been reported in the world literature.[6] Neuhauser and associates[7] first described a congenital bronchobiliary fistula in a 5 month old female in 1952. In every reported incidence, the fistula arose from the proximal portion of the right main stem bronchus, a short distance below the carina. In some patients, the distal end of the fistula joined the biliary tree at the level of the left hepatic ductal system. Two possible embryologic malformations may explain this anomaly. The first is a union of an anomalous bronchial bud with an anomalous bile duct, and the second is a duplication of the upper gastrointestinal tract. Although Neuhauser[7] favored the duplication theory of embryogenesis, the histologic appearance of the fistulous tracts makes their presence compatible with either explanation.

Trauma

Traumatic injury of the biliary ductal system significant enough to form a fistula may result from either external or iatrogenic sources. In the case of external trauma, penetrating injuries may produce partial or complete severance of ductal continuity, depending on the direction and velocity of the missile. It is rare to find isolated trauma to the ductal system. Accordingly, the severity of the overall injury dictates exploration and repair before significant bile peritonitis or fistulization can occur. Inspection and recognition of biliary tract discontinuity is the key to appropriate treatment.[38, 39]

In the case of nonpenetrating or blunt trauma, even fewer examples exist. Under these circumstances, the extrahepatic bile ducts are more likely to be injured, since they are relatively more fixed at the superior edge of the pancreas and at the liver hilum than are adjacent structures, making them subject to avulsion injury. Delay in diagnosis is common when such injury is unassociated with other intraperitoneal damage. Often the presence of ascites, mild jaundice, and elevated temperature along with inanition, acholic stools, and recurrent abdominal pain may prompt appropriate diagnostic studies to establish the nature of the injury.[8] (For further details on trauma to the biliary tract refer to Chapter 41.)

In the case of iatrogenic biliary fistulae, it is well established that an external biliary fistula may follow any operation on the biliary tract, and the cause may be related to the nature or extent of the biliary tract disease or distortion or injury resulting from the surgical procedure.

Fistula after cholecystectomy is indicative of obstruction distal to the cystic duct, in most instances by stone, scar, or injury. When a biliary fistula follows cholecystostomy, it is probable that stones in the gallbladder were overlooked, obstructing the return flow of secretion into the common duct. When the gallbladder or any significant amount of mucosal lining is not removed, a fistula that discharges mucus, or mucus and bile, may develop. Jaundice preceding the discharge of bile usually indicates obstruction and possible interruption of the common bile duct. If there has been no preceding jaundice, the discharge of bile is more likely to be the result of an unligated cystic duct or a defect in the wall of the common bile duct resulting from operative injury. Division of small bile ducts leading from the liver to the ampulla of the gallbladder may give rise to a subhepatic accumulation of bile and then to a fistula. The amount of bile usually decreases gradually over a matter of 10 to 20 days, and the fistula closes. Injury to the intrahepatic ducts, either in the area of the gallbladder bed or elsewhere within the operative field by improper retraction, may also lead to fistula formation. These fistulae, too, are usually of short duration and require no surgical intervention.

DIAGNOSIS

Age and Sex

In light of the fact that most biliary fistulae are associated with gallstone disease or malignancy, it is in keeping to note that these occur more commonly in older patients. In the Mayo Clinic series of 424 cases, the patients averaged 67 years of age, with the oldest being 78 years and the youngest 31 years.[9] Patients of Drs. Glenn and Mannix at The New York Hospital averaged 56 years of age, with 24 being over 60 years and only six being under 50 years.[3] In both series, as in many others, about 70 to 75 per cent of the lesions were found in women. The only types of fistula in which male incidence equaled or exceeded female incidence were traumatic lesions and those secondary to peptic ulcer disease. In all series, approximately 90 per cent of the lesions were attributable to cholelithiasis and cholecystitis, approximately 5 per cent being related to peptic ulcer disease, 4 per cent to intra-abdominal malignant disease, and the remainder to external or iatrogenic trauma and congenital problems.

Clinical Presentation

Only 30 per cent of all fistulae are diagnosed prior to surgical exploration or autopsy. This may be due to failure to consider this diagnosis but is more likely due to the varied and nonspecific symptoms of the disease process.

Karotkin[10] divided the clinical manifestations of biliary fistulae into the following categories:

1. In a small minority of cases, the diagnosis is readily apparent through the occurrence of unmistakable signs. An example would be the vomiting or coughing of gallstones or the passage of gallstones in fecal debris. Rivers and Mason[11] suggested that a stone larger than 0.5 cm in diameter appearing in the feces indicates the presence of an internal biliary fistula, since stones of such size are extremely unlikely to have passed through the ampulla of Vater. Severe abdominal symptoms may suddenly disappear at the time of development of an internal biliary fistula. A probable mass in the right upper quadrant may vanish abruptly, and the sudden discharge of septic material into the bowel can result in symptoms of duodenal irritation or acute diarrhea. Remission of illness related to fistula formation is usually very brief, and new or recurrent symptoms appear reasonably promptly.

2. The largest group of patients present with a symptom complex that is highly suggestive but not pathognomonic. An individual with a history indicative of long-standing biliary tract disease should always be considered a candidate for biliary fistula. The patients commonly complain of recurring episodes of biliary colic or right upper guadrant pain associated with chills, fever, vomiting, jaundice, and weight loss. The symptoms are generally more severe in persons who have developed a biliary fistula than in those with uncomplicated chronic gallbladder disease. Hematemesis occurring with or following acute cholecystitis should arouse suspicion of an internal biliary fistula. The presence of a large concentration of bile in the gastric juice on gastric analysis led to the diagnosis of internal biliary fistula in a case reported by Rankin.[12]

3. One may group a variety of instances in which the clinical history provides no direct clues to suggest the presence of a biliary fistula. The diagnosis may be disclosed incidentally during the roentgenologic studies or surgical exploration. A large group of patients will have the usual symptoms of chronic cholecystitis with no extraordinary complaints to suggest internal biliary fistula. The patient whose illness seems fully explained by recognized disease, such as peptic ulcer or carcinoma, falls into this category. Most choledochoduodenal fistulae occur in the course of chronic duodenal disease without the appearance of additional symptoms. The patient with intestinal obstruction due to gallstone ileus may fall into this category.

4. There remains a small group of patients with a biliary fistula who are asymptomatic and unable to relate a past illness suggestive of biliary tract disease. It is thought that this group is not as large as most series indicate and that previous symptoms would be detectable in many such patients if more attention were given to the history.

TYPES OF FISTULA

In reviewing the approximate incidences of the more common types of internal biliary fistula, Karotkin[10] found 60 per cent to be cholecystoduodenal, 24 per cent to be cholecystocolic, 10 per cent to be choledochoduodenal, and 6 per cent to be cholecystogastric. The remaining types comprised less than 1 per cent. In Hicken and Coray's study of 272 cases of all types,[4] the gallbladder was involved in 88 per cent, the common duct in 11 per cent, the duodenum in 69 per cent, the colon in 26 per cent, and the stomach in 4.4 per cent. Rarely are these fistulae multiple. As we have controlled ulcer disease more successfully, the incidence of ulcer-related (choledochoduodenal) fistulae appears to be diminishing, creating a relative increase in gallstone-related cholecystoenteric communications, noted in recent small series.

Biliary-Duodenal

The most common form is the cholecystoduodenal connection, usually a sequela of acute obstructive cholecystitis.[41] In addition, perforation of a duodenal ulcer into the gallbladder, either directly or through an abscess cavity, may produce this lesion. Hutchings and associates[13] reported 23 such cases from the literature and added 5 of their own. Marshall and Polk[14] noted two additional examples. Cholecystoduodenal communication is also found in association with primary carcinoma of the gallbladder.

Choledochoduodenal fistulae are secondary to penetrating duodenal ulcer in over 80 per cent of cases. The majority of these patients are males with long histories of ulcer disease. Hoppenstein and colleagues[15] noted American literature reports of 67 cases and added one of their own. When choledochoduodenal fistula is due to erosion of a common duct stone, there is usually a history of prior obstructive jaundice. The jaundice may disappear with establishment of the fistula. A choledochoduodenal fistula in a patient with no history of antecedent jaundice should suggest a primary duodenal origin, such as ulcer or cancer.

Biliary-Colonic

Primarily related to gallstone disease,[43] fistulae of this type may arise from carcinoma of the gallbladder or a primary malignancy in the hepatic flexure of the colon. Of the large series in the American literature, the Mayo Clinic[2] noted 7 of this type in 84 biliary-enteric fistula patients; the New York Hospital,[3] 3 of 40 cases; the Boston City Hospital,[16] 3 of 30; Ohio State University,[17] 6 of 22; and the University of Iowa,[18] 10 of 92. Cholangitis with chills and fever, diarrhea, and pronounced weight loss developed in about half these patients.

Biliary-Gastric

This type of fistula is, again, a product of cholelithiasis. Occasionally, one encounters vomiting of gallstones as a striking feature of this communication. Malignant tumors may also be responsible for an infrequent fistula. Fewer of these fistulae were noted by Safaie-Shirazi et al.[18] in a series of 92 fistulae; the largest number, 21, were reported among 424 internal fistulae treated at the Mayo Clinic.[9]

Intrabiliary

The most common fistula encountered in this group connects the gallbladder and common duct, always in association with long-standing cholelithiasis. Essentially all patients have choledocholithiasis, and most require reconstruction over a T-tube. Lasala and Saporta[19] reported eight cases.

Biliary-Bronchial

These are infrequent sequelae of ductal obstruction (usually stone), intrahepatic abscess (trauma and/or stone), or rare congenital anomalies. A subhepatic accumulation of pus, secondary to acute cholecystitis with perforation, may erode through the diaphragm and extend into the lung. Primary liver abscesses (amebic, echinococcic, or pyogenic) may follow a similar course. The presence of a biliary-bronchial fistula may be suspected when an exacerbation of biliary tract disease is followed by an irritating cough and expectoration of bile or, occasionally, calculi. Ferguson and Burford[20] reviewed these problems in seven patients at Barnes Hospital, St. Louis.

Other Rare Fistulae

Communication between the biliary tract and the kidney pelvis, vagina, urinary bladder, or an ovarian cyst occurs rarely and is the result of acute obstructive cholecystitis with direct extension of inflammation to the adjacent organ or indirect extension through an abscess cavity. Malignancy must also be suspected in these situations. Hemobilia may result from fistulae connecting the biliary tract with a blood vessel. They may occur spontaneously (rupture of an aneurysm of the hepatic artery into a bile duct) or from trauma. The triad of severe right upper quadrant pain, upper gastrointestinal hemorrhage, and elevated bilirubin value suggests such a lesion.[21]

Three areas of symptomatology deserve additional comment. These are *volume depletion* and *hyponatremia, cholangitis*, and *diarrhea*.

A persistent external biliary fistula or continued bile peritonitis can lead to severe electrolyte depletion if this potential is not quickly recognized. The gallbladder reduces hepatic bile to about one tenth of its original volume by absorption of isotonic sodium chloride and bicarbonate. If leakage of large amounts of bile occurs or if loss of bile is not carefully replaced, a considerable loss of sodium chloride will ensue, with the development of a typical low sodium syndrome. The magnitude of the problem can be made clear by noting that bile volume may easily reach 1000 ml or more per day in the presence of any type of partial common duct obstruction, as must be anticipated in the patient with a biliary fistula. The sodium concentration of hepatic bile does not fall as the plasma sodium decreases, and thus the loss from the bile continues. In several studies, sodium loss through a bile fistula has ranged from 150 to 260 mEq/day despite severe sodium depletion. However, many patients do quite well because they unconsciously supplement their diets with salt and experience problems only when acute illness prevents adequate sodium intake.

The clinical picture is usually one of an older patient with an external biliary fistula in whom the consequences of loss of bile (i.e., metabolic acidosis and sodium depletion) have been neglected. Such patients may grow progressively weaker and, if the situation is not recognized, may even go into coma. Measurement of serum electrolytes will quickly point the correct way to the clinician. The serum sodium level will be low, in the range of 110 mEq/l; azotemia may be present; and the serum potassium value may be elevated. A low CO_2 reflects metabolic acidosis. Knochel and associates[22] have outlined the electrolyte derangements and secondary cardiovascular and renal abnormalities associated with biliary fistula.

Cholangitis is noted in between 15 and 20 per cent of cases of biliary fistula. However, the incidence is over 50 per cent in those patients with cholecystocolic fistulae. In addition to the fact that there are many more virulent microorganisms present in the colon, the size of the fistulous tract seems to be important. As explained by Wangensteen and others,[4, 23] it is apparent that cholangitis develops in the presence of biliary bacteria only when a significant degree of outflow obstruction is present. Certainly, the absence of cholangitis in patients with biliary-intestinal anastomoses tends to confirm this finding. Thus, it can be assumed that the inflammatory response and the small diameter of the cholecystocolic fistula is compatible with the Wangensteen concept.

Diarrhea may be produced by biliary-enteric fistulae in two ways. A diarrhea-like effect is produced by the passing of the daily volume of bile directly into the intestinal tract, particularly at the colonic level. In addition, the cathartic properties of bile salts are well known; when such volume is introduced as to make it difficult for the enterohepatic circulation to reabsorb it from the small intestine, diarrhea is accentuated.

RADIOLOGIC DIAGNOSIS

Carman,[24] in 1917, reported the first case of biliary fistula diagnosed by x-ray. He was able to see barium pass through the duodenum into the biliary tract. Radiographic study offers a precise method of clinical diagnosis of biliary fistulae. Unfortunately, good roentgenologic studies are not obtained in the majority of patients in most large series.

Radiologic criteria for the diagnosis of biliary fistulae include (1) gas in the biliary passages, (2) delineation of the fistula or biliary tract by contrast medium, and (3) demonstration of laminated or faceted stone in the gastrointestinal tract or other extrabiliary structures. In addition, a presumptive diagnosis of fistula may be entertained when there appear to be mucosal changes in the duodenum, stomach, or colon at the site of a suspected fistula.

In two conditions, emphysematous cholecystitis and incompetent sphincter of Oddi, air may be seen in the biliary tree on x-ray examination. These conditions, however, are extremely rare, so much so that visualization of air in the biliary passages should be considered due to biliary fistula unless proved otherwise.

It should be noted that an internal biliary fistula may fail to admit opaque material unless pressure in the gastrointestinal tract is raised. Thus, compression of the barium-filled duodenum for a period of time may be necessary to produce filling of the biliary passages. Further, interval films following barium studies will demonstrate retained barium in the biliary tree that was obscured on routine films.

Sedlack and associates[25] noted the presence of gas in the biliary tract in 74 patients. In reviewing the literature, Borman and Rigler[26] found that of 267 fistulae, only 86 were recognized preoperatively, and in each instance the diagnosis was made by the radiologist. In their personal series of 24 cases, they made a correct radiologic diagnosis in only 37 per cent. When the diagnosis of internal biliary fistula has been established, the radiologist should make an attempt to determine the patency of the intestinal tract. Such information is invaluable, for the surgeon cannot hope to correct the biliary fistula while the intestinal tract is obstructed to any degree. The obstructive complication requires primary consideration. Before an external fistula actually forms, a diagnosis of abscess can be made by ultrasonography or CT scan. Sonographic findings include demonstration of a sonolucent mass with echogenic material adjacent to the anterior abdominal wall. Gallstones may occasionally be seen within this mass or in the gallbladder. Once the fistulous tract is formed, CT is superior to sonography, since it can better delineate the tract and its communication with specific organs.[27, 28, 44]

External biliary fistulae can also be diagnosed by radionuclide imaging. In these patients, the bile flow can be traced by serial ^{99m}Tc-IDA imaging.[40] Leakage of bile from the ducts,[29] gallbladder perforation,[30, 31] cholecystocolic fistula,[32] and gastrobiliary fistula[33] have been correctly diagnosed using this method.

SURGICAL MANAGEMENT

Patients with biliary fistulae are not good surgical risks. Dehydration, acidosis, toxemia, and hypoproteinemia, all combined with coexisting cholangitis, pancreatitis, and biliary obstruction, tend to depress liver function. It may require days of a carefully planned preoperative regimen before these patients can safely assume the added burdens of an operation. To ignore this essential preparation is to invite a high morbidity and mortality rate, as noted in reported series. There is no single procedure that can be used to correct all these abnormal biliary communications. The remedial procedures must be selected according to the viscera involved, the size and location of the fistulous orifices, and the presence of obstructive pancreatitis, cholangitis, subhepatic abscesses, and common duct stones. Each case must be individualized. The management of a biliary fistula should be considered in sequential steps.

1. Preoperatively, when possible, it is appropriate to determine the anatomy of the fistula. In the case of an external fistula, this can be done by insertion of a catheter into the cutaneous opening, with injection of contrast material for delineation of the site of origin of the fistula and the nature of the tract. In the case of an internal fistula, attempts to define the anatomy should be made through x-ray studies (upper gastrointestinal series, barium enema, cholangiography, bronchography, or cystography).

2. If it is possible, the cause of the fistula should be ascertained. Studies such as endoscopy of the upper gastrointestinal tract; radioactive scanning of the liver; ultrasonography of the liver, gallbladder, and common duct region; and cytologic evaluation of a variety of aspirated specimens may be helpful. Very often, however, only surgical exploration will reveal the true nature of the fistula.

3. Since infection is one of the major complications of fistula, appropriate antibiotic therapy must be instituted. Cultures of bile, if obtainable, are helpful in making the best choice of antibiotics. In general, agents with a high degree of enterohepatic recirculation and effectiveness against gram-negative bacilli are ideal. Such drugs as gentamicin, clindamycin, chloramphenicol, and ampicillin are good choices.

Particular attention should be directed toward possible sodium depletion. Further, the chronic nature of the illness should prompt the correction of nutritional problems with high protein and high caloric oral intake or intravenous hyperalimentation.

When one believes the patient to be in optimal condition for operative intervention, one can then consider the surgical procedure.

The Operation

There is great variation in the findings at operation, with no two situations quite alike. However, certain objectives may be stated:

1. The condition of the patient must receive overriding consideration in determining the extensiveness of the procedure.

2. Because stones and debris are often

present in the common duct and its distal portion is compressed either by inflammatory reaction or by a component of the fistula, *choledochotomy, bile duct exploration,* and *visualization* should be a planned part of any operation.

3. The fistula should be dismantled and excised insofar as this is possible.

4. The intestinal defect should be closed without compromise of luminal size.

5. When involved in the inflammatory process, the gallbladder should be removed.

6. The etiologic basis of the fistula should be corrected.

Operations for cholecystoduodenal and cholecystocolonic fistulae caused by biliary tract stone disease follow a relatively standard pattern when there are no related complications and the patient is in good general condition. The first step is to dissect and separate the components, then close the relatively small intestinal defect without luminal compromise, and finally explore the common duct and remove any obstructing material within it. The gallbladder is then excised and T-tube drainage of the common duct established.

In those instances in which the fistula involves the colon, the sequence of these steps may be changed to reduce peritoneal contamination. Accordingly, exploration of the common duct is performed first, followed by cholecystectomy, with the cholecystocolic fistula left intact until it is divided and the defect inverted in the wall of the colon.

Since only about 30 per cent of fistulae are recognized preoperatively, it is important to reiterate that the general condition of the patient is the limiting factor in the extensiveness of even the standard procedures. Most patients with fistula are elderly, have had long-standing biliary tract disease as well as potential or real liver damage, and, when the colon is involved, also have the hazard of infection emanating from an unprepared large bowel. Additionally, if the common duct is involved or compromised by the fistula, there may be an intense inflammatory response in the area. Under any or all of these circumstances in the elderly, it may be better to provide common duct decompression and withdraw to return when preoperative planning ensures optimal conditions. Lesser compromises in selected instances include substitution of cholecystostomy for cholecystectomy, establishment of a diverting right-sided colostomy, or modification of areas of excision when malignant disease is associated with the fistula.

When *biliary intestinal fistulae are caused by duodenal ulcer disease,* primary attention must be given to correction of the ulcer diathesis. When technically possible, distal gastrectomy (antrectomy) and vagotomy with closure or Welch catheter drainage of the duodenal stump and Billroth II reconstruction (gastrojejunostomy) are recommended, as this both diverts and markedly diminishes acid production and gastric secretion. The fistula is then excluded from the gastrointestinal stream. If the inflammatory reaction has produced obstruction to the flow of bile, this must be alleviated, if only by catheter drainage of the bile ducts. In some instances, the inflammation may have resulted in fibrosis with permanent stricture of the common bile duct. These cases may require choledochoduodenostomy or choledochojejunostomy. It is important to emphasize that the biliary tree should be carefully assessed by operative cholangiography for the presence of calculi and the anatomy of the fistula. Under ideal circumstances it may be possible to divide the fistula, repair the duodenal defect, and correct the disease or defect in the biliary tree. Again, individualization based on operative findings and the patient's condition is the basic consideration.

A small number of *duodenal and gastric ulcers* (benign) perforate anteriorly into the adherent gallbladder, creating a *cholecystoduodenal* or *cholecystogastric fistula.* In these instances, the eradication of the ulcer diathesis (vagotomy and antrectomy or partial gastrectomy) with diversion, when possible, is important. Cholecystectomy, with closure of the duodenum or as part of the gastric resection, is a second goal. Finally, the inflammatory response may be so great as to produce common duct obstruction, and this must be evaluated and relieved where noted. Staging, related to patient condition, deserves much consideration.

When *gastric malignancy extending into the gallbladder* exists, the invasive process is often so extensive that resection is not feasible. The neoplastic process has usually compressed the common bile duct, and the cholecystogastric fistula affords the only escape for the static bile. To molest the fistula is to invite catastrophe. Most often, gastrojejunostomy proximal to the obstructing gastric tumor (usually a pyloric or prepyloric cancer) will reduce the reflux of irritating stomach contents into the biliary tree and render the patient essentially asymptomatic with regard to cholangitis. This is an excellent palliative technique.

If one temporarily or permanently diverts offending secretions, especially infected materials, from the fistula site, it is amazing how frequently the fistula closes.[34] One then need only follow the patient carefully to ensure that stricturing is not permanent.

External fistulae are generally easier to define; they require exploration to provide freedom from distal obstruction within the biliary system (usually choledochotomy, ductal exploration, and either removal of stones or bypass of the strictured area). If biliary obstruction is caused by gallstones, endoscopic papillotomy may be all that is needed to restore the patency of the bile duct and cure the fistula.[35] The fistula invariably heals spontaneously once patency of the ductal system is accomplished. The older technique of dissection of the fistulous tract and its implantation into the gastrointestinal tract is fraught with failure and is not recommended for either external or internal fistulae.

Traumatic fistulae to the pleural, bronchial, and pericardial areas require an aggressive surgical approach. Early thoracotomy with adequate subdiaphragmatic drainage of all pockets of accumulation of bile-stained material is mandatory. Next, the fistulous tract through the diaphragm is located and closed securely with nonabsorbable sutures. The elective diaphragmatic opening is then repaired, and, in the case of pleurobiliary fistula, a decortication with drainage is done. If the original problem involved a pericardial collection, this is evacuated and a window left in the pericardium for permanent drainage into the pleural space. If an established bronchobiliary communication exists, lobectomy of the involved area will probably be necessary, since that lobe is usually severely infected. Fistulae associated with amebic, echinococcic, or tuberculous disease are rare in the United States. The principles of treatment remain the same, with the addition of specific antimicrobial therapy directed against the causative organism and maintained pre-, intra-, and postoperatively.

Congenital bronchobiliary fistulae require early surgical intervention, including thoracotomy, division of the fistula at its connection to the bronchial tree, and excision of that portion of the tract amenable to removal through the chest and diaphragm (preferably all of the tract). Since the biliary tree is not diseased, only visualization to ensure this fact preoperatively or operatively is necessary.

Fistulae from the biliary tree to structures within the peritoneal cavity, such as the urinary tract and genital area, are treated by correction of the biliary tract disease (obstruction) and division or excision of the fistula. The operative treatment of biliary fistula associated with intestinal obstruction is discussed in Chapter 17. When the fistula is not attacked at the primary operation for intestinal obstruction, it should be considered for repair at a second procedure in light of the potential for recurrent biliary tract symptoms and complications, including recurrent bowel obstruction from stones.

Natural History of Biliary Fistulae as a Consideration in Surgical Treatment

Almost every reported series of patients with biliary fistulae contains a small number of individuals who, for a variety of reasons, have not undergone definitive surgical therapy. Some have been lost to follow-up, but others have survived in relative good health for years. Added to this is autopsy evidence of the presence of biliary fistulae in patients dying of unrelated causes without documented notation of biliary or obstructive symptoms.

Does this mean that one can treat a biliary fistula expectantly or with occasional medication directed at specific symptoms? A closer analysis of the literature helps resolve this problem. It is apparent that the majority of patients with fistulae are, in fact, symptomatic with their gallstone disease, with their ulcer disease, or with whatever basic causative illness exists, and at least one third to one half are at risk for future problems.[36] It is essentially only a matter of time until there is an escalation of the difficulty. The number who actually go on to close their fistula spontaneously is small.

Real judgment then lies in the balancing of continued and perhaps progressive symptoms with the risk of operation. Some guidelines are helpful in making this decision. One should recommend operation if (1) stones or debris are still present in the biliary tree on x-ray or ultrasonography; (2) cholangitis or diarrhea appears or recurs; (3) the fistula is of the external type; (4) the fistula persists over months; (5) biliary stone or ulcer symptoms recur; (6) there is evidence of progressive liver damage; or (7) evidence of ductal obstruction is present.

Given an elective situation (obstruction and/or overwhelming sepsis not present), the mortality of operation for correction of fistula is related almost entirely to the presence of severe systemic illnesses, such as arteriosclerotic vascular disease, chronic obstructive pulmonary disease, and so forth. Thus, operation, whether one-stage or multiple procedures, within the tolerance of the elderly and systemically diseased, seems a much more reasonable approach in all but the few patients with incurable or extremely advanced associated problems.

RESULTS

Operations for correction of biliary fistulae carry a relatively high morbidity and mortality because of the nature of the problem, the age and degree of infirmity of the patients, and the association with multiple trauma.

The mortality rate in those series that considered only operations for fistulae without intestinal obstruction ranged between 0 per cent[2, 17, 37] and 30 per cent,[4] with most in the 10 to 15 per cent area. The more recently reported patients have been operated upon with a mortality of less than 10 per cent.

In addition, there appears to be a high incidence of wound infection and abscess formation associated with operation—15 to 20 per cent. Other less common but troublesome nonfatal complications noted regularly include stress bleeding from the upper gastrointestinal tract and pulmonary infection. With better preoperative preparation and a better understanding of the problem, it is anticipated that the mortality and morbidity of operations for correction of biliary fistula can be reduced to less than 5 per cent.

SUMMARY

Biliary fistulae are relatively unusual lesions. Most are related to gallstone disease, a smaller number being associated with ulcer diathesis, trauma, neoplasia, or congenital problems. Almost all are symptomatic and progressive. Suspicion of the existence of a communication is important in diagnosis; a history of symptoms plus the use of radiologic diagnostic techniques is most helpful in confirmation. Operative treatment is recommended and must be tailored to the anatomy and causative factors of the fistula. Results are good and are improving. Gallstone ileus, an obviously associated entity, is discussed in Chapter 17.

REFERENCES

1. Puig-Sureda J: Fistulas biliares internas espontaneas. Quatorzième Congrès de la Société Internationale de Chirurgie. Paris, Septembre 23–29, 1951 (Bruxelles Imprimerie Médicale et Scientifique [S.A.], 1952, pp 601–608).
2. Epperson DP, Walters W: Spontaneous internal biliary fistulas. Proc Staff Meet Mayo Clin 1953; *28*:353.
3. Glenn F, Mannix H Jr: Biliary enteric fistula. Surg Gynecol Obstet 1957;*105*:693.
4. Hicken NF, Coray QB: Spontaneous gastrointestinal biliary fistulas. Surg Gynecol Obstet 1946;*82*:723.
5. Hoffman L, Beaton H, Wantz G: Spontaneous cholecystocutaneous fistula. A complication of neglected biliary tract disease. J Am Geriatr Soc 1982;*3*:632.
6. Sane SM, Sieber WK, Girdany BR: Congenital bronchobiliary fistula. Surgery 1971;*69*:599.
7. Neuhauser EBD, Elkin M, Landing B: Congenital direct communication between the biliary system and the respiratory tract. Am J Dis Child 1952; *83*:654.
8. Fletcher WS: Nonpenetrating trauma to the gallbladder and extrahepatic bile ducts. Surg Clin North Am 1972;*52*:711.
9. Remine WH: Biliary-enteric fistulas: natural history and management. *In* Hardy JD, Zollinger RM (eds): Advances in Surgery. Vol 7. Chicago, Year Book Medical Publishers, 1973.
10. Karotkin L: Spontaneous internal biliary fistula. Med Ann Dist Columb 1981;*27*:623 and 1959;*28*:22.
11. Rivers AB, Mason JB: Cholecystoduodenal fistula. Med Clin North Am 1932;*15*:1571.
12. Rankin JO: Gastrocholecystic fistula; case report. Am J Surg 1932;*15*:109.
13. Hutchings VC, Wheeler JR, Puestow CB: Choledochoduodenal fistula complicating duodenal ulcer. Arch Surg 1956;*73*:598.
14. Marshall SF, Polk RC: Spontaneous internal biliary fistulas. Surg Clin North Am 1958;*38*:697.
15. Hoppenstein JM, Medoza CB, Watne AL: Choledochoduodenal fistula due to perforating duodenal ulcer disease. Ann Surg 1971;*173*:145.
16. Byrne JJ: Biliary fistulas. Annu J Surg 1953;*86*:181.
17. Stoll JR, Thomford NR: Biliary intestinal fistula. Am J Surg 1970;*120*:27.
18. Safaie-Shirazi S, Zike WL, Printen KJ: Spontaneous enterobiliary fistulas. Surg Gynecol Obstet 1973; *137*:769.
19. Lasala AJ, Saporta JA: Biliobiliary fistulae. Arch Surg 1960;*80*:486.
20. Ferguson TB, Burford TH: Pleurobiliary and bronchobiliary fistulas. Arch Surg 1967;*95*:380.
21. Sandblom P: Hemorrhage into the biliary tract following trauma—traumatic hemobilia. Surgery 1948;*24*:571.
22. Knochel JP, Cooper EB, Barry KG: External biliary fistula: a study of electrolyte derangements and secondary cardiovascular and renal abnormalities. Surgery 1962;*51*:746.
23. Morgenstern L, Shore JM: Selection of an optimal procedure for decompression of the obstructed common bile duct. Am J Surg 1970;*119*:38.
24. Carman RD: The Roentgen Diagnosis of Diseases of the Alimentary Canal. Philadelphia, WB Saunders, 1917, pp 368–369.
25. Sedlack RE, Hodgson JR, Butt HR, et al: Gas in the

biliary tract: clinical and experimental observations. Gastroenterology 1961;*41*:551.
26. Borman CN, Rigler LG: Spontaneous internal biliary fistula and gallstone obstruction with particular reference to roentgenologic diagnosis. Surgery 1937;*1*:349.
27. Ulreich S, Henken EM, Levinson ED: Imaging in the diagnosis of cholecystocutaneous fistulae. J Can Assoc Radiol 1983;*34*:39.
28. Frick MP, Feinberg SB, Stenlund RR, et al: Evaluation of abdominal fistulas with computed body tomography (CT). Comput Radiol 1982;*6*:17.
29. Weissman HS, Chun KJ, Frank M, et al: Demonstration of traumatic bile leakage with cholescintigraphy and ultrasonography. AJR 1979;*133*:843.
30. Brunetti JC, Van Heertum RL: Preoperative detection of gallbladder perforation. Clin Nucl Med 1980;*5*:347.
31. Mesgarzadeh M, et al: Diagnosis of clinically unsuspected gallbladder perforation in an obese patient by Tc99m-IDA cholescintigraphy. J Nucl Med 1983;*24*:1028.
32. Edell SL, Milunsky C, Garren L: Cholescintigraphic diagnosis of cholecystocolic fistula. Clin Nucl Med 1981;*6*:303.
33. Henderson RW, Telfer N, Halls JM: Gastrobiliary fistula: pre- and postoperative assessment with 99mTc-PIPIDA. AJR 1981;*137*:163.
34. Smith EE, Bowley N, Allison DJ, et al. The management of post-traumatic intrahepatic cutaneous biliary fistulas. Br J Surg 1982;*69*:317.
35. O'Rahilly S, Duignan JP, Lennon JR, et al: Successful treatment of a post-operative external biliary fistula by endoscopic papillotomy. Endoscopy 1983;*15*:68.
36. Warshaw AL, Bartlett MK: Choice of operation for gallstone intestinal obstruction. Ann Surg 1966; *164*:1051.
37. Porter JM, Mullen DC, Silver D: Spontaneous biliary-enteric fistulas. Surgery 1970;*68*:597.
38. Posner MC, Moore EE: Extrahepatic biliary tract injury: Operative management plan. J Trauma 1985;*25*:833.
39. Zeman RK, Lee CH, Stahl R, Viscomi GN, et al: Strategy for the use of biliary scintigraphy in noniatrogenic biliary trauma. Radiology 1984;*151*:771.
40. McPherson GAD, Collier NA, Lavender JP, Blumgart LH: The role of HIDA scanning in the assessment of external biliary fistulae. Surg Gastroenterol 1984;*3*:77.
41. Alberti-Flor JJ, Hernandez M, Dunn GGD, Gomez E: Cholecystoduodenal fistula. Am J Gastroenterol 1985;*80*:655.
42. Kurtz RJ, Heimann TM, Beck AR, Kurtz AB: Patterns of treatment of gallstone ileus over a 45-year period. Am J Gastroenterol 1985;*80*:95.
43. Pangan JC, Estrada R, Rosales R: Cholecystoduodenocolic fistula with recurrent gallstone ileus. Arch Surg 1984;*119*:1201.
44. Harkavy LA, Balthazar EJ, Naidich DP: CT diagnosis of cholecystoduodenal fistula. Am J Gastroenterol 1985;*80*:569.

ALFRED A. DE LORIMIER, M.D.
MICHAEL R. HARRISON, M.D.

39

Congenital Biliary Atresia

INTRODUCTION

Prolonged jaundice in early infancy may be due to a great variety of diseases. Of concern to the surgeon are those that require operative attention. The differential diagnosis of direct hyperbilirubinemia persisting beyond 2 or 3 weeks of age includes the following:

1. Systemic infections: viral, bacterial, or parasitic (congenital or transplacental infection).
2. Genetic-metabolic diseases: $alpha_1$-antitrypsin deficiency, galactosemia, hereditary fructosemia, hereditary tyrosinemia, cystic fibrosis, Niemann-Pick disease, Byler's disease, Aagenaes syndrome.
3. Neonatal hepatitis (idiopathic cholestatic jaundice of infancy).
4. Intrahepatic biliary atresia or hypoplasia.
5. Extrahepatic biliary atresia or hypoplasia.
6. Choledochal cyst.
7. Bile plug syndrome.
8. Spontaneous perforation of bile ducts.
9. Bile duct stenosis or stricture.
10. Bile duct compression.
11. Parenteral alimentation cholestasis.

The clinical characteristics and diagnostic studies used to identify infections, and genetic and metabolic diseases are outlined in Tables 39–1 and 39–2.[1] Neonatal hepatitis is a catchall term for cholestatic jaundice with patent extrahepatic and intrahepatic bile ducts, the cause of which is unknown.

DEFINITIONS

The terms *atresia, hypoplasia,* and *intrahepatic-extrahepatic atresia* are potentially confusing and frequently misunderstood. The following definitions will help clarify the subsequent discussion.

Biliary atresia is defined as obliteration of the intrahepatic and/or extrahepatic bile ducts. Indirect evidence suggests that the ducts were originally present but were destroyed by a process as yet unknown. Biliary atresia is usually classified into intrahepatic and extrahepatic types, depending on the part of the biliary tract principally affected.

In *intrahepatic biliary atresia* the extrahepatic ducts are patent, but the liver biopsy shows no intrahepatic bile ducts and little fibrosis. When occasional ducts are seen at biopsy, *intrahepatic biliary hypoplasia* is present. Intrahepatic biliary atresia and hypoplasia probably result from the same process. Intrahepatic biliary atresia usually occurs as an isolated defect and constitutes less than 5 per cent of cases of cholestasis in infants. It may occur in association with infections (e.g., congenital rubella), trisomy 17–18, or $alpha_1$-antitrypsin deficiency, and it may be familial.[2–4] Alagille's syndrome consists of intrahepatic biliary atresia or hypoplasia associated with peripheral pulmonary stenosis and, occasionally, vertebral anomalies, typical facies, and retarded physical, sexual, and mental development.[5–7] These patients do not manifest progressive hepatic fibrosis, and they have a long life expectancy.[8] The distinction between intrahepatic and extrahepatic atresia may be blurred if serial liver biopsies show progressive disappearance of intrahepatic ducts during the course of extrahepatic biliary atresia.

Extrahepatic biliary atresia is characterized by destruction of part or all of the extrahepatic ducts. In place of the ducts or gallbladder there are dense fibrotic strands and an inflammatory reaction. Extrahepatic biliary atresia almost invariably extends into the intrahepatic biliary tree. The liver biopsy usu-

Table 39–1 INFECTIONS LEADING TO CONJUGATED HYPERBILIRUBINEMIA IN EARLY INFANCY

Agent	Usual Mode of Infection	Other Manifestations	Screening Tests in Both Mother and Infant	Definitive Diagnosis
Cytomegalovirus	Transplacental	Low birth weight, micro- or hydrocephaly, intracranial calcifications, chorioretinitis, enteritis, pneumonitis, thrombocytopenia, hemolytic anemia, myocarditis.	CF antibody in serum.	Isolation from urine and from liver. Demonstration of virus in liver by IF. Specific IgM antibody.
Rubella virus	Transplacental	Low birth weight, congenital heart disease, cataracts, microphthalmia, glaucoma, deafness, bone lesions, microcephaly, thrombocytopenia, anemia.	CF and HI antibodies in serum.	Isolation of virus from nasopharyngeal secretions. Demonstration of virus in liver by IF. Specific IgM antibody.
Hepatitis B virus	Intrapartum, transfusion	No other systemic involvement reported as yet in young infants.	Hepatitis B antigen in infant; antigen and antibody in mother.	As for screening, plus demonstration of HB antigen in liver by IF and EM.
Herpes simplex	Intrapartum or immediate post partum	Skin or mucous membrane vesicles, encephalitis, cerebral calcifications, chorioretinitis, keratoconjunctivitis, pneumonitis, thrombocytopenia, coagulopathy.	Perinatal herpes in mother, or attendants. Serology and demonstration of virus in herpes-like lesions.	Isolation or demonstration of virus from superficial lesions and liver. Specific IgM antibody.

Table continued on opposite page

ally shows proliferation of bile capillaries or cholangioles, and progressive fibrosis typically develops in the periportal areas during the course of the disease.[9–12]

Three-dimensional reconstructions of the bile duct–like channels from liver biopsies and resected extrahepatic atretic ducts show a lack of arborization of normal-diameter ducts.[13–15] Instead, interconnecting ductules form a labyrinth of blind channels. The success of biliary-intestinal reconstructive procedures depends on establishing communication between the liver cells and the intestine by way of these channels.

The term *extrahepatic biliary hypoplasia* refers to cases in which the hepatoduodenal ligament contains channels of varying size lined by bile duct epithelium surrounded by fibrosis and chronic inflammation. The bile ducts between the liver and the duodenum are narrow, thickened, and fibrotic.[17] Cases of patent but small ducts that have subsequently become obliterated (resulting in typical biliary atresia) have been described.[18] More commonly, the extrahepatic ducts are narrow because they are unused, owing to lack of bile flow. Whether biliary hypoplasia is a disease of the ducts per se or whether the ducts are simply collapsed from disuse because of intrahepatic cholestasis may be answered only by following the course of the disease.[8, 19, 20]

The word "atresia" is reserved for cases with complete obliteration of bile duct remnants.[16] Hypoplasia is probably an interval stage in the evolution of biliary atresia; the clinical course of patients with hypoplasia and atresia is essentially the same.

In 15 per cent of infants with biliary atresia, there is cystic dilatation of the extrahe-

Table 39–1 INFECTIONS LEADING TO CONJUGATED HYPERBILIRUBINEMIA IN EARLY INFANCY *Continued*

Agent	Usual Mode of Infection	Other Manifestations	Screening Tests in Both Mother and Infant	Definitive Diagnosis
Coxsackie B virus	Transplacental	Meningoencephalitis, myocarditis, thrombocytopenia.	Serology of very limited value. Isolation from respiratory secretions and feces.	Isolation of virus from liver.
Varicella-zoster virus	Transplacental	Varicella rash, pneumonitis, other visceral involvement.	CF antibody in serum. Demonstration of virus in superficial lesions.	As for screening, plus demonstration of virus in liver by IF and EM.
Bacterial sepsis (*E. coli*, other enteric bacteria, *staphylococcus*, and so forth)	Intrapartum or postnatal	Lethargy, labile temperature, fever, weight loss, pallor, anemia, vomiting, diarrhea, pyuria, meningitis, and so forth.	High white blood cell count, shift to left, pyuria, anemia without reticulocytosis.	Blood culture, urine culture, CSF culture.
Treponema pallidum	Transplacental	Rhinitis, rash, bone lesions, lymphadenopathy, anemia.	VDRL or TPI, particularly in mother.	Darkfield examination of exudates for *Treponema*.
Toxoplasma gondii	Transplacental	Micro- or hydrocephaly, intracranial calcifications, chorioretinitis, microphthalmia, thrombocytopenia, anemia, skin hemorrhages.	CF antibody in serum; Sabin-Feldman dye test, titer in excess of 1:1000.	Rising antibody titers in infant. Isolation by culture from liver, CSF, eye. Specific IgM antibody.

CF = complement fixing; HI = hemagglutination inhibition; IF = immunofluorescence microscopy; EM = electronmicroscopy.
From Sass-Kortsak A: Pediatr Clin North Am 1974; *21*:777.

patic ducts in the hepatoduodenal ligament.[16–24] This kind of choledochal cyst is a different condition from cystic bile duct dilatation encountered after the neonatal period (see Chapter 40). In biliary atresia the dilated duct is rarely lined by ductal epithelium, and the wall consists of dense fibrotic tissue. Some authors prefer to call these structures bile lakes.[22] The dilated "duct" probably results from a dissection of bile into the periductal tissue of the hepatoduodenal ligament, which produces a cystic configuration.[22, 24] Bile cysts associated with biliary atresia are no larger than several centimeters in diameter. The cholangiolar proliferation and periportal fibrosis in the liver are identical to what is seen in biliary atresia without cyst formation. Although these cases have been termed correctable because the cystic structure can be anastomosed to bowel, the response to surgical treatment and the prognosis in these infants are the same as in biliary atresia without cystic changes.[22] Therefore, we consider infants with this form of choledochal cyst who present with jaundice in the first few months of life to have biliary atresia, and we refer to this entity as *cystic biliary atresia*.

The *bile plug syndrome* is defined as cholestatic jaundice due to plugging of the extrahepatic ducts with bilirubin sludge.[27, 28] Obstructive jaundice appears within the first months of life. Usually the infant has had an episode of hemolysis (e.g., erythroblastosis) or severe hemoconcentration, which has resulted in bilirubin precipitation in the extrahepatic ducts. The distal common bile duct is obstructed by the sludge, and the proximal ducts are dilated. The abdomen should be explored, a cholangiogram obtained, and the

Table 39–2 GENETIC-METABOLIC DISEASES LEADING TO CONJUGATED HYPERBILIRUBINEMIA IN EARLY INFANCY

Conditions	Mode of Inheritance	Additional Clinical Manifestations	Screening Tests	Definitive Diagnosis
Alpha$_1$-antitrypsin deficiency	Autosomal recessive	Neonatal hepatitis syndrome.	Serum protein electrophoresis: absent alpha$_1$-globulin peak.	Protease inhibitor typing. Quantitative α_1-AT measurement in serum.
Galactosemia (transferase deficiency)	Autosomal recessive	Failure to thrive, gastrointestinal symptoms, cataracts, renal tubular defect, hypoglycosemia.	Reducing sugar in urine identifiable as galactose while patient on milk feeding.	Red cell galactose-1-PO^4 uridyl transferase assay.
Hereditary fructose intolerance	Autosomal recessive	Onset of vomiting, diarrhea, weight loss with introduction of fructose (fruit and/or sucrose) in diet. Renal tubular defects, hypoglycosemia.	Reducing sugar in urine identifiable as fructose while patient receives fructose or sucrose.	Fructose tolerance test (dangerous). Liver fructose-1-PO^4 aldolase activity.
Hereditary tyrosinemia	Autosomal recessive	Failure to thrive, vomiting, diarrhea, rickets, renal tubular defects, hypoglucosemia.	High plasma tyrosine and methionine, aminoaciduria, tyrosyluria.	p-Hydroxyphenyl-pyruvic acid oxidase in liver(?)
Fibrocystic disease	Autosomal recessive	Failure to thrive, meconium ileus, malabsorption, pulmonary infections.	Digestive enzymes in feces or duodenal juice.	Sweat chloride concentration.
Niemann-Pick disease, (Types A and B)	Autosomal recessive	Failure to thrive, cherry-red spots; CNS symptoms later.	Foam cells in bone marrow.	Sphingomyelinase assay in leukocytes, cultured fibroblasts, liver tissue.

From Sass-Kortsak A: Pediatr Clin North Am 1974; *21*:777.

sludge irrigated from the duct. Recovery is prompt and permanent. Most previously reported instances of bile plug syndrome in which the extrahepatic ducts were patent but liver biopsy showed bile pigment in the periportal canaliculi were actually other forms of cholestatic jaundice.

Spontaneous perforation of the bile duct in neonates is manifested by bile ascites.[29, 30] Bile is resorbed from the peritoneal cavity, producing direct hyperbilirubinemia. The perforation is usually located at the junction of the cystic, hepatic, and common bile ducts. The etiology is unknown but may be related to an anomalous communication between the bile duct and pancreatic duct proximal to the ampulla of Vater, as occurs in patients with congenital choledochal cysts.

Other rare causes of bile duct obstruction include congenital inflammatory stenosis of the distal extrahepatic ducts and extrinsic compression.[31]

Infants who have been receiving prolonged intravenous alimentation may develop cholestatic jaundice,[32, 33] which in most cases is caused by a defect in the hepatocellular transport of bilirubin. However, some fasted babies who are receiving intravenous alimentation develop jaundice associated with a dilated gallbladder and bile ducts. The bile is viscous and may contain sludge, possibly as a result of low bile secretion and stasis. Both conditions usually resolve when the patient is allowed to eat and the parenteral nutrition is cut back.

INCIDENCE

Persistent cholestatic jaundice after the age of 2 weeks occurs about once in 5000 births. All forms of neonatal hepatitis occur approximately once in 8000 births. Extrahepatic biliary atresia affects 1 per 10,000 to 15,000 births, and intrahepatic biliary atresia about 1 per 70,000 births.[34]

The incidence of biliary atresia varies with race.[34] In Hawaii, where the weather is fairly uniform and the diet is similar, a comparison of racial groups showed the following incidence of biliary atresia:

Racial Group	*Rate/10,000 Newborns*
Caucasian	0.6 ± 0.2
Japanese	0.8 ± 0.3
Filipino	2.0 ± 0.9
Chinese	3.0 ± 1.6

Although many cases of biliary atresia have been reported from Japan, the incidence of biliary atresia in Sendai was 0.9 per 10,000 births, about the same as for Japanese in Hawaii. However, the number of cases of biliary atresia treated at children's hospitals in Japan is four to six times that in the United States. This discrepancy is probably the result of more accurate reporting owing to greater awareness and referral of patients with this condition to specialized surgical centers in Japan.

In some series, there is a marked difference in the sex incidence of biliary atresia, choledochal cyst, and other causes of neonatal jaundice.[35] Females are found to have biliary atresia and choledochal cyst one to two times as often as males, while males develop neonatal hepatitis twice as often as females. The reasons are unknown.

Among infants with jaundice that persists for 1 month, two thirds will have some form of neonatal hepatitis, and one third will have biliary atresia.[36–38] Approximately 20 per cent will have hepatitis from acquired intrauterine infection (cytomegalic inclusion virus, toxoplasmosis, syphilis, and so forth). About 10 to 15 per cent of these infants will have alpha$_1$-antitrypsin deficiency. Galactosemia accounts for 5 per cent of cases, while hereditary fructose intolerance and tyrosinemia are very rare.[1, 36, 38] Although initial studies may suggest one of these nonsurgical causes for cholestasis, it must be remembered that biliary atresia may also occur in infants with alpha$_1$-antitrypsin deficiency, galactosemia, rubella, or cytomegalic inclusion disease.[35, 36, 39]

ETIOLOGY

The etiology of biliary atresia is unknown. Some of the more popular theories are (1) failure of recanalization of embryonic bile ducts, (2) an association of anomalies, (3) evolution from hepatitis, and (4) damage from liver or bile duct toxins.

Occlusion or failure of recanalization of the bile ducts during intrauterine development probably does not occur. The biliary tract does not undergo a "solid cord" epithelial proliferative phase of development as does the duodenum.[40] If it did, one would expect biliary atresia to be associated with duodenal atresia or stenosis, which almost invariably affects the duodenum at the level of the ampulla of Vater.[41] Furthermore, experimental occlusion of the bile ducts in fetal animals produces jaundice at birth with elevated serum levels of conjugated bilirubin.[42] The placenta can transport unconjugated bilirubin but not conjugated bilirubin. With rare exceptions, jaundice in a newborn infant who eventually develops biliary atresia is mild, transient, and associated with increased levels of unconjugated bilirubin. If biliary atresia were caused by congenital obstruction of the bile ducts, it would be difficult to explain the presence of bile-stained meconium when the patient is a neonate. Finally, biliary atresia is rarely found in autopsies of newborn infants. Thus, although biliary atresia may be congenital, the bile duct obliteration is not evident until several weeks after birth.

Congenital or familial factors probably contribute to the development of biliary atresia. The effect of race on the incidence of biliary atresia has already been mentioned. Trisomy 17–18 is associated with both biliary atresia and giant cell hepatopathy.[36] Associated anomalies occur in about 10 per cent of cases and include congenital heart disease, meningomyelocele, malrotation, Down's syndrome, and polysplenia syndrome.[37, 43] These same anomalies also occur with even greater frequency in infants with neonatal hepatitis.[36] Although consanguinity has been described, familial cases are rare. There are a number of instances in which neonatal hepatitis and biliary atresia have occurred in siblings.[35]

Some authors have hypothesized that hepatitis may be a precursor of biliary atresia. Transplacental passage of virus from a mother who was a carrier of infectious hepatitis was identified in one infant with neonatal hepatitis, but, in general, neither biliary atresia nor viral hepatitis occurs in infants of mothers who acquire acute hepatitis during pregnancy.[44] Biliary atresia and neonatal hepatitis have been associated with congenital rubella, *Listeria* infection, and Epstein-Barr virus infection.[45, 46, 96] Other infectious agents are associated with neonatal hepatitis,[1] but they could be only rare causes of biliary atresia. Therefore, other organisms or agents, as yet unidentified, must be found to explain most cases.

An attractive theory to explain the etiology and clinical course of biliary atresia is the excretion of a bile duct toxin by the liver.[47] Experimentally, monohydroxylated bile acids have been shown to produce hepatocellular injury and intrahepatic bile duct proliferation similar to that seen in human infants with cholestasis. Lithocholate fed to pregnant and nursing hamsters produces liver damage with bile duct proliferation in the newborn animals.[48] It is possible that infants with biliary atresia have an inborn metabolic defect that results in the formation of a toxic bile salt or an inability to detoxify some other hepatotoxin. This theory would explain the postnatal delayed onset of biliary atresia after an initial period of normal bile flow. The histologic findings in biliary atresia, particularly the bile duct proliferation and hepatic fibrosis, are far more exaggerated than those associated with simple bile duct obstruction. Babies with biliary atresia who are treated by bile duct to intestine drainage procedures before 3 months of age have a better prognosis than those in whom the operation is performed later. This may mean that toxins formed in the liver must be drained early to prevent intrahepatic retention and increasing bile duct destruction. It must be emphasized, however, that these are only speculations, and the cause of biliary atresia is still undetermined.

CLINICAL FINDINGS

Jaundice, consisting predominantly of conjugated hyperbilirubinemia, is the initial manifestation of biliary atresia. Typically, pregnancy and delivery were uneventful, and birth weight was normal. There may be transient indirect hyperbilirubinemia that resolves within a week.[36] The baby feeds and grows normally, but then in the second and third week of life he becomes jaundiced. The stools are usually white, but they may be yellow or green or even be normal-colored after jaundice has appeared.

In the differential diagnosis, one must consider many syndromes associated with conjugated hyperbilirubinemia before assuming that the infant requires surgery. The infectious and genetic-metabolic diseases that must be considered are listed in Tables 39–1 and 39–2.[1] During the physical examination one should search for features presented in Tables 39–1 and 39–2 that characterize nonsurgical forms of jaundice. The syndrome of biliary hypoplasia includes characteristic facies, vertebral and cardiac malformations, and retarded development, findings that should be apparent on physical examination.[5–7]

Aagenaes described a hereditary syndrome

consisting of cholestatic jaundice and lymphedema of the extremities.[49] Danks et al. reported one baby with this syndrome,[38] and we encountered a family of non-Scandinavian ancestry in which two girls had intrahepatic cholestasis and lymphedema of all four extremities. Therefore, the presence of lymphedema in a jaundiced infant, particularly when there is a family history of the syndrome, suggests a nonsurgical cause of cholestasis.

In the first 30 to 60 days of life, infants with biliary atresia may have mild hepatomegaly, but the liver edge is well defined. With increasing age, progressive fibrosis and cholestasis result in an enlarged, hard liver with a sharp edge, in which the indentations of the gallbladder fossa and ligamentum teres are easily felt. The liver in hepatitis tends to be enlarged earlier, the consistency is soft, and the liver edge is blunt.

Splenomegaly occurs with equal frequency in biliary atresia and nonsurgical liver diseases.

A mass from a choledochal cyst is very rarely palpable in the first weeks of life.

Liver function studies are of limited help in defining the cause of the jaundice. If the serum bilirubin is predominantly unconjugated, bile duct disease is unlikely. About 90 per cent of infants with biliary atresia, but only 50 per cent of infants with hepatitis, have conjugated bilirubin levels exceeding 4 mg/dl.[36] Most often the total bilirubin concentration is less than 15 mg/dl, but among the few patients with values between 15 and 20 mg/dl, the incidence of biliary atresia and neonatal hepatitis is about equal. When more than 30 per cent of the total bilirubin is conjugated, mechanical obstruction of the bile duct is likely. In spite of complete ductal obstruction, the total and direct-reacting bilirubin concentration may fluctuate by as much as 3 to 5 mg/dl, so a decrease in the bilirubin concentration should not be misinterpreted as indicating a patent biliary tract.

The serum leucine aminopeptidase concentration is consistently elevated in infants with biliary atresia, whereas in patients with hepatitis it is normal.[1] An occasional patient with hepatitis has such a marked elevation of the SGOT that it is diagnostic, while others have a high alkaline phosphatase value more characteristic of a lesion of the ducts. However, study of biliary excretion is almost always required to diagnose ductal obstruction irrespective of the serum enzyme values.

The duodenum may be intubated and its contents aspirated and analyzed for the presence of bile.[50] After instillation of magnesium sulfate (10 to 15 ml of a 25 per cent solution) to stimulate bile flow, continuous aspiration over 24 hours gives the most accurate results.[52] Bile is detected in more than 80 per cent of infants with intact bile ducts, but no bile is found in those with biliary atresia.

Hepatic uptake and excretion of radioactive labeled compounds are used to assess liver function and the patency of the bile ducts. ^{99m}Technetium-labeled iminodiacetate (IDA) compounds (e.g., HIDA, PIPIDA, DISIDA) and ^{131}I rose bengal are commonly used.[53, 54, 98–100] Technetium is a gamma emitter with a half-life of 6.5 hours and can give scintigraphic images with good resolution. Because of the short half-life, phenobarbital (5 mg/kg/day) is given for 5 days before the study to enhance the rate of bile excretion.[53] After injection of 1 mCi of ^{99m}technetium, anterior images of the abdomen are obtained at frequent intervals up to 24 hours to identify excretion of the nuclide in the bowel. If hepatic uptake is poor, indicating severe impairment of liver function (hepatitis), excretion of isotope is not expected. A ^{99m}technetium sulfur colloid liver scan may demonstrate widely dilated intrahepatic ducts associated with extrahepatic bile duct obstruction (Fig. 39–1).

Because of its longer half-life, ^{131}I rose bengal can be used to measure the percentage of an intravenous dose that is excreted

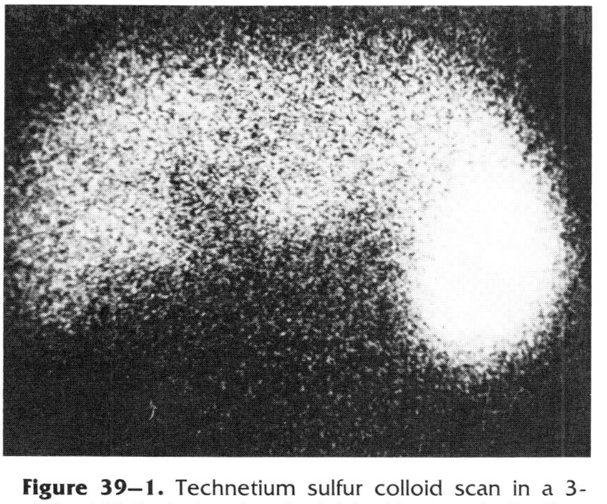

Figure 39–1. Technetium sulfur colloid scan in a 3-month-old infant, showing diminished isotope in the liver hilum due to dilated intrahepatic bile ducts associated with biliary atresia. Note the greater uptake of isotope in the spleen than in the liver as a result of impaired liver function.

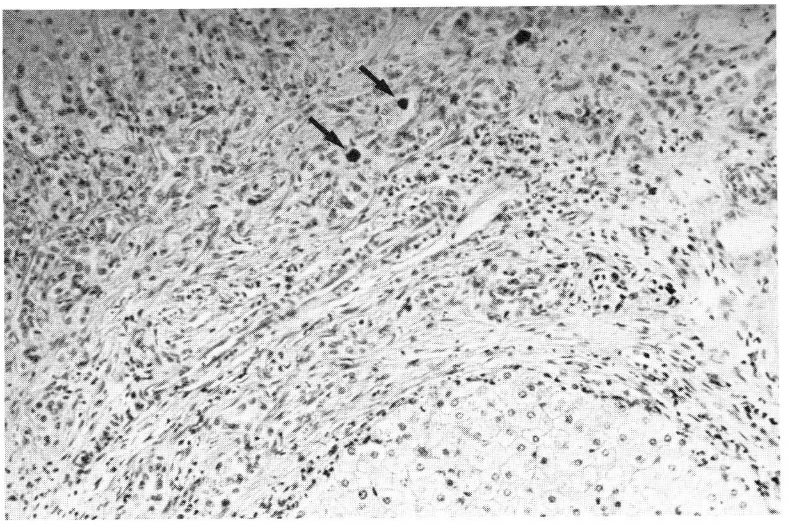

Figure 39–2. Liver biopsy from a 2-month-old infant with biliary atresia. Note the periportal fibrosis and proliferation of bile ductules. Bile pigment is present in the cholangioles (*arrows*). The architecture of the liver lobule is preserved.

in the stool over a 72-hour period. Infants with biliary atresia rarely excrete more than 10 per cent of the radioiodine into the bowel. About 15 to 20 per cent of infants with hepatitis excrete less than 10 per cent, however, so this test does not completely distinguish hepatitis from biliary atresia.[1] Because the isotope is excreted in the urine, it is imperative to separate urine from stool. Usually, the infant must be kept in a metabolic bed, and females require insertion of a bladder catheter.

An upper gastrointestinal series is not usually done. However, a bile cyst or distention of the gallbladder may produce an impression on the duodenum. The best method for demonstrating a dilated gallbladder or choledochal cyst is abdominal ultrasonography.

Other tests that have been advocated to differentiate atresia from hepatitis are the ratio of serum bile salts, the serum alpha fetoprotein level, red cell fragility tests (reflecting vitamin E deficiency), and serum levels of lipoprotein X. All these tests are too nonspecific to be of much value.[55–58, 97]

Percutaneous needle biopsy of the liver may be useful even when performed within the first several months of life.[59,60] Biliary atresia is characterized by preserved liver lobules surrounded by widened periportal areas containing proliferating bile ductules and bile lakes, increased fibrous tissue proliferation, and an inflammatory infiltrate (Fig. 39–2). Neonatal hepatitis is characterized by areas of hepatic cell necrosis, disorganized liver cords, inflammatory cells within the liver parenchyma and portal area, and giant multinucleated liver cells (Fig. 39–3). Although

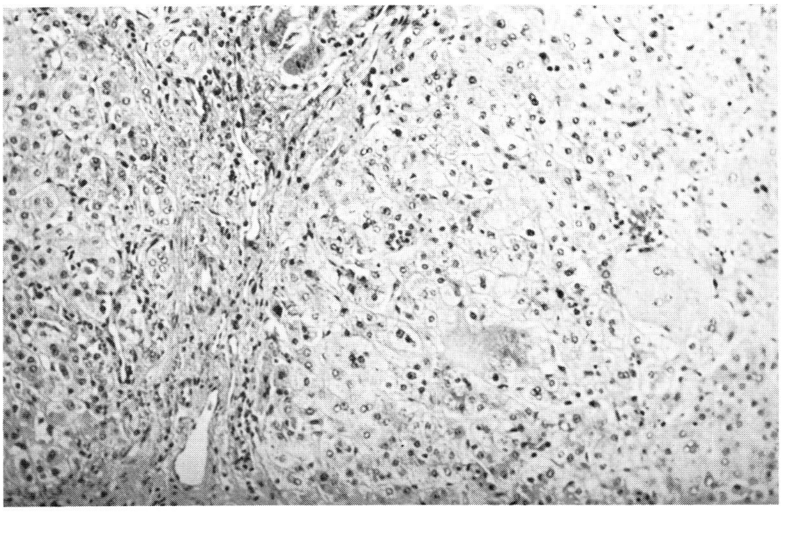

Figure 39–3. Liver biopsy from an infant with neonatal hepatitis. Note the inflammatory cells, multinucleated giant liver cells, hepatic cell necrosis, and poorly defined liver lobules.

giant cell transformation is characteristic of neonatal hepatitis, about one half of infants with biliary atresia also have giant cells. Overall results show that the biopsy diagnosis correlates with operative findings in 60 per cent of cases, is equivocal in 16 per cent, and is incorrect in 25 per cent.[61]

Percutaneous transhepatic cholangiography is not used because the ducts are so small that they can rarely be entered, and the study requires a general anesthetic.

Ultrasound and CT scans have been useful; they may show dilated bile ducts in patients with extrahepatic obstruction from stricture, extrinsic pressure, or a choledochal cyst.[62] A cystic structure in the hepatoduodenal area without a dilated gallbladder is characteristic of biliary atresia. If the gallbladder is also distended, the obstruction is more distal and probably represents distal duct atresia or bile plug syndrome.

SURGICAL DIAGNOSIS AND TREATMENT

When the clinical and laboratory studies cannot eliminate extrahepatic bile ductal obstruction, surgical exploration is indicated. Ideally, the operation should be performed before the infant is 70 days of age (see further on). Preoperative preparation should include correction of clotting defects, administration of prophylactic antibiotics, and optimal hydration and nutrition. Vitamin K (2 mg intramuscularly) should be given preoperatively. Our antibiotic regimen consists of ampicillin (50 mg/kg every 6 hours intravenously) and gentamicin (1.5 mg/kg every 8 hours). The latter is infused over 20 minutes to avoid blood levels greater than 12 ng/ml, which could produce renal toxicity and ototoxicity. Ampicillin and gentamicin should not be mixed in the same solution. Preoperatively, feedings should not be withheld for more than 4 hours in order to maintain an optimal glycogen level, which will lessen liver stress during anesthesia or hypotension.

After the patient is anesthetized, a secure peripheral or central venous catheter is placed for infusion of 5 per cent dextrose in Ringer's lactate solution (usually given at 10 ml/kg/hour intraoperatively). The abdomen is explored through a transverse upper abdominal incision, slightly cephalad to the liver edge. The gallbladder is identified, and a fine catheter is passed into the fundus. The presence of bile in the gallbladder indicates that the diagnosis is hepatitis. A cholangiogram is obtained by injecting 2 to 3 ml of 20 per cent Hypaque. The injection should be gentle and the solution diluted to minimize the chance of injuring the bile duct. A wedge biopsy should be obtained from the liver edge. Biliary atresia is probably present if the liver is deeply fissured at the gallbladder fossa and ligamentum teres, or if the surface of the liver is finely granular and firm. The liver is green-brown in both biliary atresia and hepatitis.

If the gallbladder is thick-walled or if its lumen is obliterated, biliary atresia is present. If contrast material passes into the duodenum but does not reflux into the proximal ducts, it may be necessary to place a rubber-shod bulldog clamp across the distal hepatoduodenal ligament and repeat the injection. If the common and right and left hepatic ducts cannot be opacified, they are probably atretic and must be explored. If a cystic structure is found in the hepatoduodenal ligament or at the porta hepatis, it can be cannulated to obtain a cholangiogram. Examples of cholangiographic findings are shown in Figure 39–4.

In 1959 Dr. Morio Kasai described the technique of hepatic portoenterostomy, which was first presented in English in 1968.[63] This operation does not require the presence of grossly patent ducts for a successful repair. The gallbladder is dissected from its fossa and mobilized to the junction of the cystic duct and common bile duct. The obliterated common duct is transected at the level of the duodenum and is mobilized proximally to the hilum of the liver. Usually only scar and inflammation are present, and only the fibrous remnants of the bile duct can be found. The scarred contents of the hepatoduodenal ligament are dissected off the portal vein and hepatic artery to the porta hepatis.

There are various ways of performing the dissection at the porta hepatis. The point of transection may be supraportal, portal, or infraportal.[64] In a supraportal transection, a 1 cm to 3 cm core of liver is resected in addition to removing the fibrous extrahepatic duct remnants. A portal transection is defined as being at the level of Glisson's capsule, and an infraportal dissection transects the fibrous mass proximal to the porta hepatis. The intent is to expose patent branches of the right and left hepatic ducts within or at the surface of the liver. One should dissect

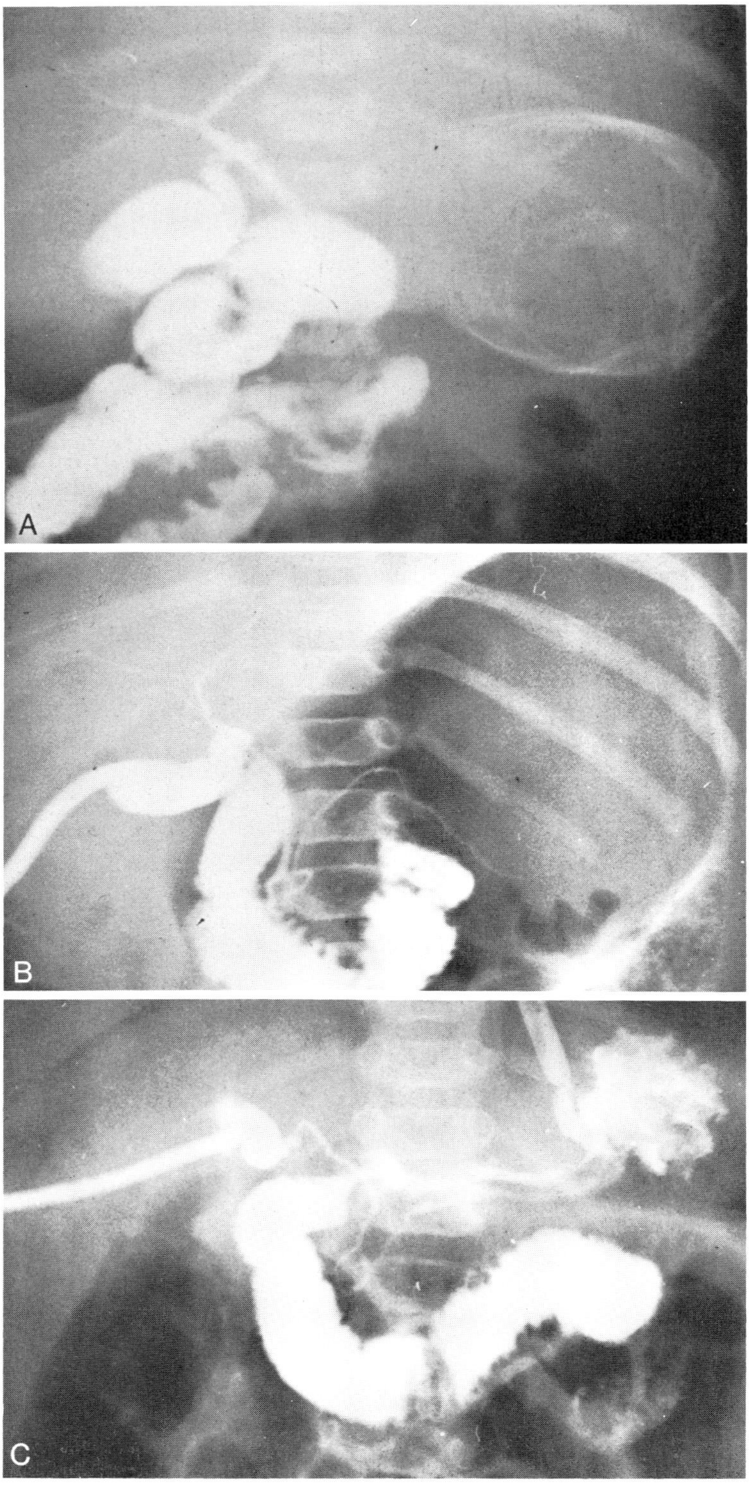

Figure 39–4. Examples of operative cholangiogram findings. *A*, Infant with jejunal atresia who developed cholestatic jaundice from intravenous alimentation. Although cholestasis would result in diminished bile production, the ducts are probably of normal size. *B*, Infant with neonatal hepatitis showing small (unused) bile ducts emptying into the duodenum. The pancreatic duct is also opacified. *C*, Infant with biliary atresia affecting the right, left, and common hepatic ducts. The gallbladder is small, the cystic duct is patent, and the common bile duct empties into the duodenum.

Illustration continued on opposite page

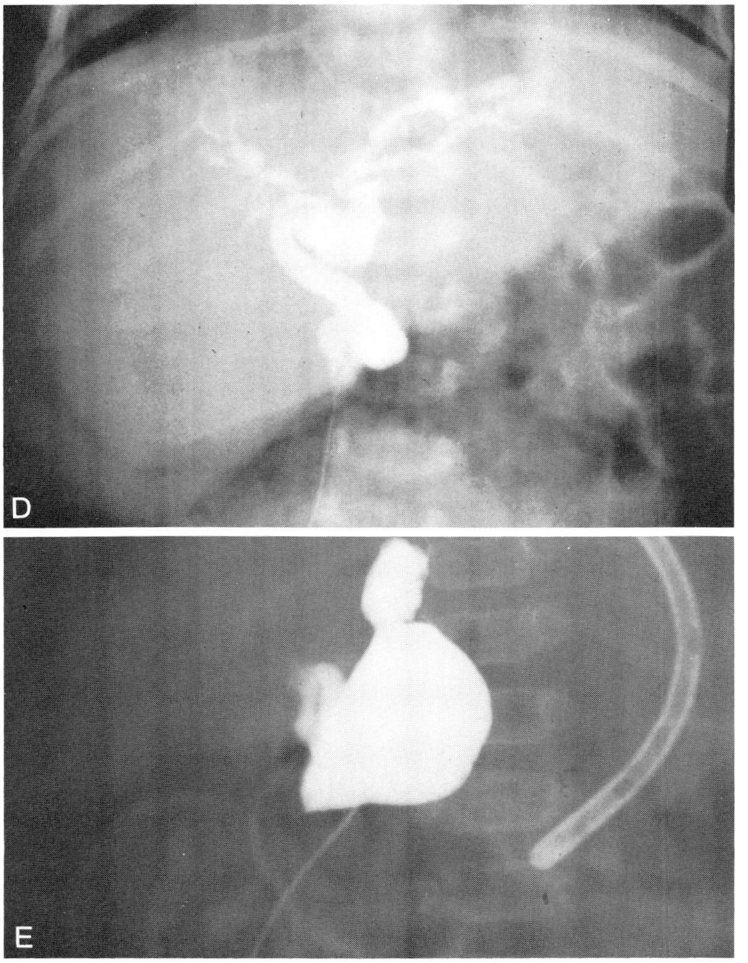

Figure 39–4 *Continued. D,* Cystic biliary atresia with obliterated common bile duct. The gallbladder was injected with contrast. It communicated with dilated "cyst" at the hilum. The "cyst" has no epithelial lining. The intrahepatic ducts were dilated with numerous areas of stenosis. *E,* Cystic biliary atresia showing a common hepatic duct but no intrahepatic bile ducts. The gallbladder and cystic ducts were obliterated. The dilated "cystic common bile duct" had no epithelial lining, and it presumably developed from dissection of bile into the hepatic duodenal ligament.

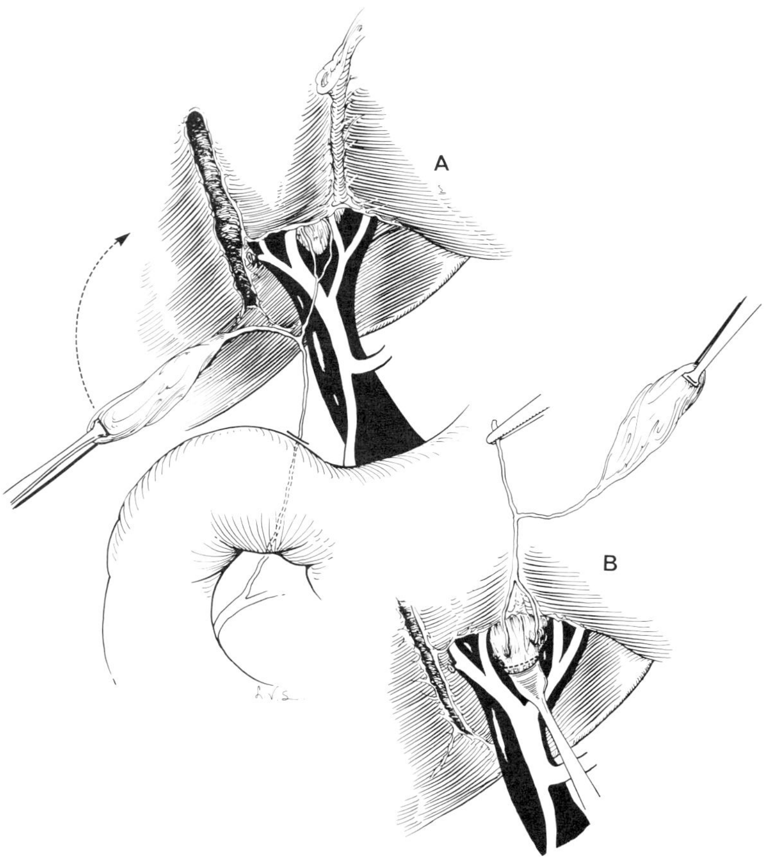

Figure 39–5. Drawing of the contents of the hepatoduodenal ligament, showing Kasai's technique of dissecting the atretic gallbladder, common bile duct, common hepatic duct, and right and left hepatic ducts to the liver hilum. The bifurcation of the right and left portal vein branches must be retracted to obtain proper exposure of the porta hepatis, where the ducts will be transected and the Roux-en-Y hepatojejunostomy accomplished.

the fibrous tissue posteriorly in the porta hepatis by retracting the bifurcation of the right and left portal veins (Fig. 39–5).[15] The point of transection of the fibrous mass is then at the level at which the portal veins enter liver parenchyma. Of the three levels of transection, the portal one gives the best results.

An operating microscope may facilitate identification of patent ductal structures and precise coagulation of small blood vessels.[65] Electrocautery and deep suture ligation should not be used for hemostasis in order to avoid injuring the small patent ducts.

Bile drainage is provided through a Roux-en-Y jejunostomy. The transected distal end of the jejunum is oversewn, and a small incision (just large enough to encompass the porta hepatis) is made near the end. An anastomosis is made between the intestine and either the edge of the transected fibrous tissue or Glisson's capsule about the porta hepatis. Continuous 5-0 chromic catgut is used, placing the sutures through all layers of the bowel. An outer row of interrupted 5-0 silk sutures is used to secure the intestine to the liver capsule. In the original Kasai procedure the proximal limb of jejunum was sutured to the side of the Roux-en-Y limb approximately 30 cm from the point of portojejunostomy. Penrose drains are placed near the hepatic anastomosis, and the wound is closed.

One of the most troubling complications of portoenterostomy is ascending cholangitis. One of the causes for this is reflux of bowel contents into the biliary ducts. Some surgeons have noted episodic reflux of food from the end of an externalized isoperistaltic Roux-en-Y limb—even when the limb is more than 25 cm long. To minimize cholangitis, the Roux-en-Y reconstruction has been modified by creating a temporary jejunostomy stoma to decompress the jejunal limb (Fig. 39–6).[66,67] Sawaguchi uses an isolated segment of jejunum 40 cm long, in which the proximal

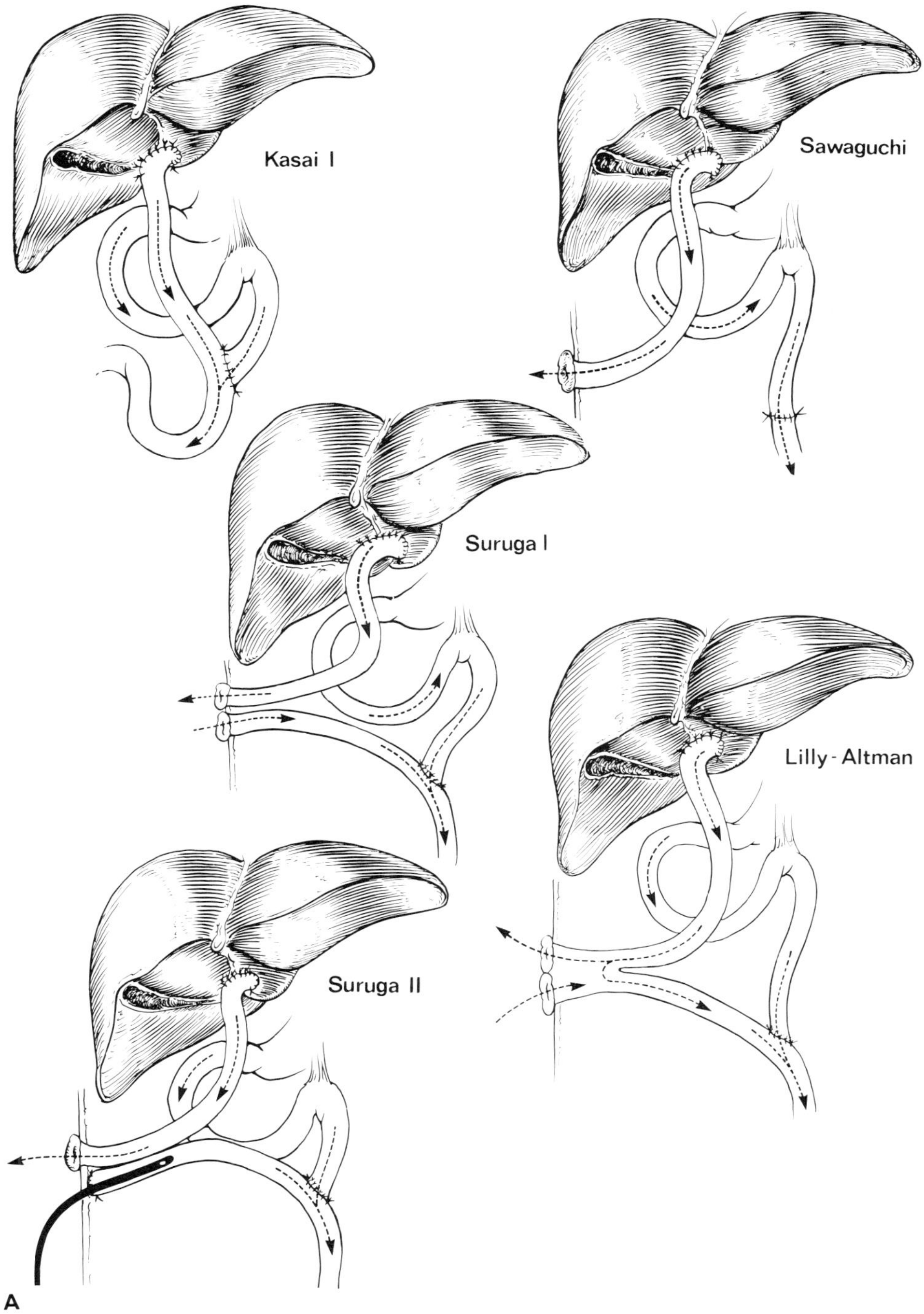

Figure 39–6. *A* and *B*, Drawings of ten operative procedures advocated for drainage of the porta hepatis with the intent of minimizing postoperative ascending cholangitis. In the Kasai II procedure, the letters designate the length of each limb of the jejunostomy (see text).

Illustration continued on following page

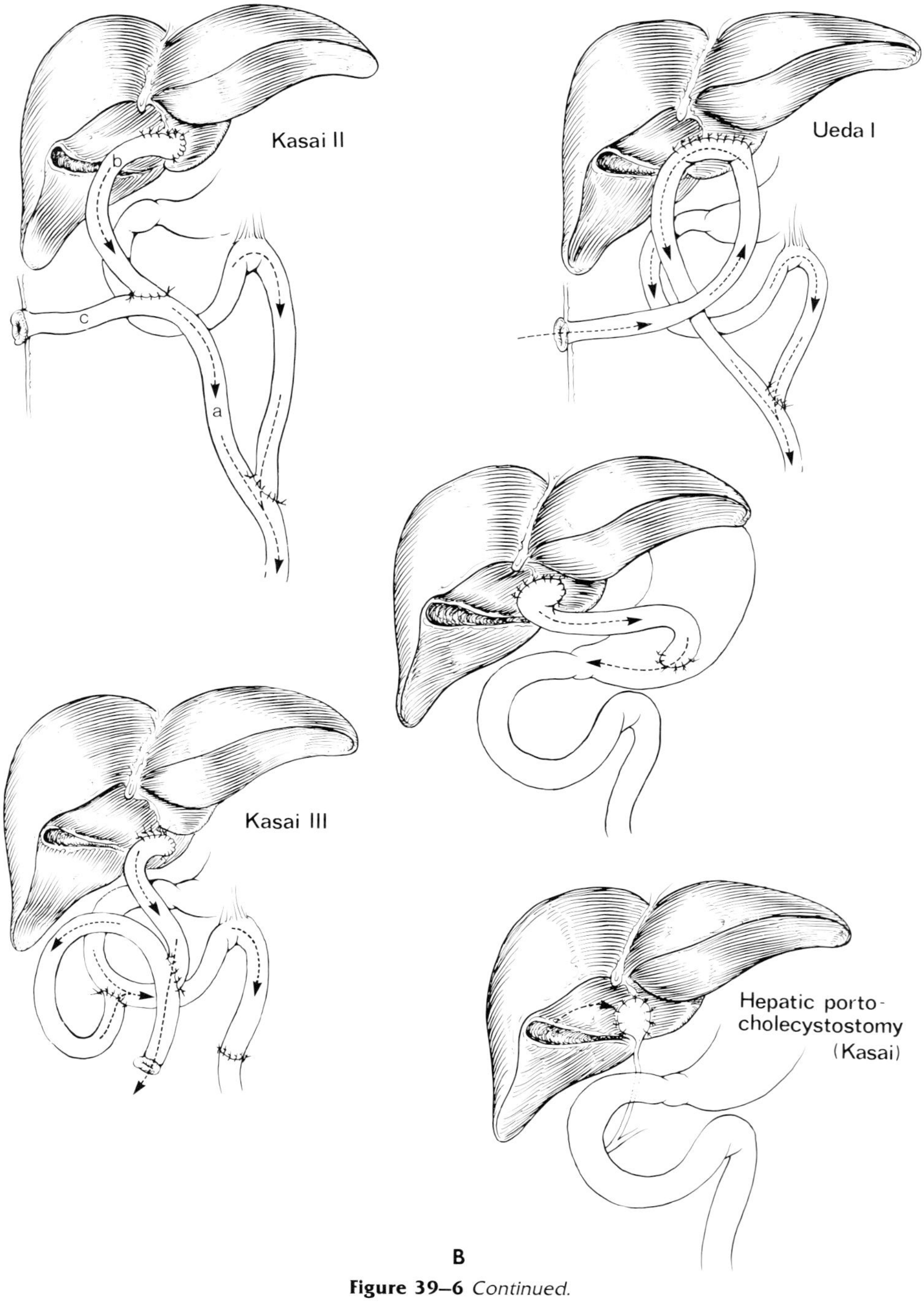

B

Figure 39–6 *Continued.*

end is sutured to the porta hepatis and the distal end is brought out through the abdominal wall as a jejunostomy.[68] Three months later the jejunostomy is taken down and sutured end-to-side to form the Roux-en-Y. This technique seems to decrease the incidence of cholangitis, but fluid and electrolyte losses have been excessive in some infants and have caused the death of at least one. Other surgeons instill the bile through the distal jejunostomy limb of an interrupted Roux-en-Y. The second stage, in which the Roux-en-Y is formed, has been followed by the development of cholangitis in some infants.

In Suruga's technique, the Roux-en-Y is interrupted as a double-barreled Mikulicz jejunostomy.[65] Lilly and Altman divide the Mikulicz spur, using a spur-crushing clamp.[69] The risk of fluid losses from the proximal jejunostomy fistula remains, but if the Mikulicz spur is divided, some of the bile passes into the distal bowel. Kasai developed a double Y modification (Kasai II) of the Roux-en-Y to decompress the portal area and at the same time to avoid excessive fluid losses.[22]

Based on the results of experiments in dogs, Kasai recommends that the external fistula limb (c) should be 8 cm, the portojejunostomy limb (b) should be 15 cm, and the jejunum between the proximal and distal Y loops should be 20 cm (Fig. 39–6). This seems to minimize enteric reflux and excessive fluid and electrolyte losses. A number of other modifications have been devised, including a gastric tube conduit (Fig. 39–6).[66, 67] Ueda described a method in which the transected end of the jejunum is brought through the abdominal wall as a stoma, and the anastomosis to the porta is placed more toward the Roux-en-Y connection.[66]

At present, most pediatric surgeons use the original Kasai Roux-en-Y and do not construct an external fistula. There is no good evidence that a jejunostomy really decreases the incidence of cholangitis, although it provides a means of studying bile production and the excretion of drugs in bile.[69, 70] Antibiotics are given for long periods to minimize cholangitis.

Approximately 15 to 25 per cent of infants have obliterated right and left hepatic ducts but a patent gallbladder and common bile duct. To avoid cholangitis in these patients, Kasai performs a hepatic portocholecystostomy (Fig. 39–6).[15, 22] The atretic right and left hepatic ducts are excised. Preserving the cystic artery, the gallbladder is mobilized, opened, and sutured to the porta hepatis.

OPERATIVE FINDINGS

Gross described the various types of abnormalities found in the extrahepatic bile ducts and defined three types of "operable" and four types of "inoperable" atresia (Fig. 39–7).[21] It was soon recognized that an occasional patient who was termed "inoperable" based on findings at laparotomy recovered postoperatively, with resolution of the jaundice and return of liver function to normal, even though no corrective procedure had been done. None of these patients had a cholangiogram to confirm the absence of a duct lumen. Such cases made surgeons reluctant to explore the ductal structures for fear of injuring small patent ducts. However, it is now appreciated that the risk of injuring the duct is remote if the operative cholangiogram is abnormal, and before adoption of operations that entailed a systematic dissection of the hepatoduodenal ligament, the results of surgery were uniformly poor. In many series, only 5 per cent of the "operable" types of biliary atresia improved postoperatively.

The notion that there are "operable" and "inoperable" forms of biliary atresia is no longer accepted. The procedures now in use result in good bile drainage and long-term survival in more than one third of cases, and it is not possible to predict with any precision which patients will improve and which will not.

Biliary atresia is now classified from gross and pathologic findings, including (1) the site of obstruction, (2) the status of the common bile duct, and (3) the appearance of the hepatic radicles at the porta hepatis.[65] Sawaguchi's 78 cases were classified as shown in Table 39–3.

In Kasai's 172 cases, Type I atresia occurred in 16 per cent, Type II atresia in 17 per cent, and Type III atresia in 67 per cent.[15] Histologic sections of the Type I and Type II cases with a "choledochal cyst" containing bile (previously referred to as "correctable" atresia) showed thick fibrotic walls and absence of an epithelial lining. Kasai postulated that these areas result from dissection of bile into the fibrous tissue, where the ducts become obliterated. Examination of the "noncorrectable" cases usually shows one or more channels, ranging in diameter

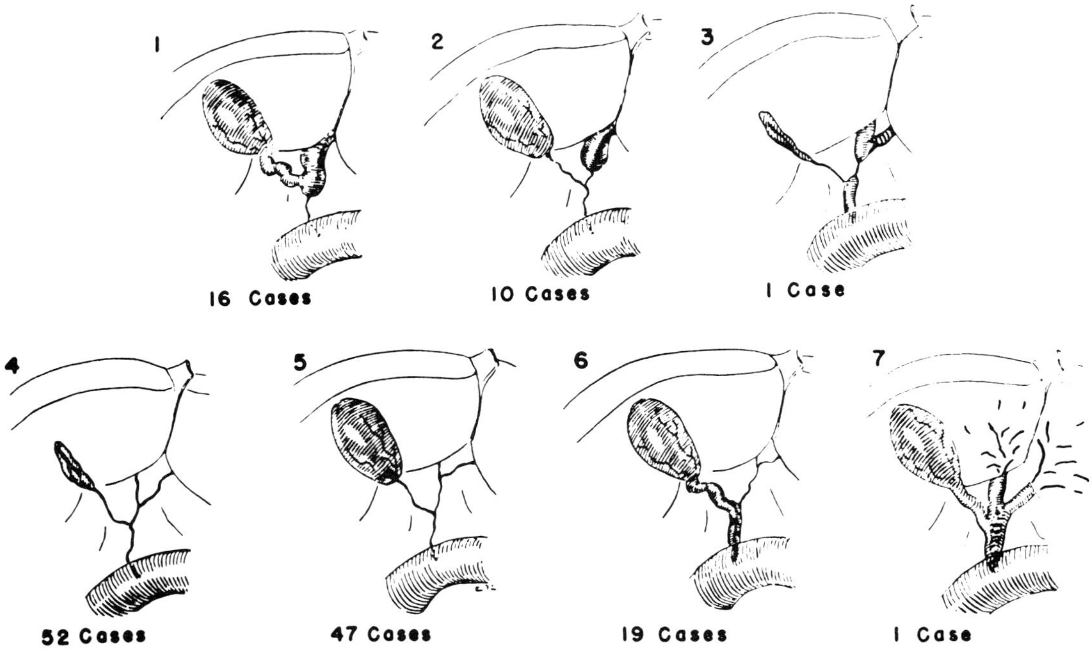

Figure 39–7. "Correctable" biliary atresia is represented in examples 1–3; "uncorrectable" surgical findings are identified by examples 4 to 7. The procedure of portoenterostomy has made the designations "correctable" and "uncorrectable" biliary atresia obsolete, since excellent bile drainage and long-term survival can be achieved in infants having "uncorrectable" types of atresia. (From Gross RE: The Surgery of Infancy and Childhood. Philadelphia, WB Saunders, 1953.)

from 10 to 80 μ, lined by bile duct epithelium.[15, 22] The size of these duct remnants correlates with the chance of obtaining good bile drainage.

Table 39–3 CLASSIFICATION OF BILIARY ATRESIA (SAWAGUCHI)[66]

Classification		Per Cent of Cases
Site of Obstruction		
Type I:	common bile duct	12
Type II:	hepatic duct	8
Type III:	ducts at the porta hepatis	80
Status of Common Bile Duct		
Type a:	patent	24
Type b:	fibrous cord	40
Type c:	aplasia	32
Type d:	miscellaneous	4
Appearance of Hepatic Radicles at the Porta Hepatitis		
Type (alpha):	dilated hepatic channels	9
Type (beta):	hypoplastic hepatic radicles	13
Type (gamma):	bile lake	9
Type (mu):	fibrous hepatic radicles	37
Type (nu):	fibrous mass	13
Type (omicron):	aplasia of hepatic radicles	17

RESULTS

In the past, the results of treatment of biliary atresia were dismal. Although the "correctable" form of atresia was found in 5 to 10 per cent of cases, satisfactory long-term results were rare.[71] The longest reported survivor is a 25 year old woman who had anastomosis of patent right and left hepatic ducts to the duodenum at the age of 12 weeks.[72]

This led some to question the advisability of early operation in jaundiced infants, because if neonatal hepatitis was found instead of atresia, the patient often became worse.[73] One suggestion was that surgical exploration be deferred for 3 to 4 months on the theory that those with hepatitis would improve, leaving only those with atresia as candidates for operation. However, expectant management of hepatitis results in the development of cirrhosis in 35 per cent of patients and death in 25 per cent, and the incidence of these complications in patients with hepatitis following a negative laparotomy is about the same. This indicates that the disease, not the operation, is responsible for the problems in patients with hepatitis who have had a diagnostic laparotomy.[73, 74]

Table 39–4 OPERATIVE RESULTS IN RELATION TO AGE AT OPERATION (KASAI)[15]

Age at Operation (Days)	Number of Patients	Good Bile Excretion
60	11	10 (91%)
61–70	18	10 (56%)
71–90	14	6 (43%)
91 or more	6	27 (55%)

The older procedures (i.e., other than hepatic portoenterostomy or portocholecystostomy) used for "correctable" biliary atresia resulted in good bile excretion in one half of patients, but only 5 to 10 per cent were considered cured.[21, 70] Portoenterostomy has greatly improved the results. For example, of infants with "uncorrectable" biliary atresia, 38 per cent were jaundice-free more than 1 year postoperatively.[75] Of 99 patients more than 3 months old at the time of exploration, one third had good bile excretion, but only 7 per cent were considered cured. Of the 116 infants less than 3 months old at the time of exploration, 61 per cent had good bile excretion and 43 per cent were apparently cured when evaluated later.[75] The latest tabulation of Kasai's results in relation to age at the time of operation is shown in Table 39–4.[75]

The relationship of site of obstruction to outcome of portoenterostomy is shown in Table 39–5. Although the cure rate among the entire group was only 30 per cent, it increased to 55 per cent among the patients treated from 1961 to 1977.[15, 22]

Kasai has also noted a correlation between the size of the bile ducts in the resected specimen and the likelihood of re-establishing bile excretion.[22] When the bile ducts were greater than 200 μ in diameter, fair to excellent excretion was noted in 17 (77 per cent) of 22 patients, and 10 patients were cured. In only 4 of 17 patients with ducts less than 200 μ was bile flow noted, and only one was cured. Others have seen this correlation, but

Table 39–5 RELATIONSHIP OF SITE OF OBSTRUCTION TO OUTCOME OF PORTOENTEROSTOMY[15]

Type of Atresia	Number of Patients	Disappearance of Jaundice	
I	27	14	(52%)
II	30	5	(17%)
III	115	33	(29%)
Total	172	52	(30%)

good bile excretion may also be achieved in some infants with no visible bile ducts.[15, 64, 65, 67, 74, 76] Matsuo et al. studied the fibrous remnants of porta hepatis at the level of the portoenterostomy in 30 patients, using a computer picture analyzer. They found that the degree of postoperative bile drainage did not correlate with the number of ductules or the size of the largest ductule observed but with the total area of all bile ductules. Effective bile flow was achieved in all patients who had at least 50,000 μ^2 and, with the exception of four patients, was not seen in those with less than 50,000 μ^2.[95]

The results of treatment vary in reports from countries other than Japan. Campbell was unable to obtain good bile drainage in any of 13 patients treated by portoenterostomy.[77] They all developed cirrhosis, and the mortality rate was high. However, Lilly and Altman had results comparable to those of the Japanese authors.[69] Of 111 cases reported by Odievre et al., 34 had sustained bile flow for at least 1 year.[78] The age at operation ranged from 5 weeks to 11 months and was less than 4 months in 26 patients. The 3 year survival in a series reported by Hitch et al. was 52 per cent.[79]

Among Kasai's nine patients treated by portocholecystostomy, six became free of jaundice, and five survived more than 5 years.[15] Altman performed portocholecystostomy in eight patients, six of whom had relief of cholestasis; five required conversion to portojejunostomy, however, because of persistent leakage of bile from the anastomosis.[80] Odievre et al. reported that four of ten patients treated by portocholecystostomy died of bile peritonitis from an anastomotic leak.[78] The problem responsible for this complication is probably a high resistance to bile flow in the distal fibrotic and narrowed ducts. Cholangitis has been rare, but the common bile duct becomes progressively narrower in some patients, and the reconstruction must be converted to a portoenterostomy. Two of Lilly's four patients treated by portocholecystostomy required reoperation because of obliteration of the common duct.[81] Thus, it appears that in many patients the process remains active and results in more widespread atresia postoperatively.

The survival of infants who have not had a biliary drainage procedure averages about 16 months.[82, 83] There is little doubt that survival is substantially improved in those who have a good immediate response to surgery. Unfortunately, however, some patients who have a good initial response later manifest progressive obliteration of the portal and intrahepatic ducts and recurrent jaundice.

Altman re-explored a group of infants who failed to respond to portoenterostomy and resected a core of liver or residual fibrous ductal structures at the porta hepatis. Two of the seven patients were improved. The poor outcome among the others might be attributed to the fact that reoperation was performed so late (the mean age at the time of reoperation was 100 days).[80]

LONG-TERM MANAGEMENT

Bile Drainage

Although some bile may be seen at the porta hepatis during the operation, little increase in bile excretion occurs for a week or more postoperatively, and usually 6 weeks to 7 months elapses before the serum bilirubin reaches normal levels. There is no standard approach for reporting the late results of surgery. Some pediatric surgeons define a good result as a decrease in the total serum bilirubin level of 50 per cent or more or the disappearance of clinical jaundice. We believe that quantitative tests, such as the stool content of intravenously injected ^{131}I rose bengal, are more meaningful. Ideally, one would desire complete resolution of cholestasis, return of liver function studies to normal, and histologic regression of fibrosis and distorted lobules. Unfortunately, complete recovery in these terms is unusual.

Other means of enhancing bile flow, such as administration of choleretic drugs (e.g., dehydrocholate [Decholin], florantyrone [Zanchol]), have been tried. Lilly and Hitch noted that administration of florantyrone increased the bilirubin concentration in the bile of five patients.[84] Kasai et al. prescribe dehydrocholic acid, using 3 ml of a 10 per cent solution diluted with 7 ml of 5 per cent glucose, given intravenously every 12 hours for 4 weeks.[15] Dehydrocholic acid and ursodeoxycholic acid (0.3 to 0.4 gm) each are given by mouth for several years thereafter.[15] There are no data to support the efficacy of these regimens.

Phenobarbital is known to stimulate conjugation and excretion of bilirubin, bile salts, and other anions, such as Bromsulphalein and rose bengal.[85] Use of phenobarbital in doses of 14 to 25 mg/kg, three to four times per day, increases bile flow and bile salt excretion in various cholestatic syndromes, and it may provide relief of pruritus in some patients.[85]

Cholestyramine has also been given to chelate bile salts in the intestinal lumen and block their return to the liver and re-excretion in bile. This would give an effect opposite to that of feeding bile salts, but whether it would help the patient is unclear.

Kasai prescribes corticosteroids starting on the sixth postoperative day, after wound healing is under way. The goal is to inhibit inflammatory edema and scar formation in the little ducts. Betamethasone (0.5 mg) is given daily for 2 to 3 weeks. Of course, the drawback of corticosteroids is that they probably increase the risk of developing cholangitis.

Cholangitis or Post-Portoenterostomy Intrahepatic Infection (PPII)

Cholangitis is a major problem following portoenterostomy.[84, 86–88] The clinical findings include high spiking fever, tachycardia, varying degrees of prostration, abdominal distention, perfusion abnormalities, a tender liver, hepatosplenomegaly, recurrent jaundice, and decreased bile flow and bilirubin clearance through the portoenterostomy. The most common presentation consists of high fever without other physical findings. Leukocytosis is usually present, and anemia is common. Changes in liver function tests are minimal, but the serum transaminase and alkaline phosphatase levels usually increase slightly. Continued infection results in intrahepatic abscess formation and death.

Most authors have considered the process to entail reflux of enteric organisms into the biliary tract (i.e., "ascending cholangitis").[84, 86–88] The infection probably results from seeding of organisms from the intestine, which is supported by the following observations: (1) The syndrome was not encountered in the era when "uncorrectable" cases were not treated with an enteric anastomosis; (2) the infection is far more prevalent in infants who develop bile drainage than those who do not, suggesting that a patent communication between the ducts and the intestine is necessary; and (3) infection is more common in infants with portoenterostomy than in those with portocholecystostomy. Paradoxically, the problem seems to be more severe in patients with large, patent intrahepatic ducts than in those with tiny ducts.

The ducts are abnormal in every infant with biliary atresia. Figure 39–8 shows two examples of readily correctable cystic biliary atresia, but postoperatively each of these infants died of overwhelming biliary sepsis despite the administration of antibiotics. In one patient, a postoperative cholangiogram showed decompression of the dilated intrahepatic ducts. The mechanism of intrahepatic sepsis in these cases may involve collapse of the abnormal beaded ducts, which are composed of multiple strictures alternating with dilated saccules. Stagnation of bile in the dilated segments allows the bacteria to proliferate. Others have postulated that the infection originates from bacteria distributed through the systemic or portal venous blood.[89, 90]

The possibility that infection of the hepatoportal lymphatics is a major factor has been considered.[66, 91] When the bile ducts become obstructed, the lymphatics become hypertrophied and engorged, and lymph flow in the porta hepatis increases. Dissection of the porta hepatis disrupts the lymphatics, and some of the bilirubin excreted into the portoenterostomy probably comes from these lymphatics. Hirsig et al. believe that PPII is a form of intrahepatic lymphangitis, and they advise suturing the omentum (omentopexy) to the porta hepatis at the time of portoenterostomy to enhance collateral lymphatic drainage.[91] This may help prevent immediate postoperative hepatic infection, but Lilly has shown that flow of lymph from the liver to the cisterna chyli is ample 6 weeks postoperatively.[92] However, of 19 patients studied by Odievre 1 year postoperatively by percutaneous transhepatic cholangiography, bile ducts were opacified in only 3 patients, and the lymphatics were opacified in the other 16.[93] In this latter group, the lymph flow seemed to be blocked at the porta hepatis in each case. Theoretically, enteric organisms could enter these lymphatics and cause the infection that has been assumed to be cholangitis. However, cholangitis was a common sequela of operations, such as choledochoduodenostomy, that did not disrupt the lymphatics.

Bacterial infection is clearly present in all cases; to accommodate the various theories of origin, the syndrome might best be termed PPII—postportoenterostomy intrahepatic infection. Thirty to 80 per cent of infants who have complete or nearly complete clearing of jaundice will experience PPII. The incidence seems to be inversely related to the age of the patient at the time of the initial operation.[66] When PPII occurs immediately or within 1 month of operation, it is particularly lethal (the mortality is 80 per cent). The mortality from PPII occurring more than 1 month postoperatively is only 5 per cent.[94] Kasai reported the incidence of PPII following his original hepatic portojejunostomy (Kasai I) to be 68 per cent. Other surgeons report an incidence of 39 to 62 per cent following the Kasai I procedure.[66]

Assuming that PPII is due to reflux of enteric organisms, Kasai and others have devised a number of ingenious variations of portoenterostomy (see Fig. 39–6).[66] The frequency of PPII following these operations is shown in Table 39–6. Kasai and Odievre reported an incidence of PPII following the Kasai II double Y portojejunostomy procedure of 35 per cent and 56 per cent, respectively.[15, 78] The Mikulicz double-barreled portojejunostomy and Sawaguchi's procedure were associated with the same incidence of PPII.[67, 68] At present there is no evidence that the incidence of PPII, which averages 57 per cent, is truly lower after any of the variations compared with the original Kasai I procedure.

When a venting enterostomy is used to avoid reflux of intestinal contents, it is usually kept open for 3 months to a year or more. It has been suggested that some of the episodes of cholangitis in patients following this procedure occur as a result of closure of the jejunostomy or development of stenosis at the skin level of the Mikulicz jejunostomy.[84] Infection in such cases has been arrested by re-establishing the proximal cutaneous jejunostomy. When no bile flow has appeared after 3 months, the jejunostomy is closed to avoid the nuisance of caring for the stoma. If good bile flow occurs, the jejunostomy is closed 2 to 3 years later.

Table 39–6 shows that portocholecystostomy is rarely followed by PPII, whereas double Y portojejunoduodenostomy is frequently followed by PPII.

More experience is necessary before it can be determined if any of the various kinds of portoenterostomy gives better results than the others. At present the Roux-en-Y hepatic portojejunostomy without a venting stoma seems to provide as good bile drainage as

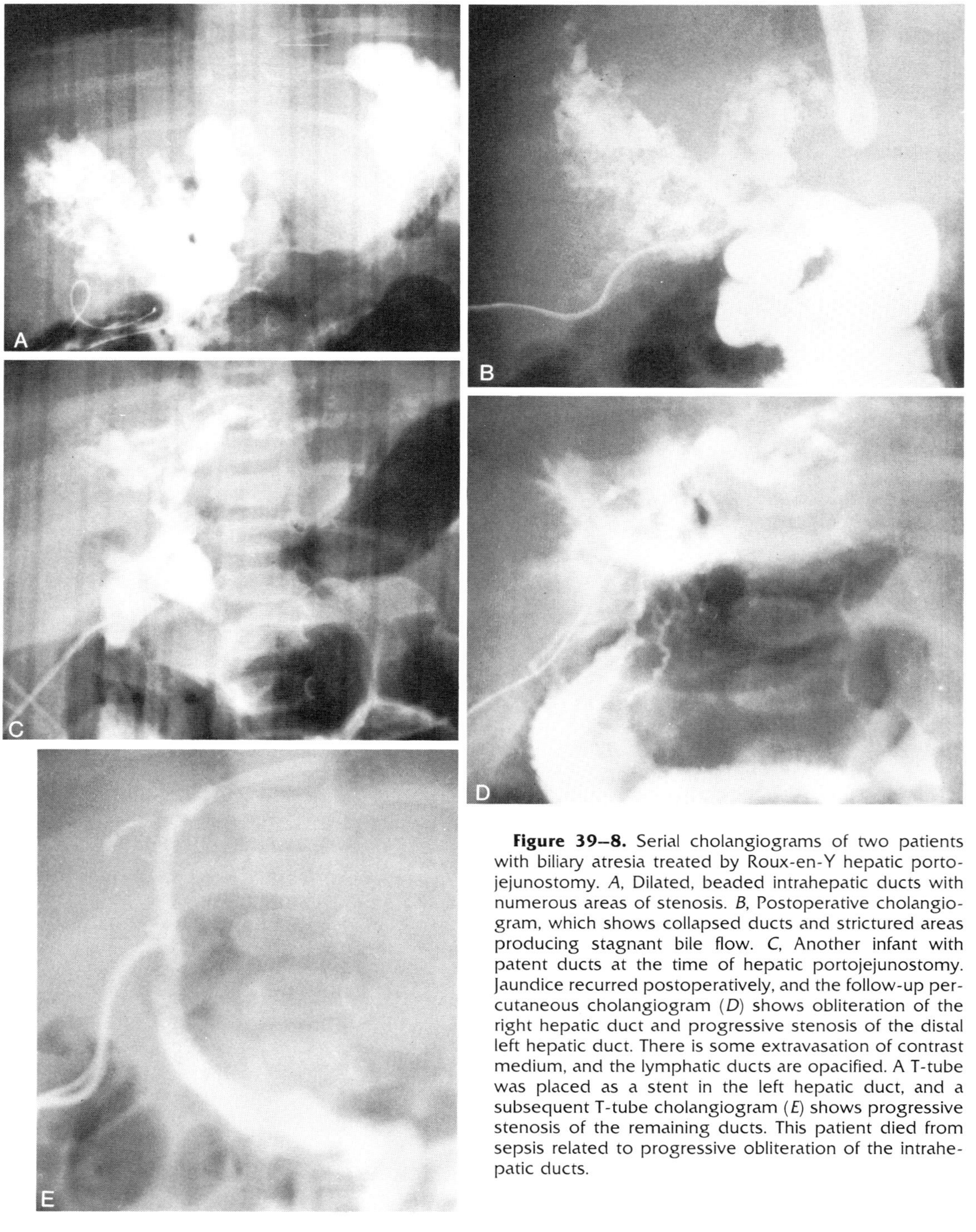

Figure 39–8. Serial cholangiograms of two patients with biliary atresia treated by Roux-en-Y hepatic portojejunostomy. *A*, Dilated, beaded intrahepatic ducts with numerous areas of stenosis. *B*, Postoperative cholangiogram, which shows collapsed ducts and strictured areas producing stagnant bile flow. *C*, Another infant with patent ducts at the time of hepatic portojejunostomy. Jaundice recurred postoperatively, and the follow-up percutaneous cholangiogram (*D*) shows obliteration of the right hepatic duct and progressive stenosis of the distal left hepatic duct. There is some extravasation of contrast medium, and the lymphatic ducts are opacified. A T-tube was placed as a stent in the left hepatic duct, and a subsequent T-tube cholangiogram (*E*) shows progressive stenosis of the remaining ducts. This patient died from sepsis related to progressive obliteration of the intrahepatic ducts.

Table 39–6 INCIDENCE OF PPII FOLLOWING VARIOUS KINDS OF PORTOENTEROSTOMY

	Kimura[66]			Kasai[63]			Sawaguchi[68]			Odievre[78]			Lilly[81, 84]		
	Surgical Procedure	*Cholangitis*	*Per Cent*	*Surgical Procedure*	*Cholangitis*	*Per Cent*	*Surgical Procedure*	*Cholangitis*	*Per Cent*	*Surgical Procedure*	*Cholangitis*	*Per Cent*	*Surgical Procedure*	*Cholangitis*	*Per Cent*
Roux-en-Y hepatic portojejunostomy (Kasai I)	23	9	39	22	15	68	26	16	62	49	25	51			
Portocutaneous jejunostomy (Sawaguchi)							24	11* (5)	46 (20)						
Double Y hepatic portojejunostomy (Kasai II)				17	6	35				9	5	56			
Hepatic portocholecystostomy (Lilly)	1	0		7	0	0				10	0	0	4	0	0
Mikulicz portojejunostomy													25	11	44
Double Y portojejunoduodenostomy				12	11	92									
Portoduodenostomy	15	6	40												

*Six of 11 had closure of the jejunostomy.

any procedure and avoids the problems of a cutaneous jejunostomy (i.e., excessive bile loss, bleeding, and the need for an appliance); a stoma, however, does have some advantages for assessing the volume and character of bile secretion.

The extent of hepatic fibrosis in liver biopsies correlates with the incidence of PPII.[66] Since there is a relationship between cholangitis and survival, it is curious that Hitch et al. did not find a relationship between the severity of hepatic fibrosis and survival.[79]

When blood cultures are positive, they usually contain enteric organisms similar to those found in the jejunum. The concentration of organisms is higher in exteriorized bowel segments of patients who have a bilirubin clearance greater than 25 ml/hour than in those with little drainage.[88] The incidence of the different bacterial species cultured from the jejunostomy is listed in Table 39–7. Unfortunately, no attempt was made to correlate

Table 39–7 INCIDENCE OF BACTERIAL SPECIES CULTURED FROM JEJUNOSTOMY

Organism	Per Cent
Escherichia coli	85
Klebsiella	71
Streptococcus Group D	70
Pseudomonas	63
Proteus	27
Bacteroides	13
Enterobacter	6

the results of the cultures with the results of blood cultures or liver biopsies in the same patients. Kobayashi et al. identified the same spectrum of bacteria from hepatic abscesses as from the Roux-en-Y segment of jejunum in autopsy specimens.[86]

Patients with PPII should be given antibiotics effective against the kinds of organisms listed in Table 39–7. Hitch and Lilly found that aminoglycoside antibiotics were not detectable in the bowel conduits, although they were present in the hepatic interstitium.[88] Penicillin was excreted in the bile, but trimethoprim-sulfamethoxazole and cephalosporins were concentrated in bile.[88] In theory, prophylactic use of these antibiotics might be expected to reduce the risk of PPII. Nevertheless, aminoglycosides have been recommended for treating acute cholangitis because of their high concentration in the liver. There is no correlation between the number, concentration, or types of bacteria in the jejunal conduit and changes in volume and bilirubin concentration of the bile. Danks and Smith performed simultaneous blood and liver needle biopsy cultures in a series of 84 episodes of PPII and found positive blood cultures in 49 and positive liver cultures in 32.[87]

The incidence of PPII displays two peaks.[84] The early peak occurs between 6 and 9 months and the late peak between 1 and 2 years postoperatively. Patients who develop

PPII immediately postoperatively have a severe disease, usually with a fatal outcome.[86, 88] The longer the infant copes with the infection, the less frequent and the less severe are the episodes. Presumably, the edema at the porta hepatis impedes bile drainage. As time passes and the inflammation subsides, bile secretion increases, which flushes organisms from the liver, an effect similar to that from passage of chyme on the intestinal flora. The late rise in the incidence of PPII may reflect progressive stenosis at the porta hepatis or within the liver.

Recurring attacks of PPII must contribute to fibrosis of the bile ducts and liver. To minimize this problem, most pediatric surgeons recommend administration of prophylactic antibiotics. Immediately after operation, ampicillin, gentamicin, or a cephalosporin (singly or in combination) is given parenterally. When oral intake is resumed, trimethoprim-sulfamethoxazole is given for at least 1 year. This combination seems to be the most effective regimen for controlling infection and produces the least amount of antibiotic-induced diarrhea.[78, 84] If PPII recurs, the patient should be hospitalized and parenteral antibiotics (e.g., aminoglycoside, a cephalosporin, and carbenicillin) restarted.

Repeated PPII, particularly when associated with jaundice, suggests that stenosis of the portoenterostomy has developed, a diagnosis that may be confirmed by transhepatic cholangiography. If a stricture is demonstrated, the anastomosis should usually be revised.[80]

Hepatic Fibrosis and Portal Hypertension

The natural history of untreated biliary atresia consists of progressive hepatic insufficiency manifested by slowly increasing jaundice, hypoalbuminemia, hypoprothrombinemia, ascites, splenomegaly, and portal hypertension. The most common cause of death is infection, usually involving pneumonia, meningitis, or sepsis. We have not been able to detect a specific immune defect in patients with biliary atresia. Rather, the infections occur relatively late in the course of the disease and seem to be a consequence of severe malnutrition from decreased appetite, malabsorption, impaired protein synthesis, and so forth. Curiously, hepatic failure associated with encephalopathy is rare. The outcome in infants who remain jaundiced following portoenterostomy is similar to that in patients managed expectantly.

In 1975, Kasai et al. reported 14 children living without jaundice 2 to 18 years following portoenterostomy.[90] Their serum bilirubin levels were all less than 1 mg/dl, and in most of them the serum transaminase levels were normal. The alkaline phosphatase value remained elevated in all but a few. Liver biopsies 2 to 10 years postoperatively showed improvement in all respects, including periportal fibrosis. Regression of fibrosis was slow and took 2 to 3 years to identify. Three patients had cirrhosis at 11 years of age, but only one had portal hypertension. It is not clear whether the hepatic fibrosis predisposes to PPII, but a correlation between the frequency of cholangitis and fibroplasia has been noted.[90] Undoubtedly, the abnormal intrahepatic ducts with segmental stenoses are a source of bile stasis and infection.

Most patients who have survived for many years have hepatic fibrosis, and portal hypertension with splenomegaly and esophageal varices is occasionally seen.[90]

LONG-TERM RESULTS

Hays and Kimura analyzed 84 patients with a survival of 5 years or more who had been treated by portoenterostomy before May 1973.[66] The operation had been performed before the patient had reached age 90 days in 85 per cent of these survivors. The incidence of ascending cholangitis, portal hypertension, and recurrent jaundice is given in Table 39–8. There was no correlation between the age at operation and the occurrence of PPII or recurrent jaundice, but the incidence of portal hypertension late after operation was greater among those who were older at the time of operation. Hepatomegaly was found in 37 per cent and splenomegaly in 17 per cent of the survivors.[66] Ten per cent of these patients required an operation to treat complications of portal hypertension. Most of these individuals were attending school or were employed, and few had any restriction of activity.

Odievre reviewed 111 patients with "uncorrectable" biliary atresia who underwent portoenterostomy between 5 weeks and 11 months of age.[93] The overall growth and development of the 34 survivors (30 per cent) were normal. In the 1 to 6½ years of follow-up on these 34 survivors, 85 per cent were

Table 39–8 PATIENT AGE AT OPERATION IN RELATION TO COMPLICATIONS AMONG 84 LONG-TERM SURVIVORS (1978)

Age at Surgery (Days)	Number of Patients*	Complications†		
		Cholangitis	*Portal Hypertension*	*Recurrent Jaundice*
40–49	7	—	—	—
50–60	18	6	3 (1)	1
61–70	17	5	4 (1)	1
71–80	14	6	3 (3)	2
81–90	15	5	4 (2)	1
91–100	5	—	2 (1)	—
101–110	7	2	—	—
111–120	1	—	1 (1)	—
Totals	84	24	17 (9)	5

Parentheses indicate those patients requiring operation for variceal hemorrhage or hypersplenism.
*Patients who survived more than 5 years following a Kasai-type procedure for biliary atresia.
†Clinically evident during the 5 years following operation.
Data from Hays DM, Kimura K: Biliary Atresia: The Japanese Experience. Cambridge; Harvard University Press, 1980.

free of jaundice, 56 per cent had one or more episodes of cholangitis, and 76 per cent had splenomegaly (presumed to be due to portal hypertension). Varices were found in 20 patients (60 per cent), but only five patients had bled. Varices seemed to have disappeared in four patients.

Hitch et al. studied the determinants of survival in 18 of 41 patients who survived for several years or more after portoenterostomy.[79] The actuarial survival at 4 years was 42 per cent, and the favorable prognostic factors were as follows: (1) age at operation less than 8 weeks, (2) male sex, (3) the presence of a large duct in the porta hepatis, (4) secretion of bilirubin greater than 17.5 $mg/m^2/24$ hours, (5) a bile to serum bilirubin ratio greater than 1, and (6) a bilirubin clearance greater than 25 ml. Survival was not related to whether hepatic fibrosis was present in the initial liver biopsy, the extent of bile duct proliferation, the degree of portal hilar inflammation, or the number of bile ductules in histologic sections of the portal area.

In the series of Alagille, 44 of 121 patients (36 per cent) operated on for biliary atresia survived for a minimum of 5 years, and 77 per cent of the survivors were anicteric. Alagille performed surgical wedge biopsies in 20 of these children followed 5 to 8 years after portoenterostomy. None was jaundiced, and none had recurrent episodes of cholangitis. Gross evidence of cirrhosis was present in all children, and histology showed micronodular cirrhosis in 13 and macronodular cirrhosis in seven. Besides cirrhosis, the most notable change was the absence of biliary ducts or ductules in many specimens. Therefore, despite satisfactory bile drainage and normal growth pattern, cirrhosis is almost always seen in long-term follow-up of patients who were treated with portoenterostomy.[101]

Long-term survival (30 to 40 per cent) following portoenterostomy is much better than survival following exploration and no portoenterostomy (2 per cent).[79, 82–84] Careful follow-up is important to detect and treat postportoenterostomy infection, impaired biliary drainage from anastomotic stricture, hepatic fibrosis, and portal hypertension with hypersplenism and esophageal varices. In patients with failed hepaticoportoenterostomies, Saito et al. have tried a second portoenterostomy with some success. These authors believe that, in the patients who did well, a deeper dissection at reoperation may have allowed the surgeon to reach deeper, rudimentary biliary radicles that were not previously draining.[98]

LIVER TRANSPLANTATION FOR PATIENTS WITH BILIARY ATRESIA

When all large series are combined, the success of the Kasai procedure averages 30 to 40 per cent. Ninety per cent of patients with failed portoenterostomies are dead before they reach 5 years of age.[90, 101, 108] In addition, some patients in whom adequate biliary drainage is achieved with the Kasai procedure later develop hepatic failure from progressive scarring due to cholangitis, or continued periportal fibrosis secondary to the primary disease.[90] These unfortunate young patients also die from liver failure. Hepatic transplantation offers a new alternative in these cases.

Between 1963 (when the first human orthotopic liver transplantation was done) and 1983, 540 patients underwent liver transplantation in four large centers in the United States and Europe. Of these, 83 patients received the transplant for biliary atresia.[107] Although more than two thirds of these procedures have been done by a single group (Starzl's),[102] enthusiasm is now growing in other centers of the United States and Western Europe.[104, 105, 108] In fact, hepatic transplantation in children had been held back in these centers, in great part because of the toxic side effects of long-term corticosteroid therapy. The introduction of cyclosporin A, which can be used alone, made it possible to offer liver transplantation to a larger number of infants. For example, in Starzl's series, the 1 year survival in children who received transplants for biliary atresia doubled following the introduction of cyclosporin A.[102] In Hannover, liver transplantation in children was not done at all prior to the development of cyclosporin. Of ten children undergoing liver transplantation since 1981, nine were alive and well at the time the series was published and one had reached 1 year of age.[105]

The best timing for liver transplantation in these children has not yet been defined. Pediatric donors, particularly those weighing less than 10 kg, are difficult to locate, and, in general, the larger the patient, the greater the ease with which the transplant is performed. Thus, whenever possible, it is best to wait until the child weighs between 7 and 10 kg. This is not always possible, as children with biliary atresia often stop gaining weight in spite of adequate nutritional support. A great deal of consideration must be given to the nutritional status of the patient. Negative nitrogen balance is often associated with ascites and coagulopathies, both of which increase the operative risk. Daily infusion of fresh frozen plasma, exchange transfusions, cryoprecipitate, and platelets prior to transplantation help correct some of the problems associated with liver failure in these children.[108]

Previous operations for biliary atresia (i.e., Kasai portoenterostomy) do not preclude successful grafting, and in fact, a Kasai procedure may provide some relief while a suitable donor is sought.[103] Biliary atresia does not recur in the transplanted liver, and, provided that rejection is controlled, the patient should be cured.

Survival of patients with biliary atresia treated with liver transplantation has improved year by year; in Starzl's series it is better than for any other etiology or age group.[102] The oldest living patient who underwent hepatic transplantation for biliary atresia is now 18 years old and is living a relatively normal life. Survival probability, calculated from the data published in 1983 from the four centers with the greatest experience in this field, indicates that nearly two thirds of the patients who undergo transplantation for biliary atresia are expected to be alive and well at 1 year.[107] This is higher than the survival for any adult group ever published and appears to brighten the very poor prognosis of patients with failed portoenterostomies.

Liver transplantation has also been used in children with inborn errors of metabolism. These include Wilson's disease, alpha$_1$-antitrypsin deficiency (17 patients in Starzl's series), tyrosinemia, and Niemann-Pick disease.[102, 108–110] When the primary metabolic defect resides in the liver, as in Wilson's disease, this disappears after a successful transplant. Liver transplantation thus appears to be a promising alternative for patients in whom a portoenterostomy was not possible or did not provide adequate biliary drainage. The precise indications and the timing will remain uncertain until more experience and long-terms results with this form of therapy are available.[108]

SUMMARY

Untreated biliary atresia is a progressive obliterative process of the bile ducts that develops shortly after birth. Before 1970, the results of surgical management of biliary atresia in North America were very discouraging. Only 10 per cent of infants were considered to have a "correctable" form of atresia, in which an identifiable patent duct could be recognized in the liver hilum. When the intestine was anastomosed to this duct, fewer than half these infants improved. Hepatic portoenterostomy and its variations result in good bile drainage and long-term survival in approximately one half of patients previously considered to have "uncorrectable" biliary atresia. The success of the operation depends on early treatment, the size of the residual biliary ducts at the porta hepatis, and the occurrence of postoperative intrahepatic infection. Hepatic fibrosis resolves in long-term survivors, and the incidence of portal hypertension is low. Recurrent intrahepatic infection is a serious problem in many patients. Discovery of the pathogenesis and prevention of biliary atresia will be the only completely effective form of management. However, the results following the Kasai portoenterostomy are good enough that any patient with persistent postnatal jaundice must be evaluated for biliary atresia and referred promptly for surgical therapy when appropriate. Liver transplantation should be considered for patients who have a failed portoenterostomy or in whom a Kasai procedure cannot be done.

REFERENCES

1. Sass-Kortsak A: Management of young infants presenting with direct-reacting hyperbilirubinemia. Pediatr Clin North Am 1974;*21*:777.
2. Sass-Kortsak A, Bowden DM, Brown RJK: Congenital intrahepatic biliary atresia. Pediatrics 1956;*17*:383.
3. Strauss L, Bernstein J: Neonatal hepatitis in congenital rubella. Arch Pathol 1968;*86*:317.
4. Odievre M, Martin JP, Hadchonal M, et al: Alpha-1 antitrypsin deficiency and liver disease in children: phenotypes, manifestations and prognosis. Pediatrics 1976;*57*:226.
5. Porter SP, Soper RT, Tidrick RT: Biliary hypoplasia. Ann Surg 1968;*167*:602.
6. Alagille D, Odievre M, Ganteor M, et al: Hepatic ductular hypoplasia associated with characteristic facies, vertebral malformations, retarded physical, mental and sexual development and cardiac murmur. J Pediatr 1975;*56*:63.
7. Riely CA, La Brecque DR, Ghant C, et al: A father and son with cholestasis and peripheral pulmonic stenosis. J Pediatr 1978;*92*:406.
8. Jones EA, Rabin L, Buckley CH, et al: Progressive intrahepatic cholestasis of infancy and childhood: a clinical pathologic study of a patient surviving to the age of 18 years. Gastroenterology 1976;*71*:675.
9. Bennett DE: Problems in neonatal obstructive jaundice. Pediatrics 1964;*3*:735.
10. Haas JE: Bile duct and liver pathology in biliary atresia. World J Surg 1978;*1*:561.
11. Kasai M, Yakovac WC, Koop CE: Liver in congenital biliary atresia and neonatal hepatitis. Arch Pathol 1962;*74*:152.
12. Smetana HG, Edlow JB, Gluny PR: Neonatal jaundice. Arch Pathol 1965;*80*:553.
13. Hanai M, Idriss F, Swenson O: Bile duct proliferation in atresia and related hepatic diseases. Arch Surg 1967;*994*:14.
14. Ohi R, Kasai M, Takahashi T: Intrahepatic biliary obstruction in congenital bile duct atresia. Tohoku J Exp Med 1969;*99*:129.
15. Kasai M, Suzuki H, Ohashi E, et al: Technique and results of operative management of biliary atresia. World J Surg 1978;*2*:571.
16. Koop CE: Progressive extrahepatic biliary obstruction of the newborn. J Pediatr Surg 1975;*10*:169.
17. Longmire WP: Congenital biliary hypoplasia. Ann Surg 1964;*159*:335.
18. Holder TM: Atresia of the extrahepatic bile duct. Am J Surg 1964;*107*:458.
19. Lilly JR: Surgery of biliary hypoplasia. J Pediatr Surg 1976;*11*:815.
20. Lilly JR: Surgical jaundice in infancy. Ann Surg 1977;*186*:549.
21. Gross RE: The Surgery of Infancy and Childhood. Philadelphia, WB Saunders, 1953, pp 508–523.
22. Kasai M: Treatment of biliary atresia with special reference to hepatic portoenterostomy and its manifestations. Prog Pediatr Surg 1974;*6*:5.
23. Longmire WP, Manfiola SA, Gordon HE: Congenital cystic disease of the liver and biliary system. Ann Surg 1971;*174*:711.
24. Lilly JR: The surgical treatment of choledochal cyst. Surg Gynecol Obstet 1979;*149*:36.
25. Saito S, Ishida M: Congenital choledochal cyst. *In* Bill AM, Kasai M (eds): Progress in Pediatric Surgery. Baltimore, University Park Press, p 63.
26. Valayer PJ, Alagille D: Experience with choledochal cyst. J Pediatr Surg 1975;*10*:65.
27. Bernstein J, Braylan R, Brough A Jr: Bile plug syndrome: a correctable cause of obstructive jaundice in infants. Pediatrics 1969;*43*:273.
28. de Lorimier AA: Jaundiced infants: problems of surgical management. Correspondence. N Engl J Med 1973;*289*:1143.
29. Lilly JR, Weintraub WH, Altman PR: Spontaneous perforation of the extrahepatic bile ducts and bile peritonitis in infancy. Surgery 1974;*75*:664.
30. Prevot J, Babut JM: Spontaneous perforations of the biliary tract in infancy. Prog Pediatr Surg 1971;*3*:187.
31. Hardy JD: Congenital bile duct stenosis. Intrahepatic cholangiocholecystectojejunostomy (Roux Y) with removal of intrahepatic stones. J Pediatr 1961;*59*:265.
32. Rogers BM, Hollenbeck JI, Donelly WH, et al: Intrahepatic cholestasis with parenteral alimentation. Am J Surg 1976;*131*:149.
33. Touloukian RJ, Downing SE: Cholestasis associated with long-term parenteral alimentation. Arch Surg 1973;*106*:58.
34. Shim WKT, Kasai M, Spence MA: Racial influence on the incidence of biliary atresia. *In* Bill MA, Kasai M (eds): Progress in Pediatric Surgery. Urban, Scharzenberg, 1979.
35. Landing BH: Considerations of the pathogenesis of neonatal hepatitis, biliary atresia and choledochal cyst—the concept of infantile obstructive cholangiopathy. Prog Pediatr Surg 1974;*6*:113.
36. Mowat AP, Psacharopoulos HT, Williams R: Extrahepatic biliary atresia versus neonatal hepatitis. Review of 137 prospectively investigated infants. Arch Dis Child 1976;*51*:763.
37. Rickham PP: Neonatal biliary obstruction. *In* Rickham PP, Johnston JH (eds): Neonatal Surgery. New York, Appleton-Century-Crofts, 1978.
38. Danks DM, Campbell PE, Jack I, et al: Studies of the etiology of neonatal hepatitis and biliary atresia. Arch Dis Child 1977;*52*:360.
39. Robertson AF: Case report: the coincidence of biliary atresia and the heterozygous state of galactosemia. Pediatrics 1965;*35*:1008.

40. Boyden EA, Cope JC, Bill AH: Anatomy and embryology of congenital intrinsic obstruction of the duodenum. Am J Surg 1967;*114*:190.
41. Reid IS: Biliary tract abnormalities associated with duodenal atresia. Arch Dis Child 1973;*48*:952.
42. Holder TM, Ashcraft KW: The effects of bile duct ligation and inflammation in the fetus. J Pediatr Surg 1967;*2*:35.
43. Chandra RS: Biliary atresia and other structural anomalies in congenital polysplenia syndrome. J Pediatr 1974;*85*:649.
44. Schweitzer IL, Wing A, McPeak C, et al: Hepatitis and hepatitis-associated antigen in 56 mother-infant pairs. JAMA 1972;*220*:1092.
45. Shinhoj P, Sardemann H, Cohn J, et al: Hepatitis associated antigen (HAA) in pregnant women and their newborn infants. Am J Dis Child 1972; *123*:380.
46. Becroft DMO: Biliary atresia associated with prenatal infection by *Listeria monocytogenes*. Arch Dis Child 1972;*47*:656.
47. Palmer AK, Heywood R: Pathological changes in the rhesus fetus associated with the oral administration of chenodeoxycholic acid. Toxicology 1974;*2*:239.
48. Silverberg M, Salomon L, Ehrlich JC: The hepatotoxic effects of lithocholic acid in the newborn hamster. Gastroenterology 1971;*60*:753.
49. Aagenaes O: Hereditary recurrent cholestasis with lymphoedema—two new families. Acta Paediatr Scand 1974;*63*:465.
50. Kasai M, Kobayashi A, Ohbe Y: Jpn J Pediatr Surg 1978;*10*:629. Cited by Hays DM, Kimura K.[66]
51. Hashimoto S, Tsugawa C, Kuimura K: J Jpn Soc Pediatr Surg 1978;*14*:889.
52. Greene HL, Helinek GL, Moran R, et al: A diagnostic approach to prolonged obstructive jaundice by 24-hour collection of duodenal fluid. J Pediatr 1979;*95*:412.
53. Majo M, Reba RC, Altman RP: Effect of phenobarbital on ^{99m}Tc-IDA scintigraphy in the evaluation of neonatal jaundice. Semin Nucl Med 1981;*11*:194.
54. Hayden PW, Rudd TG, Christie DL: Rose bengal sodium I 131 studies in infants with suspected biliary atresia. Am J Dis Child 1979;*133*:834.
55. Javitt NB, Keating JP, Grand RJ, et al: Serum bile acid patterns in neonatal hepatitis and extra-hepatic biliary atresia. J Pediatr 1977;*90*:736.
56. Zelter PM, Neerhout RC, Fonkalsrud EW, et al: Differentiation between neonatal hepatitis and biliary atresia by measuring serum alpha-feto-protein. Lancet 1974;*1*:373.
57. Melhorn DK, Gross S, Izant RJ: The red cell hydrogen peroxide hemolysis test and vitamin E absorption in the diagnosis of jaundice in infancy. J Pediatr 1972;*81*:1082.
58. Poley JR, Smith EI, Boon DJ, et al: Lipoprotein-X and the double 131 I–rose bengal test in the diagnosis of prolonged infantile jaundice. J Pediatr Surg 1972;*7*:660.
59. Brough AJ, Bernstein J: Liver biopsy in the diagnosis of infantile obstructive jaundice. Pediatrics 1979;*43*:519.
60. Bennett DE: Problems in neonatal obstructive jaundice. Pediatrics 1964;*33*:735.
61. Hays DM, Wooley MM, Snyder WH: Diagnosis of biliary atresia: relative accuracy of percutaneous liver biopsy, open liver biopsy and operative cholangiography. J Pediatr 1967;*71*:598.
62. Yamaguchi M, Sakurai M, Takeuchi S, et al: Observation of cystic dilatation of the common bile duct by ultrasonography. J Pediatr Surg 1980; *15*:207.
63. Kasai M, Kimura S, Asakura Y, et al: Surgical treatment of biliary atresia. J Pediatr Surg 1968;*3*:665.
64. Kimura K, Tsugawa C, Kubo M, et al: Technical aspects of hepatic portal dissection in biliary atresia. J Pediatr Surg 1979;*14*:27.
65. Suruga K, Kono S, Muzano T, et al: Treatment of biliary atresia: microsurgery for hepatic portoenterostomy. Surgery 1976;*80*:558.
66. Hays DM, Kimura K: Biliary Atresia: The Japanese Experience. Cambridge, Harvard University Press, 1980.
67. Hays DM: The current management of biliary atresia: lessons from Japan. Surgical Rounds, 1980, pp 33–39.
68. Sawaguchi S, et al: Two stage operation for congenital biliary atresia: A temporary external biliary fistula with a jejunal segment. Fourth Annual Meeting, Pacific Association of Pediatric Surgeons, Vancouver, Canada, 1971.
69. Lilly JR, Altman RP: Hepatic portoenterostomy (the Kasai operation) for biliary atresia. Surgery 1975;*78*:76.
70. Lilly JR, Javitt NB: Biliary lipid excretion after hepatic portoenterostomy. Ann Surg 1976; *184*:369.
71. Krovetz LJ: Congenital biliary atresia. I. Analysis of thirty cases with particular reference to diagnosis. II. Analysis of the therapeutic problem. Surgery 1960;*47*:453.
72. Berenson MM, Garde AR, Moody FG: Twenty-five year survival after surgery for complete intrahepatic biliary atresia. Gastroenterology 1974;*66*:260.
73. Thaler MM, Gellis SS: Studies in neonatal hepatitis and biliary atresia. I. Long-term prognosis of neonatal hepatitis. II. The effect of diagnostic laparotomy on long-term prognosis of neonatal hepatitis. Am J Dis Child 1968;*116*:257.
74. Lawwon EE, Boggs JD: Long-term follow-up of neonatal hepatitis: safety and value of surgical exploration. Pediatrics 1974;*53*:650.
75. Bill AM: Introduction: biliary atresia and choledochal cyst. New concepts of cause and treatment. Prog Pediatr Surg 1974;*6*:1.
76. Gautier M, Johan P, Odievre M: Histologic study of biliary fibrous remnants in 48 cases of extrahepatic biliary atresia: correlation with post-operative bile flow restoration. J Pediatr 1976;*89*:704.
77. Campbell DP: Hepatic portoenterostomy indicated or not in treatment of biliary atresia. Am J Dis Chil 1975;*129*:1427.
78. Odievre M, Valayer J, Razeman-Pinta M, et al: Hepatic portoenterostomy or cholecystectomy in the treatment of extrahepatic biliary atresia. J Pediatr 1976;*88*:774.
79. Hitch DC, Shikes RH, Lilly JR: Determinants of survival after Kasai's operation for biliary atresia using actuarial analysis. J Pediatr Surg 1979; *14*:310.
80. Altman RP: Results of re-operations for correction of extrahepatic biliary atresia. J Pediatr Surg 1979;*14*:305.
81. Lilly JR: Hepatic portocholecystostomy for biliary atresia. J Pediatr Surg 1979;*14*:301.
82. Hays DM, Snyder WH: Life-span in untreated biliary atresia. Surgery 1963;*54*:373.

83. Adelman S: Prognosis of uncorrected biliary atresia: an update. J Pediatr Surg 1978;*13*:389.
84. Lilly JR, Hitch DC: Post-operative ascending cholangitis following portoenterostomy for biliary atresia: measures for control. World J Surg 1978;*1*:581.
85. Stiehl A, Thaler MM, Admirand WH: The effects of phenobarbital on bile salts and bilirubin in patients with intrahepatic and extrahepatic cholestasis. N Engl J Med 1971;*286*:858.
86. Kobayashi A, Utsomomiya T, Ohbe Y, et al: Ascending cholangitis after successful surgical repair of biliary atresia. Arch Dis Child 1973;*48*:697.
87. Danks DM, Smith AL: Invited commentary. World J Surg 1978;*2*:585.
88. Hitch DC, Lilly JR: Identification, quantification, and significance of bacterial growth within the biliary tract after Kasai's operation. J Pediatr Surg 1978;*13*:563.
89. Danks DM, Bishop RF: Bacterial antibodies in liver disease. Lancet 1972;*1*:846.
90. Kasai M, Watanabe I, Ohi R: Follow-up studies of long-term survivors after hepatic portoenterostomy for "noncorrectible" biliary atresia. J Pediatr Surg 1975;*10*:173.
91. Hirsig J, Rickham PP, Briner J: Hepatic lymph drainage in experimental biliary atresia. Effect of omentopexy on prevention of cholangitis. J Pediatr Surg 1979;*14*:142.
92. Lilly JR: Letter to the editor. J Pediatr Surg 1978;*13*:559.
93. Odievre M: Long-term results of surgical treatment of biliary atresia. World J Surg 1978;*2*:589.
94. Akiyama H, Saeki M, Ogafa T: Jpn J Pediatr Surg 1978;*10*:673. Cited by Hays DM, Kimura K.[66]
95. Matsuo S, Ikeda S, Nakagawara A et al: Histological study of the remnant of porta hepatis in patients with extrahepatic biliary atresia—a computed picture analysis of 30 cases. Z Kinderchir 1984;*39*:46.
96. Weaver LT, Nelson R, Bell TM: The association of extrahepatic bile duct atresia and neonatal Epstein-Barr virus infection. Acta Paediatr Scand 1984;*73*:155.
97. Matsusue S, Kashihara S, Maetani S: Differentiation of congenital biliary atresia and neonatal hepatitis by statistical methods. Prog Pediatr Surg 1984;*17*:189.
98. Saito S, Tsuchida Y, Honna T: Reoperation for biliary atresia after hepatic portoenterostomy—experience in 29 cases with a report on the longest survivor in Japan. Z Kinderchir 1984;*39*:99.
99. Wynchank S, Guillet J, Leccia F, et al: Biliary atresia and neonatal hepatobiliary scintigraphy. Clin Nucl Med 1984;*9*:121.
100. Majd M, Reba RC, Altman RP: Effect of phenobarbital on ^{99m}Tc-IDA scintigraphy in the evaluation of neonatal jaundice. Semin Nucl Med 1981;*136*:1075.
101. Alagille D: Extrahepatic biliary atresia. Hepatology 1984;*4*:7S.
102. Starzl TE, et al: Analysis of liver transplantation. Hepatology 1984;*4*:47S.
103. Williams R, Mac Dougall BRD, Calne RY: Liver transplantation: Current status. Compr Ther 1982;*8*:24.
104. Rolles K, Williams R, Neuberger J, Calne R: The Cambridge and King's College hospital experience of liver transplantation, 1968–1983. Hepatology 1984;*4*:50S.
105. Pichlmayr R, et al: Experience with liver transplantation in Hannover. Hepatology 1984;*4*:56S.
106. Ascher NL, Najarian JS: Hepatic transplantation and biliary atresia: Early experience in eight patients. World J Surg 1984;*8*:57.
107. Scharschmidt B: Human liver transplantation: Analysis of data on 540 patients from four centers. Hepatology 1984;*4*:95S.
108. National Institutes of Health Consensus Development Conference Statement: Liver transplantation—June 20–23, 1983. Hepatology 1984;*4*:107S.
109. Malatack JJ, Zitelli BJ, Gartner JC, et al: Pediatric liver transplantation under therapy with cyclosporin A and steroids. Transplant Proc 1983; *15*:1292.
110. Zitelli BJ, Malatack JJ, Gartner JC, et al: Orthotopic liver transplantation in children with hepatic-based metabolic disease. Transplant Proc 1983;*15*:1284.

ERIC FONKALSRUD, M.D.

40

Biliary Cystic Disease in Children and Adults

Cystic disease may occur throughout the biliary system, from the smallest intralobular hepatic ducts to the intraduodenal portion of the common bile duct. Regardless of the anatomic location, cystic lesions tend to be congenital, except for occasional cysts stemming from infection or acquired obstruction (e.g., trauma or calculus). The signs and symptoms caused by biliary cysts are generally related to (1) the bulk of the cyst, which may compress contiguous structures; and (2) varying degrees of biliary obstruction, with or without superimposed infection.[1] Depending on their location, cysts of the biliary tract are classified as ductal or parenchymal.

DUCTAL CYSTIC LESIONS

Extrahepatic Ductal Dilatation

Congenital dilatation of the biliary ductal system (choledochal cyst) is an uncommon malformation, as evidenced by the mere 500 reported cases collected from the English literature up to 1969.[2] For many years the condition was thought to represent a congenital cystic or aneurysmal dilatation of the common bile duct located between the gallbladder and duodenum. However, recent studies of large numbers of patients with choledochal cysts demonstrate that the malformation encompasses a wider spectrum with numerous variations, including dilatation of the intrahepatic bile ducts in approximately one third of cases.[3] The rarity of the malformation in the United States is reflected by the fact that there were but two cases of choledochal cyst among 757,000 consecutive admissions to the Presbyterian Hospital in New York City.[4] From 1923 to 1954 the Cleveland Clinic Hospital saw only two cases in 192,507 admissions.[5]

Other reports have shown a higher incidence, particularly in hospitals providing care for a large number of children, where the diagnosis exists in 1 in 13,000 admissions.[6] In Japan, Kimura and associates[7] cited the fact that one of each 1000 patients admitted to the Kobe Children's Hospital has a choledochal cyst.

The first authentic case of choledochal cyst was described in 1852 by Douglas,[8] who summarized the clinical course and post-mortem findings of a 17 year old girl who had a cyst that filled the right side of the abdomen and contained one-half gallon of yellow, thin, syrupy fluid with an offensive odor. The hepatic ducts were dilated, although the cystic duct and gallbladder were not. "The remedies which appeared most to palliate her distress were hot fomentations and purgatives. Blisters were of some service." Repeated trocar aspirations of the cyst were proposed for treatment of future cases.

Laverson[9] in 1909 discussed 28 cases, and Waller[10] in 1917 described 35 additional patients with choledochal cyst. Extensive reviews of congenital cystic dilatation of the common bile duct have been reported by Shallow et al.,[11] Tsardakas and Robnett,[5] Alonso-Lej et al.,[6] and Spitz.[12] Numerous articles summarizing substantial clinical experiences in the management of choledochal cyst have been published in the Japanese literature during the past decade, inasmuch as the anomaly appears to be more prevalent in that country.[3, 7, 13–17]

Etiology

The etiology of congenital dilatation of the extrahepatic bile ducts has not been clearly defined, although many views have been expressed in the medical literature and various hypotheses have been proposed. Congenital weakness of the bile duct wall is believed to be an essential factor; this, when associated with elevated intraductal pressure due to distal obstruction, may lead to the development of a choledochal cyst.[18] The distal obstruction may result from angulation of the duct, presence of a valvelike mechanism, inflammation, congenital or acquired stenosis, "achalasia" of the sphincter of Oddi,[19] or other factors.

Yotuyanagi[20] and, later, Von Lutzki[21] proposed one of the most plausible theories for the development of choledochal cystic dilatation of the extrahepatic bile ducts. The bile ducts and liver develop by proliferation of cells from the foregut as a solid cord, and duct formation requires the development of a lumen in this cord of cells. Yotuyanagi[20] postulated that an irregular or unequal proliferation of ductal cells occurs during the conversion from a solid cord to a duct, with resultant areas of narrowing and dilatation in the ducts. Furthermore, it has been suggested that extrahepatic biliary atresia and congenital dilatation of the bile ducts may possibly be manifestations of the same underlying process of unequal proliferation of cells composing the biliary ducts. Attar and Obeid,[22] on the other hand, pointed out that such inequalities of recanalization would lead to a multilocular cyst rather than the usual unilocular dilatation. Longmire and associates[1] have suggested that certain types of choledochal cyst, especially those with multiple cystic dilatations, might be caused by a type of sclerosing choledochitis.

Babbitt and associates[23] reported on several patients who had an anomaly in the drainage of the common bile duct into the pancreatic duct, with loss of the distal sphincter mechanism. They postulated that acquired inflammation of the distal common bile duct resulting from reflux of pancreatic juice might be a major factor causing the distal obstruction. The maximal pressure in the pancreatic duct exceeds that in the common bile duct during certain phases of digestion, allowing the free reflux of pancreatic juice in many patients.[24] These investigators further proposed that this obstruction produces dilatation in the proximal areas of congenital weakness and that the presence of pancreatic juice in the bile duct may cause mucosal injury, chronic inflammation, and weakening of the bile duct wall.[7, 13] Therefore, according to Saito and Ishida,[25] Babbitt et al.,[23] and others,[92, 93] the development of cystic dilatation requires both a congenital and an acquired defect.

Anatomic Characteristics

Congenital dilatation of the bile ducts consists of a circumferential distention of the entire common bile duct, or a segment of it, with occasional extensions involving the cystic, hepatic, or intrahepatic ducts. There are also frequent anomalies of the pancreatic ducts so that, in many cases, the condition may be considered as a complex syndrome (Fig. 40–1). The cyst usually commences 1 or 2 cm above the duodenum; however, in some instances the distention may extend down to the entrance of the common bile duct into the duodenal wall.[5] The common bile duct between the cyst and the duodenum is often smaller than normal yet frequently patent; this accounts for the typical late onset of symptoms.

A new classification of choledochal cysts was based upon 560 cases in Japan collected by Komi and associates.[3] These authors described six major types of common bile duct malformations: cystic, fusiform, cylindrical, beaded, or diverticular in configuration (Fig. 40–2). Rarely, dilatation of the proximal bile duct within the wall of the duodenum may be present as a choledochocele. In over 70 per cent of cases the gallbladder is not distended and arises from a small cystic duct at the upper end of the cyst (Fig. 40–3). However, in some patients the cystic duct may be considerably dilated and the gallbladder large and tense (Fig. 40–4). Occasionally, the cystic dilatation may be present only in the cystic duct, and the remainder of the biliary tract may be normal.[26] Stones are rarely found in the gallbladder.

Although Gross[27] noted in 1953 that in occasional instances the pancreatic ducts may open directly into the choledochal cyst, it has only recently been emphasized that as many as 33 to 42 per cent of patients with choledochal cysts may have an anomalous insertion of the pancreatic duct into the biliary tract.[3, 15–17, 28] Barraya and associates[29] reported that a common pancreaticobiliary channel above the ampulla was present in approximately 90 per cent of cases of choledochal cyst. In a review of 183 cases of choledochal cyst with anomalous arrangement of the pancreaticobiliary ducts, Komi et al.[3] have classified these deformities into three basic types

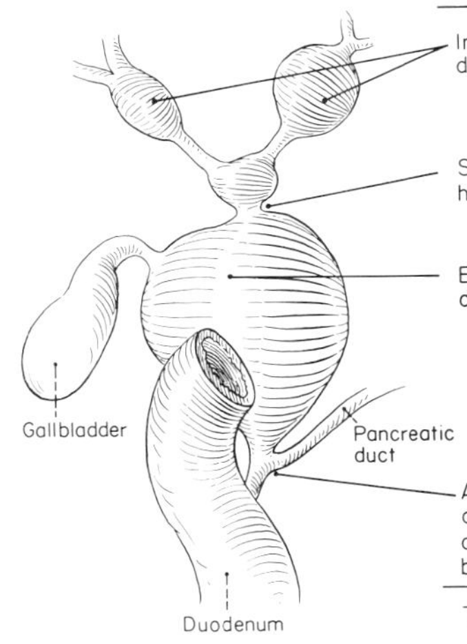

ANOMALIES	NO. CASES	%
Intrahepatic duct dilatation	236	42
Stenosis at the hepatic hilum	58	10
Extrahepatic duct dilatation	546	98
Anomalous arrangement of pancreatic-bile ducts	183	33
TOTAL CASES	560	100

Figure 40–1. The multiple variations of the choledochal cyst syndrome, based upon the detailed review of 560 collected cases from Japan.[3]

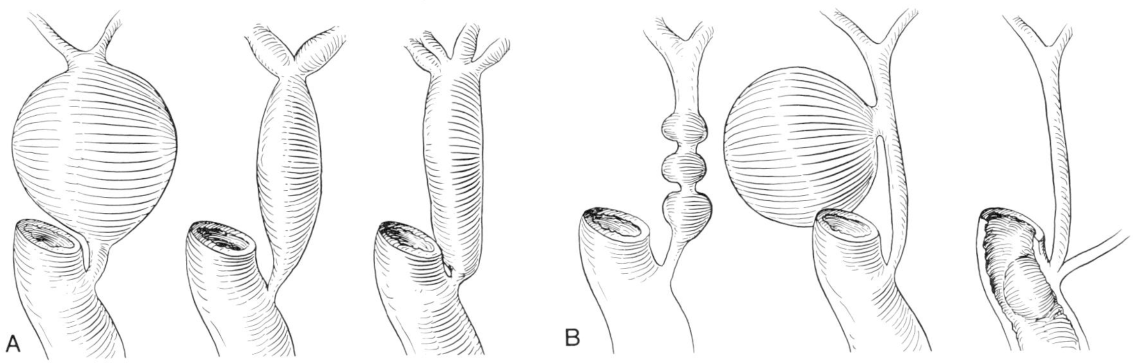

Figure 40–2. *A,* New classification of extrahepatic choledochal cysts modified from a review of 560 collected cases from Japan.[3] The cystic (54 per cent), fusiform (24 per cent), or cylindrical (15 per cent) type is present in 93 per cent of cases. *B,* The rosary, diverticular, and choledochocele varieties occur in less than 10 per cent of cases.

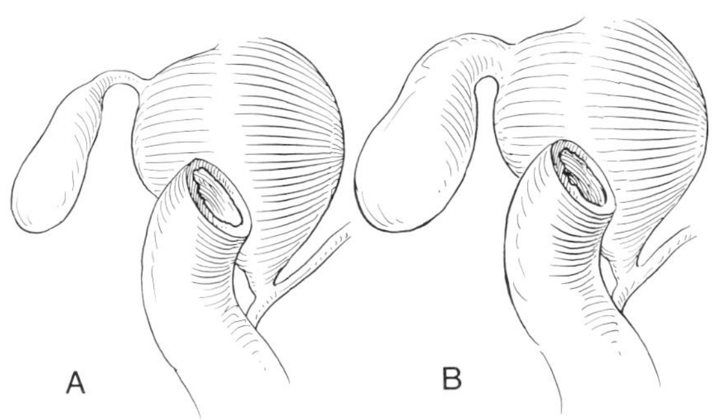

Figure 40–3. *A,* A normal-sized gallbladder arises from the wall of the choledochal cyst or from the common bile duct above the cyst in more than 70 per cent of cases. *B,* The cystic duct and gallbladder may be dilated in a small proportion of cases.

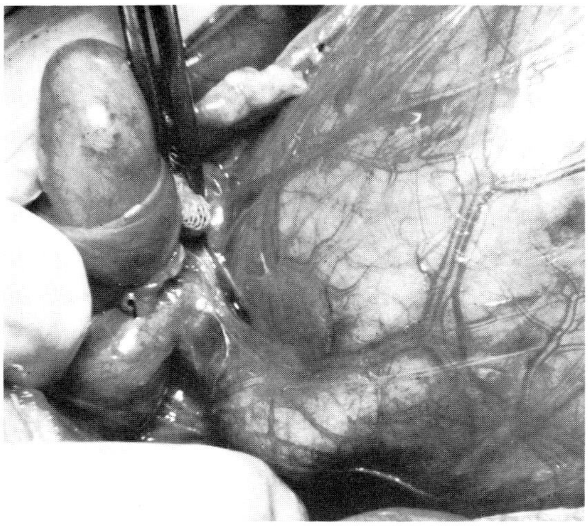

Figure 40–4. Dilated cystic duct and gallbladder arising from the side of a large cystic type of choledochal cyst.

(Fig. 40–5). It is imperative to recognize the location and type of anomalous pancreatic ducts before undertaking surgical resection of the choledochal cyst (Fig. 40–6). Babbitt and associates[23] and Kimura et al.[7] suggested that pancreatic reflux into the biliary system in patients with choledochal cyst is explained by the absence of a sphincter at the junction of the common and pancreatic ducts. Consequently, maximal pressure of the pancreatic duct exceeds that of the common bile duct during certain phases of digestion, permitting free reflux of pancreatic juice into the biliary system. This view was verified by the high amylase levels of the cystic fluid in the patients reported by Kimura et al.[7] and is supported by a growing body of clinical and laboratory findings.[14–17] Nonetheless, a common channel has not been a constant finding associated with choledochal cysts in the literature.

The wall of a choledochal cyst may vary in thickness from 1 mm to 10 mm, consisting largely of fibrous tissue with a cuboidal or columnar epithelial lining, although often there is no lining (Fig. 40–7).[30] Smooth muscle and elastic fibers are conspicuously absent in the majority of cases, which may be etiologically significant. Mucous glands, normally present in the wall, are rarely seen in choledochal cysts. The fusiform type of dilatation and the cystic dilatation that has not been exposed to recurrent episodes of cholangitis are more likely to contain a mucosal lining than are markedly distended ducts. Choledochal cysts may vary from the size of a cherry to a capacity of several liters (Fig. 40–8). The cyst usually contains green bile, which tends to be very thick and viscid; in rare cases, "white bile" may be present. Although sludge is occasionally observed, stones are uncommon.

Intrahepatic Ductal Dilatation

The frequency of intrahepatic involvement of the biliary ducts in association with cystic dilatation of the common bile duct has only recently been recognized. Caroli and associates[31] are credited with having first described the condition of intrahepatic biliary cystic dilatation. These authors proposed the following classification of intrahepatic cystic dilatation and related diseases.

1. *True polycystic disease of the liver.* The cysts occur in the parenchyma of the liver in association with typical Meyenburg complexes but do not communicate with the biliary ductal system.
2. *Mixed form of polycystic disease.* While having the same configuration as true polycystic disease, this type is accompanied by painful attacks of cholangitis. Occasional cysts contain bile and communicate directly with the biliary ductal system.
3. *Cystic dilatation of the intrahepatic biliary ducts.* These cystic lesions contain bile and have symptoms of pain and cholangitis. Meyenburg complexes are absent, but dilatation of the major bile ducts is usually observed.
4. *Congenital fibrocystic disease.* Microcysts occur in broad bands of fibrous tissue. No lesions are present within the biliary ducts. Signs of portal hypertension appear in many such patients.
5. *Multiple biliary cysts accompanied by fibro-*

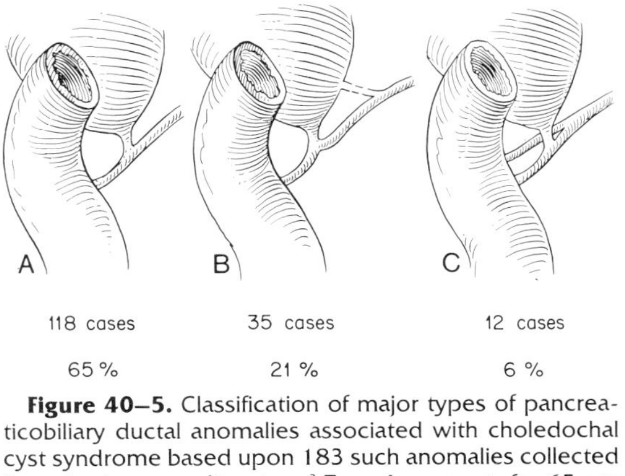

Figure 40–5. Classification of major types of pancreaticobiliary ductal anomalies associated with choledochal cyst syndrome based upon 183 such anomalies collected from the Japanese literature.[3] Type A accounts for 65 per cent of cases; Type B, 21 per cent; Type C, 6 per cent. Eight per cent had miscellaneous variations of the three basic types.

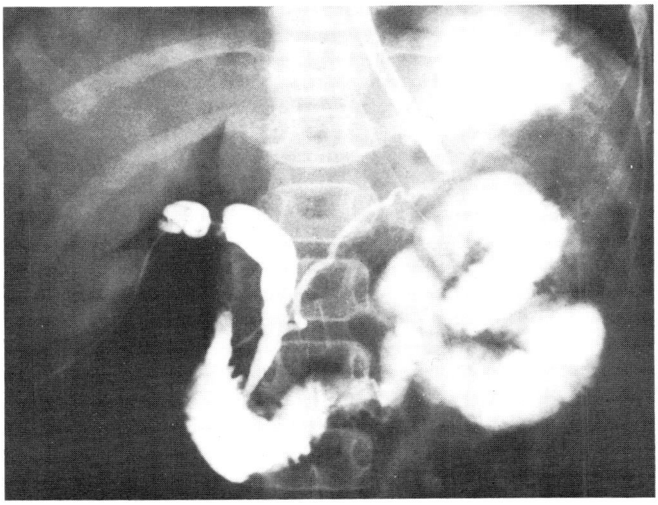

Figure 40–6. Operative cholecystogram with the upper end of a fusiform choledochal cyst occluded. This study shows the pancreatic duct entering the side of the choledochal cyst more than 1.5 cm above the ampulla.

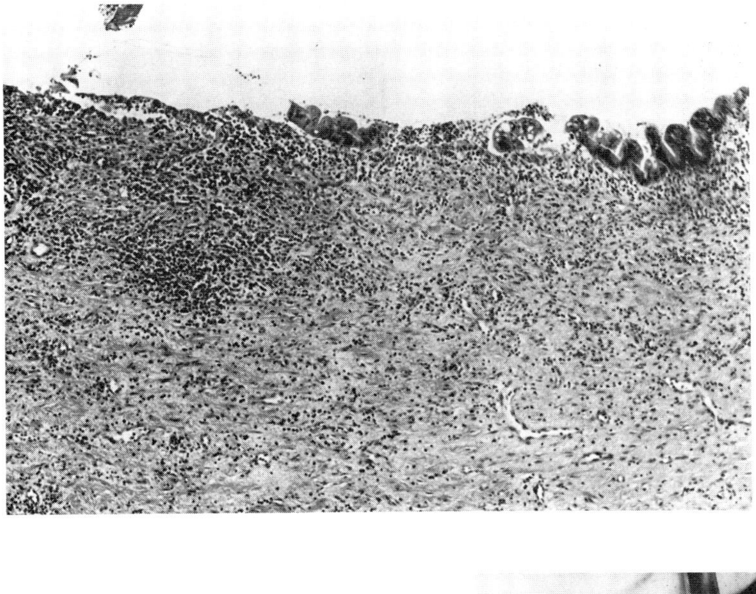

Figure 40–7. Wall of choledochal cyst, showing partial lining of columnar cells, otherwise eroded. There are chronic inflammation and fibrosis in the wall.

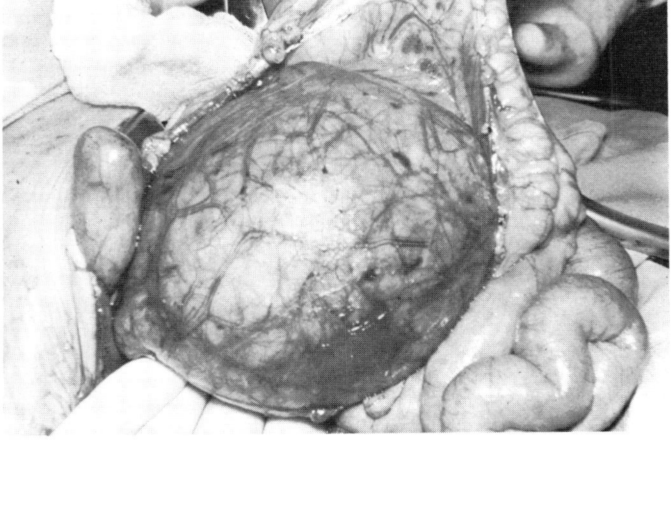

Figure 40–8. Cystic choledochal cyst in a 3-year-old girl, showing relationship to colon and gallbladder.

cystic changes. Portal hypertension is usually noted. There are cysts in the parenchyma and symptoms of cholangitis.

During the past two decades, numerous authors have identified patients with congenital dilatation of the intrahepatic ducts with or without extrahepatic dilatation. Tsuchida and Ishida[32] saw nine patients with associated intrahepatic bile duct dilatation of congenital origin and collected a total of 21 such cases from the literature. In a more recent report, Loubeau and Steichen[33] found that at least 55 of 701 reported cases of choledochal cyst evidenced combined intrahepatic and extrahepatic dilatation. A report by Saito,[13] summarizing 497 cases of choledochal cyst collected from 21 hospitals in Japan, indicated that 28 per cent of patients with extrahepatic dilatation have concomitant dilatation of the intrahepatic ducts. Komi and associates[3] noted that 236 of the 560 collected cases of choledochal cyst reviewed in the Japanese literature involved various forms of intrahepatic ductal dilatation (42 per cent). Repeated attacks of unexplained jaundice, or cholangitis starting in childhood, suggest the possibility of intrahepatic ductal dilatation.

In the majority of cases, cystic dilatation of the bile duct should be regarded as a lesion that may encompass multiple areas of the entire biliary tree. In 1958 Caroli et al.[31] reported that in the pure form of this lesion, the common duct frequently shows moderate dilatation, although in his syndrome the more peripheral ducts were primarily affected. Several anatomic configurations of intrahepatic dilatation have been described in various publications (Fig. 40–9). The diffuse cylindrical dilatation and the fusiform varieties are most common, although occasional patients may have diverticular dilatations. However, dilatation may occur throughout the major intrahepatic bile ducts in both lobes of the liver, although not always with the same type of dilatation. In many patients the dilatation appears to be confined to one lobe, generally the left lobe just above the confluence of the left and right hepatic ducts. Often there is a constriction of the duct just below the cystic area. Complete operative cholangiography with visualization of the intrahepatic ductal system is essential to establish the extent and type of intrahepatic ductal anomaly (Figs. 40–10 and 40–11). Bile stasis usually occurs, which results in the development of sludge and, in some cases, stones.

Recurrent cholangitis is common and sometimes difficult to resolve once it has developed. Intrahepatic abscesses are not infrequent. In severe diffuse disease, an extensive bacterial cellulitis of the liver develops, which requires intensive medical treatment with bed rest, antibiotics, nasogastric suction, and intravenous fluids. It is apparent from the most recent literature[3, 35] that intrahepatic ductal dilatation is typical of patients with choledochal cyst, whereas Caroli's disease, or primary intrahepatic ductal dilatation without a choledochal cyst, is rare. In the adult, a choledochal cyst appears to be the most obvious manifestation of a widespread pancreaticobiliary anomaly. For example, using ERCP, Rattner et al. have shown a high

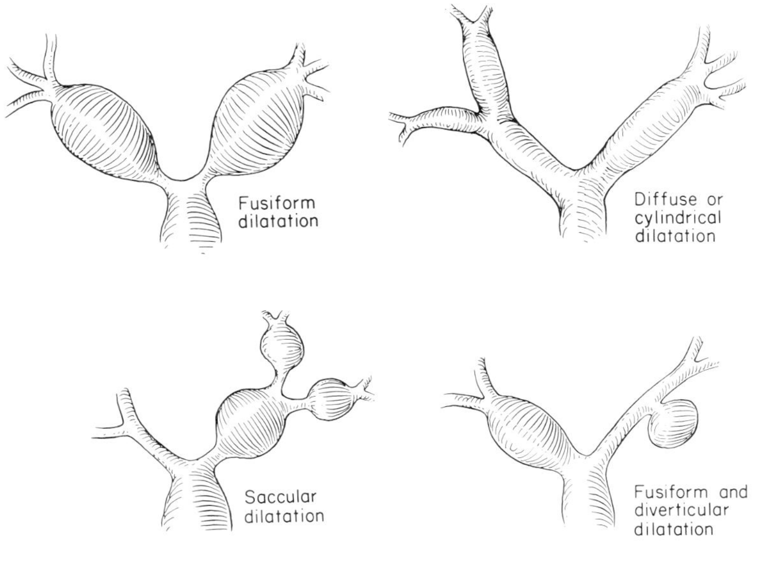

Figure 40–9. Classification of varieties of intrahepatic biliary ductal dilatation based upon reviews from several authors.[3, 12, 27, 29, 30] The approximate frequency of each type has not been determined.

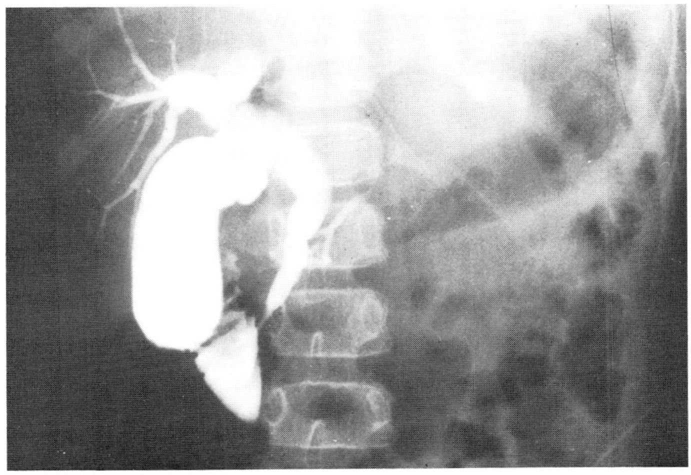

Figure 40–10. Operative cholecystogram showing large gallbladder, fusiform choledochal cyst, and fusiform dilatation of major intrahepatic ducts. Note stenosis of the common hepatic duct and anomalous entry of the pancreatic duct into the common bile duct. (Courtesy of Dr. Eitoku Arima, Kagoshima City, Japan.)

incidence of associated pancreatic duct abnormality in patients with choledochal cysts.[36] Although there is a very low incidence of associated malformation in patients with choledochal cyst, a report by Tsuchiya et al.[37] cites the occurrence of intrahepatic cystic dilatation with the Laurence-Moon-Bardet-Biedl syndrome.

Occasional clinical evidence of a diffusely dilated intrahepatic and extrahepatic ductal system with a history of multiple episodes of cholangitis, stasis, and stone formation has been referred to as congenital hypotonia of the duct wall by Longmire and Mandiola.[38] A long history of biliary disease, dating back to childhood in some of these patients, suggests a congenital origin. The diffuse fusiform dilatation, sometimes no more than 2.5 to 3.0 cm in diameter, may be easily overlooked and may cause attacks of obstructive cholangitis with stone formation. Because of the presence of the mucosal lining in this condition, these authors have recommended wide lateral decompression by anastomosis of the dilated area to the jejunum.

Symptoms

Congenital cystic dilatation of the common bile duct may produce symptoms at any time from early infancy to old age; however, 12

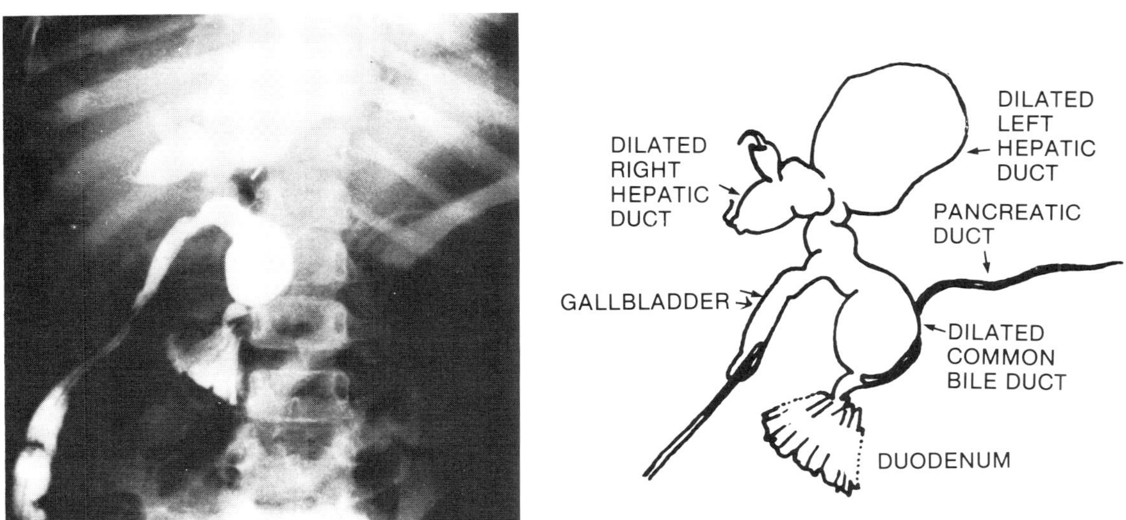

Figure 40–11. Operative cholecystogram showing cystic dilatation of both the extrahepatic and the intrahepatic bile ducts. Note the close proximity of the pancreatic duct to the cystic portion of the common bile duct. (Courtesy of Dr. Ken Kimura, Kobe, Japan.)

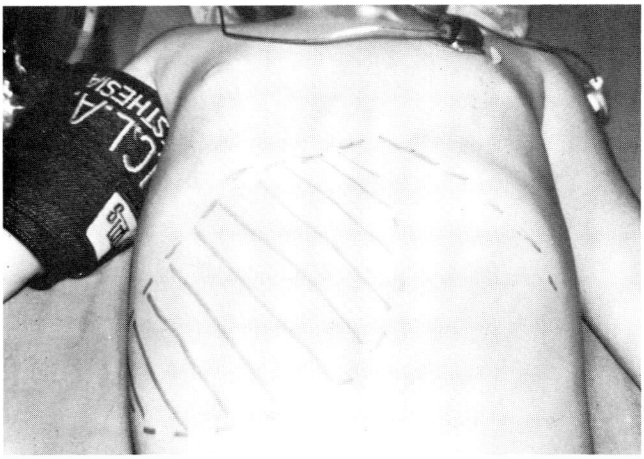

Figure 40–12. Right upper abdominal discrete cystic mass in a 4-year-old girl with the cystic type of choledochal cyst.

per cent of those afflicted are diagnosed younger than 1 year of age, and at least 59 per cent are recognized before the age of 20 years.[6, 39] It is common for a patient to manifest mild symptoms for years before the diagnosis is established. The anomaly is approximately three times more common in females than in males, and Orientals appear to be particularly affected.[6] Although congenital, this condition may not become symptomatic until the second or third decades of life, or even later in unusual cases.

Abdominal pain, jaundice, and the presence of an abdominal mass have been recognized as the clinical triad of symptoms present in more than half of patients with choledochal cyst; over two thirds of them are likely to have one or more of the three diagnostic features.[6]

The pain accompanying a choledochal cyst is typically located in the right upper abdomen but may radiate to the epigastrium, to the right lower quadrant, or to the back. The discomfort may be colicky and difficult to localize, particularly in infants and young children. The pain is believed to stem from distention of the cyst wall, often related to partial obstruction of the common bile duct or to cholangitis. Acute episodes of pain may occur when the cyst enlarges rapidly, and the pain may cease spontaneously as the cyst empties its contents into the duodenum. Pancreatitis has been reported in association with attacks of pain in patients with a choledochal cyst,[5] which is not surprising in view of the high incidence of pancreaticobiliary ductal malformations. Pancreatitis may be one of the initial manifestations of a choledochal cyst, but without laparotomy can be difficult to distinguish from a pancreatic cyst. It has been estimated that more than two thirds of all patients with choledochal cyst have some degree of pain.[5, 89, 90]

Jaundice may be absent, slight, intermittent, or long-standing and has been observed in over 70 per cent of patients with choledochal cyst.[6] Liver function tests initially are usually consistent with an obstructive process; however, after repeated episodes of cholangitis and long-standing partial biliary obstruction, cirrhosis may develop. Acholic stools, dark urine, and pruritus may accompany episodes of intense jaundice. In infants, obstructive jaundice and occasional emesis are frequent.

A mass has been found in the right upper abdomen in approximately 60 per cent of cases (Fig. 40–12).[6] Characteristically, the mass is soft, discrete, nontender, slightly mobile, and often recognizable as separate from the edge of the liver, although larger cysts are more likely to compress adjacent viscera. The size of the mass (which may not correlate directly with the degree of symptoms) and its configuration may vary during periods of cystic enlargement. A cystic mass in the right upper abdomen of a young female strongly suggests the presence of congenital cystic dilatation of the common duct.

Approximately one third of patients with choledochal cyst experience emesis, usually due to compression of the adjacent duodenum. Nausea and vomiting may occur in relationship to episodes of complete biliary obstruction when there are colicky pains. In some patients, colicky pain may terminate after vomiting of bilious fluid caused by drainage of the cyst contents into the duodenum.

Intermittent fever, present in at least one

third of cases, is believed to stem from cholangitis, which often occurs during acute obstructive episodes.

In older children, portal hypertension may develop as a result of compression of the portal vein by the adjacent choledochal cyst or of cirrhosis secondary to long-term biliary obstruction. An occasional patient with cirrhosis experiences variceal hemorrhage as the initial manifestation of the malformation.[39, 40]

On rare occasions, a neonate may develop bilious ascites with or without peritonitis as the initial manifestation of an anomaly of the common bile duct with spontaneous or traumatic rupture.[41] Lilly and associates[42] have observed that spontaneous perforation of the common bile duct in neonates rarely accompanies a choledochal cyst, although a large pseudocyst may appear surrounding the common bile duct. These infants tend to experience abdominal distention, due to bile ascites and failure to thrive, for a month or more, but the majority have unobstructed biliary tracts. Anastomosis of the surrounding pseudocyst to the intestine has been associated with a high incidence of complications. These authors concluded that simple drainage of the perforation without insertion of a T-tube into the duct and without intestinal anastomosis is usually followed by spontaneous closure of the perforation. An operative cholecystogram permits precise identification of the common duct pathology. The catheter may be left in the gallbladder and brought out externally to visualize the biliary tract again during the postoperative period. The etiology of spontaneous perforation of the common bile duct in neonates is unclear. It has been postulated that these perforations may possibly be caused by portal bacteremia localizing in the venous plexus surrounding the luminal diverticula and glands of the common duct.[41]

Malignant Potential

The incidence of carcinoma arising in bile ducts with congenital dilatation of long standing has been reported to be as high as 2.4 per cent, or approximately 20 times that in the general population.[43, 44] The incidence of carcinoma varies in relation to age at the initial appearance of symptoms. A child whose symptoms first appear before 10 years of age has a very low risk (0.7 per cent) of subsequent malignant degeneration compared with an individual in the second decade (6.8 per cent) or older (14.3 per cent).[45] Kasai and associates,[46] the first to recognize the increased incidence of carcinoma arising in choledochal cysts, have therefore advocated primary excision of the cyst whenever feasible.

Thirty cases of carcinoma associated with congenital biliary cystic disease were reviewed by Tsuchiya and coworkers in 1977[47]; the average age at diagnosis in their series was 32 years, with a range of 17 to 70 years. In most patients who developed cancer, onset occurred more than 2 years after the initial operation. In fact, delayed diagnosis of cancer has been common because the symptoms resemble those caused by narrowing of the cystoenteric anastomosis. The predominant site of carcinoma origin was the choledochal cyst wall. Adenocarcinoma was the most common histologic cell type (17 cases), with squamous cell carcinoma, cholangiocarcinoma, and anaplastic carcinoma being less frequent.[47, 48] The prognosis for patients with secondary carcinoma of a choledochal cyst is not hopeless, and resection should be undertaken in the majority of cases, when feasible. Patients with isolated dilatation of intrahepatic biliary ducts (Caroli's disease) also have a high risk of developing cholangiocarcinoma.[49]

Differential Diagnosis

Choledochal cyst should be considered in the evaluation of an infant or child found to have a mass in the right upper abdomen. Intravenous pyelography usually assists in distinguishing the most prevalent upper abdominal masses of childhood (Wilms' tumor, neuroblastoma, and multicystic or hydronephrotic kidney) from a choledochal cyst. Hepatic neoplasms are more difficult to identify without performing specific diagnostic studies, such as liver scan, diagnostic ultrasound (Fig. 40–13), intravenous cholangiogram (when jaundice is absent), computerized axial tomography (CAT scan), or selective hepatic arteriogram. Oral cholecystograms have occasionally been helpful in establishing the diagnosis, but they usually do not allow visualization. After the first few years of life, transjugular venous or percutaneous transhepatic cholangiography may help delineate the malformation, particularly in patients with intrahepatic ductal dilatation. Kimura and associates[7] found that in 5 of 15 patients undergoing either operative or en-

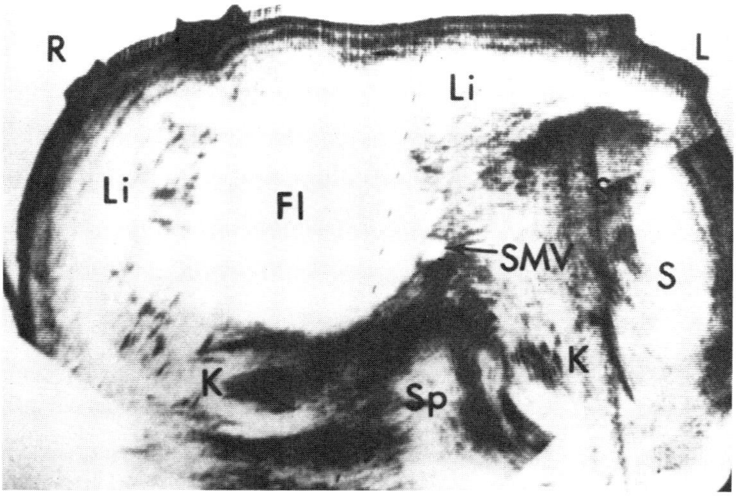

Figure 40–13. Diagnostic ultrasound scan of upper abdomen showing a large cystic choledochal cyst in a 3-year-old girl. (Li = liver, Fl = fluid, K = kidney, Sp = spine, SMV = superior mesenteric vein, St = stomach, S = spleen). (Courtesy of Dr. Fred Sample, Department of Radiology, UCLA School of Medicine, Los Angeles, California.)

doscopic retrograde choledochopancreatography (ERCP), reflux of contrast material from the biliary system into the pancreatic duct occurred. The amylase value in the choledochal cyst fluid was elevated in 4 of the 15 cases.

In patients with large cysts, an upper gastrointestinal series often shows displacement of the stomach anteriorly and inferiorly (Fig. 40–14). Hepatic function tests give evidence of obstructive jaundice during the course of the disease in approximately 86 per cent of cases.[2] Moreover, these studies can assist in establishing the diagnosis as well as indicating the extent of cirrhosis and hepatic parenchymal disease. It is imperative to relieve the obstruction in jaundiced patients, particularly during the first year of life, before advanced cirrhosis and portal hypertension become prominent.

Treatment

Treatment of choledochal cyst is surgical, consisting of drainage into the intestine as soon as the diagnosis is established. Nonoperative treatment implies an almost certain fatal outcome. Among the 232 cases reviewed by Tsardakas and Robnett,[5] of 30 patients managed nonoperatively, 29 died.[5] Considerable controversy remains, however, regarding the optimal type of surgical procedure for the management of patients with choledochal cysts.

Because external drainage as a primary procedure carries a mortality rate of more than 65 per cent, it should be avoided if at all possible.[5] Nonetheless, external drainage as the initial step in managing a patient by a two-stage operation, under rare circumstances in which there is a very large cyst, may be efficacious.[1, 50] Choledochorrhaphy, or excision of a portion of the cyst, with attempted reconstruction of a normal-sized lumen of the common bile duct may appear feasible. However, the procedure is technically difficult, and this form of reconstruction is followed by a high incidence of obstruction, leakage, and other serious complications.[51] While internal biliary drainage through the gallbladder by means of choledochoduodenostomy or cholecystojejunostomy has provided adequate decompression for short periods in occasional patients with dilated cystic ducts, long-term drainage is rarely satisfactory, and recurrent inflammation, stasis, and persistent cystic dilatation are common.

Marsupialization, aspiration, and cystogastrostomy are methods that have been utilized for biliary cystic drainage in the past, but they are now only historically interesting inasmuch as they involve numerous complications and recurrent symptoms.

For many years, choledochocystoduodenostomy was the operation of choice for managing cystic dilatation of the common bile duct, and occasional surgeons continue to recommend its use. This procedure, technically the easiest method of internal drainage, may be performed with a minimal risk of mortality as well as low early postoperative morbidity. The close proximity of the common bile duct to the duodenum makes this operation particularly appealing. Despite the fact that a large anastomosis can be performed in the majority of cases, long-term follow-up examination has indicated at least a 65 per cent incidence of morbidity due to anastomotic complications and reflux during the first 5 years after operation.[41]

Although repeated episodes of reflux of duodenal contents into the choledochal cyst have been incriminated as a major factor causing cholangitis and anastomotic stricture, it is likely that persistent inflammation in the cyst wall, gradual contraction of the cyst following drainage, and absence of peristalsis and sufficient pressure within the common bile duct to permit adequate drainage are important factors leading to anastomotic stricture with secondary failure of adequate cyst drainage and recurrent cholangitis.

Among patients followed for at least 5 years after cystoduodenostomy, 40 per cent have required a later operation, usually to revise a stricture of the cystoduodenal anastomosis.[51] Cholangitis is common, and a few cases of sudden death, presumably related to sepsis, have been observed several years later. Regardless of the size of the anastomosis, continued reflux of duodenal contents into the cyst appears to promote cholangitis, with or without anastomotic stricture. When cholangitis occurs, broad-spectrum antibiotics should be given, and early surgical revision of the anastomosis with conversion to a Roux-en-Y jejunal segment, with or without excision of the cyst, usually is necessary.

Roux-en-Y cystojejunostomy takes slightly longer than cystoduodenostomy to perform, but the 5-year follow-up indicates a lower incidence of morbidity and mortality, therefore making it the better procedure. In most patients, it is possible to excise a large wedge of tissue from the anterior wall of the cyst and thus perform a large anastomosis to the jejunal segment at least 4 or 5 cm in diameter. Most surgeons generally prefer doing a two-layer anastomosis.[1, 52]

Primary excision of the cyst with anastomosis of the common hepatic duct to the end of a Roux-en-Y jejunal segment and oversewing of the lower common duct remnant has been recommended by the majority of Japanese surgeons during the past decade (Fig. 40–15).[3, 12, 14, 16, 43, 54, 55] The reluctance of many American surgeons to use this procedure until recently stems largely from the classic review by Alonso-Lej and associates,[6] in which a 15 to 40 per cent mortality for operative resection of choledochal cyst was reported. However, in a 1975 collective review, Flanigan[56] reported a mortality of only 7 per cent associated with cyst resection. Subsequent reports from the United States endorse total excision of the cyst as the preferred mode of treatment.[36, 57–61, 88, 91, 93]

The frequent occurrence of pancreaticobiliary duct anomalies in combination with choledochal cyst makes total cyst excision somewhat more hazardous than wide drain-

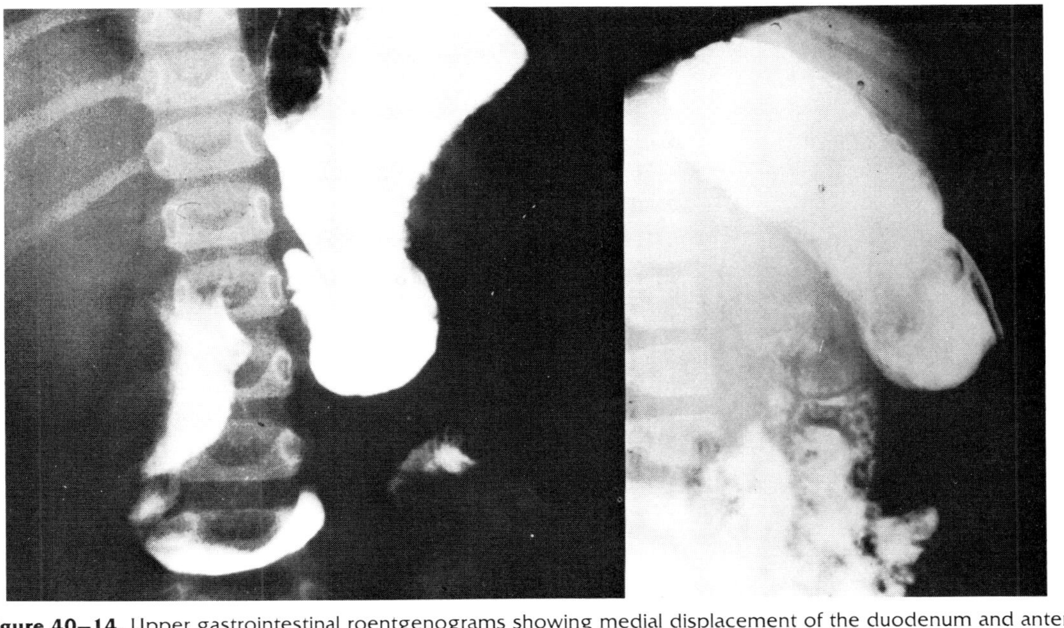

Figure 40–14. Upper gastrointestinal roentgenograms showing medial displacement of the duodenum and anterior displacement of the stomach by a large choledochal cyst.

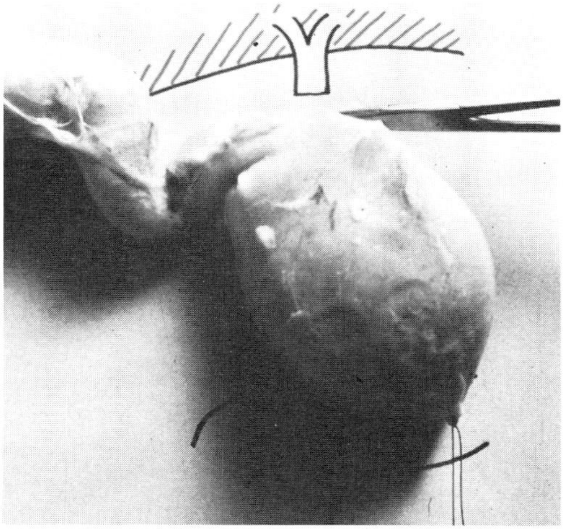

Figure 40–15. Choledochal cyst and gallbladder excised from a 3-year-old girl with a choledochal cyst. A Roux-en-Y jejunal anastomosis was constructed to the common hepatic duct. (Courtesy of Dr. Ken Kimura, Kobe, Japan.)

age into a jejunal segment. Nevertheless, certain cysts lend themselves particularly well to excision, especially those in which a stricture is present at the junction between the cyst and the common hepatic duct. Total cyst excision is also recommended by most authors for patients with associated intrahepatic cystic dilatation in order to provide the best ductal drainage. Resection of the cyst lining, leaving the back wall of the cyst intact, is the favored procedure if a large cyst is to be excised (Fig. 40–16).[35] Complete excision of the cyst may be a formidable task, and attempts to separate the portal vein and hepatic artery from an inflamed cystic wall may lead to inadvertent injury and extensive hemorrhage. Perhaps the most compelling reason for the use of cyst excision, when feasible, is that the incidence of carcinoma in the wall of the common duct is approximately 20 times higher than normal in patients with choledochal cyst.

Trout and Longmire,[51] on the other hand, have pointed out that cyst excision requires a substantial amount of dissection in a critical area and leaves the surgeon with few options in case of technical failure or late complications. They suggest that this procedure be reserved as a second possibility if cyst drainage fails.

At the time of abdominal exploration, an operative cholangiogram is essential to delineate the extent of the cyst and to determine whether or not intrahepatic dilatation is present (Figs. 40–17 and 40–18). The relationship

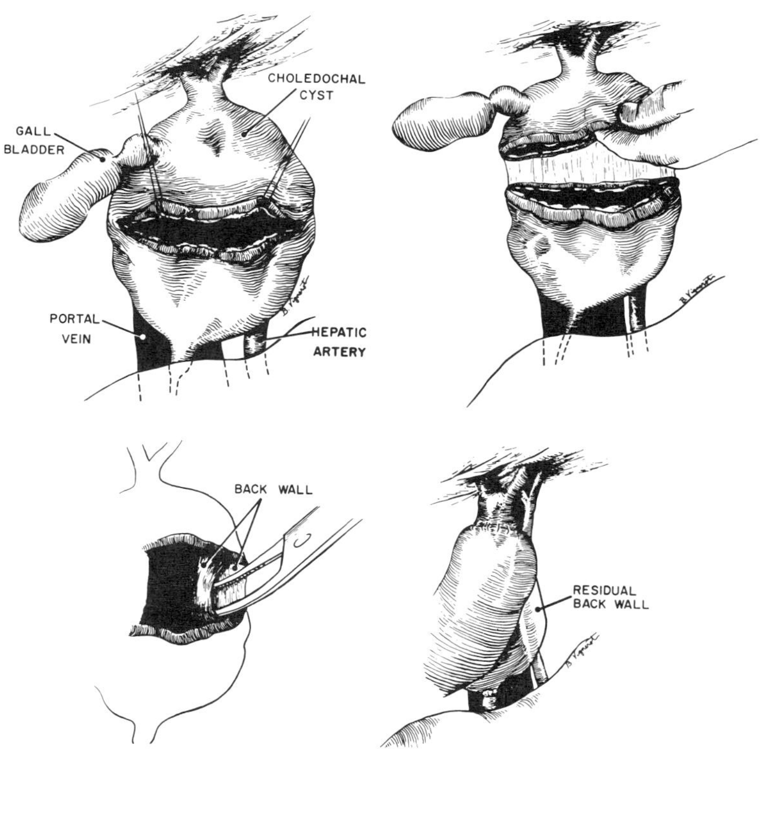

Figure 40–16. Surgical technique recommended for resection of large choledochal cyst, consisting of "shelling out" inner lining and leaving the posterior wall of cyst adjacent to portal vein, hepatic artery, and pancreatic duct. The Roux-en-Y jejunal segment is anastomosed to the common hepatic duct, and the lower end of the remaining duct is oversewn. (From Lilly JR: Surg Gynecol Obstet *149*:36, 1979. Used by permission.)

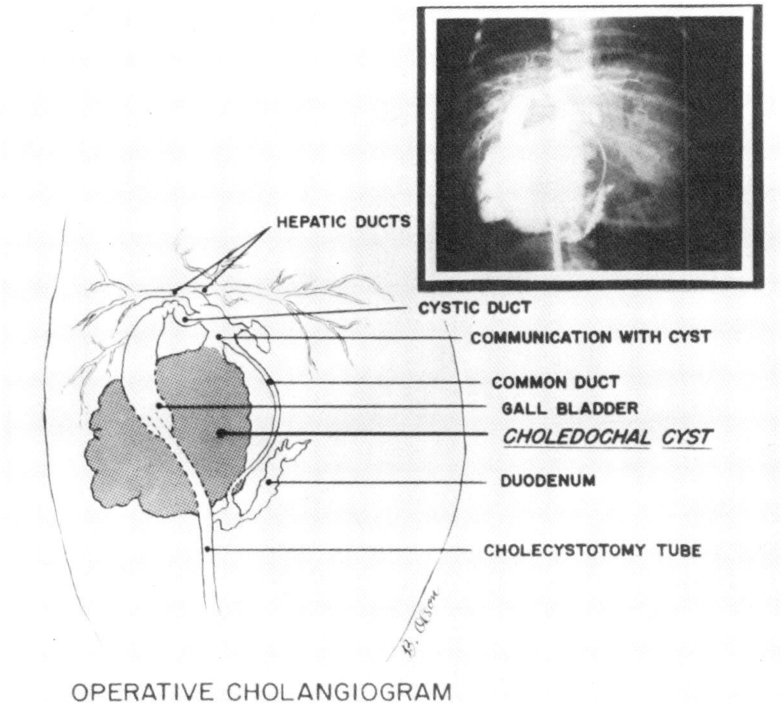

Figure 40–17. Operative cholangiogram from a 2-year-old girl, showing diverticular type of choledochal cyst with narrow common bile duct and normal intrahepatic ducts. (From Fonkalsrud EW, Boles ET: Surg Gynecol Obstet *121*:733, 1965. Used by permission.)

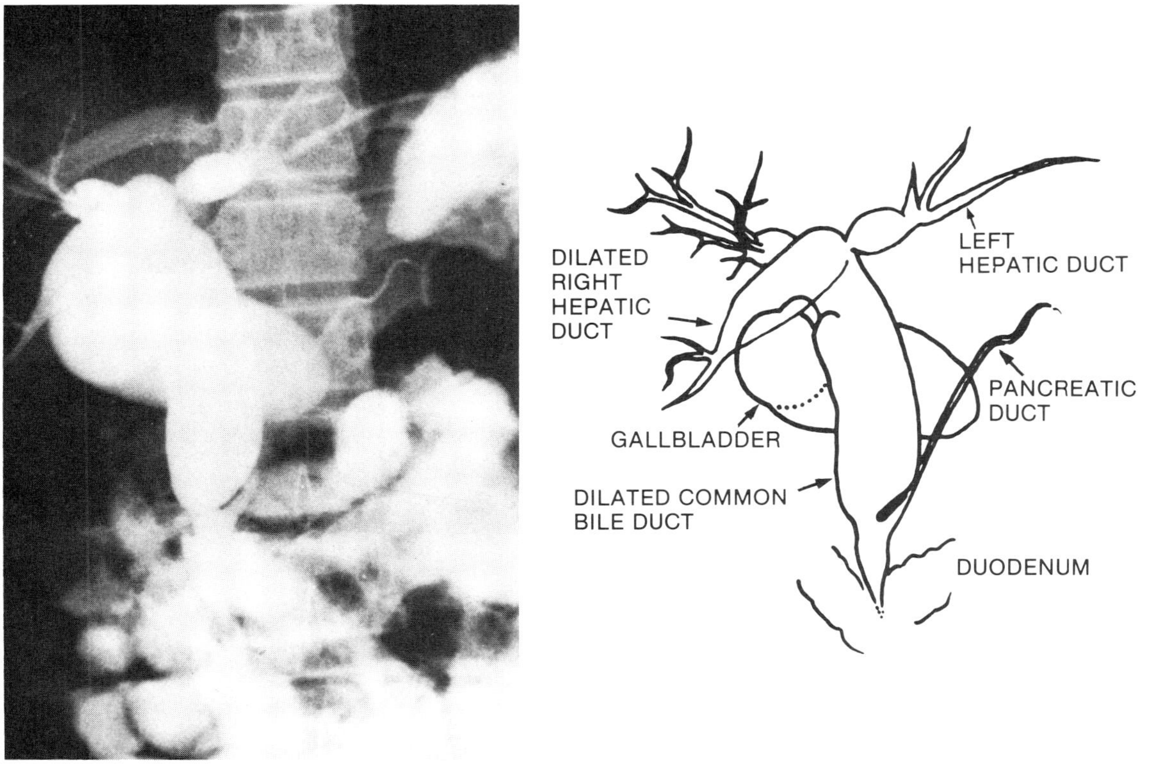

Figure 40–18. Operative cholangiogram showing cylindrical dilatation of a common bile duct, with intrahepatic fusiform dilatation and narrowing of the junction between the common bile duct and the major hepatic ducts. Note the dilated gallbladder and anomalous entry of the pancreatic duct into the lower common bile duct. (Courtesy of Dr. Ken Kimura, Kobe, Japan.)

of the pancreatic duct may also be more clearly identified by injecting contrast material into the lower portion of the cyst while temporarily occluding the midportion of the common duct. Concomitant cholecystectomy at the time of cystoenteric anastomosis is advisable, since subsequent cholecystitis and cholelithiasis can develop in patients who have had choledochointestinal anastomosis. Morgenstern and Shore[62] have shown that if the gallbladder is left in situ, decompression of the common bile duct by means of an intestinal anastomosis leads to progressive biliary tract inflammation and ascending infection, whereas if the gallbladder is removed, the reflux into the biliary tract is well tolerated.

Although a 10 per cent incidence of late peptic ulceration has been reported to occur after choledochojejunostomy,[63] this problem rarely occurs after jejunal drainage for choledochal cyst. Wheeler and Longmire[64] recently recommended interposition of an isolated jejunal segment between the common duct and the duodenum as a method of lowering the incidence of peptic ulceration while still providing adequate drainage of the common bile duct and avoiding the likelihood of reflux cholangitis.

The operative management of intrahepatic cystic dilatation remains a matter of controversy, since optimal drainage is often very difficult to establish. An operative cholangiogram will demonstrate whether there is a large peripheral intrahepatic cyst that should be drained directly (like a liver) or not. Mercadier and associates[65] in 1968 presented a case of cystic dilatation of the intrahepatic duct and reviewed the management of six other patients previously reported. Left hepatectomy with anastomosis of the jejunum to the right ductal system or the common duct appears to give the best results. This form of treatment, however, is available only to patients with dilatation confined to one lobe. For those with bilateral intrahepatic ductal dilatation, choledochoduodenostomy has not been adequate to provide sufficient drainage. Choledochojejunostomy has proved to be the most effective procedure in establishing drainage, although repeated episodes of pyogenic cholangitis and stone formation may develop in patients who have multiple cystic or diverticular lesions. A high anastomosis to the hepatic duct is particularly important in patients who have a stricture in the high common bile duct, as indicated by Komi et al.[3]

Inasmuch as the mortality for patients with Caroli's disease is high despite various forms of internal drainage, largely owing to stasis in the hypotonic ducts, it may be necessary to utilize a Silastic U-tube in certain cases when adequate ductal drainage cannot be obtained by other means. Irrigation of the intrahepatic ducts with antibiotic solution may be helpful in removing sludge in occasional patients with persistent cholangitis. Cholangitis has led to portal fibrosis and progressive loss of liver function in some patients, often complicated by recurrent suppurative cholangitis that may resist antibiotic therapy despite absence of obstruction of the common bile duct.

INTRAHEPATIC CYSTS

In 1856, the first report of a solitary hepatic cyst appeared in the literature.[66] It described a 60 year old man who died 8 days after an attack of diarrhea; the finding at autopsy was a large liver cyst the size of a 4 year old child's head. Since then, over 300 cases of solitary, nonparasitic liver cysts have been reported.[67]

Embryology

The liver develops from the embryonic hepatic diverticulum extending from the primitive foregut at the level of the caudal portion of the septum transversum. It has therefore been suggested that aberrant or dilated bile ducts, or a failure of excess intralobular hepatic ducts to involute properly and develop appropriate connections with the interlobular ducts, may lead to congenital hepatic cysts. An overgrowth or abnormal inclusion of connective tissue may be the cause of hamartomas. The observation that occasional liver cysts are lined with respiratory or ciliated epithelium may be related to the fact that the lungs and the liver develop from diverticula of the foregut in near proximity. The rare congenital tracheobiliary fistula[51] may also be explained, in part, by this common embryologic derivation of the lungs and the liver.

Classification

The following classification of cysts of the liver has been proposed by Warren and Polk:[69]

1. Congenital
   a. Solitary unilocular cyst
   b. Polycystic disease
   c. Cystic dilatation of common bile duct
2. Parasitic
3. Traumatic
4. Inflammatory

The congenital solitary cysts are further classified on a histologic basis into the following categories: (1) lymphatic cyst, (2) endothelial cyst, (3) retention of cyst of bile ducts, (4) degenerative cyst containing blood, (5) dermoid cyst, and (6) proliferative cyst.

In the most definitive review, Edmondson[70] classified congenital cystic lesions of the liver in infancy and childhood into two basic categories: the cystic mesenchymal hamartomas and the nonparasitic cysts. He noted that while teratomas and mesenchymomas may have cystic components, they are basically solid tumors. The hamartoma is characterized by marked overgrowth of mesenchymal or connective tissue of varying degrees of maturity, with a strong tendency to cystic formation. The mesenchyme may contain minor remnants of liver cells, duct cells, or even portal triads. The connective tissue may contain angiomatous and hematopoietic foci. The cysts may be without lining or may be lined with flattened cells thought to be mesothelial cells. The relative proportion of mesenchymal tissue to cysts is highly variable, so that some lesions are mainly cystic and others are solid with small cysts. The most characteristic feature, however, is the overgrowth of connective tissue.[71]

The cystic mesenchymal hamartoma was previously classified as a lymphatic or endothelial cyst. Names formerly used for a hamartoma include cavernous lymphangiomatoid lesion, lymphangioma, or bile cell fibroadenoma. Although this lesion is benign, it can be difficult to differentiate from malignant lesions of the liver without surgical resection (Figs. 40–19 and 40–20).

The nonparasitic cyst is usually solitary and may vary in diameter from a few centimeters to the size of a grapefruit. In 1906, Moschocowitz[72] was the first to suggest that solitary liver cysts arose from aberrant bile ducts, when he observed a bile duct remnant in Glisson's capsule. The inner surface is smooth and lined with columnar, cuboidal, and, occasionally, stratified squamous or ciliated epithelium. The wall is relatively thin and composed of mature connective tissue, the outermost layer of which is hyalinized. Small remnants of liver tissue or ducts may be found in the wall.

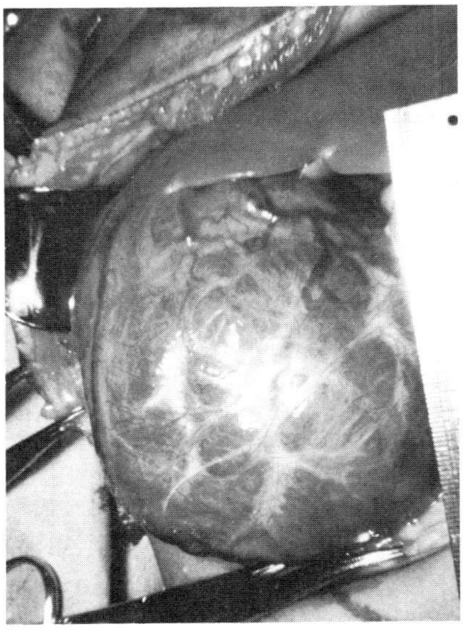

Figure 40–19. Cystic hamartoma in right lobe of the liver in a 1-year-old boy.

Clinical Features

The infrequency of solitary liver cysts is indicated by the fact that only 38 cases were encountered at the Mayo Clinic between 1906 and 1954.[73] Twelve of these cases were symptomatic relative to the cyst, while 26 were found incidentally at operation. In 1955, Geist[74] published an excellent review of the literature, reporting only 193 solitary cysts of the liver. These cysts are three to four times more prevalent in females, and they are also seen more frequently among Caucasians. The average age at which such cysts are detected is the fourth to fifth decade.

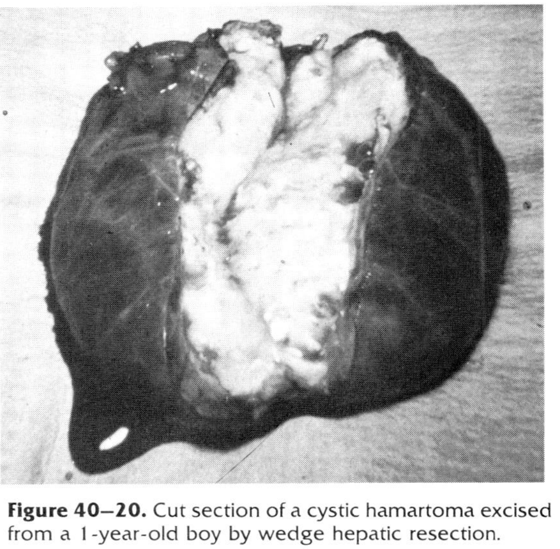

Figure 40–20. Cut section of a cystic hamartoma excised from a 1-year-old boy by wedge hepatic resection.

There is considerable variability in the location of solitary hepatic cysts. Beattie and Robertson[75] reviewed the location of 62 simple liver cysts, noting that 20 were present in the right lobe, 10 in the left lobe, and 6 in both lobes. Generally, solitary cysts are located on the inferior portion of the right hepatic lobe. They may occur completely intrahepatically, and they have even been observed to arise from the hepatic ligament.

The largest cyst reported in the literature contained an estimated 17,000 ml of fluid.[75] Although most cysts are unilocular, an occasional one may be multilocular. Davis[76] noted that of the 197 solitary cysts in his study, only 20 were multilocular. The external surface of the cyst is usually smooth and glistening, with a bluish hue. The wall, which varies in thickness, is seldom more than 8 mm and contains three microscopically distinct layers. The innermost layer is composed of epithelial cellular elements, the middle layer usually contains vascular elements, and the outer layer tends to be collagenous, often containing some muscle fibers, bile ducts, and compressed hepatic cells. Unlike the parasitic cyst, the nonparasitic type has a low internal tension and its fluid is usually slightly cloudy, although it may vary from clear to brownish. The fluid often contains albumin, cholesterol, blood cells, mucin, and epithelial elements; sometimes bile is also present. The fluid has a specific gravity varying between 1.007 and 1.024.[77]

Hepatic cysts are typically slow-growing and asymptomatic and thus are often discovered incidentally at operation. The chief presenting complaints are pain and/or an abdominal mass. The pain is described as a dull, aching sensation aggravated by motion or change of posture, probably from distention of the liver capsule and traction on the liver ligaments. Occasionally the pain is acute and sharp, as the result of hemorrhage into the cyst or torsion of a cyst on its pedicle. Other symptoms include bloating, indigestion, constipation, diarrhea, emesis, and flatulence, most of which stem from extrinsic pressure of the cyst on the gastrointestinal tract. Jaundice rarely occurs with solitary hepatic cysts; when it does, it is usually secondary to external pressure on the extrahepatic biliary system. Abscess formation is likewise uncommon, although some cysts may communicate with the biliary ductal system and become infected.

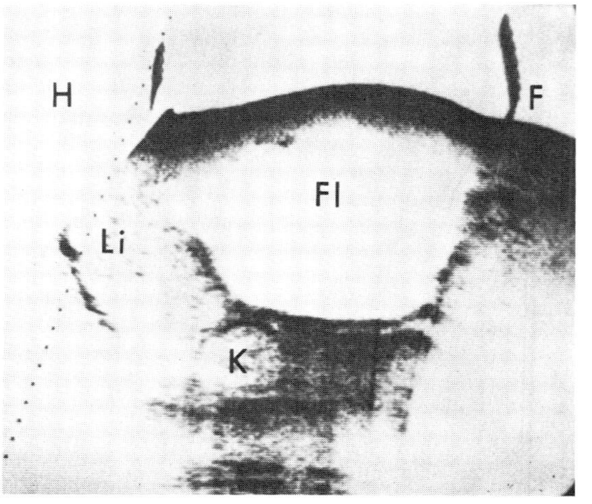

Figure 40–21. Longitudinal diagnostic ultrasound scan of right upper abdomen, showing solitary intrahepatic cyst. (H = head, Li = liver, K = kidney, Fl = fluid). (Courtesy of Dr. Fred Sample, Department of Radiology, UCLA School of Medicine, Los Angeles, California.)

Accurate preoperative diagnosis of a simple solitary hepatic cyst is difficult inasmuch as differentiation from parasitic cysts, choledochal cysts, or cystic disease of the kidney, pancreas, ovary, and mesentery may be very challenging. Liver scan and diagnostic ultrasound are useful procedures in localizing the lesion (Fig. 40–21). Eosinophilia and/or a positive Casoni skin test may differentiate a hydatid cyst from a solitary congenital cyst. An intravenous cholangiogram may give further information regarding the location of the cyst and its relationship to the intrahepatic bile ducts. However, selective hepatic arteriography is seldom necessary.

Treatment

The preferred treatment for symptomatic, nonparasitic cysts is complete extirpation (Fig. 40–22). Insertion of a needle into the cyst is not recommended because if the cyst is parasitic, its contents could leak into the peritoneal cavity and cause extensive soilage. Removal of the cyst is ideally achieved by stripping out the thin lining of the cyst in toto from its hepatic bed, particularly if the cyst is typically superficial. Major branches of the hepatic artery or portal vein may be in close proximity to such cysts, and care must be taken to avoid injuring them. It will sometimes be impossible to find a proper plane of cleavage, in which case it may be necessary to excise as much of the cyst as possible and to oversew the remaining cyst wall in order

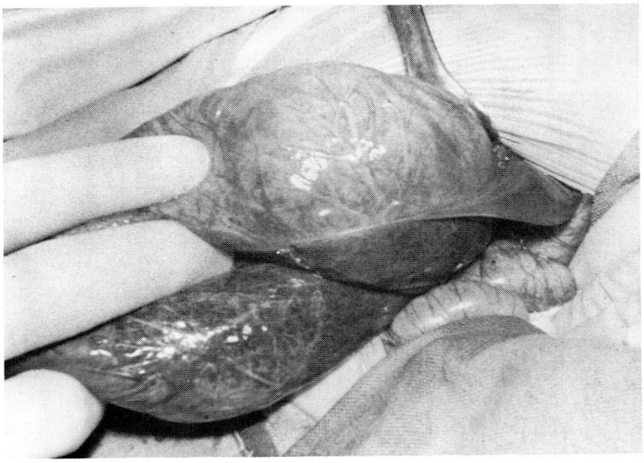

Figure 40–22. Large solitary nonparasitic cyst of the right lobe in the liver in an asymptomatic 2-year-old boy.

to maintain hemostasis and prevent bile leak (Fig. 40–23). Occasional solitary intrahepatic cysts may communicate with the biliary ductal system; it is imperative to identify and oversew such communications during cyst removal to avoid postoperative bile peritonitis or subphrenic abscess. The absence of bile within the cyst at the time of operation is strongly suggestive that there is no communication with the biliary ductal system, although this factor does not preclude the possibility.[1] If the cyst fluid is not crystal-clear, infection or bile leak must be suspected, and anastomosis to a Roux-en-Y loop, rather than simple cyst excision, should be considered. Infected cysts should be drained externally, followed by excision or internal drainage into the jejunum.

Hepatic lobectomy or partial hepatectomy may be advisable in special circumstances, particularly if a recurrence should develop after simple excision or if the cyst resides within the hepatic parenchyma, although these cysts often extend across interlobular planes and cannot be excised by an anatomic lobectomy.[1, 52, 69, 78, 79] Recurrence of a cyst generally results from failure to remove all the segments of a multiloculated cyst. Complications of untreated solitary cysts include perforation, spontaneous hemorrhage, infection, and torsion of the pedicle of a pedunculated cyst.

When multiple congenital hepatic cysts are present, the mean diameter has been reported to be 1.2 cm.[80] Excision of a major portion of the lesion is considered to be unwarranted, since the hepatic cystic disease is rarely a serious threat to the patient.

Flagg and Robinson[81] in 1967 were unable to find any reported cases of malignant degeneration occurring in solitary hepatic cysts and found only one reported case in a patient with polycystic liver disease.

Miscellaneous Hepatic Cystic Disease

Polycystic disease of the liver is a condition in which multiple small cysts are distributed throughout the liver (Fig. 40–24). Scattered cysts of varying size may appear to almost replace the entire liver. In approximately half the patients, this condition is related to polycystic disease of the kidneys, but in the remainder, normal hepatic function is preserved over many years despite extensive involvement of the liver. Although patients as young as 5 months have been identified, most cases are not diagnosed until the fifth and sixth decades.[1] This form of cystic liver disease is believed to be incidental and unimportant in the course of the patient's illness, and no specific surgical therapy is

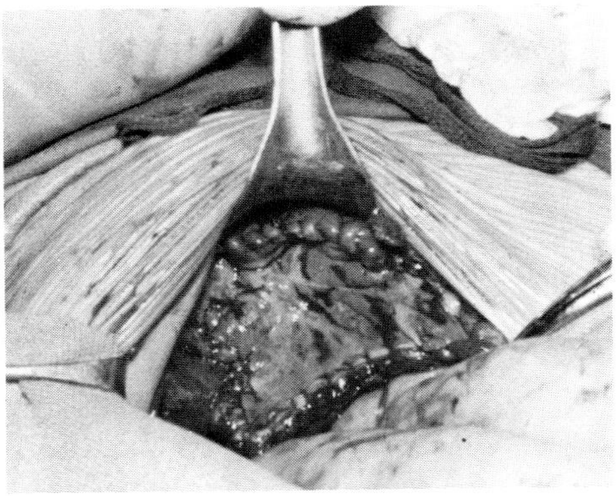

Figure 40–23. A solitary cyst of the right lobe of the liver has been excised, and the margin at the liver edge has been oversewn.

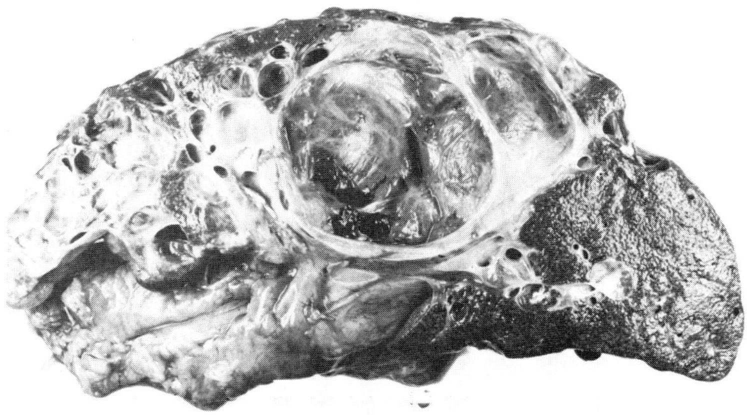

Figure 40–24. Cut section of the liver from a patient with moderately severe polycystic disease of the liver. Hepatic function was near-normal. This patient also had polycystic disease of the kidneys and developed fatal renal failure.

recommended. However, the associated polycystic renal disease is far more likely to be symptomatic and to cause serious complications. For polycystic disease of the liver, no treatment need be performed unless a very large dominant cyst is present, in which case treatment is the same as for large solitary cysts (i.e., unroofing, excision, or internal drainage).

Kerr and associates[82] have emphasized that congenital hepatic fibrosis often occurs in patients with congenital polycystic disease of the liver and kidneys. Foulk[83] suggested that although Meyenburg complexes and intrahepatic fibrosis are frequently present in patients with polycystic hepatic disease, the condition is not identical to congenital hepatic fibrosis.

Intrahepatic biliary cysts have been observed in as many as 40 per cent of patients with "uncorrectable" biliary atresia at the time of post-mortem examination.[84] In an extensive review of the clinical manifestations, Fonkalsrud and Arima[85] noted that these intrahepatic cysts were not identified in patients younger than 6 months of age coming to autopsy (Fig. 40–25). They postulated that these intrahepatic cystic "bile lakes" are dilated ductal spaces resulting from mucosal secretions accumulating over many months. Injection of these bile lakes with dye under pressure at post-mortem examination failed to show communication with other intrahepatic bile ducts. It is the current view, therefore, that such bile lakes do not represent intrahepatic cysts, which, if drained surgically through the intestinal tract, will provide active biliary drainage. By the time the bile lakes are large enough to be identified, the patients invariably have such severe cirrhosis that they will not live much longer regardless of the type of treatment provided.

Intrahepatic cysts with an endothelial lining, which are very rare, may represent an

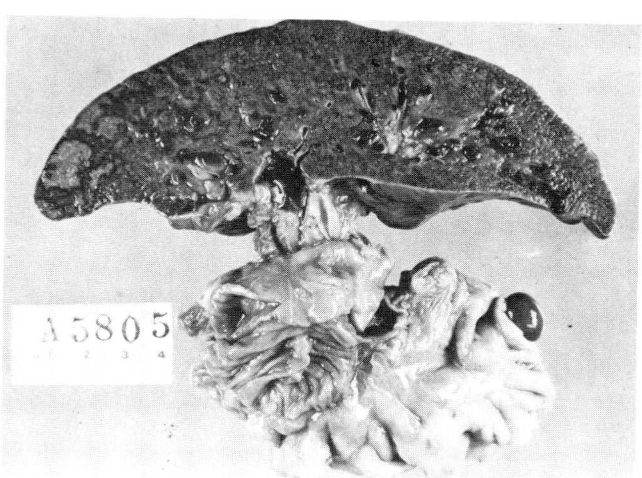

Figure 40–25. Multiple intrahepatic "bile lakes" or cysts in the hepatic parenchyma of an 18-month-old girl, who died as a result of intra- and extrahepatic biliary atresia.

organized hemangioma localized to a single area of the liver. It has also been suggested that occasional patients with intraparenchymal hemorrhage may develop a localized cyst, although this would be highly unlikely. Such cysts may contain degenerated blood elements. Although surgical treatment is rarely necessary, resection was performed for a hemangiomatous cyst as early as 1918.[86]

Teratomas of the liver, which have been reported in a few instances, correlate with the category of dermoid cysts.[71] The only proliferative or neoplastic lesion likely to be cystic is the mesenchymoma. Wellwood and associates[87] described one patient who had a cystic hepatoma and another with a localized cystic cystadenocarcinoma of the liver, both of whom died within 10 years of diagnosis. Hepatic resection, whenever feasible, is the preferred treatment for these lesions.

Symptoms from intrahepatic parenchymal cysts are usually nonspecific; these cysts are discovered accidentally or when the masses become large enough to produce pressure symptoms. Granulomatous cysts, which are surrounded by a thick fibrous capsule and filled with fibrin, clot, and amorphous debris, may represent the end stage of an old nonviable echinococcal cyst. Calcification in the cyst wall is often present under these circumstances. Cyst excision, or occasionally hepatic resection, is preferred to mere evacuation or marsupialization.

REFERENCES

1. Longmire WP Jr, Mandiola SA, Gordon HE: Congenital cystic disease of the liver and biliary system. Ann Surg 1971;*174*:711.
2. Lee SS, Min PC, Kim GS, et al: Choledochal cyst: a report of nine cases and review of the literature. Arch Surg 1969;*99*:19.
3. Komi N, Udaka H, Ikeda N, et al: Congenital dilatation of the biliary tract; new classification and study with particular reference to anomalous arrangement of the pancreaticobiliary ducts. Gastroenterol Jpn 1977;*12*:293.
4. Smith BC: Cyst of the common duct. Arch Surg 1942;*44*:968.
5. Tsardakas E, Robnett AH: Congenital cystic dilatation of the common bile duct. Arch Surg 1956;*72*:311.
6. Alonso-Lej F, Rever WB Jr, Pessagno DJ: Congenital choledochal cyst, with a report of 2, and an analysis of 94 cases. Surg Gynecol Obstet 1959;*108*:1.
7. Kimura K, Tsugawa C, Ogawa K, et al: Choledochal cyst: etiological considerations and surgical management in 22 cases. Arch Surg 1978;*113*:159.
8. Douglas AH: Cases of dilatation of the common bile duct. Monthly J Med Sci (Lond) 1852;*14*:97.
9. Laverson RS: Cysts of the common bile duct. Am J Med Sci 1909;*137*:563.
10. Waller E: Idiopathic choledochus cyst. Ann Surg 1917;*66*:446.
11. Shallow TA, Eger SA, Wagner FB Jr: Congenital cystic dilatation of the common bile duct: case report and review of the literature. Ann Surg 1943; *117*:355.
12. Spitz L: Choledochal cyst. Surg Gynecol Obstet 1978;*147*:444.
13. Saito S: Surgical treatment and long-term follow-up results of congenital dilatation of the biliary ducts. Presented at International Symposium on Cholestasis in Infancy—Its Pathogenesis, Diagnosis, and Treatment. Sendai, Japan, June 7–9, 1978.
14. Yamaguchi M: Congenital choledochal cyst. Analysis of 1,433 patients in the Japanese literature. Am J Surg 1980;*140*:653.
15. Miyano T, Suruga K, Suda K: The choledochopancreatic long common channel disorders in relation to the etiology of congenital biliary dilatation and other biliary tract disease. Ann Acad Med 1981;*10*:419.
16. Miyano T, Suruga K, Chen S-C: A clinicopathologic study of choledochal cyst. World J Surg 1980;*4*:231.
17. Ohkawa H, Sawaguchi S, Yamazaki Y, et al: Experimental analysis of the ill effect of anomalous pancreaticobiliary ductal union. J Pediatr Surg 1982;*17*:7.
18. Gross RE, Ladd WE: Abdominal Surgery of Infancy and Childhood. Philadelphia, WB Saunders, 1941, p 278.
19. Shah RC, Mehta AB, Haribhakti JB: Choledochal cyst. Am J Gastroenterol 1969;*51*:227.
20. Yotuyanagi S: Contributions to aetiology and pathogeny of idiopathic cystic dilatation of common bile duct with report of three cases: new aetiological theory. Gann 1936;*30*:601.
21. Von Lutzki A: Cystic dilatation of the common bile duct (Zystische Erweiterungen des Ductus choledochus) ZBL, Chir 1886;85, as reported in Surg Gynecol Obstet 1961;*112*:461.
22. Attar S, Obeid S: Congenital cyst of the common bile duct—a review of the literature and report of two cases. Ann Surg 1955;*142*:289.
23. Babbitt DP, Starshak RJ, Clemett AR: Choledochal cyst: a concept of etiology. Am J Roentgenol Radium Ther Nucl Med 1973;*119*:57.
24. Komi N: Pancreaticobiliary anomaly in congenital cystic dilatation of the bile duct. Operation 1975:*29*:73.
25. Saito S, Ishida M: Congenital choledochal cyst (cystic dilatation of the common bile duct). Prog Pediatr Surg 1974;*6*:63.
26. Bode WE, Aust JB: Isolated cystic dilatation of the cystic duct. Am J Surg 1983;*145*:828.
27. Gross RE: Idiopathic dilatation of the common bile duct. *In* Surgery of Infancy and Childhood. Philadelphia, WB Saunders, 1953, p 254.
28. Babbitt DP: Congenital choledochal cyst: new etiological concept based on anomalous relationships of common bile duct and pancreatic bulb. Ann Radiol 1969;*12*:231.
29. Barraya L, Pujor-Solor R, Yvergneaux JP: Quoted by Eaton SB, Ferrucci JT. *In* Radiology of the Pancreas and Duodenum. Philadelphia, WB Saunders, 1973.
30. Ravitch MN, Snyder GB: Congenital cystic dilatation of the common bile duct: special reference to radiographic studies. Surgery 1958;*44*:752.

31. Caroli J, Soupault R, Kossakowski J, et al: La dilatation polykystique congénitale des voies biliaires intra-hépatiques. Sem Hop Paris 1958;*34*:488.
32. Tsuchida Y, Ishida M: Dilatation of the intrahepatic bile ducts in congenital cystic dilatation of the common bile duct. Surgery 1971;*69*:776.
33. Loubeau JM, Steichen FM: Dilatation of intrahepatic bile ducts in choledochal cyst: case report with follow-up and review of the literature. Arch Surg 1976;*111*:1384.
34. Turnberg LA, Jones EA, Sherlock S: Biliary secretion in a patient with cystic dilatation of the intrahepatic biliary tree. Gastroenterology 1968;*54*:1155.
35. Lilly JR: Total excision of choledochal cyst. Surg Gynecol Obstet 1978;*146*:254.
36. Rattner DW, Schapiro RH, Warshaw AL: Abnormalities of the pancreatic and biliary ducts in adult patients with choledochal cysts. Arch Surg 1983;*118*:1068.
37. Tsuchiya R, Nishimura R, Ito T: Congenital cystic dilatation of the bile duct associated with Laurence-Moon-Biedl-Bardet syndrome. Arch Surg 1977; *112*:82.
38. Longmire WP Jr, Mandiola S: Nonobstructive dilatation of the common duct. Surg Clin North Am 1970;*50*:1099.
39. Fonkalsrud EW, Boles ET: Choledochal cysts in infancy and childhood. Surg Gynecol Obstet 1965;*121*:733.
40. Gillis DA, Sergeant CK: Prolonged biliary obstruction and massive gastrointestinal bleeding secondary to choledochal cyst. Surgery 1961;*52*:391.
41. Hyde GA Jr: Spontaneous perforation of bile ducts in early infancy. Pediatrics 1965;*35*:453.
42. Lilly JR, Weintraub WH, Altman RP: Spontaneous perforation of the extrahepatic bile ducts and bile peritonitis in infancy. Surgery 1974;*75*:664.
43. Todani T, Watanabe Y, Narusue M, et al: Congenital bile duct cysts: classification, operative procedures, and review of 37 cases including cancer arising from choledochal cyst. Am J Surg 1977; *134*:263.
44. Lorenzo GA, Seed RW, Beal JM: Congenital dilatation of the biliary tract. Am J Surg 1971;*121*:510.
45. Voyles CR, Smadja C, Shands WC, et al: Carcinoma in choledochal cysts. Age-related incidence. Arch Surg 1983;*118*:986.
46. Kasai M, Asakura Y, Taira Y: Surgical treatment of choledochal cyst. Ann Surg 1970;*172*:844.
47. Tsuchiya R, Harada N, Ito T, et al: Malignant tumors in choledochal cysts. Ann Surg 1977;*186*:22.
48. Chaudhuri PK, Chaudhuri B, Schuler JJ, et al: Carcinoma associated with congenital cystic dilation of bile ducts. Arch Surg 1982;*117*:1349.
49. Dayton MT, Longmire WP Jr, Tompkins RK: Caroli's disease: a premalignant condition? Am J Surg 1983;*145*:41.
50. Witlin LT, Gadacz TR, Zuidema GD, et al: Transhepatic decompression of the biliary tree in Caroli's disease. Surgery 1982;*91*:205.
51. Trout HH III, Longmire WP Jr: Long-term follow-up of patients with congenital cystic dilatation of the common bile duct. Am J Surg 1971;*121*:68.
52. Hays DM, Goodman GN, Snyder WH Jr, et al: Congenital cystic dilatation of the common bile duct. Arch Surg 1969;*98*:457.
53. Ishida M, Tsuchida Y, Saito S, et al: Primary excision of choledochal cyst. Surgery 1970;*68*:884.
54. Todani T, Watanabe Y, Mizuguchi T, et al: Hepaticoduodenostomy at the hepatic hilum after excision of choledochal cyst. Am J Surg 1981;*142*:584.
55. Todani T, Watanabe Y, Fujii T, et al: Congenital choledochal cyst with intrahepatic involvement. Arch Surg 1984;*119*:1038.
56. Flanigan DP: Biliary cysts. Ann Surg 1975;*182*:635.
57. Nunez-Hoyo M, Lees CD, Hermann RE: Bile duct cysts. Experience with 15 patients. Am J Surg 1982;*144*:295.
58. Oldham KT, Hart MJ, White TT: Choledochal cysts presenting in late childhood and adulthood. Am J Surg 1981;*141*:568.
59. Powell CS, Sawyers JL, Reynolds VH: Management of adult choledochal cysts. Ann Surg 1981;*193*:666.
60. Shafie ME, Cindo R, Mash M, et al: The changing trends in the management of choledochal cysts. Contemp Surg 1983;*23*:55.
61. Lilly JR: The surgical treatment of choledochal cyst. Surg Gynecol Obstet 1979;*149*:36.
62. Morgenstern L, Shore JM: Selection of an optimal procedure for decompression of the obstructed common bile duct. Am J Surg 1969;*119*:38.
63. McArthur MS, Longmire WP Jr: Peptic ulcer disease after choledochojejunostomy. Am J Surg 1971; *122*:155.
64. Wheeler ES, Longmire WP Jr: Repair of benign stricture of the common bile duct by jejunal interposition choledochoduodenostomy. Surg Gynecol Obstet 1978;*146*:260.
65. Mercadier M, Clot JP, Mellière D, et al: Nouvelle observation de dilatation congénitale des voies biliaires intra-hépatiques (maladie de Caroli). Sem Hop Paris 1968;*44*:3283.
66. Michel J: Kyste de la face postérieure du foie. Gaz d Hop 1856;*29*:397; as reported by Geist DC: Solitary nonparasitic cyst of the liver; review of the literature and report of two patients. Arch Surg 1955;*71*:857.
67. Clark DD, Marks C, Bernhard VM, et al: Solitary hepatic cysts. Surgery 1967;*61*:687.
68. Stigol LC, Traversaro J, Trigo ER: Carinal trifurcation with congenital tracheo-biliary fistula. Pediatrics 1966;*37*:89.
69. Warren KW, Polk RC: Benign cysts of the liver and biliary tract. Surg Clin North Am 1958;*38*:707.
70. Edmondson HA: Differential diagnosis of tumor and tumor-like lesions of liver in infancy and childhood. Am J Dis Child 1956;*91*:168.
71. Johnston PW: Congenital cysts of the liver in infancy and childhood. Am J Surg 1968;*116*:184.
72. Moschocowitz E: Nonparasitic cysts (congenital) of the liver, with a study of aberrant bile ducts. Am J Med Sci 1906;*131*:674.
73. Henson SW Jr, Gray HK, Docherty NB: Benign tumors of the liver: solitary cysts. Surg Gynecol Obstet 1956;*103*:607.
74. Geist DC: Solitary nonparasitic cyst of the liver: review of the literature and report of two patients. Arch Surg 1955;*71*:867.
75. Beattie DA, Robertson HD: Case of simple cyst of liver with analysis of 62 other cases. Lancet 1932;2:674.
76. Davis CR: Nonparasitic cysts of the liver. Am J Surg 1937;*35*:590.
77. Ackerman FD, Rhea LJ: Solitary nonparasitic cysts of the liver: their clinical and pathologic aspects. Br J Surg 1931;*18*:648.
78. Minton JP, Kinsey DL: Surgical management of a recurrent solitary multilocular nonparasitic cyst of the liver. Am J Surg 1961;*102*:710.
79. Schrumpf E, Bergan A, Blomhoff JP, et al: Partial hepatectomy in Caroli's disease. Scand J Gastroenterol 1981;*16*:581.

80. Sanfelippo PN: Cystic disease of the liver. Rev Surg 1973;*30*:375.
81. Flagg RS, Robinson DW: Solitary nonparasitic hepatic cysts: report of oldest known case and review of the literature. Arch Surg 1967;*95*:964.
82. Kerr DNS, Harrison DV, Sherlock S, et al: Congenital hepatic fibrosis. Q J Med 1961;*30*:91.
83. Foulk WT: Congenital malformations of the intrahepatic biliary tree in the adult. Gastroenterology 1970;*58*:253.
84. Danks DM, Campbell PE: Extrahepatic biliary atresia: comments on the frequency of potentially operable cases. J Pediatr 1966;*69*:21.
85. Fonkalsrud EW, Arima E: Bile lakes in congenital biliary atresia. Surgery 1975;*77*:384.
86. Lowenburg AM: Congenital unilocular cyst of the liver (hemangioma). Arch Pediatr 1918;*35*:285.
87. Wellwood JM, Madara JL, Cady B, et al: Large intrahepatic cysts and pseudocysts: pitfalls in diagnosis and treatment. Am J Surg 1978;*135*:57.
88. Nagorney DM, McIlrath DC, Adson MA: Choledochal cysts in adults: clinical management. Surgery 1984;*96*:656.
89. Heikkinen ES, Salminen PM: Congenital choledochal cyst opening into the intraduodenal part of the common bile duct and complicated by cystolithiasis and acute pancreatitis. Acta Chir Scand 1984; *150*:183.
90. Venu RP, Geenen JE, Hogan WJ, Dodds WJ, et al: Role of endoscopic retrograde cholangiopancreatography in the diagnosis and treatment of choledochocele. Gastroenterology 1984;*87*:1144.
91. Takiff H, Stone M, Fonkalsrud EW: Choledochal cysts: results of primary surgery and need for reoperation in young patients. Am J Surg 1985; *150*:141.
92. Ohkawa H, Sawaguchi S, Khalil B, et al: Cholangiovenous reflux as a cause of recurrent hyperamylasemia in choledochal dilatation with anomalous pancreaticobiliary ductal union: an experimental study. J Pediatr Surg 1985;*20*:53.
93. Cheney M, Rustad DG, Lilly JR: Choledochal cyst. World J Surg 1985;*9*:244.

CHARLES E. LUCAS, M.D.

41

Trauma to the Biliary Tract

The gallbladder and bile ducts are infrequently injured by blunt trauma, probably because of the protection afforded these structures by the overlying liver and rib cage, the pancreas, the duodenum, the vertebral column, and the paravertebral muscles.[1, 2] Once present, however, gallbladder and bile duct injuries are a major challenge to surgical acumen.[2, 3, 44–47, 53, 55] Blunt biliary tract injury is probably the most frequently overlooked intraperitoneal injury. Awareness of subtle physical signs and recognition of uncommon roentgenographic findings facilitate early diagnosis and treatment.

CLOSED BILE DUCT INJURY

Fizeau, in 1806, described the first patient with closed common bile duct injury; Battle, in 1894, made the first English language report.[1, 4] Battle's patient, a young man, was run over by a hansom cab. Laparotomy revealed a common duct injury that was treated by simple drainage. The patient died in the early postoperative period. The frequency of bile duct injury rose with the advent of the automobile. Lee and Wherry collected 43 cases in a literature review up to 1961,[5] and Moyle and Karl added 21 cases in 1969.[6] Currently, this injury occurs in less than one patient in a thousand with blunt abdominal injury.

Bile duct injury usually occurs during an automobile accident. The driver, being thrust against the steering wheel, is the usual victim. Seat belts may decrease but certainly do not eliminate the potential for bile duct injury; insufficient data are available to determine the preventive potential for airbags as they relate to biliary tract injury.[7]

Site of Bile Duct Injury

The common duct is the most frequently injured extrahepatic bile duct. Twenty-eight of 45 patients with bile duct injury described by Lee and Wherry had common duct injury[5]; 14 of 20 patients reported by Maier and coworkers had common duct injury (Table 41–1).[8] These authors noted that common hepatic duct injury was next in frequency (17 patients), followed by injury to the right hepatic duct (4 patients), left hepatic duct (2 patients), cystic duct (2 patients), and unknown causes (5 patients). Zollinger et al. reported the only patient with closed rupture of both the right and the left hepatic ducts; this patient had both hepatic ducts disrupted immediately proximal to the common hepatic duct.[9]

The common bile duct may be anatomically subdivided into three continuous portions. The first third lies cephalad to the duodenum along the free border of the lesser omentum and forms the anterior border of the epiploic foramen; the second portion lies posterior to the duodenum, immediately anterior to the portal vein, and lateral to the gastroduodenal artery; the third portion curves laterally and

Table 41–1 SITE OF BLUNT BILE DUCT INJURY

Location	Number of Patients	Per Cent
Common bile duct	42	58.3
Common hepatic duct	17	23.6
Right hepatic duct	4	5.5
Left hepatic duct	2	2.8
Cystic duct	2	2.8
Unknown	5	6.9
Total	72	100

Tabulated from data of Maier et al.,[8] and Lee and Wherry.[5]

lies embedded within the head of the pancreas, where it joins the pancreatic duct before terminating as the ampulla of Vater. Most common bile duct injuries occur at the junction of the second and third portions of the duct at the superior border of the pancreas. Occasionally, when the injury is circumferential, the distal segment of the common bile duct retracts within the pancreas and cannot be located.[2]

Mechanism of Bile Duct Injury

Several theories have been advanced to explain the mechanism of bile duct injury. Some authors have considered it to result from a rapid increase in intraluminal pressure caused by sudden compression of the gallbladder, which forces bile into the common duct and produces a *blowout* injury.[2, 10] Fletcher, however, could not produce bile duct rupture by a rapid intracholedochal insufflation of air sufficient to raise intraluminal pressure to 750 lb/sq inch.[1] This author concluded that the air escaped into the duodenum so fast that intraductal pressure could not reach a level that would rupture the duct. Moyle and Karl reported two patients with common duct rupture following a previous cholecystectomy.[6] Spasm of the ampulla of Vater has been said to occur in traumatized patients; if so, this might interfere with decompression of the duct into the duodenum, creating a situation in which common duct pressure might increase enough to cause a blowout.[12] One would think, however, that this type of injury would be distributed randomly throughout the duct, rather than occurring just at the superior border of the pancreas, as it usually does.

A more plausible theory postulates that the common bile duct, which is mobile in the porta hepatis but fixed within the head of the pancreas, can be *sheared* at the junction of its fixed and mobile segments by rapid deceleration.[8, 13]

A less popular but attractive theory holds that common duct injury results from *excessive stretching* at the time of impact.[8] When a individual is thrust against a steering wheel, the force received against the anterior abdominal wall causes a sudden decrease in the anterior-posterior diameter. The liver is pushed cephalad, and the pancreas is pushed caudad. The sudden stress applied to the noncompliant common duct may either rupture the duct or injure its blood supply, which, in turn, may result in ischemia, necrosis, and delayed rupture.

Both the *shearing* and the *stretching* theories are compatible with the site of injury being most often located along the superior border of the pancreas. The stretching theory is also compatible with delayed rupture, a common sequela. A fourth theory, that the common bile duct may be *crushed* between the steering wheel and vertebral column, is unlikely to explain many cases, since the duct is well protected by other viscera and lies to the right of the vertebral column.[13, 14, 54] A combination of mechanisms may be operative in some patients.

Regardless of how the bile duct is injured, associated injury to the hepatic artery or portal vein is almost nonexistent, probably because these vessels are so much more elastic and tortuous than the bile duct.[3, 15, 55] They are also more mobile than the duct, which is anchored below by the pancreas.

Diagnosis of Bile Duct Injury

The clinical picture of bile duct rupture varies with the presence or absence of associated intra-abdominal injuries. Patients with associated hemoperitoneum or peritonitis normally undergo early laparotomy, at which time the biliary tract injury is discovered incidentally. Thorough exploration of the porta hepatis is mandatory in any patient with a hematoma or even minimal bile staining in the portal triad in order to avoid overlooking a bile duct injury.[2, 3, 53–55] The wary surgeon knows that *free* intraperitoneal bile is seldom present in patients with bile duct injury when laparotomy is performed early for some other indication.[2]

However, bile duct rupture usually occurs without other significant intraperitoneal injuries, and diagnosis must be based upon recognition of the signs and symptoms, which, unfortunately, are often subtle. Shortly after injury, the patient with an isolated bile duct injury manifests mild to moderate shock.[2, 6, 44, 53–55] The etiology of the shock is not clear, since the blood loss is insignificant. It may be neurogenic. The hypotension responds quickly to an infusion of fluids, and it rarely recurs. Since many patients with blunt abdominal trauma have consumed excessive amounts of alcohol immediately before the injury, one may be tempted to dismiss the early hypotension as an aftereffect of alcohol. In fact, alcohol alone may be responsible for post-traumatic hypotension that is responsive to intravenous fluids even in the absence of major abdominal injury or plasma depletion. Following resuscitation, the patient may or may not complain of mild upper abdominal pain; if present, the pain usually subsides within 6 hours. Routine abdominal and chest roentgenograms show no abnormalities. Paracentesis, if performed, is usually negative. Since the patient usually improves clinically, remains stable, and is free of pain within 6 hours of injury, he is often discharged with the reassurance that "everything is all right."[16]

Once home, the patient may be able to eat at first, but by the second day, abdominal discomfort, nausea, vomiting, abdominal fullness, and low-grade fever ensue. Examination 4 to 5 days later most often reveals jaundice, adynamic ileus, and mild to moderate right upper quadrant tenderness.[1–3] Physical signs of peritonitis are infrequent. The patient may have noted the presence of light-colored stools and dark urine. Although this quiescent period averages 4 to 5 days, it may vary from 1 to 12 weeks. Abdominal roentgenograms may show a suggestion of a right upper quadrant mass, but more often the picture is that of adynamic ileus alone. In addition to hyperbilirubinemia, laboratory tests may show elevated values of SGOT, SGPT, and alkaline phosphatase, but these abnormalities are nonspecific and may not suggest the correct diagnosis.[17] Maier and coworkers[8] reported that some patients manifest hypernatremia and hyperchloremia owing to absorption of sodium and chloride from bile within the peritoneal cavity, but this is uncommon, and the serum electrolytes are usually normal.

If the patient is hospitalized at this stage, the combination of previous abdominal injury, postinjury hypotension, symptom-free interval at home, late adynamic ileus, and jaundice should alert the physician to the likelihood of biliary tract injury (Table 41–2). Continued doubt about the need for exploratory laparotomy at this point is best resolved by paracentesis or peritoneal lavage, which will yield bile.[2, 48] Intravenous cholangiography is unreliable, since even in the presence of a significant injury, the duct may be opacified and appear to be intact. Ultrasound may demonstrate the presence of an abnormal fluid collection in the region of the bile duct or in the gallbladder wall.[38, 39] The increased use of CT scanning in the evaluation of the trauma patient has also proved useful in the detection of bile duct trauma.[37, 51] Over the last few years, cholescintigraphy with ^{99m}Tc-HIDA has become the method of choice to diagnose bile leakage from injured bile ducts.[26, 33, 43, 46, 49, 50, 55–57] Alternatively, if a diagnostic laparotomy is performed for nonspecific right upper quadrant tenderness, adynamic ileus, or jaundice of undetermined cause, the diagnosis will be made.

Table 41–2 DIAGNOSTIC PENTAD FOR BLUNT BILIARY INJURY

History of recent blunt abdominal trauma
Early postinjury hypotension
Probable neurogenic origin
Responsive to intravenous fluids
Symptom-free interval
Mean duration is 5 days
Late postinjury adynamic ileus
Jaundice on readmission to hospital

Exploratory laparotomy reveals 1 to 6 liters of free intraperitoneal bile. Ordinarily, this has caused little or no inflammatory reaction, and the patient is neither septic nor toxic with bile peritonitis. This coincides with the general observation that bile in the peritoneal cavity does not produce peritonitis unless it is infected.[2, 18]

Operation, whether performed immediately or after a quiescent interval, reveals a hematoma or bile staining in the porta hepatis or the retroperitoneal planes posterior or lateral to the duodenum.[54, 55] The nature of the injury is usually difficult to discern, and it may be obvious only after thorough exploration of the porta hepatis and mobilization of the duodenum (Kocher maneuver). Any remaining doubt about the integrity of the bile duct must be resolved by an operative cholangiogram performed through the gallbladder or common bile duct. Postoperatively, one must be sure to check the prothrombin time and administer vitamin K if it is abnormal.

Bile Duct Reconstruction

The type of reconstruction that should be performed varies with the site and severity of the ductal injury.[44, 47, 54, 55] As long as both ends can be mobilized and approximated without tension, a clean, sharp transection of the common bile duct along the superior border of pancreas is best treated by an end-to-end anastomosis. A T-tube should be inserted through a proximal choledochotomy, with the transverse arm of the T used to stent the anastomosis.

A ragged or ischemic tear of the duct should not be managed by primary end-to-end repair. These injuries are best treated by end-to-side choledochoduodenostomy or Roux-en-Y choledochojejunostomy. Although there is debate on this subject, there is no evidence that choledochojejunostomy has any long-term advantages over choledochoduodenostomy or primary end-to-end anastomosis in patients without previous biliary tract disease.[47, 53] For example, Moyle and Karl could find no patients who manifested cholangitis late after various types of common bile duct reconstruction for blunt trauma regardless of the type of reconstruction.[6] We feel that one should perform the simplest operation that results in a tension-free anastomosis. Thus, an end-to-end repair or an end-to-side choledochoduodenostomy can be successfully accomplished in most patients.[6]

Often the caudad portion of a severed common bile duct retracts within the head of the pancreas and cannot be found.[2] Extensive dissection of the pancreas to ligate or oversew the lost distal end is unwarranted because it may result in severe hemorrhage or pancreatitis; if the distal duct is left open, the worst that will result is a temporary fistula that closes within a few days.

Dorton[16] and others[54, 55] recommended that prophylactic cholecystectomy be performed after choledochoduodenostomy to prevent cholecystitis from developing in the gallbladder, which now does not fill and empty normally because sphincter function is lost. In practice, however, this has been an uncommon sequela.[6] Furthermore, the gallbladder may be useful for later biliary-enteric reconstruction if the original anastomosis proves to be unsatisfactory.[3, 19] The T-tube may be removed 3 weeks after reconstruction if there is no bile fistula and if a T-tube cholangiogram demonstrates an intact anastomosis with free flow of bile into the intestine.

Distal Common Bile Duct Injuries

Discussion of injuries of the distal third of the common bile duct must take into consideration concomitant injury to the head of the pancreas, which is so often present. Injury to the distal or intrapancreatic segment is manifested by hyperamylasemia, abdominal pain, tenderness, and guarding due to retroperitoneal extravasation of pancreatic enzymes.[13, 53, 55] Severe injury to the main pancreatic duct may be identified during exploration by noting leakage of pancreatic juice and bile from the site of injury or from extraductal extravasation of contrast medium during an operative cholangiogram. Duodenotomy and retrograde cannulation of the ampulla of Vater permit intraductal injection of radiopaque contrast medium or a solution of colored dye, which stains the pancreas and surrounding tissues if the duct is ruptured. Alternatively, peroral endoscopic retrograde cannulation of the ducts may be performed during laparotomy.

The treatment of an injury of the distal common bile duct and the head of the pancreas depends upon the severity of damage to the bile and pancreatic ducts. If the main pancreatic and bile ducts are totally disrupted, the procedure of choice is pancreaticoduodenectomy.[44] When the surgeon is unable to determine whether the ducts are disrupted, duodenal diverticularization should be performed and the risk of a postoperative pancreatic and biliary fistula accepted. Duodenal diverticularization consists of vagotomy, hemigastrectomy, gastrojejunostomy, tube duodenostomy, and placement of soft rubber (Penrose) drains near the head of the pancreas (Fig. 41–1).[20] When performed for injury to the head of the pancreas and distal common bile duct, this procedure allows the patient to be nourished through the gastrojejunostomy while fistulae of the pancreas or bile duct are healing. If a biliary-cutaneous fistula develops and the patient is not yet ready to be fed, intravenous hyperalimentation should be instituted, which puts the pancreas and liver at rest during healing of the fistulae. Recent advances in all aspects of patient care, and especially in nutrition, have greatly improved chances of survival with a post-traumatic pancreatic or biliary fistula.

A less common problem, avulsion of the papilla of Vater from its insertion into the duodenum, usually causes enough peritonitis shortly after injury that it can be diagnosed during exploratory laparotomy. When the avulsion is fresh and the margins sharp, the papilla should be reimplanted into its original position and stented with a T-tube inserted through a proximal choledochotomy. If the avulsion has produced a ragged injury, the

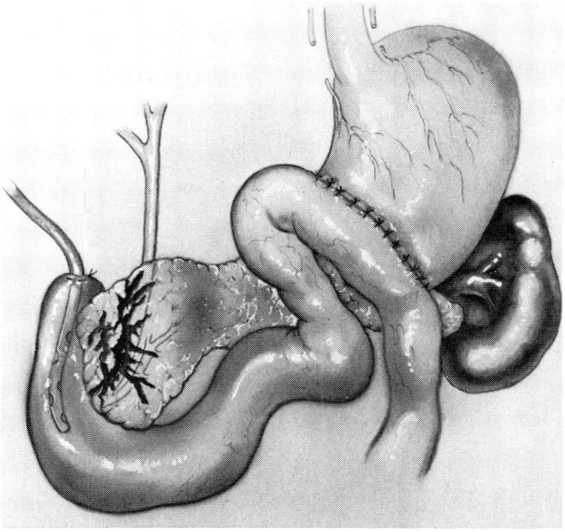

Figure 41–1. The duodenal diverticularization procedure for combined injury to the terminal bile duct and head of the pancreas allows for continued nutrition and decreases the risk of stress gastric bleeding in patients with temporary biliary cutaneous fistulae.

patient must be managed according to the guidelines outlined previously for distal common duct trauma (i.e., by diverticularization), making sure that both biliary and pancreatic flow are re-established into the gastrointestinal tract.

CLOSED GALLBLADDER INJURY

Blunt injury to the gallbladder is infrequent and difficult to diagnose. Schechter was able to find only 110 cases in a review of the literature in 1969.[21] The gallbladder is well protected, cradled between the right and left lobes of the liver. When it is injured by blunt trauma, other viscera are usually uninvolved, and the clinical findings reflect the nature of the gallbladder lesion. Three types of gallbladder injury may occur (Table 41–3).[11, 22] With *complete rupture,* bile spills into the abdomen immediately. The perforation is classically located in the fundus and is probably caused by a sudden increase in intraluminal pressure. Since most patients have been drinking alcohol shortly before injury, it is possible that the choleretic effects of alcohol contribute to rupture by distending the gallbladder with a large volume of bile at the time of impact.[17] Discharge of uninfected bile into the peritoneal cavity produces few immediate signs and symptoms, and, therefore, the nature and significance of the injury is often overlooked for a day or two.[18, 22]

Avulsion of the gallbladder from the liver bed is the most common form of trauma to the gallbladder. This injury, termed traumatic cholecystectomy,[22, 52] probably stems from uneven deceleration of the liver and gallbladder, which causes the gallbladder to be stripped from the liver. When this happens, the gallbladder is attached only by the cystic duct and cystic artery; thereafter, volvulus of the gallbladder is possible, although it is uncommon.[22] Avulsion of the gallbladder usually produces hemoperitoneum due to oozing from the liver bed or to an associated hepatic laceration between the falciform ligament and the gallbladder fossa. Occasionally the cystic artery is also avulsed from the right hepatic artery, leaving only the cystic duct and a few remaining areolar attachments between the gallbladder and liver. In this case, the gallbladder undergoes ischemic necrosis, which results in signs of peritonitis and a clinical syndrome resembling acute cholecystitis.

The mechanism of injury in *incomplete perforation* is probably the same as in complete rupture, except that the increase in intraluminal gallbladder pressure is insufficient to completely disrupt the gallbladder wall. Instead, the fundus is temporarily stretched to the point at which its vasculature is attenuated; it becomes ischemic and then ruptures several days or weeks later. In some cases, an intramural hematoma develops in the gallbladder. The delayed rupture itself may be precipitated by gallbladder contraction in response to eating.[22, 45]

Clinical Features of Gallbladder Injury

Injury to the gallbladder in association with other intraperitoneal injuries is usually found incidentally during exploratory laparotomy for treatment of the more obvious problems.

Table 41–3 TYPES OF BLUNT GALLBLADDER INJURY

Complete Blowout Rupture of Fundus
Progressive early bile ascites—early laparotomy
Early seal of perforation with delayed rupture—late laparotomy
Avulsion from Hepatic Fossa
Usually associated hemoperitoneum—early laparotomy
Contusion or Incomplete Blowout
Minimal early symptoms with quiescent interval
Late rupture of ischemic, weakened fundus

When first examined, patients with an isolated perforation of the gallbladder may have mild hypotension that responds quickly to intravenous fluids; it is not due to volume depletion but could be neurogenic.[22] Following resuscitation, abdominal tenderness and guarding are often absent, and roentgenographic and laboratory data are usually normal. A completely ruptured gallbladder may temporarily become sealed by omentum or adjacent organs and present later as a delayed rupture, with a course similar to that following gallbladder contusion. Continued leakage of bile into the peritoneal cavity from an unsealed perforation eventually produces bile ascites, which is detected by paracentesis or cholescintigraphy.[30, 31, 49, 50] The diagnosis is then usually completed at laparotomy.[17]

Contusion of the gallbladder that is destined to evolve into a late perforation is the most difficult type of gallbladder injury to diagnose in the early postinjury period.[45] After the initial resuscitation, physical findings are minimal or absent. The patient is usually discharged from the hospital and experiences a symptom-free interval of several days, during which he is able to eat and function comfortably before delayed perforation occurs. The manifestations after perforation consist of nausea, vomiting, adynamic ileus, abdominal distention, jaundice, and ascites.[22] The pentad of previous abdominal injury, transient hypotension that responded to fluid administration, a symptom-free interval at home, late adynamic ileus, and jaundice is almost pathognomonic for biliary tract injury (see Table 41–2). The patient may also have noted light-colored stools and dark urine immediately before readmission. Even when the diagnostic pentad has been fully elicited, however, the correct diagnosis is usually not made before laparotomy unless a paracentesis has demonstrated the presence of bile in the abdomen or cholescintigraphy has shown the extravasation of bile.[30, 31, 49, 50] Abdominal x-rays are usually noncontributory, although Fielding and Strachan described a patient in whom a right upper quadrant mass, consisting of bile and inflammatory fluid, displaced the hepatic flexure of the colon inferiorly.[17] More often, abdominal x-rays show only the hazy appearance that results from ascites. Ultrasonography and CT may occasionally show an intramural or intraluminal gallbladder hematoma.[37–39, 51]

Avulsion of the gallbladder from the liver bed is usually associated with bleeding and is diagnosed at the time of a laparotomy performed for hemoperitoneum. Occasionally, however, bleeding is not significant, in which case the diagnosis is made only if the patient develops torsion of the gallbladder with the signs and symptoms of acute cholecystitis.[22]

Post-Traumatic Acute Acalculous Cholecystitis

The differential diagnosis of delayed gallbladder rupture includes post-traumatic acute acalculous cholecystitis, a condition often encountered following recent trauma to some other area.[23, 40–42] Most patients with acalculous cholecystitis have been jaundiced and septic as a result of the remote injury before the onset of right upper quadrant pain, tenderness, and guarding. Laparotomy often reveals necrosis and localized perforation of the fundus of the gallbladder. Cultures of the bile and gallbladder wall are usually positive.[24] Presumably, the responsible bacteria are blood-borne during the period of bacteremia and sepsis. This syndrome may be difficult to distinguish from delayed rupture of the gallbladder following blunt trauma in patients who have associated nonabdominal injuries with suppurative complications. Occasionally, accumulation of blood clots within the gallbladder following trauma may result in acute cholecystitis.[29, 34]

The following case illustrates many of the difficulties inherent in distinguishing between these two syndromes and demonstrates the pitfalls in making the diagnosis of gallbladder rupture in a patient with associated nonabdominal injuries and sepsis.

This 43 year old musician presented to the Detroit General Hospital Emergency Room at 3 A.M. after being thrust against the steering wheel when his car hit an abutment. He was intoxicated, confused, and disoriented. Blood pressure was 105/80 mm Hg, and pulse rate was 120/min. Rapid fluid replacement restored the blood pressure to 150/100 mm Hg and dropped the pulse rate to 95/min. Physical examination and x-rays revealed multiple superficial lacerations and abrasions, a right mandibular fracture, bilateral rib fractures, an underlying lung contusion, dislocation of the right femoral head, a right acetabular fracture, and hematuria (Figs. 41–2 and 41–3). An intravenous pyelogram showed contusion of the right kidney but no extravasation of urine. As sobriety returned over the next 6 hours, the patient began to complain of mild abdominal pain and fullness. Peritoneal lavage at this time was negative.

Initial therapy included balanced skeletal trac-

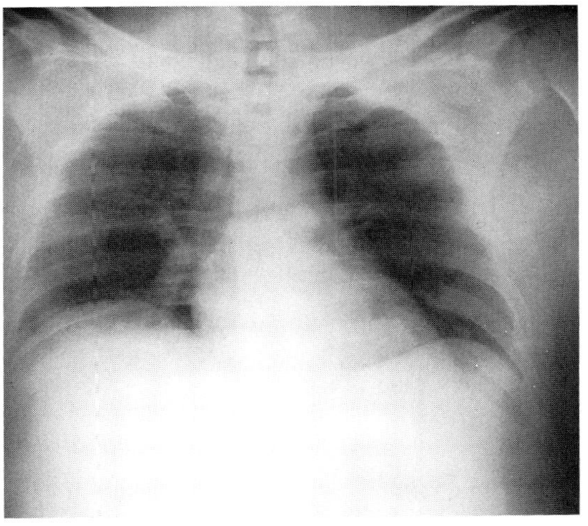

Figure 41–2. Chest x-ray taken shortly after hospital admission following a motorcycle accident. It shows bilateral rib fractures with no pneumoperitoneum or hemothorax.

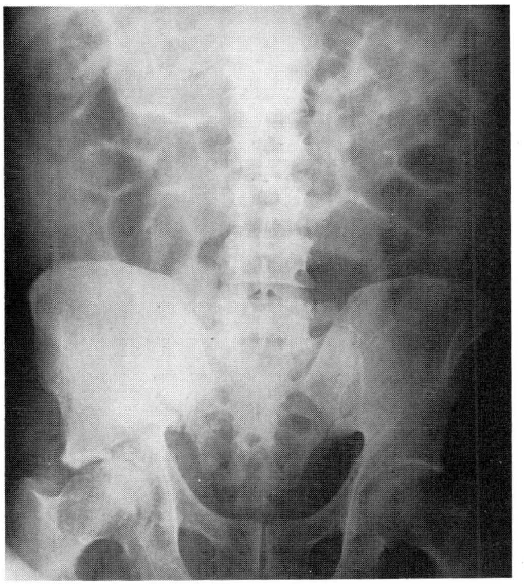

Figure 41–4. Abdominal x-ray taken 18 hours following a motorcycle accident shows an adynamic ileus. Peritoneal lavage at this time was negative.

tion to his right femur, intravenous fluids, and nasogastric decompression. Between 12 and 20 hours after injury the patient became progressively dyspneic and required intubation and ventilatory support. Abdominal roentgenograms showed an adynamic ileus (Fig. 41–4). During the next 6 days he became progressively worse and required high concentrations of inspired oxygen, administration of digitalis, and finally a tracheostomy. Chest roentgenograms suggested fluid overload and contusion and pneumonitis of the right lung. Another paracentesis 7 days after admission revealed straw-colored fluid with a total protein of 1 gm/dl, an amylase level of 51 units, a bilirubin concentration of 1.9 mg/dl, a glucose concentration of 91 mg/dl, a specific gravity of 1.022, and an electrolyte pattern similar to that of interstitial fluid. The serum bilirubin at this time was 2 mg/dl. The straw-colored fluid was thought to represent a transudate related to diffuse sepsis originating in the lungs. The patient remained septic, required large quantities of intravenous fluids to maintain vital signs, and received broad-spectrum antibiotics to cover a mixed bacterial flora cultured from the tracheostomy site and the blood. His general condition improved by the twelfth day after admission; the respiratory failure had improved, the adynamic ileus had resolved, and he had become afebrile.

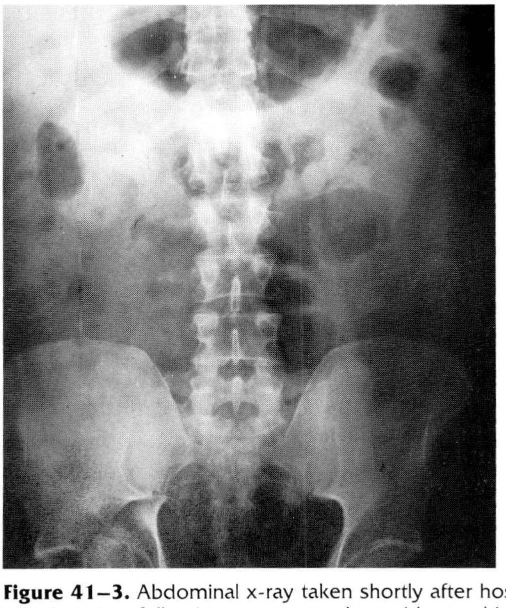

Figure 41–3. Abdominal x-ray taken shortly after hospital admission following a motorcycle accident, which shows a nonspecific gas pattern and no evidence of intra-abdominal injury. The patient had a fracture of the right acetabulum.

On the seventeenth day after admission a second episode of severe sepsis occurred, which was manifested by high fever, leukocytosis (20,000/mm^3), ileus, and the need for large volumes of intravenous fluid. An emergency upper gastrointestinal series was normal. Massive ascites developed within the next 24 hours, which was shown by paracentesis to consist of dark green bile. The serum bilirubin concentration was 5.5 mg/dl. Laparotomy revealed 6 liters of intraperitoneal bile, which had drained through a 1.5 cm ragged laceration in the fundus of the gallbladder (Fig. 41–5). Multiple adhesions between small bowel loops were easily separated by finger dissection. The peritoneal reaction was remarkably minimal considering the duration since injury. The gallbladder perforation was closed in two layers, a tube cholecystostomy was inserted, and the subhepatic space was drained with soft rubber drains. The peritoneal cavity was irrigated with 10 liters

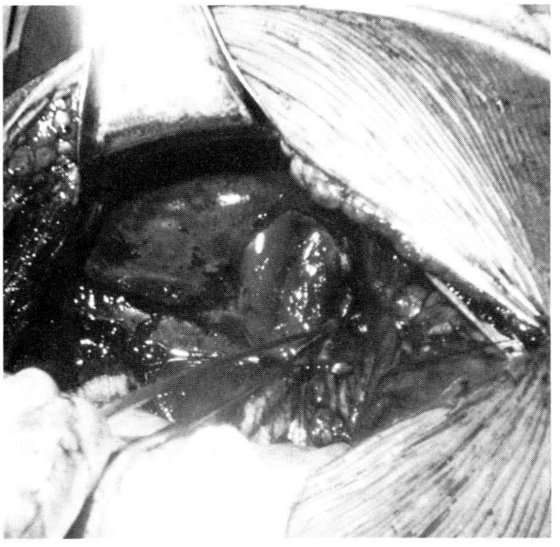

Figure 41–5. Laparotomy performed 18 days following motorcycle accident shows a 1.5 cm ragged tear in the fundus of the gallbladder (end of forceps) and diffuse bile staining with little inflammatory reaction.

of normal saline containing kanamycin, and the abdomen was closed.

Postoperatively, the patient improved rapidly. The tracheostomy was removed 1 week later. The ileus resolved, and the serum bilirubin decreased to 1.3 mg/dl. The patient was transferred to the orthopedic service 1 week later and was discharged ambulatory with a walker after 5 weeks. The cholecystostomy tube was removed 3 months after injury, and a subsequent oral cholecystogram showed good opacification of the gallbladder. One year after the injury the patient was asymptomatic.

Comment

This patient undoubtedly had a gallbladder perforation at the time of his admission. The negative peritoneal lavage was misleading and caused the delay in performing an exploratory laparotomy. The gallbladder injury had probably been sealed by the omentum or some other intra-abdominal viscus in the early postinjury period, and the seal became dislodged shortly before the marked increase in ascites developed. Gallbladder perforation is a more likely explanation for the findings than is acalculous cholecystitis because the rent in the gallbladder was large, there was no necrosis adjacent to it, and there was no gallbladder or peritoneal suppuration.

Treatment of Gallbladder Injury

Cholecystectomy is the treatment of choice for all types of gallbladder injury if the patient's condition is stable and the procedure is technically safe.[29, 45, 52, 55] When the patient is unstable, tube cholecystostomy and drainage of the subhepatic space are adequate. Closure of the perforation plus tube cholecystostomy away from the site of the perforation permits the placement of a more secure pursestring suture around the cholecystostomy site. This approach is also indicated for patients with too much inflammation in the porta hepatis to permit a safe cholecystectomy. Obviously, cholecystectomy is mandatory for patients with gangrene due to volvulus of an avulsed gallbladder.[22, 52]

Some authors prefer a more conservative approach to gallbladder injury. Penn recommends primary repair of a free perforation of the gallbladder (using nonabsorbable sutures) when the injury is clean, is located in an accessible site such as the fundus, and is less than 2 cm.[22] This approach was used by Penn in a 3 year old boy with delayed gallbladder perforation. A postoperative oral cholecystogram in this patient showed normal opacification.[22] There are no data on the incidence of cholelithiasis after primary repair.

Paracholecystic Hematoma

Blunt abdominal injury may produce a linear tear of the liver adjacent to the falciform ligament and extending inferiorly into the gallbladder fossa. Blood from this wound may dissect around the gallbladder and mimic an intramural or intraluminal hematoma of the gallbladder.[34, 37–39] Cholecystectomy is recommended for this type of injury both to exclude an intramural hematoma and to provide exposure of the liver laceration for surgical hemostasis.[25]

PENETRATING WOUNDS OF THE BILIARY TRACT

Because of their position in relation to other viscera, the gallbladder and bile ducts are comparatively well protected from blunt abdominal trauma; they possess no such advantage in the event of penetrating injury, however.

Diagnosis

The criteria for performing a laparotomy in patients with knife or gunshot wounds to the abdomen are controversial. We recommend a laparotomy for all patients with penetrating gunshot wounds of the abdomen. If doubt exists about whether the missile penetrated the peritoneal cavity, this can be resolved by performing peritoneal lavage; if the lavage fluid contains blood, missile penetration is verified, and the chance of a visceral injury is about 98 per cent.[48] If there is no blood in the lavage fluid, the patient can be managed expectantly. Sequential laboratory data, isotopic scans, and ultrasound or CT scan may be of diagnostic help. The last two may show a fluid collection near the bile duct or a liver laceration. Scintigraphy with ^{99m}Tc-HIDA is useful to show a bile leak.[26, 30, 31, 56, 57]

When laparotomy is performed, any sign that the missile passed close to the gallbladder or common duct is an indication for thorough exploration and direct inspection of these structures. If there is any question about whether the missile has injured the intrapancreatic portion of the distal common bile duct, a cholangiogram should be obtained.

Although some surgeons perform laparotomy for all penetrating knife wounds of the abdomen, most observe the patient and explore the abdomen only for signs of peritonitis or bleeding. In these patients, cholescintigraphy offers an easy and noninvasive method to rule out a bile leak.[49, 50] At the time of laparotomy, a thorough exploration should be made of the porta hepatis, common bile duct, and gallbladder for a hematoma or bile staining. Most patients with a penetrating wound of the biliary tract have an associated injury of the liver or some other organ that has caused hemoperitoneum. Perforation of the intraperitoneal portion of the gallbladder is easily recognized (Fig. 41–6). Perforations adjacent to, or within, the hepatic fossa are less apparent but usually are manifested by the presence of blood in the hepatic fossa or the wall of the gallbladder. This injury is similar to paracholecystic hematoma following blunt trauma, and it is treated in the same general way. Cholecystectomy should be performed to rule out perforation of the superior wall of the gallbladder and to provide direct access to the underlying liver injury.[25]

Treatment of Penetrating Wounds of the Biliary Tract

Patients with penetrating wounds of the gallbladder should be treated by cholecystectomy if technically feasible. Penetrating knife wounds of the extrahepatic bile ducts can usually be repaired primarily, and gunshot wounds can usually be managed by primary repair or resection of the wound plus an end-to-end anastomosis. Often the major problem is an associated injury to the portal vein or hepatic artery, with life-threatening hemorrhage.

Repair of a normal-sized bile duct may be technically difficult. The closure may be performed with one layer of interrupted sutures when the duct is less than 5 mm in external diameter (Fig. 41–7). A T-tube stent, inserted either proximal or distal to the injury, is indicated in most cases. I use 5-0 interrupted chromic sutures to repair a partial transection of the bile duct caused by a stab wound, and

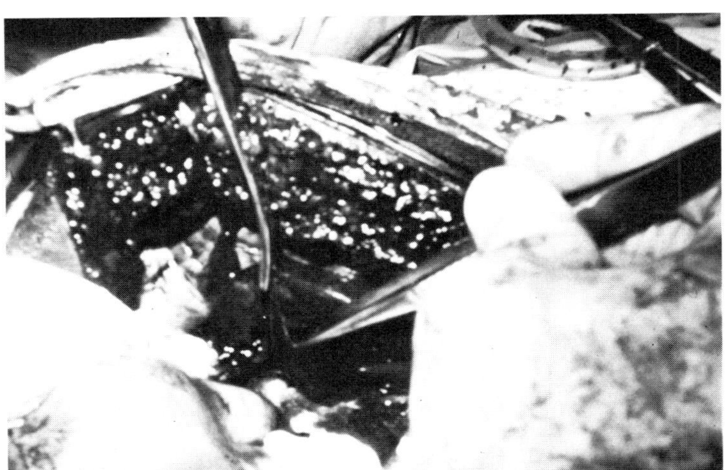

Figure 41–6. Laparotomy for penetrating gunshot wound of the abdomen shows a through-and-through perforation of the gallbladder (end of pick-ups). The bullet then entered the liver near the gallbladder fossa.

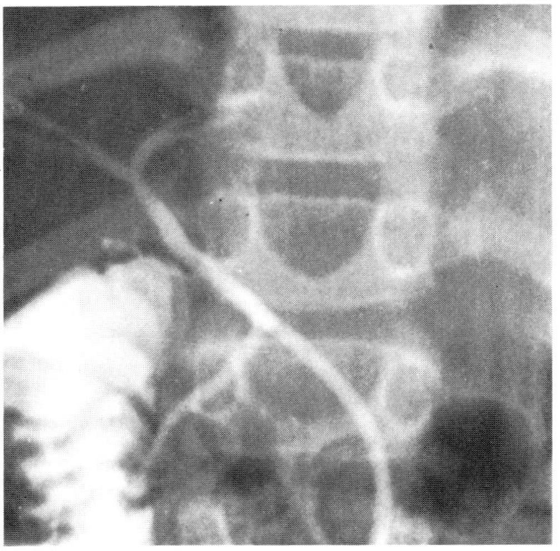

Figure 41–7. T-tube cholangiogram shows a patent common bile duct 3 weeks following an end-to-end anastomosis performed with one layer of interrupted sutures. The diameter of the bile duct was 3 mm.

one layer of interrupted 5-0 chromic or silk sutures to repair a transected duct. Any temporary bile leakage from the repair is easily managed by a soft rubber Penrose drain placed near the anastomosis. After drainage has stopped, the drains can be removed.

If the injury requires excision of 1 cm or more of the bile duct, a direct end-to-end anastomosis cannot be performed satisfactorily. Reconstruction in these cases can be by choledochoduodenostomy or Roux-en-Y choledochojejunostomy.[27] For an end-to-side choledochoduodenostomy with a normal-sized common bile duct, I prefer a one-layer anastomosis using interrupted sutures of 5-0 silk. A T-tube stent is inserted through a proximal choledochotomy. A large duct can be anastomosed to the intestine in two layers. I prefer a continuous 5-0 chromic internal layer and an interrupted 5-0 silk external layer.

Penetrating injuries of the intrapancreatic portion of the distal common bile duct are managed in the same fashion as blunt injuries of this area.[44, 55] The principal difference is that penetrating wounds are often complicated by severe bleeding from the portal vein or superior mesenteric vein behind the pancreas, which may require extensive mobilization of the pancreas and duodenum to obtain the exposure necessary for surgical hemostasis. Persistent bleeding from these structures is one of the few indications for pancreaticoduodenectomy for penetrating injuries of this area. Most patients with a major injury of the intrapancreatic bile duct can be successfully treated by diverting the intestinal flow with a Billroth II gastrectomy and draining the site of the injury. Postoperatively, there may be some bile leakage from the injured distal bile duct, but this generally stops after a few days and is of no immediate consequence unless it cannot escape from the abdomen.[13]

POSTOPERATIVE CARE

The principles of postoperative care for patients with an injury of the gallbladder or extrahepatic bile duct are similar to those for patients with other kinds of trauma. One must pay close attention to the ventilatory status, intake and output records, and function of other organs, particularly the lungs and kidneys. Nasogastric suction is important to treat postoperative ileus and gastric distention and to avoid their effects on ventilation. Broad-spectrum antibiotics are recommended for 3 days postoperatively.

Specific complications that may follow injuries of the gallbladder and extrahepatic bile ducts include subhepatic abscess caused by pooling of inadequately drained blood and bile, biliary-cutaneous fistulae from an anastomotic leak, adynamic ileus, and respiratory insufficiency from sepsis.

Most biliary-cutaneous fistulae will close spontaneously if they are well drained. If the gut is intact and working, the patient may be fed. In more complex situations, total parenteral nutrition may be necessary for a few weeks.

Patients with bile fistulae should not be given their bile to drink, nor do they need supplemental bile salts orally. The extent of malabsorption resulting from a total biliary fistula rarely exceeds 25 per cent, which is compatible with weight gain and good health. There is no indication for dietary restrictions of any kind (e.g., low-fat diet). Absorption of fat-soluble vitamins is affected to a greater extent than is absorption of triglycerides, however, and supplemental doses of vitamins A, D, and K are usually indicated.

Hemobilia

Hemobilia usually results from liver injury in which an intrahepatic hematoma decompresses into the biliary tract and blood passes through the bile ducts into the duodenum. Occasionally, bile may pass into an injured hepatic vein, resulting in marked increase in the serum level of conjugated bilirubin.[33] The manifestations of hemobilia include a history of abdominal or liver injury; right upper quadrant abdominal pain, followed by hematemesis or melena, which gives relief of the abdominal pain; and cholestatic liver function tests. Hepatic arteriography may be diagnostic if it shows an aneurysm within the liver that intermittently builds up pressure and then decompresses into the biliary tract.[28, 32, 36] The spectrum of treatment for post-traumatic hemobilia includes ligation of the artery to the involved segment of liver; hepatotomy and intrahepatic ligation of the injured branch of the hepatic artery; hepatic artery embolization using microspheres, Gelfoam, or autologous clot; or resection of the involved liver segment.[28, 32, 33] Hemobilia may also occur following a penetrating wound that extends through the substance of the liver and the gallbladder bed into the lumen of the gallbladder.[29, 34, 37, 38] Recommended treatment consists of cholecystectomy, at which time the injury to the gallbladder bed will be exposed and the bleeding can be controlled.

REFERENCES

1. Fletcher WS: Non-penetrating trauma to the gallbladder and extrahepatic bile ducts. Surg Clin North Am 1972;*52*:711.
2. Turney W.H, Lee JP, Raju S: Complete transection of the common bile duct due to blunt trauma. Ann Surg 1974;*179*:440.
3. Moffat RC, Lucas RJ: Transection of the common bile duct as an isolated injury following blunt trauma. Can J Surg 1969;*12*:334.
4. Battle WH: Traumatic rupture of the common bile duct. Trans Clin Soc Lond 1894;*27*:144.
5. Lee JG, Wherry DC: Traumatic rupture of the extra-hepatic biliary ducts from external trauma. J Trauma 1961;*1*:105.
6. Moyle WD, Karl RC: Rupture of the extrahepatic biliary duct by external blunt trauma. J Trauma 1969;*9*:623.
7. Spitz L, Von Blerk RJP: Transection of the common bile duct and pelvi-ureteric tract due to seat belt. J Trauma 1971;*11*:226.
8. Maier WB, Lightfoot WP, Rosemond GP: Extrahepatic biliary ductal injury in closed trauma. Am J Surg 1968;*116*:103.
9. Zollinger RM Jr, Keller RT, Hubay CA: Traumatic rupture of the right and left hepatic ducts. J Trauma 1972;*12*:563.
10. Mason L B, Sidbury JB, Guiang S: Rupture of the extrahepatic bile ducts from nonpenetrating trauma. Ann Surg 1954;*140*:234.
11. Steward R, Silan W: Traumatic rupture of the common bile duct. Arch Surg 1961;*82*:387.
12. Mohardt JH: Traumatic rupture of the common bile duct; report of a case and review of the literature. Quart Bull Northw Univ Med Sch 1956;*30*:16.
13. Lucas CE: Diagnosis and treatment of pancreatic and duodenal injury. Surg Clin North Am 1977; *57*:49.
14. Neely WA, Hardy JD: Traumatic severance in the common bile duct. Ann Surg 1961;*154*:874.
15. Rydell WB: Complete transection of the common bile duct due to blunt abdominal trauma. Ann Surg 1970;*100*:724.
16. Dorton HE: Complete division of the common bile duct due to blunt abdominal trauma. Am Surg 1965;*31*:333.
17. Fielding JWL, Strachan CJL: Jaundice as a sign of delayed gallbladder perforation following blunt abdominal trauma. Injury 1975;*7*:66.
18. Cohn I Jr, Cotlar AM, Atik M, et al: Bile peritonitis. Ann Surg 1960;*152*:827.
19. Mast WH, Oz M: Complete severance of the common bile duct due to external blunt trauma to the abdomen. J Int Coll Surg 1960;*34*:726.
20. Beane CJ, Donavan AJ, White EJ, et al: Duodenal diverticulization for duodenal and pancreatic injury. Am J Surg 1974;*127*:503.
21. Schechter DC: Solitary wounding of the gallbladder from blunt abdominal trauma. NY State J Med 1969;*69*:2895.
22. Penn I: Injuries to the gallbladder. Br J Surg 1961–1962;*49*:636.
23. Winegarner FG, Jackson GF: Post-traumatic acalculus cholecystitis: A highly lethal condition. J Trauma 1971;*11*:567.
24. Lucas CE, Walt AJ: Acute gangrenous acalculus cholecystitis in infancy: Report of a case. Surgery 1968;*64*:847.
25. Lucas CE, Ledgerwood AM: Factors influencing outcome after blunt duodenal injury. J Trauma 1975;*15*:839.
26. Weissmann HS, Chun KJ, Frank M, et al: Demonstration of traumatic bile leakage with cholescintigraphy and ultrasonography. Am J R 1979;*133*:843.
27. Busuttil RW, Kitahama A, Cerise E, et al: Management of blunt and penetrating injuries to the porta hepatis. Ann Surg 1980;*191*:641.
28. Sandblom P: Hemobilia: Biliary Tract Hemorrhage. Springfield, Il., C C Thomas, 1972.
29. Saad SA, Rush BF Jr, Devanesan JD, et al: Traumatic hematocele of the gallbladder with hemobilia. J Trauma 1979;*19*:67.
30. Mesgarzadeh M, et al: Diagnosis of clinically unsuspected gallbladder perforation in an obese patient by Tc^{99m}-IDA cholescintigraphy. J Nucl Med 1983;*24*:1028.
31. Brunetti JC, Van Heertum RL: Preoperative detection of gallbladder perforation. Clin Nucl Med 1980;*5*:347.
32. Sandblom P, Saegesser F, Mirkovitch V: Hepatic hemobilia: hemorrhage from the intrahepatic biliary tract. A review. World J Surg 1984;*8*:41.
33. Struyven J, Cremer M, Pirson P, et al: Posttraumatic bilhemia: diagnosis and catheter therapy. AJR 1982;*138*:746.
34. Lewis J, Varma V, Tice H, et al: Hepatobiliary scanning in hemobilia-induced acute cholecystitis. Gastrointest Radiol 1982;*7*:169.
35. Nielsen SL, Mygind T, Miskowiak J: Blood pool scintigraphy and arterial embolization in traumatic hemobilia. Eur J Nucl Med 1982;*7*:389.

36. Olsen WR: Late complications of central liver injuries. Surgery 1982;*92*:733.
37. Daneman A, Matzinger MA, Martin DJ: Posttraumatic hemorrhage into the gallbladder. CT 1983;*7*:59.
38. Grand EG, Smirniotopoulos JG: Intraluminal gallbladder hematoma: sonographic evidence of hemobilia. J Clin Ultrasound 1983;*13*:348.
39. Gottesman L, Marks RA, Khoury PT, et al: Diagnosis of isolated perforation of the gallbladder following blunt trauma using sonography and CT scan. J Trauma 1984;*24*:280.
40. Gately JF, Thomas EJ: Acute cholecystitis occurring as a complication of other diseases. Arch Surg 1983;*118*:1137.
41. Howard RJ: Acute acalculous cholecystitis. Am J Surg 1981;*141*:194.
42. Orlando R, Gleason E, Drezner AD: Acute acalculous cholecystitis in the critically ill patient. Am J Surg 1983;*145*:472.
43. Rozran RS, Preston DF, McMillan JH: Hepatobiliary imaging for demonstration of bile leaks. Clin Nucl Med 1984;*9*:189.
44. Oreskovich MR, Carrico CJ: Pancreaticoduodenectomy for trauma: a viable option? Am J Surg 1984;*147*:618.
45. Wiener I, Watson LC, Wolma FJ: Perforation of the gallbladder due to blunt abdominal trauma. Arch Surg 1982;*117*:805.
46. Zeman RK, Lee CH, Stahl R, et al: Strategy for the use of biliary scintigraphy in non-iatrogenic biliary trauma. Radiology 1984;*151*:771.
47. Saber K, El-Manialawi M: Repair of biliary duct injuries. World J Surg 1984;*8*:82.
48. Burney RE, Mueller GL, Mackenzie JR: Evaluation of experimental blunt and penetrating hepatobiliary trauma by sequential peritoneal lavage. Ann Emerg Med 1983;*12*:279.
49. Sty JR, Starshak RJ, Hubbard AM: Radionuclide evaluation in childhood injuries. Semin Nucl Med 1983;*13*:258.
50. Weissmann HS, Byun KJ, Freeman LM: Role of Tc-^{99m} IDA scintigraphy in the evaluation of hepatobiliary trauma. Semin Nucl Med 1983;*13*:199.
51. Federle MP: CT of abdominal trauma. CRC Crit Rev Diagn Imaging 1983;*19*:257.
52. Fotheringham GH: Traumatic avulsion of the gallbladder. S Afr J Surg 1983;*21*:125.
53. Weil PH: Management of retroperitoneal trauma. Curr Probl Surg 1983;*20*:540.
54. Khodadadi J, Mihich M, Finally R, et al: Avulsion of common bile duct after blunt abdominal injury: a review of the literature. Injury 1983;*14*:447.
55. Kitahama A, Elliott LF, Overby JL, et al: The extrahepatic biliary tract injury: perspective in diagnosis and treatment. Ann Surg 1982;*195*:536.
56. Sty JR, Starshak RJ, Hubbard AM: Radionuclide hepatobiliary imaging in the detection of traumatic biliary tract disease in children. Pediatr Radiol 1982;*12*:115.
57. Caride VJ, Gibson DW: Noninvasive evaluation of bile leakage. Surg Gynecol Obstet 1982;*154*:517.

PHILIP SANDBLOM, M.D.

42

Hemobilia

Hemorrhage into the biliary tract has been termed "hemobilia" or sometimes "hematobilia" from the Greek *haima,* blood, and the Latin *bilis,* bile (thus, another linguistic hybrid). It occurs when disease or trauma opens a communication between blood vessels and bile ducts, either within the liver or within the extrahepatic biliary tract.[1]

Hemobilia is analogous to hematuria in urinary tract disease. The two syndromes would be expected to have a close resemblance, as they occur in similar systems consisting of a large excreting parenchymal mass and an outflow tract connected to a collecting bladder and controlled by a distal sphincter. Whereas hematuria is a well-established sign of urinary tract disease, hemobilia is a syndrome that long remained obscure. This is not only because hemobilia occurs less often than hematuria but also because bleeding into the biliary tract is harder to recognize. If the urine becomes bloody, it is noticed immediately, but if blood enters the intestine through the papilla of Vater, it will come to light only as hematemesis or melena, and its origin may easily be mistaken or go unidentified. A surprising number of cases of hemobilia have, for this reason, been treated inadequately. While hematuria is a reliable sign of urinary tract disease, hemobilia usually must be differentiated from other more common bleeding sources in the gastrointestinal tract. This may be difficult, as absence of biliary tract symptoms frequently leaves the clinician without a clue. Hematuria is rarely of such magnitude that the blood loss requires treatment. Hemobilia, on the other hand, is often not only a symptom but also a dangerous, sometimes life-threatening complication that may constitute the main reason for treatment.

Because of its apparent rarity, hemobilia was slow to become an acknowledged entity. It was repeatedly discovered, only to be forgotten again. As early as 1654, Francis Glisson,[2] in the first detailed description of the anatomy of the liver, discussed the possibility of hemorrhage through the biliary tract in the following words (Fig. 42–1):

> Quod mihi argumento eſt, vaſa fellea nonnunquam aliuun humorem (ſi forte obvenerit) præter bilem, in inteſtina deferre: arbitrorque, læſo ex contuſione aliqua hepate, ſequi poſſe, per vomitum aut alvum, ſanguinis ejectionem; quod nimirum porus bilarius (magno ægri commodo) partem aliquam ſanguinis hepar opprimentis in ſe recipiat, & ad inteſtina deducat; unde vel motu periſtatico inverſo, ſurſum; vel eodem regulariter ſe habente, deorſum feratur.

I believe that if the liver is injured by a contusion, it may lead to blood leaving the body by way of vomit or the stool for there is no doubt that the biliary tract takes unto itself (to the great good of the patient) some of the blood issuing into the liver and leads it down to the intestines. From there it is either impelled upwards through reverse peristalsis or downwards the normal way.

Hemobilia was formerly regarded as a medical curiosity, but it is now being diagnosed with increasing frequency, owing to more widespread knowledge of the syndrome and to improved diagnostic methods.[3–6] There may, in addition, be an absolute increase in frequency because of the rising number of traffic accidents and the use of diagnostic and therapeutic techniques that result in liver injury.[3, 7–9]

ETIOLOGY

Common causes of hemobilia are trauma (either in connection with an accident or iatrogenic), inflammatory processes, gallstones, tumors, and vascular disorders. Their relative frequency is shown in Figure 42–2. The proportion noted in the diagram relates to massive or major hemobilia in a series of over 500 cases collected from the world literature.[1] Hemobilia is rather uncommon, and most surgeons will probably see only a few cases during their careers. If, on the other hand, cases of minor or occult hemobilia are included, gallstone etiology constitutes the overwhelming majority, since passage of gallstones through the biliary tract is nearly always accompanied by minute bleeding from the injured mucosa.[10, 11] In the era before cholecystography, the occurrence of microscopic melena after attacks of biliary colic was one of the main diagnostic signs of gallstone disease.

PATHOPHYSIOLOGY

Bleeding in hemobilia can be of varying degrees, from profuse violent hemorrhage causing shock and eventually death from exsanguination, to occult bleeding, which, if continued, may result in chronic secondary anemia. Most hemorrhage of consequence is arterial in origin. When only veins are injured, the bleeding is slight; in fact, the abnormal communication between the bile ducts and a hepatic vein may result in passage of bile into the venous circulation rather than blood into the bile ducts.[12] In patients with portal hypertension, venous injuries may lead to substantial hemobilia.

Hemobilia has been of greatest interest to clinicians when it occurs as profuse bleeding with massive hematemesis or melena, while minor hemobilia, though much more frequent, has been unjustly neglected.

Biliary colic and jaundice, the cardinal symptoms of hemobilia, reflect the formation of blood clots in the biliary tract that pass through or obstruct the ducts. Clot formation is influenced by the quality and quantity of bleeding. The development and fate of clots depend on whether they are dissolved, expelled into the intestine, or retained in the tract. To allow investigation in vitro of the course of events, a model of the biliary tract was constructed with bile flowing through it.[13] Blood was injected into this system in various ways. When introduced forcefully to imitate a major hemorrhage (Fig. 42–3*A*), the blood mixed with the bile and formed mushy clots that ultimately dissolved spontaneously owing to the fibrinolytic quality of bile. It was of great interest to note that when the blood was injected slowly to imitate minor hemobilia (Fig. 42–3*B*), it did not mix but instead flowed to the lowest level, where it formed a solid clot of pure blood. This finding contradicts the widespread idea that in minor hemobilia the blood remains fluid and flows unobtrusively into the intestine; it demonstrates how, even in these cases, clots may form that may be mistaken for gallstones.[14]

The pure clots are more solid and tenacious than the mixed ones. In either case, when clots are subjected to flowing bile, they eventually dissolve; if they are protected from the bile stream, however, they remain intact. Through its fibrinolytic properties, bile plays the same role as urine and saliva; namely, it clears the ducts of fibrin deposits. A clinical example of the rapidity and efficiency of this process is given in Figure 42–4. Following a percutaneous liver biopsy, the resulting hemorrhage gave rise to a long coagulum nearly filling the right hepatic ducts. At operation 12 hours later, only small fragments of this clot were encountered.

If, on the other hand, the bile flow is diverted or obstructed, the clots remain. In one case (Fig. 42–5), a common duct drain was left in place for 4 weeks, with the result that a solid clot remained and was misinter-

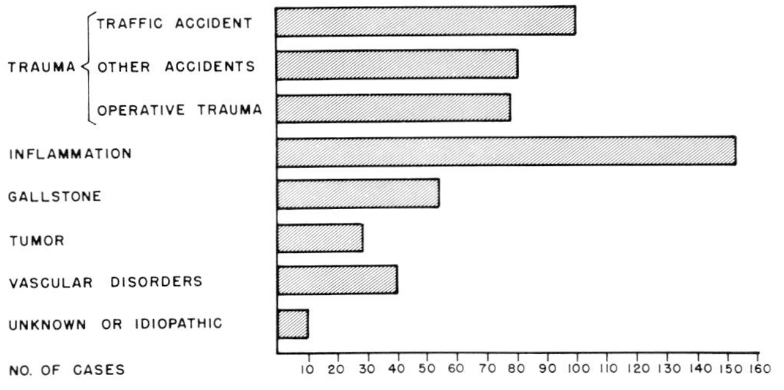

Figure 42–2. Distribution of 545 published cases of hemobilia with respect to cause.

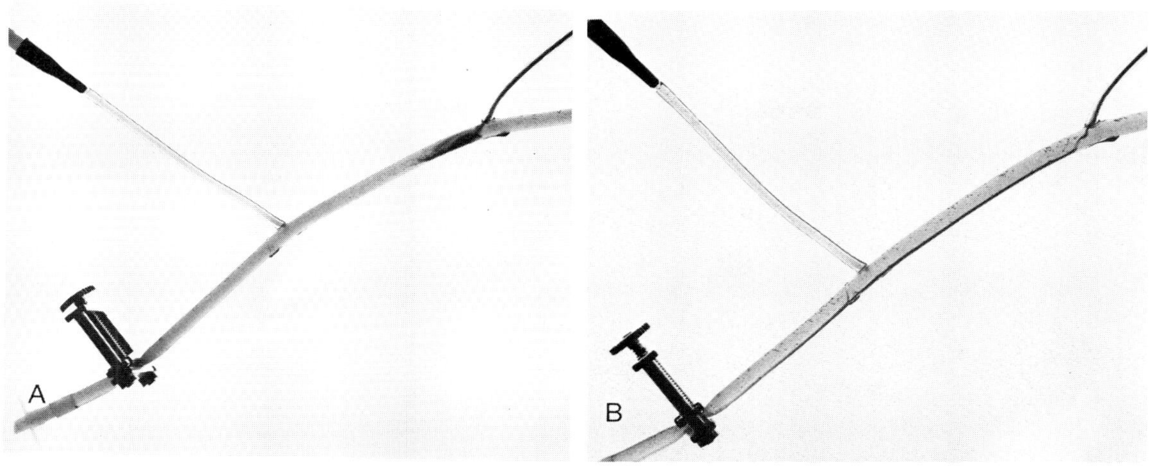

Figure 42–3. Polyvinyl chloride tubing model of the extrahepatic bile ducts. The upper tube on the left provides an outlet for the bile flow and represents a common duct drain (or the cystic duct). The clamp on the left represents a closed sphincter. Blood is injected into bile streaming through the system. *A*, When injected forcefully to imitate major hemobilia, it causes turbulence and mixes with the bile. *B*, When injected slowly to imitate minor hemobilia, it flows immiscibly to the lower portion and forms a pure coagulum.[13]

preted as a retained stone. In another case (Fig. 42–6), a solid clot totally obstructed the ampullary region and was thus unaffected by any bile flow; it had to be removed by operation for relief of the obstructive jaundice.

These clinical and experimental observations show how important it is for the surgeon to remember that a free body in the biliary tract is not always a stone. It may be a fibrin deposit or a blood clot, even if no hemobilia has been observed. If this is the case, operation will not be necessary—the fibrinolytic effect of the bile will generally suffice to clear the biliary tract. The surgeon

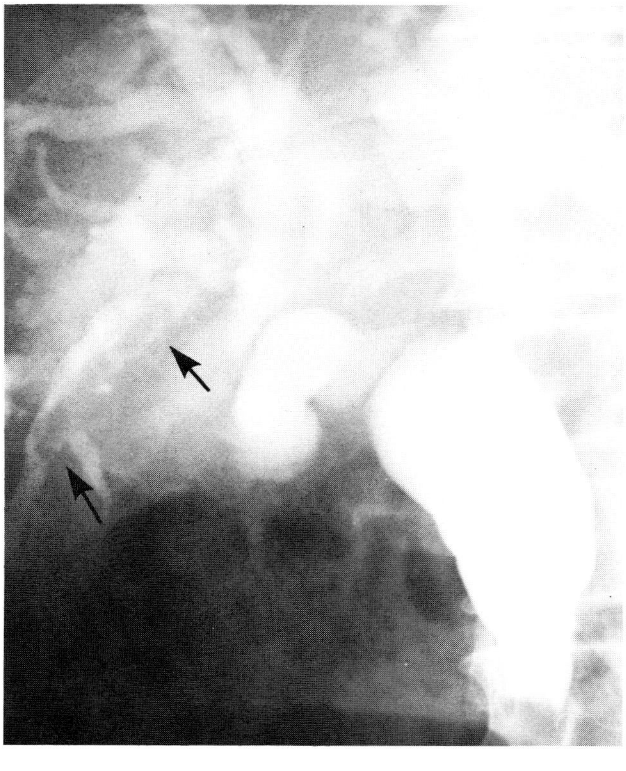

Figure 42–4. Transhepatic cholangiogram 30 minutes after liver puncture in a patient with obstructive jaundice. There is an impacted stone at the ampulla and a defect 4 cm long in the intrahepatic bile duct representing a coagulum (between the arrows). At operation (24 hours later) it was found that the coagulum had been nearly totally dissolved. (Veterans Administration Hospital, San Diego.)

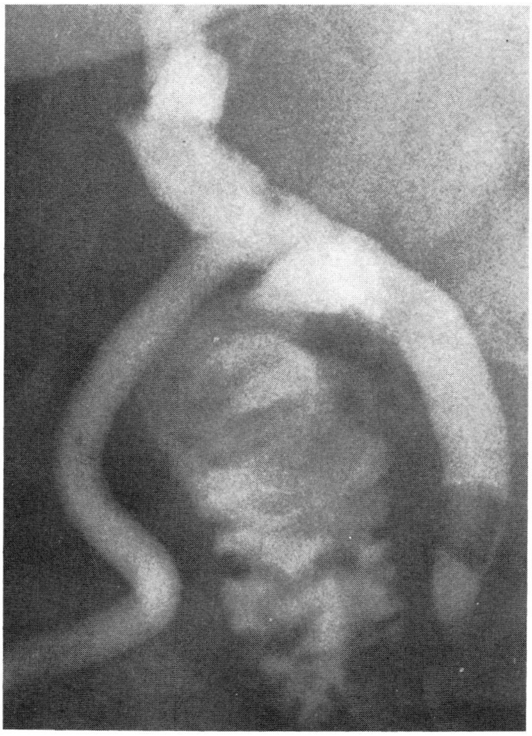

Figure 42–5. Cholangiogram 4 weeks after choledocholithotomy. A defect thought to represent a remaining stone is observed; at re-laparotomy a blood clot corresponding to the defect was extracted, whereupon repeated cholangiogram was normal. (University Hospital, Lausanne, Switzerland.)

must avoid measures that prevent the bile from exerting this action. If a suspected clot still remains, perfusion or washouts with bile or streptokinase may be tried. If a clot continues to cause a total obstruction that helps it to escape fibrinolysis, it will eventually have to be extracted.[15, 16]

Bearing in mind the fibrinolytic effect of bile, reports of successful dissolution of "remaining stones" through perfusion with various media should be reassessed—it might occasionally just have been a question of fibrinolysis and expulsion of clots.[13]

CLINICAL SIGNS

The pathognomonic symptom triad of hemobilia includes *gastrointestinal bleeding* (melena in 90 per cent of the patients and hematemesis in 60 per cent), *biliary colic* (in 70 per cent), and *jaundice* (in 60 per cent). Gastrointestinal hemorrhage in connection with biliary symptoms should always awaken suspicion of hemobilia. Hemobilia is known for its periodic appearance and does not often cease spontaneously—hence the need for treatment. Minor hemobilia may run an entirely symptomless course, but it also may, as demonstrated earlier, show all the signs of solid clot formation.

DIAGNOSIS

Because of the characteristic and consistent symptom triad, the diagnosis of hemobilia is easy to suspect, provided that one is aware of the syndrome. Far too many cases of hemobilia have been diagnosed too late (e.g., at autopsy)[3, 11, 17, 18] or after undue delay, following one or more inappropriate or inadequate operations, such as "blind gastric resection."

The best way of verifying a suspected diagnosis of hemobilia is by *selective arteriography* of the hepatic artery, which will reveal the source of bleeding in most cases (Fig. 42–7).[19] Passage of contrast medium into the biliary tract during arteriography is seen in approximately 25 per cent of patients and confirms the diagnosis.[4] Arteriography usually defines and localizes the arterial lesion even if contrast material is not seen passing into the bile ducts.[5, 20, 21] This procedure is of special value in discovering central liver lesions, which may be difficult or impossible to localize even at exploratory laparotomy. *Cholangiography* may reveal a lesion either by contrast agent filling a cavity or by displace-

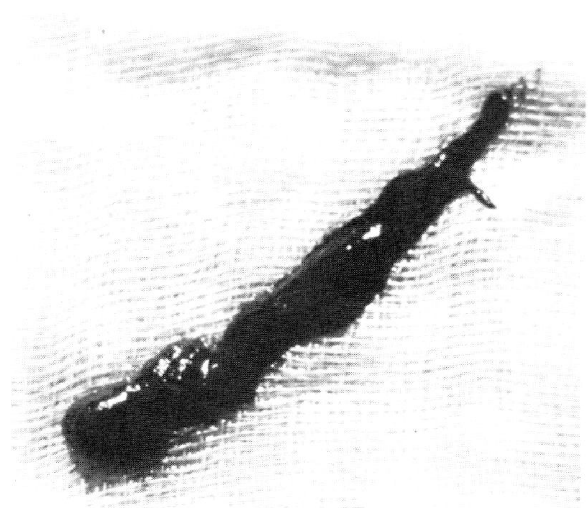

Figure 42–6. Blood clot extracted from the common duct in a case of traumatic hemobilia. Note the impression of the sphincter with a cast of the confluence of the duct of Wirsung. (L. Räf, Serafimerlasarettet, Stockholm).

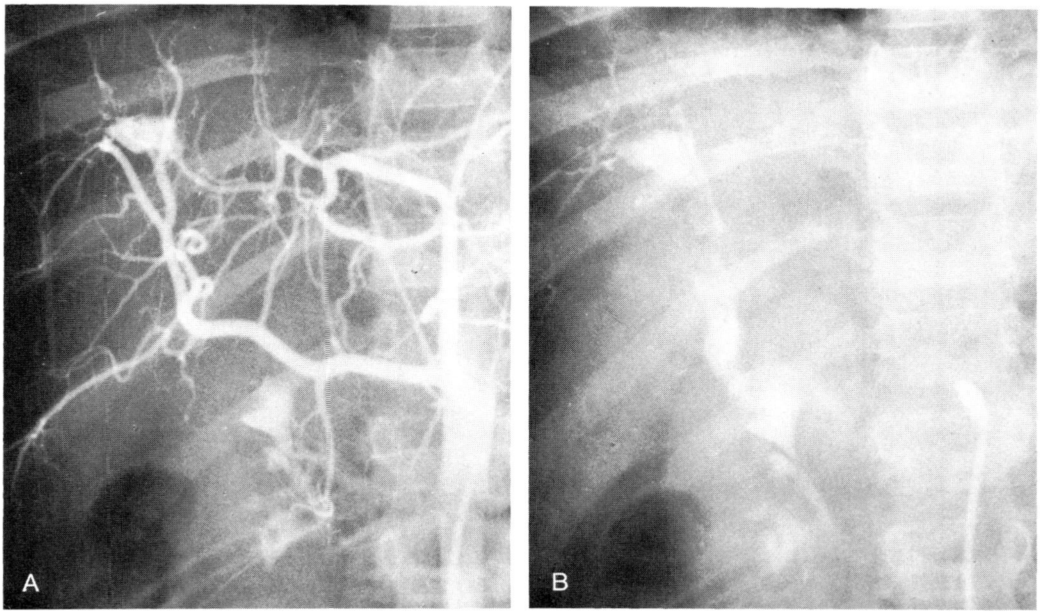

Figure 42–7. Selective angiograms of the hepatic artery in a case of central liver puncture. The radiologist has managed to catch the passage of blood and contrast medium from the artery through the central lesion and down into the common duct.[19] *A*, The pooling of contrast medium in the center of the right lobe shows the site and size of the cavity. *B*, A few seconds later, the right hepatic duct fills with contrast medium directly from the lesion. (Courtesy of T. Enge, Oslo.)

ment of the ducts. *Ultrasonography* has become of great value because even small lesions may be discovered. Thus, a small intrahepatic hematoma[4] and even an intrahepatic arteriobiliary fistula[22] may be diagnosed. The presence of clots in the gallbladder may be seen on ultrasonography as heterogeneous dependent echogenic formations without acoustic shadows.[23] *Computerized tomography* is useful in identifying intrahepatic hematomas, which present as areas of decreased density.[24–26]

Tc-99m scintigraphy may also identify intrahepatic hematomas.[27–29] *Gastrointestinal endoscopy* is a beneficial diagnostic procedure in these patients, as most present with upper gastrointestinal bleeding. The endoscopist can eliminate many alternative diagnoses and may be fortunate enough to see blood coming from the ampulla of Vater.[11, 30] Endoscopic papillotomy may also be used to relieve the common duct obstruction caused by a clot.[15, 16, 31]

CHARACTERISTICS OF THE DIFFERENT ETIOLOGIC GROUPS

Trauma

There is a great difference in the clinical manifestations of liver lesions that tear the liver capsule and those that do not (i.e., subcapsular or central liver rupture). The former produce dangerous, violent intra-abdominal hemorrhage and generally require an emergency operation to save the life of the patient. Hemobilia is rare with this lesion, as the blood flows more readily into the low-pressure peritoneal cavity than down through the biliary tract. Traumatic hemobilia is found more often in patients with a central liver rupture causing less acute and more obscure symptoms.

While the mechanism with penetrating trauma is evident, it is more complicated in blunt trauma. If the liver is compressed, the fragile and inelastic parenchyma tears easily (Fig. 42–8). The disrupting force is greatest in the middle of the organ, which explains the high frequency of central liver rupture. This is often combined with smaller superficial rifts caused by the direct force. When the surgeon sees these rifts at emergency exploration, he is apt to be satisfied that they represent the major injury, and he may miss a central cavity that is not grossly visible. The surgeon may even create a defect that predisposes to hemobilia if he superficially sutures a deep laceration.[32] Hemobilia may then appear as an unpleasant surprise later (See Fig. 42–10).[9]

Central liver ruptures may vary in size

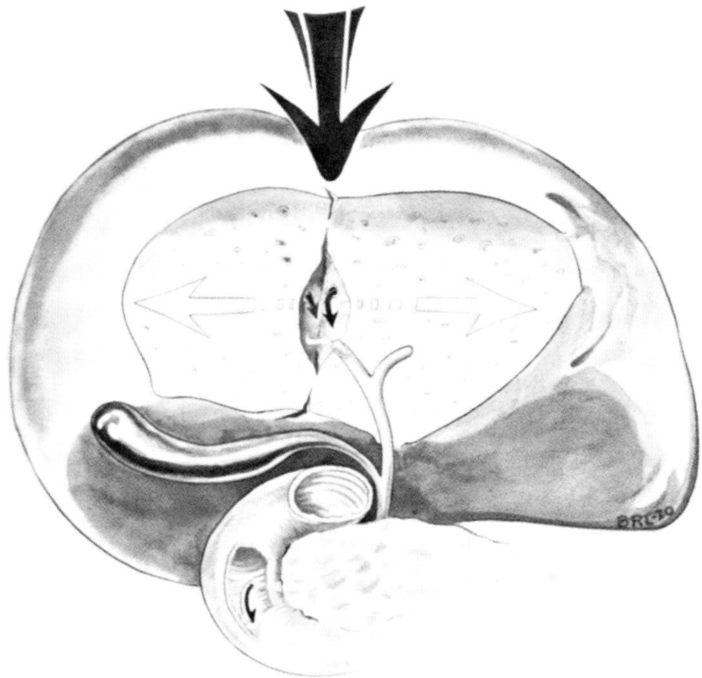

Figure 42–8. Schematic drawing of a liver injury. Traumatic compression of the liver (black arrow) results in disruptive forces (white arrows), thereby producing both superficial rifts and internal rupture. The inflowing blood leaves with the bile through the bile ducts.[1]

from large cavities extending into both lobes to small arteriobiliary fistulae. Occasionally, no bleeding, or only temporary bleeding, occurs, but most often there will be a longstanding hemobilia. The course of events in these cavities accounts for the typical clinical history of patients with traumatic hemobilia. The rupture tears bile ducts, arteries, and veins, which fill the cavity with bile and blood. If a larger artery is torn, exsanguinating gastrointestinal hemorrhage may occur, necessitating emergency surgery to save the patient's life. Usually, however, the cavity fills slowly, and the escape of bloody bile will be delayed by coagulation in the cavity or in the duct, assisted by contraction of the sphincter of Oddi. Finally, after days, weeks, or even months, the pressure in the cavity will suddenly force the clot down the tract into the intestine, followed by a gush of blood and bile.

During these events, the patient first experiences an increasing, dull pain over the liver. Sometimes hepatomegaly can be detected, and there may be signs of obstructive jaundice. Eventually the patient experiences intense biliary colic followed by hematemesis and melena. Sometimes he vomits long clots that are casts of the biliary tract. Unfortunately, relief is usually only temporary; the events will be repeated over months and years. The syndrome is characterized by periodicity, and there is little hope for spontaneous healing. A long interval between trauma and clinically manifest hemobilia may obscure the causal relationships—this may be one of the reasons why hemobilia is reported to be so uncommon following liver trauma.

The explanation for the curious course of traumatic hemobilia lies in the fact that the liver regenerates quickly but heals slowly. Animal experiments[33] have yielded an explanation for this paradox. Liver wounds inflicted from the peritoneal cavity heal promptly (Figure 42–9*A*), whereas those made through the gallbladder, which contains bile, heal slowly or not at all (Fig. 42–9*B*). It is the presence of bile in the hemobilia cavities that inhibits healing. When treating liver lesions, surgeons should consequently make an effort to prevent bile from leaking into the liver wound.

Ultrasound and CT scans are useful to diagnose the intrahepatic hematomas,[4, 24, 25] and angiography provides the definitive diagnosis in most cases.[5, 20] Since spontaneous healing is rare, the only hope for cure is adequate surgical treatment.

Although major hemobilia from liver trauma is considerably less frequent than minor hemobilia, it is still common enough that every surgeon should be able to diagnose

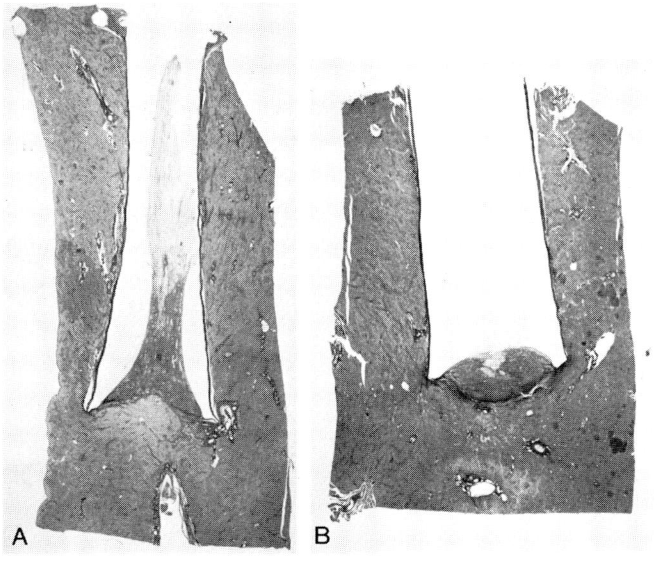

Figure 42–9. The healing of liver wounds 3 months after lesion. *A*, Wound open to the peritoneal cavity. *B*, Wound through the gallbladder containing bile shows a marked delay in healing.[33]

and treat it, especially since appropriate surgery will substantially decrease the mortality and morbidity rates.

Adequate handling of a liver lesion at the primary emergency laparotomy in patients who have sustained trauma to the liver may prevent later hemobilia. Simple packing or drainage is not sufficient.[34] The operation should include careful exploration of cavities, precise hemostasis, and suture of open bile radicles before drainage and closure. If this does not suffice, or if hemobilia occurs in spite of these efforts, a more radical procedure, preceded by arteriography, will be necessary. The choice is then between hepatic resection[32] and hepatic artery occlusion[35] (Fig. 42–10). (For details, see Chapter 41, Trauma to the Biliary Tract.) The decision depends on the location of injury, as the results of either treatment are satisfactory (Fig. 42–11).

For peripheral and well-localized lesions, resection is preferred. For those close to the hilum, where resection would be difficult or impossible, ligation of the hepatic artery or one of its branches may be the treatment of choice. A prerequisite for this procedure is free flow of blood through the portal vein. An alternative noninvasive method of arterial interruption is angiographic embolization.[36] Abnormal communications between the branches of the hepatic artery and the biliary tract can be selectively occluded by large particulate material, such as Gelfoam sponge, polyvinyl alcohol foam (Ivalon), or detachable balloons or coils.[37]

Successful treatment of hemobilia by arterial embolization was first reported by Walter et al. in 1976.[38] Embolic occlusion of the hepatic artery soon became the treatment of choice for patients with hemobilia following percutaneous liver biopsy.[39, 40] Today, hepatic artery embolization is the treatment of choice for patients with hemobilia from trauma who do not require operative treatment for associated injuries.[20, 21, 27, 41–43]

Curet's collected series reflects the increased use of noninvasive techniques in the treatment of hemobilia. Of 73 patients treated between 1976 and 1981, only 4 patients required hepatectomy, which was successful in each case. Sixteen patients were treated by ligature of the hepatic artery, which was successful in 13, and 28 patients underwent embolization, which was successful in 24.[4] Several advantages make embolization preferable to surgery in the treatment of hemobilia. Embolization requires no general anesthetic; can be readily performed; can be directed to the segmental branches of the hepatic artery, reducing the risk of hepatic necrosis; and can be repeated safely if hemobilia recurs as collateral vessels develop.[4, 5]

Iatrogenic Injury

During biliary tract surgery, the hepatic artery may be damaged by a suture or by the dissection, which may result in an arteriobiliary fistula or in a false aneurysm leaking or

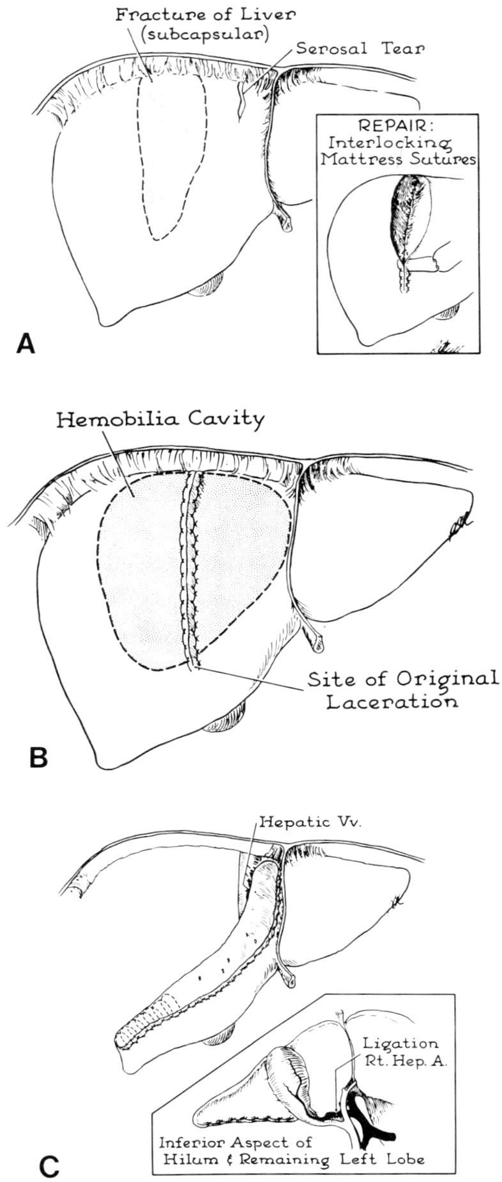

Figure 42–10. *A,* A subcapsular liver fracture is treated with a superficial suture but without proper attention to deep tears of blood vessels and bile ducts. A superficial tear is also seen. *B,* The resulting hemobilia cavity. *C,* Liver resection did not suffice to stop the bleeding, and a right hepatic artery ligature had to be added. This case illustrates the three main methods of surgical treatment: primary local measures, hepatic resection (both insufficient in this case), and arterial ligature. (From Poulos E, et al: Arch Surg *88*:596, 1974. Used by permission.)

eroding into the extrahepatic bile ducts.[44–46] Intrahepatic lesions are caused more commonly by instrumentation of the biliary tree. Instruments often damage the walls of the intrahepatic ducts, and minor bleeding often results from such procedures; however, hemorrhage usually ceases spontaneously, and the clots promptly dissolve.[3, 4] Not all surgeons are aware of the vulnerability of the intrahepatic ducts, and efforts to extract intrahepatic calculi may seriously injure the ductal wall. As the hepatic arteries are nearby, there is a risk of causing an intrahepatic hematoma if an artery is torn. The result may be profuse hemobilia, which often exits through the T-tube (Fig. 42–12).

Percutaneous instrumentation of the liver sometimes gives rise to hemobilia (see Fig. 42–4), although macroscopic hemobilia is rare if a fine-caliber needle is used. Nevertheless, with the increased use of percutaneous needle biopsy and percutaneous cannulation of the biliary ducts for cholangiography or drainage, the number of patients with iatrogenic traumatic hemobilia has markedly increased.[6–8, 47–50] Whereas iatrogenic hemobilia accounted for 17 per cent of all cases of hemobilia in a review concluded in 1972,[1] it was found to be the cause in 50 (68 per cent) of 73 patients reported between 1976 and 1981.[4]

Iatrogenic hemobilia may be seen immediately following the procedure or a few days later. The former is the result of a direct communication between the branches of the hepatic artery and the biliary tract caused by the needle or the catheter used. The latter may result from the evacuation of an intrahepatic hematoma or by secondary rupture of an intrahepatic arterial aneurysm (caused by the original trauma) into the bile ducts.[4, 7, 51] In a series of 300 transhepatic biliary catheter placements, Sarr et al. reported nine patients with hemobilia. Of these, five patients had hepatic artery pseudoaneurysms, three had arterioportal venous fistulae, and in one the cause could not be established by angiography. Seven patients were treated successfully with embolization.[52]

The formation of a pseudoaneurysm following percutaneous biliary catheter placement may be more common than previously recognized.[45] Indeed, Hoevels et al. found that 25 per cent of 83 patients who had routine angiography after percutaneous transhepatic cholangiography had developed intrahepatic vascular lesions from the catheter (14 had pseudonaneurysms, six had arterioportal fistulae, and one had an arteriohepatic vein fistula).[50] Intrahepatic hematomas have been reported in 7 per cent of patients undergoing percutaneous liver biopsy;[48] in one series, severe hemorrhage was noted among 6.4 per cent of patients undergoing percutaneous biliary drainage.[49]

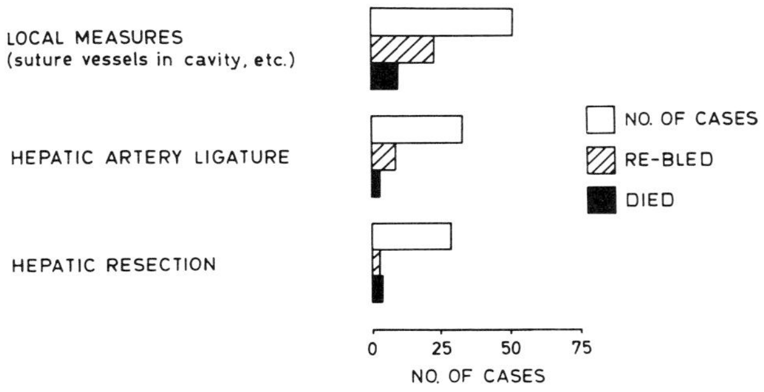

Figure 42–11. The results of the three main types of operative procedures for liver rupture causing hemobilia, with regard to rebleeding and mortality.

In patients who have indwelling biliary catheters, hemobilia may be arrested by manipulation of the catheter. Occasionally, pushing the catheter farther into the biliary ducts or removing the catheter may stop the hemorrhage.[52] Laser photocoagulation of the tract has also been used successfully.[10] Major hemobilia after operation or liver puncture may cease spontaneously. When more active intervention is necessary, embolization of the bleeding artery is the treatment of choice.[4, 37, 52–54] With this technique, hemobilia can be arrested in over 95 per cent of patients. Arterial ligation deprives an unnecessarily large amount of parenchyma of arterial blood supply.

Inflammation

The large number of inflammatory cases has a peculiar geographic distribution—all originate in the Orient (China, Vietnam, and Korea). The causative agent in this category is *Ascaris,* a nematode with a tendency to invade the bile ducts, where it frequently

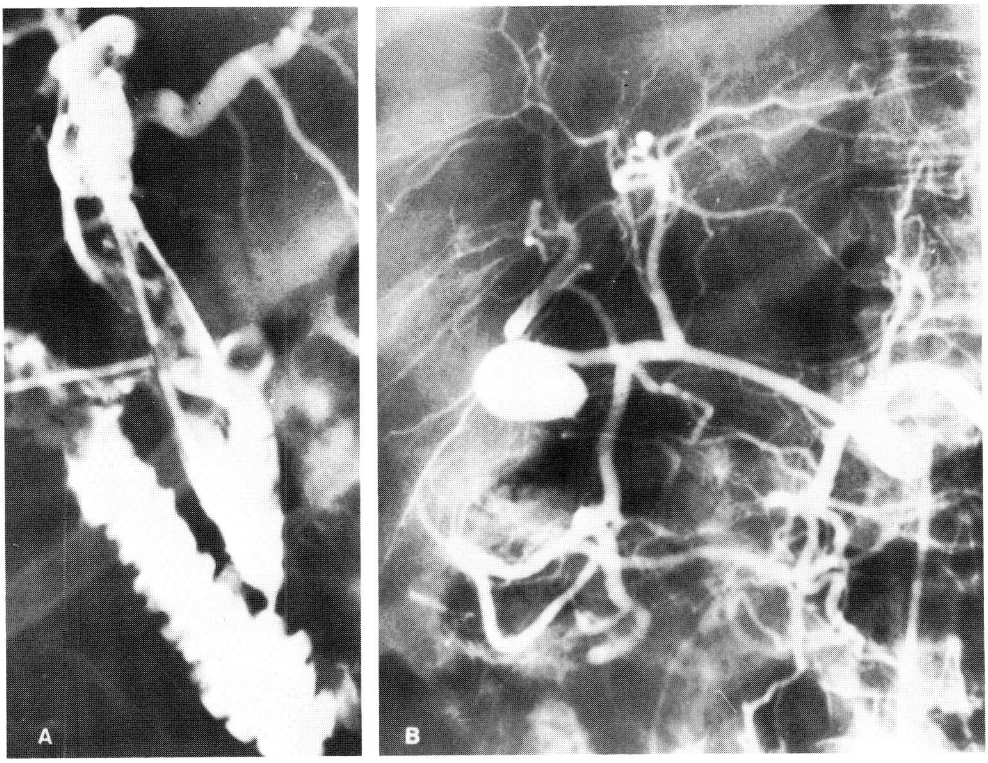

Figure 42–12. Cholangiogram and arteriogram in a patient with an operative lesion of the bile ducts. *A,* Postoperative cholangiogram after profuse hemobilia; the large filling defects represent clots. *B,* Hepatic arteriogram showing the source of the bleeding: a false aneurysm in the right hepatic artery, caused by instrumental lithotomy. Successful treatment with ligature of the responsible artery. (University Hospital, Lund, Sweden.)

produces bleeding. This so-called tropic hemobilia is a common problem in surgical departments in the Far East.[55, 56]

Gallstones

In gallstone disease, microscopic hemorrhage is frequent and can be proved in about 30 per cent of cases.[11, 14] The bleeding occurs when the stones injure the mucosa, especially in connection with biliary colic. Macroscopic hemobilia is rare, with only 50 cases reported in the literature.[3] It generally occurs when a large stone erodes the cystic artery or penetrates an adjacent viscus. Minor hemobilia is common in connection with common duct stone removal. It generally stops after suture of the common duct, but the presence of clots in the duct may occasionally cause diagnostic difficulties.[14, 57]

Tumor

As has been mentioned, tumors are an insignificant source of bleeding in the biliary tract. This is especially striking when compared with the urinary tract, where tumors are the major cause of hematuria. Tumors are relatively infrequent in the gallbladder, whereas they are common in the urinary bladder.

The common tumors in the liver are not prone to bleed into the bile ducts. The hepatomas that cause hemobilia are of the more unusual kind that arise from the ductal epithelium. Benign hemangioma has been the source of bleeding in a few cases. Metastatic tumors in the liver do not usually bleed, but hemobilia has been described as the presenting symptom of a metastatic melanoma,[58] and from metastases in such rare locations as the gallbladder wall.[1] If excision of the tumor is not possible, embolization is the treatment of choice.[59]

Vascular Disease

Vascular disease, formerly a common cause, is now responsible for only 10 per cent of cases of gross hemobilia. The frequency of true aneurysms of the hepatic artery rupturing into the biliary tract is diminishing with the disappearance of mycotic aneurysms, leaving only those of atherosclerotic origin[60] (Fig. 42–13). Vascular lesions associated with arterial hypertension sometimes give rise to hemobilia. The structure usually affected is the gallbladder, and the disorder is then designated as "apoplexy of the gallbladder" or "hemocholecyst."

Coagulopathy

Like hematuria and epistaxis, hemobilia may result from coagulopathy or anticoagulant therapy (Fig. 42–14). The increasing frequency of the latter will probably result in a number of cases of minor hemobilia with formation of clots that imitate stones. Knowledge of the risk may prevent unnecessary surgery.[14]

Hemobilia has become a generally recognized syndrome. It is not as rare as it was once thought to be. With increasing use of angiography, the number of misinterpreted cases is decreasing. Embolization of the bleeding artery is now the treatment of choice in most cases. Surgical treatment is occasionally necessary when the hemorrhage is substantial; when an adequate operation is performed with the aid of preoperative angiography, the mortality rate is low.

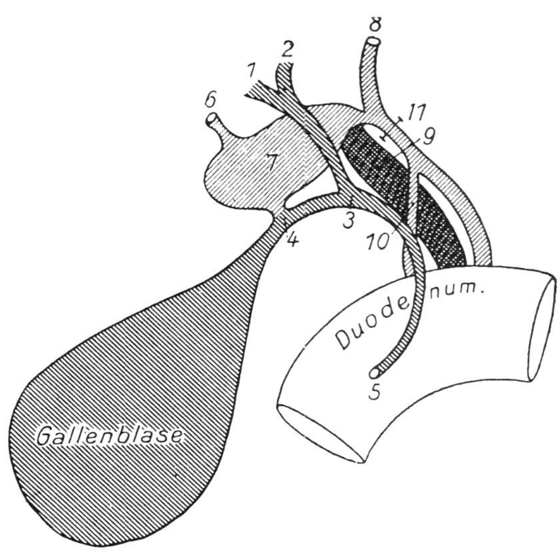

Figure 42–13. A case of true aneurysm in the right hepatic artery that ruptured into the gallbladder, causing massive hemobilia. In 1903 the German surgeon Kehr[35] operated on this patient with ligature of the main hepatic artery. This represents the first successful operation for hemobilia. The drawing is Kehr's original.

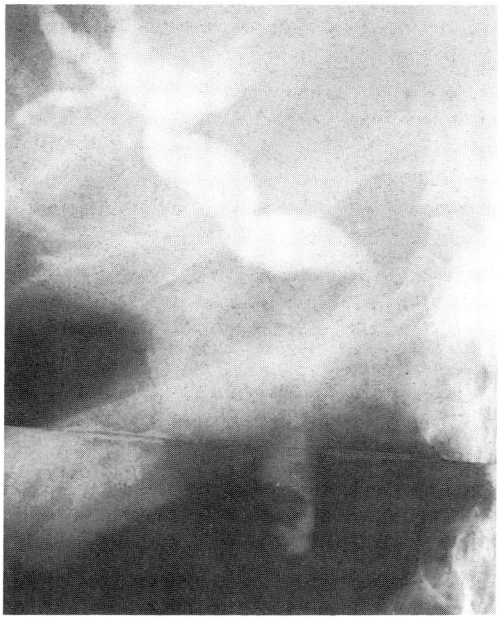

Figure 42–14. Obstructing blood clot, resulting from minor hemobilia in an otherwise normal biliary tract during anticoagulant therapy. Note the attachments to the ductal mucosa that characterize clots in the ducts.

REFERENCES

1. Sandblom P: Hemobilia. Springfield, IL, CC Thomas, 1972.
2. Glisson F: Anatomia Hepatis. Amsterdam, 1654.
3. Sandblom P, Saegesser F, Mirkovitch V: Hepatic hemobilia: hemorrhage from the intrahepatic biliary tract, a review. World J Surg 1984;*8*:41.
4. Curet P, Baumer R, Roche A, et al: Hepatic hemobilia of traumatic or iatrogenic origin: recent advances in diagnosis and therapy, review of the literature from 1976 to 1981. World J Surg 1984;*8*:1.
5. Larson DE, Farnell MB: Upper gastrointestinal hemorrhage. May Clin Proc 1983;*58*:371.
6. Goodnight JE Jr, Blaisdell FW: Hemobilia. Surg Clin North Am 1981;*61*:973.
7. Nilsson U, Evander A, Ihse I, et al: Percutaneous transhepatic cholangiography and drainage. Risks and complications. Acta Radiol 1983;*24*:433.
8. Stambuk EC, Pitt HA, Pais SO, et al: Percutaneous transhepatic drainage. Risks and benefits. Arch Surg 1983;*118*:1388.
9. Olsen WR: Late complications of central liver injuries. Surgery 1982;*92*:733.
10. Carpenter CM, Bowers JH, Luers PR, et al: Neodymium yttrium aluminum garnet laser treatment of hemobilia via a percutaneous biliary catheter track. Radiology 1983;*148*:853.
11. Balldin G, Cronstedt J: Bleeding birth of a gallstone from a hanging papilla of Vater. Endoscopy 1983;*15*:36.
12. Struyven J, Cremer M, Pirson P, et al: Posttraumatic bilhemia: diagnosis and catheter therapy. AJR 1982;*138*:746.
13. Sandblom P, Mirkovitch V, Saegesser F: Formation and fate of fibrin clots in the biliary tract. Ann Surg 1977;*185*:356.
14. Sandblom P, Essinger A: Stones or clots in the biliary tract. Acta Chir Scand 1981;*147*:673.
15. Worobetz LJ, Passi RB, Sullivan SN: Hemobilia after percutaneous liver biopsy: role of endoscopic retrograde cholangiopancreatography and sphincterotomy. Am J Gastroenterol 1983;*78*:182.
16. Jensen AR, Matzen P: Hemobilia with jaundice: treatment by endoscopic papillotomy. Am J Gastroenterol 1982;*77*:162.
17. Good AE, Mutchnick MG, Weatherbee L: Duodenal ulcer, hepatic abscesses, and fatal hemobilia with Behçet's syndrome: a case report. Am J Gastroenterol 1982;*77*:905.
18. De Risi D, Spier N, Holyoke ED: Report of a rare case of significant hemobilia and review of this entity. J Med 1982;*13*:323.
19. Enge I, Knutrud O, Norman T: Central rupture of the liver with traumatic haemobilia. A pre- and postoperative angiographic study. Br J Radiol 1968; *41*:789.
20. Kadir S, Ernst CB: Current concepts in angiographic management of gastrointestinal bleeding. Curr Probl Surg 1983;*20*:281.
21. Hirsch M, Avinonch I, Keynan A, et al: Angiographic diagnosis and treatment of hemobilia. Radiology 1982;*144*:771.
22. Greenberg M, Rubin JM, Crass JR: The ultrasound appearance of an arterio-biliary fistula. J Clin Ultrasound 1983;*11*:323.
23. Grant EG, Smirniotopoulos JG: Intraluminal gallbladder hematoma: sonographic evidence of hemobilia. J Clin Ultrasound 1983;*11*:507.
24. Krudy AG, Doppman JL, Bissonette MB, et al: Hemobilia: computed tomographic diagnosis. Radiology 1983;*148*:785.
25. Vujic I, Stanley JH, Tyminski L, et al: Computed tomographic demonstration of hemobilia. CT 1983;*7*:219.
26. Daneman A, Matzinger MA, Martin DJ: Posttraumatic hemorrhage into the gallbladder. CT 1983;*7*:59.
27. Nielsen SL, Mygind T, Miskowiak J: Blood pool scintigraphy and arterial embolization in traumatic hemobilia. Eur J Nucl Med 1982;*7*:389.

28. Lewis J, Varma V, Tice H, et al: Hepatobiliary scanning in hemobilia-induced acute cholecystitis. Gastrointest Radiol 1982;7:169.
29. Winzelberg GG, Wholey MH, Ismail-Beigi F: Hemobilia detected by Tc-99m labeled red blood cells. Clin Nucl Med 1982;7:36.
30. Kar P, Sharma MP, Singh NK, et al: Diagnosis of haemobilia by duodenoscopy. Br J Surg 1983; *70*:186.
31. Mee AS, Turner JA, Gow NM: Recurrent acute pancreatitis due to haemobilia from a hepatic artery aneurysm. Postgrad Med J 1983;*59*:590.
32. Poulos E, et al: Traumatic hemobilia treated by massive liver resection. Arch Surg 1974;*88*:596.
33. Sandblom P, Mirkovitch V, Gardiol D: The healing of liver wounds. Ann Surg 1976;*183*:679.
34. Madding GF, Kennedy PA: Trauma to the Liver, II. Philadelphia, WB Saunders, 1971.
35. Kehr H: Der este fall von ergolgreicher unterbindung der Art. Hepatica propria wegen Aneurysm. Munch Med Wochenschr 1903;*50*:1861.
36. Eggink WF, Perlberger RR, Van Urk H: Angiographic control of traumatic hemobilia by selective arterial embolization. Br J Surg 1977;*64*:635.
37. Kadir S: Athanasoulis CA, Ring EJ, et al: Transcatheter embolization of intrahepatic arterial aneurysms. Radiology 1980;*134*:335.
38. Walter JF, Paaso BT, Cannon WB: Successful transcatheter embolic control of massive hematobilia secondary to liver biopsy. AJR 1976;*127*847.
39. Merino–de Villasante J, Alvarez Rodriguez RE, Herrand-Ortiz J: Management of post biopsy hemobilia with selective arterial embolization. AJR 1977; *128*:668.
40. Perlberger RR: Control of hemobilia by angiographic embolization. AJR 1977;*128*:672.
41. Lieberman DA, et al: Arterial embolization for massive upper gastrointestinal tract bleeding in poor surgical candidates. Gastroenterology 1984;*86*:876.
42. McDougal EG, Mandel SR: Traumatic hemobilia. Successful nonoperative treatment in two cases. Am Surg 1984;*50*:169.
43. Todo S, Kishkawa T, Toyoda K, et al: Management of massive hemobilia with angiographic embolization. Jpn J Surg 1983;*13*:348.
44. Manenti A, Cortesi N: Hemobilia: a complication of biliary surgery. Report of 3 cases. Acta Chir Belg 1983;*83*:52.
45. Chen MF, Chou FF, Wang CH, et al: Hematobilia from ruptured hepatic artery aneurysm. Report of two cases. Arch Surg 1983;*118*:759.
46. Raines LA, Wool NL, Economou SG: Massive hemobilia: a complication of hemoclips. IMJ 1982; *161*:272.
47. Mueller PR, VanSonnenberg E, Simeone JF: Fine-needle transhepatic cholangiography. Indications and usefulness. Ann Intern Med 1982;*97*:567.
48. Raines DR, Van Heertum RL, Johnson LF: Intrahepatic hematomas: A complication of percutaneous liver biopsy. Gastroenterology 1973;*67*:284.
49. Monden M, Okamura J, Kobayashi N, et al: Hemobilia after percutaneous transhepatic biliary drainage. Arch Surg 1980;*115*:161.
50. Hoevels J, Nilsson U: Intrahepatic vascular lesions following nonsurgical percutaneous transhepatic bile duct intubation. Gastrointest Radiol 1980;*5*:127.
51. Mueller PR, Van Sonnenberg E, Ferrucci JT Jr: Percutaneous biliary drainage: technical and catheter-related problems in 200 procedures. AJR 1982;*138*:17.
52. Sarr MG, et al: Management of hemobilia associated with transhepatic internal biliary drainage catheters. Surgery 1984;*95*:603.
53. Hultcrantz R, Isberg B, Nilsson LH: A case of haemobilia following percutaneous liver biopsy treated by selective arterial embolization. Acta Chir Scand 1983;*149*:441.
54. Kelley CJ, Hemingway AP, McPherson GA, et al: non-surgical management of post-cholecystectomy haemobilia. Br J Surg 1983;*70*:502.
55. Tôn-Thât-Tùng: Les hémobilies tropicales. Chirurgie 1972;*98*:43.
56. Lloyd DA: Hepatobiliary ascariasis in children. Surg Annu 1982;*14*:277.
57. Sandblom P, Mirkovitch V: Minor hemobilia. Ann Surg 1979;*190*:254.
58. McArthur MS, Teergarden DK: Metastatic melanoma presenting as obstructive jaundice with hemobilia. Am J Surg 1983;*145*:830.
59. Asmat P, Beckmann CF: Transcatheter embolization of the liver for control of massive hemobilia in a patient with adenocarcinoma of the gallbladder. Am J Gastroenterol 1983;*78*:761.
60. van Vugt AB, Van Det RJ, Sier JC: Hepatic artery aneurysm. Presentation of a case of haemobilia and review of the literature. Vasa 1983;*12*:179.

ANDREW L. WARSHAW, M. D.

43

Miscellaneous Causes of Bile Duct Obstruction

INTRODUCTION

Previous chapters have concentrated on the more common causes of obstructive jaundice, especially gallstones and tumors of the biliary tree. This chapter is concerned with uncommon, unusual, and frankly extraordinary causes of bile duct obstruction. Its purpose is to alert the reader to conditions that he may not have encountered previously so that he may nonetheless be prepared—by obtaining the appropriate preoperative studies, by having made correct therapeutic decisions, and by having the requisite resources and skills.

BENIGN OBSTRUCTION AT THE LEVEL OF THE AMPULLA

Papillitis

Benign intrinsic obstruction of the outlet of the common bile duct may occur from inflammation, fibrosis, or muscular hypertonicity, conditions that have been variously called papillitis, stenosis of the sphincter of Oddi, or ampullary fibrosis. Much confusion has surrounded this condition; in fact, its existence has even been questioned. Because objective criteria for diagnosis have generally been lacking, the results of therapy have not been entirely satisfactory. The current state of our understanding suggests that much of the confusion has been generated by the failure to separate at least three discernible entities[1]: (1) common duct obstruction due to fibrotic stenosis of the papilla, (2) recurrent pancreatitis, and (3) recurrent right upper quadrant pain without jaundice or pancreatitis.

The range of histopathologic changes in the papilla includes fibrosis, acute inflammation and ulceration, chronic inflammation, and glandular hyperplasia.[2, 3] The pathogenesis of these changes is obscure. In some cases, gallstones passing down the common duct may traumatize the ampulla, producing inflammation and, ultimately, scarring. Many patients with papillary stenosis have no gallstones, however, and in them the mechanism of injury remains unknown.

Ampullary stenosis may be associated with an impacted common duct stone, or it may present, rarely, as obstructive jaundice without choledocholithiasis (Fig. 43–1). It may be further complicated by acute cholecystitis or cholangitis, with or without choledocholithiasis. Once infection has been controlled, the diagnosis can be established preoperatively by percutaneous transhepatic (PTHC) or endoscopic retrograde (ERCP) cholangiography. Intravenous cholangiography is generally inadequate to define the ampullary region. Intraoperative cholangiography can be used when preoperative cholangiography has not been performed. Inability to pass a catheter larger than 8F from the common duct into the duodenum confirms the presence of stenosis. Treatment is usually aimed at opening the stenotic orifice by transduodenal sphincterotomy or sphincteroplasty. Choledochoduodenostomy is preferred by some surgeons if the common duct is dilated enough (>2 cm) to allow a wide open anastomosis. If cholecystectomy is not required, endoscopic papillotomy is usually preferable to surgical sphincterotomy.[4–6]

The variant of papillitis responsible for recurrent pancreatitis must be distinguished from pancreatitis due to alcoholism or passage of gallstones. Patients with pancreatitis

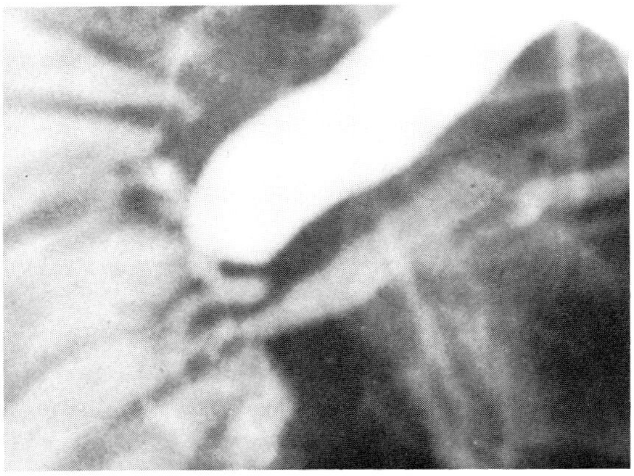

Figure 43–1. Retrograde cholangiogram and pancreatogram in a patient with papillitis and abdominal pain, whose serum bilirubin value was 1.8 mg/dl. The common duct is slightly dilated and bulbous just above its narrow intramural terminal segemnt.

due to papillitis may also have gallstones; most of the rest will be found to have chronic cholecystitis. These observations have suggested that disease of the sphincter of Oddi may sometimes cause gallstones, the reverse of the more common sequence.[7] Stenosis of the pancreatic duct orifice may also occur without associated papillitis.[8] The morphine-prostigmine test, which has defenders[3, 9] and detractors,[10] may help identify patients with this form of pancreatitis, but the most reliable clues are provided by ERCP. If the orifice of the duct of Wirsung is stenotic, it is difficult or impossible to cannulate.[9] The cannula may have to be pressed against the duct orifice in order to obtain a pancreatogram, but the resulting pancreatogram usually appears normal. Sphincteroplasty of the pancreatic duct orifice (transampullary septectomy) to relieve the stenosis of Wirsung's duct, plus a standard sphincteroplasty, appears to be effective treatment.[8, 11]

Patients with the third form of papillitis are the most difficult to diagnose. They complain of recurrent epigastric or right upper quadrant pain, which may radiate through to the right scapula and is often accompanied by nausea or vomiting. Many of these patients have had a prior cholecystectomy with only temporary or no relief of symptoms. They tend to be labeled as neurotics or as examples of the postcholecystectomy syndrome. Among the patients with these symptoms, many of whom have functional problems or pain of nonbiliary origin, are some who truly have disease of the papilla or sphincter of Oddi. Rarely, their serum alkaline phosphatase values may remain elevated, suggesting biliary stasis, or endoscopic examination and biopsy of the ampulla will confirm the presence of inflammation. More commonly, there are no such abnormalities. The morphine-prostigmine test has been of little use. Objective data are now beginning to accumulate suggesting that patients with this condition have abnormal sphincter *function* but normal *morphology*. Although the common duct may be of normal caliber or only slightly dilated on cholangiography, it may empty slowly, retaining the contrast agent for more than 30 minutes (Fig. 43–2).[5] *Common duct* pressures may be normal or elevated,[4, 5] but *sphincter of Oddi* pressures have been reported to be high.[12, 13] Dynamic flow measurements through the sphincter made at the time of common duct exploration tend to support the concept of increased resistance at the ampulla.[14] This condition may thus be one of sphincter hypertrophy, hypertonicity, or inability to relax. In properly selected patients, surgical sphincteroplasty is curative, but surgical therapy is gradually being replaced by endoscopic sphincterotomy.[6, 15–18]

Duodenal Diverticulum

Duodenal diverticula are demonstrable in about 2 per cent of barium meal studies of

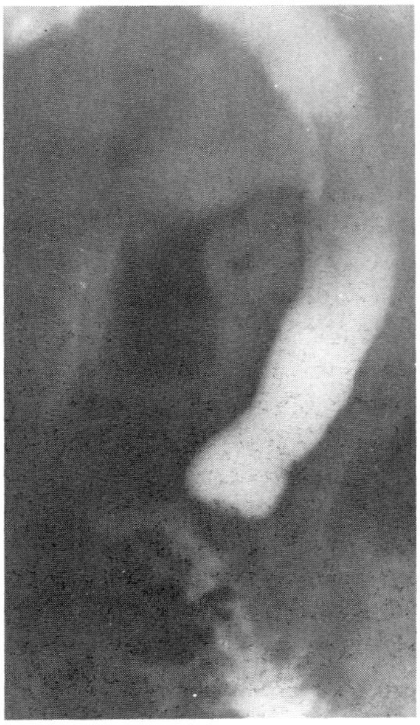

Figure 43–2. Contrast medium remaining in the common bile duct 30 minutes after retrograde filling by endoscopic catheterization. The prolonged retention implies ampullary stenosis.

the upper gastrointestinal tract and in up to 22 per cent of autopsies.[19, 20] Ninety per cent occur on the medial wall of the duodenum, and two thirds are juxta-ampullary. The ampulla may be adjacent to the diverticulum or may empty into it (Fig. 43–3). Most duodenal diverticula are wide-mouthed and have dependent orifices; stasis within a diverticulum is uncommon. Only a few patients are symptomatic and only a small minority of these require surgery, usually for the complications of perforation, hemorrhage, duodenal obstruction, or recurrent pancreatitis.[21, 22]

Perhaps the rarest complication of a duodenal diverticulum is obstructive jaundice, which may be caused by one of two mechanisms: (1) If the ampulla is located within the diverticulum, chronic inflammation of the walls of the diverticulum may cause fibrosis, which eventually narrows the ampullary orifice, a form of papillitis. Recurrent pancreatitis due to involvement of the pancreatic duct orifice may also occur.[20, 23–25] (2) If the ampulla is adjacent to the diverticulum, filling and distention of the diverticulum may compress the intramural portion of the lower common duct. One should be wary, however, of attributing biliary obstruction to a duodenal diverticulum. It is much more likely that the diverticulum is innocent and that the jaundice is due to a more usual cause, particularly gallstones.[26] If stones are found in the duct, it is generally safer to assume that the duodenal diverticulum is a coincidental finding, unrelated to the biliary obstruction, and to leave it alone.

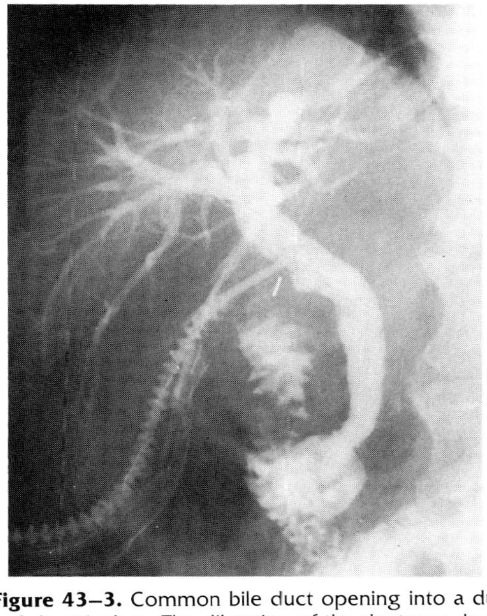

Figure 43–3. Common bile duct opening into a duodenal diverticulum. The dilatation of the duct was due to passage of gallstones and was not related to the diverticulum.

Surgery upon the diverticulum should be reserved for instances in which the diverticulum is clearly the cause of the problem. In the case of biliary obstruction or recurrent pancreatitis, evidence of ampullary stenosis should be sought by cholangiography and by operative calibration of the ampulla. It should be possible to pass a catheter larger than 8F through a nonstenotic orifice.

Many reports have emphasized the dangers of operating upon duodenal diverticula.[19–22] The mortality rate is excessive after dissection of the diverticulum from its bed in the head of the pancreas, owing to breakdown and leakage from the duodenal suture line, pancreatitis, and hemorrhage from the operative site. The most successful approach[21, 22, 24] is a combination of sphincteroplasty, diverticulectomy, and repair of the duodenal muscular defect, all performed from within the duodenal lumen. A catheter is left in the duct of Wirsung to prevent the development of pancreatitis from postsurgical edema.

Duodenal Ulcer

Despite the juxtaposition of the duodenum and the biliary tree, there are several reasons that the common duct is rarely injured by penetrating duodenal ulcers: (1) The pancreas, which intervenes between most of the lower common duct and the duodenum, acts as a protective barrier. (2) Most duodenal ulcers occur within 2 to 3 cm of the pylorus, whereas the common duct meets the duodenum beyond this vulnerable area. To reach the common duct, an ulcer would have to penetrate either the posterior or the superior wall of the distal duodenal cap. (3) The ampulla and intramural portions of the common duct are generally 7 to 10 cm from the pylorus, a site rarely involved with peptic ulcer disease.

Nevertheless, peptic ulcers occasionally cause obstructive jaundice, and as of 1975, 85 cases had been reported.[27] At the Mayo Clinic, 155 of 4250 patients with jaundice were found to have duodenal ulcers, but in only 6 of these individuals was the jaundice caused by the ulcer (0.14 per cent).[28] The ulcer disease in such patients tends to be virulent. Most of the Mayo Clinic patients had concomitant gastric outlet obstruction and had had previous complications as well.

The mechanisms of biliary obstruction include periduodenal and pancreatic edema, chronic fibrosis and contraction around the ulcer, compression of the common duct by walled-off abscesses following perforation of the ulcers, and erosion into the common duct with secondary cholangitis (Fig. 43–4).[27–30] Actually, the last complication (choledochoduodenal fistula) usually does not lead to jaundice or cholangitis and may even ameliorate the ulcer disease, presumably by alkalinizing the ulcer.[31] Obstruction, if due to fibrosis, may be chronic and may produce secondary biliary cirrhosis.[32] Most of these patients have initially had prominent ulcer symptoms, followed later by the onset of jaundice. Less often, jaundice may be the presenting feature, either with acute cholangitis or with an insidious onset mimicking cancer.[32] The diagnosis is made by upper gastrointestinal barium meal and cholangiography. The distinction between benign peptic ulcer disease and periampullary carcinoma may be difficult roentgenographically, endoscopically, and even at operation. Treatment is directed at the ulcer disease and in the precimetidine era generally required surgery. Vagotomy and a drainage procedure (pyloroplasty or gastrojejunostomy) is safer in most instances than attempting to dissect out the inflamed duodenum with the attendant risk of common duct injury. As the inflammation from the ulcer heals, the biliary complications clear.[28] Temporary biliary decompression with a T-tube may be advisable in the interim.

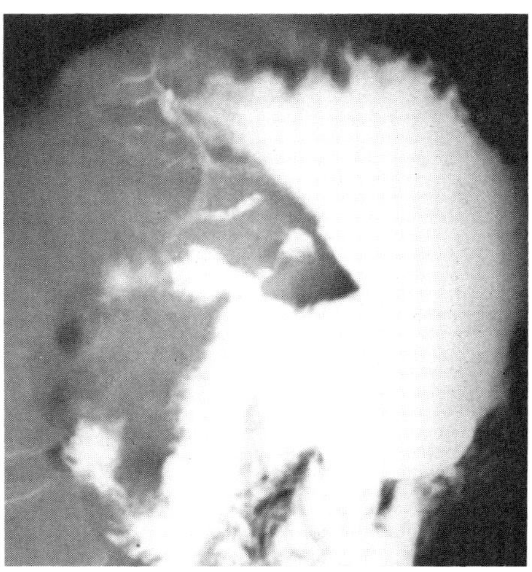

Figure 43–4. Choledochoduodenal fistula caused by a duodenal ulcer that penetrated into the common duct. Transient fever and mild hyperbilirubinemia responded to antibiotic therapy.

Successful treatment of the ulcer with cimetidine and antacids may suffice in some cases.[29, 33]

Benign Duodenal Tumors

Benign adenomatous polyps arising from the mucosa in the periampullary region may obstruct the outflow of bile or pancreatic secretions. The most common example is a mucosal polyp or papillary (villous) adenoma of the ampulla itself.[30, 31, 34, 35] The tumor is often multilobular (Fig. 43–5) or even multicentric, and it may be difficult to distinguish from a low-grade carcinoma, even on frozen section examination. Because inflammatory changes are common in the polypoid tissue, it has been suggested that some of these lesions may arise as a hyperplastic response to inflammation. If true, this type of polyp could represent a variant of papillitis.

As rare as these lesions are, even rarer are other para-ampullary mobile tumors, such as Brunner's gland adenomas,[36] which may block bile flow by falling over the ampullary orifice. Lipomas and leiomyomas, which may also be polypoid despite their submucosal origin, do not have this tendency.

Patients with ampullary polyps may present with obstructive jaundice (either intermittent or stable), biliary colic, or relapsing pancreatitis. If the diagnosis is suspected preoperatively, upper gastrointestinal contrast studies, preferably hypotonic duodenography, are useful to define the location and extent of the tumor. Multiple biopsies should be obtained via the endoscope to determine whether the tumor is benign or malignant. Since these tumors also may extend along the biliary mucosa, transhepatic cholangiography should be performed to evaluate the lower common duct.

The surgical treatment is local excision, when possible. Great care must be taken to protect and reconstruct the ends of the bile duct and pancreatic duct, a procedure that involves sphincteroplasty and postoperative intubation of both ducts to ensure adequate drainage. When the lesion is too extensive or when a serious question of malignancy remains, pancreaticoduodenal resection is required.[35]

Crohn's Disease

Crohn's disease (regional enteritis) is characterized by chronic inflammation and scar-

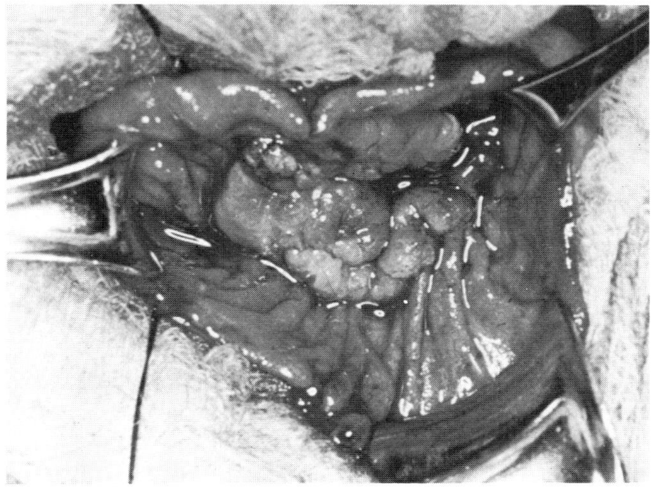

Figure 43–5. Benign villous adenoma of the ampulla that presented with obstructive jaundice. The tumor was too extensive for local excision, even with sphincteroplasty, and required pancreaticoduodenal resection.

ring. Duodenal involvement commonly produces enough swelling and stricture formation to obstruct the duodenal lumen.[37] The entire duodenum, including the ampullary region, is potentially at risk,[37] but surprisingly, biliary obstruction is rare. Instead, the ampulla damaged by Crohn's disease tends to become patulous and incompetent, allowing reflux of duodenal juice into the biliary tree (Fig. 43–6), which is of no clinical significance. Jaundice in a patient with Crohn's disease is usually due to pericholangitis, steatosis, or cirrhosis.[38, 39]

Surgical treatment of Crohn's disease of the duodenum is by gastrojejunostomy. Vagotomy is unnecessary.[37]

OBSTRUCTION OF THE INTRAPANCREATIC COMMON BILE DUCT

Acute Pancreatitis

Hyperbilirubinemia occurs in 20 to 30 per cent of patients in the initial phase of acute pancreatitis.[40–42] The causes include (1) pancreatic edema compressing the intrapancreatic portion of the common bile duct (Fig. 43–7); (2) common duct obturation by a gallstone, which may also be the cause of the pancreatitis; (3) pre-existing pancreatic disease (e.g., chronic fibrosis, pseudocyst, cancer); and (4) concomitant nonobstructive liver disease. The level of serum bilirubin, which

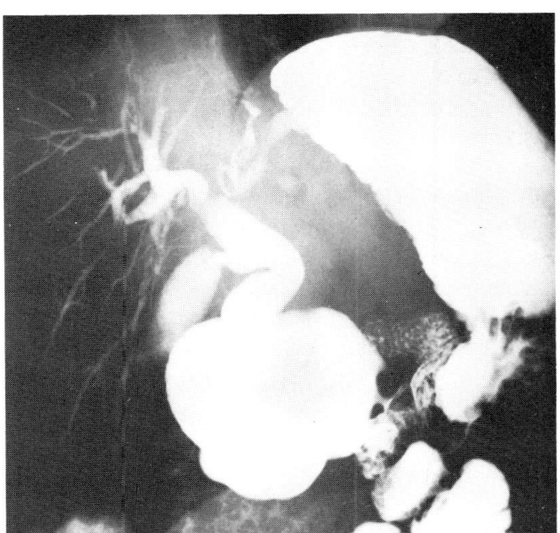

Figure 43–6. Barium contrast study in a patient with Crohn's disease involving the duodenum. There is free reflux through the ampulla into the biliary tree. Despite the bile duct dilatation, the serum bilirubin remained normal.

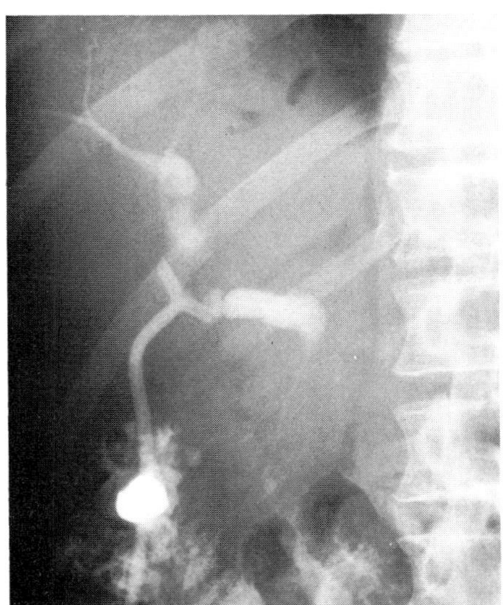

Figure 43–7. T-tube cholangiogram in a patient who developed acute pancreatitis after common duct exploration. The entire segment of the bile duct within the swollen pancreas is stenotic.

is generally under 4 to 5 mg/dl but may reach 8 mg/dl, is of no help in differentiating extraluminal compression of the bile duct by edema from intraluminal obstruction by a stone.[41] Serum alkaline phosphatase and transaminase levels also rise in patients with biliary obstruction but are of no additional diagnostic value.

Radiologic methods have little to offer. Oral cholecystography and intravenous cholangiography almost never opacify the gallbladder or bile ducts in patients with jaundice caused by pancreatitis. Retrograde cholangiography is difficult when the duodenum is deformed and edematous, and it may be dangerous because of the risk of aggravating the pancreatitis if the medium is injected unintentionally into the pancreatic duct. Transhepatic cholangiography theoretically should be effective and safe, but there has been little experience with its use in patients with acute pancreatitis.[43]

Ultimately, the major question is what to do for the jaundice. The answer depends upon the cause of the jaundice and the clinical course of the patient. Jaundice due to parenchymal liver disease is treated expectantly with nutritional support and avoidance of hepatotoxic drugs. Jaundice caused by pancreatic edema is usually temporary and subsides in most cases within a few days or weeks. The development of cholangitis or chronic obstruction requiring surgery is virtually unheard of as a consequence of uncomplicated pancreatic swelling. Jaundice later in the attack is likely to herald the appearance of a new problem, most often pancreatic necrosis and abscess formation.[44] The jaundice in these cases is produced by extrinsic common duct compression or by the adverse effects of bacterial sepsis on liver function. Pseudocysts may also cause biliary obstruction at this phase. The treatment of each of these conditions is surgical.

Most surgeons treat acute gallstone pancreatitis just as they would if there were no stones. In a few cases, the attack does not subside or it becomes progressive and life-threatening. Emergency drainage of the common duct with a T-tube, and occasionally even sphincterotomy for an impacted stone, may be required.[45] Fortunately, in most instances acute pancreatitis abates during nonoperative therapy despite the presence of a common duct stone. Cholecystectomy and common duct exploration are deferred until the acute illness has subsided, but the operation should usually be performed during the same hospitalization. Occasionally surgery is deferred for 4 to 6 weeks, until pancreatic swelling decreases. Serial examinations by ultrasonography may be helpful in the timing of surgery. Operation performed this late is easier, safer, and more likely to allow an effective search for stones.

A few surgeons advocate immediate common duct exploration, with an intent to minimize the severity of the pancreatitis by removing the common duct stone (its inciting factor).[46] This view presupposes that most cases of pancreatitis are due to the passage of gallstones[47] or that it is possible to select out those that are. This approach has not been widely accepted because it would lead to surgery in many patients whose common ducts have no stones, and because it would incur the risks of a difficult operation with attendant chances for injuring the bile ducts.

There is, however, a little-recognized group of patients with findings that may help reconcile the disparate views already described. These individuals present with abdominal pain and tenderness in the epigastrium or right upper quadrant and with elevated serum amylase and bilirubin levels. Because of the hyperamylasemia, the diagnosis of pancreatitis is almost automatic. Yet these patients have no real clinical, chemical, or radiographic evidence of pancreatic inflammation, and even at laparotomy the pancreas appears normal.[41] Their symptoms improve rapidly with little treatment. These patients have common duct stones, but not really pancreatitis. The hyperamylasemia, like the elevated bilirubin, SGOT, and alkaline phosphatase levels, is a manifestation of mechanical pancreatic duct obstruction without parenchymal inflammation.[41] If these patients could be distinguished from those with genuine pancreatitis, they could be operated upon safely within a few days of onset of the illness. In the absence of reliable, objective criteria, the decision must be based on imprecise clinical and radiographic features, such as the apparent mildness of the attack, the rapidity of clinical and chemical improvement, and the absence of radiographic evidence of pancreatic edema by upper gastrointestinal series.[48] Lesser and Warshaw[41] suggested the use of the amylase:creatinine clearance ratio, which rises when there is acute pancreatic inflammation but not when the serum amylase is elevated for other reasons (including common bile duct obstruction),[49] to select patients for early operation. Using this index, they were successful in identifying patients who had common duct stones without pancreatitis. The pancreas inspected at operation within a few days of the onset of illness appeared normal. Choledochotomy and stone extraction were carried out uneventfully.

Chronic Pancreatitis

In chronic pancreatitis, the intrapancreatic portion of the common bile duct can become compressed and distorted by fibrosis in the surrounding pancreas.[50–58] The result is a long stricture of the distal duct with dilatation proximally (Fig. 43–8). Transhepatic and retrograde cholangiograms have shown stenosis of the bile duct in about one quarter of patients with chronic alcoholic pancreatitis,[51] in a few with nonalcoholic pancreatitis, but not in those with biliary pancreatitis.

These strictures eventually cause cholestasis, which is initially manifested by chronically elevated levels of serum alkaline phosphatase[50–58, 138] and later of bilirubin. The bilirubin level may fluctuate, with periods of normality interspersed with rises during exacerbations of pancreatitis[50, 51] or cholangitis.[50, 52] Eventually, prolonged chronic obstruction may cause secondary biliary cirrhosis.[50, 51, 53]

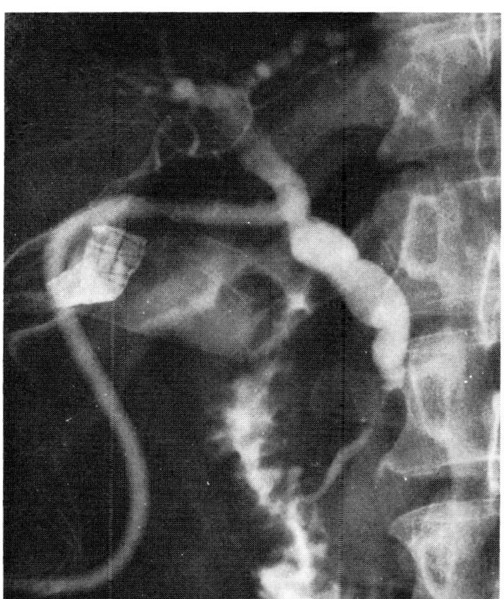

Figure 43–8. Stricture of the intrapancreatic portion of the common duct in chronic alcoholic pancreatitis.

The symptoms are variable, but generally patients exhibit one of the following patterns[50]: (1) asymptomatic; (2) intermittent jaundice, sometimes related to bouts of excessive alcohol intake, associated with abdominal pain and low-grade fever; (3) persistent jaundice, with or without pain; (4) chronic pain without jaundice, difficult to distinguish from pancreatic inflammation; or (5) acute cholangitis. These syndromes may resemble those of cholelithiasis, pancreatic cancer, cirrhosis, alcoholic hepatitis, relapsing pancreatitis, and chronic pancreatitis.

Cholangiography, either PTHC or ERCP, is diagnostic. Intravenous cholangiography is inadequate. The stricture is seen to be long, smooth, and tapered and is usually characteristic enough to be distinguished from cancer.[50–58] ERCP is preferred to PTHC because a pancreatogram can also be obtained, which confirms the diagnosis of chronic pancreatitis and helps identify pancreatic pseudocysts or ductal dilatation. If the patient has active cholangitis, cholangiography should be deferred until the infection has been controlled with antibiotics.

Surgical treatment is indicated whenever the stricture has produced chronic cholestasis or its complications. Persistent elevation of alkaline phosphatase levels, even with normal bilirubin levels, is a sufficient indication for surgery; if the cholestasis is not relieved in this situation, secondary biliary cirrhosis may result.[53] Persistent jaundice is a definite indication for surgery, but it may be mistakenly attributed to liver disease in alcoholic patients.[50] Recurrent jaundice with intervening jaundice-free periods may stem from transient pancreatic swelling during attacks of acute pancreatitis without a fixed stricture. A persistently elevated alkaline phosphatase level between attacks may also reflect transient swelling aggravating a pre-existing subclinical stenosis. Cholangiography during a quiescent interval will provide the answer.[138] It should be recognized that the acute symptoms may represent cholangitis, not just acute pancreatitis: At surgery, bile cultures in more than half the patients reveal enteric bacteria. Acute cholangitis and liver abscesses also occur.[50, 52] Pain may be associated with the stricture, with or without cholangitis, which may be indistinguishable from that of the underlying chronic pancreatitis. When considering methods of relieving pain in chronic pancreatitis, one should note that correction of the bile duct obstruction may be more important than operating upon the pancreas itself. Cholangiography (especially ERCP) is essential preoperatively in any candidate for surgical treatment of chronic pancreatitis to sort out these possibilities.[138]

The treatment of biliary strictures within the pancreas is by choledochojejunostomy, choledochoduodenostomy (preferred), or cholecystojejunostomy.[50, 52, 54–58] Transduodenal sphincteroplasty cannot be extended high enough to open the long stenotic segment.

Serious consideration should be given to performing a choledochoenterostomy whenever an intrapancreatic stricture is found during common duct exploration, even when there have been no symptoms due to the stricture. This is especially important if cholangiography shows dilatation of intrahepatic biliary radicles or if the alkaline phosphatase level has been chronically elevated. If the stricture is ignored, it may divert bile preferentially through the T-tube postoperatively, which could give rise to a permanent biliary fistula and the need for a second operation.[50]

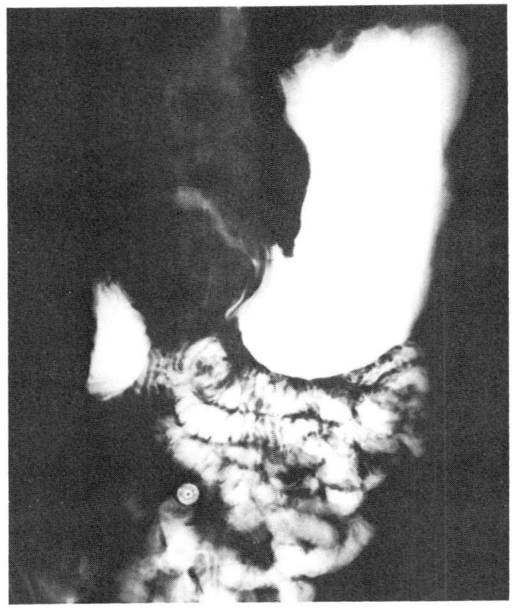

Figure 43–9. Distortion of the proximal duodenum by a pseudocyst in the head of the pancreas. The patient presented with obstructive jaundice (serum bilirubin value of 8 mg/dl).

Pancreatic Pseudocyst

As with any mass lesion situated near the head of the pancreas, pseudocysts can compress and obstruct the common bile duct. Jaundice has been reported in 8 to 17 per cent of patients with pseudocysts, but in only a few has the pseudocyst been proven to be the cause.[59] Falko et al. collected 13 examples in 1975,[59] and a few more have been added since.[60–63] Most of these patients present with manifestations suggesting pancreatic inflammatory disease, most often pain and hyperamylasemia.[64] Pancreatic calcifications are usually evident on abdominal radiographs. An occasional patient may have only painless jaundice, raising the alternative diagnosis of pancreatic cancer.[59]

Barium meal studies of the stomach and duodenum demonstrate a mass distorting the duodenal loop (Fig. 43–9). Mucosal edema and spiculation may suggest an inflammatory lesion, but its cystic nature is best demonstrated by ultrasonography or CT scanning (Fig. 43–10). Proof that the common duct is being compressed by the pseudocyst depends upon cholangiography, either ERCP (Fig. 43–11) or PTHC. It is critically important to establish a cause and effect relationship, for pseudocysts occur most often in patients with pre-existing chronic pancreatitis, which is an independent cause of common duct obstruction.[62] Figure 43–12 shows an ERCP in which the bile duct *seems* to be extrinsically compressed by an adjacent pseudocyst. However, successful drainage of the pseudocyst did not prevent the patient's return 6 weeks later with biliary obstruction and cholangitis due to the persistent *stricture*.

The treatment of biliary obstruction by pseudocyst is internal drainage of the pseudocyst.[60, 63, 69] After the pseudocyst is opened, pressure in the distended gallbladder should decrease noticeably. If the duodenum is open at the time, a sudden efflux of bile from the

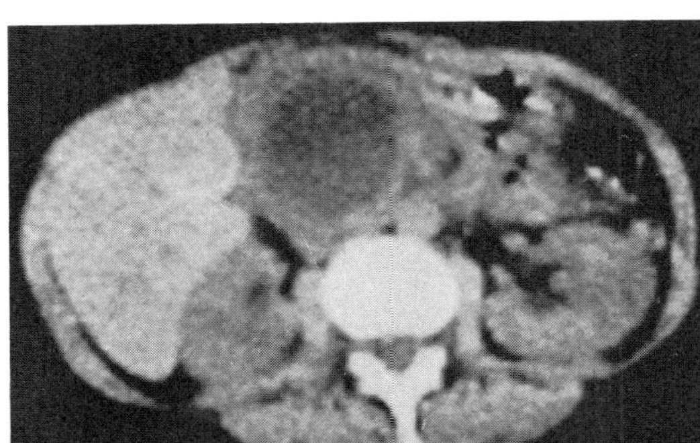

Figure 43–10. CT scan of a pseudocyst in the head of the pancreas (same patient as in Figure 43–9).

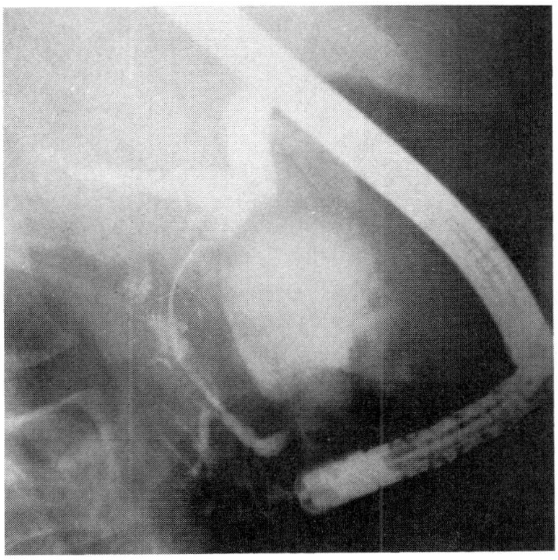

Figure 43–11. ERCP study of the patient shown in Figures 43–9 and 43–10. There is filling of the pseudocyst and of the common bile duct, which is compressed and distorted by it. Drainage of the pseudocyst relieved the biliary obstruction.

ampulla may be witnessed. While these observations suggest that drainage of the pseudocyst has relieved the biliary obstruction, it is wise to perform an operative cholangiogram to verify the change for the better. If there is a persistent stricture, a choledochoenteric bypass should be added.[62] Drainage of the cyst is often sufficient by itself, however.[63]

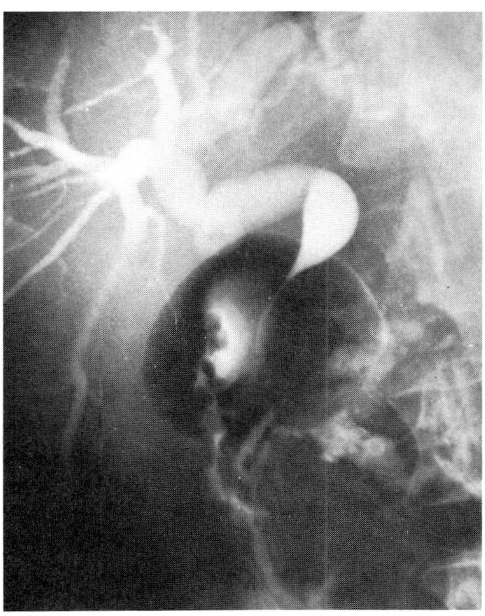

Figure 43–12. Common duct stenosis with a smooth, tapered curve, suggesting compression by the pseudocyst known to be adjacent (see Fig. 43–11). In this case, drainage of the pseudocyst did *not* relieve the biliary obstruction, which was caused by a fibrous stricture. (From Warshaw AL, et al: Gastroenterology *70*:562, 1976.)

Annular Pancreas

Annular pancreas is a congenital abnormality in which faulty rotation and development of the two embryologic anlagen of the pancreas leave pancreatic tissue embedded in the duodenal wall, usually proximal to the ampulla. Inflammation and fibrosis of the pancreatic remnants of the duodenum may lead to duodenal stenosis (the most common form of presentation) or to peptic ulceration proximal to it. Most cases are diagnosed in early childhood, but some do not become symptomatic until later.[65]

A rare sequel of annular pancreas, obstructive jaundice,[66, 67] may be due to (1) recurrent pancreatitis in the head of the gland, causing edema or fibrosis that constricts the bile duct within the pancreas, or (2) fibrosis of the duodenal wall, through which the terminal portion of the bile duct passes. The ampulla itself is distal to the annulus in most cases.[68]

The diagnosis may first be suspected after barium meal examination demonstrates a stricture of the second portion of the duodenum. Transhepatic cholangiography is required to define the level and nature of the biliary obstruction. PTHC is preferred over ERCP because duodenal distortion often interferes with passage of the endoscope. There is no evidence that because of chronic biliary stasis, gallstones are more prevalent in this disease, but, if present, gallstones also require treatment.[66] Ultrasound examination of the gallbladder is the best way to demonstrate gallstones if the patient is jaundiced.

Treatment of the obstructive jaundice entails a biliary-enteric bypass. The biliary end of the anastomosis may utilize the gallbladder, if it is not diseased, or the common bile duct. The anastomosis should be to jejunum, not duodenum, which is fibrotic, inflamed, and stenotic. The annulus itself should not be divided, a procedure that is ineffective and dangerous.[69] The duodenum is bypassed by gastrojejunostomy or duodenojejunostomy. Vagotomy is added to protect against peptic ulcer disease, which is common in patients with annular pancreas. Recurrent pancreatitis associated with annular pancreas is relieved by this operation in most patients. Rarely, a Whipple resection of the pancreatic head and duodenum is necessary to treat chronic pancreatitis.

Hydatid Cyst

Most hydatid cysts are found in the liver and lung. Only 0.1 to 0.3 per cent of cases affect the pancreas. Two instances of common bile duct obstruction by hydatid cysts in the head of the pancreas have been reported.[70, 71] They were treated by excision of the lining membrane after the cyst was emptied of its contents. One patient required choledochojejunostomy; the other did not. Hydatid cysts that rupture into the bile ducts may cause biliary obstruction. This form of biliary obstruction is discussed in Chapter 37.

BENIGN EXTRINSIC COMPRESSION OF THE COMMON DUCT

Renal Masses

The right kidney lies posterior and lateral to the second portion of the duodenum, a relationship that allows right renal masses to produce biliary obstruction. Only nine cases have been reported, however.[72–77] The primary lesions were cysts (three), hydronephrosis (two), postoperative pararenal pseudocysts or "urinomas" (three), and a perinephric abscess. The fluid collection constituting the mass in each case exceeded 2000 ml.[76]

The most common symptoms, in addition to jaundice, are nausea and vomiting due to duodenal obstruction and, less frequently, right upper quadrant pain. The second portion of the duodenum is displaced anteriorly and medially, as demonstrated by upper gastrointestinal series.[76] Urography will be part of the radiologic evaluation of the mass, but the biliary tree also must be studied to rule out gallstones, tumors, and so forth. Figure 43–13 demonstrates hydronephrosis of the right kidney in a patient who presented with obstructive jaundice. Percutaneous catheter drainage relieved the hydronephrosis and eliminated the mass, but the jaundice persisted. Transhepatic cholangiography demonstrated choledocholithiasis.

Treatment of a renal mass causing bile duct obstruction is drainage of the fluid. Nothing need be done directly to the biliary tract.[76]

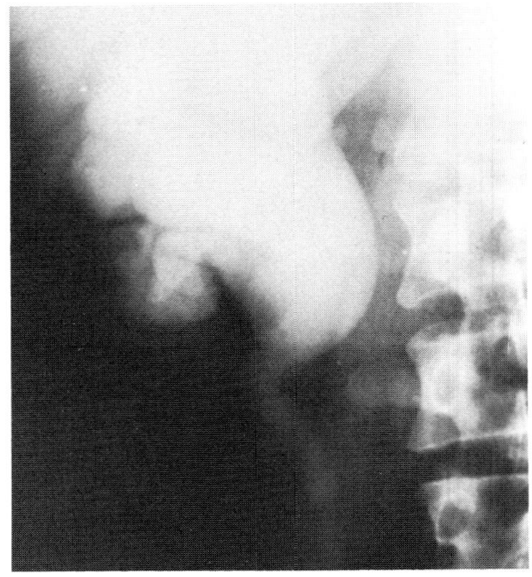

Figure 43–13. Retrograde pyelogram in a patient with concomitant obstructive jaundice. The jaundice, which failed to subside with drainage of the hydronephrosis, was caused by gallstones.

Visceral Artery Aneurysms

Visceral artery aneurysms may involve the splenic artery (53 per cent), hepatic artery (28 per cent), superior mesenteric artery (11 per cent), proper gastric arteries (5 per cent), pancreaticoduodenal artery (2 per cent), and gastroduodenal artery (1 per cent).[78] There are no reported inferior mesenteric artery aneurysms. In a few cases, more than one visceral aneurysm has been present. Atherosclerosis is the major cause, with bacterial infection (mycotic aneurysm) and trauma accounting for most of the remainder.[78–81] Adjacent abscesses, acute pancreatitis, tuberculosis, syphilis, and periarteritis nodosa have also been cited.[78–80] Aneurysms of the hepatic,[79–84] pancreaticoduodenal,[85] and gastroduodenal[78, 86] arteries have caused obstructive jaundice, either from compression of the bile ducts by the aneurysm (Fig. 43–14) or from intraluminal obturation by blood clots if the aneurysm has ruptured into the duct.

Hepatic artery aneurysms, which are situated close to the bile ducts, present with jaundice in 50 per cent of cases.[79, 80, 82, 84] The other major symptoms are right upper quadrant abdominal pain (70 per cent) and hemorrhage (60 per cent). The complete triad of hemobilia occurs in 30 per cent of cases.[82] Compression of the duodenum by the lesion may cause nausea and vomiting. Bleeding after rupture of the aneurysm may be retroperitoneal, intraperitoneal, intraluminal

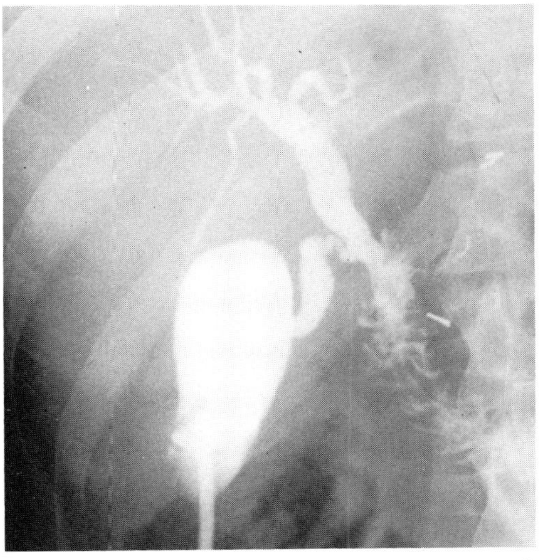

Figure 43–14. Operative cholangiogram in a patient who presented with painless obstructive jaundice, suggesting pancreatic cancer. The lower common duct is obstructed by a mass in the head of the pancreas, which was pulsatile (see Fig. 43–15).

into stomach or duodenum, or directly into the biliary tract.[80] Eighty-five per cent of hepatic artery aneurysms are diagnosed only after rupture, which is associated with a mortality rate of 32 per cent.[79] Forty-five per cent rupture into the peritoneal cavity or retroperitoneum, and most of these patients die. If the rupture is into the bile ducts or gallbladder, bleeding is intermittent and slow, at least for a time.[83] In a rare and interesting variant, the aneurysm ruptures into the portal vein and produces portal hypertension with bleeding varices.[80]

Pancreaticoduodenal artery aneurysms may also cause pain and may rupture, but only 10 per cent obstruct the bile duct.[85] They are usually located sufficiently caudad in relation to the bile duct to avoid biliary obstruction. Gastroduodenal artery aneurysms, only five of which have been reported,[78, 86] have caused jaundice in two cases. The location of the mass in these patients may initially suggest a diagnosis of cancer.

The diagnosis of jaundice due to visceral artery aneurysms is difficult to make. The gallbladder, as in other forms of lower common duct obstruction, may be distended and palpable. The pain and tenderness, although not specific, may suggest impending rupture; signs of blood loss should suggest the possibility of a ruptured aneurysm. Unfortunately, a palpable mass, thrill, or bruit, which would be more suggestive, is infrequent.[80]

The walls of the aneurysm contain enough calcium in some cases to be visible on plain abdominal x-rays. Barium studies usually show evidence of extrinsic pressure on the duodenal wall. Transhepatic cholangiography may suggest the presence of neoplastic obstruction of the duct.[84] Arteriography delineates the lesion in detail (Fig. 43–15), defining tributaries and collaterals as well as the aneurysm, information that is of value in planning the operation. Superimposing the arteriogram on the transhepatic cholangiogram may provide the clearest demonstration of the problem.[84]

Most visceral artery aneurysms can be obliterated either by ligation of the feeding vessels or by endoaneurysmorrhaphy. This is especially true of pancreaticoduodenal and gastroduodenal aneurysms, which have abundant collaterals. It was previously believed that ligation of the hepatic artery was safe proximal to the gastroduodenal artery, but that distal ligation threatened the viability of the liver. If the aneurysm involved the origin of the gastroduodenal artery or the proper hepatic artery, continuity was restored by end-to-end anastomosis, vein graft, or prosthetic graft.[80] This is now known to be incorrect.[87] Hepatic artery ligation at any level is safe,[79, 82, 83] rarely is hepatic artery reconstruction indicated, and excision of the walls of the aneurysm is unnecessary and hazardous. Hepatic artery ligation is the surgical solution for the 25 per cent of hepatic

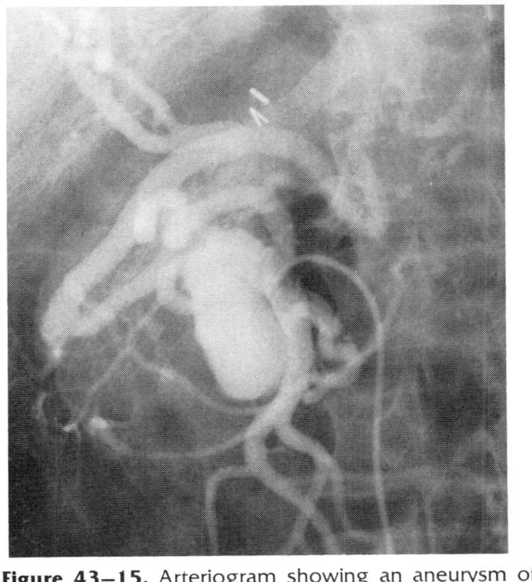

Figure 43–15. Arteriogram showing an aneurysm of the pancreaticoduodenal artery, which caused obstructive jaundice (same patient as in Figure 43–14).

artery aneurysms that are intrahepatic, but angiographic embolization of the aneurysm is simpler than surgery and is usually effective.[88]

Ligation of the aneurysm may relieve the biliary obstruction in uncomplicated cases,[78] but biliary-enteric bypass is often performed to ensure certainty. This may be accomplished by cholecystojejunostomy, choledochoduodenostomy, or Roux-en-Y choledochojejunostomy. Reconstruction using the last of these procedures is necessary when the aneurysm has eroded into the common duct.[79, 83, 89] It is wise to treat even asymptomatic visceral artery aneurysms, because the risk of rupture is great and the mortality rate after rupture is high. Pain associated with the aneurysm is an urgent signal of approaching rupture.

Tuberculosis

Even when tuberculosis was rampant, obstructive jaundice was one of its rarest complications.[90, 91] The obstruction is caused by tuberculous infection in lymph nodes in the porta hepatis or the retroduodenal area that compresses the bile duct.

Amputation Neuroma

Postcholecystectomy pain has sometimes been attributed to neuromas forming in the region of the cystic duct stump. Neuromas may also constrict the bile duct and produce jaundice. There are a few cases with histologic documentation in which the jaundice occurred several years after cholecystectomy.[92, 93] The same treatment used for other forms of common duct stricture is applicable to these lesions.

Idiopathic Retroperitoneal Fibrosis

This rare disorder is characterized by formation of a dense plaque of fibrous tissue in the retroperitoneum. The fibrotic process may invade organs, but it more commonly constricts and compresses retroperitoneal structures, especially the ureters, vena cava, aorta, and mesenteric vasculature. The extrahepatic bile duct,[94] duodenum, and pancreas may also become involved. The clinical presentation may simulate pancreatic cancer with obstructive jaundice. Surgical decompression is difficult and likely to be fruitless. Insertion of stents may be the only option.

Polycystic Liver Disease

Jaundice is an unusual feature of polycystic liver disease. In an occasional patient, cysts near the hilus of the liver may compress the bile ducts, and the resulting stasis may cause secondary stone formation.[95] Decompression or excision of the cysts as well as removal of any intraluminal debris is the appropriate treatment.

Intermittent Dislocation of the Liver

Periodic jaundice and abdominal pain have been reported in a 23 year old man in whom the diaphragmatic attachments of the right lobe of the liver were congenitally absent.[96] This defect apparently allowed the right lobe of the liver to rotate into the left upper quadrant. Biliary obstruction was presumed to result from stretching and torsion of the bile duct. Relief of these symptoms followed surgical fixation of the liver to the diaphragm.

MALIGNANT EXTRINSIC COMPRESSION OF THE COMMON DUCT

Metastases to Periductal Nodes

The nodes in the porta hepatis and along the common duct may be involved by metastases from a variety of tumors. Pancreatic, gallbladder, and gastric carcinomas metastasize there directly. The route of access from more distant primary sites is less obvious and may exemplify blood-borne metastases to lymph nodes. Occasionally, enlargement of the nodes compresses the adjacent bile duct, obstructing it and causing jaundice. The tumor may also break through the capsule of the lymph node and invade the wall of the common duct directly. In addition to the tumors already mentioned, extrahepatic biliary obstruction has been reported in patients with cancer of the colon.[97] breast,[98] and lung,[99] as well as in those with melanoma,[100–101] myeloma,[102, 103] and testicular teratoma.[104] Of these, tumors of the colon and breast are the only ones that occur often enough to be more than curiosities. The remainder of this section will discuss these two neoplasms.

Jaundice appearing in the course of cancer of the colon or breast usually signifies extensive hepatic metastases. This is a grave development with a median survival of 33 days in patients with colon cancer.[105] Death is from hepatic failure. The rare patient whose jaundice is caused by extrahepatic biliary obstruction most often has *only* extrahepatic metastases, and the liver is uninvolved.[97, 106] Surgical treatment can correct the cholestasis and extend the patient's survival.

Colon and breast cancers respond to palliative therapy more often than gallbladder, gastric, and pancreatic cancers do (Fig. 43–16). Once metastases occur in these last three lesions, death is only months away, at best. In comparison, the median survival of patients who have metastases from colon cancer confined to lymph nodes is 23 months,[107] and survival with even more advanced colon cancer exceeds that of comparable stages of other intra-abdominal cancers.[108] Metastatic breast cancer may pursue an indolent course and may respond to a variety of hormonal or chemotherapeutic treatments.

The interval between resection of the primary cancer and the onset of obstructive jaundice averages 13 months in colon cancer[97] and 2 to 3 years in breast cancer.[106] Most patients are otherwise asymptomatic, well nourished, and without pain. Their apparent good health may suggest a diagnosis of hepatitis instead of metastatic cancer. Cholangiography demonstrates the biliary obstruction, but the test may not be ordered because biliary obstruction is not seriously considered. Transhepatic cholangiography is more likely than is retrograde cholangiography to give a full definition of the upper biliary tract (Figs. 43–17 and 43–18), including the intrahepatic radicles, and is preferable for planning surgical therapy.

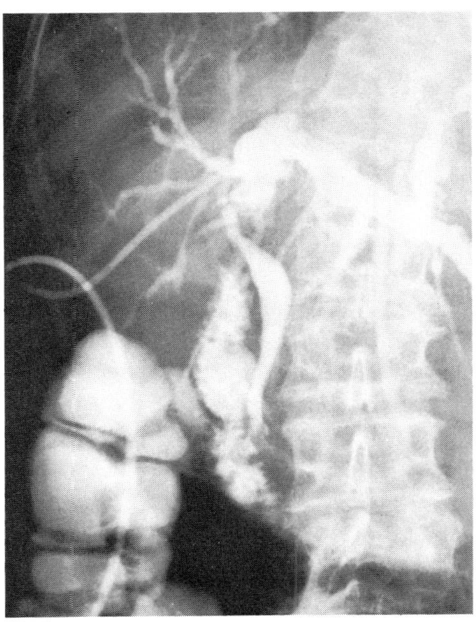

Figure 43–16. Transhepatic cholangiogram in a patient with obstruction at the hepatic duct bifurcation due to metastases from gallbladder cancer. The tumor was locally far advanced, and the patient died within 3 weeks despite transhepatic biliary drainage.

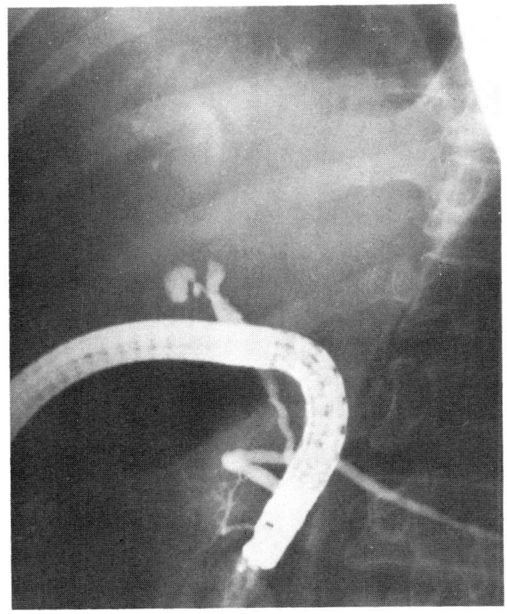

Figure 43–17. Retrograde cholangiogram in a patient with metastatic colon cancer obstructing the bile duct at the level of the porta hepatis. Note the failure to define the biliary tree above the obstructing point. (From Warshaw AL, Welch JP: Ann Surg *188*:593, 1978.)

The involvement of the periductal nodes follows three patterns: (1) obstruction by a small group of nodes high in the porta hepatis (Fig. 43–19); (2) obstruction of the lower duct by lymph nodes behind the duodenum (Fig. 43–20); or (3) enlargement of nodes along the entire length of the common duct (Fig. 43–21). Cancer in the lower nodes may also obstruct and invade the duodenum.[97]

The choice of treatment depends on the pattern of duct obstruction and the kind of tumor. Decompression is a necessary first step in most cases because the jaundice tends to progress rapidly. In approximately 40 per

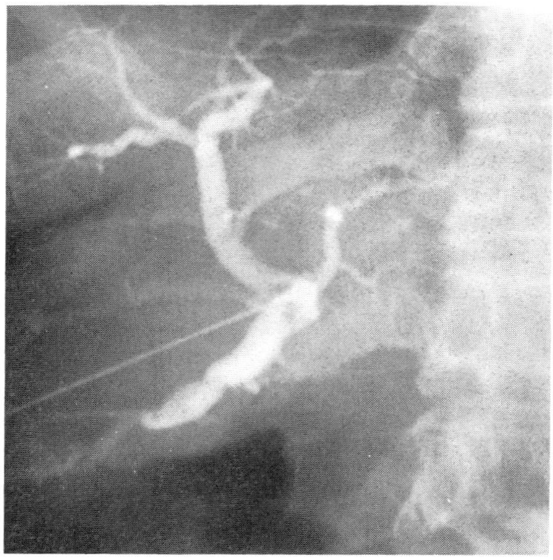

Figure 43–18. Transhepatic cholangiogram defining the biliary tree above the point of obstruction (same patient as in Figure 43–17).

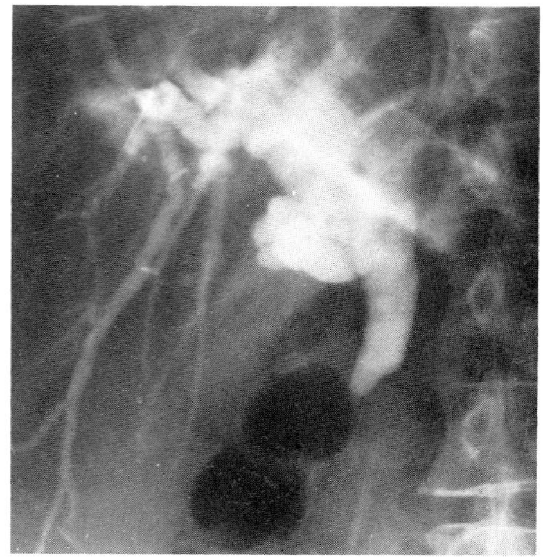

Figure 43–20. Obstruction of the lower common duct by metastatic colon cancer. The dilated common duct in this instance is suitable for choledochojejunal bypass.

cent of cases the block is low enough to permit bypass from the extrahepatic bile ducts.[97] Even in these cases, however, encroachment upon the cystic duct may obviate the use of the gallbladder.[97] In general, it is preferable to bring a Roux-en-Y limb of jejunum to a point high on the common duct to be sure of establishing effective biliary drainage above the tumor. Anastomosis to the duodenum should be avoided, because the latter may become involved by tumor.

If the extrahepatic bile ducts are unavailable because the block is in the porta hepatis, several alternatives exist. Surgical bypass can be created by bringing the Roux-en-Y loop of jejunum up to the left hepatic duct, which

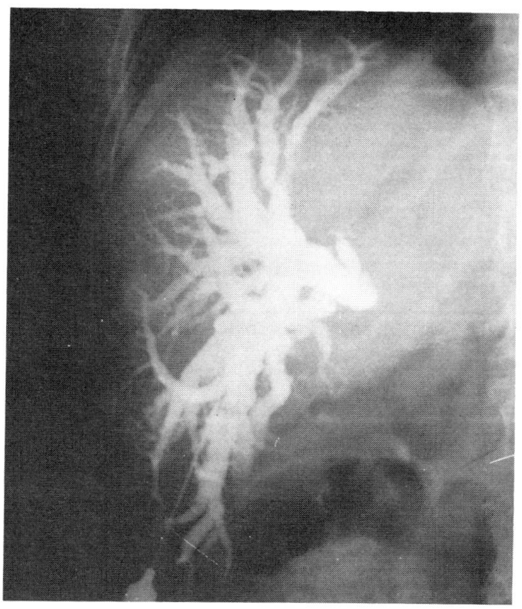

Figure 43–19. Transhepatic cholangiogram showing intrahepatic biliary dilatation and obstruction at the hepatic duct bifurcation by metastatic colon cancer. The right hepatic duct was used for anastomosis to a jejunal loop. (From Warshaw AL, Welch JP: Ann Surg *188*:593, 1978.)

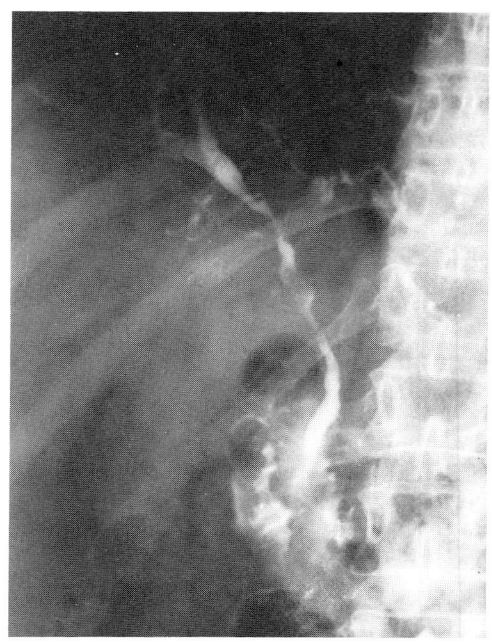

Figure 43–21. Extrinsic compression along the entire common duct from nodes filled with metastatic breast cancer.

is the most accessible of the large intrahepatic branches.[109] If the common duct is free below the tumor (see Fig. 43–17), the tumor can be bypassed by an intraluminal transhepatic stent. Originally, it was suggested that the lower end of the stent be brought out through the common duct to the skin; this "U-tube" (Fig. 43–22) could then be changed, if it plugged, by tying its replacement to one end and drawing out the other.[110] Newer techniques have made this obsolete: The lower end of the tube can now be left within the common duct or in the duodenum (Fig. 43–23)—a position allowing more efficient drainage through the end of the tube—and one less tube exits from the patient. The tube can be replaced by passing a new one over a guide wire.[111] The upper end of the tube is clamped at the skin, and bile drains out the lower end into the duodenum. For further details on transhepatic percutaneous drainage, refer to Chapter 10.

At the time of laparotomy, the margins of the tumor should be marked with metal clips to facilitate radiotherapy planning.[112, 113] If the duodenum is threatened with involvement by the tumor,[97] a gastrojejunostomy should be added.

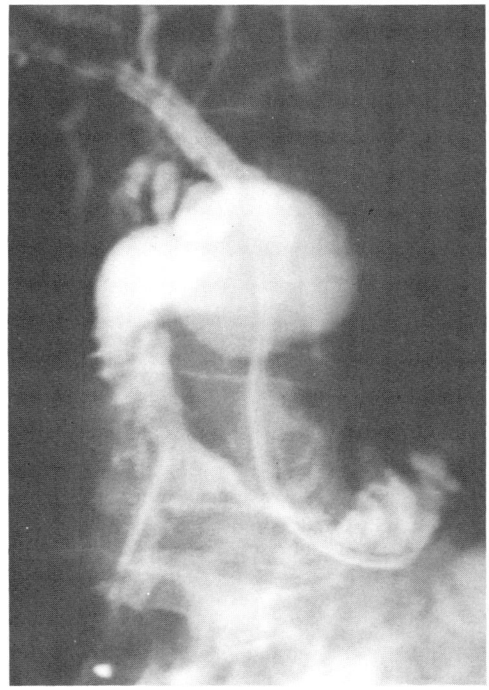

Figure 43–23. Transhepatic placement of a biliary drainage catheter past the segment of bile duct compressed by extrinsic tumor. When the proximal (percutaneous) end of the catheter is clamped, there is prograde flow of bile into the duodenum.

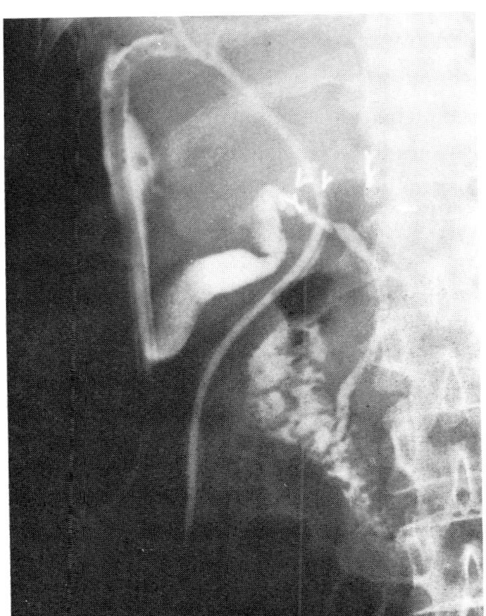

Figure 43–22. U-tube drainage of the biliary tree. The obstruction is high in the porta hepatis (same patient as in Figure 43–17). Injection of contrast into the upper end shows that the intrahepatic bile ducts are not dilated and that there is free drainage endoluminally into the duodenum. Note the metallic clips that have been placed around the tumor to target it for radiation therapy.

When obstruction is at the level of the porta hepatis, it is preferable to avoid a laparotomy in favor of transhepatic stenting under radiologic control.[114, 115] A tissue diagnosis can be obtained by percutaneous aspiration biopsy of the lesion under ultrasound or CT guidance.

Biliary bypass in patients with biliary obstruction from metastatic colon or breast cancer provides palliation and appears to prolong life. Six of eight colon cancer patients described by Warshaw and Welch[97] survived at least 1 year after biliary decompression, and two of them survived more than 3 years (Fig. 43–24). This experience contrasts with that following relief of biliary obstruction in patients with pancreatic and periampullary cancer, in whom median survival is 3 to 5 months.[108, 116] The outlook is not as good with metastatic breast cancer.[106]

After relief of biliary obstruction, other problems inevitably develop owing to progression of the cancer. Local invasion of the duodenum leads to obstruction, ulceration (Fig. 43–25), and either acute or chronic bleeding.[97] It has been suggested that bypassing the duodenum by suturing or stapling

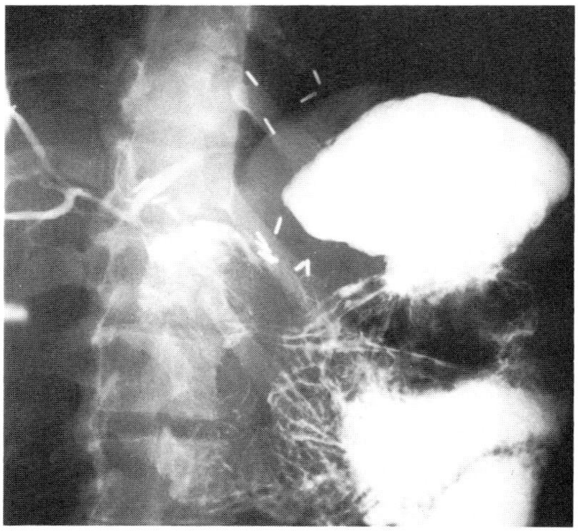

Figure 43–24. Patent choledochojejunostomy 3 years after bypass of obstructing metastatic colon cancer. (From Warshaw AL, Welch JP: Ann Surg *188*:593, 1978.)

the pylorus closed, plus gastrojejunostomy, may reduce blood loss.[97]

The experience with radiotherapy of metastases causing biliary obstruction as an adjunct to decompression is too limited to know for certain its efficacy. There is some interest in using radiotherapy as primary treatment for malignant biliary obstruction,[112–113] but surgery is necessary in most cases because several weeks must pass before the effects of irradiation shrink the tumor. Personal observations at the Massachusetts General Hospital suggest that periportal metastases from breast cancer may be more responsive to radiation therapy than those from colon cancer. Systemic chemotherapy and hormonal therapy are used in an attempt to control the tumor, but they have not been relied upon to open the blocked biliary tree.

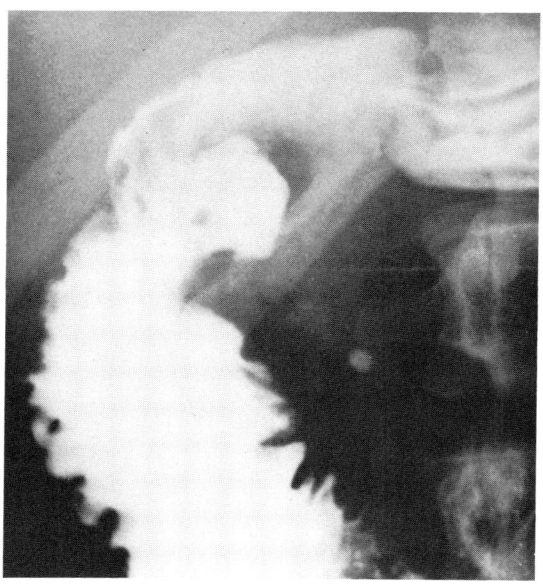

Figure 43–25. Bleeding ulcer in a mass of cancer that eroded into the duodenum from nodes behind it. The primary tumor had been in the cecum, resected 1½ years previously. (From Warshaw AL, Welch JP: Ann Surg *188*:593, 1978.)

Lymphomas and Other Lymphoid Tumors

The reported incidence of jaundice in patients with lymphomas varies from 3 to 57 per cent[117]; it averages 13 per cent for Hodgkin's disease, lymphosarcoma, and reticulum cell sarcoma.[118–120] Most often it is due to infiltration of the liver parenchyma, especially around portal tracts, or to liver dysfunction from other causes. Extrahepatic bile duct obstruction, which occurs in only a small percentage of patients,[117–122] is caused by enlarged lymph nodes, by tumor masses near the common duct, or by infiltration of the wall of the common duct. Hodgkin's disease is most likely to cause obstruction by nodal enlargement,[117, 118] reticulum cell sarcoma by infiltration of the duct wall,[121] and lymphosarcoma by periportal tumor masses or ductal infiltration.[120] Pancreatic involvement is common, but it only rarely contributes to biliary obstruction.[121] Bile duct obstruction has also been reported from enlarged nodes in a case of subleukemic lymphocytic leukemia[123] and from masses of extraosseous plasmacytoma in multiple myeloma.[124]

Obstructive jaundice caused by lymphoma generally presents not as an isolated abnormality but as part of a systemic disease involving other sites. Chemotherapy is the preferred treatment. Local irradiation of the hilus of the liver may be used adjunctively.[122] If pruritus is troublesome, percutaneous intubation of the bile ducts for decompression and drainage may be used temporarily while the effects of the other treatment are awaited. Although the obstruction may be at the lower end of the common duct,[121] surgical bypass is not indicated. A possible exception to this occurs when the diagnosis of obstructing lymphoma is first made at laparotomy; if the disease is relatively localized, biliary enteric bypass and marking of the margins of the tumor with metal clips are appropriate.

Eosinophilic Granuloma

Although multifocal eosinophilic granuloma is technically a histiocytosis rather than a malignancy, its behavior is often malignant, and the process relentlessly infiltrates tissues until the patient dies. Invasion and obstruction of the common bile duct have been reported.[125] Temporary relief has been achieved by drainage of the bile duct with a tube.

INTRALUMINAL OBTURATION

Tumor Emboli

The clinical manifestations of primary hepatocellular carcinoma are abdominal pain, weight loss, ascites, and a palpable right upper quadrant mass. Elevated serum bilirubin levels, present in about 40 per cent of patients with hepatoma, are usually due to liver failure with or without pre-existing cirrhosis.[126] A picture of extrahepatic biliary obstruction with pruritus is encountered in only 2 per cent of patients and is generally caused by direct compression or invasion of major bile ducts by tumor.[127] A rare variant occurs when fragments of hepatoma break off within the lumen of the bile duct and cause obstruction. Fewer than 40 such cases have been reported.[127–130] Some of these patients have presented with cholangitis.[129] Others have had occult blood in their stools or hemobilia.[128–131] The intraluminal debris may be a mixture of tumor and blood clot.[128]

The diagnosis is difficult to make. Hepatoma should be suspected in a patient with cirrhosis whose liver function suddenly declines for no obvious cause; however, as noted earlier, jaundice in this setting is expected. Angiography and radionuclide scans of the liver will show the mass but not the cause of the obstruction Transhepatic or retrograde cholangiography will demonstrate the intraluminal material (Fig. 43–26), but it is not easy to distinguish the tumor fragments from gallstones.[129] Sonography, which may differentiate between stones, blood clots, and solid tissue, may help in this regard.[132] The diagnosis is often not made before the duct is opened during an exploration.

The optimal treatment must take into account the biliary obstruction, the hemobilia, the potential for additional tumor emboli in the future, and the hepatoma. Ideally, if the patient were not already in end-stage liver disease, all these objectives would be accomplished by removing the embolized fragments from the common duct (Fig. 43–27) and by resecting the tumor (Fig. 43–28).[133]

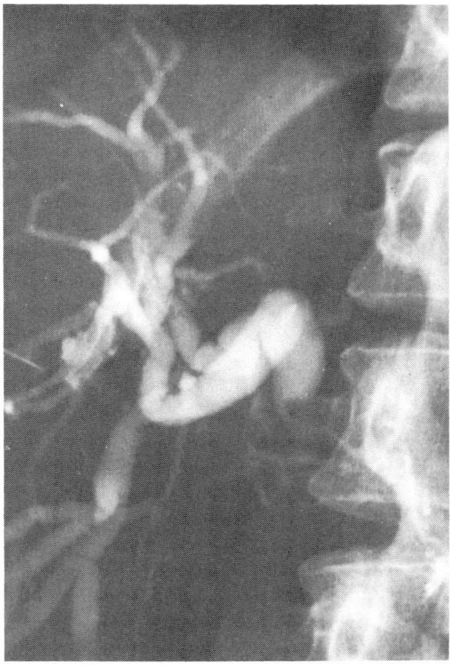

Figure 43–26. Transhepatic cholangiogram showing obstruction near the hepatic duct bifurcation by an intraluminal mass.

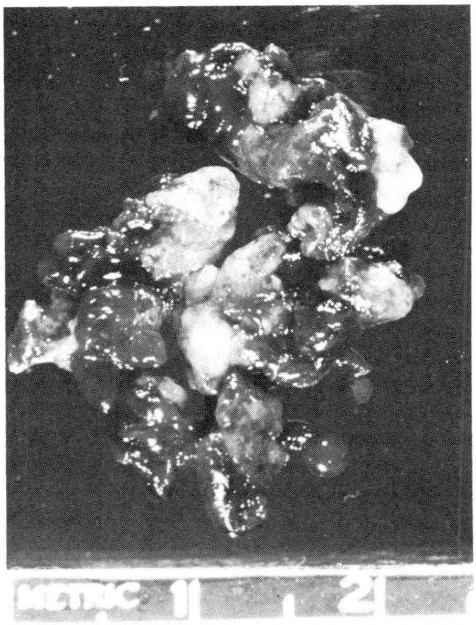

Figure 43–27. Free-floating fragments of hepatoma mixed with blood clot, removed from the common duct of a 50-year-old woman who presented with painless obstructive jaundice (same patient as in Figures 43–26 and 43–28).

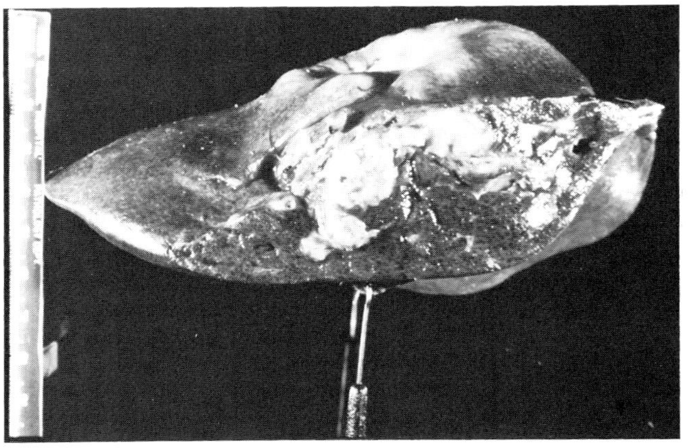

Figure 43–28. Cut section of the resected lateral segment of the left lobe of the liver, which contains a hepatoma. Fragments of the tumor, which fills and distends the bile ducts, had broken off and embolized down the lumen of the common duct (see Figs. 43–26 and 43–27).

Unfortunately, the case illustrated in Figures 43–27 and 43–28 is quite unusual because, unlike this example, hepatomas that embolize to the duct are usually too centrally located to resect.[129] A compromise treatment plan may be necessary, consisting of common bile duct exploration plus right or left hepatic artery ligation to control the hemobilia. If the patient survives long enough to have recurrent tumor emboli, it may be possible to facilitate their passage into the duodenum by endoscopic sphincterotomy.

Clonorchiasis

Infestation of the biliary tract by *Clonorchis sinensis* (Chinese liver fluke) is common in the Orient but rare in the West.[134] There is no effective medical treatment. Surgical treatment is reserved for complications, such as biliary obstruction, due not only to the parasites themselves but also to secondary formation of stones and acute cholangitis. Some patients present with pancreatitis, presumably caused by passage of the stones or the worms. In addition to cholecystectomy and clearing the bile ducts of stones and flukes, improved biliary drainage by choledochoduodenostomy or transduodenal sphincteroplasty is thought to reduce the rate of recurrent biliary obstruction, which otherwise exceeds 40 per cent.[134]

The diagnosis should be considered especially in Chinese patients with cholangitis or pancreatitis. The material retrieved from the common bile duct at operation should be submitted for immediate microscopic examination by a pathologist: The flukes may not be recognizable to the inexperienced naked eye but will be obvious among the sludge and debris under the microscope.

Foreign Body

Intraluminal biliary obstruction by a foreign body is very rare. Bullets or shrapnel may first lodge in the liver and then migrate down the duct. Rarely, entry into the duct is by direct transmural erosion.[135]

Gastric Heterotopia

Heterotopic gastric tissue has been reported to cause episodic jaundice in several patients.[136, 137] Treatment in one case entailed resection of a 2.5 cm segment of common hepatic duct and was effective.[136] The other patient seemed to improve in response to cimetidine.[137]

REFERENCES

1. Partington PG: Twenty-three years of experience with sphincterotomy and sphincteroplasty for stenosis of the sphincter of Oddi. Surg Gynecol Obstet 1977;*145*:161.
2. Acosta JM, Nardi GL: Papillitis: inflammatory disease of the ampulla of Vater. Arch Surg 1966;*92*:354.
3. Nardi GL, Acosta JM: Papillitis as a cause of pancreatitis and abdominal pain: role of evocative test, operative pancreatography and histologic evaluation. Ann Surg 1966;*164*:611.
4. Koch H, Roosch W, Schaffner O, et al: Endoscopic papillotomy. Gastroenterology 1977;*73*:1393.
5. Safrany L: Duodenoscopic sphincterotomy and gallstone removal. Gastroenterology 1977;*72*:338.
6. Shapiro HA: Endoscopic diagnosis and treatment of biliary tract disease. Surg Clin North Am 1981;*61*:843.

7. Bartlett MK: Might gallstones and recurrent pancreatitis have a common cause? Arch Surg 1967;*95*:887.
8. Acosta JM, Nardi GL, Civantos F: Distal pancreatic duct inflammation. Ann Surg 1970;*172*:256.
9. Gregg JA, Taddeo AE, Milano AF, et al: Duodenoscopy and endoscopic pancreatography in patients with positive morphine prostigmine tests. Am J Surg 1977;*134*:318.
10. LoGiudice JA, Geenan JE, Hogan WJ, et al: Evaluation of the morphine-prostigmine test in patients with suspected papillary stenosis. Gastrointest Endosc 1978;*24*:204.
11. Moody FG, Berenson MM, McCloskey D: Transampullary septectomy for post-cholecystectomy pain. Ann Surg 1977;*186*:415.
12. Geenan JE, Hogan WJ, Shaffer RD, et al: Endoscopic electrosurgical papillotomy and manometry in biliary tract disease. JAMA 1977;*237*:2075.
13. Bar-Meir S, Halpern Z, Bardan E, et al: Frequency of papillary dysfunction among cholecystectomized patients. Hepatology 1984;*4*:328.
14. White TT, Waisman H, Hopton D, et al: Radiomanometry, flow rates, and cholangiography in the evaluation of common bile duct disease. Am J Surg 1972;*123*:73.
15. Editorial: Endoscopic sphincterotomy. Lancet 1981;*2*:453.
16. Arendt R, Bosseckert H, Rogos R, et al: Experience with endoscopic sphincterotomy in the GDR. A collective study of 6 centres. Endoscopy 1983; *15*:173.
17. Viceconte G, Viceconte GW, Pietropaolo V, et al: Endoscopic sphincterotomy: indications and results. Br J Surg 1981:*68*:376.
18. Mazzeo RJ, Jordan FT, Strasius SR: Endoscopic papillotomy for recurrent common bile duct stones and papillary stenosis. A community hospital experience. Arch Surg 1983;*118*:693.
19. McSherry CK, Glenn F: Biliary tract obstruction and duodenal diverticula. Surg Gynecol Obstet 1970;*130*:829.
20. Wilk PJ, Mollura J, Danese CA: Jaundice and pancreatitis caused by a duodenal diverticulum. Am J Gastroenterol 1973;*60*:273.
21. Scudamore CH, Harrison RC, White TT: Management of duodenal diverticula, Can J Surg 1982;*25*:311.
22. Manny J, Muga M, Eyal Z: The continuing clinical enigma of duodenal diverticulum. Am J Surg 1981;*142*:596.
23. Nall R: The complications of primary duodenal diverticula. Aust N Z J Surg 1968;*37*:289.
24. Pinotti HW, Tacla M, Pontes JF, et al: Surgical procedures upon juxta-ampullar duodenal diverticula. Surg Gynecol Obstet 1972;*135*:11.
25. Thomas E, Reddy KR: Cholangitis and pancreatitis due to a juxtapapillary duodenal diverticulum. Endoscopic sphincterotomy is the other alternative in selected cases. Am J Gastroenterol 1982;*77*:303.
26. Lotveit T, Foss OP, Osnes M: Biliary pigment and cholesterol calculi in patients with and without juxtapapillary duodenal diverticula. Scand J Gastroenterol 1981;*16*:241.
27. Fuller JW, Christensen JA, Sherman RT: Common bile duct obstruction secondary to peptic ulcer. Am Surg 1975;*41*:640.
28. Orstad GR, Christensen NA, Smith LA: Jaundice as a complication of duodenal ulcer. Surg Clin North Am 1971;*51*:885.
29. Michowitz M, Farago C, Lazarovici I, et al: Choledochoduodenal fistula: A rare complication of duodenal ulcer. Am J Gastroenterol 1984;*79*:416.
30. Fernando DCJ, Gopichandran TD, Kendrick RG: Duodenal ulcers causing obstructive jaundice and a mucocele of the gallbladder. Br J Radiol 1981;*54*:72.
31. Constant E, Turcotte JG: Choledochoduodenal fistula: the natural history and management of an unusual complication of peptic ulcer disease. Ann Surg 1968;*167*:220.
32. Farrell JT, Rella AJ, Conte AJ: Obstructive jaundice secondary to duodenal ulcer. Am J Gastroenterol 1966;*46*:391.
33. Feller ER, Warshaw AL, Schapiro RH: Observations on management of choledochoduodenal fistula due to penetrating peptic ulcer. Gastroenterology 1980;*78*:126.
34. Griffen WO Jr, Schaefer JW, Schindler S, et al: Ampullary obstruction by benign duodenal polyps. Arch Surg 1968;*97*:444.
35. Sobol S, Cooperman AM: Villous adenoma of the ampulla of Vater. An unusual cause of biliary colic and obstructive jaundice. Gastroenterology 1978; *75*:107.
36. Weinberger HA: The interpretation and management of duodenal lesions other than benign ulcer. Surg Gynecol Obstet 1977;*145*:329.
37. Farmer RG, Hawk WA, Turnbill RB Jr: Crohn's disease of the duodenum (transmural duodenitis): clinical manifestations. Am J Dig Dis 1972;*17*:191.
38. Dordal E, Glasgov S, Kirsner JB: Hepatic lesions in chronic inflammatory bowel disease. Gastroenterology 1967;*52*:239.
39. Law DH: Regional enteritis. Gastroenterology 1969;*56*:1086.
40. Lukash WM: Complications of acute pancreatitis: unusual sequelae in 100 cases. Arch Surg 1967;*94*:848.
41. Lesser PB, Warshaw AL: Differentiation of pancreatitis from common bile duct obstruction with hyperamylasemia. Gastroenterology 1975;*68*:636.
42. Jacobs ML, Daggett WM, Civetta JM, et al: Acute pancreatitis: analysis of factors influencing survival. Ann Surg 1977;*185*:43.
43. Coppa GF, LeFleur R, Ranson JHC: The role of Chiba-needle cholangiography in the diagnosis of possible acute pancreatitis with cholelithiasis. Ann Surg 1981;*193*:393.
44. Warshaw AL: Inflammatory masses following acute pancreatitis: phlegmon, pseudocyst, and abscess. Surg Clin North Am 1974;*54*:621.
45. Salzman EW, Bartlett MK: Pancreatic duct exploration in selected cases of acute pancreatitis. Ann Surg 1963;*158*:859.
46. Acosta JM, Rossi R, Galli OMR, et al: Early surgery for acute gallstone pancreatitis: evaluation of a systematic approach. Surgery 1978;*83*:367.
47. Acosta JM, Ledesma CL: Gallstone migration as a cause of acute pancreatitis. New Engl J Med 1974;*290*:484.
48. Hermann RE, Hertzer NR: Time of biliary surgery after acute pancreatitis due to biliary disease. Arch Surg 1970;*100*:71.
49. Warshaw AL, Fuller AF Jr: Specificity of increased renal clearance of amylase in diagnosis of acute pancreatitis. New Engl J Med 1975;*292*:325.
50. Warshaw AL, Schapiro RH, Ferrucci JT Jr, et al: Persistent obstructive jaundice, cholangitis, and biliary cirrhosis due to common bile duct stenosis in

chronic pancreatitis. Gastroenterology 1976;*70*: 562.
51. Scott J, Summerfield JA, Elias E, et al: Chronic pancreatitis: a cause of cholestasis. Gut 1977; *18*:196.
52. Schulte WJ, LaPorta AJ, Condon RE, et al: Chronic pancreatitis: a cause of biliary stricture. Surgery 1977;*82*:303.
53. Littenberg G, Afroudakis A, Kaplowitz N: Common bile duct stenosis from chronic pancreatitis: a clinical and pathologic spectrum. Medicine 1979;*58*:385.
54. Wisloff F, Jakobsen J, Osnes M: Stenosis of the common bile duct in chronic pancreatitis. Br J Surg 1982;*69*:52.
55 Segal I, Lawson HH, Rabinowitz B, et al: Chronic pancreatitis and the hepatobiliary system. Am J Gastroenterol 1982;*77*:867.
56. Gadacz TR, Lillemoe K, Zinner M, et al: Common bile duct complications of pancreatitis: evaluation and treatment. Surgery 1983;*93*:235.
57. Aranha GV, Prinz RA, Freeark RJ, et al: The spectrum of biliary tract obstruction from chronic pancreatitis. Arch Surg 1984;*119*:595.
58. Newton BB, Rittenbury MS, Anderson MC: Extrahepatic biliary obstruction associated with pancreatitis. Ann Surg 1983;*197*:645.
59. Falko JM, Mekhjian HS, Thomas FB: Silent pancreatic pseudocyst: an unusual cause of extrahepatic biliary obstruction. Am J Dig Dis 1975;*20*:583.
60. Chawla SK, Chawla K, Sossi AJ, et al: Uncommon presentation of pancreatic pseudocyst. Am J Gastroenterol 1977;*68*:154.
61. Loludice TA, Jarmolych J, Buhac I: Pancreatic retention cyst: a cause of obstructive jaundice. JAMA 1977;*238*:889.
62. Warshaw AL, Rattner DW: Facts and fallacies of common bile duct obstruction by pancreatic pseudocysts. Ann Surg 1980;*192*:33.
63. Skellenger ME, Patterson D, Foley NT, et al: Cholestasis due to compression of the common bile duct by pancreatic pseudocysts. Am J Surg 1983;*145*:343.
64. Gonzales LL, Jaffe MS, Wiot JF, et al: Pancreatic pseudocyst: a cause of obstructive jaundice. Ann Surg 1965;*161*:569.
65. Ravitch MN: Anomalies of the pancreas. *In* Carey LC (ed.): The Pancreas. St. Louis, CV Mosby, 1973.
66. Morrell MT, Keynes WM: Annular pancreas and jaundice. Br J Surg 1970;*57*:814.
67. Merrill JR, Raffensperger JG: Pediatric annular pancreas: twenty years' experience. J Pediatr Surg 1976;*11*:921.
68. Dodd GD, Nafis WA: Annular pancreas in the adult. Am J Roentgenol 1956;*75*:333.
69. Whelan TJ, Hamilton GB: Annular pancreas. Ann Surg 1957;*146*:252.
70. Brown C: Hydatid cyst of the pancreas presenting as obstructive jaundice. Br J Clin Pract 1974; *28*:418.
71. Morton PCG, Terblanche JT, Bornman PC, et al: Obstructive jaundice caused by an intrapancreatic hydatid cyst. Br J Surg 1981;*68*:474.
72. Beirstein SS: Obstructive jaundice in a case of hydronephrosis. J Urol 1948;*59*:157.
73. Javadpour N, Ireland GW, Hakim A, et al: Giant hydronephrosis in horseshoe kidney, presenting as right upper quadrant mass and jaundice. Chicago Med School 1970;*29*:37.
74. Boltuch RL, Straffon RA: Obstructive jaundice: unusual complication of postoperative pararenal pseudocyst. Urology 1974;*3*:759.
75. Pontes JE, Pierce JM Jr: Obstructive jaundice complicating pyeloplasty. J Urol 1975;*114*:524.
76. Sannella NA, Stanton RH, Langevin RE Jr: Obstructive jaundice and renal masses. Arch Surg 1976;*111*:585.
77. Boardman KP: Duodenal and common bile duct obstruction with a pyelo-duodenal fistula caused by renal calculous pyonephrosis. Br J Urol 1976;*48*:6.
78. Bassaly I, Schwartz IR, Pinchuck A, et al: Aneurysm of the gastroduodenal artery presenting as common duct obstruction with jaundice. Am J Gastroenterol 1973;*59*:435.
79. Croom RD III, Frantz PT, Thomas CG Jr, et al: Aneurysms of the hepatic artery. South Med J 1976;*69*:1013.
80. Guida PM, Moore SW: Aneurysm of the hepatic artery. Report of five cases with a brief review of the previously reported cases. Surgery 1966; *60*:299.
81. Mojab K, Lim LT, Esfahani F, et al: Mycotic aneurysm of the hepatic artery causing obstructive jaundice. Am J Roentgenol 1977;*128*:143.
82. Collier RL, Fox TA: Aneurysm of the hepatic artery as an unusual cause of obstructive jaundice. Henry Ford Hosp Med Bull 1966;*14*:421.
83. Ariyan S, Cahow CE, Greene FL, et al: Successful treatment of hepatic artery aneurysm with erosion into the common duct. Ann Surg 1975;*182*:169.
84. Lewis DR Jr, Kung H, Connon JJ: Biliary obstruction secondary to hepatic artery aneurysm: cholangiographic appearance and diagnostic considerations. Gastroenterology 1982;*82*:1446.
85. Verta MJ Jr, Dean RH, Yao JST, et al: Pancreaticoduodenal arterial aneurysms. Ann Surg 1977;*186*:111.
86. Goffin M, Fuhrman M: Aneurysm of the gastroduodenal artery as a cause of obstructive jaundice. A case report. Am J Gastroenterol 1972;*58*:493.
87. Flint LM, Mays ET, Aaron WS, et al: Selectivity in the management of hepatic trauma. Ann Surg 1977;*185*:613.
88. Goldblatt M, Goldin AR, Shaff MI: Percutaneous embolization for the management of hepatic artery aneurysms. Gastroenterology 1977;*73*:1142.
89. Gracey L: Jaundice due to hepatic artery aneurysm. Proc R Soc Med 1970;*63*:1311.
90. Gale GL: Some serious complications of tuberculous lymph nodes: fatal hemoptysis, false aneurysm, occluded cisterna chyli, and obstructive jaundice. Am Rev Tuberc 1954;*70*:610.
91. Crowson MC, Perry M, Burden E: Tuberculosis of the pancreas: a rare cause of obstructive jaundice. Br J Surg 1984;*71*:239.
92. Bartlett MK, McDermott WV Jr: Amputation neuroma of the bile ducts with obstructive jaundice. New Engl J Med 1954;*251*:213.
93. Larson DM, Storsteen KA: Traumatic neuroma of the bile ducts with intrahepatic extension causing obstructive jaundice. Hum Pathol 1984;*15*:287.
94. Renner IG, Ponto GC, Savage WT III, et al:

Idiopathic retroperitoneal fibrosis producing common bile duct and pancreatic duct obstruction. Gastroenterology 1980;*79*:348.
95. Wittig JH, Burns R, Longmire WP Jr: Jaundice associated with polycystic liver disease. Am J Surg 1972;*136*:383.
96. Miller T, Thompson NW: Intermittent dislocation of the liver. A syndrome associated with volvulus of the transverse colon and stomach and obstructive jaundice. Arch Surg 1977;*112*:658.
97. Warshaw AL, Welch JP: Extrahepatic biliary obstruction by metastatic colon carcinoma. Ann Surg 1978;*188*:593.
98. Hunsicker RC, James PM Jr, Strawtiz JG: Findings at autopsy of 65 patients with mammary cancer correlated with clinical treatment. Am Surg 1971;*37*:313.
99. Berkowitz D, Gambescia JM, Thompson CM: Jaundice with signs of extra-hepatic obstruction as the presenting symptom of bronchogenic carcinoma. Gastroenterology 1952;*20*:653.
100. Cole HS, Freston JW: Recurrent melanoma presenting with obstructive jaundice. Rocky Mt Med J 1973;*70*:42.
101. McArthur MS, Teergarden DK: Metastatic melanoma presenting as obstructive jaundice with hemobilia. Am J Surg 1983;*145*:830.
102. Bell HG, David R, Shamsuddin AM: Extrahepatic biliary obstruction and liver failure secondary to myeloma of the pancreas. Hum Pathol 1982;*13*:940.
103. Lake G, Schade RR, Van Thiel DH: Extrahepatic biliary tract obstruction due to plasmacytoma. J Clin Gastroenterol 1983;*5*:273.
104. Rentsch I, Gartner U, Muller P, et al: Endoscopic retrograde cholangio-pancreaticography (ERCP) in obstructive jaundice caused by metastatic testicular teratoma. Endoscopy 1977;*9*:101.
105. Jaffe BM, Donegan WL, Watson F, et al: Factors influencing survival in patients with untreated hepatic metastases. Surg Gynecol Obstet 1968;*127*:1.
106. Warshaw AL, Popp J, Schapiro RH: Extrahepatic biliary obstruction by metastatic breast carcinoma. Ann Intern Med 1979;*91*:568.
107. Silverman DT, Murray JL, Smart CR, et al: Estimated median survival times of patients with colorectal cancer based on experiences with 9,745 patients. Am J Surg 1977;*133*:289.
108. Brown PW, Terz JJ, Lawrence W Jr, et al: Survival after palliative surgery for advanced intra-abdominal cancer. Am J Surg 1977;*134*:575.
109. Bismuth H, Corlette MB: Intrahepatic cholangioenteric anastomosis in carcinoma of the hilus of the liver. Surg Gynecol Obstet 1975;*140*:170.
110. Terblanche J, Louw JH: U-tube drainage in the palliative therapy of carcinoma of the main hepatic duct junction. Surg Clin North Am 1973;*53*:1245.
111. Cameron JL, Skinner DB, Zuidema GD: Long term transhepatic intubation for hilar hepatic duct strictures. Ann Surg 1976;*183*:488.
112. Hudgins PT, Meoz RT: Radiation therapy for obstructive jaundice secondary to tumor malignancy. Int J Radiat Oncol Biol Phys 1976;*1*:1195.
113. Kopelson G, Harisiadis L, Tretter P, et al: The role of radiation therapy in cancer of the extrahepatic biliary system: an analysis of thirteen patients and a review of the effectiveness of surgery, chemotherapy, and radiotherapy. Int J Radiat Oncol Biol Phys 1977;*2*:883.
114. Nakayama T, Ikeda A, Okuda K: Percutaneous transhepatic drainage of the biliary tract. Gastroenterology 1978;*74*:1978.
115. Ferrucci JT Jr, Mueller PR, Harbin WP: Percutaneous transhepatic biliary drainage: technique, results, and applications. Radiology 1980;*135*:1.
116. Tepper J, Nardi G, Suit H: Carcinoma of the pancreas: Review of MGH experience from 1963 to 1973. Analysis of surgical failure and implications for radiation therapy. Cancer 1976;*37*:1519.
117. Ochoa JI, Keene WR: Obstructive jaundice in Hodgkin's disease due to infiltration of the biliary ducts. J Fla Med Assoc 1970;*57*:21.
118. Levitan R, Diamond HD, Craver LF: Jaundice in Hodgkin's disease. Am J Med 1961;*30*:99.
119. Bouroncle BA, Old JW Jr, Vazques AG: Pathogenesis of jaundice in Hodgkin's disease. Arch Intern Med 1962;*110*:872.
120. Rosenberg SA, Diamond HD, Jaslowitz B, et al: Lymphosarcoma: a review of 1269 cases. Medicine 1961;*40*:31.
121. Ehrlich AN, Stadler G, Geller W, et al: Gastrointestinal manifestations of malignant lymphoma. Gastroenterology 1968;*54*:1115.
122. Friedman CJ, Lambert MJ III: Obstructive jaundice as initial presentation of non-Hodgkin's lymphoma: value of internal percutaneous transhepatic biliary drainage. South Med J 1981;*74*:1005.
123. Bower JS, Coca-Mir R: Jaundice in acute subleukemic lymphocytic leukemia due to obstruction of the common duct by portal nodes. JAMA 1951;*146*:987.
124. Derechin MM, Goldberg LS, Herron L: Extraosseous plasma-cytomas causing extrahepatic cholestasis and cardiac tamponade. A unique case of multiple myeloma. Scand J Haematol 1970;*7*:318.
125. Jones MB, Voet R, Pagani J, et al: Multifocal eosinophilic granuloma involving the common bile duct: histologic and cholangiographic findings. Gastroenterology 1981;*80*:384.
126. Ihde DC, Sherlock P, Winawer SJ, et al: Clinical manifestations of hepatoma: a review of 6 years' experience at a cancer hospital. Am J Med 1974;*56*:83.
127. Nonomura A, Ohta G, Kanai M, et al: Hepatocellular carcinoma presenting extrahepatic biliary obstruction. Acta Pathol Jpn 1983;*33*:789.
128. Brand SN, Brandt LJ, Sprayregan S, et al: Extrahepatic biliary obstruction secondary to a hepatoma-containing blood clot in the common bile duct. Am J Dig Dis 1970;*21*:905.
129. Wind G, Futterman S: Obstructive jaundice secondary to hepatoma: case report and literature review. Am J Gastroenterol 1977;*67*:80.
130. Lee NW, Wong P, Siu KF, et al: Cholangiography in hepatocellular carcinoma with obstructive jaundice. Clin Radiol 1984;*35*:119.
131. Johns WA, Zimmerman A: Biliary obstruction due to hemobilia caused by liver cell carcinoma. Ann Surg 1961;*153*:706.
132. Maffessanti MM, Bazzochi M, Melato M: Sonographic diagnosis of intraductal hepatoma. J Clin Ultrasound 1982;*10*:397.
133. Tsuzuki T, Ogata Y, Iida S, et al: Hepatoma with obstructive jaundice due to the migration of a

tumor mass in the biliary tract: report of a successful resection. Surgery 1979;*85*:593.
134. Sullivan WG, Koep LJ: Common bile duct obstruction and cholangiohepatitis in clonorchiasis. JAMA 1980;*243*:2060.
135. Klein E, Schneebaum S, Feuchtwanger MM, et al: Shell splinters in the common bile duct: a rare cause of obstructive jaundice. Am J Surg 1981;*141*:376.
136. Kalman PG, Stone RM, Phillips MJ: Heterotopic gastric tissue of the bile duct. Surgery 1981;*89*:384.
137. Blundell CR, Kanun CS, Earnest DL: Biliary obstruction by heterotopic gastric mucosa at the ampulla of Vater. Am J Gastroenterol 1982;*77*:111.
138. Brinton MH, Pellegrini CA, Stein SF, Way LW: Surgical treatment of chronic pancreatitis. Am J Surg 1984;*148*:754.

INDEX

Page numbers in *italics* refer to illustrations; page numbers followed by t indicate tables.